458- 464
682-688

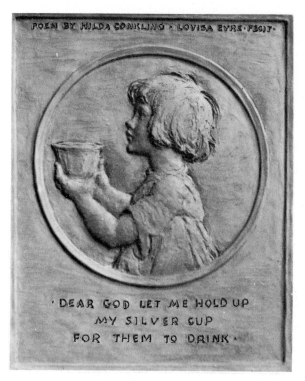

POEM BY HILDA CONKLING · LOVISA EYRE · FECIT·

·DEAR GOD LET ME HOLD UP
MY SILVER CUP
FOR THEM TO DRINK·

FRONTISPIECE BY LOUISA EYRE

The Identifying Symbol of the
Children's Hospital of Philadelphia

*Courtesy of Mrs. deLanux, Louisa E. Norton and
Edwards F. Leiper, Jr., Attorney-at-Law*

textbook of
PEDIATRIC NURSING

Fifth Edition

DOROTHY R. MARLOW, R.N., Ed.D.

Formerly, Dean and Professor of Pediatric Nursing,
College of Nursing, Villanova University;
Associate Professor of Pediatric Nursing,
University of Pennsylvania School of Nursing

W. B. SAUNDERS COMPANY/PHILADELPHIA/LONDON/TORONTO

W. B. Saunders Company: West Washington Square
Philadelphia, PA   19105

1 St. Anne's Road
Eastbourne, East Sussex BN21 3UN, England

1 Goldthorne Avenue
Toronto, Ontario M8Z 5T9, Canada

Textbook of Pediatric Nursing   ISBN   0-7216-6099-1

Last digit is the print number: 9   8   7   6   5   4   3

To the Children of the World

The children of the past,
The children of the present,
and
The children yet unborn.

In Memoriam

Mr. William Marlow and Mrs. Lillian Marlow
Parents

and

Mrs. Margaret M. Adams
Teacher, Counselor, and Friend

FOREWORD

A foreword can serve a number of purposes, and it has not been an easy task to decide toward which of these this particular foreword should be directed. Much could be said which primarily would pay tribute to the author. The pages of this book, for example, convey a warmth of feeling for children and an understanding of them seldom achieved in the printed word, and even less often in a textbook. This characteristic is so pervasive it cannot but infect the reader even to the extent of exciting like feelings. The book speaks so clearly for the author, however, in this and in other respects that this purpose was discarded.

These introductory remarks might serve the purpose of orienting the reader to the rich and varied accumulation of knowledge and its systematic organization to be found in these pages. Undoubtedly this volume is rare among texts in the scope and completeness with which the many-faceted aspects of child life are discussed. But this fact, too, will quickly be self-evident, and a second purpose was rejected.

A foreword in the form of a book review offered a highly tempting, if inappropriate, possibility. The unusual features of both the content and its organization demand critical analysis and discussion. A book review would not only misuse the opportunity this foreword offers, but also would probably be of greater interest to the teacher of pediatric nursing than to the student. In any case, it must be left for the columns of the professional journals.

What, then, can this foreword provide? Precisely, because of the nature of this book, the most useful function of a foreword may be a brief guide to the student on how to get the most out of the great deal that it offers. Chapter-by-chapter reading in textbooks is not always fruitful. The student may be searching for general understanding, and specific details are offered—about procedures, about particular situations, or about a group of diseases affecting a particular organ system. Because the information needed is scattered, the student may have difficulty bringing together knowledge of people, of their health problems when their defenses fail, and of the kind of nursing care required. The student must, however, correlate and integrate this knowledge to give appropriate and helpful nursing care. This difficulty will not be encountered in this text.

Within three consecutive chapters of this book it is possible to acquire a comprehensive picture of the child—his growth and development, his care, and his health problems—at each developmental period. Age and developmental stage are clearly seen as important influences on the occurrence of illness and on its treatment; this fundamental basis for nursing care is obvious. The meaning and significance of illness and hospitalization to the child and to his family are also related to development and make for increased understanding of this problem. The disease conditions commonly found in a given age period become readily apparent, serving not only to sharpen observations, but also to clarify the interrelations between maturation and specific kinds of illnesses.

Read carefully, then, chapter by chapter, for a general understanding of the field of pediatric nursing, for an appreciation of its scope and complexity, for an awareness of the many factors involved in nursing care, and for comprehensive knowledge of the child and his health problems. The possibility for learning does not end here, however. Selected kinds of rereading will be effective in furthering your knowledge and understanding.

Read and study consecutively and carefully each of the chapters on growth, development, and care, in each of the developmental periods. The dynamic process of growth from birth through adolescence emerges, and a text within a text is found. In a similar fashion a text devoted to the health problems of infants and children which are acute or short-term in nature evolves; or one concerned with those problems which require long-term care can be segregated. The presence of several possible texts in one volume makes it relatively easy for you to develop and expand your knowledge of the field on a longitudinal as well as on a cross-sectional basis.

There is another facet of this book to be studied. Nursing is an applied science and of necessity draws heavily upon the basic sciences and other applied sciences for its content. This knowledge is then synthesized and extended to provide a basis for nursing practice. Nursing care practices, general and specific, and the rationale underlying these practices are discussed in some detail throughout this book. You may wish to find another text within a text by delineating those general nursing care practices, together with the supporting knowledge, which can be adapted to a number of age levels and to many disease conditions.

In the final analysis, what you gain from this textbook depends upon you. It cannot give you wisdom, but it offers a foundation for the development of wisdom. It cannot give you understanding of an individual child in the real world of nursing, but it provides the kind of knowledge through which that understanding is made possible. It cannot give you skill in the practice of pediatric nursing, but it offers you the tools with which to work. It cannot give you faith in yourself or in the patients you serve, but it can lead you to the threshold of such faith.

DOROTHY E. JOHNSON, R.N., M.P.H.

Professor of Pediatric Nursing
University of California
Los Angeles

PREFACE

The care of children has changed during recent years owing to the rapid expansion of knowledge. Research carried on in disciplines such as psychology, sociology, anthropology, and medicine has contributed increased understanding of the growth and development of children in various cultural and socioeconomic groups, the meaning of parent-child relations, the effects of deprivation on the child, the effects of family disruption, and the place of the child and the adolescent in our changing world. Medical research has led to the introduction of successful methods of prevention and therapy in the areas of genetics, drugs, surgical techniques, and psychiatric care.

The role of the pediatric nurse has been influenced by these findings and also by research carried on within the nursing profession itself. The nursing profession has accepted the belief that an understanding of the healthy, developing individual is the basis for preventive care and an understanding of the individual who is ill. Because this is the foundation of the philosophy of modern health care, a new chapter has been included in this text on nursing assessment, a vital part of the responsibilities of the nurse.

The concept of assessment of the level of adaptation is important in providing care to patients and their families. Each child or parent with whom the nurse interacts is a biopsychosocial being who is located at some point on the health-illness continuum. Wherever the person is on that continuum, stimuli act upon him, requiring him to adapt. The function of the nurse is to promote and support the individual in this adaptation process, freeing him to respond to other stimuli. In order to do this, the nurse must observe and assess the person's status on the health-illness continuum, his strengths and weaknesses, and the effectiveness of his coping mechanisms. The nurse must intervene as needed to promote his adaptation to attain, retain, or regain his health. Evaluation of the effectiveness of these actions is essential.

The pediatric nurse is a team member, working with a variety of professionals toward the welfare of the child and his family: in maintaining the integrity of each family, in offering anticipatory guidance, in preventing illness, and in providing skilled nursing care for children when they are well and when they are ill. Since health services in the future will be focused more and more in the community setting, this book is intended to help the reader view the care of the child in the broadest sense.

Because of the increasing numbers of pediatric nurse practitioners, as well as the increasing numbers of men providing nursing care for children, the focus in this edition has shifted from an emphasis on "nursing care" given by female nurses to the broader concept of the "responsibilities of the nurse" in this expanding and more demanding nursing role.

In order to assume this role, the pediatric nurse must be dedicated not only to understanding and helping others, but also to self-understanding, both of which are of vital importance in responding to the child and family who look to the nurse for compassion in their therapeutic relationship. Much has been written concerning the need for better communication of feelings between individuals in our world of today. In this text I have attempted to assist the inexperienced practitioner in exploring personal feelings regarding the care of the child and his family and in communicating respect for the emotions and the uniqueness of each person involved. Through reciprocal trust, established in honest and meaningful communication with others, the nurse can practice the art and science of the nursing profession, and the patients and their families can gain love's greatest gifts—compassion, understanding, and empathy.

While considering recent research in nursing and related fields, the changing role and responsibilities of the pediatric nurse, and the basic principles of teaching and learning, this textbook has been arranged using the growth and development of the child as a basis for care.

In the opening chapters I have attempted to give the student a broad historical perspective of child care and a generalized view of the areas of knowledge that must be understood in order to provide care for children today; an overview of the concepts and principles of growth and development—physical, emotional, mental, sexual, social, and spiritual; a general discussion of the care of the child when well and ill, at home or in the hospital; and a review of the role of the pediatric nurse. A new chapter has been included in Unit I on the nursing process in the care of children. Examples of this process are given in the Appendix. Threads of knowledge introduced in this beginning unit are woven through and enlarged upon in subsequent chapters.

After this survey, the remainder of the book is organized into units, following the specific growth and development and care of well children from the neonatal period through adolescence. An understanding of growth and development and the way the child views his life, and the way the parents view the child, is vital to the nurse because efforts are directed primarily to nursing the child in his family, not his disease. After the student has developed an understanding of the healthy child, consideration is given to the effects of illness on children in each age group. Physical and emotional illnesses requiring short-term or immediate care and long-term care are discussed. The various conditions included in each age period have been selected either because they are related to the growth and development process or because their incidence is greatest during that particular age span. Increased emphasis has been placed in this edition on the scientific reasons why certain conditions predominate in each age group. Although many of these conditions may affect children of varying ages, I believe that if nurses understand the growth and development of children of various ages and the nursing care of a child having a particular condition at one age, they will be able to transfer this knowledge to the care of children of different age groups.

Few conditions have been included for which there is no discussion of the care to be given in the home or in the hospital, by the parents, the nurse in the hospital, or the community or public health nurse. Not every disorder that may be seen in the pediatric years is included here. On the other hand, I have included some conditions which were not common in the past, but which today are being seen with increasing frequency. Examples of such conditions include necrotizing enterocolitis, fetal alcohol syndrome, echovirus infection, obesity in infancy, familial dysautonomia, neurocutaneous syndromes, "nursing-bottle mouth" syndrome, sinusitis, systemic lupus erythematosus, dyslexia, peptic ulcer, Reye's syndrome, genital herpes, atherosclerosis, and clear cell adenocarcinoma of the vagina.

Additional new material has been included on parenting, preparation for parenthood, genetic counseling, immunity, diagnostic examinations for neurologic conditions, primary care, observation of the primal scene, sexual molestation, identification of rashes in dark skin, child care in the emergency room, incest, sexual aggression against the child, guidance of the adolescent, concerns of the adolescent, rape, and the use of contraceptives. Increased emphasis has been placed on current research in the areas of genetics, embryology, and fetology. In the discussion of each condition appropriate concepts related to the areas of nutrition, mental health, prevention of illness, habilitation or rehabilitation, and community health are considered. Details of the pathogenesis of diseases have been included in order to enable the student to understand better the nursing care of children. Further discussion of pathologic processes may be found in the publications listed at the end of each chapter. Information has been provided on many of the newer forms of therapy utilized in the care of ill and handicapped children, but I have not discussed in detail the use of machines and equipment usually found in speciality units of the hospital. Since many types of equipment are being produced, it would seem wise for the student to learn to use those available where care is being given.

In this edition emphasis has been placed on the role of the nurse in providing emotional support for the child and members of his family, both in the hospital and in community settings. The manner in which the nurse can help the parents support the child in his normal psychologic development and the manner in which the nurse can support and counsel the child and the adolescent are discussed. Increased emphasis has been placed on parent (mother and father)-child-professional nurse relations; the development of love for the child; the importance of the nurse's role in communication with parents to achieve depth of understanding and to change attitudes; the parents' role in the observation and care of the child; the cultural aspects of child care; and the team concept in child care, including the role of the pediatric nurse practitioner and the role of the nurse in research. Suggestions are also given concerning the way in which the nurse can help the parents prepare their child for hospitalization and support him when he is physically or emotionally ill. Included is a more comprehensive discussion of the responsibilities of the nurse in helping parents and children face crisis situations such as prolonged illness and death. The reactions of the nurse in these situations are also reviewed.

Pictures illustrating the growth and development of children as well as those illustrating children with various pathologic conditions have been included. A series of illustrations shows the actual steps in the growth and development of one girl from birth to 17 years of age. In order to compare briefly the steps in growth and development of the two sexes, pictures of a boy from two to four years of age are included. Illustrations of certain less common conditions have been included because nurses may not have the opportunity to care for children having such conditions during their clinical experience. Further additions include new tables of mortality rates of children of various ages, the most recent schedules for immunizations published by the American Academy of Pediatrics, new graphs showing the incidence of various conditions in children, and four color plates showing various conditions affecting children.

It is my belief that learners should be involved in independent study as part of the educational process if they are to become creative, self-directing and responsible nursing practitioners who can adapt to change. For this reason, the listings of teaching aids and other information and references, including publications and periodicals, at the end of each chapter have been completely revised and brought up to date. A listing of audiovisual media has been included at the end of each chapter in order to help teachers select materials that students can use to further their learning in class or in individual study in an audiovisual laboratory. For the most part all these learning aids present current knowledge in medical, nursing, and related disciplines. Included in these listings are materials primarily intended for lay persons, the consumers of health care. Nurses can profit from knowing what children and their families are learning from such sources. Articles presenting original research findings are included, because I believe that beginning practitioners should become acquainted with the value of such investigations and may perhaps be stimulated to begin creative studies of their own.

At the end of each unit the reader will find Clinical Situations and Guides to Further Study, which will serve as a review of the content of the unit. The study questions have been included for the purpose of helping the learner bring together the material presented on the care of children in each age group. Some of these questions involve the understanding of factual material, while others require the reader to use judgment in answering situational questions. More cross references than in former editions have also been provided in order to assist the learner to understand the content of the clinical area of pediatric nursing.

The material in this text was submitted to several professional persons for their opinions and suggestions. Their appraisals and contributions have helped the author to clarify or expand important areas of content. Changes of this nature have also been made on the basis of comments received from readers, including teachers, students, and practitioners of nursing.

Former editions of this textbook, while primarily intended for students and professional nurses, have also been used by other members of the health team such as physiotherapists and occupational therapists among others. Such sharing of knowledge of the area of pediatric nursing by other disciplines can ultimately lead to a closer relationship among health team members dedicated to the care of children.

Learning comes either through direct experience or through the experience and language of others. The role of the author, as of the teacher, is to bring knowledge to the learner and to interpret this knowledge in its most intelligible form. Not only must specific knowledge be transmitted, but the author or teacher must also guide the student to other sources of knowledge and to an appreciation of how new knowledge is gained through research.

It has been my hope to make this textbook representative of current thought and practice in the area of pediatric nursing. The aim has been to make it of value in the learning process of students and later as a reference when they practice nursing or become parents. I welcome all comments and suggestions from reviewers, teachers, students, and practitioners so that this text can further help nurses contribute their best efforts to the care of children and find deep personal satisfaction in working with them and their families.

DOROTHY R. MARLOW

ACKNOWLEDGMENTS

Many professional persons have contributed their knowledge and support to make the creation of this book possible.

A special tribute should be accorded those who by their faith in my endeavor encouraged me in my efforts: Dr. Theresa I. Lynch, Professor Emeritus and former Dean of the School of Nursing, University of Pennsylvania; Dr. Gladys Sellew, former Professor of Nursing of Children, University of Maryland, and Lecturer at the School of Nursing, University of Pennsylvania; Dr. Lutie Clemson Leavell, Professor Emeritus, Teachers College, Columbia University; Dr. Mildred L. Montag, Professor Emeritus, Teachers College, Columbia University; Dr. Marcia A. Dake, Director of Program Development, Nursing and Health Programs, American National Red Cross; Rosemary Johnson, Professor of Nursing, College of Nursing, Arizona State University; and Dr. B. Louise Murray, Dean, College of Nursing, University of New Mexico.

The author is very appreciative of the contributions of Evelyn N. Behanna, R. N., M.S.N., Associate Professor, Nursing of Children, and Acting Dean, College of Nursing, Villanova University, and Sheila M. Pringle, R.N., M.S. in Hygiene, Assistant Professor, Nursing of Children, College of Nursing, Villanova University, and a doctoral candidate at Temple University. Chapter 3, The Nursing Process in the Care of Children, and Appendix I were prepared by these colleagues.

It is impossible to express adequately the appreciation of the author for the generous assistance of the physicians and members of other professions in the preparation of this text:

Mary D. Ames, M.D., Professor of Pediatrics, School of Medicine, University of Pennsylvania, and Director of Ambulatory Services and Coordinator of the Department of Rehabilitation, Children's Hospital of Philadelphia

Lester Baker, M.D., Professor of Pediatrics, School of Medicine, University of Pennsylvania, and Director of The Clinical Research Center, Children's Hospital of Philadelphia

Joel Fort, M.D., former consultant to the World Health Organization and Lecturer (Professor), School of Criminology, University of California, Berkeley

Stanley Horwitz, D.D.S., Pedodontist, Ardmore, Pennsylvania

C. Everett Koop, M.D., Professor of Pediatric Surgery and Professor of Pediatrics, School of Medicine, University of Pennsylvania, and Surgeon-in-Chief, Children's Hospital of Philadelphia

William J. Rashkind, M.D., Professor of Pediatrics, School of Medicine, University of Pennsylvania, and Director of Cardiovascular Laboratories of the Children's Hospital of Philadelphia

Gladys H. Reynolds, Ph.D., Chief, Research Statistics Section, Venereal Disease Control Division, U.S. Department of Health, Education, and Welfare, Center for Disease Control, Atlanta, Georgia

Louise Schnaufer, M.D., Associate Professor of Pediatric Surgery, School of Medicine, University of Pennsylvania, and Associate Surgeon, Children's Hospital of Philadelphia

Luis Schut, M.D., Associate Professor in Neurosurgery, School of Medicine, University of Pennsylvania; Associate Neurosurgeon, Hospital of the University of Pennsylvania and Graduate Hospital; and Chief of Neurosurgery, Children's Hospital of Philadelphia

Mabel Smith, Acting Chief of Statistical Resources Branch, Division of Vital Statistics, National Center for Health Statistics, U.S. Department of Health, Education, and Welfare

Louis R. Will, D.D.S., Orthodontist, Radnor, Pennsylvania

The author is indeed grateful to the many members of the nursing profession—educators, graduate practitioners, and students—throughout the United States, Canada, and England who offered excellent suggestions, which have been incorporated in the revision of this textbook.

The author would especially like to express her appreciation to the following for their suggestions:

Adelaide Bash, R.N., M.A., Associate Professor, Bergen Community College, Paramus, New Jersey

Jessie Glass, R.N., M.P.H., former Maternal and Child Health Nursing Consultant, Division of Public Health Nursing, Pennsylvania Department of Health

Linda Goodman, R.N., M.S., Clinical Nursing Supervisor, Children's Hospital Medical Center, Boston, Massachusetts

Erna Goulding, R.N., M.A., Associate Administrator, Patient Care, Children's Hospital of Philadelphia

Lois Haffly, R.N., B.S.N., Public Health Nurse, Pennsylvania Department of Health, Delaware County

Jean M. Maurer, R.N., M.S.N., Assistant Professor, College of Nursing, Villanova University

Sister Carol Neuburger, R.N., M.S., Associate Professor, Pediatric and Maternity Nursing, College of Nursing, University of North Dakota, Grand Forks, North Dakota

Jane Oliver, R.N., M.A., Director of Staff and Student Education, Children's Hospital of Philadelphia

Brenda E. Ramsey, R.N., M.S.N., Assistant Professor, College of Nursing, Villanova University

I should like to express my appreciation also to the authors, publishers, and companies who have granted me permission to use their illustrations in this text. I should like to thank the personnel of H. Armstrong Roberts, Photographers, Gilbert and Ring, Medical Photographers, and James L. Dillon and Company, Inc., Photographers, for their excellent photographs of children. I would like to thank also Herr Achim Menge, Georg Thieme Verlag, Stuttgart, Germany, for permission to use the pictures shown on the color plates in this book.

A special word of appreciation should be extended to Dr. and Mrs. Robert Gens, to Mr. and Mrs. John Haffly and their children, Kim and Tommy, to Mr. and Mrs. Raymond Kersey and their son, Gregg, and to the many parents who granted permission for pictures of their children to appear in this book.

Gratitude should also be expressed to Mrs. Gerri Ossman and to Miss Christine Mruk for their secretarial assistance during the revision of this text.

The author wishes to express warm appreciation to the staff of W. B. Saunders Company for their fine cooperation, particularly Mr. Robert E. Wright, former Nursing Editor; Miss Helen Dietz, Senior Nursing Editor; Mrs. Laura Tarves, Production Manager for Nursing Titles; Mr. Raymond Kersey, Manager, Illustrations Department; Ms. Barbara Wittenberg, of the Illustrations Department; Miss Lorraine Battista, Manager, Design Department; and Ms. Lisette Cohen, Copy Editor. Without their sincere interest and support, the revision of this textbook would have been impossible.

To my parents, Mr. and Mrs. William Marlow, who encouraged me with their patience and understanding, and to my mentor and friend, Mrs. Margaret M. Adams, who inspired me with her philosophy of child care, I respectfully dedicate this book in memoriam.

DOROTHY R. MARLOW

CONTENTS

UNIT ONE

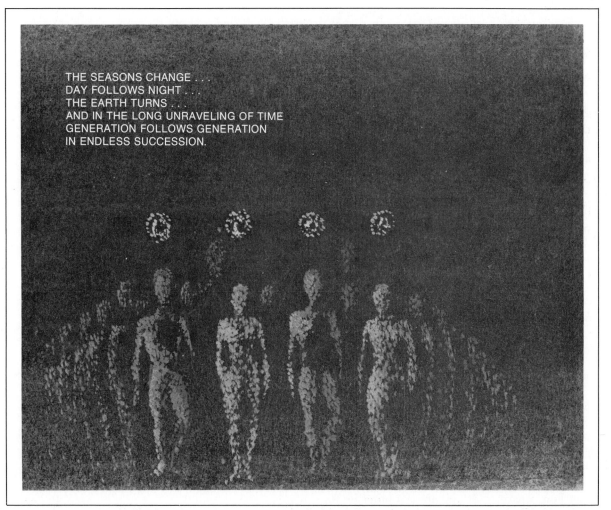

THE SEASONS CHANGE . . .
DAY FOLLOWS NIGHT . . .
THE EARTH TURNS . . .
AND IN THE LONG UNRAVELING OF TIME
GENERATION FOLLOWS GENERATION
IN ENDLESS SUCCESSION.

(Reproduced with permission from the film From Generation to Generation, Maternity Center Association, New York.)

INTRODUCTION

ON CHILDREN

And a woman who held a babe against her
      bosom said, Speak to us of Children.

And he said:
Your children are not your children.
They are the sons and daughters of Life's long-
      ing for itself.
They come through you but not from you,
And though they are with you yet they belong
      not to you.

You may give them your love but not your
      thoughts.
For they have their own thoughts.
You may house their bodies but not their souls,
For their souls dwell in the house of tomorrow,
      which you cannot visit, not even in your
      dreams.
You may strive to be like them, but seek not to
      make them like you.

For life goes not backward nor tarries with
      yesterday.
You are the bows from which your children as
      living arrows are sent forth.
The archer sees the mark upon the path of the
      infinite, and He bends you with His
      might that His arrows may go swift and
      far.

Let your bending in the archer's hand be for
      gladness;
For even as he loves the arrow that flies, so He
      loves also the bow that is stable.

Kahlil Gibran
The Prophet (1923)

Chapter One

HISTORICAL PERSPECTIVE

Just as successions of waves have broken upon the beaches of the world since the beginning of time, so have generation after generation of children been born, lived, and ultimately died since man first appeared upon the face of the earth. Whether any individual child in this multitude of children died at a young age or lived a long life was dependent upon the care he received, especially during his earliest months and years.

The manner in which children have been cared for when well or when ill has differed in accordance with how the adult members of society thought of the child, that is, his value for the preservation of the group, their religious beliefs, superstitions, migrations, and what they knew of causes of illness and its therapy. An understanding of child care since its beginning in time is essential for the nurse in order to gain an appreciation of the trends leading to our present concepts and practices in relation to children.

THE CHILD IN PRIMITIVE SOCIETIES

Little is known about life in prehistoric times, but child care is believed to have been somewhat like that among cultural groups living today in areas hardly touched by civilization. In such groups persons tend to value a child not for himself, but as a future adult. For this reason his social development according to the customs of the group is of great importance.

In early times primitive groups were nomads, who moved constantly in their search for adequate supplies of food and for safety from wild animals and hazardous weather conditions. Such groups could not be hampered by sick or weak children. The members of these groups looked favorably on those who were strong and destroyed those who were not.

When such a society ruled that a malformed or sickly infant would drain the resources of the

CHILD CARE THROUGH THE AGES

group, the infant was killed or left behind to die. Sometimes infants were killed simply because they were females who could not contribute as much productive labor to the group as could males. This practice is termed *infanticide.* Probably some infants survived, however, because their mothers protected them. Societies then as now were composed of individuals, not all of whom necessarily lived by the rules of the group.

In addition, some primitive peoples believed in superior beings who ruled not only themselves but also nature and the universe as they knew it. Perhaps, they reasoned, the forces of a storm or a period of prolonged drought was an act of a superior being who was displeased. Perhaps the birth of a deformed infant was also punishment for the previous transgressions of the parents. Such thinking did not cease with the onset of civilization.

Yet we know that the child, even in primitive tribes, had to receive at least a minimum of physical care in order to live. Whether he received also love and affection was dependent on the cultural group in which he lived and on his mother who cared for him.

THE CHILD IN ANCIENT CIVILIZATIONS

The concept of the importance of the child to his society gradually emerged as each group

3

settled on an area of fertile land instead of wandering in search of food. The child, instead of being a liability, thus slowly became an asset to his society.

Egypt. The early peoples who settled in the valley of the Nile River cared for their children, dressing even their infants in loose clothes and encouraging breast feeding. They encouraged children to learn as well as to participate in outdoor activity. As early as 1500 B.C. treatment for the diseases of childhood was prescribed, different from that given to adults.

Greece and Rome. Physical beauty was considered important to the early inhabitants of Greece; thus the children were reared so that they would have well formed bodies. The importance of the family was stressed in Rome because its function was to raise strong sons to become good warriors who could serve the state.

Hippocrates (460–370 B.C.) in his writings referred frequently to the peculiarities of disease in children. Specific treatment for the illnesses of children as opposed to that given adults was recommended by Celsus, who lived in the first Christian century.

Israel. Among the ancient Jews the hygienic measures prescribed in the Mosaic Law had a great influence on maternal and child care. The Hebrew people recognized the importance of cleanliness and nutrition. They also recognized communicable diseases and made efforts to control them. The religious ceremony of circumcision practiced on male infants also served as a health measure.

Parenthood was honored among the Hebrews, and a large family was considered a sign of God's blessing upon the parents. The greatest disappointment a Hebrew woman could have was to be childless.

THE IMPACT OF CHRISTIANITY ON THE CARE OF THE CHILD

Christianity, among other emerging religions, helped to develop a new philosophy of the sanctity of human life. Christianity taught the value of the child as an individual, not merely as a son or daughter who would cherish the parents in their old age and give them grandchildren so that the family might extend for generations to come. Furthermore, since Christianity also taught the protection of the weak by the strong and the care of the ill by the well, the helpless child and the infirm became objects of special consideration. Orphan asylums for dependent children and hospitals for the care of the sick were founded early in the history of the Christian Church.

THE CHILD IN EUROPE

Before the nineteenth century in Europe the life expectancy of human beings was short. Many parents did not live long enough to rear their children in the home. Great epidemics of contagious diseases often swept over the continent. Young men died in war or from injuries sustained while working. Women married early and had large families. The maternal death rate was high. The death rate for the total population was highest in the cities and among the poor.

The result of all these conditions was that there were many orphaned children among the poor of the growing cities. Many infants were taken to boarding homes or *baby farms*. The majority of these children were of illegitimate birth. Frequently, after the initial payment of a fee, there would be no more remuneration forthcoming; therefore it was advantageous to the owner of the "baby farm" to hasten the children's deaths.

Asylums, initially founded for the care of dependent children in A.D. 787, multiplied in number as the demands for such institutions grew. Even though the number of such institutions increased, overcrowding was still a problem. Many children died, owing to their poor condition on admission, to a lack of understanding of the principles of sanitation, nutrition or of housing, to a lack of aseptic technique when needed, and to the extremely poor quality of care which was provided. Because of these unfavorable conditions, it is estimated that half of the infants of the urban poor died before the age of five years.

Probably the darkest period in child care in Great Britain and Western Europe was the beginning years of the Industrial Revolution during the early 1800's. Children as young as six to twelve years of age worked in cotton mills for ten or more hours a day. They often fell asleep at their work, and accidents were common. But since their hands were nearly as skillful as adult hands in tying broken threads, and the cost of their maintenance (if they were apprenticed orphans) and their wages were so low, mill owners employed them in large numbers. Not until the nineteenth century was legislation passed that prohibited the worst evils of child labor.

THE CHILD IN THE UNITED STATES

Until the early decades of the twentieth century most children in the United States lived on farms or in small villages. In general this was a healthy life, although children in such areas lacked the medical care and hospital facilities that urban parents could provide. Child labor was never the problem in the United States that it was in Europe; nevertheless the children of the poor were employed in factories and stores where working conditions were unhealthy and hours far too long.

By the middle of the nineteenth century there were large slums in New York and other eastern cities. The people living there were generally from foreign countries, many of them from rural areas and not accustomed to city life. Tenements were overcrowded, unsanitary and in disrepair. Morbidity and mortality rates among infants and children were exceedingly high. Accidents in the tenements and in the streets where the children played were common.

Contaminated milk led to serious intestinal disorders among infants and children. (Dairies and stores which handled milk were not inspected, and milk was not pasteurized.) Milk from tuberculous cows caused many cases of tuberculosis among children.

The condition of neglected, abandoned and ill children aroused public and professional sympathy. The following milestones occurred in this society's effort to improve the lives of these children. While it is not the intent that the student memorize the specifics given here, these dates and events are provided as evidence of the progress made toward improvement in child care during the last two centuries.

1790. The first orphanage was established and operated at the expense of the public.
1853. The Children's Aid Society of New York was founded to move thousands of homeless children from the streets into foster homes.
1855. The Children's Hospital of Philadelphia was founded, the first hospital dedicated exclusively to the care of children.

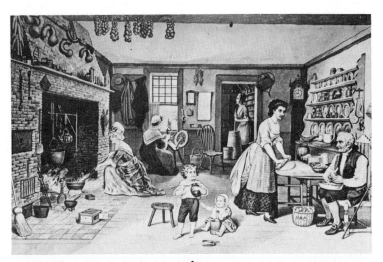

A

FIGURE 1–1. Examples of child care. A, Familial togetherness: in a colonial American kitchen. (Courtesy of The Bettman Archive.) B, "A Pastoral Visit, Virginia," by Richard Norris Brooke. (Courtesy of The Corcoran Gallery of Art.)

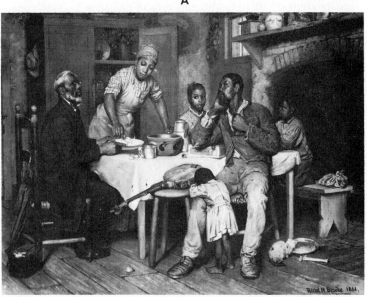

B

1860. Dr. Jacobi in New York established the first children's clinic, where he lectured to medical students on the diseases of childhood.

1875. The Society for the Prevention of Cruelty was organized in New York City.

1880. The Pediatric Section of the American Medical Association was organized.

1888. The American Pediatric Society was organized.

1899. Children's courts came into being, as distinguished from adult courts where all types of criminals appeared.

1909. The White House Conference on the Care of Dependent Children. A similar conference has been held every ten years since that time. As a result of the first conference the United States Children's Bureau was founded, under the jurisdiction of the Department of Labor, since at that time child labor was thought to be the greatest problem of childhood.

1912. The Children's Bureau was established.

1917. The first Federal Child Labor Law was passed (declared unconstitutional after nine months).

1919. The first law for the statewide care of handicapped children.

1919. The White House Conference on Child Welfare Standards. After this conference regional conferences were held to discuss the protection of the health of mothers and their children, the socioeconomic base for child welfare standards, children in need of care, and child labor.

1930. The White House Conference on Child Health and Protection. This conference produced the *Children's Charter,* which contained 19 statements concerning what the child needs for his health, education, welfare and protection. This is one of the most important documents in the history of child care.

1931. The American Academy of Pediatrics was founded.

1935. The Social Security Act of 1935, though amended many times, is basic to many of the modern efforts in health and care of children.

1940. The White House Conference on Children in a Democracy followed the great depression. Conference discussions concerned social and economic matters: what children require in a democratic way of life.

1941. A federal labor law was passed (after other attempts had been made to do so) which could successfully regulate child labor.

1946. The United Nations International Children's Emergency Fund (UNICEF) was created by the United Nations.

1948. The World Health Organization (WHO) was created by the United Nations.

1950. The Midcentury White House Conference on Children and Youth. The *Pledge to Children* was adopted. The theme of the conference was *A Fair Chance to Achieve a Healthy Personality.* The Children's Bureau subsequently published a booklet entitled *A Healthy Personality for Your Child,* a popular version of the conference's Fact Finding Digest.

1953. The Federal Department of Health, Education, and Welfare was established.

1959. The 14th General Assembly of the United Nations approved the *Declaration of the Rights of the Child.*

1960. The Golden Anniversary White House Conference on Children and Youth. The purpose of this sixth conference was to promote opportunities for children and youths to realize their full potential for a creative life in freedom and dignity.

1963. Amendments to the Social Security Act provided grants for maternal and infant care.

1965. Amendments to the Social Security Act provided funds for comprehensive health care for deprived children and youth. Medicare and Medicaid provisions were added at this time.

1967. The Child Health Act of 1967, which consists of amendments to Title V of the Social Security Act, was passed.

1969. The Office of Child Development was established with the Office of the Secretary, Department of Health, Education, and Welfare. The two major bureaus in the Office of Child Development are the Children's Bureau and the Bureau of Child Development Services which operates Project Head Start and other programs.

1970. The 1970 White House Conference on Children. For the first time the traditional White House Conference on Children and Youth was organized into two conference groups, one for those interested in the care of children and one in which the young persons themselves determined the issues and made recommendations for actions. The participants in the decennial White House Conference on Children transmitted to the President a list of 16 "overriding concerns" and 25 specific recommendations for the improvement of the care of children.

1971. The 1971 White House Conference on Youth was a unique event in the public life of this nation. For the first time a White House Conference was focused only on the concerns of young people aged 14 to 24 years. The participants truly reflected the diversity of American youth.

1972. Although Title XIX of The Social Security Act was amended in 1967 to include special provisions for the health care of financially needy persons under the age of 21 years under Medicaid, these comprehensive programs, which required early and periodic screening, diagnosis and treatment (EPSDT), were not required to be implemented in each state until 1972.

1972. The WIC (Women, Infants and Children) Program. This is a Special Supplemental Food Program to provide supplemental foods through state and local agencies to pregnant or lactating women and to infants and young children who are at risk because of inadequate nutrition and income.

1974. The Child Abuse Prevention and Treatment Act of 1974.
1974. The Sudden Infant Death Syndrome Act of 1974.
1975. Title XX was a comprehensive amendment to The Social Security Act including funds for family planning services, child care services, protective services, and foster care for children among other benefits, as well as services for adults.

Two of the most important milestones in the progress toward betterment of life for children were the White House Conferences and the establishment of the Children's Bureau.

The White House Conferences. Since the first White House Conference on Children in 1909 progress has been made in advancing and safeguarding the well-being of children in spite of a depression, hot and cold wars, and rapid change. One of the principal contributions of these Conferences has been in keeping the channels of communication open with ideas moving in both directions between the specialists, practitioners, and research workers in children's services and the parents, citizens, and youth of this country.

The Children's Bureau. In 1903 Miss Lillian Wald, founder of the Henry Street Settlement in New York City, and Mrs. Florence Kelley of the National Consumer's League saw a need for a federal organization that would endeavor to improve the conditions of children. They were especially concerned about the high mortality rate, the illegitimacy rate, the orphanages, and child labor, among other problems. News of their concern eventually reached President Theodore Roosevelt.

After the first White House Conference in 1909, a law was passed in 1912 that established the Children's Bureau. The responsibility of this new Bureau was to investigate and report "upon all matters pertaining to the welfare of children and child life among all classes of our people."[*]

The Children's Bureau is interested in the well-being of all children: the well, the sick, and the handicapped. Children from all cultural and racial groups, all socioeconomic levels, whether loved or abused, are the concern of the Bureau.

An important aspect of the work of the Children's Bureau is that of fact-gathering and reporting such statistics as the number of births, the number of children living, with their ages and family incomes, the number of sick or handicapped children, and the number of children of various ages who die. The Bureau is also interested in the number and quality of the people, programs and institutions that help children in the country.

Another aspect of the work of the Children's Bureau is that of setting standards and of building services for children in partnership with states and communities. Such federal grant-in-aid funds have provided money to help states start new services for children, to develop skilled staffs to work with children and their families, and to make possible demonstration and research projects that have led to better services.

Currently the federal government is especially interested in preventing the incidence of and improving the services to mentally retarded children, crippled children, children having long-term problems such as rheumatic fever, speech and hearing disorders, congenital heart disease, and diabetes, among others, and juvenile delinquents. The government is also concerned about children of migratory agricultural workers, those of working mothers, those who are abused or neglected, and those refugees who have no one to care for them.

The Children's Bureau also publishes pamphlets on subjects of interest to the public. The first of these bulletins, *Prenatal Care*, was published for parents in 1913. The bulletin *Infant Care* was published initially in 1914. Many more such pamphlets are listed for students at the ends of the chapters in this text.

To summarize, then, the purposes of the Children's Bureau today are

(1) develops standards and provides technical assistance to States and public and private agencies for programs relating to children and parents; (2) supports a child welfare research and demonstration grants program, and evaluates programs serving children; (3) informs the public through a Division of Public Education using all communications media and publishes a wide range of publications, including *Children Today* (formerly *Children*), an interdisciplinary journal for professionals, non-professionals, and all those interested in children.

Established with the Children's Bureau is a National Center for Child Advocacy originally including: a proposed Children's Concern Center to which parents and organizations can turn for prompt answers to inquiries about problems affecting children; an Information Secretariat, which draws together information about services for children; a Division for Vulnerable Children, which plans programs and sets licensing and other standards for services to institutionalized, handicapped, retarded and disturbed children—to children in need of adoptive or foster homes—to teenage parents and unmarried mothers; and the Community Coordinated Child Care (4–C)

---

[*] It's Your Children's Bureau, Children's Bureau, 1964, p. 4.

program, which helps local public and private child care organizations work together.*

The Children's Bureau is concerned for all children in the United States; however, it also works actively with international organizations such as the United Nations International Children's Emergency Fund, which has as its concern the children of the world.

THE CHILD IN THE DEVELOPING COUNTRIES

No one living today can think only in terms of the welfare of the children in his own town, state, or country. The speed of modern transport and the exploding world population are bringing the peoples of the world closer together than ever before. Hence health problems which were once the concern of only a small segment of the world's population today potentially threaten the whole world.

Through the international activities of the World Health Organization (WHO), the United Nations International Children's Emergency Fund (UNICEF), and other groups, assistance is being provided to developing countries in their efforts to improve their level of child care.

The World Health Organization. The World Health Organization, established as a specialized agency of the United Nations in 1948, was the first world-wide health organization in history. The headquarters of this organization are in Geneva, Switzerland.

The objective of the World Health Organization is to assist in the attainment by all peoples of the highest possible level of health. To this end this Organization acts as a director and a coordinating authority on international health work, establishes and maintains effective collaboration with governments and other interested groups, furnishes assistance to countries by providing health information and technical, educational and other services, evaluates a country's health problems when requested, stimulates and advances work to eradicate diseases and to prevent injuries, promotes improvement of nutrition, housing, sanitation and other aspects of environmental hygiene, promotes maternal and child health and welfare, and promotes mental health among its many other functions.

More specifically, the present main objectives of the World Health Organization are to control communicable diseases such as malaria, tuberculosis, leprosy, yaws, and the venereal diseases on an international scale, to build up public

health organizations in countries that have underdeveloped programs, and to educate and train medical and auxiliary personnel in the health fields.

The activities of the organization prove that nations can work together for an important cause: the improvement of human health.

The United Nations International Children's Emergency Fund. The United Nations created the United Nations International Children's Emergency Fund (UNICEF) in 1946 for the purpose of meeting the emergency needs of children, such as in times of war or other disasters in countries throughout the world. Aid to a country is given only when requested and on the basis of need without regard to race, creed or political belief.

The United Nations International Children's Emergency Fund is financed by voluntary contributions from governments, from groups, and from individuals. In the United States, children collect monies for this organization by participating in the Hallowe'en Trick or Treat effort. Also, the sale of calendars and greeting and Christmas cards by the Fund has provided monies to send medications and food to many ill and impoverished children throughout the world.

The Children of Today in the United States: Trends and Concepts Related to Their Care

Ours is a complex and changing society. Children, as they grow from infancy in a brief span of time, must learn not only to live happily for today but also to adjust rapidly to the many unexpected events they will face in their tomorrows.

The social forces that are shaping the world now and will have an impact on the future are varied. One characteristic of society today is its emphasis on speed: in its production of goods, in its mode of travel and in its energetic race to conquer space. Also, the total population in the world is increasing rapidly. This poses problems necessitating planning for all kinds of education and health and welfare services for children of all races and creeds.

At present, efforts continue to be made toward providing opportunities for every child to live, grow, and learn to his fullest potential in today's world. Individualized child-centered learning, having the support of citizen community action groups, is essential. Preserving the rights of children and fulfillment of their basic needs, including comprehensive health care when well

---

*OCD: Office of Child Development, U.S. Department of Health, Education and Welfare, 1972.

or ill, necessitates the accountability of individuals and agencies responsible for providing these services. Advocacy programs for children having *full* cultural, ethnic, racial, and sexual representation are needed from the local to the federal government levels. The involvement of children and youth as individuals and in group programs concerned with their own care and education is a goal to be sought.

Typical also of our present society are the uprooting and movement of countless family groups: the migration of families from other lands to our shores, the migration of farm laborers' families to new places of employment, the migration of rural families into the large cities, the migration of middle-class families to the suburbs, and the increase in the numbers of urban families in the lower income groups.

Partly because of these migrations, the *extended family* of a century ago, which included three generations with other relatives living in close geographic proximity, has become fragmented into small *nuclear families* composed of parents, children, and perhaps a grandparent. Whereas the extended family was tradition-bound and secure, its members being interdependent, today's small family group is largely adrift in a sea of strangers. Furthermore, even the established nuclear family, consisting of two parents, including a working father and one or more children, is changing. For any number of reasons, the decision may be made that the mother support the family and that the father stay home to care for the children. Or, both parents may feel the need to work outside the home, and the child or children may be placed in day-care centers or with another service. When parents are unmarried, separated, or divorced or when one parent has died producing a single-parent family, further adjustments are necessary in the area of child care. Attempting to prevent complete disintegration of such small family groups is the responsibility of society's agencies and society as a whole.

Stress has been placed recently on the grinding and binding effects of poverty in our society: poverty of the American Indian, the black and the Puerto Rican, as well as the Caucasian in Appalachia and other parts of our country. Federal, state, and local governments in the United States are devising ways to break the vicious cause-and-effect circle of poverty at many points. This is essential if all children are to have the opportunity to develop to their greatest potential.

Poverty has as one of its causes the bulldozing of jobs by agricultural mechanization and indus-

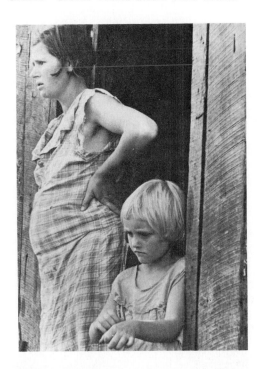

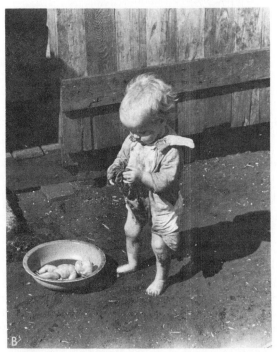

FIGURE 1–2. A, Acute and chronic diseases often occur among the poor today. (Courtesy U.S. Department of Health, Education and Welfare, Public Health Services Administration.) B, A child of migratory workers washes her doll. (Courtesy of Marion C. Wolcott.)

trial automation. This increase in mechanization and automation opens new opportunities for technicians and scientists, but results in a dearth of employment for the unskilled labor pool in

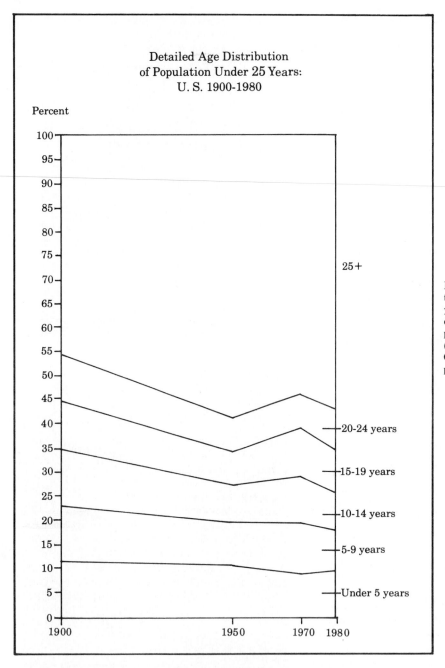

Detailed Age Distribution
of Population Under 25 Years:
U. S. 1900-1980

FIGURE 1–3. Detailed age distribution of population under 25 years: U.S. 1900–1980. As in prior decades at least one-fourth of the population will be under age 15. (1970 White House Conference on Children: *Profiles of Children*, page 14, 1970.)

which some youth without a higher education will stagnate.

Furthermore, the rapid increase in scientific knowledge in the areas of growth and development of children and the causes of illness places the burden especially on the members of the medical profession, who are expected to implement this knowledge with appropriate action. With the current manpower shortage of physicians, nurses, and other members of the medical team, adequate implementation for the welfare of all children can hardly be expected to occur.

Federal legislation in the areas of health, wel-

fare, and education has snowballed in recent years in an attempt to implement some of the results of the White House Conferences, 1970 and 1971. The federal government has and will continue to expand federally aided programs, will provide even greater support for state services, and will encourage community action on behalf of our children and youth.

In view of these several social forces, the nursing profession has a responsibility with other medical disciplines to create a world in which all children in health and illness will receive optimum care in a secure environment.

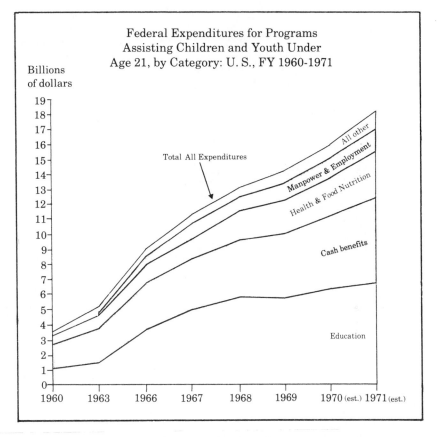

Federal Expenditures for Programs Assisting Children and Youth Under Age 21, by Category: U. S., FY 1960-1971

FIGURE 1–4. Federal expenditures for programs assisting children and youth under age 21; more federal funds are being spent to assist children and youth. (1970 White House Conference on Children: *Profiles of Children*, page 18, 1970.)

Some of the ways by which this end can be achieved will be discussed in this text.

THE CHILD IN THE COMMUNITY

It is important for the nurse to recognize the great strides that have been made in the improvement of child care in the community. Such an understanding is essential not only as a nurse, but also as a future potential parent and community member.

Part of the support which young parents gained from an extended kinship family is now being supplied by federal agencies and privately supported programs. The Children's Bureau has played a vital role in the development of many of these efforts.

Among the most important movements in the provision of comprehensive health care in the United States has been the widespread development of federal and other government programs for culturally deprived children, especially the young. *Project Head Start* has tried to improve the health of preschool children, to correct physical defects, and thus to improve their readiness for school and academic achievements. The goals of this program have not been fully realized.

Other government-sponsored programs have attempted to lower the incidence of complications associated with pregnancy and to provide services to high-risk infants in the form of early treatment to prevent or lighten defects. There have been attempts to find effective, yet imaginative ways of meeting the health needs, through comprehensive health services for children and youth from disadvantaged families, and education, encouragement, and support of their families to become aware of both the health needs of their children and of the resources available to meet them. These programs have made strides toward achieving these goals in the areas where they have been in operation.

During recent years local public assistance departments have also been attempting to extend the range of services available to children and their families. These services include foster child care, adoption services under public auspices, family counseling, homemaker services, family day care, and protective services for abused or neglected children. Thus it can be seen that the impact of federal, state and local legislative efforts on the services to children during health and illness has been varied. The goals of some programs must be more clearly stated, and more careful community planning must be done to bring about uniformly successful results.

The pressing need of American Indians and Alaskan natives for health services has been an-

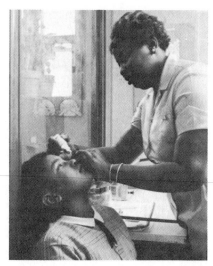

FIGURE 1–5. The prevention of blindness is an important part of the comprehensive health care program for children. (U. S. Public Health Service.)

swered in large part through the efforts of the Division of Indian Health of the United States Public Health Service. This Division is responsible for hospitals, clinics, and school health centers. Services provided include public health nursing, dental care, guidance in nutrition, medical social service, and special treatment clinics.

Since the Indian population especially is a young one, its most pressing health problems are those of infants and children. The principal health problems of these children include accidents, gastrointestinal diseases, tuberculosis and other respiratory diseases, and communicable diseases. The problem of infant and child health is due to the high incidence and severity of infectious disease, delay in obtaining treatment resulting in secondary complications, and the difficulty in providing preventive medical services. Malnutrition, anemia and poor general environment contribute to the incidence and severity of disease.

Children of migrant farm families are often deprived culturally as well as physically, intellectually, and socially. Because of repeated migrations these children have complex needs which can be met only through programs of education, social welfare, and medical services. The initial need of the parents of migrant farm families is for day-care centers where they can leave their children while they work on the farms. The health services provided at these centers depend on local need, interest, professional services, and availability of facilities. The common medical needs of these children are for immuni-

zations, improved feeding habits, physical examinations and testing if the children are ill, and correction of problems resulting from ignorance and poverty.

Although most children in the United States are born to citizens of this country, many are being brought into the United States through the process of *intercountry adoptions.* Children who are homeless and face rejection in their native land, such as Vietnamese-Caucasian and Vietnamese-Negro children, may be adopted by American families. Adoption of a child who has probably lacked security in his early life, has lived without one or both of his parents to care for him, places a great responsibility on his newfound parents as he faces a new world, a different language, and a strange culture. Such adopted children can bring added love and joy to a family group if emerging problems are handled with patience and compassion. (Adoption is discussed in Chapter 19.)

School health programs vary, depending on the locale and size of the school. The school nurse or school nurse practitioner may function alone, or may be a member of the health team consisting also of a physician, child psychologist, guidance counselor, and social worker. The nurse's functions may vary from being responsible only for providing first-aid care for children during school hours, to assisting with physical examinations and conducting hearing, vision and tuberculosis screening tests, to checking on immunizations to determine adequacy, to caring for children who have problems such as diabetes or epilepsy, to carrying out sex education programs for children and sometimes parents as well, to being a health counselor for the families represented by the children in school. The school nurse, then, may be a public health nurse who spends only a brief time in the school, or she may be a full-time nurse whose total responsibility is the care of the children enrolled in a particular school.

Camps where well children may go in the summer for wholesome recreation are located in almost all sections of the country. During the last several years camps have been established also for children having diabetes, cystic fibrosis, orthopedic handicaps, and other conditions. In each camp at least one nurse should be on duty in case of accident or illness. In the camps for the handicapped child, closer medical and nursing supervision is essential for the welfare of the campers.

Since many children having pediatric conditions which required hospitalization a few years ago are now cared for in the home, nurses have a vital role to play in the health of a community's youngest members. Especially needed are nurses who are able not only to give direct care to children, but also to teach such care effectively to the responsible adults in each situation.

Another responsibility which nurses assume with other members of the health team is that of implementing the concept of preventive pediatrics. This entails the maintenance of Child Health Conferences (see Chapter 13), immunization against preventable communicable diseases (see Chaps. 13 and 20), education for the prevention of accidents and poisonings (see Chap. 17), case-finding of children evidencing early emotional disturbances so that they can be referred to child guidance clinics or private physicians, and the case-finding of children showing signs of physical illness so that they can be referred to the appropriate source for help.

In some communities, centers for the treatment of special conditions have been established, e.g., Poison Control Centers (see Chap. 17), premature infant centers (see Chap. 9), heart centers (see Chaps. 12 and 24), and centers for the diagnosis and treatment of mentally retarded children (see Chap. 21).

In an effort to decrease fragmentation of health services for children, comprehensive health care programs are being organized within the states. Methods planned or utilized include regionalization; extension of clinic services in densely populated areas; centers having a single entry for persons seeking health or social service; increased community representation in patient-centered care systems; and liaisons between universities and teaching hospitals in order that these facilities may be community or regional health resources.

From the preceding discussion the nurse can understand that he or she has an important role to play in organized community action in collaboration with other members of the health team, in coordination of the services of various members of the nursing team, and in carrying out his or her responsibilities in direct nursing intervention in the hospital, clinic, school, home or elsewhere in the community where children or parents have health or counseling needs.

The nurse may use his or her abilities as a health educator, a teacher, an advisor, a research worker, a case finder, and as a compassionate and skilled nurse of the sick.

The Nurse of Today in the United States: Trends and Concepts in the Nursing Care of Children

From the previous discussions it is apparent that the nurse has an important role to fulfill in the nurturing of children. Consideration of the impact of societal, community, and professional forces upon the delineation of an individual professional role, the nursing of children, is of tremendous importance in order to understand how that role is ultimately fulfilled. The following forces are not discussed in order of importance, but as a constellation of factors having an influence not only on the nurse but on the nursing role in society.

CHANGES IN THE DELIVERY OF CARE

As seen earlier in this chapter, federal, state and local *governments* have committed themselves to providing improved care for mothers and children. This is especially true for those at high risk or those at the low-income or poverty level of existence. More specifically, as has been seen, funds have been allocated for the care of mothers and for the care of well children through improved nutrition, immunization programs, well-child conferences, and other services. Funds have also been allocated for the extension of screening and detection programs for hereditary disorders, the support of various clinics and health-related services for ill children, and the stimulation of research.

The trend toward *regionalization* of health care has been accelerated in recent years. The reasons for this have been the problem of economics and community demands for quality health care. Costly physical facilities and medical and nursing personnel can no longer be duplicated in agencies having close proximity to each other. Small pediatric units in general hospitals are closing because a surplus of pediatric beds has led to underutilization of departments that are uneconomical.

The specialized strengths of a medical center for children as a regional resource can be dramatically illustrated in the use of a neonatal intensive care unit. An emergency transport system can immediately bring its services to an infant in distress over a wide geographic area and speed him back to the intensive care unit. Many infants who formerly would have died thus have an improved chance for survival.

The *Health Maintenance Organization*, although not specifically for the care of children and youth, can influence their care. The Health Maintenance Organization Assistance Act of 1973 authorized federal expenditures to provide assistance and encouragement for local and state governments, nonprofit organizations, insurance companies, and agencies to change the health delivery system so that improved care could be provided.

Nurses have been involved in the implementation of these programs, but their efforts and leadership are increasingly needed. More specifically, nurses can push forward in the fight against such emerging concerns as unplanned pregnancies, learning and developmental disabilities, child abuse, emotional illness, addiction, and suicide among the young. In established health facilities as well as in free clinics or wherever children and youth are found, nurses can play a pivotal role in providing family health care and health teaching, and in coordinating multiple health resources to achieve their goals.

WORKING WITH POOR AND DEPRIVED FAMILIES

Much is being written and spoken today about *poverty* and its effects on those who are poor. Poverty in a family many times seems to perpetuate itself through the generations. The inability of a family to obtain sufficient financial resources results in inability to secure adequate nutrition, clothing, housing, health care, and educational advantages, not to mention the luxuries of life. If a family or the individuals in a family cannot break the poverty cycle, energies can be exhausted, hope can be lost, and the dire results of inadequate financial resources continue to affect the next deprived generation.

A common misconception is that persons for whom the government provides care exist only among minority groups in the ghettos of large metropolitan areas. This is certainly untrue, since deprivation also exists in rural areas, particularly among migrant farm workers. Deprivation can also exist among the temporarily poor, those individuals or families from the middle socioeconomic group who are poor because they are seeking advanced education, because they are working at low-level employment to gain experience, or because the breadwinner is unemployed. The difference between these groups is that in the first instance the family may not know what it needs, copes with what is available, and has little influence over its own destiny; in the case of the temporarily poor, the family usually knows what it needs, is attempting to make do with only the essentials for a known period of time, but can usually influence its ultimate destiny.

Although human dignity and a sense of personal worth are precious attributes guaranteed to all, in our modern society these qualities are often ignored. During recent years human contact on a personal level between the health care provider and the client has often deteriorated because of a lack of staff and mountains of paper work to be done by the caring individuals.

Nurses many times find that among the deprived families they serve, interest in health care seems to be lacking. There are several reasons why this may be so. Such families may not understand the worth and value of the health services offered. They may feel that the reception they receive at the hospital or other health agency is cold and uncaring and that the amount of time spent waiting for care at the first or subsequent appointment is too long. They may lack appropriate clothing to wear to a health facility and sufficient money for transportation, even when available. Finally, there may be a lack of child care services in the neighborhood in which their children could be placed during parental absences from home. Unless the nurse understands these problems and assists in their resolution, the nurse too may be considered an unhelpful individual.

Whether or not persons in poverty use the services nurses have to offer even in local neighborhood health centers or free clinics depends on whether the nurse can locate such individuals, whether the nurse can interpret to them on their level what is offered such as comprehensive care, and whether they believe and trust the nurse. If such potential clients believe that what the nurse says is real and indeed possible, if they can identify with the nurse, and if in the process they do not trade off their own self-worth and self-esteem, they may cooperate to their fullest ability.

In order for nurses to communicate with the poor, both the nurse and client must speak the same language. If nurses just say simply what is meant instead of attempting to sound professional, they will communicate. Using a word a person will comprehend is not talking down to that person. For instance, if the nurse asks Susie, a deprived child in a school, whether she is nauseous, Susie may not know how to respond because she does not understand the meaning of the word. On the other hand, if the nurse were to say, "Do you want to throw up?" the child would probably respond immediately.

The nurse who seeks to care for people must adapt care to them as individuals within families and communities. Understanding their socioeconomic level, health status, and attitudes toward health care is essential if productive communication is to result in improvement of their level of well-being.

ATTITUDES TOWARD TODAY'S CHILDREN

Other influences on the nurse in caring for children are the changing (and unchanging) attitudes toward the younger members of our society. The downswing in birth rate in this country that began in the 1960's and early 1970's has continued. This, the result in many instances of self-imposed population control, has and will result in a decreased need for maternity and pediatric units, schools, and businesses devoted to the production and marketing of child care products.

In spite of the decrease in family size, some nightmarish problems that existed in the past, namely, infanticide, neglect, and the abuse or maltreatment of children, still exist. The concept that persons who create may destroy what they have created can be found in old Roman law. Although such an attitude is not condoned intellectually in modern society, the practice of killing infants or children or inhibiting their normal growth and development through neglect and abuse persists.

Recently a change in attitude toward some children in our society has developed. Parents who stood, proud and hopeful, at the hospital nursery windows ten to twenty years ago, making plans for their soft-skinned newborns, could hardly have bargained for sons and daughters who reject them in favor of stereo headphones or the car, who openly declare to them, "Do you know how much I hate you?" or who act with condescension and contempt or even pity to their parents' attempts to understand their behavior. It is difficult to believe that these individuals were ever infants, locked now behind tough, "cool," insulated shells. Instead of boasting of the accomplishments of their children, parents speak of them as strangers. But is this due to something completely out of the parents' control? Does the fault lie entirely with the Devil, or the drugs, or the music, or the guru, or this horrible world? While it is true that no parents should take the full blame for the behavior of their child, the idea that a parent has *no* control over determining the kind of person his child will become is dangerous. Nurses involved in the care of children are aware that this is among the most pressing problems of our time.

INCREASED HEALTH AWARENESS BY CONSUMERS

Topics related to child behavior and health are abundant in consumer media. No longer are the members of the medical and nursing professions the sole conveyers of child care and health information. The consumer may have changed his view of these professional persons as allwise and knowing individuals and may see them as mere persons available to serve his needs, about which he already knows a great deal. The consumer is aware of what should be available to him and is demanding services that will fulfill his needs. He is a more vocal individual and can express his feelings about any perceived or real inadequacies in the health care system. The consumer is becoming more assertive in making decisions concerning his own and his family's care.

Nurses alert to consumer media can assist those with whom they work to use such information in a helpful and intelligent way. They also need to look for the concealed messages directed to health care workers. When consumers learn from television that the birth of a baby is an important event in a family's life, they do not want to be made to feel that it is a privilege to be permitted to deliver a newborn at 3 A.M. when the delivery unit has a minimal nursing staff! To understand adequately what the consumer is telling the nursing profession when there is a rise in home deliveries, each nurse must listen, read what the consumer is reading, see what the consumer is seeing, and anticipate the results of these messages. If nurses are not aware of what is happening, the public will meet their own needs in ways that may be harmful to all.

THE WOMEN'S MOVEMENT

There are radical changes occurring in the definition of femininity today. Although the first purposeful efforts to redefine the role of women began a century ago at a time when women were considered decorations, essentially both speechless and mindless, and biologically inferior to men, a small but influential group viewed women not only as wives and mothers, but as human beings with lives of their own. Over the years, the idea that all human beings achieve happiness and self-acceptance only when free to fulfill their own potentials has become more widely accepted. Individuals should be free to discover who they are and their abilities, and to strive toward their goals. With increased emphasis on self-awareness has come an increased emphasis on human sexuality. Changes in the concept of marriage, and indeed of total lifestyle, are occurring rapidly. The force of the population crisis of a few years ago and the availability of effective contraceptives have permitted women to separate recreational sex from procreational sex. While it is not the intent in this text to discuss the moral issues involved in the individual's decisions, the student should understand present trends and their impact on the nurse.

The women's movement has had an influence not only on nurses as men and women and as individuals in society, but on the physician (predominantly male)-nurse (predominantly female) relationship in respect to health care. This change can be seen in some universities where students of medicine and nursing share certain courses and experiences and thus tend to develop a common language and a better appreciation of each other's abilities and potential as future professionals.

CHANGES AND ADVANCES IN HEALTH CARE

Because physicians and nurses in many hospitals and other health care agencies are using the *problem-oriented medical record* (POMR), health personnel are evaluating and treating the client as a whole. The nurse's role in assessment of a client, interpretation of findings and direct services to a client, including the technical aspects, is assuming increased importance in health care today.

The care of children has changed dramatically for both physicians and nurses during recent decades, owing to advances in medical knowledge and to a deepened understanding of the emotional responses of children. Such advances include, among others, the discovery of various immunization measures to prevent illness and of antibiotics and other drugs that have curative value in many illnesses, and the use of public health measures and public education, which can prevent or shorten periods of hospitalization. Thus children who require hospitalization are less often isolated for prolonged periods for infectious diseases, have more frequent opportunities for early ambulation, and have shorter convalescences than in the past. Today, some children may still require long hospitalization for complicated diagnostic or therapeutic measures, some of which have been discovered only during recent years.

Advances in the understanding of human development and the stages of personality development throughout the life cycle have led to a better understanding of the needs of all family members, especially parents during the childbearing years and their children, whether in health or illness. Since the child and his family are interdependent, health team members are aware that the anxieties of the parents as well as those of the child need to be considered if a constructive response and adjustment to the experience of illness are to be made. Such understanding has led to preparation for hospitalization for both parents and child, extended visiting hours during the child's hospital stay, parental care of the child during his stay in the hospital, and many other changes, which will be discussed later.

Today many more clients than ever before require *supportive health measures*. This has increased the demand for nursing services and has augmented the nurse's role in the system of health care. In addition, since consumers are demanding more education as part of their comprehensive health care services, the nurse's role on the health care team has assumed increased importance, especially in the area of preventive and restorative care. For example, because of the increased emphasis on human sexuality, clients are asking for more and more counseling in sexual matters such as contraception for unmarried adolescents. Nurses may find it necessary to examine their own sexual attitudes and values before assistance can be given.

For all these reasons *the relationship of the physician to the nurse* has undergone alterations. The relationship is changing from one of independence of the usually male physician and dependence of the usually female nurse; it is changing to a relationship of collaboration and interdependence, a relationship having colleague status. In like manner the roles of these health professionals are being reassessed and realigned.

While the roles of the members of the helping professions are changing, *the concepts of health and illness* are changing also. One formerly accepted definition of health declared that it is a state of being in the absence of illness, implying organic illness. Presently this statement might be amplified to say that health exists when a person can meet the minimum physical, physiologic, intellectual, psychologic, and social requirements needed in order to function appropriately for his or her given age, sex, and level of growth and development. Illness, then, becomes a situation in which an individual has a disturbance in any of these areas that prevents functioning at the appropriate level of role performance. Attention is thus directed to the psychosocial characteristics as well as the physiologic characteristics of health and illness.

Emphasis has shifted during recent decades from a consideration that only the diagnosis and treatment of the ill were of importance to a position that *the promotion of health and the prevention of illness are of equal if not greater significance*. The concept of primary care has grown along with this change in emphasis or focus. *Primary care* can be defined broadly as that spectrum of services necessary to meet the large majority of routine personal health needs. More specifically, primary care can refer to a client's first contact with the health care system, leading to a decision concerning the means to resolve his problem. It also refers to the continuation of that care, including the maintenance of health, the diagnosis and treatment of symptoms, and the appropriate referrals to other sources of help. An important point that needs emphasis is that one professional assumes the responsibility for such care. This professional is aware of the client's level of health and health problems and can plan, provide, or refer to other health professionals or services, and coordinate the necessary health care and services as necessary. Professional nurses assuming these responsibilities thus function independently with clients and their families and interdependently with their colleagues in nursing as well as in other disciplines. This increased responsibility necessitates a broadening of the nursing role.

CHANGE AND EXPANSION IN THE NURSING ROLE

Important in a consideration of primary care is the *nursing process* including the taking of a history and the completion of a physical examination of the client. Completion of these responsibilities leads to a judgment or interpretation such as defining the problem or making a nursing diagnosis. Although a medical diagnosis identifies usually a discrete pathologic entity, a nursing diagnosis, which covers the entire physical and psychosocial health-illness continuum, is considerably more complex. The process by which a nurse makes a nursing diagnosis requires a clear understanding of the nature of such a diagnosis, the clear identification of the factors contributing to it, and an outline of objectives for the client, the family, and the nurse. For an expanded discussion of the nursing process, see Chapter 3.

Primary care is given in both *episodic and distributive settings*. Episodic care emphasizes the curative and restorative aspects of patient care. This usually involves patients having either acute or chronic disease, who are cared for in the hospital or other in-patient facility. Distributive care is primarily designed to maintain health and prevent disease. This type of care is more likely to be continuous in nature and to occur in the community setting with largely ambulatory patients, whether in the home, institutional or satellite clinic, school, or neighborhood health center. If the total needs of children and parents are to be met, the concepts of episodic and distributive care cannot be considered mutually exclusive.

Other aspects of the health care of children are child and family health education, including anticipatory guidance, support and counseling, health promotion and maintenance, and disease prevention, including the provision of immunizations, when appropriate. The pediatric nurse is prepared to care for the healthy child as well as for the child with short-term and long-term illnesses involving the physical as well as the psychosocial aspects. In all these areas the nurse manages the nursing care and coordinates it with the care of other members of the health team.

Child and family advocacy has gained increased importance in recent years. When the National Center for Child Advocacy was established in the Office of Child Development (OCD) in 1971, its efforts were based on the idea of advocacy as an organizing principle for constructive action for children. One impediment in improving the lives of America's children is the myth that ours is a child-oriented society and that we are doing all that needs to be done for the youngest members of our population. Actually, the participants of the 1970 White House Conference on Children included in their report an indictment of what we are doing poorly or not at all for our children. Indifference, neglect, and abuse of America's children is widespread. The problem of poor health care, lack of adequate immunizations, and faulty nutrition of the children in this country is not confined to the impoverished groups. The professional nurse who emphasizes child health maintenance, the importance of growth and development to an optimal level, the prevention of disease and its complications, and who assists children to return early to their maximum level of functioning following illness is a *child advocate*. As the nurse carries out the nursing process, is a liaison with other personnel, and functions as a teacher and consultant, the full role of child advocate will be accomplished.

The goal of *family advocacy* is to assist families and individual members to develop and function at their optimal level of ability. The advocate nurse thus becomes a coordinator, not relying on a single method or technique of intervention, but tailoring an approach to the particular problem at hand. In this kind of approach the family's access to and use of other services is important. Ultimately, a family advocate aims at providing families and the individuals within them with the technical and psychologic resources to solve their own problems. Such an effort involves a commitment on the part of the nurse to strengthen family life by helping to break through blocks that prevent family members from receiving appropriate care.

In order to fulfill adequately many of the responsibilities discussed here, the individual nurse must function increasingly not only in areas of episodic or distributive care but in *broader community efforts* as well. In such activity the nurse can become involved in a collaborative way with consumers, community officials and planners, and professionals such as lawyers, educators, and other members of the health professions. Such involvement may occur as a continuous committee effort or as participation on an ad hoc committee when problems present themselves on a local, state, or national level. Indeed, in pertinent areas of concern the professional could very well assume the leadership role in such groups.

Accountability is the mark of the true professional. Accountability in the nursing profession means that nurses must be responsible to the patient or client, whether in the hospital or the community, to themselves as people, and to nursing colleagues. The rights and privileges of nurses must be balanced with an equal array of obligations. When a nurse assumes the responsibility for intervening in the care of others, that nurse must be willing to be held accountable for the quality of care provided; that is, giving evidence of the level of care provided when compared to an agreed-upon standard or model of practice. In broad terms, accountability means a commitment to the improvement of care and to professional practice itself through research, practice, and education. The current emphasis on *quality assurance* in health care provides an opportunity to develop and use methods of quality control based on accountability that will assist in the improvement of nursing care.

If nursing needs are to be met in society, a wide range of functions on a continuum from simple to complex in a great variety of environments must be fulfilled. The consumer who desires quality health care for all people is necessitating an expansion of health care further into the community, innovative practices in health care, and a part in the evaluation of the care rendered. Such demands for increased services and involvement are being joined by demands that the skills of each member of the health team, including nurses, be used to their maximum potential.

In order to meet these needs, nurses have responded with an *expansion of the role of the nurse.* In the area of pediatric nursing there has emerged a multiplication of titles: pediatric clinical specialist, pediatric nurse master clinician, and pediatric nurse practitioner among others. The problem facing the profession now is identifying which activities specifically belong to each group. Since certain functions and responsibilities usually thought to belong to physicians have been and are being transferred to nurses, the problem becomes increasingly complex. The matter of delineating for these groups, their specific functions, and the educational preparation

necessary for fulfilling their responsibilities will have to be solved before their full contributions to the care of children can be made. In the *Joint Statement of the American Nurses' Association Division on Maternal and Child Health Nursing Practice and the American Academy of Pediatrics, Guidelines on Short-Term Continuing Education Programs for Pediatric Nurse Associates, 1971,* a method for achieving the goal of more innovative methods of utilizing the skills of the professional nurse was discussed. Since that time others have attempted to define educational requirements, roles, and responsibilities of these various groups, but confusion continues to exist.

Delineation of the boundaries of nursing has been further clouded by the conflict over the introduction of the *physician's assistant* into the health-care system. Some nurses have become indignant over this move, because they believe that although nurses have given competent assistance to physicians in the past, they are now fulfilling some of their responsibilities without receiving adequate status and compensation for their contributions.

Yet another move has been to affirm still larger boundaries of nursing through the expansion of programs for nurse midwives and primary-care nurses among others. Some nurse educators are now considering whether or not all basic preparatory programs for registered nurses should include expanded role concepts. Should the graduate of a baccalaureate program be prepared to conduct extensive health assessments, to make nursing diagnoses, and to provide treatment? The answer to these questions may be found in the future.

As the traditional responsibilities of the nursing role have become confused, so have the *legal aspects* surrounding licensing of the various nursing categories become blurred. The basic nursing practice acts of each state must be reviewed carefully. Nurses have become deeply involved in such reviews. Basically, the licensing laws have been and are written to protect the health care consumer from harmful, unsafe, or unprepared health care providers. Consumers are now also looking at these laws to determine whether, in fact, they are fulfilling this need.

The risk of malpractice action may or may not be increased as a result of the changing role of the nurse. Nurses are responsible for their own actions. The law imposes on everyone the responsibility to use reasonable care in actions directed toward others. Perhaps only when the responsibilities of those practicing in expanding nursing roles are tested in courts of law will the answers be found.

Society has been said to be a demanding master. Yet, we as health professionals have committed ourselves to serve society. When society changes, patterns of health care change, leading to a revamping of the roles of nurses. Nurses, then, must be committed and creative in their approach to care, in this case the care of children and their families.

PARENT-CHILD-PROFESSIONAL NURSE RELATIONS

The emphasis on the child has progressed from consideration of him as a miniature adult to our present belief that his physical body, his emotional processes, his intellectual functioning, and therefore his needs during health differ in many ways from those of the adult. The value of the child to society today lies not only in his potential worth as an adult—a parent or a participant in the national economy, in the arts and sciences, and in war. The value of the child lies too in his being a child. Also, his care during illness, originally disease-centered, as was the care of the adult, is now primarily preventive in nature and family- and child-centered in focus. These differences make child study a separate discipline in which scientific knowledge in many branches of learning is applied to his care.

Whether the young child is well or ill, he needs care in order to survive. This care may be provided by adults in his extended family or his nuclear family, by his parent's group of friends, or by adults in the community agencies mentioned in this text. Although his parents may wish to provide for his total care, others may assist where appropriate to foster the optimum physical and emotional growth and development of the child. *Good parent-child relations are based not on the amount of time they spend together but rather on the quality of the relation while they are together.*

Although the care of a child requires an understanding of his particular stage of growth and development and his individual ways of thinking, feeling, and coping with his environment, it is essential also for the caring adult or the nurse to understand his or her own feelings and attitudes and to realize the coping methods used as reactions to problem areas. Children provide maturing experiences for all adults who care for them. An adult is not mature in the fullest sense of the word until he has developed a capacity for parental love, an unselfish love which finds satisfaction in the happiness of the loved ones. Caring for children can provide an opportunity for adults to develop this form of love.

Few adults working with a child are successful in making a child happy unless they themselves find happiness in being with the child. This happiness, however, should not come from adopting the role of parent-substitute. They should provide for the child a sense of love and security which comes from being with an adult friend who, like a parent, does for the child what he cannot do for himself. The nurse who usurps the role of parent to the child, instead of caring for the child only when the mother or father is unable to provide such care, is not fulfilling the child's real need for the maintenance of close parent-child relations.

When the nurse has a genuine wish to engage in a human endeavor, a real sense of responsibility toward the child for whom care is provided and for his parents, judgments will not be made for them. Instead, the nurse will observe behavior and respond to the adults and the child, if he is old enough to participate, in a manner of respect, seeing them as they are, and assisting them in making their own decisions. If the nurse perceives other human beings realistically, without the colored glasses of stereotyping and prejudice, each can be seen as an irreplaceable human being and each can be respected for what he is as an individual. Thus will the nurse cease to have a self-perception as an authority figure, a mother or father substitute, and will become aware of and involved with the feelings of pain and joy of living, and the plans and actions of other human beings.

The nursing of children can be one of the most gratifying or one of the most terrifying experiences a student can have during the educational process, depending on the perception of experiences. Many students discover that cuddling of infants and young children and guiding older ones are very gratifying experiences. At the same time they may feel inadequate in their ability to care for seriously ill infants and children. Students many times are disturbed by the crying of their young patients, believing that they are doing something wrong to hurt them or that they lack the skill to satisfy their physical or psychologic needs. Students sometimes admit to feelings of inadequacy in helping parents older than themselves and in providing care for their children. They may have feelings of rejection when a child prefers other people to themselves, or the nurse may feel both enjoyment and guilt when a child prefers him or her to his parents. Sometimes students feel rejection toward parents who do not meet with their own criteria for self-control, cleanliness, and love for their children. In summary, some of the adverse feelings that students may have in response to the new experience of caring for children include inadequacy, fear of rejection, guilt, frustration, and lack of confidence.

Since students tend to view others who have had experience in caring for children as more expert than themselves, they fail to see that they still have something to contribute in their own way. Students, like others who experience anxiety, cannot reason well in anxiety-provoking situations. They need the support and guidance of experienced professional persons in the immediate environment. They also need the reassurance that can be gained by talking about their problems individually or in a group with a more experienced professional person who knows how they feel. After students learn their own beginning capabilities, recognize the correlation between their experiences in caring for adults and for children, can draw on their own knowledge, and have the support and guidance of their instructor or others with whom they can share any doubts, they will then move through graduated enjoyable experiences in providing care for children and support for their parents.

The young adult who has known a happy home life, looks forward to marriage, and rates homemaking as of equal value with professional success, is likely to be successful in caring for children. Today there are more parents in professions and more fathers and mothers who are professional people than there were a generation ago. Young people today look forward not to the choice between marriage and a profession, but to a combination of marriage and a profession.

One result of the better and more widespread understanding of the emotional life of children and that of adults is a fuller appreciation of the importance of parent-child-professional nurse relations. This, as concerns the nurse, is discussed throughout this book.

TEACHING AIDS AND OTHER INFORMATION*

American Academy of Pediatrics

Child Health and Community Health Centers in the Americas.
Migrant Health—A Review.
Nurses and Pediatricians Collaborate.
Standards of Child Health Care.
The Pediatrician and Indian Health.

American Nurses' Association

Accountability of the Nurse, 1973.
ANA Certification: Pediatric Nurse Practitioner in Ambulatory Health Care.
Bishop, B. E., and Roth, A. V.: Pediatric Nurse Practitioners: Their Practice Today, 1975.
Building for the Future, 1975.
Nurses in Health Maintenance Organizations, 1975.
Scope of Practice for the Pediatric Nurse Practitioner, 1974.
Standards of Maternal/Child Health Nursing Practice, 1973.

Consumer Product Information

Medicaid/Medicare, 1975.

Department of National Health and Welfare, Ottawa, Canada

Preparation of Nurses for an Expanded Role in Canadian Health Services.

National League for Nursing

Ozimek, D., and Yura, H.: Who Is the Nurse Practitioner? 1975.
The Changing Role of the Professional Nurse: Implications for Nursing Education, 1975.

Public Affairs Committee

Block, I.: The Health of the Poor.
Doyle, N.: Woman's Changing Place: A Look at Sexism.
Ogg, E.: La Población y el Futuro Norteamericano (Population of the American Future).
Stewart, M. S.: Hunger in America.

Southern Regional Council, Inc.

Comprehensive Health Care: A Southern View.

United States Government

America's Children, 1976.
Child Advocacy Programs 1975, 1976.
Child Health in America, 1976.
Comprehensive Emergency Services: A System Designed to Care for Children in Crisis, 1976.
Head Start: A Child Development Program, 1976.
Indian Health Care, 1974.
International MCH Projects; Research to Improve Health Services for Mothers and Children, 1975.
Maternal and Child Health Programs, 1975.
National Health System in Eight Countries, 1975.
OCD: Office of Child Development, 1975.
O'Keefe, R. A.: Home Start: Partnership With Parents, 1973.
Pechman, S. M.: Seven Parent and Child Centers, 1972.
Promoting Community Health, 1975.
Publications of the Office of Child Development, 1976.
Report of a National Conference on Home Start and Other Programs for Parents and Children, 1976.
Research Relating to Children, No. 35, 1975.
Research to Improve Health Services for Mothers and Children, 1974.
Responding to Individual Needs in Head Start, Working With the Individual Child, 1974.
The American Indians in Transition, 1975.
The Children and Youth Projects, Comprehensive Health Care in Low-Income Areas, 1972.
The Excluded Child: A Case for Child Advocacy.
The Maternal and Child Health Service Reports On: Promoting the Health of Mothers and Children, FY 1972, 1973.
The Maternity and Infant Care Projects: Reducing Risks for Mothers and Babies, 1975.
This Is HEW, 1975.
WIC Program Survey, 1975, 1975.

---

*Complete addresses are given in the Appendix.

REFERENCES

Books

Abdellah, F., Beland, I., Martin, A., and Matheney, R.: *New Directions in Patient-Centered Nursing. Guidelines for Systems of Service, Education and Research.* New York, The Macmillan Company, 1973.

Adair, J., and Deuschle, K. W.: *The People's Health: Medicine and Anthropology in a Navajo Community.* New York, Appleton-Century-Crofts, 1970.

Andreopoulos, S. (Ed.): *National Health Insurance: Can We Learn From Canada?* New York, John Wiley & Sons, Inc., 1975.

Auerbach, S. (Ed.): *Child Care: A Comprehensive Guide.* Vol. I: Rationale for Child Care — Program vs. Politics. Vol. II: Model Programs and Their Components. New York, Human Sciences Press, 1976.

Bellak, L.: *Overload: The Human Condition.* New York, Human Sciences Press, 1975.

Branch, M. F., and Paxton, P. P. (Eds.): *Providing Safe Nursing Care For Ethnic People of Color.* Appleton-Century-Crofts, 1976.

Bremner, R. H. (Ed.): *Children and Youth in America: A Documentary History.* Cambridge, Mass., Harvard University Press, 1970.

Bullough, B., and Bullough, V. L.: *Poverty, Ethnic Identity, and Health Care.* New York, Appleton-Century-Crofts, 1972.

Commission on Emotional and Learning Disorders in Children: *One Million Children: A National Study of Canadian Children with Emotional and Learning Disabilities.* Toronto, Canada, Celdic, 1970.

Demone, H. W., and Harshbarger, D.: *A Handbook of Human Service Organizations.* New York, Behavioral Publications, 1974.

French, R. M.: *The Dynamics of Health Care.* 2nd ed. New York, McGraw-Hill Book Company, 1974.

Golden Anniversary White House Conference on Children and Youth, March 27-April 2, 1960: *Conference Proceedings.* Washington, D.C. Golden Anniversary White House Conference on Children and Youth, Inc., 1960.

Gumbiner, R.: *The Health Maintenance Organization: HMO, Putting It All Together.* St. Louis, The C. V. Mosby Company, 1975.

Hernandez, C., Haug, M., and Wagner, N.: *Chicanos: Social and Psychological Perspectives.* 2nd ed. St. Louis, The C. V. Mosby Company, 1976.

Ishwaran, K.: *The Canadian Family.* Toronto, Holt, Rinehart and Winston, 1971.

Kahn, A. J., Kamerman, S. B., and McGowan, B. G.: *Child Advocacy: Report of a National Baseline Study.* New York, Columbia University School of Social Work, 1972.

Land, H.: *Large Families in London.* Toronto, Clarke, Irwin and Company, 1969.

Leininger, M. (Ed.): *Barriers and Facilitators to Quality Health Care.* Philadelphia, F. A. Davis Company, 1975.

Midcentury White House Conference on Children and Youth: *A Healthy Personality for Every Child.* Fact Finding Report. Raleigh, N.C., Health Publications Institute, Inc., 1951.

Milio, N.: *The Care of Health in Communities; Access for Outcasts.* New York, The Macmillan Company, 1975.

National Council of Organizations for Children and Youth: *America's Children 1976.* Washington, D.C., National Council of Organizations for Children and Youth, 1976.

Newell, K. W.: *Health by The People.* Geneva, World Health Organization, 1975.

UNICEF: *Children of the Developing Countries: A Report by UNICEF.* Cleveland, Ohio, World Publishing Company, 1963.

Wallace, H. M. (Ed.): *Health Care of Mothers and Children in National Health Services.* Philadelphia, Ballinger Publishing Company, 1975.

Wallace, H. M., Gold, E. M., and Lis, E. H.: *Maternal and Child Health Practices: Problems, Resources, and Methods of Delivery.* Springfield, Ill., Charles C Thomas, 1973.

White House Conference on Children and Yourth 1970–71: *Government Research on the Problems of Children and Youth.* Washington, D.C., White House Conference on Children and Youth 1970–71, 1971.

White House Conference on Children, 1970: *Profiles of Children.* Washington, D.C., White House Conference on Children 1970, 1971.

White House Conference on Youth, 1971: *Profiles of Youth.* Washington, D.C., Government Printing Office, 1972.

Periodicals

American Nurses' Association Division on Maternal and Child Health Nursing Practice and the American Academy of Pediatrics: A Joint Statement — Guidelines on Short-Term Continuing Education Programs for Pediatric Nurse Associates. *American Journal of Nursing,* 71:509, 1971.

Arboleda-Florez, J.: Infanticide: Some Medicolegal Considerations. *Canadian Psychiatric Association Journal,* 20:55, February 1975.

Brown, M. S., O'Meara, C., and Krowley, S.: The Maternal-Child Nurse Practitioner. *American Journal of Nursing,* 75:1298, August 1975.

Burnip, R., et al.: Well-child Care by Pediatric Nurse Practitioners in a Large Group Practice. A Controlled Study in 1,152 Preschool Children. *Am. J. Dis. Child,* 130:51, January 1976.

Clark, A. L., Howland, R., Affonso, D., and Uyehara, J.: "MCH in American Samoa." *American Journal of Nursing,* 74:700, April 1974.

Cochran, L. T., and O'Kane, J. M.: Population Explosion? — A Dissenting View. *Nursing Forum,* XIV:328, 1975.

Collins, R. C.: Toward a Future Strategy for Child Development. *Children Today,* 4:11, July-August 1975.

Daniel, J. H., and Hyde, J. N.: Working with High-Risk Families: Family Advocacy and the Parent Education Program. *Children Today,* 4:23, November-December 1975.

DeMause, L.: Our Forebears Made Childhood a Nightmare. *Psychology Today,* 8:85, April 1975.

Eliot, M. M.: Six Decades of Action for Children. *Children Today,* 1:2, March-April 1972.

Ferro, F.: Addressing Children's Needs. *Children Today,* 2:12, November-December 1973.

Goldstein, H.: Child Labor in America's History. *Children Today,* 5:30, May-June 1976.

Greenberg, R. A., et al.: Primary Child Health Care by Family Nurse Practitioners. *Pediatrics,* 53:900, June 1974.

Kadushin, A.: Child Welfare Services — Past and Present. *Children Today,* 5:16, May-June 1976.

Lambertsen, E. C.: Perspective on the Physician's Assistant. *Nursing Outlook,* 20:32, 1972.

Lawrence, R.: Exploring Childhood on an Indian Reservation. *Children Today,* 5:10, September-October 1976.

Lourie, N. V.: Funding Child Care Programs Under Title IV-A. *Children Today,* 1:23, July-August 1972.

MacKay, R. C.: Parents' Attitudes Toward the Nurse as Physician Associate in a Pediatric Practice. *Can. J. Public Health,* 64:121, March-April 1973.

Marker, G., and Friedman, P. R.: Rethinking Children's Rights. *Children Today,* 2:8, November-December 1973.

Mauksch, I. G., and Rogers, M. E.: On the Health Care Horizon: Nursing Issues. Nursing Is Coming of Age — Through the Practitioner Movement. *American Journal of Nursing,* 75:1833, October 1975.

O'Brien, M., Manly, M., and Heagarty, M. C.: Expanding the Public Health Nurse's Role in Child Care. *Nursing Outlook*, 23:369, June 1975.

Perkins, Sr. M. R.: Does Availability of Health Services Ensure Their Use? *Nursing Outlook*, 22:496, August 1974.

Reid, J. H., and Phillips, M.: Child Welfare Since 1912. *Children Today*, 1:13, March-April 1972.

Silver, H. K.: A Blueprint for Pediatric Health Manpower for the 1970's. *The Journal of Pediatrics*, 82:149, January 1973.

Solnit, A. J.: Changing Psychological Perspectives About Children and Their Families. *Children Today*, 5:5, May-June 1976.

Wagner, D.: Nursing in an HMO. *American Journal of Nursing*, 74:236, February 1974.

Waserman, M.: An Overview of Child Health Care in America. *Children Today*, 5:24, May-June 1976.

Wedge, P.: The National Children's Bureau in Britain. *Children Today*, 5:24, July-August 1976.

Word, S. A.: Components of a Child Advocacy Program. *Children Today*, 1:38, March-April 1972.

Zigler, E. F.: The Unmet Needs of America's Children. *Children Today*, 5:39, May-June 1976.

Zigler, E. F.: Project Head Start: Success or Failure? *Children Today*, 2:2, November-December 1973.

AUDIOVISUAL MEDIA*

Carousel Films

Hunger in America, Parts I & II
  54 minutes, 16mm, 2 reels, sound, color.
  Series: A CBS Reports Program.
  From the Mexican-Americans in San Antonio to the starving tenant farmers who live just outside of the nation's capital, this study reveals the inequities of food programs which permit 10 million men, women, and children to go hungry every day. Emphasizes the effects of starvation and malnutrition on mothers, babies and children.

United States Government

Four Children
  Producer USOEO
  20 minutes, 16mm, sound, black and white.
  Shows four Head Start children, so alike as human beings, so different as people. An intimate look at the children and the homes that influence them.

Poverty in Rural America
  Producer USDA
  29 minutes, 16mm, sound, black and white.
  Takes you where the 'Hidden Americans' live—into the mountain hollows, to the end of the rutted dirt roads, and into the bypassed communities. The people, the story of their problems, their privations, and their hopes.

The Allen Case
  Producer USSRS
  25 minutes, 16mm, sound, black and white.
  Shows a mother receiving aid for dependent children. Demonstrates how Mrs. Allen is helped to cope with her problem and how social workers can increase their skill in treatment-oriented interviewing. Useful in teaching crises intervention concepts.

---

*Complete addresses are given in the Appendix.

Chapter Two

WHAT CHILDREN MEAN TO THEIR PARENTS

GROWTH AND DEVELOPMENT OF CHILDREN

Couples plan to have children for a variety of reasons, not the least of which is that children are perceived as necessary to the happiness of the family. Children satisfy some of the parents' emotional, psychologic, social and even spiritual needs. Children enliven family life. While they are growing up they provide entertainment for the parents and they satisfy some of the parents' needs for affection. Children, in other words, may prevent loneliness and boredom in what may be an otherwise dreary life.

One or more children provide the means by which parents can perpetuate their own existence and thus conquer personal death. As long as human beings like themselves well enough to want to continue the human species, there will be children. Children prolong the parents' existence into the future. They may also be depended upon to care for their parents in old age.

The number of children desired depends on the cultural background and socioeconomic status of the parents. If the desire is to educate the children well, the more children there are, the fewer financial resources there will be to give them all higher education. How much a child actually costs his parents is dependent on where and how the family lives.

The cost of raising a child is great even in a financially secure family of the middle or upper class. But the pride that such parents take in the child and the psychologic satisfaction they derive from educating him, are worth the cost to the parents. Such a child is loved for himself; he is not seen as a measure of security for the parents.

In low-income families living in an area where unemployment and illness are everpresent, children are seen not so much as a financial burden (since not much money is devoted to their care), but as a form of social security as the

parents become older. Children in such families learn rapidly that they must earn their own way in life.

In rural environments, although children may be a financial burden during their younger years, they provide hands to help with the farm work and they can be viewed as providers for their parents later in life.

The preferred sex of children varies from one culture to another. In many societies male children are preferred because they ensure continuity of the family by carrying the family name. They may also be depended upon to provide for their parents in old age. Daughters, on the other hand, may be desired because they can participate in household duties, helping a mother who may be occupied in the care of other children. Once daughters are married, however, the support they provided earlier may lessen or cease.

Financial resources and social standing are important in determining the number of children a family has. Abstract ideas such as avoiding overpopulation or reducing the food supply may have some impact on population growth, but more personal reasons usually determine the size of an individual family.

Having a baby is a tremendous responsibility. Potential parents, in fact, may consider not hav-

23

ing any children rather than accept a responsibility that they really do not want.

PARENTING

Education for parenthood begins with the general education of the child for responsibilities in family living. More specifically, parents help the child to prepare for parenthood by helping him to understand the role of parents and of sexuality in his life and the lives of others. How the child is treated determines in large measure how he will treat his children. Thus one of the best ways to prepare to be a good parent is to grow up in a family having good parents.

The child also learns about parenting in introductory classes such as "Preparation for Family Life" in high school. Courses on parent education are also offered in undergraduate college and adult education programs. Discussion groups for young wives who are pregnant and for their husbands include discussion of the physical and emotional needs of infants and how these needs can best be met. The emotional needs are as important as the physical needs, for lack of affection has an adverse influence on personality development. Among these needs is contact with a soft, warm human body and the slight motion that comes from gentle handling and cuddling in a parent's arms.

The philosophy of life, knowledge, values, attitudes, and emotions of the mother and father concerning a child determine their ability in the area of parenting. This ability is learned beginning in their own childhood and is modified during their years of development. Good parenting depends upon the level of self-esteem of the parents as individuals, their level of maturity, and the kind of infant born to them. As was mentioned before, how they feel about their own parents is of great importance in determining parenting behavior when their own child is born. After the infant is delivered, parenting becomes a changing, dynamic behavioral process that is modified to adjust to the child's continued growth and his developing relations with his parents.

With the rapid changes in lifestyles occurring today, mother is no longer stereotyped as the only one who cares for the baby, and father may not be the sole financial support of the family. The lifestyles of the parents, whether the mother works and father cares for the family or whether there is only a single parent who does both, determines how the parenting role is viewed.

THE CHILD GROWS WITHIN A FAMILY

Growth and development of the child occur as a result of his cultural and hereditary backgrounds and the care and love which adults, usually his family, bestow upon him. Although brief mention was made in Chapter 1 of the extended kinship family and its division into smaller nuclear family groups, this concept requires further explanation. More than 200 years ago in this country the child of the pioneer most often grew up within a family which gained its livelihood from the wilderness and from the soil. In such a family several generations lived in the same home or in homes not too distant from each other. The members of the different generations were interdependent; each family member was recognized as an individual who contributed to the good of all. There was a continuity to life. The young child lived by the rules of his family and of his society. The mores, the values, the traditions were passed from one generation to the next as the children matured.

Although certain members of families remained in rural areas, gradually other family members migrated from the farms to small towns and, as cities grew, moved on to become city dwellers. Over the last few decades some city dwellers have moved out of the congested metropolitan areas and back to the more rural suburbs. This mobility tended to disintegrate the extended families, to submit smaller families and individual family members to a kind of stress unknown to the original, large, self-sufficient family. The stress resulted not only from mobility but also from the external forces of a changing social and economic order.

Likewise, small families or individual family members who immigrated to this country during past decades from other lands having different values, mores, customs, traditions and perhaps even language have met with similar kinds of stresses in their adjustment to their new cultural environment.

The cultural characteristics of a group, in this case the family, have a decisive role to play in shaping the behavior of each family member. This is especially true in the case of a child who comes to believe at an early age that what his family is, does, and values is right or "normal" for everyone. If the child lived in a completely homogeneous society there would be no great problem, but in this country, few children do. As soon as a child is able to travel beyond his home, he learns that others are different as a result of age, sex, race, religion, national origin, educational level, and income level, as well as being different in other factors such as cultural attitudes and beliefs.

The cultural patterns of our present-day society may be defined through broad, overlapping generalizations.

THE HOME

Cultural Patterns: Ethnic Group, Locality, Class, Occupation. When attempting to understand the behavior of individuals, their cultural backgrounds should always be considered. At the same time, one must use caution in stereotyping or jumping to conclusions based on limited knowledge. While it is perhaps true that certain groups may tend to have characteristic cultural patterns, these general patterns may not apply to any one particular individual in a group. Each person is unique, and to judge him without adequate knowledge would be grossly unfair.

When we speak about the Irish, Italians, blacks, Jews, Catholics, Protestants, or any other racial, religious, or ethnic group, we must perceive what each group includes. There may be several variables: young, old, males, females, first-generation Americans retaining old-world ties, second-generation Americans rejecting old-world beliefs, educated, uneducated, religious, non-religious, wealthy, or poor, as well as others within a group. There is, in other words, no homogeneous cultural group. In reality, people of differing cultural backgrounds who live in a geographic area may have more in common with other groups in the same area than they have with people of their own culture group living in a different geographic area. For instance, blacks who live in a ghetto in a large metropolitan area may have more in common with their immigrant neighbors than they have with blacks living in the rural south who are not living in poverty. Although members of a cultural group may manifest certain behavior that distinguishes them, still they may be changed by other outside influences.

There are ethnic groups represented by the few remaining Chinatowns of our large cities, by Cubans in Florida, and by the Puerto Rican and Mexican communities in New York, Chicago, and other metropolitan centers, as well as French-Canadian villages in the New England states. The cultural patterns of the middle, southern, eastern, and western states differ. Large cities, towns, villages, crossroad neighborhoods, and the open country with scattered farms all have characteristic cultural patterns.

In the democratic United States we do not like to speak of people as belonging to an upper, middle, or lower class, although there is general recognition that there are class cultures. In general, traits found among college-educated persons are not those of the uneducated.

As professional persons, many nurses are limited in their knowledge of the needs of the poor. The child born into a family of the upper or middle class is, because of the socioeconomic status of his family, likely to have more advantages of good physical care than a child born into a poverty-stricken home. Because of their probable lack of adequate education, parents in the lower-income group are likely not to provide as clean an environment or as adequate care of food substances, with the resulting increased rate of infection and diarrhea, as parents who have had the advantage of better education. Likewise, parents who cannot afford the material advantages of life for their children many times cannot afford adequate medical care for themselves or for their children. Others do not seek assistance even when they know where they can get help at no cost to themselves. The parents and children therefore may suffer from illnesses which could be easily treated if diagnosed early enough. This is not to say that children who do not receive adequate physical care do not receive adequate love. Many times such children during their early years are secure in the knowledge that their parents love them. Unfortunately, the effect of poverty on the life of a child may be most intense when he is old enough to venture outside his own home. It is during his years in school that he may compare himself, to his own disadvantage, with others who appear to him to be more fortunate than himself.

Parental characteristics and behavior in general are modeled on those of their group and, specifically, their parents. For instance, physical punishment was characteristically inflicted on their children by immigrants from many countries of Europe, but seldom used among the Chinese or Japanese in places where they retained their native culture. The position of the father and of the mother in the family varies with the customs of the group.

The culture of the ethnic group, the geographic area, urban or rural location, and social class all influence the parents, but are redefined by the *family* itself, that small, closely knit unit of society into which the child is born and in which he is brought up. It is the home culture that is influential in determining the child's growth and development. As he grows older and leaves the home and play group for school and the gang, team, club, or clique, home culture is increasingly modified by that of the community.

Types of Families. In families in which the father is away from home for long periods—e.g., men in military service and traveling salesmen—or working in other areas where it would be impracticable to have their families with them, the mother is likely to be the head of the household. In a modified form the mother as decision maker is found in new settlements on the fringes of large cities. In such families the children rarely see their fathers except on weekends.

The democratic family, in which both parents, and children when they are old enough, participate in making decisions, is the modern type. In this type both parents may work to support the family on a higher level of living than would be possible on the father's salary alone. In an increasing number of youthful marriages the wife works to support or help in the support of the family while her husband finishes his professional education. In former generations a man whose wife worked while he did not was blamed for his behavior and was pitied by her friends. Today it is understood that his education is part of his work—a job which in the long run will provide a standard of living he could not achieve without further preparation.

Another community of young married people has sprung up around military bases. The length of stay at any base is so uncertain that these homes have little of the stability found in civilian community life. But common interests are strong, and such groups are closely knit, often in a town which seldom welcomes them to full participation in its social life.

Young married couples want children and are willing to make many sacrifices in order to start their families. Both parents help in the housekeeping and in the care of the child, fitting their hours of work or study into a schedule which provides for one or the other to be home with the baby throughout the 24 hours of the day. When the baby is old enough, he may be placed in a day nursery while his mother is working.

Finally, there are families with a common source of support. Such families are dependent upon some industry and are found in certain sections of many cities. Members of such groups are likely to have many similar social traits.

Many children do not live in the kind of family built on the love felt between a man and a woman who marry and live to care for their children. There are one-parent families as the result of the death or divorce of a marital partner or as the result of children being born out of wedlock. A woman who wants one or more children may not wish to marry the father, choosing instead to raise them alone. There are families living in communes in which several young adults are available to care for the child or children who may or may not be born in wedlock. There are families in which no parents are present in the home, the children being reared by older siblings, grandparents or other relatives. There are children who are cared for by foster parents temporarily or who spend most of their childhood in institutions. Regardless of the relation of the adults to the children, they provide for the young a social and cultural heritage, and a physical climate in which to live. Each member of such a group needs to develop more or less of an understanding of the others and to give and receive love and care from them in order for full development to occur in the individuals and in the group. It is essential for the nurse who seeks to understand the growth and development of any family member, adult or child, to know the identity and role of each member of the group and the interrelation between the individual members.

THE COMMUNITY

The general community pattern of child rearing undoubtedly influences the personality of the older child. He is likely to rate his home, and the way his parents or other adults who care for him treat him, by group standards, and if the home differs widely from the general pattern, he knows it. If all parents inflict physical punishment, the child is apt to accept it as part of the usual parent-child relations. But if he is whipped and none of his friends is physically punished, he is likely to blame his parents and feel that they do not love him, that he is abused.

It is in warm home life that the child first learns the meaning of love, of giving up his pleasure because he wants the approval of loving parents. He learns to obey those who are better able than he to understand what should be done in different situations. He transfers this attitude toward authority to his baby-sitter, to neighbors, nursery school workers, nurses, and teachers. He adjusts to adult-child relations in a constantly broadening area of social contacts.

THE NURSE AND THE FAMILY

The nurse who interacts with many younger and older family members may find it impossible to be familiar with the attitudes and practices of each cultural and subcultural group with which contact is made. The nurse should, however, understand the concept of culture and its impact on the family members and sensitively attempt to understand the characteristics of culturally different groups in the local geographic area.

The cultural background of the nurse is also

important. Every culture not only has its own set of customs and values but also evidences varying attitudes toward health and illness and varying degrees of emotional control, stoicism, and reactions to pain. The cultural background of the nurse as well as of family members becomes of great importance in determining the quality of care given each individual.

THE NURSE'S UNDERSTANDING OF GROWTH AND DEVELOPMENT

The period of growth and development extends throughout the life cycle; however, the period in which the principal changes occur is from conception to the end of adolescence. It is important for the nurse to understand the total life cycle of an individual in order to better understand the behavior of parents and other adults who provide care for the child.

The principal period of growth and development is a complex one in which two cells joined as one normally become a thinking, feeling person who eventually takes his responsible place in society. The nurse should understand this process of growth and development for several reasons.

The nurse must know what to expect of a particular child at any given age and at what age certain kinds of behavior are likely to emerge in more mature forms. She uses this knowledge to observe and to judge each child in terms of norms for specific levels of development. A child may be guided into more mature behavior if the sequence of developmental behavior is understood.

In order for the nurse to help in formulating the plan for total care for each child, what is expected of different age groups and the developmental sequence which occurs throughout childhood and adolescence must be understood.

A knowledge of growth and development is important to the nurse in order to better understand the reason for particular conditions and illnesses which occur in various age groups.

When the nurse has gained experience in applying the study of growth and development in child care, mothers can be taught how to observe and to use their knowledge in order that they may help their own children to achieve optimal growth and development.

This chapter, as well as later chapters devoted to growth and development, presents concepts, principles and facts which would be helpful for the nurse to know in order to adapt care to the needs of children in different age groups. Most ranges of norms for growth and development were established in the past on samples of presumably middle-class Americans. *When average achievement levels are presented for the various age groups, the student must not interpret them as specific for the development of any one child of a given age. Each achievement may occur normally within a range of time.* The age of a specific achievement given in various tables is usually in the approximate middle of such a range. For example (see p. 508), a toddler walks alone at 14 months, but actually may normally walk alone at any time in the range between nine and 18 months of age. The student will probably find it easier to remember specific ages for levels of achievement than trying to remember the limits of ranges within which such achievement can occur.

HEREDITY, EUGENICS, AND EUTHENICS

The relatively typical physical pattern of growth and development is influenced by heredity, environment and the child's state of health. The *heredity* of a man and a woman determines that of their children. For this reason the health history of several generations of the families of each of the parents is studied to determine the hereditary traits likely to exist in the child.

Eugenics is the science that deals with influences that improve inborn or hereditary qualities of the race. Applied eugenics would influence men and women in the selection of marriage partners, helping them to avoid those unions which presumably would produce children below an accepted normal standard and encouraging those which would be likely to produce children above this standard. A few diseases are hereditary, and a tendency to a number of diseases is genetically determined. As has been pointed out, the family history or pedigree rather than the condition of the child's parents must be studied to determine the probability of a tendency toward a specific disease. Such a study is difficult among the lower-income group, whose health histories are carried by word of mouth, and among some groups whose attitude toward health and illness may be culturally influenced. With the expansion of health work in schools, clinics, public health agencies, and occupational health programs, family health histories may become more reliable than they are at present.

Also recently the procedures of amniocentesis and blood tests have been used as a means of determining some genetically determined problems (see Chap. 10).

Euthenics, in contrast to eugenics, deals with measures to promote health. It concerns itself with healthy intrauterine conditions for the developing fetus and with a wholesome environment, not only for children but also for all age groups.

In community health agencies, including hospitals, mothers as well as students are taught the general principles of child growth and development. They are taught that *each child has a different genetic potentiality for growth which cannot be exceeded, but may be hampered at any stage.* A child who deviates too far from the normal range of height, weight, physical development, or behavior should be referred to a physician. The most common cause for concern about a child is a sudden slowing up, not typical for his age, in any aspect of his development. Anticipatory guidance should be given to mothers about changes in the rate of growth and development that can be expected at certain ages.

CHARACTERISTICS OF GROWTH AND DEVELOPMENT

Growth and development are terms often used interchangeably. Each depends upon the other, and in a normal child they parallel each other. But they are not the same. *Growth* refers to an increase in physical size of the whole or any of its parts and can be measured in inches or centimeters and in pounds or kilograms. *Development* refers to progressive increase in skill and capacity of function. The term "maturation" is often used as a synonym for development. *Maturation* has the more limited application, however, of referring to the development of traits carried through the genes. Development is *orderly*, not haphazard; there is a direct relation between each of its stages and the next.

Every child is an individual and should never be considered a typical boy or girl, one unit of a group who are all alike. Each child has his own *rate of growth*, but the *pattern of growth* shows less variability. For example, an infant will be able to sit before he can stand alone. The age at which he as an individual achieves these skills may, as has been mentioned before, occur at any point in a range of time.

Although growth and development—physical, mental, social, emotional, sexual, and spiritual—proceed at different rates, they are so *interrelated* in the majority of children that the result is a progressive development of the whole child, from infancy to adulthood. Only when growth in any aspect is unusually slow or advanced is this interrelation disturbed so that the child appears abnormal. For example, a boy who at 14 years of age grows to a height of 6 feet may appear to be physically a man, but emotionally, socially, and intellectually he may achieve at a normal pubescent level. Whatever the cause, if a child is notably different from others of his age, he is likely to need help in order to make a good adjustment to home and community life. The child with a long-term illness or a handicap of body or mind also differs from his peers and will need help.

TEAM APPROACH TO FOSTER INTERRELATEDNESS OF GROWTH AND DEVELOPMENT

The concept of interrelatedness of growth and development is important in the care of the well child. In addition to the parents, who provide for the basic physical and emotional care of the child, there are other adults whose main concerns are on other aspects of care, such as health supervision (physicians and other members of the health team and nurses and other members of the nursing team), intellectual development (teachers and other school personnel from nursery school throughout formal education), social development (leaders in school groups and clubs in the community) and spiritual guidance (ministers, priests, rabbis or other spiritual advisors).

The concept of interrelations in growth is also true for the hospitalized child or one under medical supervision in the home. This is one reason why professional teamwork is important in the care of the ill child. The whole team is needed to foster progression in all areas of development in the hospitalized or home-bound child. Thus the hospital has the schoolteacher to encourage mental development, and the child care worker (the Play Lady) to create situations in which there may be pleasant social interaction. The psychologist and the psychiatrist help the nurses with the emotional problems of sick children. The dietitian, the physical therapist, and all the other members of the team work together, each focusing on a different facet of growth, toward the full development of the whole child. In the home there is the school teacher (visiting teacher), public health nurse, actually all the members of the health team, as found in the hospital. Many members of the health team work through the community or public health nurse. The health team also functions in helping the child make the transition from home to hospital to home.

Stages of Growth and Development

All children go through a normal sequence of growth, but not at the same rate. Nor is the rate the same in all areas. In general, there is a positive correlation between physical growth and mental, emotional, and sexual development. This may not be true in individual children, of course, and we have learned the danger of attempting to force a child into a standard pattern of growth. There are far too many variations in genetic traits and in the environment to make this possible. The strain upon the child may react upon his personality and even his physical health.

Adults who have a clear understanding of the stages of growth and development can apply their knowledge when caring for children. These stages, listed here, are considered in detail in the chapters on the nursing care of various age groups.

1. Fetal or embryonic—from conception to birth
2. Newborn (neonatal)—from birth to two to four weeks
3. Infancy—from two to four weeks to one year
4. Toddler—from one year to three years
5. Early childhood (preschool)—from three to six years
6. Late childhood (school)—from six to twelve years or puberty
7. Adolescence—from puberty to the beginning of adult life.

Norms of Growth

In order to find norms of physical growth we may study age groups by the *cross-sectional technique* and make a comparison of their average weight, height or other evidence of growth. Consider, for instance, the average height of five-year-olds and six-year-olds. The difference between these averages is taken as the average growth of a child during his sixth year. In a *longitudinal study* of growth, height and weight of children are followed from birth throughout childhood. Such studies show periods of accelerated growth which correlate with the individual child's stage of maturation. *Spurts of growth* are related to pubescence, which occurs earlier in some children than in others. This acceleration in rate may begin in girls as early as ten years and in others as late as 14 years; corresponding ages for boys are 12 and 16 years. An early acceleration in growth is indicative of early puberty. Since the rate slows down a year or two after the onset of puberty, a boy who is late in maturing and ashamed of his small stature and plumpness at 13 years of age can be told that he is more likely to continue growing than his friend who matured early and is inches taller than he. But a boy who matures early and is shorter than the average for his age is likely to remain short.

The mental, emotional, social, and sexual aspects of development show the same variations, but are much more influenced by environmental factors than is physical growth. Under conditions of great deprivation, however, as in wartime starvation or prolonged illness or hospitalization, physical growth might be more influenced by environmental factors than other types of development.

Norms or averages of growth must be used with caution, for not only do some children mature early and others late, and thus achieve early or late acceleration in the rate of growth, but also body build and potential height are inherited traits. Because of their heredity some children are short and fat, others of muscular build or medium height, and still others may be tall and slender. Separate norms for each of these three types of body build are of more value than single tables for all children in general.

Study of Growth and Developmental Patterns

The cross-sectional study of age groups antedated the longitudinal study. From these studies averages were readily compiled. There are disadvantages, however, in their use. These studies did not take into account body build or early and late maturation. At best, in using these schedules, a decision of normality is based on only two gross characteristics: weight and height. These are inadequate criteria for measuring a child's potential development under existing environmental conditions.

In any consideration of a child's growth the *expected rate of gain* is of greater value than a single measurement taken at any one time. Two examples of growth charts are the *Iowa Growth Chart* and the *Grid-Graph*.

The staff at the University of Iowa produced a series of six charts showing weight-age and height-age for males and females in the age groups of 0 to 12 months, 0 to six years, and five years to 18 years, based on thousands of observations of children. Figure 2–1 provides an example of an Iowa Growth Chart. The name and birth date of the child are inserted when the record is started. Each time the child is examined, his height and weight are recorded and plotted on the chart. The weight-age is shown in the section at the top of the page, and the height-age at the bottom. The child's progress can be seen in comparison with other children of his height and weight. These forms are easier to use and to read than the more complex Grid-Graph.

In order to measure graphically a child's growth in height and weight, and to record changes in body contours as well, the Grid-Graph was devised. It is based on the assumption that physical development proceeds along regular channels for different body types. The two Grid-Graphs are the Wetzel Grid and the Baby Grid. The Baby Grid is for use with infants from birth to three years, and the other form is for use with children from two to 18 years of age.

The Baby Grid (Fig. 2–2) is a height-weight gauge of the progress of the individual child. It has two parts. On the left side of the page is a channel system on which height is plotted against weight. This represents various graduations of build from slender on the right to heavy build on the left. At regular intervals of 10 these channels are crossed by horizontal "developmental level lines," which are actually increment units for development, such as Follows, Smiles, Head Control, through various levels to Speech. On the right side of the page is a grid on which can be plotted developmental levels against chronologic age with a series of curves or auxodromes which indicate the speed or rate of development for premature, normal and advanced infants. If an infant is healthy and is developing normally, his record will travel

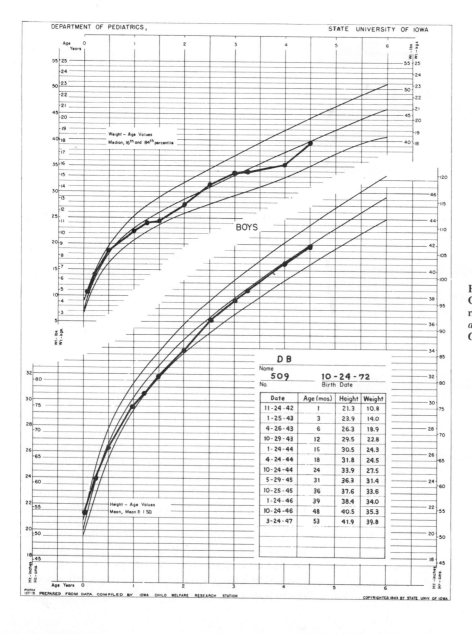

FIGURE 2–1. Iowa Growth Chart. (From M. E. Breckenridge and M. N. Murphy: *Growth and Development of the Young Child.*)

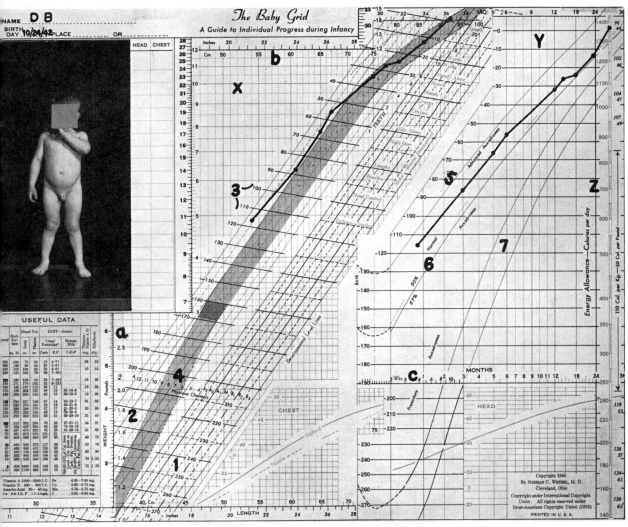

FIGURE 2-2. The Baby Grid, one of the forms of the Grid-Graph.

channel-wise and will parallel one of the auxodromes.

With the use of the Grid it is possible to evaluate how the child is developing in view of his own unique pattern, regardless of his physique and growth rate. Thus each child's progress may be predicted from his previous standards, and the physician quickly becomes aware that something is amiss when the growth pattern is distorted. If the infant shifts from one channel to another or lags in his development, he should be examined to determine the cause. The method of use of the Grid for older children is similar to that discussed for the Baby Grid.

The newer tables show more than physical growth and development. These tables include height, weight, number of teeth erupted, carpal bone age, mental age and social age. These criteria can be plotted on a common scale. They show the correlation in measurements of physi-

cal and mental growth, i.e., the interrelatedness of growth. In normal growth there is an underlying unity, the presence or lack of which is shown on these graphs.

An adequate clinical history, in addition to the composite chart, is necessary for the proper interpretation of somatic and mental growth. Deviations from the average have no meaning unless factors such as dentition, illness, emotional health, and interaction of the social and physical environments are used in interpreting the data.

Children who have delayed development may not be diagnosed until they enter school even though many causes of deviant development could be treated if diagnosed early enough. The *Denver Developmental Screening Test* (DDST) was standardized in order to meet this need of infants and preschool children. It evaluates the following aspects of the child's functioning:

THE DENVER DEVELOPMENTAL SCREENING TEST

The Denver Developmental Screening Test (DDST) offers a simple and effective way of assessing the developmental status of children during the first six years of life. Abbreviated instructions follow:

The Denver Developmental Screening Test (DDST), a device for detecting developmental delays in infancy and the preschool years, has been standardized on a large cross section of the Denver child population. The test is administered with ease and speed and lends itself to serial evaluations on the same test sheet.

Test Materials. Skein of red wool; box of raisins; rattle with a narrow handle; small clear glass bottle with ⅝ in. opening; bell; tennis ball; test form; pencil; 8 one-inch cubical colored (red, blue, yellow, green) blocks.

General Instructions. The mother should be told that this is a developmental screening device to obtain an estimate of the child's level of development and that it is not expected that the child will be able to perform each of the test items. This test relies on observations of what the child can do and on report by a parent who knows the child. Direct observation should be used whenever possible. Since the test requires active participation by the child, every effort should be made to put the child at ease. The younger child may be tested while sitting on the mother's lap. This should be done in such a way that he can comfortably reach the test materials on the table. The test should be administered before any frightening or painful procedures. One may start by laying out one or two test materials in front of the child while asking the mother whether he performs some of the personal-social items. It is best to administer the first few test items well below the child's age level in order to assure him an initial successful experience. To avoid distractions it is best to remove all test materials from the table except those required for the test that is being administered.

Steps in Administering the Test

1. Draw a vertical line on the examination sheet through the four sectors (Personal-Social, Fine Motor-Adaptive, Language, and Gross Motor) to represent the child's chronologic age. Place the date of the examination at the top of the age line. For children who were born prematurely, subtract the number of months of prematurity from the chronologic age.

2. The items to be administered are those through which the child's chronologic age line passes, unless there are obvious deviations. In each sector one should establish the area in which the child passes all the items and the point at which he fails all the items.

3. In the event that a child refuses to do some of the items requested by the examiner, it is suggested that the parent administer the item, provided she does so in the prescribed manner.

4. If a child passes an item, a large letter "P" is written on the bar. "F" designates a failure, and "R" designates a refusal.

5. Note how the child adjusted to the examination (i.e., his cooperation, attention span, self-confidence) and how he related to his mother, the examiner and the test materials.

6. Ask the parent if the child's performance was typical of his performance at other times.

7. To retest the child on the same form, use a different color pencil for the scoring and age line.

8. Instructions for administering footnoted items are on the back of the test form.

Interpretations. The test items are placed into four categories: Personal-Social, Fine Motor-Adaptive, Language, and Gross Motor. Each of the test items is designated by a bar which is so located under the age scale as to indicate clearly the ages at which 25, 50, 75 and 90 per cent of the standardization population could perform the particular test item. The left end of the bar designates the age at which 25 per cent of the standardization population could perform the item; the hatch mark at the top of the bar 50 per cent; the left end of the shaded area 75 per cent, and the right end of the bar the age at which 90 per cent of the standardization population could perform the item. (See below.)

Failure to perform an item passed by 90 per cent of children of the same age should be considered a "delay." Such a failure may be emphasized by coloring the right end of the bar of the failed item. Performances are scored as *abnormal* if two or more sectors have two or more delays, *or* if one sector has two or more delays and one other sector has one delay and in the same sector the age line does not intersect one item that is passed; as *questionable* if any one sector has two or more delays, or if one or more sectors have one delay *and* in the same sectors the age line does not intersect an item that is passed; as *untestable* if refusals occur in numbers large enough to cause the test to be questionable or abnormal if the refusals were scored as failures; and as *normal* if the performance is not abnormal, questionable or untestable.

FIGURE 2–3. Denver Developmental Screening Test. (Test kits, manuals, and forms may be purchased from the LaDoca Project & Publishing Foundation, Inc., Denver, Colorado 80216.)

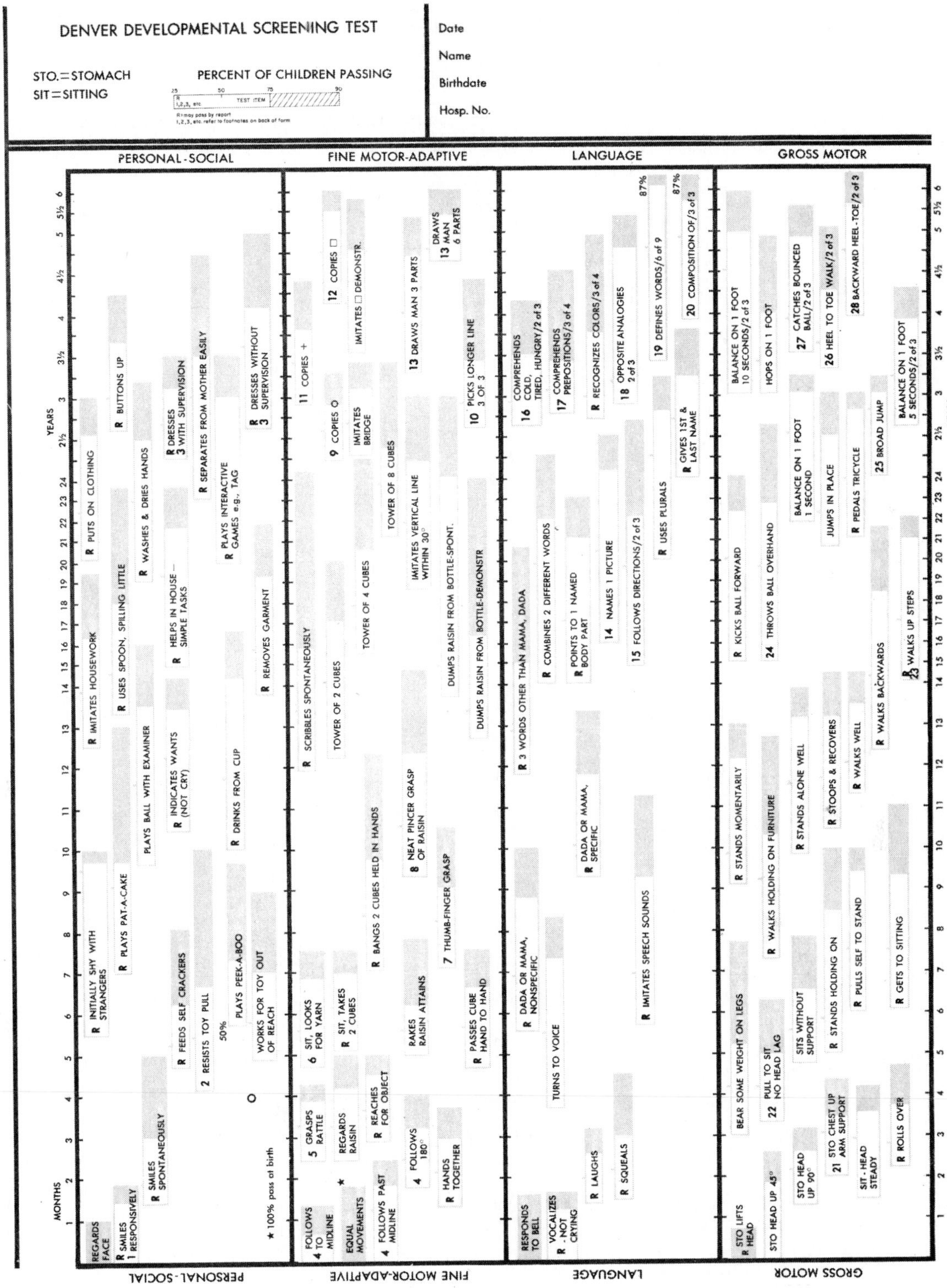

Figure 2–3. *Continued.* *Illustration continued on following page.*

gross motor, fine motor-adaptive, language, and personal-social areas. The test is simple to administer, score, and interpret and is useful for repeat evaluations of the same child (see Fig. 2–3).

Other methods for studying types of development have been devised such as that by T. Berry Brazelton, M.D., who created a tool to assess the sensory readiness and development of an infant. Another way by which physical growth pat-

DATE

NAME

DIRECTIONS   BIRTHDATE

HOSP. NO.

1. Try to get child to smile by smiling, talking or waving to him. Do not touch him.
2. When child is playing with toy, pull it away from him. Pass if he resists.
3. Child does not have to be able to tie shoes or button in the back.
4. Move yarn slowly in an arc from one side to the other, about 6" above child's face. Pass if eyes follow 90° to midline. (Past midline; 180°)
5. Pass if child grasps rattle when it is touched to the backs or tips of fingers.
6. Pass if child continues to look where yarn disappeared or tries to see where it went. Yarn should be dropped quickly from sight from tester's hand without arm movement.
7. Pass if child picks up raisin with any part of thumb and a finger.
8. Pass if child picks up raisin with the ends of thumb and index finger using an over hand approach.

  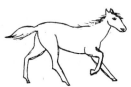 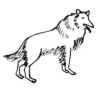

9. Pass any enclosed form. Fail continuous round motions.
10. Which line is longer? (Not bigger.) Turn paper upside down and repeat. (3/3 or 5/6)
11. Pass any crossing lines.
12. Have child copy first. If failed, demonstrate

When giving items 9, 11 and 12, do not name the forms. Do not demonstrate 9 and 11.

13. When scoring, each pair (2 arms, 2 legs, etc.) counts as one part.
14. Point to picture and have child name it. (No credit is given for sounds only.)

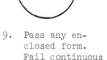   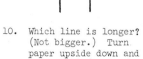 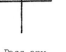   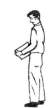

15. Tell child to: Give block to Mommie; put block on table; put block on floor. Pass 2 of 3. (Do not help child by pointing, moving head or eyes.)
16. Ask child: What do you do when you are cold? ..hungry? ..tired? Pass 2 of 3.
17. Tell child to: Put block on table; under table; in front of chair, behind chair. Pass 3 of 4. (Do not help child by pointing, moving head or eyes.)
18. Ask child: If fire is hot, ice is ?; Mother is a woman, Dad is a ?; a horse is big, a mouse is ?. Pass 2 of 3.
19. Ask child: What is a ball? ..lake? ..desk? ..house? ..banana? ..curtain? ..ceiling? ..hedge? ..pavement? Pass if defined in terms of use, shape, what it is made of or general category (such as banana is fruit, not just yellow). Pass 6 of 9.
20. Ask child: What is a spoon made of? ..a shoe made of? ..a door made of? (No other objects may be substituted.) Pass 3 of 3.
21. When placed on stomach, child lifts chest off table with support of forearms and/or hands.
22. When child is on back, grasp his hands and pull him to sitting. Pass if head does not hang back.
23. Child may use wall or rail only, not person. May not crawl.
24. Child must throw ball overhand 3 feet to within arm's reach of tester.
25. Child must perform standing broad jump over width of test sheet. (8-1/2 inches)
26. Tell child to walk forward, ⟳⟳⟳⟳➤ heel within 1 inch of toe. Tester may demonstrate. Child must walk 4 consecutive steps, 2 out of 3 trials.
27. Bounce ball to child who should stand 3 feet away from tester. Child must catch ball with hands, not arms, 2 out of 3 trials.
28. Tell child to walk backward, ◀⟳⟳⟳⟳ toe within 1 inch of heel. Tester may demonstrate. Child must walk 4 consecutive steps, 2 out of 3 trials.

DATE AND BEHAVIORAL OBSERVATIONS (how child feels at time of test, relation to tester, attention span, verbal behavior, self-confidence, etc,):

Figure 2-3. *Continued.*

Developmental delays may be due to:

1. The unwillingness of the child to use his ability
   a. Owing to temporary factors, such as fatigue, illness, hospitalization, separation from the parent, fear, etc.
   b. General unwillingness to do most things that are asked of him—such a condition may be just as detrimental as an inability to perform
2. An inability to perform the item because of
   a. general retardation
   b. pathologic factors such as deafness or neurologic impairment
   c. familial pattern of slow development in one or more areas

If unexplained developmental delays appear to be valid reflections of a child's abilities, he should be rescreened a month later. If the delays persist he should be further evaluated with more detailed diagnostic studies.

Caution. The DDST is *not* an intelligence test. It is intended as a screening instrument for use in clinical practice to note whether the development of a particular child is within the normal range.

These abbreviated instructions are amplified in the manual.

The form is copyrighted. Forms, kits, manuals and instructional films may be purchased through LADOCA Project and Publishing Foundation, Inc., East 51st Avenue and Lincoln Street, Denver, Colorado 80216.

We are indebted to the authors for permission to include the test in this volume.

Frankenburg, W. K., and Dodds, J. B.: The Denver Developmental Screening Test. J. Pediatr. 71:181, 1967.
Frankenburg, W. K., Goldstein, A. D. and Camp, B. W.: The Revised Denver Developmental Screening Test: Its accuracy as a screening instrument. J. Pediatr. 79:988, 1971.

Figure 2–3. *Continued.*

terns can be studied is through the use of *stereophotogrammetry.* Stereophotogrammetry is the production of a contour map of the hills and valleys of the whole human body; thus it is an accurate measurement of physique. This technique is used to measure and understand physiologic differences among people, to observe the growth and development of premature infants and to study the relation between mental retardation and body development. After many children have been measured in this way, a relation may be discovered between the biochemical processes controlling mental development and those controlling body growth.

The *physioprint* is similar in concept except that in this method only the face is measured. A picture is produced by a measured grid projected onto the child's face. The contours, planes, lines and curves of the facial skeletal structure and soft tissues "bend" the pattern on the face into curved lines. This results in a unique contour map of the face, different from anyone else's. The physioprint can register growth changes that can serve as a guide in tooth-straightening and denture-fitting when necessary. It can also aid in the interpretation of family-line transmission of inherited traits.

FACTORS IN GROWTH AND DEVELOPMENT

Growth and development are due not to one factor, but to a combination of many factors, all interdependent.

Heredity and Constitutional Make-up

Embryonic life begins with the cytoplasm and the nucleus of the fertilized ovum, genetically determined by both parents.

Members of families bear physical resemblances, and there is a high degree of correlation of stature with weight among siblings. The rate of growth is more alike among siblings than among unrelated persons. Some children are small not because of endocrine or nutritional disturbances, but because of their genetic constitution. Before evaluating the largeness or smallness of a child, the size of the parents should first be observed.

Racial and National Characteristics

Race. Distinguishing characteristics called racial or subracial developed in prehistoric man. As to height, there are tall and short examples among all races and subraces. Among civilized groups intermarriage has produced mixed racial types.

Nationality. We think of physical characteristics of national groups because the inhabitants of the various nations of Europe tend to be made up of homogeneous subracial groups with specific characteristics. Thus we expect children whose forebears came from the Scandinavian countries to be larger, and those from Sicily to be smaller, than the average American. Yet in America there has been so much intermingling of subracial groups that children with all the typical physical characteristics of any national group are seldom seen.

In studying the changing characteristics of the American people one must consider the influence of immigration. Immigrants frequently established themselves in the United States under conditions of extreme poverty. Their descendants of the second and third generations make up the majority of the middle and upper classes, and the lower-income group is now made up of more recent immigrants.

People from southern and eastern Europe and from Mexico and Cuba predominate among the relatively recent immigrants of the white race. The Puerto Ricans are recent arrivals, and the majority of them hold low-paying jobs. The shortness of stature among these representatives of the white race is a factor in the below-average height of children of the low-income group as compared with children of the middle- and upper-income groups. The latter, as we have noted, came from stock characterized by relatively greater height than the stock from which these more recent immigrants have come. This is not to deny the influence of good diet and of sanitation on children's height, but merely points out that different ethnic groups are likely to have different growth potentials.

Sex

Sex is determined at conception. The male infant is both longer and heavier than the female infant. Boys maintain this superiority until about 11 years of age. Then girls, who mature earlier and so reach the period of accelerated growth earlier than boys, are taller on the average than they. Boys, during the prepubertal spurt of growth and thereafter, are again taller than girls. Bone development is more advanced in girls than in boys, as shown in roentgenograms of the wrists of infants and young children. Advance in osseous development is also demonstrated by the earlier eruption of the permanent teeth in girls.

Environment

One example of the influence of environment upon potential height is found among the first and second generations of Japanese in this country. The children are generally taller than their parents because they have had the advantage of better food and living conditions than their parents, who were materially deprived when they came to the United States. A more recent example is that of children whose growth and development were stunted in concentration camps and in poverty-stricken areas in Europe during World War II and who exhibited remarkable improvement upon being removed to better conditions.

PRENATAL ENVIRONMENT

Prenatal conditions are part of the environmental climate in which the child develops and should not be forgotten in considering actual development in relation to probable optimal development.

The influence of the intrauterine environment on the child's future development is great, particularly since the uterus shields the fetus from the full impact of external adverse conditions. On the other hand, the intrauterine environment itself may be substandard. In such a case, if the fetus has reached the stage of viability, early delivery may make it possible to place the infant in a better environment than that of the uterus.

Harmful Prenatal Factors. The prenatal environment is influenced by many factors. The fetus may suffer from nutritional deficiencies when the mother's diet is insufficient in quantity or quality, regardless of her socioeconomic standard of living. There may be mechanical problems due to malposition *in utero*. The mother may suffer from metabolic endocrine disturbances, e.g., diabetes mellitus, which affect the fetus. If it is necessary for the mother to undergo radiation for cancer or other conditions, the infant may be blighted by the treatment. The mother may suffer from an infectious disease during gestation. Rubella (German measles) during the first trimester of pregnancy may lead to abnormal development of the fetus. Other infectious diseases may also affect the fetus, but there is less scientific proof of this. Toxoplasmosis and syphilis during the second and third trimesters adversely influence the fetus. Erythroblastosis fetalis due to Rh incompatibility of the blood types of the mother and the fetus may have a serious influence upon the developing fetus. Commonly, faulty placental implantation or malfunction may lead to nutritional impairment or anoxia. Recent research has shown that smoking or the use of certain drugs by the mother may result in prematurity or deformity of the child. If the mother has had good prenatal care, many of these conditions can be treated, thus ensuring a better prenatal environment for the fetus.

POSTNATAL ENVIRONMENT

An environment that provides satisfying experiences promotes growth. Since growth and development are interrelated, growth in any one

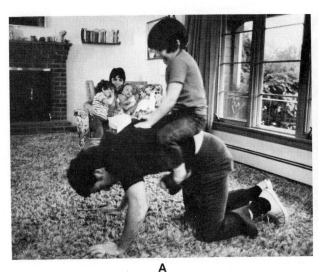 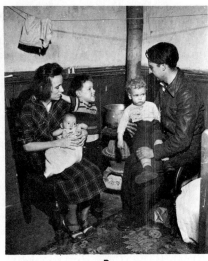

A   B

FIGURE 2–4. Children grow up in families which differ in socioeconomic status. A, Middle-class family. (From Alfred Eisestaedt, Time-Life Picture Agency. © Time, Inc.) B, Lower-class family. (H. Armstrong Roberts.)

area influences and in turn is influenced by growth in all other areas.

Factors which influence the infant's development are more likely to be of environmental origin than genetic. Among the most important environmental factors are the following.

External Environment. As was noted earlier, the family and its cultural background greatly influence the growth and development of the child during his formative years. Some of the other ways by which the family influences the postnatal environment follow.

SOCIOECONOMIC STATUS OF THE FAMILY. The environment of the lower socioeconomic groups is apt to be less favorable than that of the middle or upper groups. Parents in unfortunate financial circumstances are less likely to understand the principles of modern scientific child care, they lack money to buy the essentials of health and diet, and often they are unable, unwilling, or unsure of how to obtain medical care and hospitalization. Today, however, public health programs and health education programs in schools are gradually assisting such parents to provide better care for their children.

NUTRITION. Nutrition is related to both the quantitative and qualitative supply of food elements—proteins, fats, carbohydrates, minerals, and vitamins. But the infant's or child's use of a good diet may be impaired by faulty absorption or assimilation of food substances.

CLIMATE AND SEASON. Climatic variations influence the infant's health. This is not an important direct factor in the United States,

since the entire area lies within the temperate zone. Summer heat, however, is important when parents in the lower socioeconomic levels fail to provide adequate refrigeration of food and extermination procedures for flies and other insects. Infants in such families are prone to suffer diarrhea with subsequent dehydration.

The seasons of the year influence growth rates in height and weight, especially in older children. Weight gains are lowest in spring and early summer and greatest in late summer and autumn. The greatest gains in height among children in the United States occur in the spring.

ILLNESS AND INJURY. Illness and injury, with their accompanying debility and nutritional impairment, have a great influence on weight and some influence on growth.

EXERCISE. Exercise promotes physiologic activity and stimulates muscular development, and fresh air and moderate sunshine favor health and growth. Prolonged exposure to sunshine, especially in extremely warm areas such as the southwestern section of the United States, may cause tissue damage and even more serious consequences if the child is unprotected from the rays of the sun.

ORDINAL POSITION IN THE FAMILY. The child's position in the family is a factor in development for several reasons, among them the following: (1) Children learn from older siblings, and this is an advantage which an only child or the oldest child lacks. (2) The youngest child may be relatively slow in certain areas of development because he is given little encouragement to express himself. He is the baby and is petted by the whole family. (3) The only child is likely to develop more rapidly along intellectual lines than the average child because he is constantly with adults and is mentally stimulated by their companionship. Like the youngest child of a family, he may be slow in motor development, however, because he has so much done for him. When he is old enough to do things for himself, his parents and other relatives may not permit him to do so.

Internal Environment. INTELLIGENCE. Intelligence is correlated to some degree with physical development; i.e., the child of high intelligence is likely to be better developed than the less gifted child. Intelligence influences mental and social development.

HORMONAL BALANCE. Hormonal balance in the young child is important. Normal secretions of the endocrine glands promote normal growth of the body.

EMOTIONS. Emotional disturbances influence growth, since the disturbed child neither sleeps nor eats as well as one who is happy and contented.

TYPES OF GROWTH AND DEVELOPMENT

Physical Growth

Physical growth includes many things, among them the following.

Changes in General Body Growth. Changes result from different rates of growth in different parts of the body during the consecutive stages of development. For example, the infant's head size is one fourth of the entire length of the body at birth, whereas the adult's head size is only one eighth of his length. Growth during childhood is primarily linear; growth in adolescence is both linear and in the nature of a filling-out process until adult proportions are reached.

The pattern of general physical growth and types of organic growth are shown in Figure 2–5. From this illustration it can be seen that the rate of growth in general is most rapid during infancy and during puberty and adolescence. The rate of neural growth is most rapid before school age, when it gradually levels off. The rate of growth of lymphoid tissue is rapid until approximately the age of 12 years, when it gradually declines. The rate of genital growth is slow until puberty and adolescence, when it increases rapidly.

Head Circumference. The circumference of the head is important, since it is related to in-

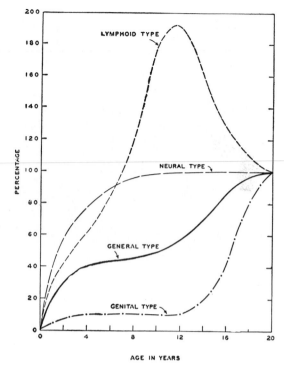

FIGURE 2–5. Main types of postnatal growth of the various parts and organs of the body. (After Scammon: *The Measurement of the Body in Childhood, The Measurement of Man.* University of Minnesota Press.)

tracranial volume. An increase in circumference permits an estimation of the rate of brain growth. This measurement has a relatively narrow normal range for a particular age group.

Thoracic Diameter. Chest measurements increase as the child grows and the shape of his chest changes. At birth the transverse and anteroposterior diameters are nearly equal. The transverse diameter increases more rapidly than the anteroposterior diameter; i.e., the width becomes greater than its depth.

Abdominal and Pelvic Measurements. The abdominal circumference is not fixed by a bony cage as is the chest and consequently is affected by the infant's nutritional state, by muscle tone, gaseous distention and even the phase of respiration. The pelvic bicristal diameter (the maximal distance between the external margins of the iliac crests) is not affected by variations in posture and musculature. The pelvic bicristal diameter is a good index of a child's slenderness or stockiness.

Weight. Weight is influenced by all the increments in size and is probably the best gross index of nutrition and growth. There is a wide variation within normal limits for each year of childhood. Excess weight in relation to the height and pelvic diameter is as abnormal as underweight. It may be the result of a glandular

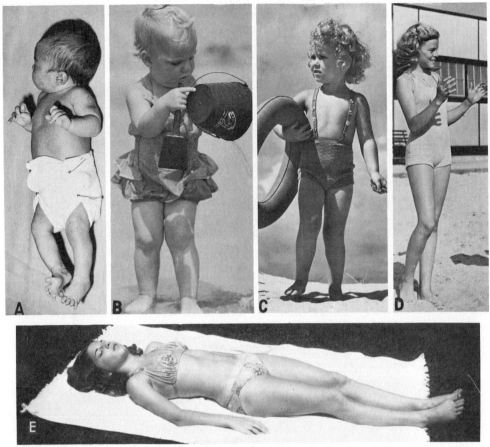

FIGURE 2–6. Body proportions change during the period of growth. The head size, trunk length and extremity length differ in (A) the newborn, (B) 18-month-old, (C) 3-year-old, (D) 11-year-old and (E) 18-year-old. (B, C, and D by H. Armstrong Roberts.)

deficiency, but is more likely to be due to overeating or to a diet containing too much starch and fat and too little protein.

Height. Yearly increments in height diminish from birth to maturity. The pubescent spurt is the only exception to this downward trend in the rate of growth. There is great variation in the yearly increases in stature among children of the same age. Some children reach adult height in their early teens, but others continue to grow throughout late adolescence. The periods of most rapid growth are infancy and puberty.

DEVELOPMENT OF MUSCULAR CONTROL

Muscular control does not develop evenly throughout the body. In human beings it follows

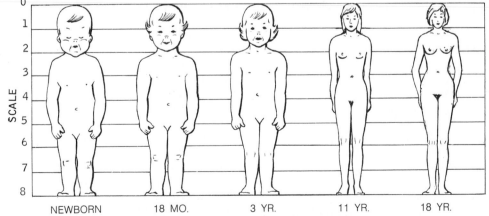

FIGURE 2–7. Scale showing changes in body proportion from birth to physical maturity.

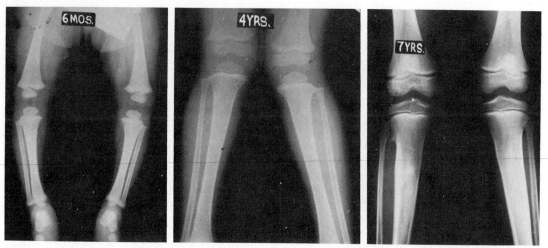

FIGURE 2–8. Roentgenogram shows "normal" progression from bowlegs through knock-knees to a balance between the two. (Courtesy of Charles E. Shopfner, M.D.: Man Is Not a Straight-legged Animal: Avoid Unnecessary Therapy. *J.A.M.A.*, 207:29, January 6, 1969.)

the spine downward—*cephalocaudal*—and in addition proceeds from the *center of the body to the periphery*. The result is that the child holds up his head before he sits. The large muscles of the arms and legs are subject to voluntary control sooner than the fine muscles of the hands and feet. As the child matures, *general movements become specific*. For example, he can use the whole hand before he can pick up a small

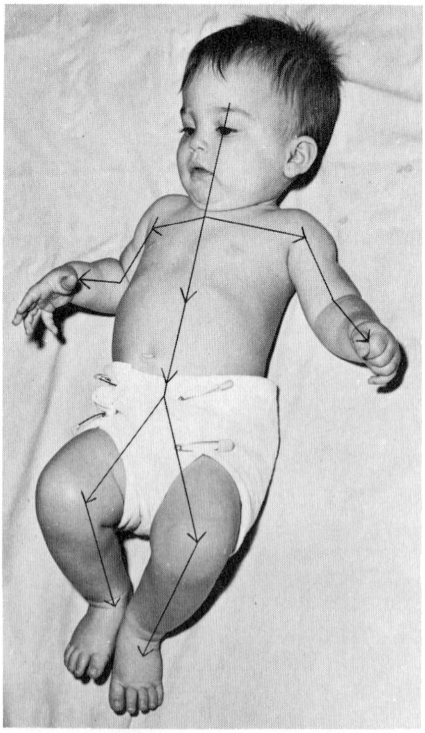

FIGURE 2–9. The development of muscular control proceeds from head to tail (cephalocaudal) and from the center of the body to the periphery.

object with the pincer grasp, i.e., between thumb and forefinger.

There is a normal sequence in the development of manual dexterity and for the stages of locomotion, just as there is for mental development and for emotional and social adequacy. A child should be given the opportunity for learning—by either experience or instruction—whenever he is ready to acquire the skill or learn by indirect experience through instruction from others. If these opportunities are presented prematurely and the child is urged to make use of them, he is apt to learn slowly; if too late, he is apt to learn rapidly, but may never acquire the same skill or proficiency he might have had if the opportunity for learning had occurred at a more auspicious time. Coincidental acquisition of a skill along with others of his age group is probably more important to a child's personality development than his ultimate proficiency in that particular skill. For example, the child who is physically unable to walk until six years of age has been an atypical child among other children and in his relations with adults. This influence on his personality may be more important than its final effect on his ability to walk, run, dance, and perform other activities.

On the other hand, disability during the preschool years may have no permanent effect upon a child. Children often have a remarkable resilience to factors which theoretically would hinder their normal personality development. This is often seen in children who have been denied learning opportunities because of sickness or the stultifying regimen of institutional life. An important factor which may determine the effect of a disability on a child is the attitude of the parents and others around him, those *significant persons* who influence his own attitude toward himself and his disability, and his ability to cope with the situation.

Mental Development

Tests of intelligence and mental development have been standardized, much like the standards for physical growth and development derived from longitudinal and cross-sectional studies in height and weight for children of different ages. There is no foolproof way of measuring the potential development of the genetically carried trait of intelligence, but among children with comparable environmental backgrounds such as those from the middle class the standardized intelligence tests are valuable in predicting capacity for intellectual development. Such tests are used in the school system. They are useful in determining whether achievement is comparable to innate ability.

Mental development depends on numerous factors. It is demonstrated in problem solving and in a general understanding of what to do in a given situation. It is important to let the child solve those problems which he is able to solve by himself and to teach him how to solve problems that are within his ability, but for which he lacks the necessary experience and practice. It is also important to solve for him problems too difficult for him so that the patience of both child and adult will not be affected by his lack of success. By the time the child is a year old he should be in the process of learning decision-making himself and of accepting the decisions of those adults in whose love he feels secure.

The initial problems with which a baby is confronted are physical ones and he is helped in their solution by the normal reflex actions of his body. The first problem is ingestion of milk. Sucking at the mother's breast and swallowing the milk are processes which require little or no practice to perform successfully. The newborn at the breast for the first time may have difficulty in getting hold of the nipple and may sputter and choke as the colostrum or milk begins to flow. But he soon learns, for he has many opportunities to practice sucking.

An infant learns to want a smiling mother because she does pleasant things for him. An early problem, then, is to make mother smile. He learns not to do those things which make her say in a decisive voice, "No, no," and frown on him.

A small baby is more adept at solving his problems than we are likely to realize, and the behavior which gets him what he wants becomes habitual. Habits can be broken, of course, but the process is difficult for both the infant and the adults about him. He should be helped to the correct solution of a problem, so that he finds pleasure not only in the behavior itself, but also in the social reward of having others pleased with him. Some adults believe that continuous, on-going attention to the infant is "spoiling" him. In reality this is meeting his normal needs and is helping him with his problem-solving efforts. The infant who receives an inadequate amount of real affection must cry to get it because he soon realizes that it is the only way to get attention of any kind. No child is more to be pitied than the crying child. He is robbed of the birthright of children, that of being loved by an increasingly widening circle of adults and accepted in the play groups of his peers.

Thus, although potential mental ability is inherited and fixed at birth, the rate and extent of its development, as measured by any one of the many mental tests, are very much influenced by a child's environment.

DETERMINATION OF LEVEL OF MENTAL DEVELOPMENT

As the structure of the nervous system grows during the prenatal period, rudimentary beginnings of the mind grow with it. As the child develops after birth, changes occur in his mental reactions that show progress from the ability to respond to the simplest stimuli toward functioning in more complex ways. Although mental development is continuous, it may be more rapid in one age period than in another.

Intelligence can be defined as the ability to adjust to new situations, to think abstractly or to profit from experience. Tests of intelligence are of many types. During infancy and early childhood such tests are likely to be of the performance type. The child is asked to manipulate testing materials or to demonstrate his motor ability. Such tests show the general level of intelligence, but do not accurately predict the child's later intellectual attainment.

When the child is able to communicate verbally, verbal intelligence tests may be given; when he is able to write (i.e., in the school age and adolescent groups), individual or group written tests may be used. There is a higher degree of consistency in intelligence test results from the age of five onward than for tests given during the preschool period.

Recently the use of group intelligence tests has been reevaluated in some urban areas. Group tests are thought by some not valid for use with disadvantaged students since they may be culturally biased. Also, since some school personnel may generalize and misinterpret them as measuring native ability, tests of achievement and school readiness are being used instead.

MEANING OF THE INTELLIGENCE QUOTIENT

The intelligence quotient (I.Q.) can be defined as the ratio between the child's chronologic age and his mental age as gained from an intelligence test. The formula for computing the intelligence quotient is as follows:

$$\frac{\text{Mental Age}}{\text{Chronologic age}} \times 100 = \text{I.Q.}$$

Since mental maturity is usually reached between the ages of 16 and 21 years, the mental age of the adult cannot be computed in this way. The age of 16 years has been arbitrarily chosen as the adult's chronologic age. For example, if an adult passed all the questions in the test designed for a 12-year-old child, his I.Q. would be 75. In the event of a perfect score in the 16-year test, his I.Q. would be 100, or normal. The level of intelligence can continue to increase beyond this age, however.

An I.Q. between 90 and 109 is usually considered to be normal or average. The I.Q. of individual children may range above or below this point. Children with an I.Q. of 140 or over are called gifted children, and those with an I.Q. of less than average represent retardation of varying degrees.

Theories of Development

Many theories have been devised to study the development of children. Among such theories are those of Freud, Erikson, and Piaget, and the stimulus-response and social interaction theories. The two that will be developed in this text are the theory of Piaget concerning cognitive development and the theory of Erikson about emotional development.

THE DEVELOPMENTAL PSYCHOLOGY OF JEAN PIAGET

Jean Piaget, a Swiss philosopher and psychologist who studied the intellectual development of children, was concerned with the origins of man's mental functioning and his understanding of the world surrounding him. In the hierarchy of mental structures, Piaget traces development from the newborn infant, who comes into the world with a primitive set of rigid reflexes that provide limited responses for survival, through evolution to highly complex structures that allow the individual to manipulate symbols and interact with his environment in a very flexible manner.

Piaget proposes that there are certain characteristics of development always present in some form. These *invariants*, as they are called, include the stage concept, organization, adaptation, equilibrium, and assimilation and accommodation. The *stage concept* simply means that development follows a sequence of stages and that each stage has its unique characteristics. Each stage builds upon the last stage in a sequential manner; however, there is no specific time limitation for each stage. *Organization* means that mental functioning does not occur in isolation. As a child learns one ability he combines it with others. For instance, when he learns to reach he combines this with his ability to look at that for which he reaches, thus integrating his abilities into a more effective whole. *Adaptation* means as the child develops he must move from his biologically provided reflexes at birth to a higher level of functioning in order to adapt to his environment. He must learn new behavior, a process that continues through his development. The concept of *equilibrium* is related to adaptation. When a new behavior emerges, he can use a more effective manner in handling his environment; but the constant demands of the environment will continue to cause disequilibrium until further ways of adapting are learned. *Assimilation and accommodation* are concerned with stimuli that continue to bombard each individual. With each stimulus the individual must learn new patterns of behavior in order to accommodate his environment. Thus, in order to adapt and maintain his equilibrium, the individual must assimilate his new tailor-made response patterns and accommodate his environment.

According to Piaget, there are certain signposts of maturation and growth. Although the newborn perceives his world as a vague mass in a fragmented manner, he gradually develops an integration or *coordination of the various sensory inputs* from touch, taste, smell, sight, and sound into an organized and objective understanding of reality. Also, the young child does not understand that objects he cannot see still exist. The adult knows that his home is there, even when he is not present to observe it. To the young child, the concept of *object constancy* comes slowly but is a milestone in development when it does appear. The ability to *use symbols* to represent reality is another important stage in development. The use of symbols leads the child to language development, which in turn produces greater symbolism leading to further mental development. A child less than seven years old *can focus on only one aspect of a situation* and cannot relate other information and observations to it. For instance, a babysitter who puts on a Halloween costume and a mask may very well frighten a young child. This is because the child cannot understand that even though the babysitter is dressed differently, he or she is still the same person. Advanced cognitive functioning requires that we understand that things, although superficially changing, do remain the same. Another idea important to Piaget's theory is *egocentrism.* In order for advanced cognitive functioning to occur, the child must move through various stages of differentiating himself from objects around him to learning to separate his own thoughts from those of others.

In summary, Piaget believes that intellectual change occurs in a sequential manner and that this change occurs as the result of continuous interaction between the child and his environment.

According to Piaget, there are four major stages of development that correspond in a rough way to the stages of emotional development. These include the sensorimotor stage (0 to 2 years), preoperational stage (2 to 7 years), concrete operational stage (7 to 11 years), and formal operational stage (11 to 15 years). These stages will be explored further in appropriate chapters in this text.

Emotional Development

Personality is not a specific attribute, but the total quality of any person's patterns of behavior. Two attributes of a healthy personality in adult life are the ability to love and the ability to work.

TABLE 2–1. STAGES OF PERSONALITY DEVELOPMENT

STAGE	APPROXIMATE AGE	PSYCHOSOCIAL CRISES	SIGNIFICANT PERSONS	TASKS
Infancy	0–1	Sense of trust vs. mistrust	Maternal person	Getting Tolerating frustration in small doses Recognizing mother as distinct from others and self
Toddler	1–3	Sense of autonomy vs. shame and doubt	Parental persons	Trying out own powers of speech Beginning acceptance of reality vs. pleasure principle
Preschool	3–6	Sense of initiative vs. guilt	Basic family	Questioning Exploring own body and environment Differentiation of sexes
School	6–12	Sense of industry vs. inferiority	Neighborhood School	Learning to win recognition by producing things Exploring, collecting Learning to relate to own sex
Puberty and adolescence	12–?	Sense of identity vs. identity diffusion	Peer groups and out groups; models of leadership	Moving toward heterosexuality Selecting vocation Beginning separation from family Integrating personality (altruism, etc.)
Late adolescence and young adult	—	Sense of intimacy and solidarity vs. isolation	Partners in friendship, sex, competition, cooperation	Becoming capable of establishing a lasting relationship with a member of the opposite sex Learning to be creative and productive

Based on Erikson: *Childhood and Society.*

STAGES OF PERSONALITY DEVELOPMENT

Emotional or personality development is a continuous process. In each stage of a child's emotional development there is a central problem which must be solved. These problems are never completely solved, however. If each problem is fairly well solved at the child's particular stage of development, the basis for progress to the next stage is firmly laid. Proper guidance and the solution of the sequence of problems are necessary at each stage of development if functional harmony is to be secured in adult life.

No child succeeds or fails completely in attainment of the goal to be reached at a particular point in his personality development. For example, the child does not learn to trust completely or never to mistrust. Every child leaves the period of infancy with habits of both trust and mistrust. Also, children who achieved a sense of trust initially may have periodic regressions to mistrust when unfortunate circumstances occur later in life. Health of personality is determined by the preponderance of the favorable attitudes and by the kinds of compensations a child develops to take care of his disabilities.

A general, overall view of the stages in emotional or personality development according to Erik H. Erikson, a psychologist and trained psychoanalyst, is given here. Further discussion will follow in later chapters.

Birth to One Year (Infancy): Sense of Trust. A baby learns to trust the adults who care for him, the mother or her substitute first, for it is she who is sensitive to his needs and shows her trust in him. The negative outcome is a sense of mistrust.

One Year to Three Years (The Toddler): Sense of Autonomy. The infant develops from a clinging, dependent little creature into a human being with a mind and a will of his own. If a child succeeds in the developmental task of this stage in his maturing process, he will have a degree of self-control not caused by fear, but by his feeling of self-esteem. If he does not succeed, he will doubt his own worth and that of others, and will have a sense of shyness and shame.

Three to Six Years (The Preschool Child): Sense of Initiative. The child at this age wants to learn what he can do for himself. He has an active imagination. He imitates adult behavior and wants to share in their activities. He wants the experience of following his will to the extreme limit. The adult can help prevent the accompanying sense of guilt such behavior may bring by imposing necessary limits on undesirable behavior and by providing a climate for exploring new learning experiences which are

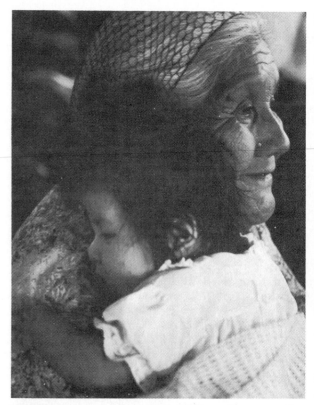

FIGURE 2–10. The bond of love bridges a three-generation gap between two Americans—a Dakota Indian baby and her great-grandmother. The baby's future, and perhaps the future of this nation and the world, may depend, in great part, on whether children can be assured the kind of early childhood conducive to healthy physical and mental development. (Courtesy of Wilbur J. Cohen: The Developmental Approach to Social Challenges, *Children*, 15:Nov.-Dec., 1968.)

desirable. The positive, maturing outcome of this force within him is a sense of initiative, delineated by conscience or superego, which is developed from parental attitudes and their examples. The negative outcome is a personality overwhelmed by guilt.

Six to Twelve Years (School Age): Sense of Industry. Children in this age group have a strong sense of duty. They want to engage in tasks in their social world which they can carry out successfully, and they want their success to be recognized by adults and by their peers. It is a calm period in which the basis is laid for later responsible citizenship. Society reaches the child directly through the school system and educates him not only intellectually, but also in the fundamental skills of living in a modern society. Children learn skills of workmanship and the ability to cooperate and to play fairly according to the rules. The danger of this period is the development of a sense of inferiority if the parents or the school expects a level of achievement which the child is unable to attain.

Twelve Years (Beginning of Adolescence): Sense of Identity. The sense of identity develops during adolescence. The adolescent wants to clarify who he is and what his role in society is to be. His attitude toward life is, "What will this mean to me?" Success in this period brings self-esteem, an attitude toward the self that is essential to the normal breaking away from dependency upon his parents and to planning for his future. The danger is self-diffusion, for he faces at the time and in his dreams of the future a life full of conflicting desires, possibilities and chances. The childhood sense of belonging because "he always has belonged" is lost in the necessity of changing from childhood dependency to adult responsibility for his own actions and those of others who are dependent upon him. He may, under adverse circumstances, develop a sense of "not-belonging."

Late Adolescence: Sense of Intimacy. After puberty, youths outgrow the "gang age," that age when they find it essential to belong to a group of their own sex and age. Boys are likely to lose interest in scouting, and girls in cliques of their own sex. In adolescence, youth develops a sense of intimacy with individuals of his own and of the opposite sex, and with himself. If a youth is not certain of his identity, he is afraid to have personal relations with others. Success in this period means union with the essence of others and a communion with their own resources. Failure to establish such intimacy results in psychologic isolation—keeping relations with others on a formal basis which lacks warmth. This is likely to result in failure in all the steps in intimacy which lead to selection of a marriage partner ("dating," courtship and engagement) and to satisfaction in marriage.

EVALUATION OF EMOTIONAL DEVELOPMENT

Tests of emotional and social development are less concrete than those dealing with physical or mental development. They are more likely to be used in therapy than elsewhere, although they are useful in planning the physical environment and the activities and qualifications of the personnel in institutions dealing with children.

Professional people working with children should be as familiar with these tests as they are with tests of physical growth and development, for a child's environment must be planned to meet all his interrelated needs, physical, mental, emotional and social.

Evaluation devices for measuring emotional or personality development are of several types. Such tests attempt to compare a child's stage of development with that of children of the same age and to show whether he is suffering from some sort of personality maladjustment. The results of such tests are not too accurate, since personality is complex and cannot be easily evaluated.

Specific examples of such devices are rating scales, self-appraisal questionnaires, projective techniques such as finger or easel painting, play activities, the Rorschach test, and others. The *Thematic Apperception Test* is one of the most inclusive tests and is frequently used in the diagnosis of generalized anxiety or behavior problems in children.

LIFE PERSPECTIVES

As an individual develops from a neonate to an adolescent and then to an adult, he develops what is known as a life perspective or a way of viewing his own life. Certainly the infant has no life perspective of his own; he is totally engrossed in the life of the present. He experiences only the moment, not reexperiencing the past or foreseeing the future. From this point the individual will formulate a life perspective as he develops through the years to adulthood. The steps in this process will be included in the later chapters on growth and development.

Social Development

Socialization, or social development, means training a child in the culture of the group. Personality traits can be divided into two classes; social and cultural. *Social traits* are those found in the well adjusted members of every group; they are traits which are necessary to group survival, such as willingness to sacrifice present comfort for future benefit, and, even more important, individual cooperation with group efforts for group benefit. This social characteristic is altruism. Love and consistency in training are necessary to socialize a child. Obviously, there are varying degrees of socialization.

Cultural traits are those which vary with the culture of different groups. Child care is a cultural trait in all groups, but the particular way in which a child is cared for is a social trait and is not exactly the same in any two cultures.

A newborn infant is not a social being. This fact may be illustrated by the few authenticated cases of children carried off by wild animals—presumably lactating and capable of carrying a child and keeping it alive. None of these children when found showed the personality characteristics of socialized human beings; they were not socialized according to the definition given above, nor did they behave according to any human culture pattern.

FACTORS IN SOCIAL DEVELOPMENT

Children learn to socialize by meeting and living with people of various ages. They learn to socialize also by participating in the activities of family life such as picnicking, traveling, and so forth, and in the activities of their peer groups.

The Play Group. Learning to live happily with adults is quite different from making friends with children of his own age. In general the adult-child relation is one in which the child learns to live within certain restrictions set by adults even though at times these restrictions may not be consistently imposed. It is probably a good thing that children do not have perfect parents, nor parents perfect children: family life would be too unrealistic.

Adults do not compete with a child on his own level for the things he wants. When children and adults disagree, it is usually a matter of the adult telling the child to do or not to do something the child does not want to do or is determined to do.

A child who adjusts well with adults may be unable to get along with other children. An only child who has no playmates finds it particularly difficult to learn the give and take of childish play. The teachers in nursery school will help him acquire the technique of getting along with other children. It may be a slow process. The adult who feels that it is easy to make the transition from being the only child in the home to being one among many others in the nursery school is mistaken. Many nursery school teachers suggest that the child's mother stay with him for the first few days until he has made friends among the other children and thinks of the school as a pleasant place to be in. Eventually he learns to be one of his group, either a leader or a follower, depending on what he can contribute to the group's success in the particular activity in which it is engaged. In the play group or team and even in the gang, leadership springs less from physical superiority—fighting, running, playing ball—than from thinking up interesting activities when the group does not know what to do with itself. The child who can think up activities agreeable to the group, "sell" his ideas to them and lead them to a successful culmination of the project is likely to become their leader.

As a child becomes engrossed in activities with his age group he does not love his parents less, but is less dependent on them for physical care, emotional support and a system of values. He becomes more self-reliant and learns how to use the resources of his group and community resources organized by adults for youth or for all age groups. He is preparing to take the responsibility of marriage and founding a home. Parents become dependent upon him as he matures and as they grow older. He slowly learns to take his place in the economic life of the country and to fulfill his role as a citizen.

Development of Sexuality

A new sexual climate of freedom in our society is emerging as a result of changing attitudes of the immediate past and current generations. Although magazine articles, books, films, and television have brought this subject into the open, many times adults as well as youth find themselves with a freedom they do not completely understand. Nurses can make an important contribution in this area, first through a knowledge of the subject and then through ease in sharing that knowledge with others.

Sexuality is an important dimension of development in the human being, a link between humans, yet it is perhaps the least understood area in the development of man. Although the sex of a child is determined genetically, at the time of conception (see Chapter 10), the development of a child's sexuality after birth is influenced by development in the physical, mental, emotional, and sociocultural areas of living. Not only is the child's sexual development colored by development in other areas, but the level of sexual maturity influences development in some of these same areas. Because of the complexity of the human in total development, parents and society, including the helping professions, have many times failed in their responsibility to counsel and guide the child through the years to adulthood.

Human sexuality is expressed in everyday life. Many persons believe erroneously that human sexuality and the act of physical intercourse are synonymous. Human sexuality is in fact fundamental to life and thus has a much broader meaning than the physical act of sex alone. It can lead ultimately to either a sustained relationship with a mate or it can be sublimated through outlets having a social value. Actually, the nurse who is married and working in this nurturing profession is using his or her own sexuality to achieve both goals.

The nurse who seeks to counsel or guide children and their parents in the important area of sexual development must understand and accept his or her own attitudes, values, and prejudices concerning sexuality, as well as having counseling skills in order to be effective. This is important because not only is knowledge transmitted through such guidance, but values and attitudes are also shared at the same time. If the nurse is judging or not comfortable with his or her own sexuality, the client may "catch" the feelings expressed on a nonverbal level to his own detriment. In other words, the information given in many instances is not as important as the attitude conveying it.

Aspects of human sexuality are discussed in the various chapters on growth and development throughout this text. The effects of certain illnesses on the sexual development of the individual are discussed in the appropriate chapters.

Play

Just as an adult works, so does a child play; it is the business of childhood. It is through play that a child grows, learns, develops, and ultimately matures. Through play the child strengthens his muscles and learns to coordinate his physical movements. Giving the child an opportunity to play creatively permits him to grow to his maximum creative potential. Giving the child an opportunity to practice imitating the adult world helps him learn to be an adult.

In order to achieve these play goals, the child needs adequate space, time, and play materials. Whether the materials are soft toys for hugging, crayons and paper for drawing, blocks for building, clay for molding, or wood for building a tree house, the child must be given the freedom to express himself as he wishes. This freedom, however, must be given in a way to ensure safety both for himself and others in order to prevent accidents.

Through play the child learns to explore his own world, to test reality against his personal powers, and to venture into the unknown. Later, through play the child learns that his own power can influence his environment and that he can respond to challenges in the real world. By observing and imitating significant others such as parents, babysitters, teachers, or scout leaders, in his environment, the child learns to live in the adult world that surrounds him.

The specific stages through which the child progresses in his play are described in the chapters on growth and development throughout this text. For example, the individual moves from solitary play during infancy to parallel play during the toddler years. Soon the child learns to play in small groups and later to select his immediate friends while at the same time responding to an ever-widening circle of acquaintances.

OBSERVATION OF PLAY

Observing children at play provides an opportunity for the nurse to understand them. Such observation is indispensable for sensitive and effective guidance and care for children. A skillful observer can develop sensitivity to the uniqueness of each child's personality and can become increasingly able to interpret the language of behavior: the significance of actions, gestures, facial expressions, and spoken words.

Children are most natural when playing. If the child is unaware of being watched, he is free to behave in his own way. If the child is aware of being observed, he may become self-conscious and react with shyness, embarrassment, frustration, or by showing off. The way an observer looks at the play of children is largely determined by his or her personal and cultural prejudices and by the kinds of childhood play previously experienced. A conscientious observer will attempt to overcome personal biases and strive for genuine empathy with the child being observed. Because the reason for observing children is to increase our understanding of them, it is of vital importance to look at the child's behavior with an open mind that is accepting, rather than judgmental.

There are three levels of observing children. The first level is observation of exactly what the child *does*. This level usually focuses on gross motor behavior and specific manipulatory activity. For instance, in reporting an observation, the nurse could write:

9:45 A.M. Christine went over to the slide, climbed the ladder, and slid down. She jumped off at the bottom and ran around to the ladder to slide down again. She did this four times.

This level of observation tells how Christine spent her time, what activity she enjoys, and for approximately how long.

In order to know more about Christine, the nurse observes and records the child's *feelings about what she does*. This second level of observation concerns the quality of behavior and the "how" of what the child does. The nurse records not only a reconstruction of the situation as it was seen, but as the child lived it and felt about it. For example:

9:45 A.M. Christine looked around and saw the slide. She climbed up the ladder and down she swooped. She giggled and jumped off at the end, bouncing back to the ladder eagerly.

The words the child says, the actions he performs and the facial and postural expressions by which he reveals his pleasure, fear, dissatisfaction, or inadequacy in reaction to events as they take place are recorded.

The first two levels of observation describe the what and how of behavior. The third level includes the *observer's impressions and interpretations of the observed behavior*. An experienced observer can report so skillfully and completely that the third step may be unnecessary because the recorded facts may speak for themselves. If an interpretation of behavior is made, it can be checked for accuracy against past and future records of observations.

Human behavior is dynamic. Because of his growth and development, the child changes in mysterious ways. As the nurse practices and develops skill in the art of observation, the child's world and its meaning for him can be explored.

SUMMARY

Heredity places limits upon development. But as we learn more about a child's needs, we are able to increase the influence of environment. A child needs an environment which provides satisfying experiences. A child desires to repeat happy experiences in which he exercises his growing ability to secure the things he wants and to do the things he strives to perform. Happiness may come only from the satisfaction of having and doing, but even at an early age happiness is likely to be influenced by the approval of other people, as shown in the smiling face, the pleasant sound of the voice, and physical caresses.

The child learns most of his fears as he connects unpleasant direct experiences with people and things, or fear is communicated to him by adults or by children who are themselves afraid. Adults may condition him to fear this or that in order to secure obedience. Common examples of this are such warnings as, "The policeman will get you if you do that," or, "You'll get sick and have to go to the doctor or, worse, the hospital if you go without your coat," and the injunction, "You will hurt yourself," often uttered to secure obedience rather than to help the child to learn prudence in his play and to exercise good judgment in new situations.

As far as possible, little children should be shielded from unhealthy sources of anger or undue anger. They need exposure to normal anger. The child and the parent can learn to discuss it and cope with it together. The child learns that it is not he that the parent does not love when the parent becomes angry, but the act of the child. He thus learns that a parent or any other person can love him and at the same time be angry with him for what he has done.

A baby learns at a surprisingly early age the consequences of his behavior in a sequence of acts within a social situation in which he may be the center of attention of both father and mother. When he wants his feeding, he cries for it, and his mother comes and gives it to him. Hunger is a physical need, but its relief is social in the

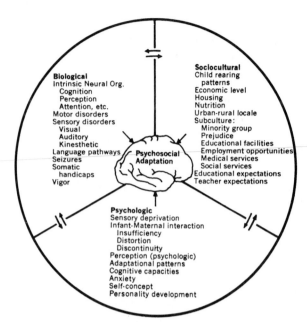

FIGURE 2–11. Multiple factors affecting psychosocial adaptation. (From Walzer, S., and Richmond, J. B.: The Epidemiology of Learning Disorders. *Pediatr. Clin. N. Am.*, 20:551, August 1973.)

sense that someone must give the baby his feeding. These social experiences are fully as important as experiences with the physical world about him—e.g., that his rattle is fun to suck and that it makes a nice sound when shaken. Both types of experience help a baby to mature mentally, emotionally and socially. Since they involve physical activity and other needs for growth, they serve to further the whole process of maturation.

As a child grows from infancy he slowly develops a concept of *body image* based on his knowledge of his own body according to his present and past perceptions of his biologic configuration, his physiologic functioning, his developmental maturation, and the social reinforcement of others. This is a dynamic process proceeding throughout life and involves giving to one's body at any point in time the characteristics of unity and distinctness from others. A child's perception of his body image during health as compared with that during illness will be discussed later.

In contacts with children, the nurse sees the result of all these factors we have considered under physical, mental, emotional, social, and sexual growth and development. Every child is an individual; no two children are exactly alike. General statements of growth and development must be modified in the light of individual characteristics. But until the nurse knows the child well enough to adapt care to his individual needs, concepts of growth and development typical of his age group will help to meet those needs.

Throughout this book general concepts are developed in relation to the various age groups—from the neonatal through the adolescent period—whose nursing care in health and in disease is under consideration.

PARENTAL ATTITUDES TOWARD GROWTH AND DEVELOPMENT

The old idea of child care was to bring up the child on a strict regimen of food, sleep, and play. He was overprotected. The strict routine protected him from accidents and health hazards, but prevented him from acquiring the ability to adapt to life outside of the area controlled by his parents. He could not build up resistance to infection. The overprotected child whose mother claimed that he had never had a cold or sore throat was likely to suffer from a series of severe respiratory infections when he entered school. He did not use good judgment when crossing the street or in climbing or in games which taxed his physical skills. He was apt to be accident-prone. He was indeed geared to a strict regimen in regard to food likes and dislikes and his sleeping habits, but this regimen was possible only at home, and he was not prepared for even a gradual entry into community life.

Parents were likely to demand that such a child, whom they had allowed little self-direction, should direct himself successfully in school and on the playground. Boys, particularly, were expected to fight their own battles and in general suddenly change from overprotected, overdirected, obedient little boys in the home to schoolboys who showed ability to get along, if not to lead, in their own group. Strange as it may seem, some children are raised in this manner even today.

This era of the authoritative, overprotective parent was followed by the trend toward permissiveness. The infant was to be placed on a self-demand schedule of feedings; he was to be offered an unlimited amount of his feeding whenever he was hungry and was to take as little or as much as he desired. The toddler was to choose his own diet from wholesome foods and was never urged to eat. Naps were to be taken when he was sleepy; he was never led, rebelling, to bed. He was never punished. The adult as far as possible permitted him to do what he wanted to do and trusted to the natural consequences of his behavior to show him what was the logical thing to do in problem situations. This attitude was likely to create an inconsiderate child, making heavy demands on the time and patience of his parents and other adults. Many youths in today's world have been subjected to this type of child rearing with sometimes disastrous results in terms of their inadequate adjustment to society.

The newer idea is that the child must be prepared to take his place in the world and to live in a state of workable adjustment with his physical and social environment. He is to be treated as an individual, but as one who has not yet developed to the point at which he can decide what is best for him or recognize the

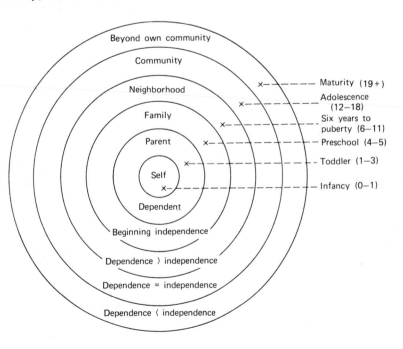

FIGURE 2–12. Psychological horizons of youth. Horizons expand in the growing years (> means greater than; < means less than). (From Rines, A. R., and Montag, M. L.: *Nursing Concepts and Nursing Care.* New York, John Wiley & Sons, Inc., 1976.)

rights of others. Behavioral psychologists believe that one method of helping a child is to reinforce his desired behavior through recognition and ignore his undesired behaviors. Explanations at his level of understanding as to why things have to be done are important, but at the same time limits must be set if necessary so that the child cannot harm himself or another person.

As a child grows, parents must learn to view him and themselves differently. Parental attitudes toward a child's growth may be poorly formed because they do not know what to expect of their child and do not know his real needs at various stages of his development. Nurses many times can interpret growth and development to parents and thus alleviate much of their misunderstanding about the process. In addition to individual teaching, some parents are seeking group counseling and are even taking parent education or training courses in an effort to understand their children as well as themselves. Nurses can assist parents by playing a larger role in this effort.

Parents are influenced also by the "child" each of them used to be. It is not easy to change each parent's view of his or her own background experiences in childhood. Some parents retain within themselves the children they used to be and see things as though their past home situations still existed. At the same time parents are also looking at the same situations through an accumulation of adult experiences. Parents then see their children as they would a blurred photograph, using a camera which was out of focus. The phases through which a parent progresses as the child grows will be discussed in appropriate chapters throughout this text.

THE NURSE'S ATTITUDES TOWARD GROWTH AND DEVELOPMENT

The attitude of the nurse toward children and the specific manner in which child growth and development are viewed are dependent, among other things, on the way the nurse was reared and on the total knowledge of and experiences with children, both within and outside the family. If

his or her own home life was reasonably happy and experiences with children were satisfying, attitudes toward children in general will probably be more positive than if an unhappy childhood and equally unhappy experiences with other children were had.

In order to work effectively with children the nurse needs to become aware of personal thinking in regard to parenthood itself, the role of parents and children, and the family as an institution. The nurse is sometimes inclined to minimize the role of the father in the family constellation and to work only with the mother when planning for the child.

The nurse also needs to recognize personal cultural attitudes. Many nurses, though able to aid effectively parents and children from the middle class, have difficulty in assisting patients and their parents from the lower socioeconomic groups. This is due to the fact that nurses themselves are primarily middle-class-oriented and have some difficulty in understanding those different from themselves.

In addition the nurse needs to be perceptive and sensitive to the specific problems of children and their families. In order to develop this sensitivity the nurse's own emotional drives must be recognized in order to effectively work with mothers of all ages. Feelings about authority versus permissiveness should be understood to work effectively with the pediatric age group. If the student finds problems in this area or feels uncomfortable in working with children, this matter can be discussed with the instructor or counselor. It is unfortunate but usually true that a student who is moody and unhappy caring for children will generally bring unhappiness to the children themselves owing to a lack of sensitivity to their needs and their sensitivity to those around them.

The student, finally, needs to develop a warm and sympathetic yet flexible attitude toward caring for children. It must be realized that in dealing with either normal or problem behavior, a solution based on the child's needs with full recognition of the student's feelings about it will usually be most satisfactory, one which will help the child in his movement along the road to maturity and the nurse in dealing with future problems in this area.

TEACHING AIDS AND OTHER INFORMATION*

American Academy of Pediatrics

An Evaluation Strategy for Assessing Individual and Population Health Status.
Child Health Record.

Growing Pains.
Human Growth Hormone.

---

*Complete addresses are given in the Appendix.

American Nurses' Association

Becoming Aware of Cultural Differences in Nursing, 1973.

Child Study Association of America

Auerbach, A. B.: The Why and How of Discipline, 1974.
Book Review Committee: Family Life and Child Development, 1975, 1976.

Child Welfare League of America, Inc.

Comer, J. P.: Beyond Black and White, 1972.

Consumer Product Information

Safe Toy Tips, 1974.
Toys: Fun in the Making, 1973.
Your Child's Emotional Health, 1973.

Department of National Health and Welfare, Ottawa, Canada

A New Perspective on the Health of Canadians.
Family Living and Sex Education: A Canadian Overview.
Family Living and Sex Education: A Guide for Parents and Youth Leaders.
Keep Your Family Safe (safety in the home).
Report on the Relationship between Income and Nutrition.
Table of Heights and Weights of Canadians.

National Association for Mental Health, Inc.

Family Life and Sex Education.
Lo Que Todo Nino Necesita Para Criarse Mentalmente Saludable (What Every Child Needs for Good Mental Health).
What Every Child Needs for Good Mental Health.

National Association for Retarded Citizens

Hunt, J. McV.: How Children Develop Intellectually.
Murphy, L. B.: Spontaneous Ways of Learning in Young Children.
Wolfe, A. G.: Differences Can Enrich Our Lives: Helping Children Prepare for Cultural Diversity.

Ross Laboratories

Children Are Different: Relation of Age to Physiologic Function, 1970.

United States Government

A Child's World.
Child Development in the Home, 1974.
Cognitive Development in Young Children, 1976.
Creative Life for Your Children, Reprinted 1972.
Exploring Childhood, 1973.
Facts About the Mental Health of Children, 1972.
How Children Grow, Reprinted 1974.
International MCH Projects: Research to Improve Health Services for Mothers and Children, 1975.
Low Income Teaching Kit, Child Development Teaching Material, 1972.
Research Relating to Children, 1975.
Russell, F. F.: Identification and Management of Selected Developmental Disabilities: A Guide for Nurses, 1975.
Safe Toys for Your Child: How to Select Them, How to Use Them Safely, 1972.
Sex-Role Attitude Items and Scales from U.S. Sample Surveys, 1975.
The Individual Child, 1973.
Toy Safety, 1972.

REFERENCES

Books

Babcock, D. E.: *Introduction to Growth, Development, and Family Life.* 3rd ed. Philadelphia, F. A. Davis Company, 1972.

Baer, M. J.: *Growth and Maturation; An Introduction to Physical Development.* Cambridge, Mass., Howard A. Doyle Publishing Company, 1973.

Berlin, I. N. (Eds.): *Advocacy For Child Mental Health.* New York, Brunner/Mazel Publishers, 1975.

Burton, B. T.: *Human Nutrition.* 3rd ed. New York, McGraw-Hill Book Company, 1976.

Caplan, F., and Caplan, T.: *The Power of Play.* New York, Doubleday Anchor Press, 1974.

Davie, R., Butler, N., and Goldstein, H.: *From Birth to Seven: The Second Report of the National Child Development Study.* London, National Children's Bureau, 1972.

Duvall, E. M.: *Family Development.* 4th ed. Philadelphia, J. B. Lippincott Company, 1971.

Erikson, E. H.: *Childhood and Society.* New York, W. W. Norton and Company, 1964.

Erickson, M. L.: *Assessment and Management of Developmental Changes in Children.* St. Louis, The C. V. Mosby Company, 1976.

Hernandez, C. A., Haug, M. J., and Wagner, N. N.: *Chicanos: Social and Psychological Perspectives.* 2nd ed. St. Louis, The C. V. Mosby Company, 1976.

Hurlock, E. B.: *Child Development.* 5th ed. New York, McGraw-Hill Book Company, 1972.

Hurlock, E. B.: *Developmental Psychology.* 4th ed. New York, McGraw Hill Book Company, 1975.

Kaluger, G., and Kaluger, M. F.: *Human Development: The Span of Life.* St. Louis, The C. V. Mosby Company, 1974.

Knobloch, H., and Pasamanick, B.: *Gesell & Amatruda's Developmental Diagnosis.* 3rd ed. New York, Harper & Row Publishers, Inc., 1974.

Lawrence, M. M.: *Young Inner City Families: Development of Ego Strength Under Stress.* New York, Behavioral Publications, Inc., 1975.

Leininger, M. M.: *Nursing and Anthropology: Two Worlds to Blend: Culture Factors in Nursing Care.* New York, John Wiley & Sons, Inc., 1970.

Lowrey, G. H.: *Growth and Development of Children.* 6th ed. Chicago, Year Book Medical Publishers, Inc., 1973.

Lubin, G. I., Magary, J. F., and Poulsen, M. K. (Eds.): *Piagetian Theory and The Helping Professions.* Los Angeles, University of Southern California, 1975.

Lynn, D. B.: *The Father: His Role in Child Development.* Monterey, California, Brooks/Cole Publishing Company, 1974.

McDonald, M.: *Not by the Color of Their Skin: The Impact of Racial Differences on the Child's Development.* New York, International University Press, 1970.

Oliven, J. F.: *Clinical Sexuality: A Manual for the Physician and the Professions.* 3rd ed. Philadelphia, J. B. Lippincott Company, 1974.

Piaget, J., and Inhelder, B.: *The Psychology of the Child.* New York, Basic Books, Inc., 1969.

Piers, M. W. (Ed.): *Play and Development.* New York, W. W. Norton and Company, 1972.

Poland, R. G.: *Human Experience: A Psychology of Growth.* St. Louis, The C. V. Mosby Company, 1974.

Sattler, J. M.: *The Assessment of Children's Intelligence.* Revised 1st ed. Philadelphia, W. B. Saunders Company, 1975.

Saul, L. J.: *Emotional Maturity: The Development and Dy-*

namics of Personality and Its Disorders. 3rd ed. Philadelphia, J. B. Lippincott Company, 1971.

Shope, D. F.: *Interpersonal Sexuality.* Philadelphia, W. B. Saunders Company, 1975.

Smith, D. W., and Bierman, E. L. (eds.): *The Biologic Ages of Man: From Conception Through Old Age.* Philadelphia, W. B. Saunders Company, 1973.

Taichert, L. C.: *Childhood Learning, Behavior, and the Family.* New York, Behavioral Publications, 1973.

Toman, W.: *Family Constellation: Its Effects on Personality and Social Behavior.* 3rd ed. New York, Springer Publishing Company, Inc. 1976.

Trantham, C. R., and Pederson, J. K.: *Normal Language Development: The Key to Diagnosis and Therapy for Language-Disordered Children.* Baltimore, The Williams & Wilkins Company, 1975.

Valadian, I., and Porter, D.: *Child Growth and Development.* Boston, Little, Brown & Company, Inc., 1976.

Wagner, N. N., and Haug, M. J.: *Chicanos: Social and Psychological Perspectives.* St. Louis, The C. V. Mosby Company, 1971.

Witmer, H. L., and Kotinsky, R.: *Personality in the Making.* The Fact-Finding Report of the Midcentury White House Conference on Children and Youth. New York, Harper and Brothers, 1952.

Periodicals

Bettelheim, B.: A Look Into Your Future . . . Child Raising. *Today's Health,* 51:56, April 1973.

Bruner, J. S.: Play Is Serious Business. *Psychology Today,* 8:80, January 1975.

Calderone, M. S.: Education in Human Sexuality for Health Professionals. *Nursing Digest,* 1:48, December 1973.

Dickerscheid, J. D., and Kirkpatrick, S. W.: Verbal Interaction Patterns of Mothers, Children, and Other Persons in the Home. *Home Economics Res. J.,* 1:83, December 1972.

Eiduson, B. T.: Looking at Children in Emergent Family Styles. *Children Today,* 3:2, July-August 1974.

Greene, D., and Lepper, M. R.: Intrinsic Motivation: How To Turn Play Into Work. *Psychology Today,* 8:49, September 1974.

Kagan, J.: Future of Child Development Research. *Nursing Digest,* 1:64, December 1973.

Kyle, J. R., and Savino, A. B.: Teaching Parents Behavior Modification. *Nursing Outlook,* 21:717, November 1973.

Lancaster, J.: Coping Mechanisms for the Working Mother. *American Journal of Nursing,* 75:1322, August 1975.

Lief, H. I., and Payne, T.: Sexuality—Knowledge and Attitudes. *American Journal of Nursing,* 75:2026, November 1975.

Luce, T. S.: Blacks, Whites and Yellows: They All Look Alike to Me. *Psychology Today,* 8:105, November 1974.

Mousseau, J.: The Family, Prison of Love. *Psychology Today,* 9:52, August 1975.

Olgas, M.: Relationship Between Parent's Health Status and Body Image of Their Children. *Nursing Research,* 23:319, July-August 1974.

Osborn, F.: The Emergence of a Valid Eugenics. *Nursing Digest,* 2:89, January 1974.

Petrillo, M., and Sanger, S.: 8 Types of Families . . . And How They Affect Your Job. *Nursing '73,* 3:42, May 1973.

Pratt, L.: Child-Rearing Methods and Children's Health Behavior. *J. Health Soc. Behav.,* 14:61, March 1973.

Reece, C.: Black Self-Concept. *Children Today,* 3:24, March-April 1974.

Sabry, Z. I., Campbell, J. A., Campbell, M. E., and Forbes, A. L.: Nutrition Canada. *Nutrition Today,* 9:5, January-February 1974.

Safran, C.: What We're Finding Out About Sexual Stereotypes. *Today's Health,* 53:14, October 1975.

Zajonc, R. B.: Dumber By The Dozen. *Psychology Today,* 8:37, January 1975.

AUDIOVISUAL MEDIA*

American Journal of Nursing Company

Heredity and Behavior
Film/videotape, 44 minute class, black and white.
Development and its dependency upon heredity and environment are discussed.

Overview
Film/videotape, 44 minute class, black and white.
The study of children is introduced by discussion and demonstration of the continuity of development through the stages of infancy, toddlerhood, preschool years, middle years of childhood, and adolescence.

Education Development Center, Inc.

Brazelton Neonatal Behavioral Assessment Scale
3 reels, 16mm, sound, black and white, manual.
Introduction—20 min.
Variations in normal behavior—20 min.
Self Scoring Exam—23 min.
These three films, along with two manuals, provide training for the evaluation of the behavior of the neonate as well as a neurological examination.

LaDoca Project and Publishing Foundation, Inc.

Denver Developmental Screening Test
4 reels, 16mm, sound, color, workbook, manual, test kits, test pads.
Denver Developmental training film for nurses—2—45 min. reels.

Denver Developmental proficiency film—30 min.
DDST/proficiency—27 min.
Based on a test developed by William K. Frankenburg, M.D., and others of the University of Colorado Medical Center. The first film, in conjunction with manuals and kits, teaches how to perform DDST with children. The second film assists in measuring the nurse's proficiency and knowledge of administering the tests. Actual examples on the third film test the nurse's skill in administering the test.

J. B. Lippincott Company

Growth and Development: A Chronicle of Four Children
16mm and Super—8mm and/or videotapes, sound, color.
This series of sound color motion pictures demonstrates the range of normal variation in social, physical, and cognitive development during the first four years of life. Holistic in approach, the films focus on each child's social and emotional development, identification behavior, motor development, habitual responses, concepts of reality, and body structure and function.

McGraw-Hill Book Company

Cognitive Development
18 minutes, color and videocassette.

Development
33 minutes, color and videocassette.

Sensory World
33 minutes, color.

Sex Role Development
23 minutes, color and videocassette.

Public Affairs Committee

We Are All Brothers
20 minutes, 54 frames, partial color, 35mm.

Ross Laboratories

Growth Charts
This collection of charts traces the physical and social development of children. Two separate sheets—one for boys, the other for girls—illustrate the normal patterns of adaptive-social and physical development from birth to 56 weeks. Characteristic crying habits, smiling behavior, socializing tendencies, and self-concepts are described as they vary throughout the 56 weeks, as are physical attributes like degree and type of hearing, eye, and hand control. A separate graph shows shifts in head circumference from birth to three years of age.

Telstar Productions, Inc.

Defenses of the Ego
28 minutes, sound, videotape
Shows internal defense mechanism plus displacement and regression.

Trainex Corporation

Growth and Development
Audio-tape cassettes—33 1/3 LP, color, 35 mm.
Provides parents with information on a number of growth patterns including head shape, sleep habits, teething, walking, and talking.

Normal Patterns of Development
Audio-tape cassettes—33 1/3 LP, color, 35 mm.

---

*Complete addresses are given in the Appendix.

Chapter Three

THE NURSING PROCESS IN THE CARE OF CHILDREN

by EVELYN N. BEHANNA and
SHEILA M. PRINGLE

The nursing process is generally accepted by professional nurses as the foundation for their practice. The nursing process is a continuous phenomenon, which is actually the application of problem-solving methodology to nursing care. Though various authors may describe the nursing process in different terminology, it is generally considered to consist of sequential steps through which the client's problems are identified and probable solutions are revealed.

The process itself is used in every helping situation, although every situation has its own unique features. When dealing with a child, for example, it is extremely important to gain his cooperation and assistance and that of respective family members. Inclusion of family members as part of the health team can assist in securing the child's cooperation in every aspect of the required health care.

The nursing process has been described by many authors as having four basic steps—assessment, problem identification, intervention, and evaluation. These basic steps can be further delineated to include additional tasks. The four basic steps, though important, do not adequately

describe the total process. Before assessment can occur, data must be collected. It is also necessary to plan the care and consider many alternative actions before intervention can take place. Nursing process, then, involves a minimum of six basic steps—data collection, assessment, problem identification, planning for care, intervention, and evaluation.

A brief description of nursing as a helping process might follow this pattern. An individual or client (in this instance a child) requires nursing assistance. As the nurse, you first collect the data, then assess it to determine the strengths and weaknesses of this individual. Nursing problems are identified from the areas of weakness. Plans for assisting the individual are made, utilizing previously determined strengths of the client. Nursing intervention then takes place and the results are evaluated in the light of the client's new health status. The steps are ongoing and are repeated until the individual returns to his optimal level of health and no longer requires nursing assistance.

Nursing process is frequently viewed as linear, i.e., patient with problem→data collection→ assessment → problem identification → plan → intervention→evaluation. The process has also been viewed as circular in nature. These are simplistic representations, which seem to deny the complex nature of individuals and their health problems. Nurses must always keep in mind that external and internal forces are constantly influencing an individual and his health problems. It might be helpful to view the individual as the central point of a matrix (Fig. 3–1).

The diagram illustrates that the individual is a unique being but is a member of a family, which is also encased in a community, with everchanging environmental stresses. In addition, the individual is influenced by needs and goals, is a participant in life's activities, and has a particular health status, with established strengths and weaknesses. When an individual requires assis-

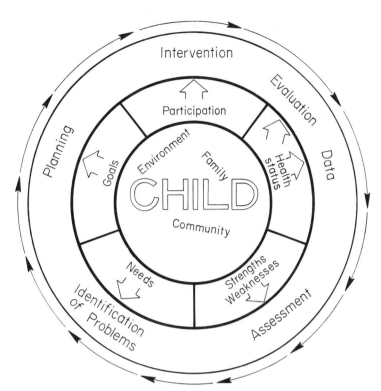

Figure 3-1. The nursing process as a matrix.

tance because of a health problem, the nursing process is usually set into motion.

The diagram demonstrates a method by which the nursing process takes into consideration the complex nature of the individual. Health status becomes part of the data; strengths and weaknesses are assessed. Needs are now expressed as problems, and goals focus on plans to meet the problems. Participation in life's activities is now channeled into implementation of the plan of action. After such a plan has been implemented, the client's health status is again evaluated.

Each of the steps in the nursing process is now discussed in greater depth.

DATA COLLECTION

Deliberate data collection is the first goal of the nurse when initiating the helping process. Data collection should be systematic and thorough. Information is gathered from all possible sources: the child, his family, data from examinations (physical and developmental), records, and other health personnel. To obtain data requires the skills of observation and communication.

Observation includes use of all five senses (sight, hearing, touch, taste, and smell) consciously and deliberately. The specific information obtained this way is more precise and more

useful than the kind gained from casual daily contacts.

Data are frequently obtained, clarified, and validated through communication skills. Verbal and nonverbal communication skills are necessary. Verbal communication includes both the written and spoken word. Nonverbal communication includes messages transmitted without using words, for example, through touch, gesture, movement, facial expression, body positions, or sounds such as groans, grunts, or sighs, giggling, or laughter.

Physical and Developmental Examination

It is essential that the nurse be able to observe and collect data in relation to the infant's or child's physical and developmental health status. What follows is an overview of significant techniques used in the physical and developmental examination of the pediatric client.

Data collection concerning the physical status is accomplished by observation and requires use of the techniques of palpation, auscultation, and percussion. More than one technique of data collection may be needed to differentiate the normal from the abnormal. These three techniques, along with interviewing (communication) and observation used during history-taking and other testing, can assist in determining the client's health problems.

The technique of applying the hands to parts of the patient's body to determine any underlying deviation from normal is known as *palpation*. *Auscultation* is the technique of listening, either with a stethoscope or the naked ear, for sounds in specific areas of the patient's body in order to differentiate normal from abnormal sounds. *Percussion* is the technique of tapping a portion of the body and noting the sounds produced and the resistance encountered.

The nurse can use instruments such as the ophthalmoscope, otoscope, flashlight, stethoscope, sphygmomanometer, percussion hammer, and tuning fork in assessing the client's physical status.

Developmental data collection is needed to provide information about whether the infant, child, or adolescent is meeting the developmental milestones appropriate for the respective age. Physical and developmental norms by age categories can be located in Chapters 7, 13, 16, 19, 22, and 25. One of the most widely used developmental tests for ages one through six is the Denver Developmental Screening Test described in Chapter 2.

Determination of the physical and developmental status of the child requires particular skills. A great deal of information can be obtained during the interview with the parent and child by merely observing the child's actions and reactions to the environment and to the individuals within this setting. When the actual physical examination begins, the nurse must be cognizant of the age of the child, and whether or not the child has had previous experience with such an examination. This information assists the nurse to determine which part of the body to inspect first and how much parental assistance will be needed.

The general appearance of the infant or child can be noted at the time of history-taking. These gross observations are concerned with whether the child appears well cared for and alert, as well as with determining the child's skin color

TABLE 3–1. STRATEGIES FOR COOPERATION

AGE	PHYSICAL STATUS DATA COLLECTION	STRATEGY PERFORMED WHILE CHILD IS
0–12 months	1. Skin color and respirations are observed 2. Vital signs are taken; auscultate heart and chest 3. Palpate anterior and posterior fontanels 4. Head circumference measurement 5. Examine eyes, ears, nose, and throat	Sleeping or quiet Positioned on parent's lap
	6. Palpate and examine abdomen 7. Examine genitalia and rectum 8. Test central nervous system development	Give a bottle or distract with a toy or rattle while on an examining table
1–3 years	1. Vital signs and blood pressure	Positioned on parent's lap
	2. Gross observation of growth and development. Examine extremities and central nervous system	Become acquainted with tongue blade, stethoscope, or other appropriate equipment
	3. Examine head, eyes, ears, nose and neck 4. Examination and auscultation of heart and chest	Positioned on parent's lap
	5. Examine abdomen 6. Examine genitalia 7. Examine rectum	Give a toy as a distraction or a security object
	8. Rectal temperature may be taken at this point	Lying on abdomen—holding parent's hands; nurse's hand on child's back
3–6 years	1. Vital signs and blood pressure; examination and auscultation of heart and chest 2. Observation of growth and development and central nervous system 3. Examine head, neck, eyes, ears, and nose	Become acquainted with the nurse and handling tongue blade, stethoscope, or other appropriate equipment; given emotional support by parent
	4. Examine abdomen 5. Examine genitalia 6. Examine rectum	Lying on an examining table with parent in attendance
6–12 years	1. Vital signs, blood pressure, examination and auscultation of heart and chest 2. Observation of growth and development and central nervous system 3. Examine head, neck, eyes, ears, and nose 4. Examine abdomen 5. Examine genitalia 6. Examine rectum	Accompanied by parent, if child desires Familiarized with examining equipment to be used. Involved with examination; gain cooperation thru conversation and receiving explanation of the procedure

and mood. While the physical examination is being performed, vital signs, height, and weight can be determined. It would be advantageous to record the height and weight on a "Growth Grid" so that the growth profile can be visualized (standard anthropometric charts: see Chapter 2). It is imperative that the nurse obtain as much information as possible while the child is calm and not threatened. There are certain strategies that the nurse can employ to gain the cooperation of the child during completion of the data collection. These strategies are listed in Table 3–1 for children of different age groups.

During the data collection step, the nurse gathers information but does not interpret it.

ASSESSMENT

In reality, assessment can begin while information is being gathered. It differs from data collection in that judgments are made about the information that has been collected.

A primary task of the nurse during assessment is to compare the collected data with established norms of growth and development. It is essential, then, that professional nurses develop a theoretical framework from which to operate. Such a framework should include knowledge about the uniqueness of the individual, expected patterns of growth and development, and the way in which the systems of the human body are interrelated in function.

After the data have been compared and contrasted, categories of strengths and weaknesses are developed.

Data must be viewed from many perspectives. When comparing data to a norm, the nurse must keep in mind that the same data can be used in other contexts. For example, a child of nine months has rolled off a bed. It is normal for a nine-month-old child to roll over, yet children of nine months should not be placed on beds without constant supervision, thus the same data can pinpoint a strength of the child (his ability to roll) and a weakness of his family (failure to provide a safe environment). The same data may therefore be categorized twice, as a strength and as a weakness.

Inherent within the assessment phase is the understanding that the professional nurse reaffirms the accuracy of the collected data before making judgments. Examples of reaffirming the accuracy of data would be taking the vital signs more than once if the nurse questions them and reviewing the client's growth and development levels if they are not within normal limits.

Data found to be within normal limits are considered strengths; findings that are abnormal are regarded as weaknesses.

At this point in the process the weaknesses are reviewed and patient problems are identified.

IDENTIFICATION OF PROBLEMS

The delineated areas of weakness provide the data to identify existing and potential health problems. Problem identification requires a deliberate intellectual approach by the health worker.

A conceptual framework that the professional nurse finds useful in identifying health problems is that of the basic needs of man. Maslow has suggested that each individual has basic human needs that must always be met. He has placed these needs in hierarchical fashion: physiologic, safety, love, self-esteem, and self-actualization. Physiologic needs are the most basic and must be met before other higher level needs appear and are fulfilled.

The nurse objectively reviews the previously categorized weaknesses to identify whether the areas of weakness might interfere with the individual's ability to meet his or her own needs. If in the nurse's judgment the weaknesses will interfere with the meeting of needs, a problem has been identified.

Clients and their families must assist in the problem identification stage. Unless there is agreement by the nurse and the client that a problem exists, it is unlikely that the client will cooperate or participate in plans to correct that problem.

PLANNING

Planning for intervention involves the nurse and the client and, when possible, the family. The focus on the nurse's plan of action must be based on principles and sound rationale. Principles that guide nursing actions are drawn from the basis of knowledge found in previous studies of the humanities and science.

The nurse's plan of action must be structured to include all of the identified problems, both actual and potential.

The problems are first reviewed for the order in which they should be met. One method would be to utilize the hierarchy of needs to determine problem selection order. For example, plan to meet problems that interfere with body equilibrium (physiologic) before planning for interferences with availability of emotional support (love) or interferences with achieving (self-actualization).

Once the order for dealing with problems has been decided, it is up to the nurse to construct short-term and long-term objectives and propose specific actions for alleviating them. The nurse then uses knowledge of the client's strengths to aid in planning intervention.

Short-term objectives are usually designed to focus attention on those aspects of identified problems that can be remedied quickly or remedied by others providing care. Long-term objectives usually focus on aspects of the problems that require the client and family to learn new skills in order to cope with the health problem when the client has returned home.

If a short-term objective is to provide comfort and rest, the nurse can plan care so that the client is disturbed as little as possible. For example, vital signs, morning care, and breakfast

TABLE 3–2. NURSING PROCESS FOR A CHILD HAVING ACCIDENTAL INJURY*

DATA COLLECTION			ASSESSMENT	PROBLEM IDENTIFICATION	PLANNING	INTERVENTION	EVALUATION
Capitola Nash (name)	History Taking and Examination	Comparison and Contrast	Strengths and Weaknesses	(possible)			
9-month-old girl	Weight: 18 lb. Height: 27 in. TPR: 99–150–40	normal normal pulse rapid; respiration rapid; temperature normal	Capitola appears to be well within normal range of growth and development except for the following weaknesses; 1. Rapid pulse 2. Rapid respiration	Head trauma, tissue and bone trauma Head trauma, possible child abuse.	1. Monitor vital signs: alteration in vital signs is an indicator of change in physical status 2. Neurologic evaluation; check for level of consciousness, unusual behavior. Alteration of level of consciousness or marked change in behavior can be indicative of increased intracranial pressure and meningeal irritation	1. Every ½ hour 6 times; then q1 hour times 24, observe for signs of respiratory distress 2. Observe for pupil reaction, response to name, observe for increased irritability, nausea and vomiting; observe for bulging fontanel	1. Vital signs stabiliz[e] within normal ran[ge] 2. Pupils remain equ[al] and react to light; [in]fant responds to name; no vomitin[g] nausea or change [in] behavior
	Heart sounds; no rales, rhonchi	normal					
	Motor: Turns over Crawls Pulls to stand Sits alone Speech: Says DA-DA and MA-MA Cries when scolded Social: Cries at strangers	normal normal normal normal normal normal normal					
Bruised area above left eye	Head: Posterior fontanel closed Anterior fontanel open 1–1½ cm. Eyes: Pupils equal and react to light Ecchymosis above left eye	normal normal normal abnormal	3. Ecchymosis above left eye in temporal area		3. Rest to permit the body time to repair itself and quiet to reduce stimuli that increase intracranial pressure	3. Plan all intervention measures to permit maximum periods of rest, i.e., bathe, feed, take vital signs at one time, then rest; position infant in other than affected areas; turn q 2 hours	3. Sleeps intermitten[t] plays with toes an[d] toys when awake.
Bruised area over left shoulder	Extremities: Ecchymosis left shoulder–scapula area. Cries when arm manipulated Right arm and shoulder: Good abduction and adduction, skin clear Legs: Manipulated freely, abduction and adduction good, skin clear Abdomen: Liver palpable 1 to 2 cm. below right costal margin Spleen: Not palpable	abnormal normal normal normal	4. Ecchymosis over scapula area	Tissue and bone trauma, possible child abuse	4. Look for old healing bruises and scars over body, as abused children frequently have unexplained healing, bruises, or scars	4. Provide range of motion to maintain function and check limitations; inspect child's body thoroughly; observe parent-child interactions	4. If bruises found [or] parent-child interaction unusual, su[s]pect child abuse, [re]fer to Social Servi[ce] Department after [dis]cussion with phys[i]cian or if addition[al] evidence found in [the] x-rays
Parents stated:	Capitola fell from kitchen table while mother was in process of changing her diaper. Capitola did not lose consciousness prior to or after the fall, but cried a great deal		5. Her physical abilities of standing alone, and sitting alone, though obviously strengths, can lead to additional accidents, therefore, should also be considered a possible weakness	Infant Safety	5. Comfort: to reduce crying and allay fears	5. Allow family members to stay	5. Note if child crie[s] when parents lea[ve] the room
			6. Parent placed infant in a place of danger and parent not aware of safety needs		6. Teaching: to prevent accidents	6. Normal growth and development pattern, safety in the home	6. Parents have discussed and writte[n] plans for improvi[ng] home safety
			7. Strength: Parents' observation of infant and seeking immediate treatment	Emotional support infant and parents	7. Reassurance and information given to allay parents, fears	7. Explain procedures and plan of care	7. Parents able to participate in car[e]

*Other examples of the nursing process appear in Appendix 1.

can be organized to use a minimal period of time and thus provide more time for rest. Comfort has been provided via morning care and breakfast. In addition, if this client has a strong family member who is usually present, include that family member in the care process. It is also advisable that the family member stay with the client to ensure quiet rest periods. If a long-term objective is more rest periods at home, then to meet this objective more data, planning, and teaching would be required.

Each action that the nurse considers for a given problem should be based on a specific reason. It is not enough to plan in terms of generalities or desirable objectives. Each action should be viewed in terms of the desired effect for this client, at this time, with this health problem. Providing comfort and rest may be the objective for clients with bronchiolitis and croup, yet the planned actions should differ. The child with croup has difficulty with inspiration. A desirable position of comfort would include semi-Fowler's position or lying on the back with the head elevated to provide full chest expansion and support to the back and head while reducing the child's efforts to breathe. The child with bronchiolitis has difficulty with expiration. A position of comfort for this child would be on his abdomen to aid in the expulsion of air. Each problem identified could have many tentative nursing actions; it is up to the nurse to decide which actions should be tried and in what order.

INTERVENTION

The planned objectives are translated into nursing intervention via the tentative actions. Just as it was essential that the client and his family were involved in identifying the problems, it is now essential that client and family participate in the actions to alleviate or correct the problem. Though it is the nurse who uses a knowledge base to frame the actions, they must involve client participation. Cooperation and improved health status are best secured when the client and family members know the reason for the actions and actively work toward the agreed upon objectives.

EVALUATION

As intervention proceeds, it is the responsibility of the nurse to gather new data, make new assessments, and use alternative actions. It may be necessary to revise plans if the actions have not brought about the desired results.

During the evaluation phase the data collected should reflect achievement of short-term objectives, health status should be improved, and health problems minimized. It is possible that as one problem is alleviated, others may appear. This is due in part to the complex nature of individuals and their health problems. As demonstrated in the matrix diagram, the individual's health status is the beginning source for the data needed to set the nursing process into motion, and a revised health status becomes the final stage of the evaluation phase of the nursing process.

Table 3–2 is an example of how the nursing process operates in the case of a child having an accidental injury. It is not meant to be all-inclusive of the care given to a client, but is meant to illustrate that data lead to assessment, problem identification, planning, intervention, and evaluation. As new data emerge, the process continues until the client achieves maximum health.

Throughout this chapter the term *client* has been used in reference to a child who is a patient. In the appendix when a nursing process example referring to an individual is given this term may be used also. Since pediatric nursing is family-centered, the term "client" may refer to a child, a mother, or a father, or another family member, depending on the person to whom professional care or help is being given. It is for this reason that the individual under discussion will usually be named throughout the other sections of this text in order to reduce confusion.

REFERENCES

Books

Alexander, M., and Brown, M.: *Pediatric Physical Diagnosis for Nurses.* New York, McGraw-Hill Book Company, 1974.

Bailey, J. T., and Claus, K. E.: *Decision Making in Nursing: Tools for Change.* St. Louis, The C. V. Mosby Company, 1975.

Bates, B.: *A Guide to Physical Examination.* Philadelphia, J. B. Lippincott Company, 1974.

Becknell, E. P., and Smith, D. M.: *System of Nursing Practice: A Clinical Nursing Assessment Tool.* Philadelphia, F. A. Davis Company, 1975.

Browning, M. H. (Compiler): *The Nursing Process in Practice.* New York, American Journal of Nursing Company, 1974.

Capell, P. T., and Case, D. B.: *Ambulatory Care Manual for Nurse Practitioners.* Philadelphia, J. B. Lippincott Company, 1976.

Chinn, P. L., and Leitch, C. J.: *Child Health Maintenance: A Guide to Clinical Assessment*. St. Louis, The C. V. Mosby Company, 1974.

Gillies, D. A., and Alyn, I. B.: *Patient Assessment and Management by the Nurse Practitioner*. Philadelphia, W. B. Saunders Company, 1976.

Little, D. E., and Carnevali, D. L.: *Nursing Care Planning*. 2nd ed. Philadelphia, J. B. Lippincott Company, 1976.

Loomis, M. E., and Horsley, J. A.: *Interpersonal Change: A Behavioral Approach to Nursing Practice*. New York, McGraw-Hill Book Company, 1974.

Marriner, A.: *The Nursing Process: A Scientific Approach to Nursing Care*. St. Louis, The C. V. Mosby Company, 1975.

Mayers, M. G.: *A Systematic Approach to the Nursing Care Plan*. New York, Appleton-Century-Crofts, 1972.

Mitchell, P. H.: *Concepts Basic to Nursing*. New York, McGraw-Hill Book Company, 1973.

Murray, R., and Zentner, J.: *Nursing Assessment and Health Promotion Through the Life Span*. Englewood Cliffs, N.J., Prentice-Hall, 1975.

Orlando, I. J.: *The Discipline and Teaching of Nursing Process (An Evaluative Study)*. New York, G. P. Putnam's Sons, 1972.

Prior, J. A., and Silberstein, J. S.: *Physical Diagnosis: The History and Examination of the Patient*. 4th ed. St. Louis, The C. V. Mosby Company, 1973.

Saxton, D. F., and Hyland, P. A.: *Planning and Implementing Nursing Intervention*. St. Louis, The C. V. Mosby Company, 1975.

Sherman, J. L., Jr., and Fields, S. K.: *Guide to Patient Evaluation: History Taking, Physical Examination and the Problem-Oriented Method*. New York, Medical Examination Publishing Company, 1974.

Sundeen, S. J., Stuart, G. W., Rankin, E. D., and Cohen, S. P.: *The Nursing Process: Personal Growth, Interpersonal Competence*. St. Louis, The C. V. Mosby Company, 1976.

Travelbee, J.: *Interpersonal Aspects of Nursing*. 2nd ed. Philadelphia, F. A. Davis Company, 1971.

Tucker, S.: *Patient Care Standards*. St. Louis, The C. V. Mosby Company, 1975.

Yura, H., and Walsh, M. B.: *The Nursing Process: Assessing, Planning, Implementing, Evaluating*. 2nd ed. New York, Appleton-Century-Crofts, 1973.

Periodicals

Alexander, M. M., and Brown, M. S.: Physical Examination: Part 16: The Musculoskeletal System. *Nursing 76*, 6:51, April 1976.

Aspinall, M. J.: Nursing Diagnosis—The Weak Link. *Nursing Outlook*, 24:433, July 1976.

Barnsteiner, J. H.: Bicentennial Forecast: Pediatric Nursing. *RN*, 39:21, November 1976.

Bircher, A.: On the Development and Classification of Diagnoses. *Nursing Forum*, 14:10, (No. 1) 1975.

Bloch, D.: Some Crucial Terms in Nursing—What Do They Really Mean? *Nursing Outlook*, 22:689, November 1974.

Brown, M. S., and Alexander, M. M.: Physical Examination: Part 15: Female Genitalia. *Nursing 76*, 6:39, March 1976.

de Tornyay, R.: Nursing Decisions 4: Experiences in Clinical Problem Solving. *RN*, 39:47, January 1976.

de Tornyay, R.: Nursing Decisions: Experiences in Clinical Problem Solving. Series 2, Number 3. *RN*, 39:51, December 1976.

Gebbie, K., and Lavin, M. A.: Classifying Nursing Diagnoses. *Am. J. Nursing*, 74:250, February 1974.

Goodwin, J. O., and Edwards, B. S.: Developing a Computer Program to Assist the Nursing Process: Phase I—From Systems Analysis to an Expandable Program. *Nursing Research*, 24:299, July-August 1975.

Hagopian, G., and Kilpack, V.: Baccalaureate Students Learn Assessment Skills. *Nursing Outlook*, 22:454, July 1974.

Jarvis, C. M.: Vital Signs. *Nursing 76*, 6:31, April 1976.

O'Connell, A. L., and Bates, B.: The Case Method in Nurse Practitioner Education. *Nursing Outlook*, 24:243, April 1976.

Roy, Sr. C.: A Diagnostic Classification System for Nursing. *Nursing Outlook*, 23:90, February 1975.

Roy, Sr. C.: The Impact of Nursing Diagnosis. *Nursing Digest*, 4:67, Summer 1976.

Ryan, B. J.: Nursing Care Plans: A Systems Approach to Developing Criteria for Planning and Evaluation. *J. Nursing Administration*, 3:50, May-June 1973.

AUDIOVISUAL MEDIA*

Harper & Row, Publishers

The Nursing Process
   Multi-media program.
   Unit 1—Overview of the Nursing Process.
   Unit 2—Observation: Tools and Factors.
   Unit 5—Communication.
   Unit 6—The Health Team as a Source of Information.
   Unit 7—The Patient as a Source of Information.
   Unit 8/9—Assessment.
   Unit 10—Planning.
   Unit 11—Implementation.
   Unit 12—Evaluating Patient Care.

J. B. Lippincott Company

A Visual Guide to Physical Examination Series
   16mm, 13 films, sound, color.
   The Head and Neck—13 min.
   The Thorax—6 min.
   The Heart—5 min.
   Pressure and Pulses—5 min.
   The Breast and Axilla—5 min.
   The Abdomen—7 min.
   The Male Genitalia, Anus and Rectum—10 min.
   The Female Genitalia, Anus and Rectum—10 min.

The Peripheral Vascular System—10 min.
The Musculoskeletal System—15 min.
The Neurological System—Part I: 20 min.
The Neurological System—Part II: 20 min.
Special Procedures of the Pediatric Physical Examination—10 min.

Medical Electronic Educational Services, Inc.

Physical Diagnosis in Patient Assessment
   5 programs of varied length, 35mm filmstrip and tape, sound, color.
   Physical diagnosis, history taking, inspection, palpation and percussion and auscultation. An overview of the logic and techniques of physical diagnosis from the standpoint of their application in ongoing patient assessment.

Wayne State University

DENT: Directions for Education in Nursing Via Technology
   30 min. lessons, videotape and videocassette, 16mm film
   Nursing Process
      I. Assessment
      II. Planning and Implementation
      III. Evaluation

---

*Complete addresses are given in the Appendix.

Chapter Four

ILLNESS AND THE CHILD

THE DIFFERENCES IN ILLNESS IN CHILDREN AND ADULTS

The child's body is building up to a maximum development rather than being at a plateau of physical fitness or in the stages of decline. The exact age of the peak of the process of bodily repair is not known, but repair does seem to decrease after 18 to 20 years of age. If the statement that physical adolescence ends with the eruption of the wisdom teeth is correct, this is a concrete example of the last of the building-up processes of the teeth. It is true, however, that decay may occur long before this time.

Even though the child's capacity for repair is greater, he lacks the reserve forces which the adult has. Such lack is shown in an easily upset electrolyte balance, sudden elevation or lowering of temperature, rapid spread of infection, and destruction of body tissue.

The differences in illness in children and adults are based on the anatomic, physiologic and psychologic differences between the immature child and the mature adult.

Anatomic differences between the newborn and the adult are obvious. Size is the outstanding difference; it influences the method and equipment used in caring for the child. A more specific anatomic difference between them is the greater size and weight of the newborn's head when compared with body length and weight. This characteristic, coupled with his immature motor development, makes handling of the infant quite different from that of the older child or adult. Injury can occur to the head of the infant from a fall due to the adult's being unable to handle the child properly.

The sutures of the skull in the newborn are not united; the brain is not protected by the skull in the areas of the open fontanels. The infant's bones are neither as firm nor as brittle as those of the older child. Thus, when intracranial pressure develops in the infant, his head simply enlarges as the sutures separate. This is not possible in the adult, who exhibits other indications of increased intracranial pressure.

The normal shape of the head and the chest of the infant can be altered by constant pressure from lying in one position. The parent or the nurse must move the infant frequently so that the child's bones will not become deformed.

In the adult, the cardiac sphincter of the stomach is usually fairly tight. In the infant it is more relaxed. This is one of the reasons why vomiting in infancy is so frequent and why so many adults have difficulty vomiting even when they are nauseated.

Certain diseases are influenced by the interaction of anatomic development with physiologic development. An example of such a disease is infection of the middle ear (otitis media), a condition often occurring in young children when they have a sore throat, because the eustachian tube is both shorter and straighter than that of the older child or adult.

The student will find many other examples of disease related to anatomic development of the child throughout the units of this text.

The differences in the *physiologic processes* of the newborn infant and of the older child or adult are less obvious than the anatomic differences. But the physiologic characteristics of an age group are more important in the adaptation of nursing care to needs than are the anatomic ones, since they are subject to greater control by medical and nursing procedures. For example, some blood values of children different from those of adults are shown in Tables 4–1 and 4–2.

Physiologic development influences the child's susceptibility to certain diseases, the symptoms of disease and the probability of lasting harm. The infant or small child requires a

TABLE 4-1. HEMATOLOGIC VALUES DURING INFANCY AND CHILDHOOD

AGE	HEMOGLOBIN GM./100 ML. %		HEMATOCRIT %		RETICULOCYTES %	WBC/MM.³ %		NEUTROPHILS %		LYMPHOCYTES % MEAN (RELATIVELY WIDE RANGE)	EOSINOPHILS % MEAN	MONOCYTES % MEAN	NUCLEATED RED CELLS /100 WBC
	MEAN	RANGE	MEAN	RANGE	MEAN	MEAN	RANGE	MEAN	RANGE				
Cord blood	16.8	13.7-20.1	55	45-65	5.0	18,000	(9-30,000)	61	(40-80)	31	2	6	7.0 (3-10)
2 weeks	16.5	13.0-20.0	50	42-66	1.0	12,000	(5-21,000)	40		48	3	9	0
3 months	12.0	9.5-14.5	36	31-41	1.0	12,000	(6-18,000)	30		63	2	5	0
6 mos.-6 yrs.	12.0	10.5-14.0	37	33-42	1.0	10,000	(6-15,000)	45		48	2	5	0
7-12 yrs.	13.0	11.0-16.0	38	34-40	1.0	8,000	(4500-13,500)	55		38	2	5	0
Adult Female	14	12.0-16.0	42	37-47	1.6	7,500	(5-10,000)	55	(35-70)	35	3	7	0
Adult Male	16	14.0-18.0	47	42-52									

All values represent compromises between a number of standard sources and published reports. Greatest variations in "normal" are seen in infancy and early childhood.

The decreases in hemoglobin and hematocrit values and in the red blood cell count which occur in all infants during the first 2 or 3 months of life have been designated "**physiologic anemia**" of infancy. The erythrocytes are normocytic and normochromic, and there is no unusual reticulocytosis. These decreases are apparently related to the relatively short life span of the fetal red cell and to the dilutional effects of the infant's expanding blood volume. The pattern is not altered by the administration of iron or other "hematinic" substances. Low birth weight accentuates this "anemia" of early infancy; in such infants hemoglobin values may fall as low as 6.0 to 7.0 gm./100 ml. Usually there are no symptoms, even with this degree of anemia, but, if the infant is failing to grow or thrive, a small (5 ml. per kg.) transfusion of sedimented compatible red blood cells may be beneficial.

Although iron medication does not prevent this "physiologic anemia" the iron stores of infants of low birth weight and of infants who have had significant perinatal blood loss should be replenished by administration of medicinal iron or by feeding of an iron-fortified milk formula.

From V. C. Vaughan, and R. J. McKay: *Nelson Textbook of Pediatrics*. 10th ed. Philadelphia, W. B. Saunders Company, 1975, p. 1110.

TABLE 4–2. NORMAL BLOOD VALUES

DETERMINATION	SPECIMEN	AGE*/SEX	NORMAL VALUE	
Bilirubin, total			Premature/Full Term	
		Cord	< 2	< 2 mg/dl
		0–1 day	< 8	< 6 mg/dl
		1–2 day	<12	< 8 mg/dl
		3–5 day	<16	<12 mg/dl
		Thereafter	< 2	< 1 mg/dl
Bilirubin, direct			0–1 mg/dl	
Calcium, total		Newborn	3.7–7.0 mEq/l	(For
		Infant	5.2–6.0 mEq/l	conversion
		Child	5.0–5.7 mEq/l	see Table
		Thereafter	4.5–5.7 mEq/l	30–11)
Carbon dioxide content (CO_2)	venous (arterial 2 mEq/l less)	Cord	14–22 mEq/l	
		Newborn	19–27 mEq/l	
		Infant	20–28 mEq/l	
		Child	18–27 mEq/l	
		Thereafter	23–29 mEq/l	
Carbon dioxide, partial pressure (pCO_2)	whole blood, arterial whole blood, venous		35–45 mm Hg 40–50 mm Hg	
Chloride		Cord	96–104 mEq/l	
		Newborn	93–112 mEq/l	
		Infant	95–110 mEq/l	
		Child	101–108 mEq/l	
		Thereafter	98–108 mEq/l	
Cholesterol, total		Cord	45–100 mg/dl	
		Newborn	45–170 mg/dl	
		Infant	70–175 mg/dl	
		Child	120–240 mg/dl	
		Thereafter	150–250 mg/dl	
Galactose		Newborn/Infant	0–20 mg/dl	
Glucose, fasting (FBS)		Premature	20– 60 mg/dl	
		Newborn	30– 80 mg/dl	
		Child	60–100 mg/dl	
		Thereafter	70–110 mg/dl	
Iron		Newborn	100–200 μg/dl	
		4 mo–2 yr	40–100 μg/dl	
		Thereafter	85–150 μg/dl	
Lipids, total		Newborn–2 yr	170– 450 mg/dl	
		2 yr–14 yr	490–1000 mg/dl	
		Thereafter	400– 800 mg/dl	
pH (37°C)[7]	whole blood, arterial	Premature (cord)	7.15–7.35	
		Premature (48 hr)	7.35–7.50	
		Newborn	7.27–7.47	
		Thereafter	7.35–7.45	
Phenylalanine			0.5–2.0 mg/dl	
Protein, total		Premature	4.3–7.6 gm/dl	
		Newborn	4.6–7.6 gm/dl	
		Child	6.2–8.1 gm/dl	
		Thereafter	5.5–7.8 gm/dl	
Sodium		Premature (cord)	116–140 mEq/l	
		Premature (48 hr)	128–148 mEq/l	
		Newborn (cord)	126–166 mEq/l	
		Newborn	139–162 mEq/l	
		Infant	139–146 mEq/l	
		Child	138–145 mEq/l	
		Thereafter	135–151 mEq/l	
Urea nitrogen (BUN)		Newborn/infant	5–15 mg/dl	
		Thereafter	10–20 mg/dl	

*Age ranges are defined as follows:

Premature	birth–1 mo	Child	2 yr–puberty
Newborn	birth–1 wk	Adolescent	puberty–adult
Neonatal	1 wk–1 mo	Adult	>18 yr
Infant	1 mo–2 yr		

Excerpted from Vaughan, V. C., III, and McKay, R. J.: *Nelson Textbook of Pediatrics.* 10th ed. Philadelphia, W. B. Saunders Co., 1975.

greater caloric and fluid intake in proportion to his weight than does the older child, because of his need to support growth, and to carry on physical activity and basic metabolic functions. Any pathologic condition which causes loss of fluid, e.g., diarrhea or fever, quickly alters the electrolyte balance. Also, when replacing the lost fluids and electrolytes intravenously, the anatomic and physiologic ability of the small child to absorb fluid slowly necessitates careful regulation of the rate of flow. If fluid were injected intravenously into the infant at the same rate it is usually given to the adult, the child would soon have pulmonary edema.

Important among the differences in the occurrence of illness in children and adults is their resistance to disease. The infant derives from his mother a short-lived immunity to certain infectious diseases. Immunization against most contagious diseases he is likely to contract must be given early in infancy, since many of these diseases may be fatal or cause permanent impairment of bodily functions.

In general, the symptoms of disease in an infant are different from those in an older child or adult, owing to the pathologic state caused by the injurious agents on tissues in different stages of development. It is important in pediatric nursing to learn the cause-effect relation of any pathologic agent to the developmental stage of the child's body, in order to give preventive and curative nursing care and to be prepared for any emergency. For instance, infants and very young children may have convulsions due to the elevation of temperature accompanying the onset of a contagious disease, whereas an older child or adult is likely to have a chill preceding the fever at the onset of an infection.

Mental and emotional reactions to illness differ in various age groups. Both objective signs (those which can be observed) and subjective symptoms (those which cannot be observed and are known only to the person who experiences them) are important in comprehensive nursing. Since the infant and the young child cannot tell how they feel, the nurse is compelled to rely solely on signs. Awareness of both what to expect and the full meaning of the observations are important.

The older the child, the more successful he is in communicating symptoms to the nurse. Although an infant cannot tell how he feels, and does not localize pain as an older child will do, he may pull at an aching ear, or cry when some part of his body is moved. Such behavior provides an objective sign of a subjective symptom. These signs are important; to learn their meaning is an essential part of pediatric nursing. An older child may use signs of discomfort or pain—whether he feels pain or not—as an attention-getting device. The infant under a year of age does not do this, and behavior indicating pain in a young infant should never be ignored.

It is the mother or father who usually notes a change in the child's behavior and reports to the physician or nurse that "Johnny is not acting the way he usually does." If the nurse is able to assess the level of reliability of the parent's observations as good, it is wise to attend to any such comments because the parent knows the child's daily behavior better than a professional person who sees the child for the first time or only infrequently. The nurse will also be able to rely on parents for further observations they might make during the course of any subsequent illness. If the parents do not seem to be able to observe the child's condition accurately, the nurse needs to determine the cause of their failure and tactfully help them in this area.

The sudden changes in the condition of a sick or injured child, coupled with this inability to express how he feels, mean that the nurse must be constantly on the alert for signs and symptoms of aggravation of or improvement in his condition. The nurse must also be alert for symptoms which may be important to the physician in making a diagnosis or altering a tentative diagnosis.

Appreciation of the psychosomatic influence on diseases peculiar to or occurring in childhood is relatively new. It ties in with advances in the study of child psychology and child psychiatry. In these circumstances the child's emotional state interacts with his physical state to a greater degree than is commonly the case. Charting of physical symptoms means little to the physician in judging the implications of a sudden change in a child's condition unless the nurse also charts his *behavior*. Description of behavior enables the physician to draw conclusions as to the cause of symptoms, which may be due to emotional rather than physical factors. Adults verbalize an emotional state; a child does not. Nurses are apt to chart behavior which causes trouble, but not that of a quiet child who has retreated within himself. The latter may be more important than the former, however, in determining the true meaning of a change in symptoms.

A child may face certain temporary anxiety-producing situations alone with no one to protect him. He may fall and hurt himself when no one is about. The injured child cries for his mother and appears to think that with her coming he will feel much better. The crisis merges then into a less fearful situation when his mother does arrive.

But some children. like some adults, do suffer generalized states of anxiety, in which a troubled past appears to be ever-present in their consciousness and present pleasures seem only a prelude to unpleasant things to come. But even the most anxious child usually knows that pleasant things sometimes happen. A realistic view includes factors which mitigate the severity of any experience. Children who are too anxious, however, need psychiatric help, in which the nurse plays an important role.

The child's attention span is short but intense. It can be shifted from his bodily discomfort to something pleasant in the environment. Naturally, his attention is soon shifted again to his physical condition, and fresh pleasant stimuli should be provided. Above all, he must not be allowed to feel that he is alone in his difficulties. This does not mean that someone must be constantly with him, but rather that he must learn from experience that someone is thinking of him and will come now and then or whenever he cries or calls for help. One advantage of hospitalization for the older children, care in an institution for convalescent or chronically ill children, or a school for handicapped children, is that he sees others who have problems not too different from his own. An egocentric younger child in such situations not only may gain no support from the presence of other children, but also may fear that what happens to them may happen to him.

Children are apt to plead a physical excuse for not doing things they do not want to do. When a child says that he has a "tummy ache" at school time, but is all right as soon as it is too late to go, he should not be scolded. The adult should view the situation as the child views it and understand that such behavior is meaningful to the child. The important thing is to determine and to resolve any problems the child might be having in relation to school attendance. Children under five or six seldom invent excuses of this kind. With them the problem is to have them report when they do feel physically ill.

Infants and little children are, in general, better patients than adults are because (1) they live in the present, easily forgetting the past and not concerned with the future; (2) their attention span is short; and (3) they are readily interested in other bodily sensations—sights, sounds, a bit of something sweet, the motion of being rocked, or sucking a finger. This apparent transience of discomfort often deceives an inexperienced nurse, who feels that the child's condition is improving. The nurse should, of course, endeavor to amuse the child, but should not necessarily regard his response as evidence that the cause of pain or discomfort has abated.

TYPES OF ILLNESSES OF CHILDREN

Many specific illnesses such as appendicitis or pneumonia seen in adults are also seen in children. But children, because of their immaturity and the various stages of growth and development through which they pass, are prone to acquire conditions not seen in adult medical practice.

Congenital anomalies such as atresia of the esophagus, imperforate anus, or omphalocele are structural anomalies present at birth, due, it is believed, to the faulty interaction between genetic and environmental factors *in utero.* Surgery is now being used successfully to treat anomalies in children who a few decades or so ago would have died. Some congenital anomalies such as polycystic kidneys are compatible with life and may not be recognized until childhood or adult life.

Conditions of the newborn such as erythroblastosis fetalis are unknown in adults because the children are either successfully treated prior to adult life, or they die before they reach maturity.

Nutritional disorders are seen more commonly in infancy than later in childhood or adulthood because of the child's rapid growth during the first year of life. Examples of deficiency diseases are rickets and scurvy.

Young children, because of their intense activity, their insatiable curiosity and their immaturity, have more *accidents* such as scalds and falls, and *poisonings* from medications or household solutions than do adults. Lead poisoning from ingestion of lead paint occurs more commonly in the toddler group because of their desire to bite on hard surfaces such as painted crib rails.

Emotional disturbances of children, whether neurotic traits, conduct disorders, psychosomatic disturbances or psychoses, appear to be increasing in incidence among the pediatric age group.

Malignancies, such as leukemia, brain tumor, Wilms's tumor or bone tumor, are seen in children, but are not as common as in the adult.

Some *illnesses related to the process of growth and development,* such as failure to thrive and acne vulgaris, are seen during the pediatric years.

Infections are extremely frequent causes of concern during childhood, since the infant and the child do not have the immunity that adults have to many infectious agents. Respiratory infections are especially frequent during the years of growth. The child is exposed to many infections when he goes to kindergarten and to school. This is not necessarily unfortunate, since he can thus build up his immunologic defenses against them at an early age.

Diseases and other pathologic states common in children of various age groups are considered in the following chapters. Some of these conditions are acute in one age group and do not ex-

TABLE 4-3. DEATHS UNDER 1 YEAR AND INFANT MORTALITY RATES BY COLOR, FOR 65 SELECTED CAUSES: UNITED STATES, 1974

MONTHLY VITAL STATISTICS REPORT

DEATHS UNDER 1 YEAR AND INFANT MORTALITY RATES BY COLOR, FOR 65 SELECTED CAUSES: UNITED STATES, 1974

[Refers only to resident deaths occurring within the United States. Excludes fetal deaths]

Cause of death (Eighth Revision, International Classification of Diseases, Adapted, 1965)	Number Total	White	All other	Rate[1] Total	White	All other
All causes	52,776	38,249	14,527	1,670.1	1,484.9	2,486.8
Diarrheal diseases---009	646	375	271	20.4	14.6	46.4
Whooping cough---033	13	11	2	0.4	0.4	0.3
Meningococcal infections---036	47	34	13	1.5	1.3	2.2
Tetanus---037	3	3	-	0.1	0.1	-
Septicemia---038	910	620	290	28.8	24.1	49.6
Viral diseases---040-079	191	148	43	6.0	5.7	7.4
Congenital syphilis---090	7	3	4	0.2	0.1	0.7
Other infective and parasitic diseases---Remainder of 000-136	149	107	42	4.7	4.2	7.2
Malignant neoplasms, including neoplasms of lymphatic and hematopoeitic tissues---140-209	115	90	25	3.6	3.5	4.3
Benign neoplasms and neoplasms of unspecified nature---210-239	61	50	11	1.9	1.9	1.9
Diseases of thymus gland---254	19	16	3	0.6	0.6	0.5
Cystic fibrosis---273.0	67	64	3	2.1	2.5	0.5
Diseases of the blood-forming organs---280-289	178	126	52	5.6	4.9	8.9
Meningitis---320	567	366	201	17.9	14.2	34.4
Other diseases of nervous system and sense organs---321-389	439	316	123	13.9	12.3	21.1
Acute upper respiratory infections---460-465	108	65	43	3.4	2.5	7.4
Bronchitis and bronchiolitis---466,490,491	189	127	62	6.0	4.9	10.6
Influenza and pneumonia---470-474,480-486	2,613	1,645	968	82.7	63.9	165.7
Influenza---470-474	36	28	8	1.1	1.1	1.4
Pneumonia---480-486	2,577	1,617	960	81.6	62.8	164.3
Other chronic interstitial pneumonia---517	27	19	8	0.9	0.7	1.4
All other diseases of respiratory system---492,493,500-516,518,519	453	319	134	14.3	12.4	22.9
Hernia and intestinal obstruction---550-553,560	497	420	77	15.7	16.3	13.2
Gastritis, duodenitis, enteritis, and colitis of noninfectious origin---535,561,563	51	32	19	1.6	1.2	3.3
Other diseases of digestive system---520-534,536,537,540-543,562,564-577	310	216	94	9.8	8.4	16.1
Congenital anomalies---740-759	8,607	7,119	1,488	272.4	276.4	254.7
Anencephalus---740	748	685	63	23.7	26.6	10.8
Spina bifida---741	455	413	42	14.4	16.0	7.2
Congenital hydrocephalus---742	362	294	68	11.5	11.4	11.6
Other congenital anomalies of central nervous system and eye---743,744	353	290	63	11.2	11.3	10.8
Congenital anomalies of heart---746	3,181	2,596	585	100.7	100.8	100.1
Other congenital anomalies of circulatory system---747	633	504	129	20.0	19.6	22.1
Congenital anomalies of respiratory system---748	656	530	126	20.8	20.6	21.6
Congenital anomalies of digestive system---749-751	382	290	92	12.1	11.3	15.7
Congenital anomalies of genitourinary system---752,753	285	236	49	9.0	9.2	8.4
Congenital anomalies of musculoskeletal system---754-756	264	223	41	8.4	8.7	7.0
Down's disease---759.3	90	76	14	2.8	3.0	2.4
Other congenital syndromes affecting multiple systems---759.0-759.2,759.4-759.9	1,015	840	175	32.1	32.6	30.0
Other and unspecified congenital anomalies---745,757,758	183	142	41	5.8	5.5	7.0
Certain causes of mortality in early infancy---760-769.2,769.4-772,774-778	28,712	20,821	7,891	908.6	808.3	1,350.8
Chronic circulatory and genitourinary diseases in mother---760	6	5	1	0.2	0.2	0.2
Other maternal conditions unrelated to pregnancy---761	256	202	54	8.1	7.8	9.2
Syphilis---761.0	2	-	2	0.1	-	0.3
Diabetes mellitus---761.1	130	112	18	4.1	4.3	3.1
Rubella---761.3	11	5	6	0.3	0.2	1.0
All other maternal conditions unrelated to pregnancy---761.2,761.4-761.7,761.9	113	85	28	3.6	3.3	4.8
Toxemia of pregnancy---762	115	84	31	3.6	3.3	5.3
Maternal antepartum and intrapartum infection---763	173	110	63	5.5	4.3	10.8
Difficult labor---764-768	413	321	92	13.1	12.5	15.7
With mention of birth injury (.0-.3)	132	102	30	4.2	4.0	5.1
Without mention of birth injury (.4,.9)	281	219	62	8.9	8.5	10.6
All other complications of pregnancy and childbirth---769.0,769.2,769.4,769.5,769.9	3,342	2,455	887	105.8	95.3	151.8
Conditions of placenta---770	1,203	966	237	38.1	37.5	40.6
Conditions of umbilical cord---771	304	247	57	9.6	9.6	9.8
Birth injury without mention of cause---772	1,792	1,301	491	56.7	50.5	84.1
Hemolytic diseases of newborn---774,775	340	295	45	10.8	11.5	7.7
Hyaline membrane disease---776.1	4,300	3,379	921	136.1	131.2	157.7
Respiratory distress syndrome---776.2	4,022	3,036	986	127.3	117.9	168.8
Asphyxia of newborn, unspecified---776.9	4,652	3,233	1,369	147.2	127.5	234.4
All other anoxic and hypoxic conditions not elsewhere classifiable---776.0,776.3,776.4	750	516	234	23.7	20.0	40.1
Immaturity, unqualified---777	4,719	3,105	1,614	149.3	120.5	276.3
Postmaturity---778.1	6	4	2	0.2	0.2	0.3
Hemorrhagic disease of newborn---778.2	588	399	189	18.6	15.5	32.4
All other conditions of newborn---778.0,778.3,778.9	1,731	1,113	618	54.8	43.2	105.8
Symptoms and ill-defined conditions---780-796	4,700	3,024	1,676	148.7	117.4	286.9
Accidents---E800-E949	1,453	1,034	419	46.0	40.1	71.7
Inhalation or ingestion of food or other object causing obstruction or suffocation---E911,E912	442	320	122	14.0	12.4	20.9
Accidental mechanical suffocation---E913	285	202	83	9.0	7.8	14.2
Other accidental causes---E800-E910,E914-E949	726	512	214	23.0	19.9	36.6
Homicide---E960-E978	166	92	74	5.3	3.6	12.7
All other causes---Residual	1,478	987	491	46.8	38.3	84.1

[1]Per 100,000 live births in specified group.

Department of Health, Education and Welfare. Public Health Service, National Center for Health Statistics, 1974.

tend into other periods of life. Other conditions have their origin during one period and extend into later life. The various conditions found in children are grouped in this book according to the age level when they most commonly occur or when they are of greatest significance to the child and his family.

The student will see that the nursing care of the child having each condition is based on (1) the anatomic, physiologic and psychologic development and the growth factor normal to the age group and on (2) the treatment (preventive or curative) of each disease. This is all the assistance which a textbook can give the student. Adaptation to the needs of the individual child is made at the bedside under the guidance of the instructor.

MORTALITY AND MORBIDITY

MORTALITY RATES

The older a child becomes, the greater are his chances for survival. The risk of dying on the first day of life is many thousands of times greater than the risk of any day during the school years. Each age group among children is particularly affected by certain factors of a bad environment, is more or less susceptible to certain diseases and is exposed to varying accident hazards. Tables 4–3, 4–4, 4–5, and 4–6 show the causes of death during infancy, and during the remainder of childhood and early adolescence for the United States and Canada.

The *infant mortality rate* is an expression of the ratio of deaths for infants under one year of age in any given period of time to the number of births during the same period. In other words, it is the number of deaths per 1000 live births. The *neonatal mortality rate* indicates the mortality rate for the first month of life.

The infant mortality rate has declined dramatically since the beginning of this century. In the United States in 1900 it was approximately 200 per 1000 live births. Notable reductions have occurred especially since 1965, when the rate was 24.7 per thousand live births, to the 1970 provisional rate of 19.8. Although this rate is relatively low, the United States still has a higher infant death rate than several other na-

TABLE 4–4. *DEATHS AND DEATH RATES FOR TEN LEADING CAUSES OF DEATH IN SPECIFIED AGE GROUPS: UNITED STATES, 1974*

RANK ORDER	AGE AND CAUSE OF DEATH	NUMBER	RATE*
	1–4 years		
	All causes	9,831	73.9
1	Accidents	3,882	29.2
	Motor vehicle accidents	1,322	9.9
	All other accidents	2,560	19.3
2	Congenital anomalies	1,191	9.0
3	Malignant neoplasms, including neoplasms of lymphatic and hematopoietic tissues	785	5.9
4	Influenza and pneumonia	619	4.7
5	Homicide	296	2.2
6	Diseases of heart	262	2.0
7	Meningitis	224	1.7
8	Enteritis and other diarrheal diseases	110	0.8
9	Cerebrovascular diseases	107	0.8
10	Anemias	90	0.7
	All other causes	2,265	17.0
	5–14 years		
	All causes	14,636	38.2
1	Accidents	7,037	18.4
	Motor vehicle accidents	3,332	8.7
	All other accidents	3,705	9.7
2	Malignant neoplasms, including neoplasms of lymphatic and hematopoietic tissues	2,001	5.2
3	Congenital anomalies	818	2.1
4	Influenza and pneumonia	489	1.3
5	Homicide	399	1.0
6	Diseases of heart	352	0.9
7	Cerebrovascular diseases	249	0.6
8	Suicide	188	0.5
9	Benign neoplasms and neoplasms of unspecified nature	138	0.4
10	Anemias	119	0.3
	All other causes	2,846	7.4

*Rates per 100,000 estimated population in specified groups.
From Department of Health, Education, and Welfare, Public Health Service, National Center for Health Statistics.

TABLE 4-5. INFANT DEATHS FOR SELECTED DETAILED CAUSES, CANADA, 1974

CAUSES	TOTAL	RATE*	CAUSES	TOTAL	RATE
All Causes	5,192	1502.1	Bronchitis, emphysema, and asthma	19	5.5
Infective and Parasitic Diseases	175	50.6	Other causes	58	16.8
Dysentery	86	24.9			
Tuberculosis	–	–	Diseases of the Digestive System	80	23.1
Whooping Cough	2	0.6	Hernia	43	12.4
Meningococcal infection	15	4.3	Intestinal obstruction without mention of hernia	5	1.4
Septicemia	42	12.2	Noninfectious gastroenteritis and colitis	8	2.3
Chickenpox	3	0.9	Other causes	24	6.9
Measles	7	2.0			
Rubella	1	0.3	Diseases of the Genitourinary System	8	2.3
Viral encephalitis	–	–			
Coxsackie virus disease	–	–	Diseases of the Skin and Subcutaneous Tissue	2	0.6
Syphilis	–	–			
Other causes	19	5.5	Diseases of the Musculoskeletal System and Connective Tissue	3	0.9
Neoplasms	23	6.7	Congenital Anomalies	1,204	348.3
Brain and nervous system	7	2.0	Brain, spinal cord, and nervous system	341	98.7
Leukemia	4	1.2	Heart	360	104.2
Other malignant neoplasms	5	1.4	Other circulatory system	77	22.3
Benign neoplasms	4	1.2	Respiratory system	76	22.0
Other neoplasms	3	0.9	Digestive system	77	22.3
			Urinary system	63	18.2
Allergic, Endocrine and Metabolic Diseases	37	10.7	Multiple systems	124	35.9
Disorders of pancreatic internal secretion, other than diabetes mellitus	2	0.6	Other causes	86	24.9
Diseases of thymus gland	4	1.2	Certain Causes of Perinatal Mortality	2,451	709.1
Avitaminoses and other nutritional deficiency	6	1.7	Maternal conditions unrelated to pregnancy	21	6.1
Other metabolic diseases	19	5.5	Maternal toxemia and infection	43	12.4
Other causes	6	1.7	Difficult labor	55	15.9
			Other complications of pregnancy and childbirth	299	86.5
Blood Diseases	20	5.8	Conditions of placenta and umbilical cord	219	63.4
Anemias	1	0.3	Birth injury	151	43.7
Coagulation defects	7	2.0	Hemolytic disease of newborn	35	10.1
Other causes	12	3.5	Anoxia and hypoxia	1,038	300.3
			Immaturity	498	144.1
Mental Disorders	2	0.6	Other causes	92	26.6
Diseases of the Nervous System and Sense Organs	74	21.4	Symptoms and Ill-Defined Conditions	427	123.5
Meningitis	27	7.8	Accidents, Poisonings and Violence	239	69.1
Cerebral spastic infantile paralysis	9	2.6	Motor vehicle accidents	25	7.2
Otitis media and mastoiditis	4	1.2	Accidental falls	8	2.3
Other causes	34	9.8	Fire accidents	22	6.4
			Inhalation and Ingestion	103	29.8
Diseases of the Circulatory System	27	7.8	Mechanical suffocation	48	13.9
			Other causes	33	9.5
Diseases of the Respiratory System	420	121.5			
Acute respiratory infections	50	14.5			
Influenza	11	3.2			
Pneumonia	282	81.6			

*Per 100,000 live births. Extracted from *Vital Statistics,* v. 3: Death, 1974. Vital Statistics Section, Health Division, Statistics Canada.

tions. Sweden, for instance, has the lowest infant death rate.

Although among the Alaskan natives a few years ago the infant mortality rate was 54.8 and among the American Indians was 35.9, still the greatest problem of infant mortality in the United States is concentrated among the non-whites in big city slums. In some ghetto districts the rate is markedly higher than it is in other areas of the country. If 50 or so of the worst areas were excluded, this country's infant mortality rate would drop abruptly.

The main causes of our failure to have a lower infant death rate are premature birth and inadequate prenatal care. Since lack of prenatal care increases the incidence of prematurity, more emphasis should be given to improved maternity care programs. Such facilities as prenatal clinics must be located in areas accessible to the lower socioeconomic groups.

Years ago the leading cause of death among infants was intestinal disturbances due to bacteria in milk and food. In hot summer weather babies from congested slums suffering from in-

TABLE 4–6. SELECTED CAUSES AND RATES* OF DEATH FOR SPECIFIED AGE GROUPS, CANADA, 1974

CAUSE	AGES 0–4		AGES 5–9		AGES 10–14	
	Number	Rate	Number	Rate	Number	Rate
All Causes	6,272	355.2	830	41.9	939	39.9
Accidents	704	39.9	494	25.0	542	23.0
Respiratory Diseases	537	30.4	25	1.3	35	1.5
Influenza and pneumonia	364	20.6	15	0.8	20	0.9
Bronchitis, emphysema, and asthma	28	3.8	4	0.3	7	0.3
All cancer (malignant neoplasms)	109	6.2	120	6.1	124	5.3
Cancer of lymphatic and hematopoietic tissue	53	2.9	71	3.6	63	2.7
Cardiovascular-Renal Diseases	47	2.5	18	0.8	34	1.3
Diseases of heart	30	1.7	7	0.4	15	0.6
Cerebrovascular disease	8	0.5	3	0.2	10	0.4
Nephritis and nephrosis	3	0.2	2	0.1	4	0.2
Cirrhosis of liver	10	0.6	2	0.1	4	0.2

*Per 100,000 population. When comparing with U. S. figures, note that U. S. figures begin at age 1 year and do not incorporate infants, as do Canadian figures.
Extracted from *Vital Statistics*, v. 3: Death, 1974.

fectious diarrheas filled the pediatric units. Many were not brought to the hospital until they were moribund. Strict control of the production and handling of milk sold by dairies and stores, inspection of food and places where food was sold or served and the availability of electric refrigeration resulted in a lessening of this once leading cause of infant mortality. Infectious diarrhea still occurs, but is not as prevalent as it once was.

Another great killer of infants was and still is respiratory infection. Morbidity and mortality from respiratory diseases following contagious diseases have been reduced through immunization programs, which have greatly decreased the incidence and severity of the contagious diseases of childhood. If a respiratory infection does occur, antibiotics are available for use against either a primary or secondary infection. Production of interferon, a protein normally produced by body cells to limit the spread of viral infections, may be stimulated by the injection of certain macromolecular substances such as double-stranded RNA.

The principal causes of infant deaths in recent years have been immaturity and other prenatal and natal causes, asphyxia and atelectasis, congenital malformations, birth injuries, influenza and pneumonia, and certain other infections.

During childhood the mortality rates gradually change for certain conditions, as can be seen in Table 4–4, from one through four years of age and from five through 14 years of age, the start of adolescence. The principal causes of deaths of children between one and 14 years of age in recent years were accidents (except motor vehicle), motor vehicle accidents, malignant neoplasms—including leukemia—congenital anomalies, and influenza and pneumonia.

MORBIDITY RATES

The *morbidity or illness rates* are, of course, much higher than the mortality rates for children in each age group. The average boy or girl in the United States has approximately three episodes of acute illness each year. Respiratory conditions are the chief cause of acute illness among children. Approximately one of five children has at least one chronic condition such as an allergy or respiratory ailment. The rate of illness from chronic conditions increases with age.

As to the hospitalization of children, nonwhite children are hospitalized much less frequently than white children, but when they do go to the hospital they usually stay longer. As the income of a family increases, the rate of hospitalization of the children increases, but the average length of stay decreases. Rural children are hospitalized less frequently than city children, but they tend to stay longer.

Dental caries is the most common physical defect among school children; however, half the children under 15 years of age have never been to a dentist. Even among those receiving dental care, many are not receiving adequate care. Again, children from white, nonfarm, and higher-income families receive more dental care than do children from nonwhite, farm, and low-income families.

The drop in the mortality and morbidity rates from contagious diseases in all age groups is proof of the value of research in medicine. Immunization is now possible against many of the former diseases of childhood. One kind of infection, however, whose incidence is seemingly on the increase is that caused by *Staphylococcus*

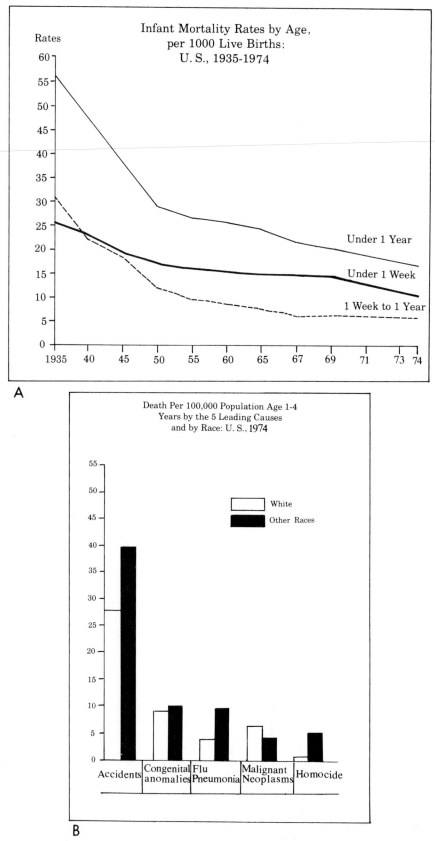

FIGURE 4–1. *A*, In the 38-year period from 1935 to 1973, death rates during the first year of life decreased sharply, especially in those who lived past the first week. *B*, In preschool children, after age one, accidents are the major cause of death. (Data from the U.S. Department of Health, Education and Welfare, National Center for Health Statistics, Washington, D.C.)

Infant Death Rates, Canada, 1935–1974

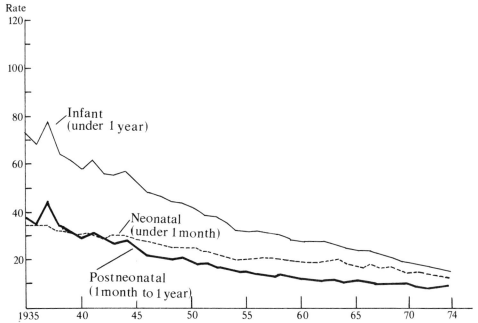

FIGURE 4–2. Infant death rates in Canada, 1935 to 1974 per 1000 live births. (Adapted from *Statistics Canada, 1974.*)

aureus. No immunization procedure has yet been found to prevent the spread of infection caused by this organism.

An illness of a long-term nature may have a wholesome or a devastating effect on the total health—physical, mental, emotional, social, sexual, and spiritual—of the family as well as on the chronically ill or handicapped child. Not only the parents may be affected because the illness may impose a burden on their marital relations as well as on their health and financial resources, but also the siblings may be directly or indirectly affected with a resultant influence on their level of development in the future. Such possible changes in the family due to the care of the chronically ill or handicapped child will be discussed later.

Statistics show that there is a class differential in morbidity and mortality rates among children.

The unhygienic environment of children in the low-income groups is reflected in the higher death rate among them as compared with that of children in the middle- or upper-income group in the same age brackets. This is due both to the parent's lack of education in matters pertaining to health and also to their inability to pay for the things that make for good health: adequate diet, good housing, clothing, recreation, and adequate medical attention. The health professions must assume the responsibility for educating these parents in the care of their children and the need for medical care when illnesses occur. Medical care and hospitalization are usually provided without charge or at a minimal fee to those unable to pay fully for them; however, many do not even today know how or will not take advantage of these opportunities to improve the health of their children.

TEACHING AIDS AND OTHER INFORMATION*

American Academy of Pediatrics

Child Health Record.
Guidelines for Child Health Care.
Standards of Child Health Care.

Canadian Mental Health Association

(In collaboration with the Hospital for Sick Children, Toronto)

Suddenly It Happens—Your Child Is Ill.

Department of National Health and Welfare, Ottawa, Canada

Nursing Resources in Canada.

————————

*Complete addresses are given in the Appendix.

Public Affairs Committee

Seaver, J.: When Your Child Is Sick.

Ross Laboratories

Children Are Different: Relation of Age to Physiologic Function, 1970.

The American Cancer Society, Inc.

Cancer Incidence: Survival and Mortality for Children Under 15 Years of Age.

United States Government

Answers to Questions About American Indians, 1974.

A Study of Infant Mortality from Linked Records by Age of Mother, Total-Birth Order, and Other Variables – United States, 1973.

Child Health in America, 1975.

Child Health in America, 1976.

Garfinkel, J., Chabot, M. J., and Pratt, M. W.: Infant, Maternal, and Childhood Mortality in the United States, 1968–1973, 1975.

Pechman, S. M.: Seven Parent and Child Centers, 1972.

Programs of the Bureau of Community Health Services, 1973.

The Maternal and Child Health Service Reports on: Promoting the Health of Mothers and Children, FY 1972, 1973.

REFERENCES

Books

Andreopoulos, S. (Ed.): *Primary Care: Where Medicine Fails.* New York, John Wiley & Sons, Inc., 1974.

Barness, L. A.: *Manual of Pediatric Physical Diagnosis.* 4th ed. Chicago, Year Book Medical Publishers, Inc., 1972.

Barnett, H. L., and Einhorn, A. H. (Eds.): *Pediatrics.* 15th ed. New York, Appleton-Century-Crofts, 1972.

Davis, J. A., and Dobbing, J. (Eds.): *Scientific Foundations of Paediatrics.* Philadelphia, W. B. Saunders Company, 1974.

Dynski-Klein, M.: *Color Atlas of Pediatrics.* Chicago, Year Book Medical Publishers, Inc., 1975.

Gellis, S. S., and Kagan, B. M. (Eds.): *Current Pediatric Therapy 7.* Philadelphia, W. B. Saunders Company, 1976.

Goss, C. M. (Ed.): *Gray's Anatomy of the Human Body.* 29th ed. Philadelphia, Lea & Febiger, 1973.

Hertzler, J. H., and Mirza, M.: *Handbook of Pediatric Surgery.* Chicago, Year Book Medical Publishers, Inc., 1974.

Horrobin, D. F.: *Physiology: An Introduction to Human Physiology.* Philadelphia, F. A. Davis Company, 1973.

Hughes, J. G.: *Synopsis of Pediatrics.* 4th ed. St. Louis, The C. V. Mosby Company, 1975.

Hutchinson, J. H.: *Practical Pediatric Problems.* 4th ed. Chicago, Year Book Medical Publishers, Inc., 1975.

Illingworth, R. S.: *Common Symptoms of Disease in Children.* 4th ed. Philadelphia, J. B. Lippincott Company, 1973.

Jones, R. K., and Jones, P. A.: *Sociology in Medicine.* New York, John Wiley & Sons, Inc., 1975.

Kempe, C. H., Silver, H. K., and O'Brien, D. (Eds.): *Current Pediatric Diagnosis and Treatment.* 3rd ed. Los Altos, California, Lange Medical Publications, 1974.

Moll, H.: *Atlas of Pediatric Diseases.* Philadelphia, W. B. Saunders Company, 1976.

Rickham, P. P.: *Synopsis of Pediatric Surgery.* Chicago, Year Book Medical Publishers, Inc., 1975.

Selye, H.: *The Stress of Life.* 2nd ed. New York, McGraw-Hill Book Company, 1976.

Silver, H. K., Kempe, C. H., and Bruyn, H. B.: *Handbook of Pediatrics.* Los Altos, California, Lange Medical Publications, 1975.

Smith, C. A. (Ed.): *The Critically Ill Child.* Philadelphia, W. B. Saunders Company, 1972.

Smith, D. W., and Marshall, R. E. (Eds.): *Introduction to Clinical Pediatrics.* 2nd ed. Philadelphia, W. B. Saunders Company, 1977.

Surgical Staff, Hospital for Sick Children, Toronto, Canada: *Care For the Injured Child.* Baltimore, Williams & Wilkins Company, 1975.

Vaughan, V. C. III, and McKay, R. J. (Eds.): *Nelson Textbook of Pediatrics.* 10th ed. Philadelphia, W. B. Saunders Company, 1975.

Waring, W. W., and Jeannsonne, L. O.: *Practical Manual of Pediatrics: A Pocket Reference for Those Who Treat Children.* St. Louis, The C. V. Mosby Company, 1975.

Wasserman, E., and Slobody, L. B. (Eds.): *Survey of Clinical Pediatrics.* 6th ed. New York, McGraw-Hill Book Company, 1974.

Periodicals

Heisel, J. S., Ream, S., Raitz, R., Rappaport, M., and Coddington, R. D.: The Significance of Life Events as Contributing Factors in the Diseases of Children. *The Journal of Pediatrics,* 83:119, July 1973.

Hunt, E.: Infant Mortality Trends and Maternal and Infant Care. *Children,* 17:88, May–June 1970.

Pearman, J. R.: Survey of Unmet Medical Needs of Children in Six Counties in Florida. *Pub. Health Rep.,* 85:189, March 1970.

McElroy, C.: Caring for the Untreated Infant. *The Canadian Nurse,* 71:26, December 1975.

Rosenfeld, A.: Thymosin: Breaking the Immune Barrier. *Nursing Digest,* 3:48, September–October 1975.

Stine, O. C., and Chuaqui, C.: Mothers' Intended Actions for Childhood Symptoms. *Am. J. Pub. Health,* 59:2035, November 1969.

Wallace, H. M., Goldstein, H., Eisner, V., and Oglesby, A. C.: Patterns of Infant and Early Childhood Mortality in the California Project of a Collaborative Inter-American Study. *Bulletin of the Pan American Health Organization,* IX:32, 1975.

Wallace, H. M.: Some Thoughts on Planning Health Care for Children and Youth. *Children,* 18:95, May–June 1971.

AUDIOVISUAL MEDIA

W. B. Saunders Company

Pediatric Conferences with Sydney Gellis

Series of six two-track tape cassettes, each approximately one hour of commentary, issued bimonthly. Dr. Gellis and his colleagues discuss current developments – many long before they reach the pages of any medical journal.

---

*Complete addresses are given in the Appendix.

Chapter Five

THE NURSE AND THE ILL CHILD

The role of the pediatric nurse has changed as research in medicine and its allied sciences has led to improvements in the medical care of children and as research in the social sciences has led to changed views about their psychologic development and needs. In this chapter the emerging role of the pediatric nurse will be explored as a background against which the growth and development of children and their care when ill can be studied.

FACILITIES FOR THE CARE OF ILL CHILDREN

There are several kinds of facilities for the care of ill children. These include the pediatric unit in a general hospital or in a children's hospital, the intensive care unit, the pediatric research center, short-term care facilities, long-term care facilities, facilities for the care of ambulatory patients, home care programs, and care of the child at home by a private physician.

THE PEDIATRIC UNIT

The pediatric unit must be built and furnished to meet the needs of children and of their parents. Children's needs can be classified under three main headings: adequate provision for care, protection from physical danger, e.g., infection and accidents, and protection from a psychologically threatening environment.

In the pediatric unit the surroundings should be homelike and cheerful and the décor scaled to the child's size. Bright colors in addition to the usual pastels can be used. When children are permitted to wear appropriate clothing rather than hospital gowns, they tend to feel more as though they were at home. Colorful attire such as pastel dresses or smocks worn by nurses tend to brighten the hospital atmosphere as well as to promote better nurse-child-parent

relations. Growing plants or small pets provide both color and also an interest for children outside themselves.

In general, the pediatric unit should have a smaller number of beds than the usual adult unit, since children need more care than adults. Informality and flexibility of design in the unit are important so that optimum use of space is possible at all times. The hospitalized child should be segregated by care requirements and by age, just as children in the community select their companions when they are well. The beds should be placed so that the children can relate to both the internal and external environments of the unit. Natural light should be available in patient areas as much as possible.

Each room or patient unit should have an adjustable hospital bed, crib or bassinet as needed, overbed table for older children, bedside cabinet, cabinet or crib bag for toys, comfortable chair, closet space, wastepaper basket, and facilities for running water. If at all possible, each patient area should have an oxygen and a suction outlet in case of an emergency. Facilities should be available on the unit or close by in order to accommodate a parent should he or she ask to stay overnight.

In multiple bedrooms, partitions or cubicles that permit visibility of all children by the nurse may be installed. The glass portions of the cubicle walls should be constructed of shatterproof

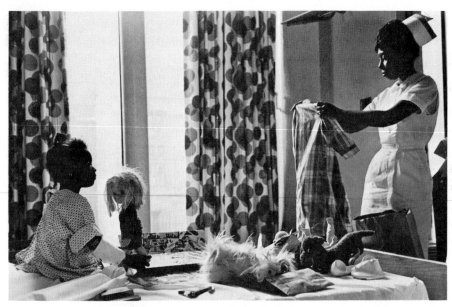

FIGURE 5-1. Familiar clothing helps the child to feel more at ease in the strange hospital environment. (From "All Rooms are Private in New Children's Hospital" by William McKillip in *Hospitals*, March 1, 1967.) (Bremen I. Johnson, Director of Bureau Publications, American Hospital Association.)

glass in order to make this visibility safely possible. Cubicles tend to separate children who otherwise might be able to play together. Cubicles do, however, demarcate areas of potential infection so that isolation precautions can be carried out. They do little to decrease airborne infection. Visitors are encouraged to visit only in their cubicle if there is a question of infection.

The nurses' station should be situated centrally within the pediatric unit. Rooms for the

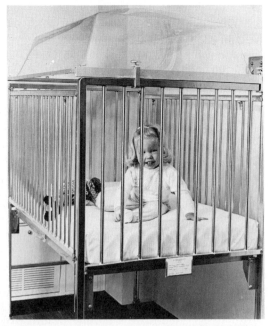

FIGURE 5-2. The sides of the crib should be sufficiently high so that the small child cannot fall when he leans against them. An extension above the crib sides can prevent the active child from falling out of bed. The Safety Dome Crib Top also prevents the active small child from climbing out of bed. (American Hospital Supply, 2020 Ridge Avenue, Evanston, Illinois 60201.)

sickest patients and young infants should be nearby. Although electronic communications systems should not be installed when human interaction is essential, if one is used, the call system should be one which can be used by younger children. A television monitoring system connected with each room is more desirable than a call system.

A waiting room for parents and friends should be located close to the elevators and stairs. This area should be clearly visible from the nurses' station.

The treatment area and the examination area could be two separate rooms or one soundproofed, well lighted room which contains all the necessary equipment for examining and treating children. The use of such a room for painful procedures is important so that other children cannot see what is happening to another child.

Playroom space and a schoolroom are essential for use as therapeutic adjuncts for patients who are ambulatory or convalescent. Children who are well enough can also be taken to these rooms on stretchers or in wheelchairs. The use of these rooms will be discussed later in this chapter.

Meals can be eaten around small tables in the play area or in the center of the pediatric unit. For children who must remain in bed, colorful overbed tables may be used.

Other areas of the pediatric unit include a consultation room providing space to talk privately with parents and children and to demonstrate care necessary after discharge, adequate bathroom facilities for both adults and children, a room which could be utilized for the education of students, and adequate storage space.

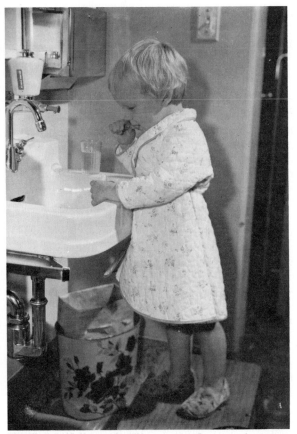

FIGURE 5–3. The hospitalized child finds the atmosphere more familiar if he is allowed to take care of his own needs. (Courtesy of Hospital Sainte-Justine, Montreal.)

INTENSIVE CARE UNIT OR NEWBORN INTENSIVE CARE UNIT

Intensive care units or newborn intensive care units for critically ill children or newborns are found in many children's hospitals and large pediatric departments in general hospitals. In some states, for example Wisconsin, care of the high-risk newborn takes place in regional centers especially equipped for this purpose. Infants who are critically ill at birth are transported from local hospitals to these centers for perinatal care.

Electronic engineering techniques must be specifically adapted to the problems of intensive care for newborns or children. Intensive care necessitates receiving and interpreting continuous information on the physiologic and biochemical status of the children who have conditions predisposing to cardiovascular, respiratory or nervous system collapse. The care of critically ill children in the intensive care unit involves the use of such equipment as cardiac monitors, pacemakers, cardioverters, defibrillators, hypohyperthermia units, suction machines, a volume respirator, and an intermittent positive-pressure respirator, among others. Drugs and surgical equipment necessary for the usual emergencies are available.

Newborns or children requiring intensive care include those with congenital anomalies or major illnesses of the newborn, coma, status asthmaticus, severe bronchiolitis and pneumonia, congenital heart disease with failure, and children undergoing major cardiovascular or neurosurgical procedures. Children who are seriously ill from poisoning or trauma are also cared for in the intensive care unit.

Until recently death was defined as the moment when the child stopped breathing. Now the child can be kept alive after the cessation of breathing, after failure of the heart and circula-

FIGURE 5–4. Mealtime is more enjoyable if ambulatory patients eat together at a common table. (Courtesy of Hospital Sainte-Justine, Montreal.)

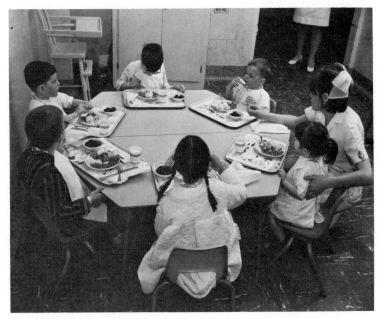

tory system, or even after functional failure of the brain and nervous system. Children can be restored to useful life after temporary failure of one of these vital systems if the gap between changes in his condition and the rapid institution of proper therapy can be minimized.

The important key to all intensive care is to be able to initiate treatment before the condition of the child becomes too critical to respond. Since the condition of a child tends to change more rapidly than that of an adult, constant observation and monitoring by nurses using electronic devices are essential to the child's survival. If a child can be supported effectively during the acute phase of his illness, he has a better chance for life than one who cannot.

In addition, a pediatric medical resuscitation team may be organized to handle medical emergencies in other areas of the hospital. Such a team may take with them a resuscitation cart on which equipment and drugs necessary for resuscitation efforts may be made available for immediate use.

One problem faced by a conscious child in the intensive care unit and easily forgotten by those caring for him is his lack of adequate rest, or sleep deprivation. A child who has been accustomed to sleeping during the night in a darkened room may be disturbed by the bright lighting and frequent need for taking vital signs over a 24-hour period. If the nurse is aware of the child's distress, an attempt can be made to provide him with a semidarkened area in which to sleep and take his vital signs at times when he will be disturbed as little as possible.

Through the effective utilization of monitoring devices, comprehensive surveillance of the child's vital systems will enable a medical team to institute supportive treatment, to control the life support system, and to determine when therapy can be discontinued.

PEDIATRIC RESEARCH CENTER

Some children's hospitals have pediatric research centers where little-understood diseases are under constant study. Pediatric research centers give nurses a new opportunity to fulfill the basic principles of child care, since the ratio of nurses to patients is high. These centers give children who are able the opportunity to have a schedule much as they followed at home. Careful planning by the nursing staff is necessary to ensure a child's contentment in spite of the painful test procedures that must be done. A dedicated group of nurses working together can minimize the potentially damaging effects of hospitalization.

Pediatric research centers also provide for nurses an opportunity to participate with other team members in the studies being done, as well as an opportunity to investigate nursing problems which may arise.

FACILITIES FOR SHORT-TERM CARE

Continuity of care for children having short illnesses can be provided through the use of hospital facilities for overnight or short-term observations of children. Such a unit forms a kind of "halfway" house as a means of avoiding prolonged hospitalization while providing care of acute illnesses on a short-term basis.

FACILITIES FOR LONG-TERM CARE

Children having handicaps may be cared for in long-term hospitals and other facilities instead of at home. Such facilities are important for the care of children whose parents could not provide adequate care and whose homes would not be conducive to a restful, prolonged convalescence, such as the child having a severe cardiac problem. Available facilities outside the home include public or private hospitals or homes for the convalescent or chronically ill child, residential schools for the handicapped, and summer camps for children having similar diagnoses, such as those having diabetes. Placement of a child into one of these facilities should not be done lightly, since it means taking the child from his parents. But for certain children placement may be a necessity, as will be shown later.

FACILITIES FOR THE CARE OF AMBULATORY PATIENTS

The pediatric outpatient department can make a real contribution to the hospital because of new medical developments and new social pressures. The outpatient department in many institutions is moving out into the community and toward the concept of a community health service center. The outpatient department today serves not only the indigent, but also persons of all income levels.

Increasing numbers of private physicians use the outpatient department for children having problems needing careful diagnosis and treatment such as those having complex medical or surgical problems or psychologic difficulties. Because of the awareness of the need to avoid the possible trauma of hospitalization and the possibility of cross-infection, more children having pneumonia, abscesses, urinary, or other infections can be treated on an outpatient basis if there is a responsible adult in the home. Some physicians believe that elective surgery such as a herniorrhaphy on a well infant can be done on an outpatient basis if the child is properly prepared and if the parents can provide good care for him postoperatively. One of the newer functions of the medical staff in outpatient departments is to trace hereditary conditions and do genetic counseling.

Ambulatory patients should be scheduled carefully and not have to wait in large groups prior to their appointments. Comprehensive high-quality services should be made available to all.

One function of the nurse is to provide health teaching for patients. If parents and children do have to wait to see the physician in the outpatient department or prior to admission to the hospital, the nurse can utilize the time available to provide short health lessons tailored to the patient's specific circumstances. The nurse needs to be approachable, one who listens, teaches and cares, in order to make such communication a real learning situation for the parent and child.

A parent who brings a child to the outpatient clinic may feel not only anxious about the child's condition but also guilty about his or her possible role in causing his illness. The nurse can assist such a parent to discuss feelings openly and thus alleviate some distress. A play area is essential in the outpatient clinic so that the child's attention can be diverted and the parent can have time for a conference with the nurse.

The nurse who counsels parents of children who are ambulatory or who attend an outpatient clinic assumes a very responsible role in the care of pediatric patients. Observations of the parents and children prior to their visit with the physician may help plan medical care. Also, the nurse needs to be certain that any recommendations made to the parent are completely understood so that they can be followed correctly at home. Recommendations relating to nursing procedures, medications, and the time of the next visit must be thoroughly understood by the mother and the child.

(For a discussion of free-standing surgical centers outside the hospital, see p. 650.)

HOME CARE PROGRAMS

The home care program has as its main purpose to provide comprehensive health services to children in their homes. The home care program in a pediatric unit or children's hospital is a recent innovation, although such programs have existed for the care of elderly or indigent patients. The home care program seeks to prevent or reduce the trauma of hospitalization by shortening the hospital stay and by avoiding the interruption in parent-child relations which hospitalization can produce, to provide for the care of children who can be as well or better treated in their home environments, and to utilize the assistance of appropriate community services as well as hospital facilities for children who no longer need care in the hospital.

In order for the home care program to function well, the child's home environment must be conducive to recovery, and there must be someone present in the household competent enough to cooperate with the health team between medical and nursing visits.

CARE OF THE CHILD AT HOME BY A PRIVATE PHYSICIAN

The parents who care for their child in the home in cooperation with a private physician, either a pediatrician or a general practitioner, feel more secure if they can contact the physician about any problems they may be having. For this reason many physicians set aside a specific time each day to receive such telephone calls.

The physician, in order to give advice over the telephone, must know the parents well and have faith in their accuracy in describing symptoms. The physician usually will not have such a relation with a stranger and therefore cannot be expected to assist a parent who is not known.

In order to improve the quality of care given to the children in their practices, some pediatricians have recently employed paramedical personnel, usually a specially prepared nurse, nurse practitioner, or pediatric nurse associate who visits the children in their homes, and a social worker. The nurse may be responsible among other duties for visiting all newborn infants and all infants and children having illnesses in their homes for the purpose of parent education. When the nurse makes a home call, information about the environment of the home and the activities of the family may be added to the child's record. With this kind of assistance the pediatrician is able to make more efficient use of time.

MODERN CONCEPTS IN THE CARE OF HOSPITALIZED CHILDREN

It would be difficult today to find a young adult who had not spent some time in a hospital during the childhood years. Many will remember such experiences with fear and trembling because of the loneliness and pain they felt at an age when they could not cope with these feelings alone. Needless to say, practices in use in some hospitals today have changed little over the past 20 years, but in others have gone through a period of rapid transition. This has occurred partially because of findings from research in the social sciences, partially because of newer thinking in child psychology, and partially because of social or consumer pressure.

VISITING HOURS

Many years ago when parents were permitted to visit their hospitalized child only one hour once a month, children were needlessly deprived of parental love. Today many hospitals permit visiting from 2 to 8 p.m. or from early in the morning to bedtime, while other institutions permit visiting at any time during the day or night.

The extent of visiting by the parents should be determined by their need to see the child and, more important, by the child's need for the parents. Some nurses may believe that parental visiting is upsetting to a particular child because he cries when the parent leaves. Nothing could be further from the truth, because such a child is acting normally. If he did not appear upset when the parents left him, the nurses would have need to be concerned. They might believe that such quiet behavior indicated that he had "adjusted" to the hospital routine and the care of nurses when, in reality, he had just given up in despair. A more detailed discussion of this subject will be found in the chapters dealing with illness in the various age groups.

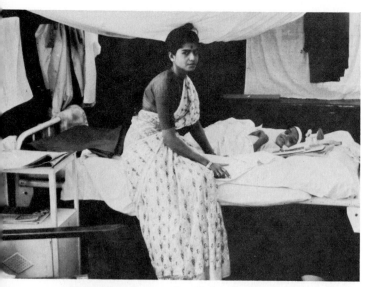

FIGURE 5–5. In a hospital in India, a mother provides nursing care as well as emotional support for her baby. (From Bell, J. B., and Bell, E. A.: *Children*, July-August, 1970, p. 156.)

ROOMING-IN

Parents should never be required to stay at a child's bedside, but neither should they be prohibited from doing this if they so desire.

For parents who stay during the daytime in the pediatric unit, some hospitals provide a comfortable lounge or waiting room where they can relax. In some institutions meals can be served to the parents in the child's room, or they may eat in the hospital cafeteria or coffee shop.

Mothers of seriously ill children especially may be encouraged to stay in the hospital all night if they desire to do so and facilities are available for their comfort. Fathers may also stay if facilities are made available for them. Various arrangements have been made for parents to stay in the hospital setting. The mother may sleep on a chair, a cot, a folding bed or a convertible chair in the child's room, if it is large enough. Some hospitals have rooms on the pediatric unit where the mothers may sleep. In case of an emergency they could be easily summoned. Other institutions have a wing of the hospital or a motel type of accommodation for parents and other relatives. In hospitals where no facilities are made for parents to stay they may be directed to accommodations close by in the community.

Some hospitals have *care-by-parent* or *family participation units* where the mother actually lives in the hospital with her child. This method of care has its roots in the Orient, where the whole family becomes involved with the care of the sick. Under this system the child gets attention when he needs it each day from a familiar person, under the supervision of the nurse. This is a good setting where nurses can gain experience in communicating nursing skills and explaining procedures to mothers. This should be done so that all mothers from various backgrounds can learn to nurse their children.

Specifically, the nurse's responsibilities in such a setting are to prepare the parent to meet the child's needs in the hospital, to help the child maintain a schedule similar to the one he had at home, to interpret medical procedures and scheduled diagnostic tests, and to do health teaching and anticipatory guidance as necessary. In the family unit the nurse can observe the parents, their skills, attitudes and techniques, and any problems in parent-child relations that may be apparent. The nurse must also observe and evaluate the physical and emotional needs of each mother so that none of them becomes too fatigued by the experience.

Some mothers may be too anxious or guilty or just may not want to participate in the care of their children in the hospital. Others may welcome the opportunity to give their children a sense of security through their presence.

The subject of parents remaining with their children during hospitalization is discussed in greater detail in the chapters on illness.

THE HEALTH AND NURSING TEAMS

Nurses who care for children see their role in terms of their relations with the parents, the child and the family group as a whole. The nurse may be described broadly not as a parent substitute, but as "Father's or Mother's friend." In this role the nurse may individually plan for and actually give comprehensive care to children or may function as a member of a nursing team.

The nurse who is a member of a *nursing team* works closely with one or more professional nurses, nursing students, licensed practical nurses, nurse attendants, and others in a joint effort. In order to function as a leader or member of this team, the nurse must understand the comprehensive care of patients assigned to the team and be willing to contribute to their optimum care.

The role of the nurse who cares for children involves not only working with the individual child, his family unit and the nursing team but also cooperating with members of the broader *health team*: physician, social worker, nutritionist, school teacher, Play Lady, public health or community nurse, religious counselor, and others as the need arises. The nurse fulfills the responsibility of the profession by being an active participating member of this team, contributing skills and knowledge to the total effort of the group.

Although the student should know the functions of most of the various members of the health team mentioned above, the functions of the recreation specialist or children's activities specialist (Play Lady) and the school teacher may not be so well understood. Both these members of the health team are important adjuncts to total patient care.

The *recreation specialist*, or *children's activities specialist (Play Lady)*, has several functions. On the basis of information gleaned about the child a plan or program for each child geared according to an evaluation of his needs can be made. Group activities can also be planned when possible to give the children safe outlets for anxieties and hostilities. Familiar playthings can be given to children postoperatively in order to reduce their fears. The recreation specialist can plan projects for the children to carry out according to their ages. A report on the activities of the children can be given to the medical and nursing staffs.

The functions of the *school teacher* are much the same as they are in classrooms in the community. Further discussion concerning the activities of the recreation specialist and the school teacher will be given later in this chapter and others throughout this text.

Other persons with whom the nurse interacts when caring for children are the *volunteers.* These are members of the community who have an interest in hospitalized children and the time to contribute to their care. One specific group of volunteers that has received well-deserved publicity in recent years is the Foster Grandparents. These men and women who have had years of experience in living can bring warmth and understanding to ill children and, in many instances, to the parents as well.

PLAY AND SCHOOL IN THE HOSPITAL

The idea of providing opportunities for play and learning activities is certainly not a recent one in institutions, but the practice of providing programs to meet these needs is new in many hospitals.

Play is a child's way of living, his daily "work." It can satisfy needs in the child for his physical, emotional, social and mental development. It is also one of childhood's most effective tools for mastering stress. Play is as essential for the sick child as for the healthy one. The sick child needs it to fill lonely hours and, by expressing his feelings through it, to reduce the trauma caused by hospitalization.

The growth of play and school programs in pediatric units of hospitals is due partly to the improved medical and nursing care which children now receive. Today children recover from their acute illnesses in a shorter time and thus have more time to recover while not on bed rest. Also the current importance placed on the emotional, social and mental aspects of a child's life in the hospital has been due to research in these areas. It is now understood that play can help a child to comprehend intrusive and surgical procedures, and also to express his fantasies, fears and anxieties.

Children can play in areas provided for this purpose or in the center of the pediatric unit. Obviously, if they play where acutely ill children are, they tend to be a disturbing factor in the environment and to be in the way of physicians and other personnel. Hospitals today are either including playrooms in their new buildings or are converting porches or other rooms to be used for this purpose. If no room is available which can be used for this specific purpose, a

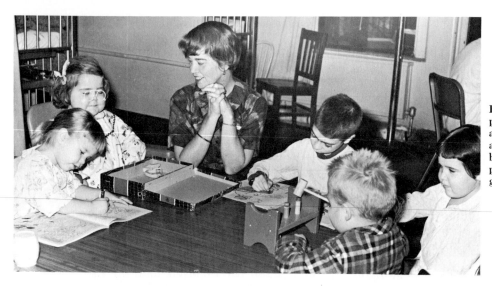

FIGURE 5–6. Children enjoy playing together under the guidance of the Play Lady. As soon as the child is able to be out of bed, he should be encouraged to play with other children in a group just as if he were at home.

toy cart can be designed which can be moved from bed to bed.

If a large room and an outdoor area are available for play, some children who are restricted to their beds, stretchers or wheelchairs can be moved so that they can participate in play activities. Certainly the children who cannot be moved should be involved in play activities at their own beds if they are able.

The nurse incorporates play activities into the daily life of each pediatric patient because play is a part of the child's total needs. The nurse must consider, when planning activities for any child, his age, his interests, the diagnosis and the limitations imposed upon him by his illness. When the child is acutely ill and unable to play actively with toys, he may enjoy listening to stories. Telling a story instead of reading it draws children into emotional involvement in it. The storyteller can ask questions, insert comments about the individual child, and thus make him feel a part of the story itself. If stories about animals or children are told, the child can pretend to be one of the characters and interject his own comments into the narration. Other activities which children in bed can do are watching a plant such as a sweet potato vine, a carrot, or herbs grow, watching an ant hill or some goldfish in a tank, or a canary or parakeet placed near the bed, or watching supervised television programs.

In the play area children who are permitted out of bed should be free to develop mental, motor, and social skills and to express themselves in a variety of art media, such as finger painting or molding with clay. Even in the hospital children enjoy playing with household equipment. They also like equipment peculiar

to the hospital which will allow them to work out their feelings about hospitalization.

Children frequently select toys such as doctor

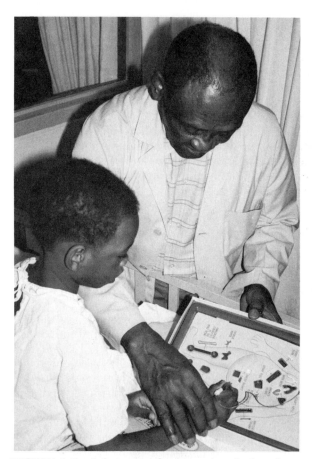

FIGURE 5–7. A foster grandparent makes the long hours seem a bit shorter for his "foster grandchild." (Courtesy of LCA/ALC Home, Augsburg Bible Studies.)

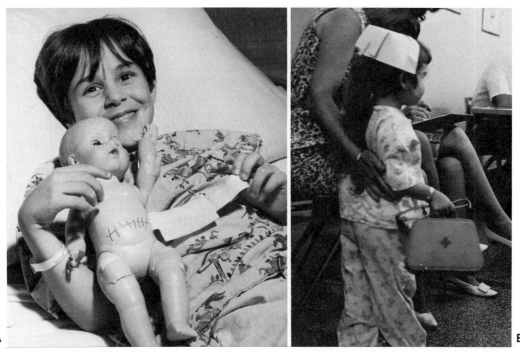

FIGURE 5-8. Play activities. *A*, Play is therapeutic for this postoperative child whose doll had abdominal surgery also. *B*, After this young child's illness, she enjoys playing "nurse." (Courtesy of Shirley Bonnem, Children's Hospital of Philadelphia.)

or nurse dolls, play syringes and stethoscopes with which they can imitate the activities they see around them. Old cloth can be used in such play to restrain a doll, to make a doll's sheet, to make bandages or to improvise a sling for a supposedly broken arm. Recently puppets have been used to demonstrate procedures to children who are to be hospitalized. Children enjoy not only seeing "the show," but also playing with the doctor and nurse puppets after it is over. Such activities are therapeutic in that they help the child to work out his feelings about his hospitalization.

Much of the equipment which is of value in the play of normal children is also necessary in the hospital play area, particularly simple craft materials, blocks, puzzles, story books, dolls, doll houses, and phonograph records. Children enjoy play telephones because they can pretend that they are calling home. They also enjoy clay, paints, puppets, and pounding boards on which they can express their anger. They enjoy tricy-

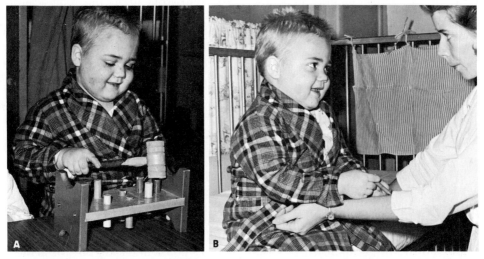

FIGURE 5-9. Angry feelings which may result from hospitalization can be worked off through the use of (*A*) a bang board or (*B*) equipment peculiar to the hospital such as a "play" hypodermic injection for his nurse.

cles, carts, and wagons through the use of which they develop or exercise their large muscles.

Other suggestions for use in the care of a child whose parents cannot or will not communicate with him are surprise boxes made of shoe boxes and filled with small wrapped toys and cards sent to him in the mail by his nurse. In this way he feels remembered by adults other than his parents.

Children's play areas cannot be kept clean and orderly as judged by adult standards. If the nurses are too concerned about the physical appearance of play areas during playtime, the children feel that the unit personnel do not approve of their play and are likely to enter only half-heartedly into their make-believe, creative work or games.

Children should be taught to take care of toys which they brought from home or were given to them by their parents. They may and indeed should let other children play with them if their social growth is to go forward in the hospital as it normally would in their homes, but a place must be provided where their toys can be safely stored. A toy bag which can be tied to one end of the child's bed or crib can be easily made by the hospital sewing room personnel or by volunteer groups. These may be taken home by the child or laundered for use by other children, depending on the policy of the hospital. As a child learns to take care of his own toys he also learns to respect those of other children.

Much can be learned from watching a child play in a relaxed environment. His approach to play and his relation to his peers, parents and other adults should be observed and recorded. Also to be noted are the degree of his activity, his attention span, his ability to tolerate frustration, his verbal ability, and his concept formation. In addition, the nurse should note the child's comments about his home and his hospitalization and his general attitude and behavior. Such observations will help the nurse to understand how the child is coping with this difficult crisis in his life. If he can handle it well, his experience may be of help in mastering problem situations in later years.

Nurses should have an opportunity to participate in the play program for hospitalized children. In this way they not only learn about children and their play, but also have an opportunity to appreciate the contribution of the recreation specialist or Play Lady to the comprehensive care of their patients.

An important member of the health team in the pediatric unit is the public school teacher, generally employed by the local Board of Education, but released from regular classroom activities to teach hospitalized children. The school teacher works particularly with the children who are in the hospital for relatively long periods of time; however, any child whose physician recommends this sort of activity for him can be taught. Even when it is obvious that the child is too ill ever to return to school, keeping up with his class is important to him as a link with the outside world. In some hospitals the teacher teaches at the children's bedsides, while in other institutions the children who are able can be brought together in a classroom set aside for this purpose. The child who is kept busy and feels useful and important, and whose mind is occupied, is a far happier child than one who is allowed to vegetate. Also, the child who keeps up with his class in their work is able to return to school with his own friends after his hospitalization.

The subjects of play and school for the child are elaborated upon in subsequent chapters.

THE ROLE OF THE NURSE IN CHILD CARE

Many nurses believe that they can accomplish their mission in child care by providing "parent love" for each child with whom they come in contact. The nurse may believe that expressions of affection, tenderness, warmth, and concern will be rewarded by the child's love in return. The nurse may believe that since the parents are not with the child constantly, whether the child is in school or in the hospital, a replacement for them in the child's affections is necessary.

Love of the parents for a child does not consist only of cuddling, feeding, and playing with the infant or child. Love also includes those interactions of parent with child that stimulate growth, perception, curiosity, investigation of the environment, independence, and achievement of age-appropriate tasks. Parental love requires that not only the total dependence of the newborn but also the increasing independence of the toddler is cause for rejoicing. As the child grows, the parents must be able to encourage further growth and to continue to love the child even though his interests are different from their own. To loving parents the ability of the child to realize his own individual capacities and potential is more important than their own expectations of the child.

Parental love is difficult to achieve. Such a capacity to love is usually based on having had similar experiences in one's own youth. As the mature adult finds a sense of achievement and pleasure in his own work, and in his relations with others, so also he wants these same satisfactions for his children. As the mature parent can accept varied feelings relating to anger, love, grief, and sex, so also can the child learn through the process of identification.

In our culture such fortunate parents and their children are relatively rare. Many parents today had serious emotional deprivation in their early lives, so that in their adult lives they strive for material things to make up for their loss. If such an adult marries another with similar problems, the children of the union may not be able to get much love from their parents because unfortunately they do not have much to give.

But the nurse cannot fill the total need for love in such a child's life. Love results, in the nursing setting, from the mutual effort of the nurse and the child to achieve his recovery. A mutual regard of child and nurse develops after repeated testing of the adult by the child and repeated efforts on the part of the nurse to gain the child's trust. Out of a prolonged interaction as in a long-term hospitalization, the nurse and the child find the capacity to love. *Love from the child is the result of the efforts of the nurse and not the initiating force in the relationship.* But even then, if the parents have not completely deserted their child, the nurse is still functioning in the role of a "kind friend" of his parents who cares for him when they are unable to do so.

Communicating with Parents

If we really want to serve the child well, we first have to communicate in an effective way with the parents, especially the mother. *Communication with the parents should be regarded as a process whose purposes are to obtain and to transmit information, to provide an opportunity for them to ventilate their feelings and relieve tension, and to motivate them in the direction of understanding and resolving their own problems.* In order to assure effective communication with either parents or children the nurse must have respect for them as human beings, and take into account their needs, problems, fears, customs and cultural backgrounds.

Furthermore, *readiness to learn* is dependent on the parents' present situation. In an acute crisis or a threatening event when they feel insecure, they need firm help. At this time they are highly suggestible and will listen to what is discussed. It is important that what is offered has a sound basis, since they will just as easily accept an irrational solution to their problem. Examples of periods in the lives of parents when they need help and guidance in relation to their child are when he is ill or hospitalized and during the difficult periods of his development as during the toilet training period or during adolescence. It is well known that though a slight increase in anxiety or fear is associated with more learning, extreme anxiety has the opposite effect.

In each communication the nurse has with the parents there should be a clearly defined purpose, yet one broad enough to allow for modification as the need arises. For instance, factual information on health care, feeding, inoculations, and so on, is important; however, the interest of the parent must be ascertained before it is given. If the parent is not interested, little will be gained from such a conference unless the nurse first ascertains what is blocking his interest.

The success of any interview depends primarily on the nurse's ability to establish and maintain a sound interpersonal relation with the parent. The attainment of such a relation is largely based on the nurse's warmth, sensitivity, objectivity and understanding. But speech alone does not transmit depth of interest and feeling. The nurse's physical appearance and movement, such as the neatness and appropriateness of the uniform or clothing, facial expression, leaning forward to show interest, looking directly at the parent to show concern, and the movement of the hands, are vitally important in furthering a good interviewing relation.

Our attitudes and behavior as nurses toward those whom we wish to help have been largely conditioned by our own relations and experience. Among other things, the age and sex of the parent, as well as physical and personal characteristics, often activate certain feelings and responses which may have no basis of reality in our experience with the particular parent. The nurse may like or dislike a child's parent, not so much because of him or her as an individual, but because the nurse is attributing to and displacing on the parent feelings which stem from identifying him or her with someone extremely close, often a parent, brother, or sister. The unresolved conflict toward key members of the family is reflected in the way the nurse relates to others in professional and personal relations. The nurse should be able to recognize and not deny feelings toward a parent or child, even though he or she may not know the specific origin of these feelings.

The nurse often represents the same sort of figure to the parents as to their child. Although the nurse can tolerate hostility, guilt, and dependency from the child, it is more difficult to do so from the parents who are more nearly the nurse's own age. He or she should nevertheless convey warm acceptance of them and genuine regard for their feelings. The nurse can provide for the parents a rare opportunity to express their feelings to someone who is understanding and not critical or moralistic.

The nurse should be aware of certain principles in establishing these relations with the parents and their child.

1. *The nurse begins to build a working relationship with the parents and child from the first contact with them, whether in their home, in the hospital or in the community.*

2. *The nurse understands that all behavior is meaningful, although the meaning may not always be too clear.*

3. *The nurse accepts the parents and their child exactly as they are,* refraining from evaluating actions as "bad" or "wrong" and from passing judgment on other human beings. This does not mean indifference to ethical values. It simply means that the aim is understanding, and therefore the interest is focused on causation.

4. *The nurse should have empathy for parents and children.* This implies an appreciation of how they feel inwardly, how things are for them, but it does not mean that their feelings or troubles become those of the nurse. He or she would like both parents and children to know that each of their problems is of importance and that the nurse is there to aid in their solution.

5. *The nurse should be willing to acknowledge the parents' right to their own decisions concerning their children.* Sometimes such decisions may be painful for the nurse to accept.

6. *The nurse permits both parents and child to express negative emotions.* When a parent or child expresses negative feelings, the nurse should be personally secure and not respond subjectively to his statements. Ability to accept him despite his expression or resentment helps convince him that he is truly understood.

7. *The nurse should ask questions limited to a single idea or reference.* If questions are too long or complex, the parent may become confused or ignore the meaning the nurse intended.

8. *The nurse should speak in language understandable to the parents.*

9. *The nurse and the physician as well as other members of the health and nursing teams must help the parents and child to feel that there is unity and strength among them.*

Many situations in pediatric nursing require a knowledge by the nurse of interviewing techniques. *A genuine expression of liking and warmth sets the tone for the parents and child and helps them to relax.* Whenever possible, listen and let the parents tell their story, then assist them to explain it more fully. The nondirective method of interviewing can be successful in some nursing situations. The main technique in the nondirective method is to reflect what the parent or child has said, either by asking a question, repeating his last words using a questioning inflection, or by rephrasing what he has said. This method in its pure form limits the nurse to a minimum of verbal activity; however, nonverbal responses in posture or expression can be used.

The principle of the nondirective method may be used when a real conflict is evident such as when discussing the fear of death or of surgery. In such situations superficial reassurance is worthless, because though it may comfort the sympathizer, it offers only temporary relief to the person who is reassured. The nurse can be helpful if a real effort is made to understand the parent and then to help him identify the reasons for his fears. It is most important to listen, making little comment, and to *be with* the parents or child at such a time.

One caution must be remembered when using the nondirective technique, however. The nurse should not be guilty of probing or leading a parent to say more than he ought or really wants to say. Such a conference might cause the parent more anxiety than he had prior to it.

When interviewing parents whose behavior indicates concern, the nurse should focus on this and try to identify and meet the immediate needs. At times, as upon admission of a child to the hospital, the nurse may find it necessary to defer the usual initial interview until later. With experience the nurse develops skill in utilizing a variety of ways of communicating with parents.

In most interviewing situations pauses will occur. The nurse must learn to tolerate them with ease. Pauses many times precede a significant turn in the conversation. Perhaps the parent or child would like to say something important and is wondering whether he can really trust the nurse. Perhaps he wants to say something, but finds it difficult to put his concern into words, or he wants to stop talking about a particular topic. Nurses should not be embarrassed by such pauses.

The nurse cannot possibly provide answers or help parents find answers to all the complex problems they and their children struggle with. If credit is given for having the capacity to arrive at their own answers, the nurse's role will be to help them get a clearer vision of the situation and an awareness of possible alternate decisions and their consequences. *The purpose of the nurse is not to solve problems, but to strengthen the parent's and child's capacity to deal with them. If the situation which either the parent or child presents is beyond the professional competence of the nurse, he or she should seek help from other members of the health team.*

ADMISSION OF THE CHILD TO THE HOSPITAL

PREPARATION FOR ADMISSION TO THE HOSPITAL

Prevention is a strong component of nursing care. The maintenance of health and the prevention of illness is a goal all nurses would like to achieve for children. Realistically, however, nurses know that some children will become ill in spite of the best health care that can be provided. Even immunizations cannot protect against all illnesses of childhood. It is essential, then, that children, especially if they are to be spared the psychologic or emotional trauma of hospitalization, be prepared for this possibility. Nurses can intervene and play a vital role in this effort.

Little can be done to prepare the infant, but for the older child more can be accomplished in terms of preparation for hospitalization. Booklets, films, puppet shows, or other creative means may be used to prepare the well child of even kindergarten-age who does not immediately require treatment in a hospital. For children who are scheduled for hospitalization, preadmission parties for prospective patients, their siblings, and parents may be given. School programs aimed at educating parents are available so they can help their children deal with hospitalization, should the necessity arise. Such programs may be planned by Parent-Teacher Associations. Plans can also be made to have well older children visit the hospital to orient them to the physical environment and to some aspects of care provided.

Preparation of children for hospitalization is of such importance that discussions on this subject in greater detail are included in later chapters of this text.

ADMISSION TO THE HOSPITAL

The philosophy of child care, whether in a hospital or other community agency, should be consistently one of concern and support for the child and his parents. The beliefs about child care held by the members of both the health and nursing teams should be clear and easily transmitted through the behavior and communication of the professional and nonprofessional personnel.

Admission of a child to the hospital can be considered in connection with the activities involved or from the standpoint of the emotional effect upon the child and his family. We shall consider first the emotional effect, because it is often mistakenly accorded less importance than the physical care given the child. The nurse's attitude is probably the most important single factor in the emotional atmosphere during the child's admission (Fig. 5–10).

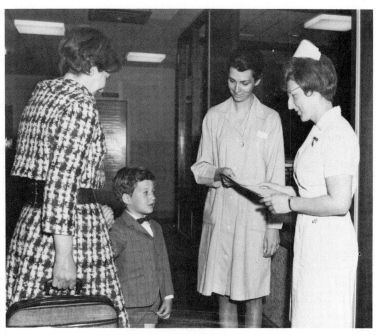

FIGURE 5–10. Admission to the hospital. The nurse must be understanding of the feelings of both child and parents, when the child is admitted to the hospital. (Courtesy of Hospital Sainte-Justine, Montreal.)

Hospitalization of children is so common today that we tend to forget its importance as a break in the unity of the family. The feelings of each member of the family must be considered if this break is to result in furthering rather than hindering the emotional and social maturity of all concerned. Although the nurse has the main role in helping the child and his parents adjust to the hospital situation, the entire health team is involved in creating the optimum emotional environment on the child's admission.

Emotional Reactions on Admission of a Child to the Hospital

PARENTAL REACTION

Parents whose child has been admitted to the hospital feel not only that he is separated from them, but also that others are taking their place and, furthermore, giving him necessary care which they, with all their intense love for him, cannot give.

Immediate operation is often necessary to save the life of an infant who is born deformed or deviates from the normal, or he may be sent home from the newborn nursery with his mother, for deferred admission to the pediatric unit when he has reached the optimum age for correction of the defect. In general the reaction of parents to such a child at birth is that he presents a threat to all their happy expectations centered on the concept of a normal baby. It is natural that when he is readmitted to the hospital they still feel anxiety, anger, fear, disappointment and possibly guilt (see p. 231 for further discussion).

Anxiety during a child's illness not only interferes with a parent's ability to provide support for the child but may also be transmitted like an infection to the child himself. The anxious parent can be recognized by his trembling, coarse or wavery voice, restlessness, irritableness, withdrawal or erratic body movements. He may also show angry, hostile and aggressive behavior toward the nurses and physicians caring for his child.

When the nurse detects anxiety in the parent, the first task is to identify the causes of the anxiety and to give whatever help possible to alleviate it.

A father or a mother, particularly with her first child, often feels that his sickness is due to some error she has committed and is her fault. If he was an unwanted baby, she may consider it punishment for not having had the normal maternal love for the child during her pregnancy and after his birth.

If the parents blame themselves for the child's illness, the nurse can explain the real cause of illness to them and convey to them her belief that they are competent. If the parents did make an error and illness resulted, the nurse can attempt to convince the parents that a mistake can be made by anyone.

If the mother is anxious because she feels that she is not competent, the nurse can give sincere praise for things she does well in order to increase her self-confidence. Having the mother guide the nurse in details of care as it was done in the home will not only increase the mother's confidence but will also be reassuring to the child.

If the parents need help with resolving their guilt beyond that which the nurse can give, they should be referred to another helpful professional person.

Specific Causes of Parental Anxiety. In addition to their feelings about the illness itself, parents may be frightened and excited by the new experience of placing their child in the hospital. Among the many factors which increase their anxiety are the following.

1. Fear of the strange environment in the hospital. If the parent is disturbed by the continuing strangeness of the hospital atmosphere, the nurse can try to explain the use of equipment in lay terminology, to make the surroundings more homelike, and to encourage the parents to ask questions. Simple answers to questions help to allay anxiety. Also, if the nurse explains to the parents what they can do for and with their child, they will tend to feel more secure in caring for him within the limits which have been established.
2. Fear of separation from the child and fear that the nurses may be unloving or that, because they are able to do so much for him, they will take his love from them. If the mother is anxious because the nurses are giving her child care, the nurse could suggest tactfully that she partially care for the child herself. Such activity would help the mother to cope in a more healthy way with her anxiety.
3. Fear of the unknown and of what will happen to the child immediately and in the future. The life of a handicapped child appears the more difficult because parents have no clear picture of what it will be like.
4. Fear that the child will suffer.
5. Fear that the condition is infectious and may spread to other members of the family.
6. Fear of unbearable financial obligations incurred through the illness. The social service worker may be able to help with such problems.

7. Fear that society will look upon the illness as a reflection of something wrong with the child's parents.

A parent's anxiety magnifies all other problems. They may enter into long discussions of problems extraneous to that of the child's illness. The nurse should accept this as natural and never feel that their dwelling on other difficulties means that they are disinterested in the child.

The majority of parents want the understanding, sympathetic support which the nurse can give and thereby gain a realistic view of the difficulties which they and the child must face. Some parents, especially mothers, may appear withdrawn, however; these are in greater need of help. To assist them to put into words their deep emotion may be too heavy a responsibility for the nurse to undertake. The psychiatrist or psychiatric social worker should be available to guide both the parents in their trouble and the nurse in contacts with them.

THE CHILD'S REACTION

Illness or a physical handicap threatens both the physical development of a child and his sense of trust in other people which is important to his emotional development. Sickness causes pain, restraint of movement, long sleepless periods and, in an infant who cannot be fed by mouth, restriction in the fulfillment of his sucking need. When he most needs his mother, he is without her, unless the hospital has provision for her remaining day and night.

Hospitalization is a completely new experience to the infant or young child. When he was taken to the private physician's office or the Child Health Conference, he made friends with physicians and nurses, but he is too young to understand that the hospital personnel are also his friends. Since his parents tend to be anxious, their feeling of fear is communicated to him. What the hospital means to the pediatric patient will depend upon his stage of maturity and upon how accustomed he was to being left with friends. It will also depend in large measure upon how well the young child was prepared for this hospitalization. If he regards the separation from his parents as punishment for wrongdoing, he will be less able to cope with it than if he knows the real reason why he is hospitalized and something of what to expect after admission.

The infant especially may be emotionally disturbed by hospitalization. Not only is he separated from his parents, but also he may suffer from sensory deprivation if the nursing personnel do not take the time to provide the loving care he needs. If the infant, on the other hand, is bright and outgoing, nurses may give him more than the usual amount of cuddling. It is important for the nurse to understand the reason for such behavior in this situation. Is the nurse meeting the needs of a particular lovable infant, or meeting personal needs by ministering to him at the risk of not providing tender loving care for the less beautiful and less responsive patient?

Sensory deprivation of the pediatric patient may also occur if the child is being cared for in an incubator, in an isolation area or in the intensive care unit. If for any reason the child does not have close physical contact with another human being, he may be traumatized emotionally to a greater degree than he is physically because of his illness.

NURSE-CHILD RELATIONS

The needs of the ill child are similar to those of the well child; however, the nurse has a responsibility for meeting part of his needs when he is hospitalized. The child needs to trust those persons responsible for his care. Since he is not able to judge the competencies of the members of the health and nursing teams, he must rely only on his perception of their relations with him. The child must feel that the adults around him know who he is, understand him, and like him as a person, different from the other children. The older infant or child usually feels more secure if the nurses call him by the name his parents use in addressing him. If his parents call him "Junior" instead of his given name of "Bruce," the hospital personnel should do the same to prevent his having to adjust to a new name during his hospitalization. The child needs understanding and physical contact also from his parents. The nurse can help the parents provide the kind of comforting support he needs. Since a child needs to continue to grow and develop while he is a patient, he needs a nurse who is aware of his pattern of behavior at home and can follow it to some degree in the hospital. And last, but not the least important, the child needs to play and come in contact with other children.

The Child's View. The child perceives this relation as one in which he receives from the nurse (1) physical care formerly given by his mother or some other member of the family, (2) new kinds of care which may be painful and frightening, (3) a sense of security in an adult's affection, and (4) the link with home and parents.

An older child realizes that in addition to the foregoing the nurse teaches him good hygiene and is a model of one of the many persons he can emulate when grown up. The child may sense, but not clearly perceive, that the nurse teaches him to adapt to his condition, physically and emotionally. He soon learns the nurse's relation with his parents and with the physicians and makes use of these contacts.

The extent to which nursing care can be given in a homelike setting is a question which each hospital decides in the light of physical resources and available personnel. By homelike physical environment is meant sunlight, color, pictures, music and television, small tables and chairs, toys, wagons, tricycles, and so on. For instance, pink or blue plastic individual bathtubs, floating toys and colored towels and washcloths make the bath more homelike.

Food can be served from a self-heated food cart decorated to look like a chuck wagon. The older child may be taken to the hospital cafeteria or snack shop to eat certain meals in order to change his environment temporarily and to remind him of past happy experiences of eating in a restaurant with his parents.

The use of a stroller instead of a wheelchair or stretcher to transport the child is another example of the introduction into the hospital setting of compatible equipment and techniques which will connect what of necessity must be strange and cause anxiety in the child with the care he received at home from his mother. Permitting a child to take a doll or other toy to the operating room or to a place where he is to be subjected to diagnostic tests is an evidence of the understanding attitude of nurses and physicians toward his fear.

More important than equipment or methods adapted to children is the rapport between the nurse and the child. Although, ideally, one nurse should give the child all the care he needs as long as he is in the hospital, realistically this cannot often be done. It is important, therefore, that as few nurses as possible be responsible for the child's care. The child should learn to know "his" nurses and they to know him as a person. If he had a few nurses he knew well, there would be sufficient stability in his relations so that he could accept relief nurses more readily. That nurses wear uniforms which in his view are similar and that they do things for him in much the same way helps him to accept new nurses among those who routinely care for him. A new friend may be pleasant when he knows that the old ones are still there.

The Nurse's View in the Care of the Child. 1. *The nurse perceives his or her role very much as the child perceives it* because the role has been defined to meet his needs. Some negligent nurses do not live up to the professional role of the nurse, and their influence is soon reflected in a change in the child's definition of the nurse-child relation. His idea that nurses are good to little children may change, and he may think nurses mean, whose role is an authoritative, punitive one, in spite of the physical care they give him according to the best technique.

But to his limited concept of their relations the nurse may add much that the child does not realize.

2. *The nurse guides the hospitalized child to better ways of living.* The nurse should offer the child opportunities to maintain good habits of hygiene or to improve upon them if possible during the usually short hospital stay. As far as possible, new ways of caring for him, new equipment, new foods in his diet, and new concepts of cleanliness should be introduced gradually. Helping the patient to substitute better habits for current or harmful ones is so much a part of comprehensive nursing that in this book such habits are taken up in connection with the nursing care of children.

Unfortunately a child may lose good habits while he is in the hospital and regress to infantile ways, or an older child may acquire undesirable habits. A case in point is that of control of urine and stool. A child's physical condition and nervousness due to his strange surroundings may make control difficult for him. But often this is not the cause of a wet and soiled bed. He has cried for a nurse to put him on the "potty" or take him to the toilet. When no one came, he stood holding on to the bars of his crib, crying more loudly, and in the end relieved himself in bed. Nurses know better than to punish or shame a child when this happens. They as well as the parents should realize that he is sick, but often they do not understand that his emotional state and physical exertion are harmful for him. If nurses are too busy with some important duty, they may think that his needs are not urgent enough. They may consider that it takes less time to change his clothing and his bed when it is convenient than to come at once when he calls. In fact, they may put diapers on a child who has worn pants for months. In consequence, when he wets himself day after day, he ceases to call the nurse and returns to his infantile habit of relieving himself whenever and wherever he feels inclined to do so. He has thus lost a good habit and regressed to earlier behavior.

3. *The nurse perceives her role as a helping person.* Illness and hospitalization cause stress or problems in adjustment for the child and his family. Parents and their children need from the nurse comfort, a source of strength, and knowl-

edge. The nurse therefore must see himself or herself as a helping person who can provide emotional support to those in need. *Nurses must realize that before support can be provided, however, they must first care about patients sufficiently to earn their confidence.* Only then can a positive emotional relation with the child and his family be developed which is the base for providing such support and strength to them. *The nurse must be aware of the feelings of both parents and children so that a response to them can be made and their resources strengthened to handle their problems.*

In the care of the acutely ill child the nurse must recognize anxiety and provide relief from it by patiently listening to complaints, showing concern about the child, and, while providing rest for him, giving him physical care which further indicates her deep interest. *Words alone will not convey to the parents that everything possible is being done to promote the child's recovery.* As the anxiety of the parents is abated, the anxiety of the child will be also, because it is a well known fact that *anxiety is contagious.*

The student nurse may not at first be able to provide the kind or amount of support that children and their parents need. The student may be so involved with personal anxiety in having to care for deformed, critically ill or dying children that the parental anxiety which is present may not even be perceived. *Pediatric nursing requires of the nurse great patience and tenderness, but it also requires great emotional strength in times of stress.*

The nurse may not be able to handle overwhelming feelings in caring for children. She or he may at first attempt to protect the self by building an impenetrable wall against patients. Nurses may even flee physically from an uncomfortable situation in which they do not permit themselves to become emotionally involved. The nurse, to whom parents and children turn for support, thus leaves them at a time when they need professional help most. If the nurse does not physically leave the situation, the interaction with patients and their families may be cut off by utilizing verbal blocks to satisfying communication. This may be done by imposing ideas in conversation instead of listening to the ideas of others, by giving weak, false reassurance, by jumping to faulty conclusions, and by changing the subject whenever the topic is uncomfortable. Before the student can reassure patients or families personal feelings must be resolved about the care of ill children. The nurse must gain spiritual strength and replenish the personal reservoir of emotional strength before helping others. Often the instructor or another faculty member can help considerably in achieving these tasks.

In order for the nurse to understand his or her own feelings and thus be better able to cope with them, the existence of such feelings must be recognized. This knowledge may help the nurse learn to use energy in a more constructive way.

NURSE-PARENT RELATIONS

It is a truism that the nurse's relation with the child's parents is based on the fact that they are the parents of the child or client for whom care is being given. He is the focal point of their relations. The father, but more frequently the mother who gives care to the child, may be more in need of the nurse's sympathetic, understanding, permissive guidance than an acutely ill child is of emotional support. The influence of the mother's attitude upon the child is so great that it is not only for the mother's sake but also for the child's, that the nurse has a serious responsibility to help the mother. In order to understand how to help mothers the student should be willing to learn from them. The nurse needs to know not only their weaknesses but also their strengths, and make the most of them in the care the child receives. Prior to entering nursing the individual is more likely to have had experience solely with children deprived of their mothers' company. But in most cases separation from the mother took place under pleasant auspices, so that neither child nor mother was seriously disturbed. (One or both might have had a moment of concern over what to do without the other. No child likes to be left behind when Mother goes out for the evening, and Mother may have some doubts as to Johnny's being old enough to go to camp. But such partings are chosen, and no great fear is involved.) If the inexperienced nurse has had extensive experience as a babysitter or camp counselor or has otherwise come in contact with children, rapport with the mother is easier to establish because they have in common a knowledge of children. On this instruction is built, drawing from a professional knowledge of sick children.

The mother knows her child far better than the nurse does. The mother may be so intent upon him that she accepts him as the prototype of all children and does not see him against a background of other children; she does not see wherein he is like them or differs from them—his limitations and assets, his potentiality. But even a mother who has a distorted view of her child can teach the nurse many things about him which will assist in understanding his behavior. Reliance on the mother as a real help in the adjustment of the child with a chronic condition or severe handicap helps the nurse in accepting his condition. To give the child physical care is usually an emotional relief to the mother and reassures the child in his strange surroundings. The nurse can teach the mother many procedures and ways of caring for the child which she will need to know when she eventually takes him home.

The nurse knows more about pathology and treatment than the mother does, but what little the mother of a child with a chronic disease or a handicap does know is in direct relation to her child and the care she has given him. Until the nurses have had time to map out a plan of comprehensive nursing for him, the mother may be better able to lift and turn him so that it does not hurt, to feed him most comfortably or to create a play situation adapted to his likes and limitations. When the nurse has had time to apply professional knowledge to the child, the mother can be taught better ways of caring for him. Both the mother and the nurse, then, have much to contribute to each other in applying the principle of quality nursing to the child patient or client.

The value of a child psychologist with whom nurses can talk over the problems they meet in human relations is generally recognized. These relations are so complex that the guidance of a specialist is often necessary. (This also applies to the nurse's handling of personal emotional problems in the social involvements which constantly occur in the pediatric area.)

It should always be remembered that the child eventually goes home to his family. To bring about changes in habits, however beneficial, which cause strained relations between the child and his parents or friends when he leaves the hospital is of doubtful value. To teach a child not to use indecent words when these same words are part of the neighborhood daily speech is a case in point. To teach a boy not to fight, if his father would punish him if he did not show this ability to care for himself among other boys, would be folly.

A hospitalized child, however, must not be permitted to harm other children even though he may be permitted to do so at home. In this situation *the nurse may condemn the act, but not the child or the teachings of his parents.* One factor in the emotional disorders of American children is that the majority in the low-income group are taught in schools, hospitals, and other institutions where the culture of the middle class is held to be the goal of socialization, that their parents' attitudes, beliefs, and ways of doing things are not up to standard. Many of the older immigrants and some of the migrants and immigrants of today have come to our cities because they want their children to have advantages they themselves did not have; they want their children to move into a social class above their own. For a son or daughter to maintain the economic and social position of the parents is not the American philosophy. If their children do not surpass them, parents are likely to feel that they did not give their offspring the advantages they should have received.

In spite of this, clashes in the home often arise between parental attitudes and behavior characteristic of a lower class and those middle-class attitudes and characteristics which professional workers are teaching children, not only because they believe in the superiority of middle-class culture, but also because they are preparing the children to move up into the middle class. It is not the child's mobility which parents resent, but rather the lack of respect for his elders which such teaching is likely to engender. The nurse should help the child to draw a distinction between superficial cultural traits in which he differs from his parents and the fundamental traits which are recognized in all classes as fine and highly desirable, e.g., courage, honesty, fidelity, truthfulness, and self-sacrifice for those one loves.

Parent Education. The discussion of nurse-parent relations leads directly into the matter of parent education. In a broad sense parent education begins in childhood, when the personality of the prospective parent is formed in the home. That is, a child from a stable home in which he participates in good parent-child-sibling relations is being educated for creating such a home when he himself marries and founds a family. In instances of juvenile delinquency or warped personality we constantly hear that the parents are to blame for their children's behavior, but we seldom stop to consider the logic of that conclusion: the parents, too, were once children and therefore were influenced by their own home environment. This is not an acceptance of the fatalistic view whereby the blame for the faults of one generation rests upon the preceding one, and so on back indefinitely. Although personality is strongly set in childhood, it can be altered, albeit with greater difficulty, at any age up to senescence. The nurse, then, must accept the parents' personalities and their attitude toward the child while guiding them to a better understanding of how to help him grow up.

The nurse in any shared nurse-parent learning situation must remember certain basic principles. First of all what the mother already knows must be ascertained. In other words, the nurse must know the level of the mother's understanding and her background of experience. The nurse must know the mother's resources at home. Does the mother have the equipment she will need or the financial resources to obtain this equipment? The nurse, realizing the mother's problems, must be willing to proceed slowly, allowing time for the mother to absorb what is to be learned. In order to make certain that the mother understands fully, the nurse should either write down what has been said or have the mother repeat what she has learned.

The pediatric nurse's role includes a *demonstration* of physical care and child guidance. That is why it is important that the nurse be prepared to teach the mother. But the nurse's influence on the mother does not always center on physical care and its psychologic components. The nurse demonstrates to the mother how to help the child handle his emotions and also to create or remove stimuli, increasing those which promote a beneficial response and decreasing those which do not.

It is essential to recognize the nurse's role in interacting with other professional personnel serving the child and parents. That is, the physician and the child psychiatrist direct the medical and sociopsychologic components of what is demonstrated and taught the parent. The nurse is likely to be the most effective member of the professional group working with the child in the constant application of the plan for parental education; the nurse demonstrates, while giving physical care, how to meet the child's emotional needs. Procedures are taught which the parents will have to continue for the child when he returns home — both what to do and its psychologic component.

The nurse helps the parents emotionally, guiding them in attitude toward the child's condition and in their concepts of themselves. Parents often blame themselves too much for the afflictions of their children. They should realize that they cannot expect perfection of themselves or of anyone else. They must also realize that child care, like all rationally directed action, is based on a weighing of pros and cons as to what is to be done for the child. Their decision must be based on the probability of the outcome. We can give statistics as to automobile accidents, certain diets and the chances of recovery from specific disease or injuries, but no one can predict with certainty about a particular child. We often hear a parent say, "We wish we had not consented to the operation." They should be encouraged to believe that they made a wise decision even if, in their particular case, it proved to be wrong.

The Nurse's Responsibilities on the Admission of a Child

At the time of admission the nurse should consciously remember that even though the procedure of admission is well known to hospital personnel, this experience is most distressing to the child and his parents. The nurse should try to see this experience through the eyes of the child and his parents and offer information and emotional support from their first meeting.

The role of the nurse in the admission procedure is complementary to that of the parents and the child. To fill this role the nurse must understand that the mother's behavior is the result of the way the child's sickness and hospitalization appear to her. The mother should never be told not to cry or that she is "really fortunate, because the situation could be worse." Such comments cause a mother to repress her feelings and to be ashamed that she spoke so openly. Repression of anxiety or feelings of guilt or inadequacy causes these feelings to increase, while expression of them diminishes their intensity.

The nurse should never be critical of a parent's attitude, however unreasonable it may appear. Such criticism leads to greater tension and possibly to hostility on the parent's part. In order to be helpful the nurse must understand what the illness means to parents, who may be misinformed as to the cause, prognosis and necessary treatment.

The following are ways in which the nurse may make the parents feel more secure and calm in the hospital, and the child less restless:

1. The parents should be taken with the child to his bed in the unit or private room. Then they know where the child is and have a mental picture of his comfortable physical environment. Reducing their anxiety reduces that of the child.

2. The nurse who admits the child should introduce the head nurse or team leader to the parents. All names should be clearly pronounced. If the child is old enough, he should be introduced to other children of his own age and to the attending personnel.

3. The parents should be given a friendly welcome and should be seated comfortably. The nurse, even if other duties need attention, must be unhurried and calm. The nurse's attitude increases the parents' trust in the hospital and medical staff which the nurse represents.

4. The admission procedure should be carefully explained, and all questions asked by the parents should be answered clearly, fully, and in a way which will not frighten them.

The specific routine of admission is as follows:

1. History of Illnesses. The nurse introduces

TABLE 5–1. EQUIVALENT TEMPERATURE READINGS (CENTIGRADE AND FAHRENHEIT)*

°C	°F	°C	°F	°C	°F	°C	°F
0	32.0	37.2	99	39.2	102.6	41.2	106.2
20	68.0	37.4	99.3	39.4	102.9	41.4	106.5
30	86.0	37.6	99.7	39.6	103.3	41.6	106.9
31	87.8	37.8	100.1	39.8	103.7	41.8	107.2
32	89.6	38.0	100.4	40.0	104	42	107.6
33	91.4	38.2	100.8	40.2	104.4	43	109.4
34	93.2	38.4	101.2	40.4	104.7	44	111.2
35	95.0	38.6	101.5	40.6	105.1	100	212
36	96.8	38.8	101.8	40.8	105.4		
37	98.6	39.0	102.2	41.0	105.8		

*To convert Centigrade readings to Fahrenheit, multiply by 1.8 and add 32. To convert Fahrenheit readings to Centigrade, subtract 32 and divide by 1.8.

From Vaughan, V. C., III, and McKay, R. J.: *Nelson Textbook of Pediatrics,* 10th ed., Philadelphia, W. B. Saunders Company, 1975, p. 1801.

the parents to the physician who will take the history of the present illness. The child should not be present, for if he is old enough, he will understand and sense his parents' anxiety. Even an infant senses tension and anxiety in his parents.

2. Vital Signs. The nurse takes the vital signs: temperature, pulse, respiration, and, if necessary, blood pressure. A temperature reading per rectum using either a glass or an electronic thermometer should be taken last, since it is likely to make the child cry. Crying influences the respiration and pulse rates, and an accurate record is not obtained. The taking of a rectal temperature represents to some children a real invasion of their bodies. It is important, therefore, to take the temperature rectally only as long as necessary.

Temperature readings may be expressed in either Centigrade or Fahrenheit degrees according to the policy of the agency.

The normal pulse and respiratory rates for children are shown in Figures 5–11 and 5–12.

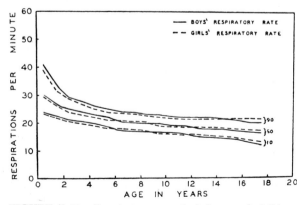

FIGURE 5–11. Respiratory rates in infants and children. (From Vaughan, V. C., III, and McKay, R. J.: *Nelson Textbook of Pediatrics.* 10th ed., Philadelphia, W. B. Saunders Co., 1975, p. 37.)

The middle lines on each figure represent the averages for the various age groups.

The blood pressure is taken if ordered by the physician on admission. Since it is difficult to obtain an accurate blood pressure reading on an infant or small child, the nurse must be careful to use the correct equipment. A large source of error in taking measurements of blood pressure is the use of a cuff of inappropriate width. The cuff should be about the same width in proportion to the arm circumference as that used for the adult or it should cover approximately two thirds of the upper arm. The same cuff should be used for each reading for accuracy. The width of the arm cuff used on children of various ages is as follows:

> Newborns — 2.5 cm.
> 2 weeks to 1 year — 5 cm.
> 1 to 13 years — 9 cm.
> Adult — 13 cm.

The child should be at rest when the blood pressure reading is made. Excitement, discomfort, or distrust of the person taking the reading affects the blood pressure so that an accurate reading cannot be made.

The average normal blood pressure readings for children are as follows:

Age	Systolic	Diastolic
Birth	40	—
1 month	80	—
4 years	85	60
8 years	95	62
12 years	108	67
16 years (boys)	118	75
20 years (boys)	120	75

As can be seen from the foregoing readings, there is a gradual rise in systolic blood pressure in both boys and girls during growth. Diastolic blood pressure rises only slightly over the age

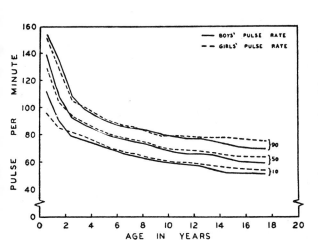

FIGURE 5–12. Pulse rates in infants and children. (From Vaughan, V. C., and McKay, R. J.: *Nelson Textbook of Pediatrics.* 10th ed., Philadelphia, W. B. Saunders Co., 1975, p. 37.)

span from six to 18 years. Until the age of 14 years there seems to be no significant sex difference. After that age the systolic pressure continues to rise in boys, but remains stable in girls. In addition to the age and sex differences in blood pressure readings, there are differences in children who are more mature than others at a given age.

3. Weight. The nurse weighs the child on admission (see p. 379).

4. Examination of the Child. One parent should undress the infant or young child and, if possible, assist with the examination. Every effort should be made by both the physician and the nurse to complete the examination without restraining the child. The nurse may have to help in restraint of an infant or young child, however, during examination of the head (eyes, ears, nose and mouth). During this part of the examination the nurse holds the child with his back against his or her chest. One hand, placed on his forehead, steadies his head, and the other arm restrains his arms. Sometimes it may be necessary to "mummy" (see p. 413) the body and further restrain the child by leaning over his body while placing the hands on either side of his head.

The nurse should speak to the child and caress him in order that restraint may not be frightening to him or to his mother.

5. Procedures. Both the infant and the older child should be prepared for treatments and unpleasant procedures, although they cannot understand the implications. This preparation in an infant may be no more than conditioning him to know that an unpleasant procedure is associated with something which brings comfort. We cannot explain the purpose or the procedure of

sticking a needle into his arm, but we can make it appear as one of the unpleasant things which he has learned to accept as part of a pleasant relation with other people. We talk to him and pet him and let him experience this procedure in a pleasant setting. He should have learned to trust others when unpleasant things are done to him in his routine care (e.g., cleaning his nose). This trust in others carries over from routine care to the unfamiliar experiences in the hospital; he cries from pain, but his fright is decreased. If his mother or a nurse to whom he is accustomed is with him, he applies this generalized experience with unpleasant procedures to this particular incident.

A child in the toddler age group or older should have all procedures which are to be done to him explained in terms he can understand. Listening to the physician's or nurse's heart through the stethoscope is a kind of explanation he understands. Not all procedures can be demonstrated in this way, but the use of such techniques gives the child a basis for understanding the general purpose of examinations and treatments. Picture books, drawings, puppets, and dolls have been used to help a child understand what will be done to him before the examination, treatment or procedure is undertaken. Since verbal explanation may not always be possible, the nurse's presence is needed to provide comfort for the child.

If the child is to have an operation, he may be terrified at the idea of anesthesia. An introduction to the anesthetist and an explanation that anesthesia is a special quiet and safe kind of sleep from which he will wake up may reduce the child's anxiety. Also, if the child can see and examine a face mask, he will not be as afraid as he would if he were not prepared for seeing it at the time of surgery. The young patient should be informed that he may take a favorite stuffed toy or doll to the operating room with him. Such a toy may be a focal point for him that spans the unfamiliar world that he has known.

Boys who have been taught that "Little men do not cry" should be given permission to cry and react to pain when necessary. Such behavior in response to acute discomfort is a normal and desirable reaction.

The postoperative period should be explained to the child prior to surgery. When the child awakens from anesthesia he may be restrained to his crib, he may have bottles of intravenous fluids or blood dangling over him, he may have tubes emerging from his body, he will see strange people in colored uniforms hurrying around the area, and he will feel lost without his parents, who he believes will never find him again. Anxiety or panic as a result of these feelings can be prevented if adequate explanations are given to the child preoperatively.

As he gradually recovers, the child may feel that his physicians and nurses have acted in a hostile manner toward him because they caused him pain, yet he cannot retaliate for fear of losing their love and care. If the child does become anxious and angry about the treatments he is receiving, the nurse can help by encouraging him to work out his feelings by performing the same procedures on his stuffed animal or doll. *Activities which reduce his tension help him to cope with the reality of the situation.*

The nurse who understands and can deal in a positive manner with personal feelings about hurting children will be able to help the child deal with his anxiety. He can develop mastery over his feelings and fantasies if the nurse can discuss them with him and help him to play them out.

If the parents become anxious even though the nurse has explained to them the necessary procedures to be done to their child, they can be informed frequently concerning his progress, his eating, toileting and sleeping habits, and his playroom or school activities.

PARENTS' CONFERENCE WITH THE NURSE OR TEAM LEADER

The Nursing History. An adequate nursing history should be obtained from the parents on admission or within the first 24 hours after admission. Data collection is an extremely important part of the nursing process. The parents may fill out the nursing history sheet, but it is essential that the nurse review it and clarify any unanswered questions. The nurse can also seek additional information based on answers already given. It is of prime importance that the nurse obtain a good data base from which to identify problems and formulate an appropriate individualized nursing care plan for the child and his family as part of the nursing process.

The discussion should center on the parent's child and not on children in general. To emphasize this the nurse should speak of the child by name rather than by some general term such as "baby" or "little boy." Such an approach leads to asking the parents for information about the child which the nurses need in caring for him. This information should be available to the whole health team. Figure 14–1 is an example of one outline used for obtaining such information according to age groups.

The nurse should tell the parents the hours when they will be allowed to visit the child and should explain why it is advisable for them to come as often as possible to see him. If a mother seems reluctant to visit frequently, she may be questioned as to the reason, but should not be made to feel guilty about not visiting. If the mother speaks of needing help which the nurse cannot give, arrangements may be made for her to talk with the physician or, with his permission, the social worker.

It should be explained to the mother that during visiting hours she may help in the child's care. There may be little she can do for a critically ill child, but gradually, as she becomes accustomed to his care and as his condition improves, she will be able to do more for him, e.g., giving him the "potty," bathing or feeding him or changing his diaper. Helping in his nursing care relieves not only the mother's sense of frustration at not being able to do everything for him, but also her sense of guilt if she feels that his sickness was caused by neglect on her part. At the same time she is learning how to give the care he will require after he has gone home.

If the hospital has written policies about visiting hours and regulations as to food, toys, the wearing of gowns and masks, and so on, this should be fully explained to the parents, who should be given a copy of the rules—if the hospital has printed copies—before leaving the pediatric area.

The parents should remain, if possible, until the child is comfortable. If they have permission from the hospital for unlimited visiting hours or if the child is in a private room, all facilities for their comfort should be explained to them: the location of the washroom, smoking room, lounge, public telephone, and the place where they may sleep and have their meals. In the majority of hospitals only breakfast is served to the parents; for their other meals they may go to the cafeteria or snack-bar. To be away from the child for these short periods gives them a needed change of environment.

If the parents intend to remain with the child during treatments, examinations, and the taking of specimens, the purpose of these procedures should be explained to them. *Although the parents may participate in the child's care, the nurse must be responsible for the total nursing care.* With the parents as assistants, the nurse has an opportunity not only to give information but also to help them to understand health teaching which will affect not only the patient but also the entire family. It is an ideal situation, for the parents learn through observation and discussion rather than through formal teaching, which is only indirectly related to the individual child.

On the other hand, when parents remain with

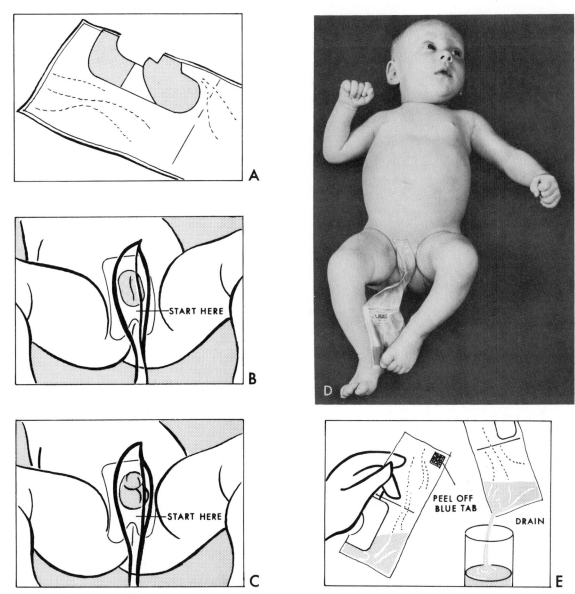

FIGURE 5–13. Hollister's pediatric urine collector for use with both sexes. *A,* Remove protective paper, exposing hypo-allergenic adhesive. *B, For girls:* Stretch perineum to remove skin all around the vagina. Be sure to start at the bridge of skin separating the rectum from the vagina and work upward. *C, For boys:* Fit bag over penis and press flaps firmly to perineum, making sure entire adhesive coating is firmly attached to skin with no puckering of adhesive. *D,* Hollister bag in place. *E, To drain:* Hold bag in left hand. Tilt bag so urine is away from blue tab. Remove tab and drain in clean receptacle. (Courtesy Hollister, Chicago, Illinois.)

their children, the nurses may actually see their patients less often than they would if the parents were not present. This tends to make the parents uncomfortable and displeased with the nursing care given. Specific guidelines for parent-child-nurse interaction and for areas of parental and nursing responsibilities should be formulated in each institution in order to prevent the occurrence of such negative feelings.

NURSING PROCEDURES AFTER ADMISSION OF A CHILD

After admission of a child to the hospital the nurse may need to carry out certain procedures,

including medical aseptic technique, collection of urine specimens, collection of blood specimens and the giving of medications. The collection of specimens of other body fluids such as cerebrospinal fluid, the giving of adequate amounts of fluids orally or parenterally, and other procedures will be discussed later.

Medical Aseptic Technique. The *purpose* of medical aseptic technique is to prevent transmission of infection from one child to another or to the personnel who care for him. It is the joint responsibility of the medical and nursing staffs to plan the procedures and techniques and to carry out medical aseptic patient care.

Medical aseptic technique is necessary whenever the patient and his belongings are considered contaminated. Those who care for him are considered to be clean when they enter his unit, but to become contaminated when they touch him or his equipment.

The *isolation unit* is an area, cubicle, room, or part of a unit in which one or more patients having the same infectious disease are given care. The furnishings in an isolation unit should be simple, as few as possible for the comfort of the patient and easily cleaned. There should be sufficient equipment for the patient's care, but excess articles should not be kept in the same area. The amount of equipment will depend upon the child's age, the kind of infection and the number of patients isolated in the unit. All furniture, the sink, walls, floor, and equipment are considered contaminated in such a unit. The area where the gown is hung is contaminated, but the inside of the gown is kept clean. A damp cloth or a wet mop is used in cleaning the room to prevent organisms from being dispersed in the air. Bedside equipment should be sterilized at regular intervals while the patient is in an isolation unit.

Admission of a patient to an isolation unit involves a number of procedures. It is customary to send the child's clothes home and give the parents instructions as to disinfection or sterilization by airing them, washing them thoroughly or boiling whatever can be sterilized in this way.

Each patient should have his own equipment, such as a thermometer and bathing equipment, in his unit. Toys brought to the hospital with the child should be of the sort that can be easily cleaned; they should be tied to the bed so they cannot drop to the floor. Care must be taken that the string or tape tying the toys to the crib cannot become twisted around the child's neck.

Visiting an isolated patient is permitted because of the importance of preserving parent-child relations. Parents must observe certain precautions, however, for their own safety and that of the child. They should be given instructions about visiting regulations for such patients. It is a good plan to have these instructions printed in order that parents may read them when they are at home and the initial anxiety over the child's hospitalization is passed.

When parents visit, they must wear isolation gowns. The parents must be supervised during visiting hours to prevent their breaking the prescribed hospital technique.

Gown and handwashing techniques are time-consuming, but are important factors in medical aseptic technique. Anyone who gives direct care involving close contact with a child must wear a gown to protect clothing from contamination.

The nurse should not give care to isolated patients if there are abrasions on the nurse's hands, since they cannot be cleansed thoroughly. Furthermore, if the patient has an infection which can be contracted through a break in the skin, the nurse might become infected with the organism.

The policies on gown and handwashing techniques adopted by the hospital or other agency should be followed by everyone coming in contact with the patient.

Mask technique is important, since infectious disease is commonly spread through droplet spray from the nose and mouth, the portals through which respiratory infection is most likely to enter the body. The wearing of masks is a controversial topic, however; some physicians believe masks to be of value, but others believe them to be ineffective. If a mask is worn, it should cover both the nose and the mouth to prevent (1) spreading of organisms present in the spray of the nose and throat of the wearer, and (2) inhalation of infectious material in the air about a patient suffering from a respiratory infection. A mask should be worn once and then discarded, for it is readily contaminated by the constant passage of air through its meshes, which trap bacteria. A mask should never be dropped loosely around the neck and then drawn up into position over the nose and mouth.

Concurrent disinfection is the destruction of pathogenic organisms carried out continuously while the child is isolated. Such articles as dishes, clothing, bedding and equipment for treatment must be disinfected. Any articles brought out of the room which were used by or have touched a patient must be disinfected before being used for another patient. Specific directions for disinfection are usually outlined by the hospital and are influenced by sewer facilities in the area.

Terminal disinfection means making the physical environment and the body of the child *clean* so that infection cannot be conveyed to others after he has ceased to be a source of infection.

Collection of Urine Specimens. Urine specimens are usually requested on admission. Collection of such specimens from older children who can cooperate with either the nurse or the mother is relatively easy, but is more difficult from infants.

The collection of urine specimens from infants involves the application of a collecting device to the perineum. Pediatric urine collectors are made of clear, pliable, plastic material

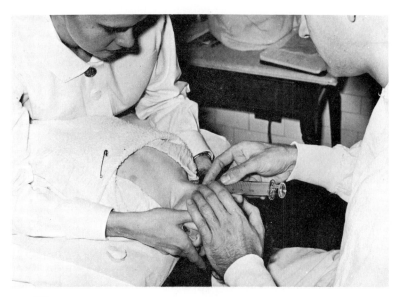

FIGURE 5–14. Procedure for the collection of a blood specimen from the external jugular vein. The "mummy restraint" (see p. 413) is used. The child's head is rotated fully to one side and extended partly over the end of the table to stretch the vein. The nurse places the palm of one hand over the occiput, the fingers of the other hand over the bones of the face. The nurse must avoid making pressure over the child's nose or mouth.

secured to a sponge ring (Fig. 5–13). After the skin has been cleaned and dried this sponge ring, coated with pressure-sensitive adhesive, is attached firmly around the genitalia. When the child voids, the plastic receptacle can be removed easily. The adhesive surfaces can be pressed together and the specimen sent in the leak-proof bag thus formed to the laboratory.

Since catheterization is rarely ordered on infants or small children, physicians usually request that a clean urine specimen be obtained. In order to obtain a clean specimen from an infant or small child the genitalia should be cleaned, using cotton balls wet with sterile soap and water and then rinsed with an antiseptic solution. When washing the female genitalia, it is important that a different cotton ball be used for each stroke made from above the clitoris downward to the anus. The strokes should cleanse the meatus first, then move outward to the perineum. After cleaning the genitalia thoroughly, a plastic urine collector should be applied as described above.

To obtain a clean specimen from a preschool or older child who can cooperate, cleanse the genitalia as described above. A girl can sit on a training chair beneath which is a sterile potty or basin, or she may void into a sterile bedpan. A boy may void into a sterile urinal or directly into the sterile specimen bottle.

Although a midstream specimen is likely to be cleaner than the urine voided initially, such a specimen is difficult to obtain from small children. If the child is able to cooperate, have him void a small amount into an unsterile container, and then void into a sterile receptacle.

The collection of a continuous or 24-hour urine specimen are discussed later.

Collection of Blood Specimens. Blood specimens are obtained for determination of the degree of illness, for diagnosis, or for evaluation of therapy.

The procedure used for adult patients is used for older children whose veins are large enough and who are able to cooperate after an explanation of the procedure has been given them. In infants and young children whose veins are small only the larger veins may be used, most commonly the femoral or external jugular veins. Since infants and small children cannot understand a verbal explanation, mummy restraint is used, and the procedure is completed as soon as possible. The assistance of the nurse in drawing blood shortens the procedure because the physician can locate the vein with more ease.

The nurse's responsibility is to restrain the child's head during jugular puncture (Fig. 5–14) or the legs during femoral puncture (Fig. 5–15).

After the needle has been removed from the jugular vein, firm pressure should be exerted over the vein for three to five minutes while the child is held in a sitting position. After femoral vein puncture firm pressure should be exerted over the vein, also for three to five minutes, in order to prevent leakage of blood into the subcutaneous tissues. While the infant is restrained, it is important that the nurse make comforting sounds during the procedure and that the infant be held or rocked after the procedure. Small children can be encouraged to play out their anger and frustration caused by the pain of the needle insertion after the procedure has been completed.

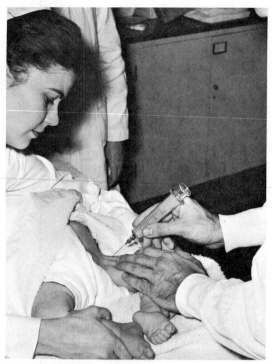

FIGURE 5–15. Procedure for the collection of a blood specimen from the femoral vein. The "mummy restraint" is used over the upper part of the child's body. The nurse spreads the child's legs apart in a frog position and holds them securely. The infant's genitalia are covered with a diaper.

Medications. The giving of medications to a child is a serious responsibility. The need for accuracy in pouring and giving medications is even greater than with adult patients. The dose varies with the size, surface area, and age of the child, and the nurse has no standard dose as is customary for adult patients. Since the dose is relatively small, a slight mistake in the amount of a drug given makes a greater proportional error in terms of the amount ordered than with the adult dose.

Every hospital has its own method of identification for patients. Identification is necessary with all patients, but is more difficult with children. The infant cannot give his name, and a small child is likely to give his nickname or only his first name. The nurse must carefully identify a child before giving him medication. Most hospitals use wristbands for identifying children, and the child's name is also marked upon his bed. A double check on the child who is out of bed and old enough to tell is to ask him his name. (The nurse should never say, "Are you Alice Jones?" but should ask, "What is your name?") The child's name is checked with that on the medicine card, as is done in giving medication to adult patients.

The nurse should give all medications in a way that helps to establish a constructive relation with the child. To tell a child that a medicine will taste good when it tastes bad destroys a child's faith in nurses.

Since the possibility of error is greater in the giving of medication to children than to adults, and since a child's reaction to a dose ordered by a physician is less predictable than an adult's reaction, the nurse must be alert to recognize undesirable effects of the medication given.

DRUG DOSAGE.   Since most drugs are put up by drug companies in a convenient form or strength for a standard adult dose, children's doses are often computed in terms of fractions of the adult dose on the basis of age or weight. Although the physician prescribes the dosage of medication, the nurse should have a general knowledge of the relation between the customary adult dose and that for children in different age groups from infancy through childhood.

Many hospitals are presently using "unit dose," a medication system that can save nursing time by having the exact doses of medication prepared by the pharmacist. It is still important, however, for the nurse to know the usually prescribed pediatric doses.

Dosages based on the child's weight or body surface area give the most accurate results. Although the nurse does not decide the dosage to be given the child, he or she must be alert to amounts of drugs customarily ordered by the physicians. If an amount ordered seems to be excessive, this fact should be called to the attention of the physician.

The nurse may locate the rules for calculating drug dosages for children in pharmacology books and pediatric medical textbooks, as well as the recommended dosages of specific drugs in literature supplied by drug companies or from sources such as the *Physician's Desk Reference.*

The nurse should know the expected action of the drug as well as the appropriate dose commonly ordered for a child the size of the patient. The nurse should also be alert to symptoms of overdosage, since the child usually does not complain, and report such symptoms at once to the physician so that quick action can be taken to counteract the effects of the drug.

ORAL ADMINISTRATION.   Infants will generally accept medication put into their mouths, provided it is in a form which they can readily swallow. The medication should be given slowly in order to prevent choking. The nurse should sit down and hold the infant, or, if he cannot be removed from his crib, raise him to a sitting position, or, if this contraindicated, elevate his head

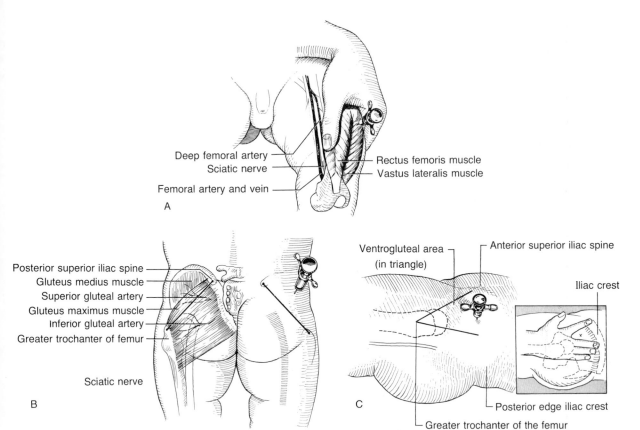

FIGURE 5–16. Intramuscular injections may be given at different sites, depending on the size and age of the child, the condition of the muscle mass, and the type of medication used. *A*, The vastus lateralis, because it is well-developed at birth and because it is not close to major nerves and vessels, is chosen in very young children. *B*, After the child has been walking for about a year, the gluteal muscles are well enough developed to be used as an injection site. *C*, The ventrogluteal site, easily accessible from all positions and containing no important nerves or vessels, is frequently recommended for intramuscular injections in children. (From Brandt, P. A., Smith, M. E., Ashburn, S. S., and Graves, J.: IM injections in children. *Am J. Nursing*, 72:1402, August, 1972.)

and shoulders. There is then less danger of his choking.

The toddler especially may rebel at taking oral medications. The nurse can help the young child to gain control of his behavior by holding him initially and, through faith in his ability to cooperate, encourage him by saying, "It is hard for you to take this medicine now, but soon you will be able to take it yourself." As the child learns to cooperate, he will slowly regain the sense of autonomy he lost when he became ill and raise his level of self-esteem.

The older child, because he is unhappy in the hospital or has had experience with bad-tasting medicines, may refuse his medication. There is no single technique for winning his cooperation. The nurse must study the situation and find the best way to get him to take the medication. The nurse's manner should be positive, firm, and kind. When the nurse gives a child a feeling of support, that his dislike of the medication is understood and that his cooperation would be appreciated, he is conditioned to take the medication. The nurse must convey in manner rather than in words that he *must take the medication.* The child should never be begged or coaxed. Children will cooperate more readily if they see other children taking medicine.

More specifically, if the older child refuses to take his medicine, he should be allowed to choose, if possible, between taking it in pill or liquid form. Also, he should be encouraged to select the kind of fluid he would like to take as a "chaser" and to hold the cup or glass as he drinks. Independence is important to the growing child. If he is given some measure of control in a situation, he will cooperate to the extent of his ability.

If the child is encouraged to talk about his feelings about medications and if the nurse accepts his feelings honestly along with any suggestions the parents have to make about the situation, a solution may be found to this problem.

TABLE 5–2. CONVERSION OF APOTHECARY'S MEASURES TO METRIC EQUIVALENTS

Weights

Apothecary	Metric Approximate	Metric More Nearly Accurate
1 grain.............................. 60 mg	0.06 gm	0.06479 gm
2 grains............................ 120 mg	0.12 gm	
3 grains............................ 180 mg	0.2 gm	
5 grains............................ 300 mg	0.3 gm	
15 grains.........................1000 mg	1.0 gm	
60 grains or 1 dram............................	4.0 gm	3.888 gm
240 grains or 4 drams, ½ oz....................	15.0 gm	
480 grains or 8 drams, 1 oz....................	30.0 gm	31.103 gm
		31.103 gm (Troy)
		28.350 gm (Avoir.)
12 oz or 1 pound....................360.0 gm		373.24177 gm
12 oz or 1 pound....................360.0 gm		373.24177 gm (Troy)
16 oz or 1 pound....................480.0 gm		453.592 gm (Avoir.)
¾ grain.......................... 45 mg		
½ grain.......................... 30 mg		
⅜ grain.......................... 23 mg		
¼ grain.......................... 15 mg		
⅙ grain.......................... 10 mg		
⅛ grain.......................... 8 mg		
1/10 grain........................ 6 mg		
1/16 grain........................ 4 mg		
1/32 grain........................ 2 mg		
1/64 grain........................ 1 mg		
1/100 grain....................... 0.6 mg		
1/250 grain....................... 0.25 mg		
1/300 grain....................... 0.2 mg		
1/1000 grain...................... 0.06 mg		

Liquid Measures

	Approximate	More Nearly Accurate
1 minim..........................	0.06 ml	0.06161 ml
3 minims.........................	0.2 ml	
15 minims........................	1.0 ml	0.92415 ml *
60 minims, 1 fl. dram............	4.0 ml	3.6967 ml
480 minims 1 fl oz..............	30.0 ml	29.5737 ml
16 fl oz or 1 pt........	500.0 ml	473.179 ml
32 fl oz or 1 qt........	1000.0 ml	946.358 ml

*1 ml is equal to 16.23 minims.

Quantity of drug prescribed in grams per 2 ounces (60 ml) gives dose in grains per dram.

From Vaughan, V. C., III, and McKay, R. J.: *Nelson Textbook of Pediatrics*, 10th ed., Philadelphia, W. B. Saunders Company, 1975, p. 1801.

Many liquid drugs are mixed by the drug companies in flavored syrups. If they are not, it is a good plan to disguise the taste of a drug by putting it in cherry syrup, Karo, or honey syrup. Pills should be crushed and the contents of capsules emptied and mixed with syrup for children too young to take bulk medication. In general, medications should not be mixed with milk or food unless specifically ordered by the physician, because the child might develop a serious dislike for that food.

Medication can be given from a medicine glass, the tip of a teaspoon or a rubber-tipped medicine dropper. Fluid medications may be sucked through bright-colored straws.

The nurse should be careful not to let personal distaste for a drug show in facial expressions, for the child will quickly adopt this attitude toward his medication.

If a child always struggles when medication is given him and his cooperation cannot be obtained, the nurse should report this to the physician. To struggle may do the child more harm than to go without his medicine. The nurse should never hold the child's nose or force the medication into his mouth, for he may aspirate the medication. Such action shows that the nurse is hostile and not helpful to the child.

If the medication is immediately vomited, the physician should be notified. Orders may be given for the dose to be repeated. Unpleasant-tasting drugs should not be given around mealtime, for they may interfere with the child's appetite.

The child is usually old enough to take pills by the age of four to six years; however, children as young as two years of age can be taught to swallow pills. The child should be told to place the pill near the back of his tongue and to drink the water, fruit juice, or milk offered him in order to wash down the pill.

A child who cooperates in taking his medicine should be praised and thereby will know that this nurse appreciates his help.

INTRAMUSCULAR INJECTIONS. The giving of the first intramuscular injection is important, because on the basis of this experience the child builds up his attitude toward future injections. The procedure using either an intramuscular needle and syringe or the jet injector is the same as for the adult.

If the child is old enough to understand, the procedure should be explained to him. He should be allowed to express his fear and resentment of needles. The child of school age and the adolescent, like the little child, should be allowed to vent their feelings of dislike or resentment.

Prior to giving an injection the nurse should spend time with the child and develop a degree of rapport with him. Then the procedure should be carried out quickly and gently. It is a good plan to have a second nurse assist, to support or restrain the child, or both. One technique helpful when giving an intramuscular injection is to provide a diversionary action by offering the child something else on which he can fix his attention. He could hold someone's hand and squeeze it when he feels the needle stick, or he could lie prone and concentrate on pointing his toes inward. By pointing his toes inward the gluteal muscles relax and the injection into the buttock is less painful. Since the injection is painful to some degree, the nurse must help him master his feeling about such necessary forms of treatment.

The upper outer quadrant of the buttocks may be used as the site for injecting medication intramuscularly; however, because serious trauma can result from administering injections incorrectly into the buttocks, many hospitals now recommend the use of the muscle in the anterolateral aspect of the thigh. If the child has sufficiently large muscles on other parts of the body, the injection site should be varied. The length of the needle used for intramuscular injections is important; it should be long enough so that the medication is given deeply into the muscle tissue in order to be absorbed properly.

After the procedure the nurse should show

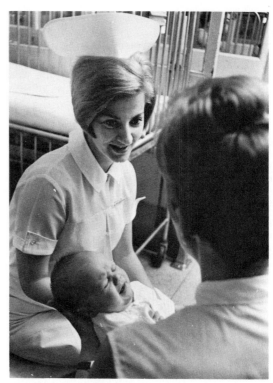

FIGURE 5–17. Discharge of a child from the pediatric unit to his parents' care requires explicit instructions given during the period of hospitalization. The calm, secure attitude of the nurse helps the mother feel more certain of her own ability to care for the child at home. (Public Relations Department, The Children's Hospital of Philadelphia.)

her approval of the infant or child for his cooperation and hold him for a few minutes so that he does not associate only pain with this ministration. He may then be given some toy to divert his attention from the experience. If he has been uncooperative, the nurse should not show disapproval. He too should be held and comforted and then given a toy.

An older child may be allowed to select the site for injection, subject to the nurse's approval, and cleanse the area for himself.

When the nurse charts medications, the site of injection is noted. This is especially important for those children who require frequent injections.

INTRAVENOUS ADMINISTRATION. Nurses in some hospitals are permitted to insert medications into bottles of intravenous solutions to be given to children. This procedure requires the utmost care for the safety of the patient. Since the policy varies in agencies, it is essential that the student be aware of the rule regarding the practice of adding medications to intravenous fluids in the hospital where this experience is gained, for the student's own safety as well as that of the children for whom care is being given.

RECTAL ADMINISTRATION. Drugs given by rectum are injected in the same manner as a retention enema. The medication may be mixed with a little water or a small amount of starch solution. It should be given slowly so that all of it is retained.

Some medications to be given rectally are also available in suppository form. In explaining this procedure to a young child it can be likened to the experience he has already had of having a rectal temperature taken. When giving a rectal suppository the nurse should open its covering immediately before inserting it. Finger cots on the thumb and index finger or a disposable glove may be used in order to insert the suppository beyond the anal sphincter. The buttocks should be held firmly together for a few minutes after insertion until the desire to expel the suppository has passed.

The Nursing Process in the Care of the Pediatric Patient

The nursing process or planning for and implementation of the plan of nursing care for an individual child or client within his family constellation and cultural background are the responsibilities of the nurse (see Chapter 3). The nursing team's understanding of the basic nursing care of children, the level of the specific child's growth and development, the knowledge concerning his illness, the goals of the health team in diagnosis and therapy, the scientific process involved in problem solving, and the kinds of observations to be made are essential as a basis for changing the plan according to changes in the needs of the child. Some of these important aspects of care are discussed in this chapter, while others are investigated throughout this textbook.

OBSERVATION OF CHILDREN

The use of observation as a means of understanding children has value for those who would work sensitively and effectively with them. Each human being has certain basic and pervasive qualities that set him apart from all others. These qualities, resulting from a dynamic interaction between his inherent nature and his total environment, are apparent very early in life. An observer can become skillful in interpreting the language of behavior through his observations of actions, gestures, facial expressions, language, and the timing of daily activities of others. Each person who observes will develop his own techniques and style of description and interpretation of behavior; however, some suggestions might be helpful in this area.

A child is most unaffected and natural when he is unaware of being watched. Since everything a child does has meaning, the observer should accurately and completely note everything he says and how he acts, everything that is done or said to him, and every facial expression, gesture and movement he makes. These notes should be rewritten in full soon after the observations are made. A conscientious nurse will be aware of personal and cultural prejudices and will do everything possible to overcome evident biases. The nurse also observes a child's behavior with an open mind that is accepting and interested and not judgmental or condemning. The nurse should review the steps for observation as given in Chapter 2.

Since the child's behavior constantly changes during health or illness, the purpose of the nurse observer is to discover clues about his physical and emotional status and behavior. The nurse who develops observational skills will be able to utilize them in providing better care for pediatric patients.

SAFETY MEASURES

Accidents are a leading cause of death among infants and small children. Great emphasis should be placed on the prevention of accidents in the hospital, both for the safety of the child and in order that parents may have a practical demonstration of how accidents common to little children may be avoided. The following discussion is concerned chiefly with accidents in the hospital, but certain of these also occur in the home.

Many safety measures deal with the construction of the building or unit and are beyond the control of the nurse. Among these are the following:

1. Fireproof, wide stairways.
2. Windows protected by locked screens and window guards and so placed that drafts do not blow upon the children when the windows are open for ventilation.
3. Gates at the entrance to rooms where small children play, so constructed that a child cannot open them or catch his fingers between the door and its frame.

Other measures for children's safety which are directly under the nurse's control are as follows:
1. The catches on the side gates of the crib should be in good condition, and the gates should always be up when the child is in bed. When administering care with the side

gate down, the nurse should keep one hand on the infant or little child to prevent his falling, especially when looking away from him or reaching for an object on the bedside table. For children who have been placed in cribs and do not require jacket restraints, the use of "bumper pads" gives them the freedom of crawling around without the danger of being caught between the mattress and the crib sides. Also, the use of a plastic bubble top on a toddler's crib will permit him to stand up but not to climb out of his crib.

2. Restraints, if used, should be applied correctly to prevent constriction of any part of the child's body. The greatest danger is that of strangulation through pressure of a jacket restraint which has slipped out of place and encircled a patient's neck.

3. Medicine cabinets should be locked when not in use, and medications should *never* be left standing on a bedside table.

4. Instruments and solutions should be kept in cabinets or on shelves where children cannot reach them.

5. *Safety pins should be closed* at once when taken from a child's clothing and put out of his reach. An infant or young child tends to put small objects into his mouth.

6. Toys should have rounded rather than sharp edges. They should never be painted with lead paint and should not have small parts which a child could remove and swallow or aspirate. Toys should never be left on the floor, since a child or a nurse who is carrying a child might trip over them. For the same reason, wet areas on the floors should be dried immediately.

7. Infants and small children should not be allowed to play with tongue depressors or applicators.

8. Electric outlets and fans should be covered when not in use, and the fans should be placed where children cannot reach them.

9. Isolation techniques should be carried out on all children with infectious illnesses. For this to be practicable, adequate facilities must be available for hand washing after caring for each child. All other isolation procedures to prevent cross-infection must be rigidly followed. In the children's units of some hospitals ultraviolet rays are used to cut down the number of airborne organisms. The nurse must be aware of symptoms indicating the onset of infectious disease in children and adults. Such symptoms should be promptly reported.

10. Nursing bottles should *never* be propped, *nor should feedings be forced* upon a little child. There is danger of aspiration, which may cause pulmonary disease or even sudden death.

11. In giving medication to an infant or a little child who will not cooperate, a second nurse is required to assist in gentle restraint. Oily medications should *never* be given orally to a child who is crying, because of the danger of aspiration (see p. 403).

12. Hot-water bottles must always be tightly stoppered and covered before being placed near a child's body or even in the bed with him. The water temperature should not be over 115° F. (46.1° C.).

13. The bulb of a thermometer should be checked to be certain that it is not cracked. If the temperature is taken rectally, the nurse must hold the thermometer in place so that it will not be dislodged and so that the child will not injure himself if he rolls over.

DISCHARGE FROM THE HOSPITAL

The physician or nurse, or psychiatrist if he is attached to the health team, should tell the parents that it is natural for an infant, or even an older child, when taken home, to show symptoms of a disturbed relation with his parents. He may be more clinging and seek more affection than before hospitalization, but the reverse may also be true, and he may withdraw from or even reject his parents. He may show his need for comfort by sucking his thumb excessively or reverting to behaviorisms which he had outgrown. His parents must accept this regression as the result of the emotional trauma produced by his separation from them and must help him to regain the normal parent-child relations by their unwavering affection.

Discharge of a child from the pediatric unit to his parents' care requires explicit instructions, especially if his mother has not stayed with him during his hospitalization. *These instructions should be given gradually during the hospitalization instead of on the day of discharge, since the parents are usually too excited to comprehend what they are being told.* Important among these are instructions in the use of any specific equipment needed in his care at home, and in the giving of medications; review of the physician's orders; time of the next clinic or physician's appointment; and description of new habits which the child has acquired since his mother last cared for him—e.g., drinking from a cup or eating from a spoon—or new developments in muscular activity. If an infant has learned to roll over, it is important that his parents know it in order to protect him from falling. These new habits change not only the parents' image of the child, but also the way in which care is given.

NURSING CARE OF THE CHRONICALLY OR TERMINALLY ILL CHILD AND HIS FAMILY

Usually when a child has a short-term illness with presumably a good outcome, the parents may be anxious, but their anxiety is not that generally felt by parents of a chronically ill child or a child having a terminal illness.

The Care of the Chronically Ill Child

The role of the nurse in helping parents deal with the problem of caring for a chronically ill child such as one having cerebral palsy, poliomyelitis, diabetes, rheumatic fever or some other long-term illness is more complex than that of one caring for an acutely ill child.

Lengthy illness during childhood tends to interfere with the healthy course of the child's development, both physically and emotionally.

The child's need for continuing attention and care makes it extremely difficult for him to achieve his goal in his struggle toward maturity and emotional independence. If the parents are not cognizant of this problem, the child will possibly remain dependent and socially immature. Prolonged illness is likely to prevent the child from developing a confidence in his own abilities and a sense of acceptability to his peer group.

Nurses must help parents to understand that they should give the chronically ill child as many of the normal experiences of childhood as possible and by so doing help the child to acquire a positive, healthy attitude toward growing up emotionally and becoming a mature adult. In order to do this successfully parents need to understand the nature of the child's illness, his treatment, and the exact limitations the condition places on his activities. Most important, parents and child should understand what the child *can* do as well as what he *cannot* do. Only by exercising his own abilities will the child be able to attain a sense of usefulness and competence.

Parents also should understand how their own reactions to the child's illness, such as great overconcern about his health status, may be a hindrance rather than a help to the child's recovery. Their positive view of his illness will help the child to accept his own limitations and strive to improve his abilities.

The Nurse and the Terminally Ill Child

For most people, even medical and nursing personnel, the phenomenon of death is a difficult event to face. It is not only difficult for the experienced professional to face, but it is also difficult to help the inexperienced nurse learn in pediatrics to help both the dying child and his grieving parents. Although words can be written on "what you should do in a particular situation," this kind of information is not likely to be of much assistance in a practical event in which the individual becomes involved. For this reason our discussion of death will concern first the perception of death, then in sequence how the nurse perceives death, what the physician can do, how the parents feel, the meaning of death to a child, and finally the role of the nurse in the care of the terminally ill child and his family.

THE PERCEPTION OF DEATH

Death is an inevitable and universal experience. But in our American culture, where the emphasis is on life, especially youthful life, the denial of how death occurs is common.

During the education of the nurse, however, death in general is gradually perceived as a natural event in life, one that in many instances is a positive phenomenon in that it relieves the patient of intolerable pain and long-lasting incapacity. Those who are religiously inclined see death as being controlled by a supernatural power, that is in fact "God's will," and is the beginning of a new life, whether this includes the idea of eternal reward or punishment or not.

Whether the nurse believes that death is a natural event or a supernaturally controlled moment in time, the belief that some control can be exerted must still be held, otherwise the lifesaving equipment readily available in hospitals would not be used. Even in hospitals controlled by religious groups, nurses tend to believe that God approves their attempt to alleviate discomfort and to prolong life.

Since death itself is an end that comes to all living things, the nurse is bound, in spite of frequent encounters with the event, in spite of religious or secular orientation, and in spite of knowledge of its causes, to have some degree of anxiety about the situation for the patient and for himself or herself. *The fear of death is the most inescapable of all the fears faced by the living.*

The way in which the event of death has been handled in many hospitals has been to remove the dying person, conscious or unconscious, to an area away from other patients. What this means to the conscious patient is that at the very time he needs people around him, he is left alone. Is it any wonder, then, that the older dying child becomes depressed? Do we do this really for the dying patient and his family's comfort, or do we do this because the unit personnel are more comfortable if they cannot see him?

The best way to improve care for the dying patient is to determine the significance of death to the person, whether nurse, physician, parents or client.

THE NURSING STUDENT PERCEIVES DEATH

The attitude of nursing students toward death is dependent on their culture, age, religion, education, perspective on living, and their own inner security. Because of their youth they have not usually had the experience with life and death that an older person generally has had. Because of their own youth and dreams of a family, students are especially vulnerable when seeing a family tragedy involving a child. This is especially difficult in pediatric nursing, where the age of the dying child may not be too far from their own age or possibly from that of one of their siblings. The student may feel as others have felt when caring for a dying child:

"I was panicky. I just knew I couldn't handle the situation alone."

"I prayed that Mary would not die while I was in the room with her. I wanted to run away."

"Jimmy was such a beautiful little boy. I cried until 3 a.m. each day I took care of him."

"After Bridget died I wondered whether I could have done any more for her. I wondered whether I could ever go through this with a child of my own or even if I wanted any children if I might have to face this."

Every student's individual reactions to death are influenced by people and significant events of the past. These influences do not stop even when a young person becomes a graduate nurse. Often a nursing student's or young graduate nurse's first contact with death is clouded by fear and an intense feeling of inadequacy. *It is important, therefore, for the nurse to recognize his or her own feelings and inadequacies and to work through them sufficiently so that he or she is able to give care to the dying child and his family.*

Since the orientation as a nurse is to save life, even an experienced nurse may be ill at ease in talking with and caring for the dying child. Perhaps this is because the nurse has never had to face the prospect of "nonbeing" personally, therefore emotional disturbance may be felt when death is faced with someone else.

It is possible for both the nurse and the physician to protect themselves from the subject of death by developing a shell around themselves, to pretend that death does not occur or that it is not their concern. Some professional persons insulate this shell to the point of callousness. But though this attitude protects the nurse from suffering, it does nothing to help the child and his parents to face the event that is to come.

The first step nursing students must take is to engage in introspection concerning their beliefs about death and about dying patients. They must understand and perhaps alter their attitudes toward the process of dying. To do this they may need help from an instructor, a religious counselor, a psychiatrist or another member of the health team. Introspection is difficult and painful, but a necessary part of the educational process. At this time students must have their religious convictions supported and their reservoir of emotional strength refilled. They must remember that they can and must be helped to understand and handle their own feelings more effectively, for only by so doing can they give emotional support to the child and his parents and share in their grief as feeling persons.

The nurse must be cognizant of the fact that during the process of the child's dying, closeness to the parents involves him or her in a crisis situation in which personal problems are stimulated by those of the parents. The nurse may become vulnerable as the parents' problems bring to the foreground personal internal conflicts. The nurse in this situation cannot support the parents without having these personal needs recognized and met. As long as the nurse is unable to accept grief realistically, he or she will be able to do nothing but inhibit the expression of grief in the parents. But if the nurse can learn to recognize his or her own underlying feelings rather than negate them, fears can be handled and what the child and parents are saying can actually be heard.

Conversation with the dying child and his parents is difficult. The child may be emaciated or disfigured. Some parents are very demanding, and the nurse may respond with anger. Some children are very likable, and the nurse may be grief-stricken by the thought of their death.

It is unfortunate when the child's and family's needs are overlooked and the needs of the nurse take precedence. The nurse should appreciate the fact that his or her attitude is of vital importance in this situation and seek to resolve personal anxieties before entering into this experience.

What the Physician Can Do

Death in an elderly person may be welcomed by the patient and his family because it puts an end to pain and disability. The family is comforted by the knowledge that the person has had a long life and has made some contribution to society. But the death of a child is unacceptable to physicians and everyone else involved. The death of a child from a congenital anomaly incompatible with life or from an automobile accident may come quickly; that from leukemia or a malignant brain tumor usually comes slowly and brings sheer agony not only to the family but to the entire pediatric unit community as well.

The physician has a responsibility for all patients to sustain life until no longer able to do so. A great deal is currently being written about the problem of when death really occurs for an individual patient. The important thing is that the nurse know of the research and philosophical exploration currently taking place concerning this problem.

The physician, in addition to medical therapy, must decide with the help of other members of the health and nursing teams whether or not the parents and child should be told that death is to be expected. Some physicians believe that parents should be told because it is their right to know what is happening to their child. The physician can tell them about the disease condition affecting their child, that nothing known presently in medical therapy can save their child's life, but that he will be protected from pain and suffering as much as possible. Even when told the truth in this manner, the family must be left with a little ray of hope. Even in malignancy in children there have been just enough unexplained remissions to justify leaving them with a little hope. Usually parents will ask the physician, "How long will he live?" or, "Can he return to school?" The physician can try to answer these questions honestly, but the answers understandably are difficult to formulate.

Most physicians realize the help the religious advisor can give at this time. With the parents' knowledge, they may invite a priest, minister, or rabbi to be present during this discussion of their child's illness. For physicians as well as nurses know that if the parents can lean on their religious advisor with confidence, they can support the child better than can the medical and nursing personnel alone.

If an older child asks the physician, "Am I going to die?" this is an even more difficult question to answer than those of the parents. If the child is very stable and mature, some physicians will say, "Yes, but we are not certain when this will be." Children many times can accept this answer better than they can an evasion. If they are old enough to ask this question, they probably have given it a great deal of thought already.

Other physicians believe that the knowledge of death by the parents and the child can only produce more anxiety and that it removes any hope to which they can cling. Actually, no general answer can be given to this question for all families. It is not even clear-cut on many occasions in an individual family.

How the Parents May Feel

Few human experiences bring with them more suffering to parents than the death of their child. If the parents are told that their child cannot live, they tend to feel limited in their ability to control the situation, and they feel trapped. They are about to lose a loved child and may react stoically or with fear, anger, regression, or denial.

Nurses may feel that parents who know the prognosis are being "good" parents when they accept the fact of death gracefully, cause no trouble on the pediatric unit, and are able to provide support for their child. If the family believes in God, they know that He is omnipotent and also that the child's fate is in His hands. Thus they are relieved of their own personal guilt and responsibility.

If the parents lose control, are demanding of the nurses' time, are angry and cry, they are likely to prevent the nurses from performing well with the child and to evoke strong feelings among medical and nursing personnel. Such parents may be avoided at a time when they themselves are most lonely and afraid. The health team members may need to have discussions about their own feelings and reactions in such a situation in order to be able to give the parents the support they need.

Some parents seem devoid of affect after being told that their child will die. They talk about the coming death with what appears to be a minimum of feeling. At that time they seem to have a lack of emotion, or a dissociation between emotion and mind and body.

Some parents, because of their own feelings of guilt and anxiety, try to satisfy the child's every whim. They feel that being permissive will prevent frustration in the child and provide a pleasant environment for his last days on earth. Actually, this behavior causes the child to regress to an excessively demanding state in which his desires become insatiable. Even the parents eventually react with hostility to such a change in their child. And so a vicious cycle is begun. The parent, knowing of his hostility toward the child, feels increasingly guilty, sets fewer limits on the child's behavior, observes increasing demands by the child, and tries even harder to satisfy these demands. The child, feeling the hostility of the parents, becomes even more insecure and demanding. The child may ultimately suffer more from the hostility of the parents thus engendered than he would have done had consistent limits been set and maintained.

Families after the initial shock may want to know whether they can have a Christmas or a birthday celebration early for the terminally ill child. If the patient is very young and without siblings, this may be done. But if he is older and does not know the seriousness of his illness, he may wonder why these celebrations are being held early. Besides, he may be alive when the events occur naturally, and he may be further confused.

If everything medically possible has been done for the child, the physician may ask the parents to help to decide whether to have the child stay in the hospital or to take him home for the remainder of his life. This decision may be based on the presence of other children in the family, the ability of the parents to care for him, and the resources of the family in terms of financial ability and housing. If the child is sent home, the aid of the members of the health team in the community, such as the public health nurse, could be very supportive and helpful to the family.

The Meaning of Death to the Child

As with other aspects of a child's normal growth and development, when he becomes older he changes in his understanding of himself and of the world in which he lives. In like manner he changes his concepts of life and death. Parents cannot really succeed in trying to keep children naive about the fact of death. The best that parents can do is to act naturally in relation to the subject, answer his questions, and thus gradually acquaint the child with this aspect of life.

To a child in the preschool period the idea of death as a physical fact is beyond his understanding. A dead person to a small child is one who has gone away as on a trip, but who may eventually return. To a young child, although the dead person he sees may not move, he still lives. Death does not usually frighten a very young child, although if he himself is very ill he may be frightened because of his excessive bleeding or difficult respirations. What frightens him when someone he loves dies is the fact that he has been left alone, that he has been separated from a source of security and love.

Often the young child will have his first real experience with death when a pet dies. At this time he learns that the pet does not return, and he grieves, but in most instances a new pet is obtained and life continues on hardly interrupted.

When the child is about five or six years of age he begins to accept the fact of death, but believes that death has a gradual process to it, that the dead person can return to life, then die again. As in other developmental stages, a child may come to this conclusion earlier or later than five to six years, but it is one stage in his movement toward a mature understanding of the meaning of death.

After they have begun school, children imagine death as personified in some form. Some children begin to conceptualize death as a person who carries living people off, especially after dark if they are "bad." Some children believe that death is the same thing as a dead person who lies in a coffin. Children between six and nine years believe in general that death is invisible, that no one can really see it until he is carried away himself.

At about nine to ten years of age children begin to understand that death is the end-point of the life of the body, that it is inevitable and that eventually every living thing must die.[*]

The thoughts of the adolescent concerning death tend to be more varied than those of younger children and are dependent on past memories, degree of belief in a religion, cultural differences, and thoughts of the future. In other words, death is viewed in terms of the individual's life perspective.

Depending on the level of maturity of the pa-

---

[*]M. H. Nagy: The Child's View of Death; in H. Feifel: *The Meaning of Death.* New York, McGraw-Hill Book Company, Inc., 1959.

tient during his terminal illness, he may progress through five stages (E. Kübler Ross).* The first of these stages is *shock and denial:* "It can't be me." When the patient can no longer say, "No, not me," he asks usually, "Why me?" The patient becomes *angry* and difficult with his family and friends as well as with the health team personnel. He is not really angry at other persons; he is angry because other persons have life while he is in the process of losing his. The nurse can help most in this situation if the patient and his family, members of which are going through stages similar to those of the patient, are encouraged to ventilate, to express their anger, to scream if it will make them feel better.

Sometimes the patient will appear to lose his anger without help. This has occurred because he has entered the stage of *bargaining.* He is bargaining with God, giving Him a promise in exchange for a lengthening of his life. One young man of 17 years said, "If God will let me live, I'll become a priest." In this stage the patient is saying, "Yes, me, but...." When he drops the "but," he acknowledges what is happening and becomes *depressed.* He may not want to talk, want no visitors, and may spend his time crying quietly. This too is difficult for members of the nursing team to cope with. The patient is grieving because he will soon lose everyone and everything he has known and loved. He will soon want only one person at the very end to sit by his side silently, without words, to hold his hand, stroke his hair, or just be there. The patient enters the stage of *acceptance,* which is a good feeling, different from resignation, which is a bitter form of giving up or defeat. Acceptance means that he has finally said and done everything he believed was unfinished business and is ready to go. The family probably needs more support at this time than the patient does.

The young person having a terminal illness has two problems. Not only is he losing his most precious possession, life, through death, but he is also losing the very close relationships that he needs. Many times the parents and friends of a dying young person are so overwhelmed by their own grief that they cannot give him the support he needs so desperately.

The way a child views death depends not only on his developmental age but also on his experiences with death in the past, especially in his own immediate family. The meaning of the death of someone close to a child may be varied, depending on his age and relation to the deceased. If a brother or sister dies, the child, no matter what his age, still has his parents on whom to depend. Yet the death of another child affects the parents, who may either turn protectively to the surviving child or children or turn from them in their grief. If the child is older when the sibling dies, he may come to the conclusion that "this may happen to me too, soon, maybe tomorrow or next week." This is a frightening thought for a child of any age. If he also was close to the dead child, he may have guilt feelings about past anger or jealousy toward the dead person or because he failed to do something that would have made him happier when he was alive.

When a parent dies, a real crisis occurs for the child. If the mother dies when the child is very young, he feels frightened by his separation from her. If he is older, he knows that life will never be the same again. If his father dies and his mother must go to work, he suffers the loss not only of his father but also of his mother, who may be away from him at work part of the day. Also, guilt feelings occur when anyone whom the child loved dies. He may have felt hostile, resentful, or jealous at some time toward the deceased. He may even have wished for the removal of the person from his life. When, in effect, his wishes come true, he may feel that what has happened was his fault alone.

The reactions that the child is likely to have concerning the death of someone in the family can be reduced if he knows what is going on and that adults are being honest with him when he asks questions. The decision as to whether or not the child should attend the funeral services depends on his age, the religious custom of the family, and the degree of anxiety which the child shows. Adults should, in general, make an effort to limit expression of their own grief in the child's presence so that their emotion will not be too frightening to the child. But the abilities of the child should be utilized as a contribution to the well-being of the family to whatever extent this is possible.

Children evidence grief in a manner different from that shown by the adult. A child who experiences a deep sense of loss will play actively, "misbehave" by adult standards, or else withdraw. A child should not be reprimanded for his behavior at such a time. This would only tend to increase the burden of guilt he may already feel.

In summary, the way a child views death, especially if he is old enough to know what his illness means, depends on his degree of maturity and the experiences with death he has had in the past.

---

*E. Kübler-Ross: *On Death and Dying.* New York, Macmillan Company, 1969.

Opinions vary when the child is terminally ill as to whether or not the child should be told honestly about his own condition and poor prognosis. It is the parents' duty with the physician to decide what to tell the child about his condition. It is also the parents' responsibility to decide who should tell the child, whether it be a religious advisor, physician or friend. The important thing for the nurse to know is what information the physician and his parents have decided he should have. Even though not agreeing with what has been told the child, the nurse should respect the wishes of the parents and the physician in this regard and not try to force personal beliefs on them. Certainly the nurse should never confuse the child by giving him information he is not able to handle.

The Role of the Nurse in the Care of the Terminally Ill Child and His Parents

The value which society attributes to a person depends on his age, social class, beauty, and personality, among other characteristics. A child who is just beginning life and has presumably more potential for making a greater contribution to society than an elderly person who "has lived his life" is valued highly. It should come as no surprise, therefore, that every kind of life-prolonging or revival technique is usually utilized to save the life of a child. It should also not come as a surprise that some nurses cannot care for children because they cannot tolerate seeing them die. These nurses have failed to resolve their own feelings, which thus get in the way of helping parents and children in crisis situations.

Death for a young infant such as a premature and for an older child dying with leukemia is different for nurses. The premature infant is not aware of his impending death, while the older child may very well be. This difference changes the way nurses talk, think and act when they are near the patient.

To nurse a child whose death is inevitable and to support the parents is indeed an art and a challenge. First, the nurse must remember that *children who are dying are also still living.* He or she must help them to live their last few days or months to the fullest, to maintain the interests they had before their illness, and to find new ones. The nurse must also remember that children derive security from having reasonable and consistent limits set on their behavior. At a time when the child feels that his body is changing and is undependable, it is especially important that his environment be completely secure.

As mentioned before, one of the serious problems in the care of the dying child is resolution of the question about how much the parents and the child should be told about the child's condition. If the physician makes this decision alone, many times he does not communicate it to the nurse, who is then left close to the family and the child without knowing how to respond to questions should they arise. A better idea for handling this situation is for parents, physician, nurse, and other appropriate members of the health team to make the decision together.

The clergy of the family's choosing should be brought into contact with the child and the family as soon as possible if the family wishes to talk with him. The nurse has learned in previous courses the role of the clergy of various religions at the time of death. If the family does not wish to see a religious advisor, the nurse should consider their wishes even though they run counter to his or her own set of values.

In the past nurses generally emphasized physical care and treatment routines in the care of the dying child and did not provide coordinated, consistent psychologic care to him and to his family. After the parents have been told about the seriousness of their child's illness they may bear it quietly and with evidence of inner strength, they may become restless and hostile, or they may become depressed and withdrawn. It is especially difficult for the nurse to help those who are withdrawn. One approach as the parents sit quietly together is to say, "This news must disturb you very much." When the parents respond affirmatively to this statement, the nurse can say, "Can you tell me how you feel about it?" If the parents can discuss their feelings, they will probably then be better able to support each other. But the nurse has no right to continue to probe if the parents give an indication that they do not wish to talk. The responsibility of the nurse is to offer his or her presence and help, to be available, and to help the parents know that they are not alone. *The helping person's strength at such a time lies in the ability to be able to experience with the parents some of the pain of the tragedy without becoming overwhelmed by it.*

When parents do not express emotion, but seem to accept the child's death too well, the nurse can gently indicate that it is "all right to cry." Such parents need support for their apparent lack of emotion or for the dissociation they feel between mind, action and emotion. The nurse can support them in their apparently unfeeling state by explaining that this is nature's protective way so that they can carry on in the face of such a loss. But the nurse should not pressure such parents to cry because by so doing she could destroy the protective mechanism they are using to hold themselves together.

The nurse should not be surprised if the parents of a dying child seem to ignore the child completely and discuss a past loss. Such experience is not lost, but is revived with another impending loss. This is especially true if the grief work was not completed in the past. The nurse can help such a parent abreact to his past grief so that when the time comes he can grieve about his child with no further need to protect himself from bringing alive old memories.

The grief of parents for a dying child is painful to watch. The nurse should understand the reactions of parents when they cannot leave the child's room as well as when they cannot enter it. The nurse should permit and assist the parents to do any bit of nursing care they wish for their child, relieving them when they appear to be tired or worn. The parents' attempt to cope with their situation may lead them to provide tender loving care for their child or to rush frantically from task to task in the child's room. They may berate the physicians and nurses or praise their efforts extravagantly. The nurse cannot be disturbed if the parents do not react as expected. Each parent's behavior reflects his attempts to handle his own feelings and as such must be accepted by the nurse.

The nurse in a helping role can give most by furnishing an opportunity for those who are pained to express their anger and fears to someone who will not be devastated by their expressed feelings. The parents should be encouraged to talk about what they want at any particular moment. The nurse should encourage parents to talk about what bothers them so that their real concerns can be delineated. They can be helped to face the reality of what is taking place. As the parents learn to know the nurse better, they sense the support available.

Families need to talk about their child. When they feel lonely and frightened, they want to talk to relatives and friends as well as to physicians and nurses. They must have a chance to be upset so that they can face the reality of what lies ahead. They need to be able to talk with their child if he is old enough to know what is happening. The nurse should be aware of the fact that anticipatory guidance or talking about the impending loss with others helps them to adjust to the impact of the loss itself.

Dying patients, whether adults or children, do not generally want to be left alone. They want frequent contact with another human being. They need the opportunity to talk, to be upset if they know the prognosis. They need to know that someone cares.

The dying child may feel very lonely if his parents do not stay with him constantly. The child therefore needs and wants his nurse to be nearby. The nurse's presence increases his sense of security in the knowledge that someone cares.

Knowing this, the nurse should encourage the parents and any other relatives to visit. The problem may then arise that the adults become so upset at the appearance of the child that they leave the room and cannot return because of their own emotion. If they have not told the child that they are leaving, or if they have told him that they would return soon, he may be disturbed by their apparent lack of honesty. Actually, if the child's visitors cannot control their emotions to some degree, it might be better if they left the room. Adults who have lost their emotional control completely may be very frightening to the child.

Dying children need about the same kind of support as other ill children the same age. For example, the greatest fear of the child under five is that of separation from the mother, while the greatest fear of the child from five to nine years is of bodily procedures and mutilation. The older the child, the more likely he is to be concerned about his own death. He will ask questions, and it is the nurse's responsibility to learn exactly what is troubling him. Is he upset because he is in pain, or is it because he saw his mother crying? Children should know that parents become upset when children are not feeling well and cannot play.

The older child, when dying, should be treated with dignity and respect as a member of the family group. His opinions should be considered in matters which affect him as an individual, e.g., whether he wants the school teacher to come to see him or whether his younger brother may ride his bicycle while he is in the hospital.

The older child, like the adult, should not be told that he looks better, when he knows that he is very ill. Honesty is important in relations with the child as with the adult.

The child who senses or knows that he is going to die fears going to sleep at night. It is a challenge for the nurse to find nursing measures and appropriate medications to give him needed rest. Night lights and the nurse's looking in on him frequently help the child to feel secure.

Constancy of personnel should be provided so far as possible for the sake of the child and his parents to counteract the feeling of loss and abandonment they may feel. Parents appreciate the same nurses who understand their child being with him. They appreciate honesty in their answers to questions and the opportunity to call at any time to learn how their child is.

In the face of grief many times the questions answered, the directions given to the hospital chapel or local church, the offer to telephone a relative or friend, the touch of a known sympathetic hand, the offer to get coffee, or just the nurse's own presence are all that is required to reassure the parents that the nurse cares.

It is important that the nurse keep the room neat, welcome the family warmly and permit as much visiting as possible. Parents or nurses should not close shades or curtains or talk in whispers in the child's room any more than they should in the room of the adult who is dying.

During the child's terminal illness providing a place that is comfortable and private for the frightened and grieving family is most important. Provision of such a place gives the family further indication that the nurse understands and cares.

Both the parents and the child should know that the child is getting the best possible care in the situation. The greatest gift the nurse can give to the dying child and his parents is to be with them when words have little meaning. Yet this is not easy for the nurse to do.

When the parents are not told about the prognosis, the nurse is placed in a difficult situation when they or the child asks questions. The nurses carry the burden of the problem, since physicians are not in frequent contact with the family members. When the child is hospitalized for only a short time and is to be "sent home to die," the problem of questioning is less likely to arise than if the child has a prolonged period of hospitalization. Both the child, if he is older, and the parents then feel more comfortable in questioning the nurse. In this situation the nurse is faced with feelings of frustration, sadness, and helplessness.

After the death of the child the nurse usually sees in the hospital setting the first shock wave of disbelief overcome the parents. The parents may then gradually become aware of what has happened to their child. The nurse rarely sees the restitution which completes the work of mourning, because this takes much longer.

When the nurse tries to help the parents after the death of the child, whatever behavior they evidence should be accepted, whether shock, denial, tearfulness, or anger. The danger of grief lies not in how the parents feel, but in their inability to tolerate the feeling, their believing that they should feel or act differently. Keeping feelings hidden at such a time as this does not mean that they will go away. They may burst forth later with surprising impact if they are not worked through.

Many times nurses who cared for a child over a period of time find that after his death they, like the parents, were unable to control their tears. They have sought refuge in linen closets, bathrooms, or locker rooms in order to prevent the family from observing their loss of control. Why should not the nurses who worked so closely with a child, giving him the best care they could, be able to express their deep emotion? Many times parents feel comforted when seeing the nurse cry, because this indicates to them not only that they are not alone in their grief, but also that the nurse as a person was deeply moved by their child's death.

Some parents wish to remain with their child for a while after death or request to see the child if they were not present at the moment of death. Such requests should be honored. The nurse should attempt to tidy the crib or bed and room; however, the most important professional function is to remain quietly with the parents and to give any support they may need. Sometimes a hand on the parent's shoulder is all that is necessary to help them know that someone cares. After the initial shock has passed, parents appreciate any comments about their ability to care for the child. A nurse's comment, "What wonderful parents you have been," will long be remembered. But many times simply being with the bereaved parents will give more solace and comfort than the nurse can know.

The question often arises concerning what to tell siblings in a family after the child has died. They should be told that the child was extremely ill and that the doctors were not able to make him better. If they have beliefs in an afterlife, the parents can say that the child has gone to heaven.

A first assignment to do postmortem body care on a child can be extremely difficult if two inexperienced nurses are sent into the room alone. It can be an invaluable experience if an inexperienced nurse is sent with a mature member of the nursing staff to carry out this procedure.

The question usually arises whether the other children in the hospital unit should be told when a child they know dies. When questions are raised by these children, they are many times told that the critically ill child was transferred to another unit, that he was taken to the operating room or was sent home. Certainly the older children on the unit have further questions about the absent child's condition, but if these questions are brought into the open, the nurses suddenly appear too busy to respond. Although the decision as to what should be done in this situation should be made by the members of the health team on the basis of the number of children involved, their ages, their diagnoses, and their closeness to the dead child among other factors, it is usually the nurse who must eventually answer the question to the children's satisfaction. If the question is not answered adequately, the children learn that death is not a subject that can be easily discussed.

Dying is not only a biological phenomenon, but also a social experience. If the parents and the child do not know the prognosis, they cannot discuss it with others, they cannot say goodbyes, nor can the parents openly plan for ways in which they will handle the situation with other children in the family once the death occurs.

The dying child and his parents present real problems for the nurse caring for them. But if each nurse works out a personal religious belief and a philosophy and feeling about death, he or she will be able to provide a human guide to the unknown for the family. The nurse will find each situation a challenge in which to practice the real art and science of the nursing profession.

SUMMARY

Throughout this book the role of the pediatric nurse outside the hospital is emphasized in the areas of maintenance of optimum health, normal growth and development, and the prevention of illness. The chapters on normal growth and development in this text speak directly to the specifics the nurse should know in order to assist families in reaching these goals. In the expanding role of the professional nurse, the pediatric nurse has a great opportunity to work with children and their families before hospitalization is required.

Since illness does unfortunately occur in the pediatric group, the importance of the problem that hospitalization presents to a child and the ways in which hospital personnel and the child's parents can help him to adjust to the situation are also discussed. There is always danger to a child's emotional development caused by long-term hospitalization with separation from parents and siblings. To avoid this, infants and young children are being treated whenever possible on an outpatient basis. Antibiotics can easily be given for certain acute infections and in order to limit complications. Outpatient treatment or ambulatory care is therefore possible in many cases for which formerly it was necessary to hospitalize the child.

In order to fulfill the nursing role in the total plan of care for every hospitalized child the nurse must think through his or her own feelings about each family. In some situations a psychiatrist is available to help, not only so that the nurse may learn how to handle personal emotional problems, but also so that what is done and said will have an immediate and beneficial influence on the parents' attitudes and on the child's condition. Of all the members of the health team, the nurse, by rejection of a child or his parents, would be the most injurious. If the nurse accepts the child, he or she will learn, while nursing him, to apply theoretical knowledge and past experience to his care. Having done this, the nurse is in a position to teach the parents.

The mother of a chronically ill child who has been cared for at home can help the nurse in this adaptation of general knowledge of pediatric nursing to the care of the particular patient. The mother should be considered a member of the health team, the one who works most closely with the nurses.

Pediatric nursing must be adapted to the wide range of development from the newborn infant through adolescence. In order to fulfill this complex role, the nurse must understand the normal physical, emotional, social, mental, sexual, and spiritual aspects of growth and development of children, and the parent-child relation as background for care of both the well child and the sick child of varying ages. Each unit of this book deals with a progressively older age group. We must consider the basic characteristics of growth and development of each group and define the general principles of pediatric nursing to meet their needs. We must then consider the diseases most commonly occurring in each age group and the nursing care involved.

GUIDES TO FURTHER STUDY

1. What is your understanding of the role of the professional nurse in providing care for a sick child? What should be the nurse's relations with the child and with his parents?

2. Make a survey in your community of various agencies which provide care for well and for sick children. List them and their specific functions.

3. Recall a hospitalization experience during childhood. (This may be your own experience or that of a sibling or friend.) Was this a positive or a negative experience? Give specific memories you have about it and propose ways by which they could have been made more pleasant.

4. Define and differentiate clearly between the following

terms: (a) growth and development and (b) eugenics and euthenics.

5. Obtain either your own, a sibling's, or a friend's "Baby Book." List the steps of growth and development recorded in it. Summarize the principles of growth and development and apply them to this record.

6. Select a well sibling or a friend's child in any of the following age groups: birth to one year, one to three years, three to six years, six to 12 years or 12 to 18 years. Discuss the growth and development and care of this child with his parents. Define the problems these parents are facing with this child. In class, each student will discuss the child who was investigated, highlighting important points about the child's home, type of family, his community, and his physical, emotional, social, sexual, and mental growth and development, and care.

7. Discuss individually with your own or a friend's grandmother and mother their attitudes about the care of children. State the differences in philosophy or child care practices expressed. What would some of the reasons be for these differences?

8. Immediately after the admission of a child to the hospital, observe the behavior of both the parents and the child. On the basis of specific observations you have made draw conclusions as to the feelings of the parents and the child. What could you as a nurse do to help the parents and child face this situation less anxiously or more positively?

9. What can you observe in the children's area on which you are working that would help a child feel more at home in the hospital setting?

10. Evaluate the unit in which you are working as to its safety for the care of the children. List your findings and make constructive suggestions for its improvement.

11. List the various personnel in the pediatric unit who provide some sort of care or guidance for children and their parents. Differentiate as clearly as you can between the functions of these persons.

12. Children and adults react differently to disease processes. Explain why this is true and what effect this understanding has or will have on the sort of care you give to children.

TEACHING AIDS AND OTHER INFORMATION*

American Academy of Pediatrics
Care of Children in Hospitals.

The American Cancer Society, Inc.
Grief, A Part of Living.

American Nurses' Association
Becoming Aware of Cultural Differences in Nursing, 1973.

Beakthru Inc.
No Togethers.

Blue Cross Association
A Foreign Language Guide to Health Care.

Child Study Association of America
Wolf, A. W. M.: Helping Your Child to Understand Death, Revised 1973.

Child Welfare League of America, Inc.
Zwerdling, E.: The ABC's of Casework with Children: A Social Work Teacher's Notebook, 1974.

The Children's Hospital Medical Center, Boston, Mass.
Rey, M., and Rey, H. A.: Curious George Goes to the Hospital.

Consumer Product Information
What About Metric, 1973.

Public Affairs Committee
Doyle, N.: The Dying Person and the Family.
Irwin, T.: How to Cope with Crises.

Ross Laboratories
The Care of Children with Chronic Illnesses.

The Touchstone Center
My Roots Be Coming Back.
Out of My Body.

United States Government
Altshuler, A.: Books That Help Children with a Hospital Experience, 1974.

United States Metric System Association
Metric Handbook for Hospitals.

*Complete addresses are given in the Appendix.

REFERENCES

Books

American Academy of Pediatrics: Care of Children in Hospitals. Evanston, Ill., American Academy of Pediatrics, 1971.
Andreopoulos, S. (Ed.): Primary Care: Where Medicine Fails. New York, John Wiley & Sons, Inc., 1974.
Azarnoff, P., and Flegal, S.: A Pediatric Play Program: Developing a Therapeutic Play Program for Children in Medical Settings. Springfield, Ill., Charles C Thomas, Publisher, 1975.
Bergersen, B. S., and Goth, A.: Pharmacology in Nursing. 13th ed. St. Louis, The C. V. Mosby Company, 1976.
Branch, M. F., and Paxton, P. P. (Eds.): Providing Safe Nursing Care for Ethnic People of Color. New York, Appleton-Century-Crofts, 1976.
Brink, P. J. (Ed.): Transcultural Nursing; A Book of Readings. Englewood Cliffs, N. J., Prentice-Hall, Inc., 1976.
Bullmer, K.: The Art of Empathy. New York, Human Sciences Press, 1975.
Carlson, C. E.: Behavioral Concepts and Nursing Intervention. Philadelphia, J. B. Lippincott Company, 1970.
Chapman, J. E., and Chapman, H. H.: Behavior and Health Care: A Humanistic Helping Process. St. Louis, The C. V. Mosby Company, 1975.
Creighton, H.: Law Every Nurse Should Know. 2nd ed. Philadelphia, W. B. Saunders Company, 1970.

deCastro, F. J., Rolfe, U. T., and Drew, J. K.: *The Pediatric Nurse Practitioner: Guidelines for Practice*. 2nd ed. St. Louis, The C. V. Mosby Company, 1976.

DeMyer, W.: *Technique of the Neurologic Examination*. 2nd ed. New York, McGraw-Hill Book Company, 1974.

Erickson, M. L.: *Assessment and Management of Developmental Changes in Children*. St. Louis, The C. V. Mosby Company, 1976.

Falconer, M. W., Patterson, H. R., and Gustafson, E. A.: *Current Drug Handbook 1976-1978*. Philadelphia, W. B. Saunders Company, 1976.

French, R. M.: *Guide to Diagnostic Procedures*. 4th ed. New York, McGraw-Hill Book Company, 1975.

Hall, J. E., and Weaver, B. R.: *Nursing of Families in Crisis*. Philadelphia, J. B. Lippincott Company, 1974.

Hardgrove, C. B., and Dawson, R. B.: *Parents and Children in the Hospital: The Family's Role in Pediatrics*. Boston, Little, Brown & Company, 1972.

Hernandez, C., Haug, M., and Wagner, N.: *Chicanos: Social and Psychological Perspectives*. 2nd ed. St. Louis, The C. V. Mosby Company, 1976.

Kron, T.: *Communication in Nursing*. 2nd ed. Philadelphia, W. B. Saunders Company, 1972.

Kubler-Ross, E.: *Death: The Final Stage of Growth*. Englewood Cliffs, N. J., Prentice-Hall, 1975.

Kubler-Ross, E.: *Questions and Answers on Death and Dying*. New York, Collier Books, 1974.

Lindheim, R., Glaser, H. H., and Coffin, C.: *Changing Hospital Environments for Children*. Cambridge, Mass., Harvard University Press, 1972.

Little, D. E., and Carnevali, D. L.: *Nursing Care Planning*. 2nd ed. Philadelphia, J. B. Lippincott Company, 1976.

Lowbury, E. J. L., et al.: *Control of Hospital Infection: A Practical Handbook*. New York, Halsted Press, 1975.

Marram, G. D., Schlegel, M. W., and Bevis, E. O.: *Primary Nursing; A Model for Individualized Care*. St. Louis, The C. V. Mosby Company, 1974.

Metheny, N. M., and Snively, W. D.: *Nurses' Handbook of Fluid Balance*. 2nd ed. Philadelphia, J. B. Lippincott Company, 1974.

Modell, W. (Ed.): *Drugs of Choice 1976-1977*. St. Louis, The C. V. Mosby Company, 1975.

Murray, R., and Zentner, J.: *Nursing Assessment and Health Promotion Through the Life Span*. Englewood Cliffs, N. J., Prentice-Hall, 1975.

Nordmark, M. T., and Rohweder, A. W.: *Scientific Foundations of Nursing*. 3rd ed. Philadelphia, J. B. Lippincott Company, 1975.

O'Brien, M. J.: *Communications and Relationships in Nursing*. St. Louis, The C. V. Mosby Company, 1974.

Oremland, E. K., and Oremland, J. D. (Eds.): *The Effects of Hospitalization on Children; Models for Their Care*. Springfield, Ill., Charles C Thomas, 1973.

Pohl, M. L.: *The Teaching Function of the Nursing Practitioner*. 2nd ed. Dubuque, Iowa, William C. Brown Company, 1973.

Robinson, C. H.: *Basic Nutrition and Diet Therapy*. 3rd ed. New York, Macmillan Publishing Company, 1975.

Schoenberg, B., et al. (eds.): *Bereavement: Its Psychosocial Aspects*. New York, Columbia University Press, 1975.

Shirkey, H. C.: *Pediatric Drug Handbook*. Philadelphia, W. B. Saunders Company, 1977.

Tabery, J. J., Webb, M. R., and Mueller, B. V.: *Communicating in Spanish for Medical Personnel*. Boston, Little, Brown & Company, 1975.

Zeligs, R.: *Children's Experience with Death*. Springfield, Ill., Charles C Thomas, 1974.

Periodicals

Aradine, C. R.: Books for Children about Death. *Pediatrics*, 57:372, March 1976.

Barker, V. L.: Rural Mobile Health Unit. *American Journal of Nursing*, 76:274, February 1976.

Bates, B.: Doctor and Nurse: Changing Roles and Relations. *Nursing Digest*, 2:70, October 1974.

Baxter, P.: Frustration Felt by a Mother and Her Child During the Child's Hospitalization. *American Journal of Maternal Child Nursing*, 1:159, May-June 1976.

Bellack, J. P.: Helping a Child Cope with the Stress of Injury. *American Journal of Nursing*, 74:1491, August 1974.

Bertucci, M., Huston, M., and Perloff, E.: Comparative Study of Progress Notes using Problem-Oriented and Traditional Methods of Charting. *Nursing Research*, 23:351, July-August 1974.

Brandt, P. A., et al.: IM Injections in Children. *American Journal of Nursing*, 72:1402, August 1972.

Brooks, M. M.: Why Play in the Hospital? *Nursing Clinics of North America*, 5:431, September 1970.

Carter, M. D.: Identification of Behaviors Displayed by Children Experiencing Prolonged Hospitalization. *Int. J. Nurs. Studies*, 10:125, May 1973.

Davitz, L. J., and Davitz, J. R.: How Nurses View Patient Suffering. *RN*, 38:69, October 1975.

Dickinson, Sr. C.: The Search for Spiritual Meaning. *American Journal of Nursing*, 75:1789, October 1975.

DiPalma, J. R.: What You Need To Know About Bioavailability. *RN*, 38:114, September 1975.

Egolf, D. B., and Chester, S. L.: Speechless Messages. *Nursing Digest*, 4:26, March-April 1976.

Elseed, A. M., Shinebourne, E. A., and Joseph, M. C.: Assessment of Techniques for Measurement of Blood Pressure in Infants and Children. *Arch. Dis. Child*, 48:932, December 1973.

Freiberg, K. H.: How Parents React When Their Child is Hospitalized. *American Journal of Nursing*, 72:1270, July 1972.

Freihofer, P., and Felton, G.: Nursing Behaviors in Bereavement: An Exploratory Study. *Nursing Research*, 25:332, September-October 1976.

Galligan, A. C.: Books for the Hospitalized Child. *American Journal of Nursing*, 75:2164, December 1975.

Gardner, G. G., and Simkins, R. A.: Does It Really Matter What Nurses Wear in the Intensive Care Unit? *American Journal of Maternal Child Nursing*, 1:239, July-August 1976.

Gold, M. R., and Rosenberg, R. G.: Use of Emergency Room Services by the Population of a Neighborhood Health Center. *Health Serv. Rep.*, 89:65, January-February 1974.

Gottheil, E., McGurn, W. C., and Pollak, O.: Truth and/or Hope for the Dying Patient. *Nursing Digest*, 4:12, March-April 1976.

Grant, D.: *VIP Treatment* Proves This Hospital Really Cares. *The Canadian Nurse*, 72:24, July 1976.

Green, C. S.: Understanding Children's Needs Through Therapeutic Play. *Nursing '74*, 4:31, October 1974.

Greenberg, R. A., et al.: Primary Child Health Care by Family Nurse Practitioners. *Pediatrics*, 53:900, June 1974.

Gyulay, J.: The Forgotten Grievers. *American Journal of Nursing*, 75:1476, September 1975.

Hardgrove, C. B., and Dawson, R. B.: Ideas, A to Z, for Personalizing Pediatric Units. *Nursing '76*, 6:57, April 1976.

Isler, C.: Helping Hospital Patients-Out. *RN*, 38:43, November 1975.

Jackson, P. L.: Chronic Grief. *American Journal of Nursing*, 74:1288, July 1974.

Jackson, P. L.: The Child's Developing Concept of Death: Implications for Nursing Care of the Terminally Ill Child. *Nursing Forum*, 14:204, 1975.

Kerr, A. H.: That's Where the Goodies Are! *Nursing '75*, 5:34, February 1975.

Kohut, S. A.: Guidelines for Using Interpreters. *Nursing Digest*, 3:55, January-February 1976.

Koocher, G. P.: Talking with Children about Death. *Am. J. Orthopsychiatry*, 44:404, April 1974.

Lees, R. E. M.: Physician Timesaving by Employment of Expanded-Role Nurses in Family Practice. *Can. Med. Assoc. J.*, 108:871, April 1973.

Lester, D., Getty, C., and Kneisl, C. R.: Attitudes of Nursing Students and Nursing Faculty Toward Death. *Nursing Research*, 23:50, January-February 1974.

Luciano, K., and Shumsky, C. J.: Pediatric Procedures: The Explanation Should Always Come First. *Nursing '75*, 5:49, January 1975.

McCaffery, M.: Patients in Pain. *Nursing '73*, 3:41, June 1973.

McGreevy, A., and Van Heukelem, J.: Crying. *The Canadian Nurse*, 72:18, January 1976.

Mackay, R. C., Alexander, D. S., and Kingsbury, L. J.: Parents' Attitudes Towards the Nurse as Physician Associate in a Pediatric Practice. *Can. J. Public Health*, 64:121, March-April 1973.

Mitchell, P. H.: A Systematic Nursing Progress Record: The Problem-Oriented Approach. *Nursing Forum*, 12:187, 1973.

Mann, S. A.: Coping With a Child's Fatal Illness: A Parent's Dilemma. *Nursing Clinics of North America*, 9:81, March 1974.

Naugle, E. H.: The Difference Caring Makes. *American Journal of Nursing*, 73:1890, November 1973.

Northrup, F. C.: The Dying Child. *American Journal of Nursing*, 74:1066, June 1974.

Nowak, M. M., Brundhofer, B., and Gibaldi, M.: Rectal Absorption from Aspirin Suppositories in Children and Adults. *Pediatrics*, 54:23, July 1974.

Ormond, E. A. R., and Caulfield, C.: A Practical Guide to Giving Oral Medications to Young Children, *The American Journal of Maternal Child Nursing*, 1:320, September-October 1976.

Perkins, Sr. M. R.: Does Availability of Health Services Ensure Their Use? *Nursing Outlook*, 22:496, August 1974.

Popoff, D.: What Are Your Feelings About Death and Dying? *Nursing '75*, 5:15, August 1975.

Rabalais, J. T.: Dangers of Accepting Stereotypes: A Boy Taught Me About Nonacceptance. *Nursing '75*, 5:43, February 1975.

Rachels, J.: Active and Passive Euthanasia. *Nursing Digest*, 4:52, Fall 1976.

Robinson, D.: Illness Behaviour and Children's Hospitalization: A Schema of Parents' Attitudes Toward Authority. *Soc. Sci. Med.*, 6:447, August 1972.

Schultz, N. V.: How Children Perceive Pain. *Nursing Outlook*, 19:670, October 1971.

Schwartz, L. H., and Schwartz, J. L.: Transference: The Hidden Element in Your Relations with Patients. *Nursing '73*, 3:37, October 1973.

Shah, C. P., Robinson, G. C., Kinnis, C., and Davenport, H. T.: Day Care Surgery for Children: A Controlled Study of Medical Complications and Parental Attitudes. *Med. Care*, 10:437, September-October 1972.

Smith, J. C.: Spending Time with the Hospitalized Child. *The American Journal of Meternal Child Nursing*, 1:164, May-June 1976.

Spinetta, J. J., Rigler, D., and Karon, M.: Personal Space as a Measure of a Dying Child's Sense of Isolation. *J. Consult. Clin. Psychol.*, 42:751, 1974.

Tripp, S. L.: What to Ask & What to Do When Parents Call About Children's Illnesses. *Nursing '74*, 4:73, June 1974.

Van Dersal, W. R.: How to be a Good Communicator—and a Better Nurse. *Nursing '74*, 4:57, December 1974.

Wallerstein, E., Marshall, C. L., Alexander, R., Cunningham, N., and Thomstad, K.: Pediatric Outreach Via Television. *Nursing Digest*, 2:74, March 1974.

Williams, J. C.: Understanding the Feelings of the Dying. *Nursing '76*, 6:52, March 1976.

AUDIOVISUAL MEDIA*

American Dental Association

The Hands that Help (Las Manos Que Ayudan)
    24 minutes, 16mm, sound, color.
    Documentary film describing a unique teaching and community service project performed by the students and faculty of the University of California School of Dentistry. Shows the design and outfitting of the buses into mobile clinics, the living conditions of the migrant population in the San Joaquin and Salinas-Santa Clara Valleys, and the dental treatment rendered.

The American Journal of Nursing Company

A Day in the Life....
    17min., sound, color.
    Film follows a young registered nurse through a typical day on a Pediatric floor of a large modern hospital. On the sound track, the young nurse expresses her thoughts and feelings about her work, and about the young patients in her care.

Pediatric Nursing
    A Conference on the Dying Child
    Participating Instructors: Alexander, C., Belniak, R., and Logue, B.
    44 minutes, 16mm film or videotape, sound, black and white, guide.
    Presented are the problems of the nurse's own emotions in caring for the dying child, how she must accept them and the emotions of the family, how the child learns the concept of death, inadvertent changes in the care of the child who is

dying, how support might be given to child and parents alike.

Nursing Appraisal of Infant Neurological Development
    Participating Instructor: Haynes, U.
    44 minutes, 16mm film or videotape, sound, black and white, guide.
    Normal neuro-motor-sensory system of the infant in the first year is discussed. Mrs. Haynes demonstrates normal reflexes of one-, three-, and nine-month-old babies with emphasis on the methods nurses should employ in observing infants for normal growth and development.

The Hospitalized Child
    Participating Instructor: Berlinger, M.
    44 minutes, 16mm film, or videotape, sound, black and white, guide.
    Introduction to Pediatric Nursing class. Difficulties, fears and fantasies of children, both very young and over five years, in accepting hospitalization are described.

Play Therapy and the Hospitalized Child
    26 minutes, black and white.
    Film describes how to aid children in coping with their hospital experience through play therapy.

Psychiatric-Mental Health Nursing
    The Crisis of Loss
    30 minutes, videotape, sound, color.
    The commonly encountered nursing problem of loss and mourning is examined within the framework of crisis theory.

---

*Complete addresses are given in the Appendix.

Charles Press–Prentice-Hall, Inc.

Death and Dying
  Jackson, E. N.
  45 minutes.
  Dr. Jackson directs his remarks to parents and to those in the caregiving professions who will ultimately shape children's attitudes toward death. Direct, honest answers to their questions on death provide a basis for a healthy philosophy that can sustain an individual throughout life.

Death and the Family: From the Caring Professions' Point of View
  Fredlund, D.
  30 minutes.
  Professor Fredlund discusses children's attitudes toward death. She underscores the need for children to be made aware of death and for them to learn to accept loss in a realistic manner.

Nursing Skills and Technique Series
  Pediatric Restraints: Arm Cuff and Crib Net
  2–5 minutes, 8mm filmloop, color, guide.
  Demonstration of two types of restraint commonly used in pediatrics.

Talking to Children About Death
  Williams, G. G.
  57 minutes.
  Dr. Williams discusses ways to open the channels of communication between parent and child on the sensitive issue of death. He offers suggestions on how to help approach the topic of death with children.

Children's Hospital, National Medical Center, Washington, D.C.

To Prepare a Child
  32 minutes, 16mm, sound, color, with study guide and bibliography.
  The purpose of this film is stated in its title. Studies have shown that the occurrence of psychological upset of hospitalization is greater in the unprepared than in the prepared child. The child care staff in the film demonstrate the quality of care children need to be well-prepared for this experience.

Concept Media

Nonverbal Communication in Nursing
  5 programs of varied length, 35 mm filmstrip/tape, sound, color, guide.
    The silent vocabulary – 16 min.
    Kinesics: the study of body language – 20 min.
    Touch – 23 min.
    Proxemics: space and human experience – 28 min.
    Interactions for study – 14 min.
  Discusses communication as a complex multisensory process which includes learned body language, touch and spatial relationships and how this can affect nursing care.

Greater Cleveland Hospital Association

Restraining the Adult and Pediatric Patient
  28 minutes, 16mm film or videotape, sound, color, guide.
  Reviews policies and legal implications related to the application of restraints, as well as indications for clinical use and the proper methods of applying restraints.

J. B. Lippincott Company

Fundamentals of Nursing Series
  Gown: Re-use Technique
  8mm film loop, color.
  Asepsis. How to put on a previously used isolation gown, remove, hang up.

Medical Electronic Educational Services, Inc.

Pediatric Nursing Series
  Medicating Children
  33 minutes, 35mm filmstrip/tape, sound, color, guides.
  Teaches the special precautions and calculations needed in medicating children.

  Prevention of Accidents to Children
  22 minutes, 35mm filmstrip/tape, sound, color, guides.
  Teaches how to provide a safe environment for the pediatric patient, paying particular attention to child's level of development.

Trainex Corporation

Admission and Orientation of the Child
  35mm filmstrips, audio-tape-cassettes, 33 1/3 LP, color.
  Examines the initial exposure to the hospital from the point of view of the child and his parents. The viewer is given an understanding of their fears and anxieties, and techniques are indicated for reducing the trauma of hospitalization. Hospital personnel are made aware of the emotional (as well as the physical) needs of the child, and the value of parental participation in the care and treatment of the child is demonstrated.

Care of the Sick Child
  35mm filmstrip, audio-tape cassettes, 33 1/3 LP, color.
  Provides important rules for the use of medicines. Also explains the importance of fever and the proper procedure for using rectal thermometers.

Parents and Their Ill Child
  35mm filmstrip, audio-tape cassette, 33 1/3 LP, color.
  Parents of children who may require diagnostic or surgical procedures in the hospital are given suggestions which will help prepare their child and themselves for the hospital experience.

Preparing the Child for Procedures
  35mm filmstrip, audio-tape cassettes, 33 1/3 LP, color.
  This program is designed to help health care personnel minimize emotional trauma that a child could experience as a result of hospitalization. It shows ways in which the child might interpret hospital surroundings and procedures, and techniques employed in helping him to make correct interpretations. Included is a discussion of the value of structured play activities.

Principles of Isolation Technique
  35mm filmstrip, audio-tape cassettes, 33 1/3 LP, color.
  Full-color photographs provide step-by-step demonstrations of those techniques basic to effective isolation: preparing the isolation unit, handwashing, putting on and removing protective apparel, discarding disposable items and wastes within the isolation unit, and, doublebagging to remove disposable and nondisposable items from the isolation unit. The principles of isolation technique taught in this program are applicable to five different types of isolation: respiratory isolation, enteric precautions, strict isolation, protective isolation, and wound and skin precautions.

Stephen Goes to the Hospital
  35mm filmstrip, audio-tape cassettes, 33 1/3 LP, color.
  A story for children told by Stephen's doctor. The filmstrip begins in Dr. Jensen's office with Stephen being examined by him. The child viewer sees the doctor using a tongue depressor, flashlight, otoscope, a stethoscope, and a thermometer. Stephen is then admitted to the hospital where he has a blood test and a chest X-ray, and is given a liquid medication and an injection. He is shown eating and sleeping in the hospital. Also depicted, is the separation from his mother as she leaves to go home for the evening. The filmstrip concludes with Stephen's discharge from the hospital.

The Psychological Impact of Isolation
35mm filmstrip, audio-tape cassettes, 33 1/3 LP, color.
This filmstrip emphasizes patient needs, feelings, and behavior at three developmental stages — adult, adolescent, and early childhood. Full-color visuals and sensitive narration combine to develop a greater awareness of the impact of isolation upon the patient and to foster an attitude of acceptance of each patient's individuality and his unique methods of coping with the isolation situation.

The Metric System
35mm filmstrips, audio-tape cassettes, 33 1/3 LP, color.
This program presents basic units of metric measurement consistently used within the health care facility. The use of prefixes to indicate larger and smaller quantities of these units is explained and illustrated. Also shown in this filmstrip is the process of converting different metric units into equivalent amounts by altering the decimal placement.

United States Government

Technical Procedures for Diagnosis and Therapy in Children
Producer: USN
27 minutes, 16mm film, optical sound, color
Gives step by step procedures for femoral venipuncture, internal jugular puncture, lumbar puncture, subdural tap, gastric lavage, scalp venipuncture, and cutdown.

Wayne State University

DENT: Directions for Education in Nursing via Technology
30 minute lessons, 16mm film, videotape and videocassette.

Nursing Care Plans
Purpose–Types of plans
Process of development
Role of nurse in process

UNIT TWO

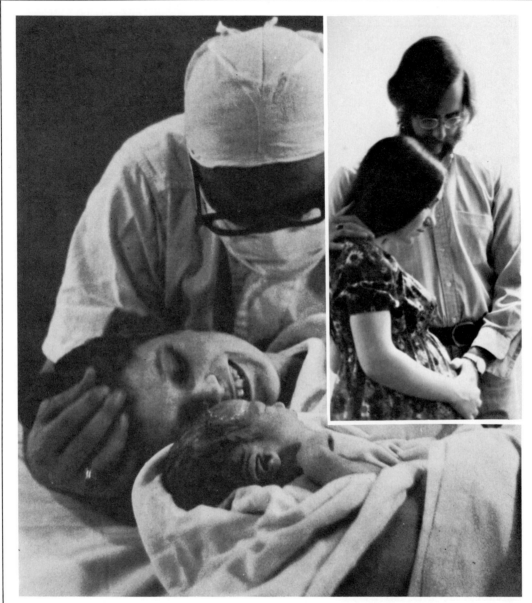

(Courtesy of M. Ciavolino, Jr. From *Baby Talk*: June, 1971; Courtesy of James A. Schaffer, Photographer, Hyattsville, Md.)

THE NEWBORN

THE NEWBORN

Our birth is but a sleep and a forgetting:
The Soul that rises with us, our life's star,
    Hath had elsewhere its setting,
    And cometh from afar:
    Not in entire forgetfulness,
    And not in utter nakedness,
But trailing clouds of glory do we come
    From God, who is our home:
Heaven lies about us in our infancy!

William Wordsworth (1770–1850),

Ode on Intimations of Immortality from
Recollections of Early Childhood
(lines 58–66)

Chapter Six

PREPARATION FOR PARENTHOOD

In most states, serologic tests for syphilis are required before a marriage license is issued to a couple. These tests are done to prevent transmission of syphilis from one partner to the other and ultimately to their children. If the family has a history of genetic disease, genetic counseling can be obtained to determine the wisdom of having children.

When pregnancy occurs, the mother-to-be requires good health care to prevent harm to herself and to her infant. Such care includes a thorough medical examination to detect and then to treat such conditions as anemia, diabetes, cardiac or renal disease, or tuberculosis. Thorough and repeated gynecological examinations during pregnancy are essential in order to obtain pelvic measurements and to note the growth of the fetus so that a safe delivery can be planned. Laboratory tests include determination of the Rh type of the mother's blood. Mothers who are Rh negative and having a first child may be treated at the time of delivery so that sensitization to the Rh factor does not occur. If sensitization has occurred in the past, special care must be given to the newborn if he has erythroblastosis fetalis.

Tests for determining the presence of syphilis and tuberculosis are done to prevent these diseases from infecting the newborn. If the mother has syphilis, proper treatment during the first half of pregnancy will prevent the infant from being born with congenital syphilis. If tuberculosis is diagnosed, the mother is treated during pregnancy for her own protection, and care is taken after delivery to prevent infection of the newborn. The mother should be protected against all viral and bacterial infections, if this is possible.

Good general hygiene, cleanliness, and adequate nutrition are important to the pregnant woman. Cleanliness helps to prevent infections,

THE NEWBORN, HIS FAMILY AND THE NURSE

and a diet containing essential nutrients including protein and vitamins contributes to the well-being of the mother and promotes optimum growth in the fetus. It is desirable that the mother avoid cigarette smoking, which may reduce her oxygen supply and thus that of the fetus.

Education and emotional support for childbearing and child rearing have been mentioned previously. During education-for-parenthood discussions parents learn that they are not alone with their anxieties, fears, and fantasies, that others share them also. With the support of other couples and the professional discussion leader, many problems can be uncovered, and relieved or resolved completely. The supportive role of the nurse discussion leader is so important that in some hospitals he or she is called to be present when the mothers in the group are admitted in labor.

But education for child rearing should not stop when the newborn is delivered. Confident child care is certainly an important contributor to a child's healthy development. The goals of such parental education include increasing the parents' knowledge of child development and methods of care, providing parents with more social contacts and role models of successful parents, and providing support in a relaxed atmosphere in which parents can explore their individual and mutual feelings about caring for a child.

ENVIRONMENT AND DEVELOPMENT OF THE FETUS

The uterus of a healthy woman is perfectly adapted to the needs of the fetus. Her body is the medium which adapts conditions outside her to the developmental immaturity of the fetus. Since her heat-regulating mechanism keeps the temperature within the uterus constant, changes in outdoor or room temperature do not affect the fetus. The amniotic fluid in the uterus acts as a sterile insulating medium in which there is no friction.

The fetus needs oxygen and nutrients in order to live and grow. These are supplied through the blood stream of the prospective mother by way of the placenta and umbilical cord. Through the placenta and umbilical cord also the fetus is relieved of the waste products of metabolism.

The fetus is completely dependent upon the mother for all vital functions because the fetal organs have not developed to the extent that extrauterine life is possible. The lungs are not inflated. The circulatory system is adapted only to intrauterine life; little blood flows through the pulmonary artery, since the foramen ovale and the ductus arteriosus are not closed as they are after birth. The digestive tract cannot reduce even the simplest foods to the state in which elements can be taken up by the blood stream.

The fetus tends to develop normally even at the expense of the mother. An accident to the woman may involve the fetus. Anything which interferes with the normal transfer of oxygen or nutriment from the maternal blood stream to that of the fetus will jeopardize its safety.

THE NEWBORN

Neonatal Hazards and Preparation

Birth is associated with the most drastic changes that ever befall a person. In extrauterine life all functions undergo a radical change. A sudden adjustment has to be made from a "topsy-turvy aquatic environment" to a so-called sane air existence. After birth the infant not only must continue the vital activities of intrauterine life, but must also initiate other extrauterine processes which his mother per-

formed for him. The normal infant is able to do this, provided he receives essential care. *If the infant is to survive the crucial neonatal period, three conditions are necessary: that he be in good physical condition, that he experience a safe delivery, and that he then receive good care.*

INFANT MORTALITY

Improvement in maternal and infant care has greatly reduced the infant mortality rate in the last 25 to 30 years, but the decrease has been slower in the neonatal period than in the remaining months of infancy. From the second to the twelfth month of life less than half as many infants die as between birth and four weeks of age. The highest infant death rate is within the first month of life, and within that month in the first 24 hours. The most critical period for the infant is the first hour of extrauterine life, when the drastic change from intrauterine to extrauterine existence occurs.

Death in the neonatal period is most commonly due to the effects of prematurity, in particular hyaline membrane disease (see also Chapter 9). Other causes of death are *congenital malformations*, which render it impossible for the infant to establish an independent existence, *birth injuries, asphyxia,* and *atelectasis.* These conditions are discussed in succeeding chapters. Here we should take note that not all causes of congenital malformations are clearly understood. The number of infants who are kept alive and whose condition is relieved or mitigated by surgery is much higher than it was in the past. Birth injuries are not as common a cause of death as they were a few decades ago. Increasing numbers of prospective mothers are receiving better prenatal care. Difficult deliveries are anticipated and arrangements made for hospitalization of the mothers. Instrumental and operative deliveries are more judicious. The educated nurse-midwife is replacing the experienced but ignorant midwife. For these reasons the percentage of infants injured during delivery has been reduced.

The development of the new science of perinatology, dealing with diseases occurring shortly before and after birth, has changed the picture in regard to the viability of premature infants. The introduction of regional perinatal care centers and high-risk newborn nurseries has meant that infants of low birth weight and premature birth are surviving in much greater numbers. Furthermore, more infants are being examined during the first month of their lives by physicians, midwives and nurses after discharge from the nursery. Thus problems arising shortly after birth can be discovered and treated promptly. Research is currently being done in an attempt to find subtle indicators of fetal distress in order to save the fetus before birth or the newborn after birth.

Consumers, however, may be displeased with the quality of care given in hospitals in spite of these medical advances leading to a safe delivery. Parents who decide that their infant should be born at home rather than in the hospital may base their decision on psychologic reasons, wishing to be intensely involved in the childbearing experience and to have the support of family and friends at the time of birth. If an obstetrical problem arises in the actual delivery of the newborn, both mother and child may be in jeopardy. In the future, sensitive family-centered maternity care should be available in both the home and the hospital so that this tragedy may be avoided.

Health and Welfare Measures for Reduction of Infant Mortality. Since 1964, federal comprehensive care programs for low-income, hard-to-reach groups of mothers and infants at high risk have been in operation. These have represented a great expansion of maternal and child health services beyond that seen in traditional preventive medicine. *There are Maternity and Infant Care projects throughout the United States for the purpose of improving services to reduce infant mortality and to promote maternal and child health.* More specifically, the goals of these programs are to increase the number of prenatal and postnatal clinics in neighborhoods where they are needed, to provide special services for patients having complications of pregnancy, and to provide hospital care for mothers and infants as needed.

The environment of a pregnant woman influences her health, which in turn creates a healthful or unhealthful environment for the fetus. Unfortunately not all pregnant women can be provided with a healthful environment, but federal, state, and local health and welfare programs have made a great difference in the conditions under which the low-income group lives. Since newborn infants are prone to infections, the death rate among them is influenced by good sanitation in the community, cleanliness and avoidance of overcrowding in the home, fresh air and sunshine.

Some pregnant women do not go to a physician early in pregnancy, or they pay little attention to his advice. To win them over to a different attitude toward their own health and safety and to create in them a desire for the infant is a challenging task for the nurse.

The young female nurse has a special role in working with these mothers. She is likely to have good rapport with the young prospective mother because as a nurse she is intensely interested in pregnancy, knows well the physical processes that are taking place and, by her own attitude toward health and confidence in the medical advice given, influences the patients in a way different from that in which the older nurse, medical social worker or even the physician influences her.

As long as the infant is well his mother can be taught to give him all the care he needs, and she probably gives it better than anyone else because of her love for him. Some mothers, of course, either do not love their children or are unable to show their love in ways that transmit security to them. The cause of this is often extremely difficult to determine. The mother may be in need of psychiatric treatment. When the mother cannot give her infant the loving care he needs, some other person must be found to serve as a mother-substitute or to supplement the care she gives.

If the baby is not gaining weight as he should or is ill, the professional services of the nurse are needed. Infants have surprising vitality, but little resistance to disease, particularly disease which interferes with electrolyte balance, such as dehydration because of diarrhea, or massive infection with or without a high fever. Mothers must be taught to take the infant's temperature. If it is elevated, he must be seen by a physician, and measures taken to prevent the condition from becoming worse.

Clinics, outpatient departments, and admitting departments of hospitals, particularly in the low-income areas of large cities, are open 24 hours a day every day in the week. Immediate availability of the physician, the nurse or the pediatric nurse practitioner, and hospitalization if necessary, are extremely important.

Even a healthy infant needs a good regimen directed by a physician who examines him at regular intervals. It is often the nurse who welcomes the mother to the physician's office or the Child Health Conference and helps her to understand the physician's suggestions. Nurses in Child Health Conferences and outpatient departments of hospitals look for signs that the infant is not gaining as he should, has some chronic condition or is in the first stage of an acute disease. They must be particularly skillful in observing symptoms and eliciting information from a mother, since the infant cannot say how he feels.

Health and Welfare programs extend care to individual children, through whom the nurse makes her great contribution to the reduction of infant mortality. Whether the nurse is caring for patients in the pediatric unit or in a public health agency, she is working with individual babies. Only by keeping each one healthy and caring for each one when he is sick or in need of operation will infant morbidity and mortality rates be reduced.

Family Responses to the Newborn

Today emphasis is being placed on viewing the family as a whole rather than as a group of individuals. In regard to the newborn it is essential that we consider the responses of each member of the nuclear family: the mother, the father and the siblings in terms of their reactions to the new family member. It is true that while the infant is being formed physically, the individual family members are creating a family psychologically.

THE MOTHER

Pregnancy is a period of crisis for a woman involving profound endocrine, somatic, and psychological changes. The mastery of this significant turning point in her life depends to a large extent on her emotional maturity. If the mother has unfulfilled needs, this may prevent the full development of the quality of motherliness essential for the well-being of her infant.

In caring for the newborn the nurse bases his or her role on much more than an understanding of the baby's physical attributes. It is the nurse's responsibility to help the parents build a happier family life through his coming. In order to do this the mutual dependency of the mother and her infant must be understood.

Immediate or early contact between the mother and the newborn after birth is extremely important to the future of the individual mother-child relationship. The mother is especially sensitized following delivery to form an attachment to her infant. By *attachment* is meant a unique, enduring emotional relationship between two persons that is specific to them. Early contact between mother and child can affect certain aspects of mothering behavior such as breast feeding and fondling, which may have significance for the later development of the child. This concept is of importance especially when considering newborns who are taken from their mothers immediately after birth, for example, those who are premature (see Chapter 9) or who have congenital anomalies incompatible with life but amenable to surgical correction (see Chapter 11). Mothers of such infants may not be able to form the degree of attachment that might otherwise have been possible.

Mother love is supposed to be the strongest emotional tie between two human beings. The influence of the endocrine glands as they function in the pregnant or lactating mother is evident even among the higher animals. They are gentle in handling their young and are likely to be fiercely protective of them. If all her offspring are taken from a mother, she will become restless, may refuse to eat, and may evidence frustration at the blocking of an instinct based

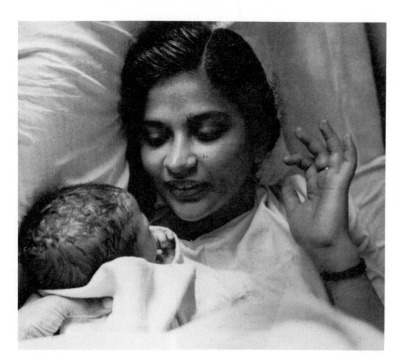

FIGURE 6–1. The love of a mother for her child is seen throughout the world. (Courtesy of the Medical Mission Sisters, Philadelphia, Pennsylvania.)

on glandular secretion. The human mother has not only this physical basis for her dependency on her infant, but also a love for him which has been developing through the long months of gestation. If she is separated from her baby, she is denied relief from an emotional need based in part on her physical condition.

Up to the child's birth there is a *symbiotic relation* between the mother and the fetus. A symbiotic relation is one of extreme closeness. Before birth the fetus existed as a parasite within his mother. The two—mother and fetus—were necessary to each other. The fetus could not live unless her body supplied his needs, and she in turn needed the product of conception to complete the physical changes which pregnancy was producing in her.

Mothers desire to continue this symbiotic relation after the child's birth, and the nurse should recognize the importance of the tie. Modern obstetrical nursing is planned to keep mother and baby together, his bassinet beside her bed. Mothers are urged to nurse their infants, since breast feeding is the closest approach to a symbiotic relation which can be achieved after the birth of the child.

Although the symbiotic relation exists, the nurse must not expect all mothers to hold their newborns comfortably at first. Some mothers will initially touch their infants only with the tips of their fingers. As the mother becomes more comfortable in her role, as her infant gradually responds to her touch, and as their attachment deepens, the mother will eventually be able to hold or enfold her child in her arms. In view of the stages through which the mother must move before being entirely comfortable in caring for her infant, the nurse must not become impatient if the mother does not adjust immediately to the process of breast feeding or rooming-in.

As the mother begins to experience responses from her baby, especially smiling in response to her smile, she is encouraged to continue in her mothering role more spontaneously. The mother, particularly with her first infant, may have difficulty in establishing a rhythm, with the result that feeding and sleeping patterns may be hard to establish. This experience needs to be a mutually satisfying one for both mother and child. The nurse can be of great assistance to the mother by assessing her needs for help and guidance and anticipating her times of feeling discouraged and dissatisfied with her new role. The new mother needs opportunities to resume activities and relationships which were a source of satisfaction for her prior to the birth of her child.

The attitudes of some mothers toward the rearing of their children may change as a result of the Women's Liberation movement, but the close relationship between a mother and her newborn child must remain if a healthy mother-child relationship is to develop.

THE FATHER

The presence of the father in the delivery room at the time of the newborn's birth, his holding his newborn in his arms, and his frequent visits to the mother's room during hospitalization help to cement family ties. The father, who all too often has been a forgotten family member, has two responsibilities in the family after the birth of his child. His first responsibility is to his wife. The hormonal changes which are inevitable after childbirth produce in many women a state of depression. The mother needs to feel at this time that she is loved so that she in turn can love her infant. The father, therefore, not only must feel love toward his wife but must also communicate this feeling to her.

The role of the father is honored in many societies. The father, like the mother, has looked forward to having a son or daughter. Half of the child's heredity is transmitted through him, and the infant is as much a continuation of himself as of his wife. In a family the children need the masculine influence as much as they do the feminine. They need a father's affection, as they need a mother's. But because of the newborn's immediate need for his mother, the father's role is likely to appear subsidiary and to be taken as a matter of course, and he may feel left out of this most important event in married life.

The newborn has a powerful impact on the father. In turn, the father becomes involved with

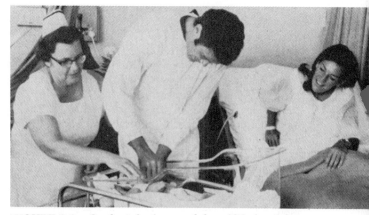

FIGURE 6–2. On the infant's second day of life, her father delicately cleans the folds of her groin before diapering her. The nurse who had demonstrated this procedure earlier supervises him. (Illustration by John Pineda, courtesy of *Tropic Medicine.*)

him through a process known as *engrossment*. Engrossment means that the father is absorbed with his child and preoccupied with his welfare. This father-infant bond leads to his focusing attention on his child, looking at and touching the infant, thinking him perfect, and caring for him. As the father becomes further involved with his infant, the level of the father's self-esteem rises.

Cultural influences may play a part in the development of engrossment. In some cultures the father is not supposed to make contact with his young infant or to give expression to his feelings if he does. Also, the mother may feel threatened if the father gives too much attention to his child. Brief counseling may be of value to such couples in helping them develop better parent-child relations.

Male nurses have an important role to play in this engrossment process. The nurse can establish a unique rapport with fathers during labor, help them to share their awakening feelings about their infants, and to give them care.

The modern father is not willing to be left out of all these new activities in the home; neither does he want to be made to feel like "mother's helper." Father wants to feel like a real contributor, an important nurturing person in the care of his family. He changes diapers and picks up and cuddles his infant as successfully as the mother. In this way he reaches the baby's consciousness and lays the basis for affection. As the infant responds, the father becomes increasingly fond of taking an active part in his care. So the coming of the baby has strengthened the parents' love for each other through their love for the newborn infant.

THE SIBLINGS

The siblings' reaction to the arrival of a new baby in the family is conditioned by their parents' attitude and the number of other members in the family. The acceptance of the infant is of such importance that in some hospitals siblings are permitted to visit their mother and new brother or sister prior to their mother's discharge. If the parents encourage siblings to share in the care of the infant and at the same time provide love and security for them as individuals, the children are less likely to consider the newcomer an intruder in their home. (See Chapter 19 for further discussion of the reaction of siblings to the birth of a child.)

The Newborn's Response to Birth

That giving birth to a child is difficult and even dangerous for the mother is common knowl-edge, but that even an easy normal birth must be a great strain upon the baby is seldom realized. His body sustains the pressure of the uterine contractions and his head the pressure of the resisting cervix. Although good obstetrical care prevents injury to the infant as well as to the mother and makes his passage through the birth canal less exhausting, birth still remains an anxiety-provoking experience. To this is added the necessity to adapt to life as a separate entity, no longer part of the mother.

As long as the fetus is nurtured through his mother's body, his health and that of his mother are the concern of the obstetrician and the obstetrical nurse. But the infant's health after birth is the concern of the pediatrician, the pediatric nurse, and the pediatric nurse practitioner.

THE WORLD AS THE INFANT EXPERIENCES IT

Since an infant's senses are not acute and discriminating at birth, the world about him must appear to be "one great, blooming, buzzing confusion." Yet the beginning of personality is there. How far personality at birth determines that of the older child or adult is not known, but it is certain that environmental factors modify personality early in infancy. The infant has two great drives: to be loved and to love. (Although the need to be loved is evident at birth, the drive to love is not manifested until later.) The physical needs of the infant who is loved are sure to be satisfied, but the unloved infant is likely to be neglected. The infant equates the relief of a need with love. Since hunger is an imperative need, it is natural that the infant loves the person who feeds him. Assured of food and cuddling, the infant develops a sense of *trust*. The implication of this is that when the mother holds her baby to her breast while he nurses or when she feeds him from the bottle, she is showing him love in a way that he can sense. The loved, contented baby forms a habit of contentment and does not easily become fretful. Anxiety-arousing stimuli should be kept from him, for a habit of anxiety can be as easily aroused as that of contentment.

Some psychologists believe that the infant is capable of fear and anger at birth. If so, these two emotions are difficult to distinguish. Sudden loss of support or a loud noise will produce a reflex startle reaction, and this is said to be evidence of fear. When he is crying loudly, we infer that he is angry. In either case he is reacting to a stimulus which he does not like and wants to have stopped. He soon learns that crying will bring someone who will make him comfortable. Since it is generally his mother who does this, he soon learns to prefer her to other people. This appears to be the basis of his love

The relations of husband and wife are like this:

Those of a husband, wife and child can be diagrammed like this:

Those of a husband, wife, and 2 children look like this:

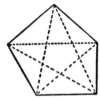

Those of a husband, wife, and 3 children look like this:

Within every family there are 2 variables which submit to precise mathematical determination. One of these is the number of members in the family, i.e., the size of the group; the other is the number of personal relations between its members. If these 2 variables are considered mathematically, what happens with the addition of each new member of the family group may be set forth in the following 2 sets of numbers:

Number of persons.... 2, 3, 4, 5, 6, 7, 8
Number of personal relations.. 1, 3, 6, 10, 15, 21, 28

FIGURE 6–3. Bossard's Law of Family Interaction. (J. H. S. Bossard: *The Sociology of Child Development.* Rev. ed. New York, Harper and Brothers.)

for his mother. She responds to his flattering preference for her with endearing attention, and so the cycle of mother-baby, baby-mother love is strengthened. Secure in her care for him, he will accept supplementary care from other people, provided it is *like* that which she gives him.

The child who is cared for by a changing group of people fails to form an affectionate attachment to anyone. He is likely to be very self-centered, and this situation, if continued, is one factor in producing the autistic child.

One principle of child care is that *the infant needs consistent loving care given by one or two people, an adequate amount of sensory stimulation based on his temperament, a minimal amount of anxiety and a maximum amount of contentment.* Only then can the infant learn to adapt to his new environment.

Role of the Professional Nurse

The nurse provides emotional support and anticipatory guidance for the parents in the care of their newborn and assesses their attitudes and their potential ability to provide an environment which will foster the development of trust in their infant. In order to carry out this responsibility effectively the nurse must be aware of cultural differences and traditional values and ideas that various groups have, whether due to poverty, language differences, educational background, skin color, or other factors.

NEEDS OF THE PARENTS

The role of the nurse in caring for the family during the postpartum period must be based not on the needs of the hospital and its staff, but on the needs of the parents and their child.

The new family relations which spring from the arrival of the baby are evidenced through all the hours of the day and night, as a new element in the former kinship within the family. The family relations before the first pregnancy were one to one, but with the birth of the first child each member is related to two others. Neither parent may now expect the entire love and attention of the other. With the second and succeeding births the change in relations becomes more complex (see Fig. 6–3). Note that the father's place in Figure 6–3 is comparable to that of the mother.

The supportive role of the professional nurse in the adjustment of the parents to their new relations to one another and to their child is enacted while giving the mother and her infant physical care. This support gives her role its peculiar significance and makes it more effective than that of the other professional members of the health team. Other team members, of course, give physical help to patients, but it is not characterized by meeting their daily recurrent needs and so is less likely to be helpful in adjustment to a new situation which involves the minute details of family life.

We are apt to concentrate attention on the mother rather than on the father. This is justified, but both parents (particularly if this is their first child) need help in making all the necessary adjustments involved in childbirth and in the care of the newborn infant. The nurse, more than any other member of the hospital staff, makes the parents feel at home. The nurse is host in the hospital and makes the first meeting of the mother and the father, after the birth of their child, emotionally satisfying. The nurse should remember that the mother will be thinking of all that was said and done in this first brief visit until her husband comes again. A satisfying visit promotes tranquil rest; an unsatisfying one, emotional disturbance.

Hospital policies control what the nurse may allow the parents. If the hospital imposes stringent rules as to visiting hours and viewing the infant, this first meeting of husband and wife may be so emotionally unsatisfying that the mother's physical condition is adversely influenced by her disappointment. In any case, however, the nurse's friendly, cordial manner is helpful.

The nurse should accept the mother's dependency needs and not expect from her all the self-care of which she is physically capable. In the early days of ambulation after delivery it is easy for the nurse to forget the emotional effect of childbirth upon a young mother. If the mother is not emotionally ready for the routine self-care customary in the hospital, the nurse should do for her what the mother feels she cannot do for herself. The mother should never be made to feel that she is failing to live up to the nurse's concept of the modern woman who accepts childbirth as a natural process which incapacitates for only a day or two. (Even the most ardent believer in natural childbirth realizes that not all women are capable of carrying it to completion without emotional trauma. This is true also of early self-care.) Nurses should accept and understand the reactions of each mother and plan her care accordingly. When both the physical and the emotional needs of the mother have been met, the mother feels secure in the hospital and can accept the rest she requires before returning to her duties in the home or on the job. Because of the close emotional union of mother and child, she will not be content unless she knows that the infant, too, is well cared for by the nurses.

The mother should be encouraged to talk over her recent experience in the delivery room and also any matter which worries her about the infant, her own condition, or her home. Past experiences are interpreted in the light of the present. If the nurse makes the mother's stay in the hospital as pleasant as possible, the mother's attitude toward future pregnancies and deliveries is likely to be optimistic.

After the birth of their newborn some parents may consider the matter of future family planning if they have not done so before. As a result of experience in maternity nursing the nurse should be knowledgeable in this area in order to provide guidance for parents to sources of such assistance if it is not possible to give this needed information at the time.

NEEDS OF THE NEWBORN

The basic needs of the newborn are those of any helpless young animal dependent upon its mother, but with these significant differences. He is the most dependent of any young creature for a longer period of time, and yet he is the recipient of the scientific knowledge which only human beings possess and is himself one of the coming generation who may add to this fund of knowledge.

The nurse's knowledge of what is normal in a newborn baby enables him or her to know what is abnormal. The nurse should observe and appraise the status of the infant when he is brought to the nursery. *Many potentially dangerous abnormalities of the newborn can be treated before a serious physiologic disturbance results. These require early recognition and diagnosis.* (See Chapter 7 for further discussion.)

The newborn is likely to be exhausted by the birth process, and gentle handling to conserve his strength is necessary. His personality is being formed by his experiences even during these first few days of life. Gentleness in caring for him is an expression of love, and makes physical care—his bath and the changing of his diaper—a pleasure to him. He likes skin-to-skin contact. His heat-regulating system is so poorly developed that he needs external warmth. A soft cuddly blanket gives him the feeling of a closed environment of even temperature such as he experienced in the uterus. He needs frequent changes of position, not merely from lying on one side to the other, but also the many minor changes which occur when he is picked up and cuddled.

Self-Demand Schedule. It is believed that the newborn responds to his needs with sleeping when his body needs sleep and with crying when his body needs nourishment. He demands sleep and feedings in accordance with his rhythm of bodily functions, a rhythm which is fairly constant from day to day. *His schedule should be planned in accordance with his demands and will vary with his physical condition.* If he has a fever, he will, of course, want water more frequently, and his sleep will be intermittent. As he matures, the interval between feedings will lengthen and he will take more at each feeding. His periods of wakefulness will be longer, and his total time spent in sleep will be less.

The self-demand schedule must be carried out in a stable environment adapted to the infant's immaturity. This environment is both physical and social. The physical environment must be hygienic, and the social environment such that he learns to associate a feeling of well-being with the care given him (for further discussion of self-demand feeding see Chapter 8).

After the traumatic experience of birth the newborn needs to acquire strength before he begins to gain in weight and vigor. This is a period of adjustment for him in which the self-demand schedule is particularly important. He should be offered the breast or bottle, but never unduly urged. From the time he enters the nursery his comprehensive nursing care includes meeting both his physical and his emotional needs; otherwise he will not reach and maintain his optimum level of well-being and feel secure in the strange environment of the nursery.

Rooming-in

An environment can be planned which will be suitable for all infants, each of whom requires environmental adaptation to meet his needs. It is extremely difficult to provide this in a nursery where one or two nurses are caring for a large number of infants. Needs are likely to be met at certain fixed times suited to the average infant's schedule for feeding, sleep and periods of placid rest. The nursery schedule is adjusted to administrative and personnel considerations as well as to the needs of the average infant. Many infants are not average, however. Also, a baby's needs vary from day to day. Furthermore, babies need affection shown in ways which are peculiar to the mother-child relation and which no nurse can reproduce in the care of a constantly changing group of babies. Rooming-in is a method which provides for infant, mother, and nurse the conditions in which each is most satisfied and can most successfully fulfill his or her role.

Rooming-in is a hospital arrangement whereby the mother has her newborn infant by her bedside and takes as much care of him as her condition permits and she desires. It is a family-centered service in the hospital situation. It is an effort to meet parents' request for more information about the care of the baby, and it gives both the parents and the baby a homelike feeling in the impersonal hospital atmosphere.

The practice of rooming-in gives the young mother an opportunity to become acquainted with her child and accustomed to his care. It relieves her anxiety as to his welfare in the nursery, where she often hears babies crying and is sure that one of them is hers. It permits the baby's father to hold or feed him or change his diaper. This is a different introduction from standing in the hall and looking through a glass window at a room full of infants while a nurse brings *the one* to the nursery side of the window.

The infant who rooms-in receives more individual attention, for his mother can reach over and pat him, change his position, give him water or replace a wet or soiled diaper. Feeding is promoted because when the mother sees her infant hungry, she is motivated to put him to the breast. If the physician approves of the infant's being on a self-demand schedule, the mother can easily feed him whenever he wants to nurse.

Some mothers, however, do not want the baby's crib beside their bed. They do not want to feed him on a self-demand schedule, nor do they want to give him care. These are likely to be the mothers of large families and have been overworked up to the time of delivery. They are in need of a complete rest and should not be forced to do more for their infants than give them the breast or, if they are bottle-fed, hold them for a few minutes each day.

There are disadvantages to rooming-in from the point of view of both the parents and the hospital. Some mothers are neither physically nor emotionally able to do their part in the rooming-in care of an infant. The physician may feel that there is danger of infection, although the infectious conditions which the newborn is most likely to contract are those which are carried from infant to infant by the hospital personnel or through the use of improperly sterilized equipment. The hospital administrator knows that rooming-in requires more well-qualified personnel and uses more floor space than does the traditional care given to newborns in a central nursery.

For rooming-in to be successful, the staff nurses must have warm, comforting personalities. They must not insist on a rigid plan of nursing care. Rather, they should promote normal relations in the family and help the parents make their own plan for the infant. This they do by sharing with them their own knowledge of child care and giving the parents reassurance in their ability to meet any problems which may arise in the care of the infant.

MODIFICATIONS OF TRADITIONAL MATERNITY UNITS

Although rooming-in would seem to be the ideal method by which the needs of both newborns and parents could be met, the practice is not widely accepted in this country.

If rooming-in is not practical in the maternity area, the same objectives may be attained in the traditional maternity unit by the following modifications in arrangement and in assignment of patients to the nursing personnel.

1. *Individual family units* may be assigned to the nurse for study and the making of a plan of care. The nurse can observe the interpersonal relations within this "family" and plan the care of mother and child with reference to their relation to the father, maternal grandmother, or other relatives who visit the patient. In this way the nurse can carry out a supporting role with the family as a whole. If attention is focused on only one member, the needs of others are likely to be forgotten, and thereby the nurse may create friction within the family which reacts adversely on the patient. Of course if the hospital policy does not permit nurses who are caring for the mothers on the maternity unit to enter the newborn nursery, this family-centered plan of nursing care cannot be carried out. Nevertheless the nurse assigned to the care of the mother and the nurse caring for the infant may unite as a team in their study of the family and confer on the needs of the family as a whole.

2. Nurses may be helped by the instructors and supervisors to establish a cooperative learning relationship with the infant's parents. Thereby (a) the parents will realize that the nurse is interested in their baby and in their ability to provide good care for him after his discharge from the hospital, and (b) the nurse makes the greatest gain in knowledge and skill from the experience in the nursing care of the infant and his mother.

3. Routines can be made more flexible so that the needs of the individual family may be met through having the nurse use good judgment in the application of hospital regulations. Mothers might be permitted to keep their babies with them longer than is required for feeding. Husbands might be encouraged to talk of their new role of father if this is the first child, or of being the father of an increasingly large family. The nurse will find that successful adjustment to the first baby differs in many ways from that to the second and later children.

With the first baby the role of a father is new and at least temporarily appears as the most important of his roles in the many groups to which he belongs. With succeeding children the role is no longer novel and now has the added element of duties and pleasures related to children of different ages and probably sex, and of working with the mother to establish proper sibling relations.

4. Group discussions may be scheduled for mothers in the maternity unit so that their specific needs can be learned and met. Such discussions may be planned by the students in nursing under the direction of their instructors.

5. If the mother has had no previous experience, she may be taught to bathe and dress her infant. Even if she is already expert in child care, she may profit by reviewing the hospital technique, and she surely needs to make the acquaintance of her baby in those situations that mean most to him, i.e., in which affection is shown in his direct physical care.

6. Parents may be told of the community resources available in case they need assistance after leaving the hospital.

SHARED LEARNING: NURSE-PARENT EDUCATION

In a narrow interpretation, parental education in the hospital is limited to teaching mothers to prepare formulas, to bathe their infants and to give them physical care. In a broader sense it is a continuation of the parental education and prenatal courses which the parents have participated in. Such courses give the information needed in making important decisions about the baby, but do not provide ready-made answers to questions about the individual baby in his family setting. It is in the application of what the mothers have already learned that the nurse is most helpful. It is a shared learning experience, for the nurse, like the mother, must apply knowledge of child care to the individual infant.

If the student nurse has had little experience in caring for infants and if the mother has had several children of her own, the nurse may learn more from the mother than the mother from the nurse. On the other hand, if the nurse has had considerable experience with children and if this is the mother's first baby, the nurse shares with the mother this greater knowledge.

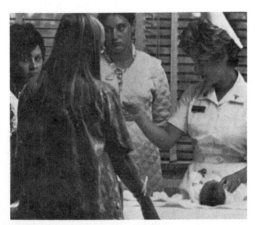

FIGURE 6–4. Nurse-parent education. (Courtesy of the Army Nurse Corps.)

The nurse should appreciate the mother's level of understanding and background of experience. This will vary with the mother's socioeconomic class and ethnic background and will also depend upon whether this is her first baby and whether she has had experience with the infants of near relatives. The mother may herself be a professional woman working in the area of child care and may be an expert in the daily care of children.

The nurse should know what sort of care will be possible in the home, the equipment available, and the level of living which can be maintained. Specific directions should be written down, or if they are given orally, the mother should be asked to repeat what the nurse has said. *Instructions should be given slowly over a period of time; a mother cannot absorb all that she is to learn of child care at one time.* Knowledge and experience should come gradually. If a mother attended prenatal classes, she has already learned much and will learn more from the physicians and nurses in the hospital. The community or public health nurse will show her the adaptation of all she has learned to the home care of her baby and its application to the immediate situation.

For inexperienced nurses working with the mother as members of the team caring for the child in the hospital, such teaching is a shared learning experience. The expression *shared learning experience* of the mother and nurse is often more truly descriptive of their relations than saying that the nurse teaches the patient.

It is simpler to teach the physical care of children than the psychologic care, and this is particularly true of infant care. The tremendous importance of happiness in infancy lies not only in the present, but also in the formation of the child's personality. The mother-child relationship is recognized as the normal center of the baby's emotional development and is therefore most important. Other members of the family and the world outside are likely to influence the infant through their effect upon his mother.

The love of a mother for her child is the great incentive to her for learning how best to care for him. Such love is likely to make her somewhat critical of instruction given in a purely professional way. The nurse's manner should be warm and friendly, convincing each mother of their joint ability to apply scientific principles to child care.

Recognition of Maternal Dependency Needs

Physical weakness after delivery of a firstborn child is likely to increase a woman's feeling of incompetency in the role of mother of an infant, who, when she leaves the hospital, will be completely dependent upon her for his care. This brings us to the problem of meeting her dependency needs so that she feels secure and confident that she will receive the help she has a right to expect from her family and the community. If she worries over the future, her relationship with her baby is influenced by her anxiety and ceases to be the happy fulfillment of her pregnancy. This will influence her ability to nurse the baby at the breast, and her insecurity for the baby and herself on leaving the hospital may be communicated to the infant. He is not likely to be a contented, happy baby.

The mother's dependency needs, both physical and emotional, influence her relations with her baby. She needs her husband's understanding love. She needs to know that he loves the baby not only for itself, but also as the common object of their affection, and that the infant strengthens the emotional bond between them. In contrast, the infant may be made the center of emotional conflicts. The presence of other children may be an emotionally sustaining influence on the one hand, but on the other hand may create many problems caused by their jealousy of the attention given the new arrival.

Probably the crucial factor in the situation is how the mother deals with her dependency needs. In the hospital she may resent being asked to undertake more self-care and more care of the baby than she feels able to undertake. At the other extreme there are mothers who are accustomed to denying the existence of their dependency needs. They find even a few days of enforced hospitalization unpleasant and want to go home too early.

Mothers who feel insecure and fear criticism of their care of the baby insist upon rules to follow or depend upon their own mother's advice in all the little day-to-day problems that arise. The mother who finds dependency humiliating may not ask for the help she needs in caring for her baby.

Nurses will find that the mother of a first baby is more likely to feel dependent, whether she acknowledges it or not, than the mother of several healthy children. The baby looks so small and his ways are so different from those of older babies whom she knows that she is afraid he is choking, suffocating or in extreme danger of some sort. Such a mother is apt to feel that his crying is caused by a condition which must be remedied at once. If she is the overdependent type, she will make many demands upon the nurses. If she is accustomed to taking responsibility and denying her dependency needs, she may force herself into the role of the self-reliant, competent mother, but with a feeling that she is not receiving the help to which she is entitled. Neither extreme leads to good mother-child relations. These women need all the help the nurse can give them.

The young nurse is close in age to many maternity patients and therefore can have a great influence on them. This closeness, which is of potential value, is likely to involve the nurse emotionally in the relations with a young mother and, in so doing, hampers service to the patient. Young nurses who are married or expect to be married soon may develop a feeling of identity with the mother which hinders rather than helps their nursing care. It is important for them to retain their professional attitude and a degree of objectivity which does not necessarily cause them to be cold or aloof.

The reaction of the mother to childbirth should be considered and her care arranged accordingly. Sending her home from the hospital within a few days after delivery may be necessary. But it is essential that she be given help in the housework and care of the baby. Her own mother or sister or a visiting housekeeper can give her the assistance she needs.

The Unloving Mother

When a mother does not love her baby—as may happen if he is born out of wedlock—the great stimulus to learn to care for him is absent (see Chapter 27). No mother should be urged to keep her child against her wishes. It would probably be far better for both if he were placed in an adoptive home where he could be loved and cherished. Such a mother need not be taught the care of the infant.

There are other mothers who are married, however, who did not want to become pregnant and who feel that the baby interferes with their professional or social life. Many such mothers find that they love the baby dearly when he is put in their arms, but others remain indifferent to him and look upon his care as an unwanted chore. In hospitals where it is routine for mothers to attend the group discussion meetings and demonstrations of child care these mothers attend with all the others. They are likely to feel guilty that they do not nurture love for the baby and as a result are overpunctilious in learning all the details of his physical care. Later at home, when the community or public health nurse sees mother and child, the baby's fine physical condition under his mother's care may generate in her a sense of achievement and pride in him which may in turn evoke love.

The unloving mother initially may provoke a negative response on the part of the nurse in the hospital and in the community. It is important, therefore, that each nurse examine his or her feelings so that further stimulation of guilt in the mother is avoided.

TEACHING AIDS AND OTHER INFORMATION*

Consumer Product Information

How a Mother Affects Her Unborn Child, 1970.
So You're Going To Be a New Father, 1973.
The Food Stamp Program, 1975.

Department of National Health and Welfare, Ottawa, Canada

Current Status of Family Planning in Canada.
Facts and Fancy about Birth Control, Sex Education and Family Planning.
Family Living and Sex Education: A Canadian Overview.
Family Planning: A Resource Guide for Nurses.

Johnson & Johnson

Auerbach, A. B.: Preparation for Parenthood Through Group Discussion: A Guide for Nurse-Leaders of Expectant-Parent Classes, 1976.

Maternity Center Association

A Baby Is Born.
For the Expectant Father.
How Does Your Baby Grow?
Maternity Center Association.
Nutrition and Birth.
Preparation for Childbearing.

The National Foundation—March of Dimes

Be Good to Your Baby Before It Is Born, 1975.
Confidential: To Fathers and Fathers-to-Be.

Planned Parenthood Federation of America, Inc.

Basics of Birth Control.
Have Your Next Baby When You Want To.
The Safe Period.
To Be a Mother . . . To Be a Father.

Public Affairs Committee

Carson, R.: Nine Months to Get Ready—The Importance of Prenatal Care.
Carson, R.: Nueve Meses Para Prepararse: La Importancia del Cuidado Prenatal (Nine Months to Get Ready).
Doyle, N.: Woman's Changing Place: A Look at Sexism.
Genné, W., and Genné, E.: Building a Marriage on Two Altars.

United States Government

Cuidado Prenatal (Prenatal Care), 1975.

*Complete addresses are given in the Appendix.

Drugs and Pregnancy, 1974.
Family Planning and Health, 1975.
NICHD Answers Your Questions About Family Planning,
Infants and Children, 1976

Prenatal Care, 1973
The Man Who Cares, 1975.
WIC Program Survey, 1975, 1975.

REFERENCES

Books

Arey, L. B.: *Developmental Anatomy.* 7th ed. Philadelphia, W. B. Saunders Company, 1974.

Arms, S.: *Immaculate Deception.* Boston, Houghton Mifflin Company, 1975.

Balinsky, B. I.: *An Introduction to Embryology.* 4th ed. Philadelphia, W. B. Saunders Company, 1975.

Barber, V., and Skaggs, M. M.: *The Mother Person.* Indianapolis, Ind., The Bobbs-Merrill Company, 1975.

Bernhardt, K. S.: *Being a Parent: Unchanging Values in a Changing World.* Toronto, University of Toronto Press, 1970.

Demarest, R. J., and Sciarra, J. J.: *Conception, Birth and Contraception:* A Visual Presentation. New York, McGraw-Hill Book Company, 1976.

Dickason, E. J., and Schult, M. O.: *Maternal and Infant Care.* New York, McGraw-Hill Book Company, 1975.

Dodson, F.: *How to Father.* Los Angeles, Nash Publishing Corporation, 1974.

Duvall, E. M.: *Family Development.* 4th ed. Philadelphia, J. B. Lippincott Company, 1971.

Garcia, C. R., and Rosenfeld, D. L.: *Family Planning.* Philadelphia, F. A. Davis Company, 1976.

Green, R. (Ed.): *Human Sexuality; A Health Practitioner's Text.* Baltimore, Williams & Wilkins Company, 1975.

Greenhill, J. P., and Friedman, E. A.: *Biological Principles and Modern Practice of Obstetrics.* Philadelphia, W. B. Saunders Company, 1974.

Hafez, E. S. E., and Evans, T. N.: *Human Reproduction: Conception and Contraception.* New York, Harper & Row Publishers, 1973.

Haire, D.: *The Cultural Warping of Childbirth.* Seattle, Washington, International Childbirth Education Association, 1972.

Hallum, J. L.: *Midwifery.* New York, Arco Publishing Company, 1974.

Johnson, M. A.: *Developing the Art of Understanding.* 2nd ed. New York, Springer Publishing Company, 1972.

Laliberta, D. (ed.): *Child Health Care in Rural Areas; a Manual for Auxiliary Nurse Midwives.* New York, Asia Publishing House, 1974.

Langman, J.: *Medical Embryology; Human Development—Normal and Abnormal.* 3rd ed. Baltimore, Williams & Wilkins Company, 1975.

Lawrence, M. M.: *Young Inner City Families: Development of Ego Strength Under Stress.* New York, Behavioral Publications, 1975.

Leboyer, F.: *Birth Without Violence.* New York, Alfred A. Knopf, Inc., 1975.

Lynn, D. B.: *The Father: His Role in Child Development.* Monterey, California, Brooks/Cole Publishing Company, 1974.

McGinnis, T. C., and Finnegan, D. G.: *Open Family and Marriage; A Guide to Personal Growth.* St. Louis, The C. V. Mosby Company, 1976.

Moore, K. L.: *Before We Are Born: Basic Embryology and Birth Defects.* Philadelphia, W. B. Saunders Company, 1974.

Moore, K. L.: *Study Guide and Review Manual of Human Embryology.* Philadelphia, W. B. Saunders Company, 1975.

Myles, M. F.: *Textbook for Midwives; with Modern Concepts of Obstetric and Neonatal Care.* 8th ed. Edinburgh, Churchill Livingstone, 1975.

Oliven, J. F.: *Clinical Sexuality: A Manual for the Physician and the Professions.* 3rd ed. Philadelphia, J. B. Lippincott Company, 1974.

Page, E. W., Villee, C. A., and Villee, D. B.: *Human Reproduction: The Core Content of Obstetrics, Gynecology and Perinatal Medicine.* 2nd ed. Philadelphia, W. B. Saunders Company, 1976.

Pierson, E. C., and D'Antonio, W. V.: *Female and Male; Dimensions of Human Sexuality.* Philadelphia, J. B. Lippincott, 1974.

Reinhardt, A. M., and Quinn, M. D. (Eds.): *Family-Centered Community Nursing: A Socio-Cultural Framework.* St. Louis, The C. V. Mosby Company, 1973.

Selye, H.: *The Stress of Life.* Rev. ed. New York, McGraw-Hill Book Co., 1976.

Shope, D. F.: *Interpersonal Sexuality.* Philadelphia, W. B. Saunders Company, 1975.

Vaughan, V. C., and Brazelton, T. B. (Eds.): *The Family—Can It Be Saved?* Chicago, Year Book Medical Publishers Inc., 1976.

Wagner, N. N.: *Perspectives on Human Sexuality: Psychological, Social and Cultural Research Findings.* New York, Behavioral Publications, 1974.

Wallace, H. M., Gold, E. M., and Lis, E. H. (Eds.): *Maternal and Child Health Practices: Problems, Resources, and Methods of Delivery.* Springfield, Ill., Charles C Thomas, 1973.

Zeitz, A. N.: *Postpartum as a Continuing Link in the Symbiotic Relationship of Parents and Child.* New York, Zanab Press, 1975.

Periodicals

Adamkiewicz, V. W.: What Are the Bonds Between the Fetus and the Uterus? *The Canadian Nurse,* 72:26, February, 1976.

Ager, J. W., Werley, H. H., Allen, D. V., Shea, F. P., and Lewis, H. Y.: Vasectomy: Who Gets One and Why? *Am. J. Public Health,* 64:680, July 1974.

Atkinson, L. D.: Is Family-Centered Care a Myth? *The American Journal of Maternal-Child Nursing,* 1:256, July-August 1976.

Clark, A. L.: Labor and Birth: Expectations and Outcomes. *Nursing Forum,* 14:412, 1975.

Clark, D., Keith, L., Pildes, R., and Vargas, G.: Drug-dependent Obstetric Patients: A Study of 104 Admissions to the Cook County Hospital. *JOGN Nurs.,* 3:17, September-October 1974.

Cronenwett, L. R., and Newmark, L. L.: Fathers' Responses to Childbirth. *Nursing Research,* 23:210, May-June 1974.

Davitz, L. J.: Childbirth Nigerian Style. *RN,* 35:40, March 1972.

Doering, S. G., and Entwisle, D. R.: Preparation During Pregnancy and Ability to Cope with Labor and Delivery. *Am. J. Orthopsychiatry,* 45:825, October 1975.

Dryfoos, J. G.: Women Who Need and Receive Family Planning Services: Estimates at Mid-Decade. *Fam. Plann. Perspect.,* 4:172, July-August 1975.

Edwards, M. E.: Unattended Home Birth. *Am. J. Nursing,* 73:1332, August 1973.

Farris, L. S.: Approaches to Caring for the American Indian Maternity Patient. *The American Journal of Maternal-Child Nursing,* 1:80, March-April 1976.

Greenberg, M., and Morris, N.: Engrossment: The Newborn's Impact Upon the Father. *Nursing Digest*, 4:19, January-February 1976.

Higdon, H.: Giving Birth... Gently. *Family Health/Today's Health*, 8:40, May 1976.

Institute of Medicine, National Academy of Sciences: Infant Death: An Analysis of Maternal Risk and Health Care. *Conn. Med.*, 38:123, March 1974.

Jacobs, D., Garcia, C., Rickels, K., and Preucel, R. W.: A Prospective Study on the Psychological Effects of Therapeutic Abortion. *Compr. Psychiatry*, 15:423, September-October 1974.

Lechtig, A., et al.: Effect of Food Supplementation During Pregnancy on Birthweight. *Pediatrics*, 56:508, October 1975.

Lubic, R. W.: Developing Maternity Services Women Will Trust. *Am. J. Nursing*, 75:1685, October 1975.

Luke, B.: A Lesson in Eating for Two. *RN*, 38:36, November 1975.

McBride, A. B.: Can Family Life Survive? *Am. J. Nursing* 75:1648, October 1975.

Marquart, R. K.: Expectant Fathers: What Are Their Needs? *The American Journal of Maternal-Child Nursing*, 1:32, January-February 1976.

May, K. A.: Psychologic Involvement in Pregnancy by Expectant Fathers. *Nursing Digest*, 4:8, September-October 1976.

Popoff, D.: What Are Your Feelings About Death and Dying? *Nursing '75*, 5:55, September 1975.

Presser, H. B.: Early Motherhood: Ignorance or Bliss? *Fam. Plann. Perspect.*, 6:8, Winter 1974.

Scott, J. R., and Bose, N. B.: Effect of Psychoprophylaxis (Lamaze preparation) on Labor and Delivery in Primiparas. *N. Engl. J. Med.*, 294:1205, May 27, 1976.

Smoking and disease: The evidence reviewed. *WHO Chron.*, 29:402, October 1975.

Sonstegard, L. J., and Egan, E.: Family-Centered Nursing Makes a Difference. *The American Journal of Maternal-Child Nursing*, 1:249, July-August 1976.

Sumner, G.: Giving Expectant Parents the Help They Need: The ABC's of Prenatal Education. *The American Journal of Maternal-Child Nursing*, 1:220, July-August 1976.

Timberlake, B.: The New Life Center. *Am. J. Nursing*, 75:1456, September 1975.

Wapner, J.: The Attitudes, Feelings, and Behaviors of Expectant Fathers Attending Lamaze Classes. *Birth Fam. J.*, 3:5, Spring 1976.

Weintraub, D. R., and Wald, S. B.: Specialized vs. Combined Clinics: Patterns of Delivery of Family Planning Services. *Fam. Plann. Perspect.*, 6:98, Spring 1974.

Williams, T. M.: Canadian Childrearing Patterns and the Response of Canadian Universities to Women as Childbearers and Childrearers. *Can. Ment. Health*, 23:6, September 1975.

Zax, M., Sameroff, A. J., and Farnum, J. E.: Childbirth Education, Maternal Attitudes, and Delivery. *Am. J. Obstet. Gynecol.*, 123:185, September 15, 1975.

AUDIOVISUAL MEDIA*

The American Journal of Nursing Company

Hospital Maternity Care: Family Centered
25 minutes, color.

How Many Children Do You Want?
15 minutes, 35mm filmstrip series, audio-tape cassettes, 33⅓ RPM records, sound, color.

Drugstore Methods and Least Effective Methods of Birth Control
Evaluates methods of birth control and explains the most common misunderstandings about contraception.

Doctor Methods of Birth Control
Provides basic information about birth control pills, IUD, diaphragm, vasectomy, tubal ligation, and hysterectomy.

How Babies Begin
A discussion of the reproductive organs and conception. These filmstrips explain various birth control methods and the reproductive process in simple terms. The filmstrips are especially valuable in patient education, and are ideal for use in health departments and hospital clinics.

Maternity Nursing
15 44-minute classes, 16mm film or videotape, audio-tape cassettes, sound, color or black and white.
Instructor: Barge, F., and Sokolski, Sr. T. A.

Normal Pregnancy
Pregnancy is discussed as a socially significant process affecting individuals, the family, and the community. The physiologic process, including signs and symptoms of pregnancy, and physical and emotional changes during the prenatal period, are explained and illustrated.

Normal Labor and Delivery
The physiology and mechanisms of labor are presented with demonstrations. Basic concepts and implications for nursing are emphasized.

Normal Puerperium
Presents the aims of postpartal care, including physiologic changes and the clinical aspects of care. Emphasizes nursing care including health guidance and parent teaching.

Antepartum Care
Participating Instructor: Alpern, W.
Presents the development of antepartum care, and current practices. Demonstrates by a patient interview the prenatal visit to the obstetrician, and illustrates the role of the nurse.

Hospital Care—Admission and Delivery
Follows a laboring mother from hospital admission through labor and delivery. Emphasizes the roles of the father, nurse, and medical team.

The First Two Weeks of Life
17 minutes, color.
Ideal for use in prenatal instruction classes for expectant parents. It is aimed specifically at reducing the levels of anxiety that are often felt by young couples about to have their first baby. In the film, the camera captures the completely spontaneous and unrehearsed excitement of childbirth and the parents' first moments witht their new daughter.

Canadian Film Institute

Purposes of Family Planning
18 minute film, color.
This is a film of the positive purposes of family planning—health, emotional stability, a child's need for individual love and attention—presented simply for all ages and income levels.

Childbirth Education Films, Inc.

First Breath
45 minutes, 16mm, color.
This film exploring the childbirth experience is appropriate for members of the health professions rather than for expectant parents or layman. Although the initial delivery

room sequence is an emotionally moving scene for any viewer, the interviews that follow with several psychiatrists, pediatricians, and obstetricians attempt to point out the benefits of "prepared childbirth," or Lamaze, on a scientific level.

Minimal fetal medication, decreased fear to lessen pain, increased ability to work with one's body, and facilitation of the second stage of labor are some of the pertinent data presented.

Harper & Row Publishers

The Biological Aspects of Sexuality
  Allen, J. M.
  35mm slides, 22 minutes each, audio-tape cassette, sound, color, guide.

Conception Control
  Major methods of contraception discussed against background of human sexual anatomy; mechanics and statistical effectiveness of each method; importance of contraception in regulating population; individual responsibility; sterilization and abortion.

Human Development
  Development of the fetus from conception to birth (drawings and photographs); the first trimester as a demonstration of concepts relating to the developmental process; the nature and process of birth.

Hospital Audio Visual Education

Becoming
  30 minutes, Super 8mm.
  This film describes the Lamaze method of natural childbirth. It deals with the physical and psychological factors of nonmedicated birth, and stresses the roles played by physician, nurse, and husband in creating and sustaining confidence within the family. The film is designed for nursing education and inservice training, childbirth educational classes, and classes dealing with family dynamics and human relationships.

International Film Bureau, Inc.

Barnet (The Child)
  48 minutes, 16mm, color.
  This beautifully photographed enjoyable film follows a young couple through a first pregnancy from conception to their return home with their new baby. The film is directed to expectant couples, as shown by the clear, simple explanations and the way care is presented. It should also be useful to introduce student nurses to the childbearing phase of family life.

Maternity Center Association

Birth Atlas
  19 charts, 14″ × 20″, bound in an easel-back book. (6th ed.)
  Classic series of charts depicting in detail fertilization, development of the embryo and fetus, labor, and birth. Pictures of the famous Dickinson-Belskie sculptures. Used throughout the world for classroom and group discussion.

Birth Atlas Slide Series
  Set of 22 slides, 2″ × 2″ cardboard-mounted, with 24-page booklet, 6 × 9.
  Shown against a variety of color backgrounds, this series is adapted from the Birth Atlas. It includes illustrations of breech labor and the male and female reproductive organs. An attractive booklet accompanies the slides.

McGraw-Hill Book Company

Maternal and Child Care
  Remillet, J. G.

Series of 3 film loops approximately 7 minutes each, Super-8mm loops or 16mm films, sound, color.
  Prenatal Care
  Postpartum Care
  Infant Appraisal
  These films instruct the nurse in the assessment of the normal newborn and the expectant and new mother in proper health care. These films can be used effectively in parent education.

Ottawa-Carleton Regional Health Unit

Hello World
  35 minutes, 16mm.
  This is designed to answer questions of prospective mothers and fathers about the birth of their child.

W. B. Saunders Company

Current Topics in Obstetrics and Gynecology
  Director: Tyson, J. E.
  Fathers in the Delivery Room

Trainex Corporation

Emergency Childbirth
  35mm filmstrip, audio-tape cassettes, 33⅓ LP, color.
  Graphically portrayed and explained are the step-by-step techniques for assisting a mother during normal childbirth. The anatomy and physiology of the pregnant woman and the fetus are reviewed and the basic principles and considerations that relate to a normal delivery are vividly presented in a delivery-room setting.

Prenatal Care, the First Trimester—Nine Months to Motherhood.
  35mm filmstrip, audio-tape cassette, 33½ LP, color.
  This program explains physical changes of the mother and development of the baby during the first three months of pregnancy. The importance of prenatal medical supervision, good nutrition, personal hygiene and appropriate exercise is emphasized. Some warning signs of possible complications are described, as well as the effects of the mother's smoking and drinking on the health of the unborn child.

Prenatal Care, the Second Trimester—Six Months to Motherhood.
  35mm filmstrip, audio-tape cassette, 33⅓ LP, color.
  A review of the first three months of pregnancy. Then an examination of the baby's development during the second three months, including the first movements felt by the mother, beginning about five calendar months before the expected birth date. Warning signs of possible complications during the fourth, fifth, and sixth months of pregnancy are described.

Prenatal Care, the Third Trimester—Three Months to Motherhood
  35mm filmstrip, audio-tape cassette, 33⅓ LP, color.
  The first six months of pregnancy are reviewed and the baby's development during the seventh month is described. Physical changes experienced by the mother, including signs of pending labor, are outlined. The differences between false labor and true labor and warning signs of complications during the seventh, eighth and ninth months of pregnancy are presented.

United States Government

Human Reproduction: How Reproduction Is Controlled
  Producer: USNMAC
  35mm filmstrip, ¼ inch audio-tape, color.
  Discusses control of conception to include the rhythm method, mechanical blockage, chemical blockage, and contraceptive pills.

---

*Complete addresses are given in the Appendix.

Chapter Seven

CHARACTER-ISTICS AND NURSING ASSESSMENT OF THE NEWBORN

uation. Whether the nurse examines the mouth, gums, palate, and facial contractions while the infant is crying or the chest and abdomen while he is sleeping, all parts of the examination are important. A detailed record of the examination is necessary if it is to be helpful to the physician and other nurses caring for the infant.

Since nurses are assuming increasing responsibilities in relation to newborn infants, in that they carry out physical assessment as well as providing care in many maternity units, they must understand the physical attributes and functional disturbances of the newborn (see Chapter 8, p. 159). Anatomically, physiologically, and psychologically the baby differs from adults and even from older children. His characteristics are those of his age group. Every baby is an individual and should never be regarded as a

Birth is a most traumatic experience for the neonate. The nurse has the important function of assuming the immediate and constant observation of his physical status, including doing a nursing assessment.

Prior to doing this examination, the nurse must review the mother's history: her age, her history of previous pregnancies, her health during this pregnancy, the complications of the pregnancy, a history of any drugs she has taken, and her Rh typing. The nurse must also review the birth history of this newborn: the gestational age, the kind and duration of labor, the type of delivery, whether sedation or anesthesia was given to the mother, the resuscitation required, the Apgar score (see Chapter 8 p. 154), the birth weight and length, and the infant's color and cry at birth. Such histories, when carefully taken, provide pertinent information about where a disorder or an abnormality may exist. The infant's temperature, pulse and respiratory rates, degree of consciousness, and general level of activity must also be ascertained.

The nurse may adapt the sequence of the examination to the individual newborn and the sit-

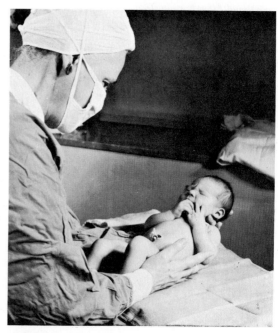

FIGURE 7–1. The infant is observed for obvious malformations before the detailed examination begins. (Courtesy of Pfizer Laboratories, Brooklyn, New York.)

typical infant, one unit of a group in which all are alike. But averages and *the range of normality should be remembered so that each baby may receive medical care if he deviates too far from the so-called normal.* It is impossible to study the infant except as a living whole; it is essential to understand his physiologic activity, which in turn is strongly influenced by his emotional state.

PHYSIOLOGIC RESILIENCE

Nature provides the fetus and the newborn with a certain physiologic resilience. The normal neonate is relatively indifferent to a range of body temperature from as low as 97° F. (36.1° C.) to as high as 100° F. (37.7° C.); in premature infants the body temperature may even drop to 94° F. (34.4° C.). By indifference is meant that the newborn does not seem uncomfortable or show the concomitant signs of low or high temperature which would appear in the adult. The infant has an unstable heat-regulating system, and his body temperature is influenced by the environmental temperature. If the room is cold, so is his body; if he is covered with too many blankets, his body temperature rises. Regulate the temperature about him, and his returns to normal.

The infant is also indifferent to abnormal levels of substances in the blood. The levels usually found in predictable concentration in the blood of normal children are less standardized in the neonate and even more unpredictable in premature infants.

Although the blood glucose level may be low, the usual hypoglycemic reaction of the adult is not seen. The infant shows some departure of the blood hydrogen ion content and carbon dioxide tension from the adult level (see p. 63). There is also an increase in the range of infants' normal values. The infant can survive without breathing for a relatively longer time than the adult, though there are limits to his tolerance for lack of oxygen.

This physiologic resilience has many obvious advantages, and because of it many infants have survived who otherwise would have died. Yet it has one great disadvantage: it conceals or minimizes physical signs of diagnostic value. For instance, infection in the newborn may not be accompanied by fever as it is in older children or adults. In other cases an infant who is moderately dehydrated may have respirations which seem to be barely perceptibly increased, yet he may have a blood pH of 7.2 or even lower without having acidotic Kussmaul respirations.

Also, infants do not conform to a pattern in their reactions to drugs; this fact makes it essential that the nurse observe infants carefully for untoward reactions.

All in all, this passive resistance of the infant is an ally. But there are limits to his resistance which cannot be safely overstepped. This is particularly true of the premature infant, who shows few defense mechanisms against unfavorable circumstances.

The first few days of life are normally a time when the infant is in a state of negative balance, e.g., postnatal weight loss, loss of body fluids, and decreases in hemoglobin, calories, nitrogen, sodium chloride, and inherited antibodies. There is danger of feeding him too much and too early in an attempt to make up for these losses.

Death on the first day of extrauterine life is not due to wasting of resources. Negative balance is normal, and only harm results from attempting to force it to positive.

LENGTH AND WEIGHT

The length of the average newborn male is 20 inches (50 cm.); of the female, 19.6 inches (49 cm.). The normal range for both sexes is from 19 to 21½ inches (47.5 to 53.75 cm.).

The weight of the normal newborn also tends to vary. About two thirds of all full-term infants weigh between 2700 and 3850 gm., or between 6 and 8½ pounds. Many infants, of course, weigh more or less than this. The average girl weighs approximately 7 pounds, the average boy approximately 7½ pounds.

During the first few days after birth the infant tends to lose about 6 to 10 ounces, or 5 to 10 per cent of his birth weight. Factors contributing to this initial loss are the withdrawal of hormones originally obtained from the mother, the withholding of water and the loss of feces and urine.

TEMPERATURE, PULSE, RESPIRATION AND BLOOD PRESSURE

The temperature, pulse and respiration of the newborn vary in an unpredictable way. He appears to have a passive resistance or resilience, within a wide range of bodily responses; yet when these limits of tolerance are exceeded, because he lacks the adult's reserve vitality, he may suddenly appear ill. *The need for constant observation is an essential of infant nursing care.* The nurse must learn from experience to

A deep flush spreads over the entire body if baby cries hard. Veins on head swell and throb. You will notice no tears as tear ducts do not function as yet.

The skin is thin and dry. You may see veins through it. Fair skin may be rosy-red temporarily. Downy hair is not unusual. Some *vernix caseosa* (white, prenatal skin covering) remains.

Head usually strikes you as being too big for the body. It may be temporarily out of shape—lop-sided or elongated—due to pressure before or during birth. A crop of thick hair or a bald head is normal.

The feet look more complete than they are. X-ray would show only one real bone at the heel. Other bones are now cartilage. Skin often loose and wrinkly.

The trunk may startle you in some normal detail: short neck, small sloping shoulders, swollen breasts, large rounded abdomen, umbilical stump (future navel), slender, narrow pelvis and hips.

Eyes appear dark blue or gray, have a blank stary gaze. You may catch one or both turning or turned to crossed or wall-eyed position. Lids, characteristically, puffy.

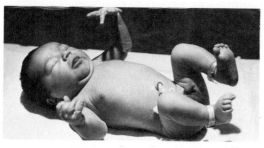

A   B

The legs are most often seen drawn up against the abdomen in pre-birth position. Extended legs measure shorter than you'd expect compared to the arms. The knees stay slightly bent and legs are more or less bowed.

Genitals of both sexes will seem large (especially scrotum) in comparison with the scale of, for example, the hands to adult size.

The face will disappoint you unless you expect to see: pudgy cheeks, a broad, flat nose with mere hint of a bridge, receding chin, undersized lower jaw.

Weight unless well above the average of 6 or 7 lbs. will not prepare you for how really tiny newborn is. Top to toe measure: anywhere between 18" to 21".

The hands, if you open them out flat from their characteristic fist position, have: finely lined palms, tissue-paper thin nails, dry, loose fitting skin and deep bracelet creases at wrist.

On the skull you will see or feel the two most obvious soft spots or *fontanels*. One is above the brow, the other close to crown of head in back. Scalp skin may be loose. Brow may be wrinkled.

FIGURE 7–2.   What a healthy newborn baby looks like. *A*, Photographer Burton Berinsky took this photograph of a newborn, just six hours old, in the nursery of Long Island College Hospital, Brooklyn, N.Y. (From *American Baby for the Mother-to-be and New Mother*, July, 1973.) *B*, This unretouched photograph taken six hours after birth at Lawrence Memorial Hospital. (From *Baby Talk*, January, 1964.)

recognize the significance of his response to sensations which he cannot let her know about in words or actions, e.g., pushing off the covers if he is too hot.

TEMPERATURE

The infant's temperature at birth is slightly higher than his mother's, since the uterus lies deeply insulated within her body. It drops immediately after birth in adjustment to the temperature of the delivery room and then rises to normal within about eight hours. His hands and feet are colder than the rest of his body, since his circulation is poor. This lack of stability, due to underdevelopment of his heat-regulating system, requires that external heat be applied. He is generally wrapped in warm blankets in the delivery room. The nurse who puts him in his crib must remember that too much heat for too long will send his temperature above normal.

PULSE

Fetal electrocardiography is used to record electrical impulses of the fetal heart *in utero.* Abnormal intrauterine conditions can thus be diagnosed and evaluated and immediately treated after birth.

The infant's pulse is normally irregular, owing to immaturity of the cardiac regulatory center in the medulla. The rate is rapid, around 120 to 150 per minute. Extreme irregularity results from any one of many physical or emotional stimuli. When the infant is startled or cries, his pulse rate not only increases, but also becomes more irregular. Irregularity of rhythm of the pulse may follow that of the respiration.

RESPIRATION

Respiration in the newborn is irregular in depth, rate, and rhythm and varies from 35 to 50 per minute. Like the pulse rate, it is readily altered by internal or external stimuli. Normally, respirations are gentle and quiet, rapid and shallow. They can be observed most easily by watching abdominal movement, since respiration in the newborn is carried on largely by the diaphragm and abdominal muscles. Dyspnea or cyanosis may occur suddenly in an infant who is breathing normally. These signs may be the first indication of the presence of a congenital anomaly or other condition from which an infant may suddenly expire if he does not receive adequate care. The nurse should notify the physician if respiration drops below 35 or exceeds 50 per minute when the infant is at rest or if dyspnea or cyanosis occurs.

The normal cry is lusty, frequent and often apparently without cause. If the infant does not cry, he should be stimulated to do so at approxi-mately hourly intervals in order to force expansion of his lungs by the concomitant deep respirations.

BLOOD PRESSURE

The blood pressure is characteristically low. It is difficult to determine accurately and may vary with the size of the cuff used (see p. 92).

THE SKIN

The skin of the Caucasian newborn is red or dark pink, in the black infant a reddish black, and in the Mongolian the color of a tea rose. It is soft, covered with lanugo and overlaid with vernix caseosa. Good elasticity or *turgor* is evidence that an infant is in good condition.

Lanugo is a slight downy distribution of fine hair over the body, most evident on the shoulders, back, extremities, forehead and temples. Since lanugo begins to appear on the fetus by about the sixteenth week of gestation and to disappear after the thirty-second week, its presence is often an evidence of prematurity. The premature infant has a heavier showing than the full-term infant. Lanugo tends to disappear during the first weeks of life.

Vernix caseosa is a cheeselike, greasy, yellowish-white substance, sometimes likened to cream cheese or cold cream, which covers the newborn's skin. It consists of secretions from sebaceous glands and epithelial cells. Its distribution over the body is variable, being heavier in the folds of the skin and between the labia. It dries or fades spontaneously and rubs off on the infant's clothing.

Tissue turgor refers to the sensation of fullness derived from the presence of hydrated subcutaneous tissue. Elasticity of the skin is demonstrated when a fold of skin is grasped between the thumb and forefinger. When released, the skin promptly springs back to form the smooth, soft surface of the body.

Observation may reveal the following additional normal findings. *Desquamation* or peeling of the skin occurs during the first two to four weeks of life. Denuded areas may occur where the delicate skin has been rubbed off the nose, knees and elbows because of pressure and erosion on the sheets. The skin of the buttocks needs special care so that it does not become chafed. A wet or soiled diaper should be changed at once.

Transient *rashes* may occur. *Milia* is a condition in which tiny white papillae occur, particularly on the nose and chin, owing to obstruction of the sebaceous glands. These blemishes disappear in a week or two. *Physiologic jaundice* becomes definite between the third and seventh days. It is likely to appear gradually on the second or third day and is seen in the majority of infants (see also p. 145).

There may be marks upon the infant's body. Some are temporary, caused by the trauma of birth; others are due to immaturity, even in the infant born at term; still others are permanent birthmarks. Among the temporary marks are *hemangiomas,* or pink spots, on the upper eyelids, between the eyebrows, and on the nose, upper lip or back of the neck. The mother may be reassured that they will disappear spontaneously. If forceps were used during delivery, temporary *forceps marks* may be left upon the part of the body or head where the blades exerted pressure. In a breech delivery there may be edema and extravasation of blood into the tissues of the buttocks and genitals due to trauma to the presenting parts. In fact, there may be *bruising of tissues* on almost any part of the infant's body as he progresses through the birth canal.

Another mark which may be present is the so-called *Mongolian spot.* These spots, which are slate colored, usually occur on the buttocks or lower portion of the back of infants whose parents are black, Oriental, or from the Mediterranean area. They fade during the preschool years without treatment.

By two weeks of age the infant should have the typical rosy, soft, dewy skin which we associate with babies. The sweat glands become active by the end of the second week.

THE HEAD

The head is proportionately large, averaging 34 to 35 cm. (13.6 to 14 inches) in circumference. The normal limits of head size are 33 to 37 cm. (13.2 to 14.8 inches). The head is one fourth the total length of the infant. In the adult the length of the head is one eighth of the total height (see Fig. 2–7). The infant's cranium is large and the face relatively small when compared with the adult cranium and face. The jaws are relatively small, and the chin is receding. The circumference of the head equals or exceeds that of the chest or abdomen.

The *fontanels* are openings at the points of union of the skull bones. These should be palpated to determine whether they are open or closed. The anterior fontanel is diamond-shaped and located at the juncture of the two parietal and two frontal bones. It is 2 to 3 cm. (0.8 to 1.2 inches) in width and 3 to 4 cm. (1.2 to 1.6 inches) in length (Fig. 7–4). The posterior fontanel is triangular and located between the occipital and parietal bones. It is much smaller than the anterior fontanel and may be nearly closed. The fontanels bulge when the infant cries or strains or if there is increased pressure within the skull. Increased intracranial pressure may be due to a number of causes, among them hydrocephalus (see p. 301). The anterior fontanel normally closes by the time the infant is 12 to 18 months old, and the posterior fontanel by the end of the second month.

The bones of the cranium are held together by membranes at the suture lines. During delivery, pressure may mold the head into asymmetrical proportions. In general the head assumes its normal shape by the time the infant is a week old.

Caput succedaneum is swelling or edema of the presenting portion of the scalp and may be localized or fairly extensive. It usually disappears by the third day (Fig. 7–5).

Cephalhematoma is an accumulation of blood between the periosteum and a flat skull bone.

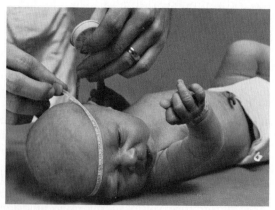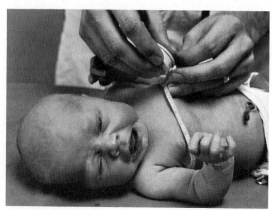

FIGURE 7–3.   The circumferences of the head and chest are measured. In the course of being examined newborns almost invariably protest. (Courtesy of Dr. Charles H. Peete, Jr., and *Baby Talk* Magazine.)

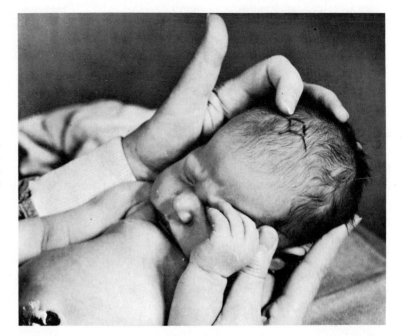

FIGURE 7–4. The size of the fontanels varies considerably from infant to infant. They are palpated to ascertain their tension. (Courtesy of Pfizer Laboratories, Brooklyn, New York.)

The collection of blood does not cross a suture line. The mass is soft, irreducible, and fluctuating. It does not increase on crying. A cephalhematoma may not be evident during the first few days of life because of the presence of a large caput succedaneum. Aspiration of this sanguineous collection should not be done because of the danger of infection and because the condition usually clears within a few weeks (Fig. 7–6).

FACE AND NECK

The infant's face is expressionless. The ears are flabby until the cartilage calcifies. The neck is short and creased. These creases, particularly in a fat infant, are deep and likely to become sore unless carefully cleaned.

In the normal infant it should be possible to turn the head freely from side to side. If there is rigidity, the sternocleidomastoid muscles may have been injured during delivery. When the infant is lying on his back and begins to cry, his head is held in the midline, and both sides of his face are mobile. Absence of symmetry in movement or contour is evidence of an abnormality.

The infant who is born with ears like the handles of a loving cup should have plastic surgery performed before he begins school in order to prevent the psychic trauma caused by

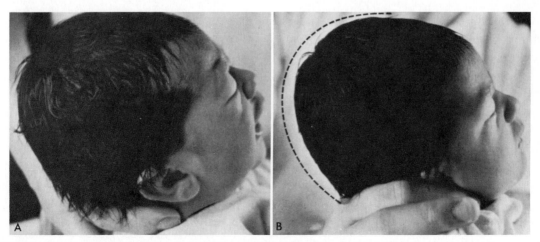

FIGURE 7–5. Caput succedaneum. A. Edema of the scalp. B. Reduction of edema. (Number Two of a series on variations and minor departures in newborn infants. Courtesy of Mead Johnson and Co.)

COLOR PLATE I

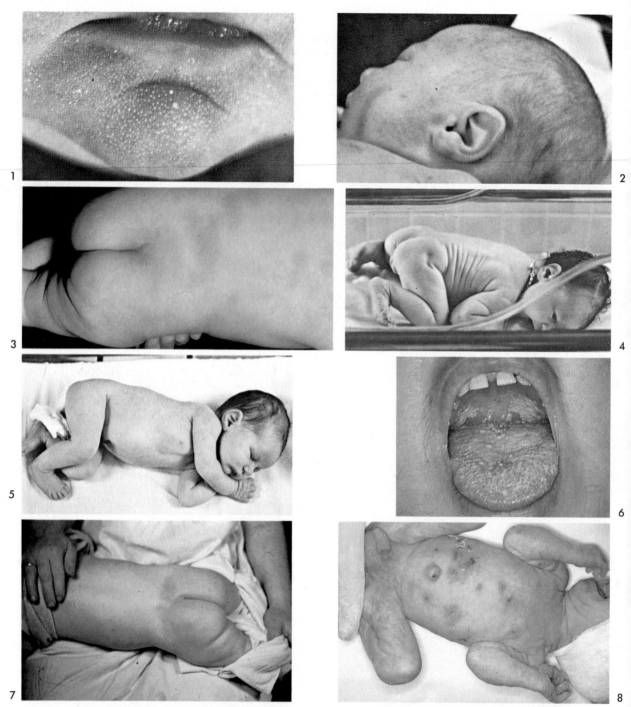

1, Tiny sebaceous retention cysts, **milia** appear as whitish, opalescent, pinhead-sized spots, mainly on and around the nose. Milia can be felt with the finger and usually disappear spontaneously within a few weeks (see p. 139). *2*, **Forceps pressure marks** on the face, usually located on the cheek and jaw area, are important only because mothers notice them and sometimes become alarmed (see p. 140). *3*, The **Mongolian spot** is a diffuse grayish-blue discoloration in the sacral area present since birth (see p. 140). *4*, **Cyanosis** of hands, feet, and sometimes lips, frequent during the early hours of life, is generally ascribed to limited development of the peripheral capillary circulation in the skin (see p. 189 and 247). *5*, **Icterus neonatorum** (physiologic jaundice). One third to one half of normal newborns develop jaundice in the first week of life. Usually noted 48 to 72 hours after birth, it disappears by the age of two weeks (see p. 145). (*1, 2, 4,* and *5* courtesy of Mead Johnson Laboratories.) *6*, **Thrush** (moniliasis of the oral cavity). This condition presents with erythema, edema, and a whitish coating of the mucous membranes (see p. 261). (*3* and *6* from *Frieboes/Schonfeld's Color Atlas of Dermatology*, by J. Kimmig and M. Janner. American edition translated and revised by H. Goldschmidt. Stuttgart, Georg Thiem Verlag, 1966.) 7, Early eczematous primary irritant **diaper dermatitis** (see p. 164). *8*, Disseminated **herpes simplex** (see p. 469) (Courtesy of Dr. Robert J. Morgan.) (*7* and *8* from *Neonatal Dermatology*, by L. M. Solomon and N. B. Esterly. Philadelphia, W. B. Saunders Co., 1973.)

142

1   2   3

4

5

6

7   8   9

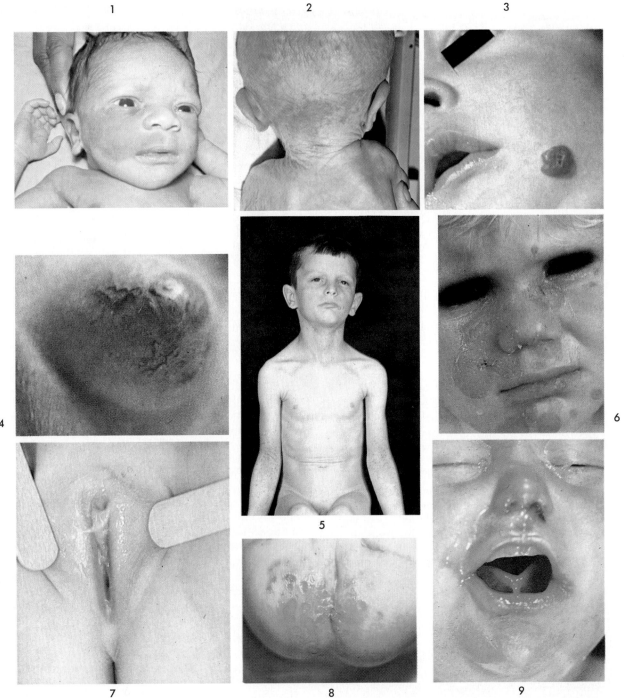

1, **Port wine stain** in distribution of trigeminal nerve. Studies should be done to rule out Sturge-Weber syndrome (see p. 273). (From Hodgman, J. E., Freedman, R. I., and Levan, N. E.: *Pediatr. Clin. N. Am.*, 18(3):Plate I, August 1971.) *2*, **Nevus flammeus** of the nape (see p. 273). (From *Neonatal Dermatology*, by L. M. Solomon and N. B. Esterly. Philadelphia, W. B. Saunders Co., 1973.) *3*, **Nevus vasculosus** (strawberry mark). Soft raised, bluish-red tumor with irregular surface and beginning central ulceration (see p. 273). *4*, **Cavernous hemangiomata** are composed of a communicating meshwork of interconnected venules, with or without a few vascular sinuses (see p. 273). (Courtesy of Mead Johnson Laboratories.) *5*, **Atopic dermatitis.** Pruritic excoriated lesions of the face and extremities (see p. 469). *6*, **Impetigo contagiosa.** Rapidly spreading circinate erythematous lesions, with thick, shiny crusts and isolated vesicles; caused by staphylococci (see p. 266). *7*, **Gonorrheal vulvovaginitis** in infancy. Edema, erythema, and purulent discharge from the vagina vestibulum, urethral orifice, and labia majora and minora. (3, 5, 6, and 7 from *Frieboes/Schonfeld's Color Atlas of Dermatology*, by J. Kimmig and M. Janner. American edition translated and revised by H. Goldschmidt. Stuttgart, Georg Thieme Verlag, 1966.) *8*, **Syphilis.** Eroded perioral maculopapular skin lesions in the newborn (see p. 262). *9*, **Snuffles** in syphilitic infant. Note split infectious papule on left (see p. 262). (8 and 9 courtesy of U.S. Department of Health, Education and Welfare.)

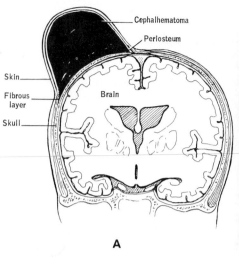

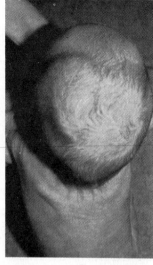

FIGURE 7–6. Cephalhematoma. *A.* The collection of blood lies between the periosteum and the skull bone. *B.* Typical limitation of cephalhematoma by clearly visible coronal, sagittal, and lambdoid sutures. (From Moll, H. Atlas of Pediatric Diseases. Philadelphia, W. B. Saunders Co., 1976.)

his being different from other members of his group.

THE CHEST

The chest is bell-shaped and at birth is approximately the same circumference as the abdomen and less than the head. For this reason it appears small. By the time the child is two years old the size of the chest exceeds that of the head, and he begins to take on more nearly adult proportions.

The thorax is almost circular. The anterior and lateral diameters are the same because of the pressure of the arms against the chest wall *in utero*. The infant does not use the thoracic cage in breathing as does the older child or adult; he uses the diaphragm and abdominal muscles to exhale and inhale.

The breasts may be swollen because of hormonal activity originating from the mother, and, pale milky fluid ("witch's milk") can be expressed. The condition disappears in two to four weeks without treatment, but as long as it lasts the breasts are tender and should be touched only when necessary and then very gently.

The *thymus* is usually proportionately large and triples its weight by the time the child is five years old; it then remains approximately the same size until he is about ten years old, when it begins to decrease. A dominant role is played by the thymus in the development of immunologic competence by the fetus and young child. It has been disproved that a large thymus is the cause of respiratory difficulty or sudden death by asphyxia. Usually some other factor is accountable for cyanosis or apnea.

RESPIRATORY SYSTEM

The mechanism of respiration is established before birth, but at birth it undergoes profound changes. Prerespiratory movements begin in the fourth month of gestation. Amniotic fluid may move in and out of the lungs as a result of these tidal movements. Oxygen is, of course, obtained through the placental circulation. The hypoxia resulting from severance of the cord assists in initiating breathing through stimulation of the respiratory center by the accumulation of carbon dioxide. The process of birth and the environmental change also stimulate the respiratory center. The first breath, usually taken within 30 seconds after birth, helps to expand the col-

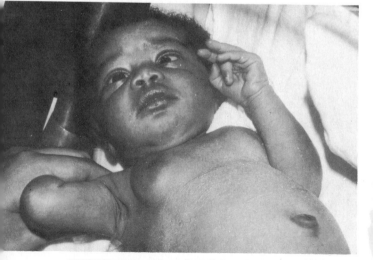

FIGURE 7–7. "Physiologic" breast engorgement. (Courtesy of Drs. David Fisher and John Paton in Solomon, L. M., and Esterly, N. B.: *Neonatal Dermatology.* (Philadelphia, W. B. Saunders Co., 1973.)

lapsed lungs, though full expansion does not occur for several days.

CIRCULATORY SYSTEM

At birth sudden changes occur in the circulatory system. The circulatory pattern must change from fetal dependency on the placenta to include the expanding lungs. The functional structures (i.e., foramen ovale and ductus arteriosus) of intrauterine life must be obliterated. The circulation of the pulmonary system is perfected, and a short time after birth oxygenated blood flows through the infant's body in the same manner as that of the adult. The foramen ovale (see Fig. 12–3) closes by the third month. The ductus arteriosus is occluded when the infant is from several weeks to four months old. Approximately 2 per cent of newborns have transitory, insignificant heart murmurs caused by blood leaking through openings not yet closed. These murmurs disappear within a few weeks.

The *vascular system* and *heart* are large in the newborn in comparison with their size in adult life. The blood volume of the newborn is about 10 to 12 per cent of his body weight. This percentage is influenced by the amount of blood received from the placenta before clamping of the cord.

BLOOD

The blood contains a relatively high number of red blood cells and a high hemoglobin level at birth (see Tables 4–1 and 4–2). These characteristics are essential to provide adequate oxygenation *in utero* and during the first few postnatal days before the lungs expand fully. Oxygenation improves during the first two weeks of life to the extent that a high red cell count and hemoglobin level are no longer necessary, and hemolysis occurs. There is a continued fall in the red cell count and hemoglobin levels during the first three months of life, resulting in a physiologic anemia.

PHYSIOLOGIC JAUNDICE (ICTERUS NEONATORUM)

Infants have an excessive amount of bilirubin in the blood at birth. Normally the breakdown of red blood cells after birth produces a higher level of bilirubin, which in turn may produce the yellow discoloration of jaundice. Red blood cells break down to form fat-soluble indirect bilirubin, which cannot be excreted by the kidneys. Indirect bilirubin is converted to direct bilirubin through the action of the hepatic enzyme glucuronyl transferase; thus it becomes water-soluble and capable of being excreted. The lack of full activity of this enzyme at birth may contribute to physiologic jaundice.

No jaundice is evident when the bilirubin remains within the circulatory system, because the hemoglobin which produces the red coloration of the skin obscures the yellow of the bilirubin. When the indirect level rises above 7 mg. per 100 ml. in term infants, the bilirubin becomes evident outside the vascular space and can be noted as jaundice. In low-birth-weight infants whose skin surface lacks subcutaneous fat deposits, the reddened coloration of the skin obscures the yellow of jaundice, which can be seen, nevertheless, by blanching the skin with pressure.

Physiologic jaundice occurs in approximately 55 to 70 per cent of all newborns, from two to three days after birth. It increases for a few days and usually disappears by the seventh day. The urine may become dark, and the infant appears sluggish, even showing anorexia. Although the normal bilirubin level is 1.0 mg. per 100 ml. or slightly higher in the newborn, hyperbilirubinemia beyond physiologic levels exists when the total serum bilirubin levels reach 18 to 20 mg. per 100 ml. during the first seven days of life.

Certain infants who are breast-fed may have jaundice for a longer time than usual, owing to the presence of pregnanediol-3a,20a in breast milk. This substance depresses the action of the hepatic enzyme glucuronyl transferase. The level of indirect bilirubin should be determined frequently in these newborns, and breast feedings may have to be discontinued until the bilirubin level drops. The mother's milk supply should be maintained so that the infant can resume breast feeding when the jaundice subsides.

Continuing jaundice indicates a pathologic condition such as obstruction of the bile ducts, syphilis, or erythroblastosis fetalis.

Treatment is rarely necessary for physiologic jaundice. Phototherapy may be used to treat the full-term newborn; since it is used mainly with low-weight, immature infants, however, it is discussed in Chapter 9.

PHYSIOLOGIC HYPOPROTHROMBINEMIA

During the first few days of life the prothrombin level decreases in all infants. Thus the clotting time is prolonged. This condition is most acute between the second and fifth postnatal days. It can be prevented to a great extent by giving vitamin K to the mother during labor or to the infant after birth. Recovery usually occurs between seven and ten days of age.

GASTROINTESTINAL SYSTEM

Sucking pads, mouth, and jaw

The sucking pads are deposits of fatty tissue in the cheeks which persist even when the infant is extremely malnourished. They disappear when sucking is no longer the only way of taking food.

The infant has a receding chin, which trembles at the slightest stimulation, especially if he is startled or whimpers. His tongue is relatively large and protrudes when the mouth is open. The newborn cannot move food from his lips to the pharynx. Later, when food is given, it must be placed at the back of his tongue so that he can swallow it. At two or three months of age salivation occurs. Since the infant has not yet learned to swallow facilely, he may drool.

Esophagus, stomach, and intestines

The cardiac sphincter is not as well developed as the pyloric sphincter. For this reason the infant should be "bubbled" several times while being fed so that air which he has swallowed may be eructed. (A little milk may come up with the air.) If the air were to remain in the stomach, there would be danger of vomiting or, if it passed into the intestine, of colic.

Occasionally the action of the pyloric valve may not be normal, and regurgitating (the vomiting of food immediately after it has been taken) may be so constant that an infant fails to gain weight (see Chapter 14).

It is difficult to measure the size of the infant's stomach. The contents are emptied almost immediately into the duodenum. When we look at the infant and the amount of milk he is taking, it is evident that the fluid is leaving the stomach before the feeding is completed. It is likely that at birth the stomach holds from 1 to 2 ounces, at two weeks 3 ounces, at five months 7 ounces and at ten months 10 ounces. The entire formula should be out of the infant's stomach in 2½ to three hours. Digestion is slowed by food high in protein or fat.

The intestinal tract functions as an outlet for amniotic fluid as early as the fifth month of intrauterine life. The normal gastrointestinal tract assumes its function readily after birth. *Meconium,* the first fecal material, is a sticky, odorless material, greenish black to brownish green, which is passed from eight to 24 hours after birth.

The nature of the *stools* changes daily in the first week. They are called transitional stools. From the third to the fifth day they are loose, contain mucus and are greenish yellow. After the fifth day the nature of the stools depends on the feeding. The stools of the breast-fed infant are yellow and pasty. The breast-fed infant will normally have from two to four stools a day. The stools of an infant fed on a formula of modified cow's milk are light yellow and hard and are passed once or twice daily. The composition of some commercially prepared formulas is so similar to that of breast milk that it may be difficult to differentiate the stools of infants fed these formulas from those of infants who are breast-fed. Later, when the infant is receiving a soft diet, the stools are brown or colored from the kind of food given him.

Abdomen

The umbilical stump begins to shrink and become discolored soon after birth and within a few days turns black (see p. 165). It sloughs off between the sixth and tenth days, but leaves a granulating area which heals in another week. The umbilical cord must be examined closely during the first 24 hours after birth and then daily for any trace of bleeding, which should be reported to the physician at once. If bleeding occurs, the cord should be clamped or retied immediately. After the first day there is less danger of bleeding, but signs of infection may appear and should be reported. Extreme care must be taken that this lesion does not become infected, since the blood vessels of the cord and their extension into the abdomen afford a potential portal of entry for organisms until the umbilical wound is completely healed. A bactericidal dye is used in many nurseries to paint the cord stump in order to help prevent infection.

Examination of internal organs

In addition to the external examination, three tests are necessary to complete the appraisal of the gastrointestinal system of the newborn. These tests are designed to uncover anomalies which prevent normal physiologic processes. *These anomalies, not obvious on general inspection, are of such importance that their early discovery and correction may mean saving the infant's life. Such anomalies include imperforate anus, omphalocele, and esophageal atresia.* (See Chapter 11 for further discussion.)

Imperforate Anus. In order to test for the presence of this condition, in the absence of a meconium stool, the physician or nurse need only insert into the infant's rectum a thermometer, a gloved finger (since the infant's rectum is very small, it is well to use the index or little finger), or a soft rubber catheter.

Omphalocele. The point of juncture of the umbilical cord with the abdomen should be examined to make certain that a loop of intestine is not protruding into the base of the cord.

Esophageal Atresia. A newborn who appears to have an excessive amount of saliva or one who drools may have esophageal atresia. In order to test for its presence a soft rubber catheter may be passed through the esophagus into the stomach. Any obstruction should be reported immediately, for the infant will be unable to take nourishment. Repair should be made before his condition is weakened by lack of nourishment or before pneumonia develops, owing to aspiration of formula.

These simple tests are not dangerous to the newborn. They may be safely performed by the student nurse under the direction and supervision of the physician or an instructor, if the policy of the agency in which care is being given permits this to be done. The nurse does not, of course, make a diagnosis of a medical condition, but through intelligent observation and description of these findings the physician can be informed of conditions which require his consideration.

ANOGENITAL AREA

The infant's buttocks are plump, firm and pink. In the anal region there should be no redness or fissures.

GENITALIA

Male Genitalia. The size of the penis and scrotum varies. The prepuce or foreskin of the penis may adhere to the glans. The testes have usually descended into the scrotum by the eighth month of intrauterine life, but in some cases they remain in the abdomen or the inguinal canal. This condition is commonly known as undescended testes or cryptorchidism (see p. 427).

Female Genitalia. The female genitalia may be slightly swollen, owing to hormone activity originating from the mother. The labia majora are undeveloped, and the exposed labia minora appear large. The vagina exudes a mucous discharge which may occasionally be blood-tinged during the first week. This is also caused by hormones transmitted from mother to infant. The condition should disappear by the second or third week.

URINE

The infant has urine in the bladder at birth and may void immediately or after several hours. In a small percentage of newborns, however, urination may be delayed until the second day. The urine is dilute because of the immaturity of the kidneys and their lack of ability to concentrate. Loss of a large amount of water may result in temporary hemoconcentration. A pink stain may be found on the diaper which is usually due to deposition of uric acid crystals.

The nurse should note on the chart the time that the infant first voids, the strength of his urinary stream and his voiding pattern. If these are not normal, urinary tract pathology may be present such as the absence of one or both kidneys or some form of urinary tract obstruction. The most common cause of failure to void in newborns is dehydration.

SKELETAL STRUCTURE

The bones of the newborn are soft because they are composed chiefly of cartilage in which there is only a small amount of calcium. The skeleton is flexible and the joints are elastic to ensure a safe passage through the birth canal.

The infant's back is normally straight and flat. The lumbar and sacral curves develop later when the infant sits up and begins to stand.

The legs are small, short and bowed or curve outward as the infant lies with his legs abducted and flexed, so that the soles of the feet nearly touch each other. The feet appear to be flat, owing to the presence of the plantar fat pad (a pad of fat in the longitudinal arch of the foot). The legs should be examined to determine whether there is any limitation of movement.

The arms, like the legs, are relatively short, and the position of the neonate is often that of the tonic neck reflex (see p. 149). The hands are plump, the fingers relatively short, and the nails are smooth and soft and extend over the fingertips. The hands are clenched in little fists. The fingers should be separated and examined.

Many of the common anomalies of infancy are noted in the extremities (e.g., clubfoot or syndactyly, the latter a union of the fingers or toes). Although these do not interfere with vital functions, as do anomalies of the heart, bladder, or other internal organs, they are a cause of great anxiety to the parents.

MUSCLES

Muscular contour in the healthy, plump infant is smooth, and his muscles, in spite of their lack of strength and his inability to control them, feel hard and slightly resistant to pressure. The nurse should note whether the infant offers normal resistance to passive movement of his extremities. If he does not, he may be suffering from cerebral injury, narcosis, or even shock. If

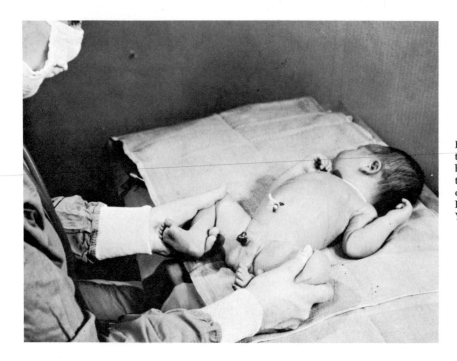

FIGURE 7–8. Congenital dislocation of the hips may be recognized by testing gross abduction of the thighs and observing for protrusion of the femoral heads. (Courtesy of Pfizer Laboratories, Brooklyn, New York.)

an infant feels limp in the nurse's hands, the condition should never be mistaken for a mere characteristic of his immaturity.

The movements of the newborn are random and uncoordinated; he wriggles and stretches. When the nurse picks him up, his back and head must be supported, for he lacks the muscular strength to hold even his head steady and would slump if placed in a sitting position.

NERVOUS SYSTEM

The nervous system of the newborn is strikingly immature. His bodily functions and responses to external stimuli are carried on chiefly by the midbrain and reflexes of the spinal cord. The cerebral influence characteristic of even the preschool child is lacking.

As soon as the nerve fibers become myelinated and make the necessary connections with one another, control from the higher cerebral centers begins, and increasingly more complex and purposeful behavior is possible. One can observe the neurologic development from week to week as it proceeds caudally from above.

REFLEXES

Certain reflexes are absolutely essential to the infant's life, and many are protective. Among these latter are the *blinking reflex*, which is aroused when the infant is subjected to a bright light, and the *reflexes of coughing* and *sneezing*, which clear the respiratory tract. The *yawn re-*

flex is in a sense protective, since thereby the infant draws in an added supply of oxygen.

A number of reflex actions are involved in feeding. The *rooting reflex* causes the infant to turn his head toward anything which touches his cheek and is his way of reaching for food. It helps the infant to locate the nipple with his mouth when the breast touches his cheek. The *sucking reflex* provides sucking movements when anything touches the lips. This reflex is normally present at birth and is accompanied by the *swallowing reflex*. The *gagging reflex* comes into play when he has taken more into his mouth than he can successfully swallow. He can also cough if a little of the fluid is "swallowed the wrong way" and enters the trachea.

The infant is not skillful in coordinating all these reflexes and requires help from the mother or nurse. He may have trouble getting the nipple into his mouth, and when he does succeed, the nipple may be under rather than on the tongue. These reflexes, essential to successful nursing, are absent or underdeveloped in the premature infant, but their absence in the full-term infant would indicate narcosis, brain injury, or mental retardation. If the sucking reflex is not stimulated, it ceases to exist.

The *grasp reflex* is present in both hands and feet. An infant will grasp any object put into his hands, hold on briefly and then drop it. At birth he may be able to hold on so securely to an adult's forefinger inserted into his fist that he may be lifted from the crib to a standing position (the "Darwinian reflex"). This grasping action in its reflex form fades. As the infant matures the action becomes conscious and purposeful and obviously is one which brings him pleasure — shaking his rattle, for instance. Although he cannot grasp with his feet, his toes react to stimulation with an attempt to get hold of the object which touches the sole of the foot or the toes (Fig. 7–9, A).

If the infant is held upright around the chest with his feet touching the examination table or crib, he will attempt prancing movements with his legs. This is called the *dancing reflex;* it soon disappears. Not until he is trying to stand and walk does he again make any attempt to move his legs as in prancing, though he gets great fun from kicking as he lies on his back.

The newborn has one great unlearned reaction to strong stimuli: the *startle reflex.* At birth or soon after this reflex is aroused by a sudden loud noise or loss of support. The reaction is a generalized, aimless muscular activity. The startle or *Moro reflex* demonstrates an awareness of equilibrium in the newborn. This reflex can best be elicited when the infant is quiet and without the restraint of clothing. A sudden stimulus such as jarring the table or bassinet will cause the infant to draw up his legs with the soles of the feet turned toward each other and the undersurface of the toes almost touching. The arms assume the embrace position. These movements, followed by a rather fixed and rigid position, normally are symmetrical. The Moro reflex is a normal reaction which is strongest during the first eight weeks or so of life; it may persist, but be increasingly difficult to elicit, until about the fifth month. In its absence the possibility of brain damage must be considered (Fig. 7–9, B).

The *tonic neck reflex* is a postural reflex in which the infant, when lying on his back, turns his head to one side and extends the arm and the leg on the side to which the head is turned at right angles from his body; he flexes the other leg and arm. He may make a fist with both hands. This position has been aptly called the infant's fencing position; it occurs in fetal life by about 20 to 28 weeks of gestation and in the newborn and infant up to about the eighteenth or twentieth week (Fig. 7–9, C).

Successful use of the reflex mechanism is evidence of normal functioning of the nervous system. If a reflex is impaired or absent, it may be that the central nervous system has sustained injury. Although it may not be possible to correct the condition, the care of the infant can and must be adapted to his disability. For instance, if he cannot suck, he must be fed by gavage.

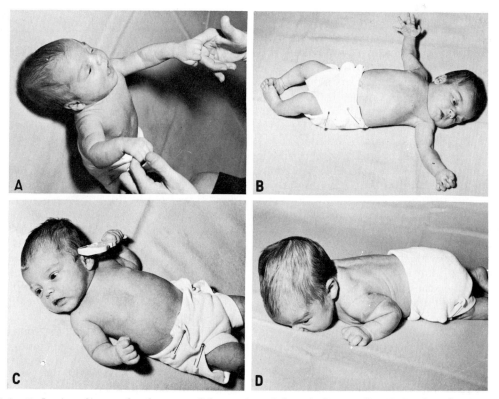

FIGURE 7–9.   Reflexes and motor development of the newborn infant. *A,* Grasp reflex. *B,* Startle reflex (Moro reflex). *C,* Tonic neck reflex. *D,* Lifts head slightly from the bed.

Certain reflexes present in the newborn disappear as he matures, and the cerebrum exercises greater control over the nervous system. This brings about changes in behavior to which the care given him by the mother or nurse must be adapted.

The Brazelton neonatal assessment scale (see p. 33) may be used in addition to a standard neurologic evaluation of the newborn. Areas that this test assesses are alertness or orienting, that is, the response of the infant to visual, auditory, inanimate, and animate stimuli; the degree of irritability; and the degree of motor maturity, meaning the smoothness of the infant's movements, the amount of tremulousness, and the frequency of occurrence of the startle reflex.

The Conditioned Reflex. This is the only way by which the infant learns, and it is largely limited to carrying over the satisfaction from feeding to the concomitants of the process. He sees the nurse's or mother's face, although it is blurred for him, and learns to like those who feed him because of their association with the relief of his hunger and the general comfort of being fed.

Motor activity

The movements of the newborn are rapid, varied and diffuse. Any specific movements he makes are simple reflex actions or are prompted by a reflex action, such as swallowing prompted by the sucking reflex. Although he begins soon after birth to learn about the world through the conditioned reflex, practically all his behavior is still due to reflex response to stimuli. His whole body is likely to be involved in his activity, and his responses appear to be aroused by some generalized state such as hunger, pain, or discomfort from lying too long in one position. He does not localize the feeling of pain or hunger.

When the infant feels that something is wrong, he reacts with his whole body and may try out reflex movements which he associates with relief. For instance, although he does not yet connect the breast or the bottle with relief from hunger, he makes sucking movements with his lips and will try to suck anything which comes in contact with them. Specific responses to specific stimuli are an outgrowth of this generalized activity; the useless movements are dropped, and the useful movements which bring him a reward are perfected through practice. This is not due primarily to practice, however, but rather to maturation of his nervous system, muscles, bones and, in fact, his entire body. Maturation does not proceed at the same rate in all the systems of the body, but the general pattern makes possible the typical behavior of infants at certain ages. Naturally they must be given opportunity to try out and practice new responses, or their behavior will be atypical.

At birth the infant can raise his head slightly when lying on his abdomen, but not when on his back. If he is pulled to a sitting position, his head falls back, and his spine is curved in a bow from shoulders to hips. At an early age the infant can make crawling movements when on his abdomen and a little later push himself up in his crib by kicking movements.

EMOTIONAL RESPONSES

Signs of emotion in the newborn are extremely difficult to interpret. Probably all that can be said is that two emotional states are evident: in one he lies peacefully, and in the other he appears in discomfort—his face is twisted, and he cries. To this could be added his emotional response to the startle stimulus.

Since vocalization shows his emotion and, increasingly as he grows older, will express *the emotion* he wishes to convey, vocalization is considered under Emotional Responses.

Vocalization

The newborn vocalizes solely by crying, and this he does in response to any discomfort or pain. He is an egocentric little person, entirely dependent upon adult care and unable to make his wants known in any other way. His birth cry is the beginning of vocalization and serves two purposes: to supply the blood with sufficient oxygen and to inflate the unexpanded lungs.

If the cry is weak, relatively high-pitched and not sustained, an abnormal condition must be suspected. It should be a lusty cry even with only the stimulation of the birth incident. No one knows whether the birth cry has any connection with discomfort or is a pure reflex evoked by his physiologic needs.

Soon crying is used to express discomfort. If crying brings the infant relief and pleasant sensations from the care given him, he soon learns through the conditioning of this reflex to cry for attention. Even within the first 24 hours the cry varies in pitch, intensity, and continuity, so that it has meaning to those who are accustomed to caring for infants.

The stimulation to cry comes from the immediate environment or from his own body. He may be hungry, in pain, or in need of exercise such as comes from being picked up and moved about. Infants often cry for unknown reasons, and the cause of their discomfort cannot be ascertained. When an infant is neither hungry nor wet, if he stops crying when cuddled, we can infer that this is what he needed, and after being quieted he may be put back in his crib. But the infant who continues to cry while he is being held and petted is probably in distress and should be watched carefully for other symptoms of illness.

Hunger is said to be the most common cause of crying, and this is an argument for putting the infant on a self-demand feeding schedule (see p. 167).

The cry is made almost exclusively from vowels produced in the front of the mouth. Soon he makes other sounds which are as important as crying as a forerunner of speech. These sounds are explosive—coos, grunts, and gurgles. They probably have no meaning other than that they occur only when he appears contented. But the next stage of vocalization—that of repetition of syllables, as in "ma-ma"—is built upon his practice in phonation.

SPECIAL SENSES

An infant shows by his general discomfort that he can feel pressure, temperature change, and pain.

TOUCH

The sense of touch is the most highly developed of the special senses and is most acute on the lips, tongue, ears, and forehead. Failure to grasp the nipple is therefore one indication of brain damage. The normal newborn responds to the touch of the hands of those caring for him from the moment of his birth.

SIGHT

The eyes are blue or gray at birth, changing to the permanent color in three to six months. Their movements are not coordinated, and both eyes momentarily may turn inward or outward.

It is difficult to know what an infant sees. His eyes are only half open, and the lids are swollen. There may be a purulent discharge from the use of silver nitrate (see p. 158). The pupils react to light, and bright lights appear to be unpleasant to the infant.

Recent research has shown that normal fullterm newborns do have the capacity to shed tears, although they are usually not obvious until the infant is three to four weeks old.

HEARING

Because of the presence of fluid in the external auditory canal and the unequal pressure within and outside of the auditory apparatus, the newborn cannot hear until after his first cry.

To test the hearing of the newborn, a bell or a commercial instrument may be sounded a little distance from his ear. If he hears it, he will respond with generalized activity of his whole body, he will cease his activity, or he will move his limbs or his eyes. The best pretest condition is when the infant is sleeping lightly halfway between feedings. In general, 90 decibels is the best intensity of tone to stimulate a behavior response.

The infant normally makes some response to sound from the third to the seventh day, and there is evidence that he hears ordinary sounds before the tenth day. By the fourth week he is likely to react to the voice of his mother or nurse more frequently than to a loud noise.

TASTE

The infant's sense of taste is more highly developed than that of sight or hearing. He accepts sweet fluids and resists acid, sour or bitter ones.

SMELL

The only evidence of the sense of smell is that many infants appear to smell breast milk and reach for the nipple. There is a wide difference among infants in their apparent ability to smell.

SKIN SENSATIONS

Sensations of touch, pressure, temperature, and pain are present soon after birth, and at the end of ten days the infant reacts violently to cutaneous irritation.

ORGANIC SENSATIONS

The infant appears to be highly sensitive to organic stimulation, since hunger and thirst are the most common causes of crying. The newborn and the very young infant are not likely to have pain from gas in the intestines, but the infant of a few weeks appears to suffer intensely if his feeding produces colic.

SLEEP

Sleep in the newborn can hardly be distinguished from tranquil rest. The neonate sleeps from 15 to 18 or 20 hours a day. Short waking periods occur every two hours, but are fewer and shorter during the night, probably because there are fewer external stimuli to arouse him. He is awakened by internal discomfort such as hunger or pain. Hunger is by far the most common cause of an infant's waking before his physiologic need for sleep has been satisfied. As he grows older the length of unbroken periods of sleep and also of wakefulness increases.

IMMUNITY

Antibodies for certain infectious diseases pass through the placenta from mother to infant. Among these antibodies are those of smallpox, mumps, diphtheria, and measles if the mother is immune to these diseases. This passive immunity lasts from a few weeks to several months. Little immunity is passed on for chickenpox or pertussis, and young infants may contract these diseases. It is not feasible to immunize very young infants, since they are not sufficiently mature to form antibodies successfully.

If an infant does contract a contagious disease, it is likely to be more severe and to be followed by more complications than in an older child.

INDIVIDUALITY

Each newborn has an individual pattern of reactivity that persists through later periods of his life. If his nurse, after assessing him and caring for him, helps his family to recognize his individuality, satisfactory development of the child can be facilitated.

TEACHING AIDS AND OTHER INFORMATION*

Alexander Graham Bell Association for the Deaf

Can Your Baby Hear?
Hearing Alert.

American Academy of Pediatrics

Hospital Care of Newborn Infants.
Joint Statement on Neonatal Screening for Hearing Impairment.
Screening of Newborn Infants for Metabolic Disease.

National Society for the Prevention of Blindness, Inc.

Your Child's Sight: How Can You Help, 1975.

Public Affairs Committee

Gould, J.: Will My Baby Be Born Normal?

Ross Laboratories

Status of the Fetus and Newborn, 1973.

United States Government

International MCH Projects: Research to Improve Health Services for Mothers and Children, 1975.
Kavanagh, J. F.: The Genesis and Pathogenesis of Speech and Language, 1971.

---

*Complete addresses are given in the Appendix.

REFERENCES

Books

Abramson, H.: *Symposium on the Functional Physiopathology of the Fetus and Neonate: Clinical Correlations.* St. Louis, The C. V. Mosby Company, 1971.
Babson, S. G., Benson, R. C., Pernoll, M. L., and Benda, G. I.: *Management of High-Risk Pregnancy and Intensive Care of the Neonate.* 3rd ed. St. Louis, The C. V. Mosby Company, 1975.
Crelin, E. S.: *Functional Anatomy of the Newborn.* New Haven, Conn., Yale University Press, 1973.
Eisen, H. N.: *Immunology.* New York, Harper & Row Publishers, 1974.
Illingworth, R. S.: *Basic Developmental Screening.* Philadelphia, J. B. Lippincott Company, 1973.
Lemire, R. J., Loeser, J. D., Alvord, E. C., and Leech, R. W.: *Normal and Abnormal Development of the Human Nervous System.* New York, Harper & Row Publishers, 1975.
Miller, A. L., Rohman, B. F., and Thompson, F. V.: *Your Child's Hearing and Speech.* Springfield, Ill., Charles C Thomas, 1974.
Moore, M. L.: *The Newborn and The Nurse.* Philadelphia, W. B. Saunders Company, 1972.
Moschella, S. L., Pillsbury, D. M., and Hurley, H. J.: *Dermatology.* Philadelphia, W. B. Saunders Company, 1975.
Park, B. H., and Good, R. A.: *Principles of Modern Immuno-*
biology: Basic and Clinical. Philadelphia, Lea & Febiger, 1974.
Schaffer, A. J., and Avery, M. E.: *Diseases of the Newborn.* 4th ed. Philadelphia, W. B. Saunders Company, 1977.
Smith, C. A., and Nelson, N. M. (Eds.): *The Physiology of the Newborn Infant.* 4th ed. Springfield, Ill., Charles C Thomas, 1975.
Smith, D. W., and Bierman, E. L. (Eds.): *The Biologic Ages of Man.* Philadelphia, W. B. Saunders Company, 1973.
Smith, J. F.: *Pediatric Neuropathology.* New York, McGraw-Hill Book Company, 1974.

Periodicals

Adams, M. M.: Appraisal of the Newborn Infant. *Am. J. Nursing,* 55:1336, 1955.
Aleksandrowicz, M. K.: The Effect of Pain-Relieving Drugs Administered During Labor and Delivery on the Behavior of the Newborn: A Review. *Merrill-Palmer Q.,* 20:121, April 1974.
Carroll, M. H.: Preventing Newborn Deaths From Drug Withdrawal. *RN,* 34:34, December 1971.
Chiswick, M. L., and Milner, R. D. G.: Crying Vital Capacity. Measurement of Neonatal Lung Function. *Arch. Dis. Child,* 51:22, January 1976.
Cohen, S. N., and Olson, W. A.: Drugs That Depress the

Newborn Infant. *Pediat. Clin. N. Amer.*, 17:835, November 1970.

Doner, F.: Blindness *Can* Be Prevented. *The Canadian Nurse*, 72:27, January 1976.

Eoff, M. J., Meier, R. S., and Miller, C.: Temperature Measurement in Infants. *Nursing Research*, 23:457, November-December 1974.

Farrar, C. A.: Assessing Individuality in the Newborn. *Nursing Digest*, 3:16, July-August 1975.

Gillon, J. E.: Behavior of Newborns With Cardiac Distress. *Am. J. Nursing*, 73:254, February 1973.

Guilleminault, C., Peraita, R., Souquet, M., and Dement, W. C.: Apneas During Sleep in Infants. Possible Relationship With Sudden Infant Death Syndrome. *Science*, 190:677, November 14, 1975.

Hardy, J. B.: Birth Weight and Subsequent Physical and Intellectual Development. *N. Engl. J. Med.*, 289:973, November 1, 1973.

Marcil, V.: Physical Assessment of the Newborn. *The Canadian Nurse*, 72:20, March 1976.

Maurer, D. M., and Maurer, C. E.: Newborn Babies See Better Than You Think. *Psychology Today*, 10:85, October 1976.

Shimek, M. L. Screening Newborns for Hearing Loss. *Nursing Outlook*, 19:115, February 1971.

Watkins, J. B.: Bile Acid Metabolism and Fat Absorption in Newborn Infants. *Pediatr. Clin. N. Am.*, 21:501, May 1974.

AUDIOVISUAL MEDIA*

American Journal of Nursing Company

Maternity Nursing Class
The Neonate
44 minutes, 16mm film or videotape, sound, color, black and white, guide.
Demonstrates the characteristics of the neonate—appearance, reflexes, and variations. Discusses parental concerns.

Respiratory Distress in Children
12 minutes, sound, color.
This film is limited to illustrations of signs of respiratory distress in children, without reference to cause or treatment. Contrasts examples of children with healthy breathing patterns to examples of infants experiencing respiratory distress.

The Examination of the Newborn
20 minutes, color.
Demonstrates appraisal of the baby, by inspection, auscultation, percussion, and palpation with examples of normal and abnormal findings.

Charles Press–Prentice-Hall, Inc.

Growth and Development: Neonate, Part I
2–5 minutes, Super-8mm filmloop, color, guide.
Overall appearance, muscle tone, movement and some reflexes of a two day old infant.

Growth and Development: Neonate, Part II
2–5 minutes, Super-8mm filmloop, color, guide.
Continued examination of appearance, muscle tone, movement and some reflexes of a two day old infant.

Pediatrics: Newborn Respiratory Tract
Nowakowski, L.
25 35mm slides, 11 overhead transparencies, guide.

A step-by-step comparison of the newborn and adult respiratory tracts for nurses, respiratory therapists, and advanced students of pulmonary anatomy.

Health Sciences Communication Center, Case Western Reserve University

The Neurological Evaluation of the Maturity of Newborn Infants
32 minutes, 16mm film or videocassette, sound, color.
Because of its complexity and detail, the neonatal neurological examination has been a difficult subject to teach. This program has been designed for, and proven effective in, teaching the Tison method to practitioners, house officers, nurses, and students. The demonstration includes the examination of a full term newborn infant, and four neonates ranging in gestational age from thirty to thirty-eight weeks. Viewer participation is encouraged through the use of the Amiel-Tison charts, which are sent with each film.

McGraw-Hill Book Company

Maternal and Child Care
Infant Appraisal
7 minutes, 16mm film or Super-8mm filmloop, sound, color.
Demonstrates the procedure for assessing the newborn and emphasizes the importance of involving the mother in the examination.

Trainex Corporation

Physical Examination of the Newborn
35mm filmstrip, audio-tape cassettes, 33 1/3 LP, color.
Provides an excellent overview of findings in examination of the newborn, illustrated with selected photographs of significant features and characteristics present in the normal newborn.

---

*Complete addresses are given in the Appendix.

Chapter Eight

CARE OF THE NEWBORN

In the delivery room the infant is inspected for any gross anomalies such as spina bifida, cleft lip and cleft palate, imperforate anus, hydrocephalus, and birthmarks, and for evidence of shock or birth trauma. Many anomalies are not immediately evident on inspection, however, and these are the concern of the physician and the nurse in the nursery.

Within 60 seconds after the infant's body has been completely born, five objective signs should be evaluated to determine the presence of asphyxia and the need for assisted ventilation: heart rate, respiratory effort, muscle tone, reflex irritability, and color. These are shown on the scoring-system chart developed by Dr. Virginia Apgar (see Table 8–1 and Fig. 8–1). Each of these signs is an index of the infant's depression or lack of it at birth and is given a score of 0, 1, or 2. The infant is in the best possible condition if his score is 10. If he has a score of 5 to 10, he usually needs no treatment. If his score is 4 or below, the infant's condition must be immediately diagnosed and treatment given. Approximately 70 to 90 out of every 100 newborns should receive a score of 7 or above one minute after birth.

The Apgar scoring test should be repeated when the newborn is five minutes old because this is an accurate way to determine neurological abnormality and provides an index to the likelihood of death.

The physician and the nurse have several responsibilities in the care of the infant immediately after his birth.

The family-centered care which the nurse provides for parents and their newborn infants is based on an understanding of the physical status of the newborn and the emotional reactions of the infant and of his parents to the process of childbirth. Soon after birth the newborn has a period of alertness that is felt to be a good time for the newborn and his parents to interact, for the parents to touch and hold their infant. Some newborns may be put to their mother's breasts while still in the delivery room. During the postpartum period the symbiotic relationship between mother and child continues.

The preceding chapter presented the physical and physiologic characteristics of the normal newborn. This chapter is concerned with his care immediately after delivery, in the nursery and after discharge from the hospital.

CARE IN THE DELIVERY ROOM

Immediate care of the newborn includes gentleness and prevention of infection, establishment and maintenance of respiration, care of the umbilical cord, care of the eyes, stabilization of his temperature, identification of the infant and maintaining a record of observations on his condition.

Establishment and Maintenance of Respiration

The infant's respiration must be established and maintained. For this it is necessary that he cry lustily periodically. Full expansion of the

TABLE 8-1. *APGAR SCORING CHART*

SIGN	0	1	2
Heart rate	Absent	Slow (less than 100)	Greater than 100
Respiratory effort	Absent	Weak cry, hypoventilation	Good strong cry
Muscle tone	Limp	Some flexion of extremities	Well flexed
Reflex irritability: skin stimulation to feet	No response	Some motion	Cry
Color	Blue, pale	Body pink, extremities blue	Completely pink

V. Apgar and others: Evaluation of the Newborn Infant—Second Report. *J.A.M.A.*, *168*:1988, 1958.

lungs provides oxygen for the blood, which until birth was supplied through the placental circulation. Removal of this source of oxygen stimulates respiratory movements within the infant's body, movements which took place in a superficial manner even during intrauterine life. Any infant who does not breathe within 30 seconds after birth is in danger of asphyxia. The need for close observation of the infant and for having everything in readiness for his resuscitation is evident.

In addition to the respiratory rate and the presence or absence of cyanosis, a method of scoring the amount of retraction present gives an estimation of the degree of respiratory difficulty in the newborn (Fig. 8–3).

Some infants need further stimulation than that provided normally through separation from the mother. Failure to cry may be due to several causes, a common one being obstruction of his air passage with mucus. In order to clear the airway, the infant may be held by his feet with the head down and the neck curved backward. The infant may also be placed in the Trendelenburg position, with a slight lateral tilt and the neck hyperextended. In these positions the mucus drains out by gravity. Drainage of mucus may also be facilitated by stroking the neck in the direction of the mouth. This is known as milking the trachea. Respiration may be further stimulated by gently rubbing the infant's back or spanking his buttocks or the soles of his feet. The mucus may be gently wiped from his mouth with the nurse's gloved finger.

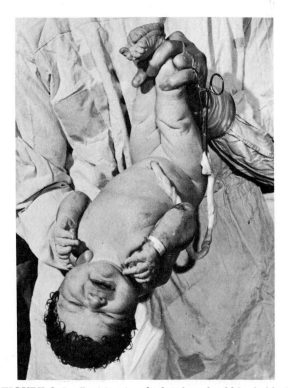

FIGURE 8-1. Dr. Virginia Apgar, originator of the Apgar score, slaps a baby's feet sharply to determine response to reflex irritability. This normal baby cries lustily. (Courtesy of the National Foundation—March of Dimes.)

FIGURE 8-2. Position in which infant should be held after delivery. If the infant's first breath occurs in the head-up position, respiratory obstruction follows. Note the identification band on the wrist. (From *Resuscitation of the Newborn Infant.* American Academy of Pediatrics.)

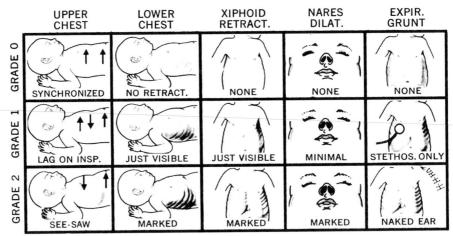

	UPPER CHEST	LOWER CHEST	XIPHOID RETRACT.	NARES DILAT.	EXPIR. GRUNT
GRADE 0	SYNCHRONIZED	NO RETRACT.	NONE	NONE	NONE
GRADE 1	LAG ON INSP.	JUST VISIBLE	JUST VISIBLE	MINIMAL	STETHOS. ONLY
GRADE 2	SEE-SAW	MARKED	MARKED	MARKED	NAKED EAR

FIGURE 8–3. Criteria of respiratory distress. Grade 0 for each criterion indicates no respiratory distress; grade 2 for each criterion indicates severe respiratory distress. Abbreviations: DILAT., dilatation; EXPIR., expiratory; INSP., inspiratory; RETRACT., retraction; STETHOS., stethoscope. (Courtesy of Mead Johnson & Company, in Vaughan, V. C., III, and McKay, R. J.: *Nelson Textbook of Pediatrics*, 10th ed. Philadelphia, W. B. Saunders Co., 1975.)

If these measures fail, it may be necessary to remove mucus by suction. A soft catheter may be used with a suction appliance, either an electrically powered suction machine or a DeLee mucus trap. (The size of the catheter used may vary, depending on the size of the infant and the procedure adopted by the individual hospital.) When the catheter is in position, gentle suction is made. Suction should not be too vigorous, so as to prevent damage to the mucous membranes. It is important that mucus be removed before the infant draws his first breath in order to prevent aspiration of mucus. When as much mucus as possible has been removed, the infant should be placed in the head-down position to induce further drainage unless this is contraindicated.

If the infant does not cry after such resuscitation measures, the physician will clamp the cord, and more drastic means of stimulating the infant to breathe will be used. The newborn's heart rate should be continuously monitored.

After the airway has been cleared, ventilation with oxygen is indicated. If the infant's tongue is lying against the posterior pharyngeal wall, thereby obstructing the airway, a properly placed small pharyngeal airway will correct the obstruction. If the infant still does not breathe adequately, the lungs may be inflated by administering oxygen under controlled intermittent pressure with the use of a snugly fitting mask. Usually pressures of 15 to 20 cm. of water are safe to use. When oxygen is being given, the physician should auscultate the chest to determine whether the gas is entering the lungs.

If the infant's lungs are still not adequately ex-panded, direct laryngoscopy should be carried out so that any obstructing foreign material can be removed. In some instances positive pressure may be applied by use of a snugly fitting no. 12 French endotracheal tube or by a few short puffs of air at high pressure. In an emergency when no mechanical devices are available, mouth-to-mouth resuscitation using only the air in the operator's mouth may be used. Air forced under too great pressure into the infant's lungs may result in rupture of them. Respiratory stimulants are not used, but a circulatory stimulant may be useful. If the heartbeat is absent after adequate oxygen has been given, closed cardiac massage should be instituted at a rate of 100 to 120 times per minute.

Care of the Umbilical Cord

Two clamps are used to compress the cord. They are placed about 2 inches from the abdomen. If possible, this is not done until the cord has stopped pulsating, for the infant will then receive approximately 100 ml. of blood from the placenta, which will provide him with a store of iron and other desirable blood constituents. He will need this iron during the first few months of life when the iron content of his diet tends to be below his needs. But if the mother has been deeply anesthetized, he may evidence signs of depression from passage of the anesthetic or analgesic agent across the placental barrier.

After the cord has been clamped, a ligature is tied in a square knot about 1 inch from the ab-

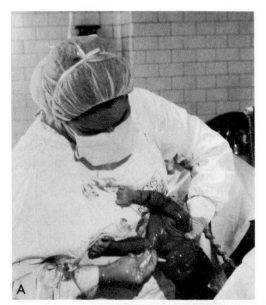

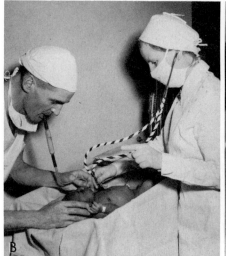

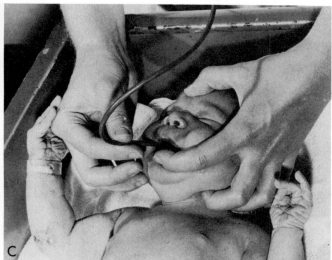

FIGURE 8–4. *A*, Aspiration of the newborn immediately after birth with a rubber syringe. *B*, DeLee glass trap and rubber catheter may be used for aspiration. Movement of nurse's finger is the silent method of indicating the heart rate of a newborn. *C*, Method of suctioning the pharynx of a newborn. (*A*, from *R.N.*, January, 1970, cover illustration. *B* and *C*, from *Resuscitation of the Newborn Infant*, American Academy of Pediatrics.)

dominal wall. After removal of the clamp, the cord should be turned back on itself and tied a second time with the same ligature. Instead of a ligature, a clamp which crushes the vessels may be placed on the cord and removed after several hours, or another kind of clamp may be left on the cord until it drops off. Some institutions favor the use of a special broad rubber band.

There is a difference of opinion as to whether an antiseptic solution and a dressing should be applied to the cord. The custom of the hospital or the physician's order should be followed. If there is a possibility that an exchange transfusion due to incompatibility of blood types may become necessary, the cord should be left a little long and covered with a sterile dressing for the first 24 hours. It should be inspected, as should all umbilical cords, for bleeding during

the first day and for the presence of infection until it comes off.

Extreme care must be taken that the cord does not become contaminated. The cord is connected with the great blood vessels of the abdomen, through which infection could be carried, with septicemia a likely result.

Care of the Eyes

If the mother has gonorrhea, the infant's eyes may be inoculated with the organism during delivery. If the eyes are not adequately treated at once, ophthalmia neonatorum is likely to develop (see p. 260). A prophylactic treatment against newborn gonococcal ophthalmia is required by state law. A germicide may be instilled into the eyes of the newborn shortly after delivery. Silver nitrate has been used for many years. Penicillin, which is a gonococcide, has been used more recently.

Silver nitrate may be dropped between the eyelids at any time after the head has been delivered until the third stage of labor is completed. The eyelids are cleansed carefully with a sterile cotton ball moistened with sterile water; wiping should proceed from the nose outward. The lower lid is pulled down, and 2 drops of a 1 per cent solution of silver nitrate are instilled into the conjunctival sac. After a minute or two the eyes are irrigated with warm physiologic salt solution; this washes out the excess silver nitrate and forms a precipitate with the remainder. In about 50 per cent of infants a chemical irritation may result from the silver nitrate. Although within a few hours a profuse discharge may appear in the eyes, there is no permanent ill effect from the treatment and the chemical conjunctivitis. Because some physicians believe that insufficient contact of the silver nitrate occurs when the eyes are irrigated, they recommend that the medication not be rinsed from the eyes.

Penicillin may be administered as a topical application in the form of penicillin ophthalmic ointment or may be given intramuscularly.

Stabilization of Temperature

The temperature of the newborn usually drops immediately after birth, especially in an air conditioned delivery room, but returns to normal in about eight hours. The temperature in the delivery room is lower than that *in utero*, and this accounts for the drop in the infant's temperature after delivery. To raise his body temperature to normal, he should be dried and wrapped in a dry, warm, sterile cotton flannel blanket immediately after birth.

The newborn is adversely affected by hypothermia, a drop in body temperature. This results in an increased metabolic rate leading to an increased need for and consumption of oxygen. This increased metabolic rate also results in an increased consumption of glucose. If untreated, hypoglycemia occurs and brain damage may result.

When the newborn is not warmed to his normal temperature, his ability to compensate begins to fail. Fatigue occurs because of increased respiratory effort. As respirations become slow and shallow, bradycardia occurs. Lack of oxygen results in pulmonary vasoconstriction, which results in less oxygen intake and further carbon dioxide retention. Respiratory

acidosis occurs along with the existing metabolic acidosis. The central nervous system becomes depressed, and reflexes and responses diminish. There may also be vomiting and abdominal distention.

Identification of the Infant

All infants must be identified in some manner before they are removed from the delivery room. Several methods are in use, the most common among them being an adhesive label bearing identification information applied to the infant's back, a name bracelet or necklace placed on the wrist or about the neck, identification tapes marked with identification numbers for both the infant and the mother placed about their wrists (see Fig. 8–2), and foot or palm prints of the infant taken while he is still on the delivery table. This last is the most "mistake-proof," but must be very carefully done in order to get clear prints. It must be done in conjunction with a form of identification which can be used in caring for the infant.

Baptism

If there is danger of death of the newborn, the majority of Christian parents wish to have their child baptized immediately. This may, of course, take place in the delivery room, but is more likely to be the responsibility of the nurse in the nursery. If the parents are Roman Catholics, a priest should be called if it appears that the infant will live until he arrives. If the parents are Protestant, a minister of their faith should be called. If death is imminent and a priest is not present, the nurse or physician may perform the baptism by pouring water on the infant's forehead while saying, "I baptize you in the name of the Father and of the Son and of the Holy Spirit." The Roman Catholic Church teaches that every fetus and embryo should also be baptized if possible. Conditional baptism can be carried out if it is not certain whether the subject is capable of receiving baptism, by saying, "If you are capable of receiving baptism, I baptize you in the name of the Father and of the Son and of the Holy Spirit." Although it is not essential to repeat the Lord's Prayer or the Apostles' Creed, or both, this is often done.

Essentials of Nursing Care

Nursing care is begun in the delivery room immediately after birth and is continued in the nursery or the mother's room if the infant rooms-in with her.

The great need for *gentleness* in caring for the newborn has already been stressed. He has undergone a difficult if not exhausting experience and is now initiating bodily functions for himself which his mother's body performed for him while he was in the uterus. He has been accustomed to his "marine bath," and even the softest fabric is irritating. Being moved about independently is a novel experience after the confinement of the uterus. Since the newborn's initial experiences with the world are through body contact and his sense of touch, the smoothness of the nurse's actions and confidence in handling him transmit to the newborn a sense of security in his new environment.

Avoidance of infection is imperative. The only source of infection before birth was through the mother's blood stream, but now there are many portals of infection. In general his nursing care is that of strict aseptic nursing. Clothing and the linen and blankets for his crib, the gown which the nurse wears, and all equipment used in his care should be surgically clean if not sterile. His bedside equipment is, of course, for his personal use only. The nurse who cares for him should never be on duty with a cold, sore throat, loose stools, or any septic skin infection. Infection which might be of little consequence in an older child or adult may cause the death of a newborn.

CARE IN THE NURSERY

The newborn, wrapped in a warm receiving blanket, is transferred to the nursery in either a warm crib or the nurse's arms. He is then dressed in a diaper, shirt, and gown, and is loosely wrapped in a blanket and placed in a warm crib. If the father has not seen him previously, the infant is shown to him as soon as possible.

One of the newer developments in the care of newborns is to place those born on the same day in a glass-enclosed room. Thus each day a different room is utilized for the new infants. As they are discharged from each room it is cleaned thoroughly. If infection does occur, it is easier to contain in a smaller unit than in a larger nursery area.

General Nursing Procedures

While the newborn remains in the hospital daily care must be provided for him. This is an intermediate step between the care given directly after birth and his care at home. Since many infant deaths occur in the first few days of life, his physical care and the observations made and charted by the nurse are fully as important as those in the first few hours of life.

Only when the nurse is aware of the physical attributes, the physiologic activities and the common functional disorders of the newborn can the newborn under care be appraised. (See Chapter 7 for characteristics of the normal newborn.)

PRELIMINARY PHYSICAL EXAMINATION

The nurse must observe the infant closely. On his admission or soon after, the nurse should appraise his physical status. This appraisal can be accurate only when what is normal and what is abnormal in the newborn is known. (There is a wide range of individual differences among normal infants.) This knowledge cannot be learned solely in class or from books; it comes only with experience in the care of the newborn. For this reason the student should be particularly careful to query the instructor or supervisor whenever in doubt about the significance of variations in an infant's physical state and behavior.

As was discussed in Chapter 7, in order for a nurse to apply the knowledge of what is normal to a particular infant, his history should be known: the mother's age, history of previous and present pregnancies, maternal Rh factor, duration of labor, color of the amniotic fluid and the infant's Apgar score.

The nurse's legal responsibility in the appraisal of the newborn is in part determined by the policy of the agency and may vary; however, the moral responsibility to provide the best care possible for the patient never varies.

The nurse must remember that the most common signs of infant distress are (1) increased rate or difficulty of respirations, (2) sternal retractions, (3) excessive mucus as when the infant drools or blows bubbles, (4) worried facial expression, (5) cyanosis, (6) abdominal distention or mass, (7) inadequate evacuation of meconium within 24 hours after birth, (8) inadequate voiding, (9) vomiting of bile-stained material, (10) unusual jaundice of the skin, and (11) convulsions. The nurse may be responsible for appraisal not only when the infant is brought to the nursery but also when he is discharged. If so, the normal maturation which takes place during the first few days of life must be understood. The standards of normality for a three-day-old infant are not the same as during his first hour of extrauterine life.

The role of the professional nurse now includes many functions which formerly belonged exclusively to the physician. This is made necessary by (1) the extreme shortage of medical personnel as compared with the increasing demand and (2) the greater competency of the modern professional nurse in assisting the physician by accurate, intelligent observation. Whatever the policy of the hospital, the nurse can best fulfill the responsibility for the infant's complete nursing care by frequent observation of his condition. This is necessary not only for the infant's safety, but also for improving the nurse's own ability to make discriminating judgments between normal and abnormal states.

In addition to appraisal of the infant in order to determine whether problems exist, the nurse may also review parts of the examination with the mother after she is rested so that she will not be worried about characteristics which are normal in the newborn, such as shape of the head or crossed eyes. Such information can prevent or dispel many anxieties which the mother may have.

CONTINUOUS OBSERVATION

General observation of an infant must be made at frequent intervals during the day and night for evidence of malfunction in vital bodily functions, including respiratory distress.

Respiratory Distress. Respiratory distress is shown by the rate and nature of an infant's respirations, his cry, color, and general behavior. If the infant appears to be choking, mucus may be found in the nose or mouth. The air passages may be cleared immediately by placing the infant with his head lower than his body and stroking his neck in the direction of his mouth. If these procedures do not give relief and the physician cannot be reached, the nurse should use an aspirator and provide oxygen if this is necessary. To meet such an emergency, equipment for aspiration and oxygen administration should always be kept in the area where newborns are cared for.

Position of the Infant. Because of the possibility of respiratory distress during the first 24 hours of life, the foot of the crib or the mattress is elevated at a 15- to 20-degree angle. The infant is placed on his side in this head-down position. He should be rotated to the other side every two or three hours, since lying constantly on one side will cause the bones of the skull to be flattened. The shape of the chest is also influenced by the position in which he lies, but seldom to the extent of deformity such as occurs in the skull. Since infants like to face the light and it is essential that they do not lie always upon the same side, the infant's head will be alternately at the "top" or "foot" of the crib.

The newborn should become accustomed to sleeping on his abdomen, but because of the danger of suffocation, he should be placed on his abdomen only when it is possible to watch him closely.

The position in which the infant is held should accord with his level of maturation, particularly that of his neuromuscular system. Even a normal infant cannot hold his head up without support until he is six weeks old. To hold an infant upright, the nurse should support his head and shoulders with one hand and his buttocks with the other. The hold upon him should be firm and steady so that he has no fear of loss of support. (Some child psychologists hold that such fear is one of the few fundamental fears of infancy.) An infant enjoys being held, and holding him gives the nurse an opportunity to help him develop a sense of trust in those who care for him.

Temperature. Proper temperature and humidity control must be maintained in the nursery or, if the infant is rooming-in, the mother's room. Room temperature and humidity are important in respiratory considerations, particularly in the newborn infant. During the day the temperature should range from 68 to 76° F. (20.0 to 24.4° C.), and the humidity from 45 to 55 per cent. The infant's heat-regulating centers are poorly developed, and he reacts quickly to any divergence in temperature of his environment. The air in the room should be fresh, but there must be no drafts. Fresh air usually has sufficient moisture to prevent drying of the mucous membranes of the nose and throat.

The body temperature of the newborn upon admission to the nursery may be subnormal (see p. 139). He should be dressed in dry clothes and external heat applied, if necessary, until his temperature is normal.

If the infant has been delivered in the home, hot-water bottles placed outside the crib covers may be used to provide an accessory heat source.

Since heat perception is poorly developed in the newborn, three precautions in the use of hot-water bottles must be remembered: (1) The temperature of the water must not be over 115° F. (46.1° C.). (2) The bag must be covered with flannel or a towel and should be checked for leakage before being used. (3) The bag must not be placed upon the infant's chest or abdomen, where its weight might interfere with respiratory movements. Ordinarily three hot-water bottles are used, one under the legs and one on each side of the body. These provide heat for the extremities, where the circulation is poor, without overheating the chest. Hot-water bottles cool quickly and need to be refilled frequently.

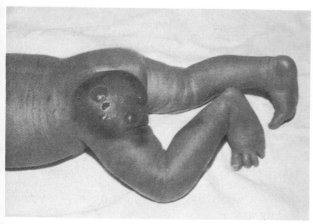

FIGURE 8–5. Second-degree burn in a newborn caused by a hot-water bottle. (Moll, H.: *Atlas of Pediatric Diseases*, Philadelphia, W. B. Saunders Co., 1976.)

If three are used, they may be filled in rotation. Electric pads should not be used, for there is always danger of overheating or of shock from faulty connections.

An incubator is the most satisfactory method of applying external heat. The incubator maintains a controlled, uniform temperature. The heat regulator should be set at 80 to 85° F. (26.7 to 27.8° C.), depending upon the procedure established by the hospital personnel. The infant's temperature must be checked frequently in order that the regulator of the incubator may be adjusted to meet his needs. An infant's temperature responds readily to external heat, and his temperature should be taken every hour until his body heat is established at normal. The average newborn may then be removed from the incubator to his crib, but those who weigh less than average or are debilitated from a difficult delivery may need longer confinement in the incubator.

The amount of clothing and covering an infant needs depends upon the temperature of the room. In general the nursery is kept at a higher temperature than the mother's room, and so the infant who rooms-in will need extra covering. Mothers tend to dress their babies too warmly because they use as their guide the temperature of the infant's hands and feet. Mothers will learn from the nurse that a more accurate way of determining whether an infant is warm or cool is observing the color of his face. If it is flushed, the infant is too warm; if pale or bluish, he is too cool. The mother may feel the arms and legs of the infant, rather than the hands and feet, to check on her observation of the color of his face. She will then have an adequate basis for determining the amount of clothing and covering he needs.

Infants cannot adjust their body temperature

to the rapid changes in environmental temperature when they are carried from the nursery through the hall to the mother's room. For this reason they are wrapped in blankets when taken to their mothers.

After the temperature of the newborn has become stabilized it is taken every four hours during the first two days and after that at periods depending on the policy established by the hospital. The temperature may be taken by either the axillary or the rectal method. Each infant should have his own thermometer to reduce the possibility of cross-infection in the nursery. If temperatures are routinely taken by rectum, care must be exercised to prevent irritation or injury to the rectal mucosa and unnecessary stimulation of defecation, causing a loss of fluid and calories. The thermometer bulb should be examined carefully for imperfections. The infant's legs should be grasped firmly with the nurse's index finger between the ankle bones. The rec-

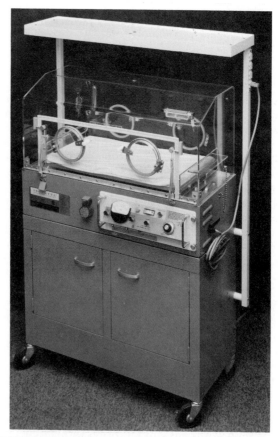

FIGURE 8–6. Isolette Incubator. The Isolette features an easy-to-clean conditioning chamber, optional humidity and oxygen control, and unequalled isolation through the use of the exclusive microfilter on the outside air adaptor. The infant can be weighed inside the incubator. A "background" air temperature of about 86° F. is maintained by the standard Isolette temperature control. (Courtesy of Isolette, A Narco Medical Company, Warminster, Pennsylvania.)

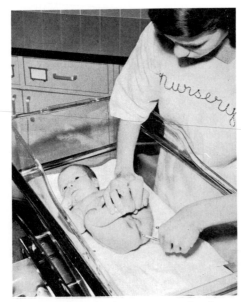

FIGURE 8-7. The infant's temperature is taken rectally. If the infant has a fever, the temperature should be taken every 4 hours. When taking the temperature, the nurse should place her index finger between the infant's ankles and hold the thermometer securely in place. (Davis and Rubin: *DeLee's Obstetrics for Nurses.* 17th ed.)

tal thermometer should be well lubricated and inserted for a period of time determined by hospital policy. A safer procedure is taking the infant's temperature by the axillary method. The thermometer must be held firmly in the axilla, with the infant's arm pressed against his side, for at least five minutes or until the mercury stops rising.

Recent research has resulted in a new temperature monitoring device consisting of a small film patch which, when applied to the abdomen above the liver, changes color, depending on the infant's temperature. The patch can be left in place for 24 hours, permitting frequent readings without disturbing the infant.

Weight. The infant is weighed at birth and each following day at approximately the same time, usually when he is given his morning care. Newborns are usually weighed completely nude in a warm nursery. A fresh sheet of paper or a diaper should be balanced on the scale before he is placed upon it.

If the infant is immature or not in good health or the nursery is not sufficiently warm, he may be weighed dressed and wrapped in his blanket. Then, when he is undressed for morning care, these articles are weighed and their weight is subtracted from the combined weight of the infant, his clothes and his blanket.

Certain types of incubators contain all necessary equipment, including scales. An infant can then be cared for and weighed without removing him to a cooler atmosphere.

The infant's weight is compared each day with that of the day before. If he loses more than the usual physiologic loss during the first few days or if, after a week, he shows little or no gain in weight, the physician's attention should be called to the weight chart.

Specific Nursing Care

Care of the newborn varies in different hospitals; however, the following generalizations can be stated.

CARE OF THE SKIN

Thorough cleansing of the body immediately after delivery is not done, for the vernix caseosa is believed to have a beneficial effect upon the tender skin. The vernix is dissipated in a few days.

The majority of pediatricians accept the theory that the less the skin is handled and abraded by even gentle friction, the better is its condition. Even under this regimen skin irritation may occur in some infants.

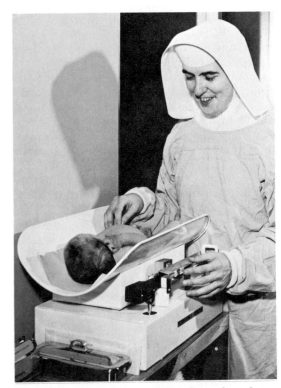

FIGURE 8-8. The nurse carefully places the infant onto the scoop basket of the scale, which is covered with sterile impervious paper. While weighing the infant, she keeps her hand over the infant's body to protect him from falling. (Fitzgerald Mercy Hospital, Darby, Pa.)

The following method is in accordance with modern concepts of child care.

1. Soon after birth the blood on the face and scalp is washed away with a very soft cloth or cotton balls and water.

2. No attempt is made to remove the vernix caseosa, which adheres to the skin and has a protective value. It has been likened to vanishing cream in its softening effect upon the infant's peeling skin.

3. The infant should not be exposed, since he would become chilled. While the nurse is wiping off the amniotic fluid and blood he should be covered with his blanket. The nurse exposes only that part of his body which is being wiped at the moment. In this way his entire body is not uncovered at any time. He is then dressed in a diaper and shirt and loosely wrapped in a fresh blanket.

4. During the first day the vernix caseosa rubs into the skin or comes off on the infant's clothing. On the second day any remnant adhering in the creases of the body may be wiped off with a soft cloth or cotton balls.

Daily Morning Care. The following technique for bathing the infant in the nursery is based on generally accepted principles and is used in many hospitals.

1. His condition is observed at bath time, since he is nude. In bathing him, special attention is given to the condition of the skin, eyes, nose, ears, mouth, umbilicus, and genitalia. The bath is a time when the infant is free of restraint from diaper or clothing, and his spontaneous movements may be observed better then than at any other time. Any unusual condition or abnormal movements should be reported.

2. The infant may be washed with a soft cloth or absorbent cotton and clear water. No soap or oil should be used. Several years ago research showed that bathing of newborns with solutions containing 3 per cent or more of hexachlorophene (which was formerly widely used to prevent staphylococcal disease during the first month of life) is unsafe. Experiments on animals have shown that this substance may be absorbed from the skin, may cause vacuolization in the white matter of the brain and thus brain damage. At present, hexachlorophene is used only when necessary according to the procedure established by the hospital and when prescribed by a physician. Other methods to prevent infection of newborns should be utilized. A soft dry cloth should be used to dry his face and body and, if cotton was used, to prevent wisps of cotton from clinging to the skin or body orifices.

3. The outer layer of skin normally peels off in minute grainy particles or in fairly large flakes. These areas may be bathed with clear water, dried and have oil applied to them. Cracks in the skin around the wrists and ankles should be cleansed and oiled. It is often difficult for a mother to believe that these lesions are normal and of no significance. Fortunately they improve readily under proper treatment.

4. Care of the buttocks and genitalia is extremely important. The area should be washed with warm water. In the male infant special attention should be given to the areas of skin contact about the scrotum and the penis. In some institutions a bland soap is used if it is difficult to remove the stool with clear water. There is a difference of opinion as to whether oil should be used on the buttocks. Some physicians believe that its use increases the danger of infection, while others order it to be applied routinely.

5. Talcum powder is usually contraindicated. Some mothers, however, believe that it prevents chafing. Its use, then, with the infant who rooms-in with his mother depends upon her insistence on its value and the policy of the hospital. The harm it may cause to the skin is slight. There is some danger that the mother may shake the can too vigorously and that some of the fine powder particles may drift so that the infant can inhale them. Even the better powders on the market may be irritating to the infant's delicate respiratory tract. Powder accumulated in the folds of skin may become saturated with body secretions. If powder is used with oil, it forms a paste which is likely to retain urine, feces, or bodily secretions and prove irritating. Zinc stearate powders should never be used because of their intensely irritating effect upon the respiratory tract. Powders made for infants do not contain zinc stearate, but the ordinary commercial powders may. Powder containing boric acid should never be used because of its poisonous effect on human beings. Powder containing hexachlorophene may be used only on a physician's order.

Other procedures included in the daily morning care are taking the infant's temperature, weighing him, changing the covering on the umbilical cord if one is used or cleaning around the cord stump (see p. 165), changing the sheets and pads of his bed, and cutting his fingernails and toenails if they extend beyond the ends of the fingers and toes. The nails should be cut square, the corners slightly rounded, so that the infant cannot scratch himself.

Skin Irritations. In spite of good care, skin irritations develop in some infants.

Probably the most common skin irritation after the neonatal period is *miliaria* (prickly heat). It is caused by a superficial bacterial action after excessive sweating during hot weather or fever. The signs are small erythematous papules and vesicles which cause itching. The treatment is cleanliness, washing with warm water and a mild soap, rinsing with clear water and drying thoroughly. Soothing lotions may be used, calamine lotion being the most common. It dries the skin as powder does and stays on the irritated area without caking. In general, miliaria is a sign that the infant has been too warmly dressed. Even in hot weather it is not likely to occur in areas freely exposed to the air.

Intertrigo, or chafing, is most often seen in infants with very sensitive skins. It occurs where two surfaces of skin are in contact—behind the ears, in the creases in the neck, axillae, and groin and, in the male, under the scrotum—and is particularly likely to occur where there is moisture from sweat, urine, feces, or milk which has dripped into a fold of skin. The condition is also caused by friction, although this is seldom the case in the newborn, whose clothing is soft and whose physical activity is limited.

The manifestations of intertrigo are raw, red, moist areas in the skin folds. The lesions do not itch, and they do not heal by forming a crust or scab. Instead, the area becomes dry and gradually assumes its normal texture and appearance. Prevention lies in cleanliness, particularly in the folds of the skin, and in keeping the skin dry and free from contact with organisms which could cause the area to become infected. The areas may need to be cleansed several times a day if they are soiled or sticky with secretions.

The nurse is not likely to see intertrigo in an infant born in the hospital, but rather in those delivered at home and brought into the hospital by mothers after a few days because of some complication which required hospital care.

There may be *abrasions* on the heels, knees, toes, and elbows from rubbing against the crib linens. These seldom occur in the healthy, well-cared-for newborn, but are frequent in a neglected undernourished infant who lies crying and engages in aimless crawling or kicking movements. Such an infant may be brought to the hospital for an illness. The irritated areas should be bandaged lightly and kept scrupulously clean.

Diaper rash is caused by irritation from urine and stool. It is seldom seen in the breast-fed infant, but is common in the infant on a formula. If the stool is irritating and the diaper is not changed immediately, the buttocks may become red, and then shiny and raw. The lesions smart when the infant urinates and are a frequent cause of crying among infants not receiving sufficient care. Treatment consists in exposure of the area to warmth and air by placing a diaper under the infant and laying him on his abdomen with his shirt folded up above the buttocks. The diaper should be changed, of course, whenever it is soiled. If possible, the area should be exposed to sunlight. When exposure to sunlight is not practicable or is insufficient therapy, a soothing ointment such as zinc oxide, A and D ointment, or methylbenzethonium chloride (Diaparene) will aid the healing process. Diaparene contains a germicide inimical to harmful bacteria which decompose urine in the diaper area and cause irritation.

Diapers which have been improperly washed and rinsed may cause a rash. If diapers are to be washed at home, they should be soaked in cold water, then washed with a mild soap, rinsed thoroughly and, if possible, dried in the sun. Commercial laundries do excellent work, and many hospitals as well as private families are using their services. Disposable diapers are being used increasingly for the care of infants in both hospital and home.

Cleanliness is the main factor in the prevention of diaper rash. Plastic pants are seldom put on infants, but, when used, may predispose to diaper rash because the diaper is likely not to be changed often enough.

CARE OF THE EYES, NOSE, EARS, AND MOUTH

Care should be given only as necessary to the infant's eyes. Any secretions that have accumulated in the corners should be washed out with a soft washcloth and clear water, stroking from the inner canthus outward. The eyes should not be irrigated even if there is a discharge unless the physician orders irrigation. If irrigation is prescribed, physiologic salt solution should be used. Boric acid should not be used, because it is harmful when taken internally. Since boric acid solutions are both odorless and colorless, they may be mistaken for water.

Because any severe discharge from the eyes may be evidence of a serious infection, the physician will probably order warm saline irrigations and isolation precautions and send specimens of the discharge to the laboratory for culture. He may prescribe antibiotic drugs or ointment to counteract the infection.

The infant's nose and ears may be cleansed externally by using a twisted cotton cone moistened in water. All excess water should be squeezed out, since it annoys the infant if it drips upon his face. Oil should never be used because of the danger of aspiration with resulting harm to the respiratory tract. No attempt should be made to cleanse the nose or ears internally. Toothpicks or wooden applicator sticks covered with cotton should not be used because of the danger of injury from deep penetration if the infant moves unexpectedly. There is also the risk that the cotton may become loose and lodge in the nose or ear; it will then be necessary for the physician to remove the cotton with instruments.

The mouth should not be cleansed except by offering sterile water between feedings. There is danger of injuring the tissues and thus predisposing to infection.

CARE OF THE GENITALIA

The Vulva. The vulva should be cleansed gently with a bland soap and warm water. Some of the vernix caseosa may be removed each day at bath time and when the buttocks are cleansed after passage of a stool. Mothers should be instructed *to cleanse the vulva from the urethra toward the anus,* using a different section of the washcloth with each stroke. With this method there is less likelihood that the urethra will become contaminated with fecal organisms, thereby minimizing the possibility of cystitis due to infection traveling up the urethra to the bladder.

The Penis. In cleansing the penis the foreskin may be retracted, when possible, each day if the infant has not been circumcised. Irritation will result if smegma, a malodorous cheeselike substance, and bacteria are not removed from beneath the foreskin. The cleansing process should be done very gently, and the foreskin should be retracted only as far as it will go without pressure. It must be returned to its normal position immediately afterward to prevent painful paraphimosis due to constriction and edema.

If the foreskin is adherent to the glans during the neonatal period, the physician may postpone retraction. Nevertheless the mother should be taught the procedure so that later, in cleansing the penis, she will be familiar with the technique.

PHIMOSIS. In this condition the foreskin is so tightly hooded over the tip of the glans that it impedes the discharge of urine and predisposes to irritation. The treatment is by circumcision — surgical removal of the foreskin. The operation is performed to prevent infection, to facilitate the discharge of urine and to make the area easier to clean. Written permission for the operation must be obtained. Although there are no valid medical reasons for circumcision in the neonatal period except phimosis, the operation may be done on the first day of life before physiologic hypoprothrombinemia occurs, or on the sixth to the eighth day, at which time the infant has recovered from physiologic hypoprothrombinemia and the bleeding and coagulation times are usually within normal limits.

Although circumcision is a minor operation, the infant needs care after it. The nurse must watch for bleeding. A soothing ointment may be applied to the raw area after the diaper has been changed (some physicians prefer that no diaper be used). Such care should continue until the area is healed.

CARE OF THE UMBILICAL CORD

During the first 24 hours after the infant's admission to the nursery the cord must be observed closely for bleeding. Sometimes the cord contains an excessive amount of Wharton's jelly. When this shrinks, as part of the normal process, a ligature or clamp which was tight becomes loosened, and there is danger of hemorrhage. Normally a clot forms at the end of the cord stump and may prevent bleeding even if the ligature or clamp is loose. But if the clot is dislodged through manipulation, bleeding will occur. To prevent further loss of blood the nurse should apply a sterile hemostatic forceps as far from the abdominal wall as possible. The physician or nurse can then apply another clamp or ligature to the cord, closer to the abdominal wall.

The cord may heal in one of two ways: by dry or moist gangrene. Dry healing is preferred because a dry area is a poor medium for the growth of bacteria. Normally, the umbilical wound is completely healed in a week.

The umbilical area may be cleansed each day with 60 to 70 per cent alcohol, which has a drying effect and promotes antisepsis. Other solutions may be used, depending on the procedure adopted by the hospital personnel. If a cord dressing is used, it should be changed promptly when soiled. If infection develops around the umbilicus, as shown by redness in the area, malodor, or moisture or discharge from the cord, the physician should be notified at once. Treatment of such infection usually consists in frequent applications of an alcohol dressing and an antibiotic applied locally or given systemically, or both, depending on the results of a culture of the area.

INANITION OR DEHYDRATION FEVER

Between the second and fourth days of life the infant may have fever as a result of his low fluid intake with normal fluid loss. His temperature may rise to 102 to 104° F. (38.9 to 40° C.). His skin becomes dry, urine output is decreased, and his face and body show that he has undergone a sudden loss in weight. Treatment consists in increasing the amount of fluid taken, giving water between milk feedings, or in administration of parenteral fluids.

Prevention of Infection

The newborn has little resistance to disease. For this reason all nurses caring for the newborn must understand the importance of aseptic technique. Probably the fundamental rule to be followed by parents and hospital personnel is that they wash their hands thoroughly before handling the infant. In the nursery this is done on entering the room. Antiseptic detergents are better for this purpose than toilet soap, and the hands should be washed under running water. No rings or wrist watch should be worn, since either may be the site of lodgment of bacteria. Even imperfect nail polish may be a source of transmission of infection. It is possible for an infant to be orally infected with organisms from his own stool. For this reason the nurse's hands should be washed thoroughly after changing his diaper and before feeding him.

In some nurseries all personnel routinely wear masks. Their value is questionable, however. If they are not changed frequently or if they become soiled when adjusted, they are a source of contamination rather than of protection to the infant.

No one who has symptoms of a respiratory, intestinal or skin infection should enter the nursery or rooms where infants are with their mothers; such persons should have absolutely no contact, direct or indirect, with the infants. If the mother acquires an infection, her infant should not be taken to her; if he rooms-in, he should be isolated from her. If she has been in contact with the infant, he should be isolated not only from her but also from the other infants in the nursery so that he may not be a source of transmission if he has contracted his mother's disease.

Infection is far more likely to be carried by direct contact with an infected person than by indirect contact through contaminated equipment. Nevertheless contaminated equipment is definitely a source of infection. Each infant should have his own personal articles for his bath and other care. These may be kept in his stand or in a drawer underneath the bassinet and taken with him to his mother's room if he is to room-in with her.

An infant in the nursery who shows signs of infection should be isolated at once. The other infants must be closely observed for symptoms of the specific infection which he has contracted. Symptoms of the most common infections are refusal of feedings, frequent loose stools, elevation of temperature, seizure behavior, drainage from the umbilicus, and discharges from the eyes or nose. Respiratory infections are first evidenced by a running nose and a rise in temperature. Skin lesions are easily observed when the infant is undressed for morning care or when the diaper is changed.

Records and Birth Registration

The nurse caring for an infant in the nursery is responsible for all notations on his permanent record. When the infant rooms-in, the mother tells the nurse of the care she has given him and her observations on his condition and behavior. This the nurse charts.

In addition to the permanent records, some nurseries have *daily record sheets* which are not permanent records. These are composite tally sheets used for the total nursery population. The auxiliary personnel as well as the nurses record on these sheets the care they have given the infants and their observations, such as morning care, feedings, stool passages, and urination. The nurse copies from these temporary daily sheets the notations about each infant onto his individual chart. In some instances the information is summarized, e.g., the number of stools during the day and the total amount of feeding taken. Important notations commonly included in the nurse's notes on individual permanent records include the following:

The infant's name, day of life, birth weight, and daily weight

Observations on his condition: his cry, respirations, temperature, the condition of the cord, mouth, eyes, and skin, frequency and nature of stools, and urine

The time of feedings and the amount taken and retained; frequency and volume of regurgitation.

Medication and treatments given

Execution of all physician's orders, such as administration of oxygen, irrigations, and the like.

The physician, midwife, nurse, or attendant who delivers the infant is responsible for the birth registration with the local registrar. The information necessary for the birth certificate includes the child's name, date and place of birth, names of each of the parents, and other data of local option. This information should be accurate and easily read, since it is filed permanently with the state Bureau of Vital Statistics. Some form of notification of the registration is sent to the parents, who should keep it as proof that the infant's birth has been registered. Proof of birth registration may be important in later life to determine whether a child is of school age, whether a youth is of legal age for employment or voting, or whether a person is old enough for Social Security benefits, and so on.

FEEDING THE NEWBORN INFANT

The infant may be hungry immediately after birth or may show no signs of needing food for the first or even the second day. The nurse should be able to recognize the signs of hunger in the newborn. He becomes restless, cries, moves his head in search of food (the rooting reflex) and makes sucking movements which, bringing no relief, are likely to end in crying.

Usually he goes to sleep for several hours after being fed, wakening when he again needs food or is uncomfortable. The most common causes of crying in a healthy infant are hunger and discomfort from a soiled diaper.

In addition to caring for the infant, the nurse has the responsibility of supporting the mother in her decision as to how to feed her child. Discussion of methods of feeding the newborn should be held during the prenatal period, but the final decision may be made either before or after the birth of the infant. Although the nurse should be able to provide information which the mother may request, the mother should not be strongly encouraged to feed the infant by either the breast or bottle on a rigid schedule or on a self-demand schedule. Guilt feelings may be aroused in the mother if she does not or cannot cooperate. For instance, a mother, because the nurse encouraged her to breast-feed her infant on a self-demand routine, tried to do so in order to follow orders. The mother failed in her attempts and felt guilty about her inability to be a "good" mother. Perhaps another mother might have refused to cooperate with the nurse, leading that mother to feel guilty also. The nurse should realize that the bodily contact a mother has with her child in whatever feeding process used is ultimately of greater importance than the method of feeding.

Self-Demand Feeding

The infant on a self-demand or self-regulating schedule nurses when he wants food. Then he sleeps until the contractions of an empty stomach waken him. He cries, but when the formula is given him, the muscular contractions cease, and he experiences a pleasant sensation of fullness. If he is fed whenever he is hungry, he will develop a good appetite. Whether he is breast-fed or bottle-fed, he will establish his own rhythm of feeding.

If an infant is on a self-demand feeding schedule, it is particularly necessary for the nurse to recognize signs of hunger in order to satisfy his demand for food, rather than use the bottle to pacify him whenever he cries.

Breast Feeding

Probably the psychologic and emotional factors are more important than the physical factors in helping a mother decide to breast-feed her infant, since satisfactory artificial feedings can be easily obtained.

Some physicians believe that the infant should be put to the breast as soon after delivery as the condition of the mother and of her infant permits. They believe that this early suckling assists in the involution of the uterus, stimulates lactation and also provides emotional satisfaction for both mother and child. Other physicians believe that nursing should be postponed until four to 24 hours after birth. This would allow time for the infant's throat to be cleared of mucus and for the infant to sleep after the exertion of birth and of being handled by physicians and nurses in the necessary care after birth. This interval also permits the mother to rest before giving her infant the breast. Because the normal newborn usually has strong rooting and sucking reflexes, his first feeding at the breast should prove satisfying for both mother and child. After his initial weight loss he should gain from 6 to 8 ounces a week.

If he is underfed, he is likely to be constipated. He may have colic, may vomit, may be irritable, and may alternate crying with sucking his fingers. Vomiting and colic are also characteristic of the overfed infant. In general, however, the breast-fed infant shows a steady gain in weight and is less prone to intestinal upsets than the infant on an artificial feeding plan.

Advantages to the Mother. The mother as well as the infant benefits from breast feeding. The infant's sucking at the breast promotes involution of the uterus after parturition. Many mothers find great emotional satisfaction in feeding the infant at the breast, for it is the culmination of the symbiotic unity which existed during the infant's intrauterine life. The fact that breast feeding saves time, trouble, and money appeals to some women.

Objections and Contraindications to Breast Feeding. For some women the advantages of breast feeding may be outweighed by other factors. The mother may have conscious or unconscious attitudes toward breast feeding which interfere with her ability to produce milk. She may have negative attitudes resulting from her own upbringing. These may cause her to have an aversion to nursing and the maternal role. The professionally educated woman many times is very eager to nurse her infant and arranges her schedule so that this is possible. If the mother works outside the home and is not self-employed or has many social engagements, it may be impossible for her to be at home promptly at feeding time, provoking infant distress and discomfort from engorged breasts. In order to provide greater freedom for the mother and to give the father an opportunity to feed the infant, breast milk may be expressed, frozen and fed at appropriate occasions. To accustom the infant to a different kind of feeding, an artificial formula may be substituted periodically for breast milk.

The great contraindication to nursing is

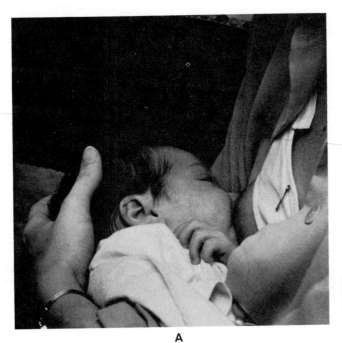

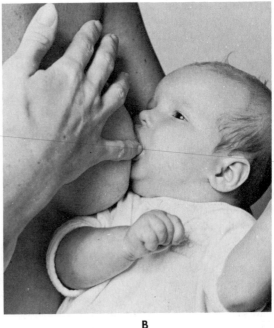

A

B

FIGURE 8–9. *A*, As to the emotional value of breastfeeding—without overstating the case—it makes it easier for the mother and for the baby to develop a close feeling. This is especially true of the baby whose first concepts of "security" are gained by touch, warmth and finally the satisfaction of food. (Courtesy Erika Stone and *Baby Talk*.) *B*, Breaking suction by placing the fourth finger at the corner of the infant's mouth before pulling him away. This prevents sore nipples. (Applebaum, R. M.: *Pediatr. Clin. N. Am.*, 17:203, 1970.) *C*, Picasso line drawing illustrating en face position and cuddling. (Courtesy of the Fogg Art Museum, Harvard University.)

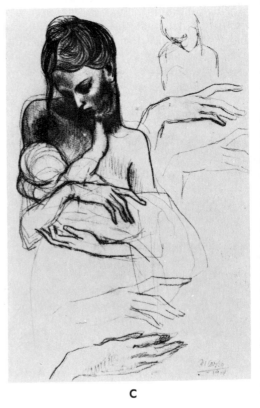

C

serious illness of the mother. If she has tuberculosis, her condition may be aggravated by lactation, and her infant would be in grave danger of contracting the disease through intimate contact. A mother may lack the vitality to nurse her infant, owing to some serious complication which developed during pregnancy. For instance, she may be anemic after excessive loss of blood.

She may have a chronic disease, e.g., cancer, heart disease, or impairment of the kidneys, which is not infectious, but which prevents her undergoing the strain of lactation. Her labor and delivery may have been complicated by an intercurrent illness or emergency operation which requires prolonged convalescence.

If her condition permits breast feeding in the

presence of intercurrent infection, her milk may be expressed, boiled and given to the infant. Thus the milk supply will be maintained until she is able to give the infant her breast.

The milk from a *mother addicted to drugs,* e.g., morphine, heroin, or codeine, will contain small amounts of the drug. The amount the infant receives may not be enough to hurt him, but it may prove habit-forming. Penicillin may be passed to an infant through breast milk and produce allergic sensitization. Various other drugs such as some anticoagulants, laxatives, antithyroid drugs, and alcohol, among others, may also pass through the breast milk to the infant.

Menstruation is not a contraindication to breast feeding unless the mother's nutrition is disturbed. *Pregnancy* is a contraindication to breast feeding only because of the strain upon the mother.

Mental illness is not in itself a contraindication to nursing, although grave danger is involved when a small infant is entrusted to a mentally disturbed patient. Since her milk is normal in amount and composition, it may be expressed and given to her child if the procedure does not disturb or aggravate the mother and if there is a probability that her condition will improve to the extent that the infant may safely be put to the breast at some future time.

Local lesions such as cracked nipples, tumors or breast abscess may contraindicate breast feeding. The milk may be manually expressed to relieve the mother's discomfort from engorgement and to maintain breast function so that she can nurse her infant if the local condition is cured. If the milk is not contaminated, it can be given to the infant.

Some mothers have so-called *inverted nipples;* i.e., the nipples do not stand out so that the infant can grasp them with his mouth. A breast shield will help the infant to attain suction and secure the milk, or the milk may be extracted with a breast pump and prepared as a bottle feeding. If a shield is used, a small amount of colostrum or milk may be expressed into it before it is applied, or it may be partially filled with sterile water.

The *infant's condition* may contraindicate breast feeding. He may be too weak to suck, or sucking may exhaust his strength. The premature infant not only may be too weak to suck but also may lack the necessary reflexes. The infant with a cleft palate or cleft lip or with facial nerve paralysis is unable to suck. For such infants the breast milk may be manually expressed and given by medicine dropper.

Erythroblastosis fetalis is not a contraindication to breast feeding, since Rh antibodies in the mother's milk are inactivated in the infant's intestinal tract.

Maternal Personality and Breast Feeding. The desire to breast-feed their infants is common among women who obtain satisfaction in fulfilling the feminine role. They do not feel that childbirth is an ordeal to be feared and consider that wives may lead domestic lives as rewarding as those of their working husbands. Wanting to breast-feed an infant appears to be closely related to motherly attitudes. Such women are likely to be successful with breast feeding. Voluntary breast feeding increases their feeling of competency in child care. They are less likely to worry about the child than the mother who has reluctantly consented to breast-feed her infant and lives in fear that her milk supply will not be sufficient to meet his nutritional needs.

Advantages to the Infant. There are many reasons why physicians hold breast feeding to be superior to even an adequate formula properly prepared and given with loving care. The most important arguments for breast feeding from the point of view of the infant's health are as follows:

Breast milk is more easily digested than cow's milk and is designed by nature to satisfy the needs of the human infant just as cow's milk meets the needs of the calf.

Breast milk is available at all times. This fact is important if the infant is to be on a self-demand schedule. Breast feeding can be used to comfort an infant, although this should not be done to excess.

Breast-fed infants have greater immunity to certain childhood diseases. Certain antibacterial and antiviral substances are believed to be transmitted in the milk which increase the infant's resistance to infectious diseases. The extent of this protection has not been proved.

Breast-fed infants are less likely to have gastrointestinal disorders and food allergies in infancy.

Breast-fed infants are less likely to suffer from colds and severe respiratory infections.

Breast-fed infants are less likely to acquire infections in homes where cleanliness is difficult to attain. This is because breast milk is sterile, and the mother's nipples are easily cleaned.

Breast-fed infants enjoy the watchfulness and close contact with their mothers' bodies and can take as much or as little milk as they desire. They can regulate the rapidity of the intake and can never be forced to take more than they want.

Breast-fed infants are less prone to anemia or vitamin deficiency.

Factors in the Supply of Breast Milk. The majority of women who have been delivered of a healthy full-term infant and are themselves in good health are capable of breast-feeding their infants.

Physical factors in the supply of breast milk include (a) an ample diet with an increased protein intake and a sufficient supply of calcium from milk and other sources.

(b) The mother requires an ample supply of vitamins, especially vitamin D, for her needs and also for the baby, since he receives vitamins through her milk.

(c) Her fluid intake should be adequate for her needs, and should supply 16 to 32 ounces of milk for the infant.

(d) The stimulus of the infant's sucking. If the infant does not fully empty the breasts, the remaining milk should be manually expressed (see p. 172).

(e) She needs normal exercise. Housework, if not too exhausting, is excellent, but she should also have exercise out of doors every day.

(f) The nursing mother should avoid fatigue. She should have from eight to ten hours of sleep at night and a nap during the day. It must be remembered that her rest is broken by the infant's night feeding.

(g) The amount of milk-producing tissue in the breasts affects the supply. Large breasts may contain a great deal of fat or supporting tissue and an inadequate amount of glandular secreting tissue.

(h) Chemical stimulation by the lactogenic hormones cannot be controlled by any known means, but since the hormones are related to pregnancy, they are in general sufficient in amount.

Psychologic factors in the supply of breast milk are extremely important. The mother needs to feel competent in her capacity to supply the feedings day and night in amounts sufficient to satisfy the infant. She needs to feel secure, happy and relaxed in her family life. Naturally she, like mothers who bottle feed their infants, will become tense or anxious at times, and the quantity of her milk may be decreased, but the quality remains unchanged. When the mother has regained her composure, her breasts will again be full. She should be told that the emotional strain of coming home from the hospital and undertaking the care of the infant may produce a state of tension which will diminish the flow of milk, but that the condition is only temporary.

Secretion and Composition of Breast Milk. The secretions of the mammary glands are under the influence of a lactogenic hormone derived from the pituitary gland and are stimulated through the influence of pregnancy.

The delivery of milk from the breasts is embodied in the milk-ejection or "let-down" reflex. The presence of the infant, his sucking or even his crying causes the release of oxytocin from the posterior portion of the pituitary, which in turn causes the contractile tissue around the alveoli to squeeze the milk into the larger ducts and then to the nipples. If the mother is tense, this reflex will be inhibited and milk present in the breast will not be brought to the nipples.

Colostrum is secreted during the first two to four days after delivery. It is yellow, and thin or watery in consistency. It has more protein and minerals and less fat and carbohydrate than breast milk. It is easily digested and has a mild laxative action.

Breast milk appears two to four days after delivery. By the end of the first four to five weeks, breast milk is constant in composition and remains so. The amount increases as the infant's need for food increases. By the end of the first week 6 to 10 ounces (180 to 300 cc.) a day is the normal amount of milk for a healthy mother to produce; by the end of the first month, 20 ounces (600 cc.), and later, 30 ounces (900 cc.) a day.

Breast milk is slightly bluish and has a relatively high sugar content. In the infant's stomach, breast milk forms a soft, flocculent curd. If the mother is taking an adequate diet, the vitamin content of her milk is sufficient, or nearly so, for the infant. Mothers should be told that if they take drugs, e.g., opiates, alcohol, belladonna, or penicillin, a small amount of the drug will be present in the milk.

Table 8–2 shows the relative composition of breast milk and cow's milk. Breast milk has more carbohydrate and easily digested protein, lactalbumin; it has less protein in the form of casein, which is difficult to digest, than cow's milk, and has approximately the same amount of fat and is of equal caloric value.

TECHNIQUE OF BREAST FEEDING

The mother should be told that the supply of breast milk will be available by the third to fifth day. During the latent period before an adequate supply of milk is available, the infant loses weight. This is a normal phenomenon and should not cause the mother anxiety. Glucose water may be given to supply the required amount of fluid.

The usual procedure is to put the infant to the breast immediately after birth or from four to twelve hours after delivery. Those physicians who advise waiting give as their reasons that the infant and his mother should be given time to rest after the birth process and that time should

TABLE 8–2. *COMPARISON OF HUMAN AND COW'S MILKS*

| | REPRESENTATIVE COMPOSITION OF MATURE MILKS | | | VARIATIONS IN COMPOSITION OF UNPOOLED MILK SAMPLES* | |
	HUMAN	COW'S	COW'S EVAP.	HUMAN	COW'S
Components (per cent):					
Water	87.6	87.3	73.0	87.0 - 89.0	83.0 - 88.0
Total solids	12.4	12.7	27.0	8.5 - 15.0	8.5 - 19.0
Proteins	1.2	3.3	7.3	0.7 - 2.0	2.8 - 3.6
Casein	0.4	2.8	6.2	0.14- 0.68	2.1 - 2.8
Whey	0.6	0.6	1.3	0.5 - 1.1	0.3 - 0.6
Lactalbumin	0.3	0.4	0.88	0.14- 0.6	0.27- 0.57
Lactoglobulin	0.2	0.2	0.44		0.14- 0.42
Lactose	7.0	4.8	10.6	5.0 - 9.2	4.0 - 5.5
Fat	3.8	3.7	8.2	1.3 - 8.3	3.1 - 5.2
Minerals (ash)	0.21	0.72	1.6	0.16- 0.27	0.64- 0.75
Minerals (per liter):					
Sodium (mEq)	7.0	25.0	55.0	2.0 - 13.0	13.5 - 93.0
Potassium (mEq)	14.0	35.0	77.0	9.5 - 17.5	9.7 - 74.0
Chloride (mEq)	12.0	29.0	46.0	2.6 - 21.0	27.0 - 40.0
Calcium (mg)	330.0	1250.0	2750.0	170.0 - 610.0	560.0 -3810.0
Phosphorus (mg)	150.0	960.0	2112.0	70.0 - 270.0	560.0 -1120.0
Magnesium (mg)	40.0	120.0	264.0	20.0 - 60.0	70.0 - 220.0
Sulfur (mg)	140.0	300.0	660.0	50.0 - 300.0	240.0 - 360.0
Iron (mg)	1.5	1.0	2.2	0.2 - 1.8	0.2 - 1.4
Zinc (mg)	1.2	3.8	8.4	0.17- 3.02	1.9 - 6.6
Copper (mg)	0.4	0.3	0.66	0.1 - 0.7	0.2 - 0.8
Iodine (mg)	0.07	0.21	0.46	0.05- 0.09	0.13- 1.8
Amino Acids (mg/liter):					
Histidine	230.0	800.0	1760.0	160.0 - 340.0	700.0 -1300.0
Isoleucine	860.0	2120.0	4664.0	460.0 -1020.0	1800.0 -2900.0
Leucine	1610.0	3560.0	7832.0	720.0 -1590.0	2400.0 -3900.0
Lysine	790.0	2570.0	5654.0	530.0 -1040.0	2200.0 -3100.0
Methionine	230.0	870.0	1914.0	90.0 - 210.0	600.0 - 900.0
Phenylalanine	640.0	1730.0	3860.0	300.0 - 580.0	1400.0 -2200.0
Threonine	620.0	1520.0	3344.0	400.0 - 760.0	1200.0 -2200.0
Tryptophan	220.0	500.0	1100.0	130.0 - 260.0	400.0 - 800.0
Valine	900.0	2280.0	4956.0	480.0 -1140.0	2100.0 -2800.0
Calories† (approximate):					
Per fluid ounce	20.0	20.0	44.0‡	18.0 - 24.0	17.0 - 25.0
Per liter	710.0	690.0	1520.0	600.0 - 790.0	570.0 - 850.0

*Values are taken from several studies; agreement is approximate, but not all components were evaluated in each.

† Calorie = large calorie = kcal = Cal. (See text.)

‡ In practice, commonly regarded as 40 calories (40 kcal).

The data are assembled from a number of sources.

From Vaughan, V. C., III, and McKay, R. J.: *Nelson Textbook of Pediatrics,* 10th ed., Philadelphia, W. B. Saunders Company, 1975.

be allowed for mucus to be cleared from the infant's throat before he attempts to suck and swallow milk. The time spent in nursing at the breast and the number of feedings are increased after the first day or two.

Healthy, supple nipples are important in making the feeding time comfortable for the mother. Erect nipples favor ease of sucking. If the nipples are flat, an ointment should be applied with a gentle, rolling motion of the fingers from the outer rim of the nipple to the tip. If the nipples are cracked and painful, they may be lubricated with petrolatum jelly, or a protective nipple shield may be used to minimize the trauma of nursing.

The breasts should be cleansed carefully once a day when the mother takes a shower. No other care of the nipples before or after feeding the infant is usually necessary.

The mother's clothing should not be too tight over the breasts. If a little milk tends to exude from the nipples, she should be careful to keep the area and her clothing clean and dry by using protective pads.

The mother should wash her hands thoroughly with soap and water before the infant is put to the breast. She should be in a comfortable position, sitting or lying on her side. Her head should be slightly elevated. In presenting the nipple to the infant and while he is sucking she should support the breast tissue away from his nostrils so that he may breathe easily.

The room should be quiet while the infant nurses, and the mother should not be disturbed in any way. A normal newborn has a "rooting" reflex, so that when anything touches his cheek when he is hungry he turns his cheek in that direction. It is important, therefore, that the nurse not touch the infant's opposite cheek to try to turn his head toward the breast. If the nipple touches the infant's cheek, he will turn in that direction to suck.

Although the infant obtains 85 to 90 per cent of his feeding in the first five to eight minutes of vigorous sucking, he should be allowed to nurse from ten to twenty minutes. He enjoys this, and the added milk he gets is to his advantage. Since sucking stimulates the secretion of milk, he should nurse from both breasts at each feeding. It is important that the infant grasp the whole nipple within his mouth; otherwise he cannot achieve adequate suction and may gulp air, since the tip of the nipple is so small that he does not close his lips closely around it.

Early in breast feeding if the milk is not sufficient to meet the infant's needs, the mother should be encouraged to nurse more often, obtain more rest, and perhaps increase her fluid intake. It is customary to weigh the infant before and after his feedings if there is doubt about the quantity of breast milk. This, however, is likely to make the mother tense and fearful that she cannot supply his needs. Her anxiety reacts on the physical process of lactation and tends to decrease the supply. Many physicians do not favor complementary feedings of modified cow's milk because if the infant is completely satisfied, he may not be hungry enough to empty the mother's breasts at the next feeding. After breast feeding is fully established, a relief bottle of artificial feeding may be offered in order to make weaning to the bottle easier after breast feeding is completed.

It is not as necessary to bubble the breast-fed infant as it is the bottle-fed one. The infant should be held over the shoulder or seated erect in his mother's lap and gently patted or stroked on the back (see Fig. 8–11). Thereby the air he has swallowed will rise to the top of his stomach and be eructated. It may be advisable with some infants to do this several times during a feeding and with all infants after the feeding, before laying them in the crib. If the infant's stomach is too full, he may spit up a little milk with each eructation or even after he has been put back in the crib. He may also hiccup. In that case he should be given a little warm water and comforted until the hiccups cease.

Sterile water may be offered between feedings, but it is not necessary for the infant to take it. He should not be urged, for water may interfere with his capacity to finish his next feeding. Giving water is an excellent way to accustom the infant to the artificial nipple so that he will nurse from the bottle in case breast feedings for some reason must be suddenly discontinued. It likewise prepares him to take orange juice in water when the physician orders it.

Infants like to cling to the breast after they have ceased to suck. To remove the infant if he does not voluntarily release the nipple, gentle pressure may be made on his cheeks, or the mother may insert her finger into his mouth. These methods allow air to enter his mouth; suction is then lessened, and he cannot maintain his hold on the nipple. This method is not painful to the mother, nor does it irritate the soft skin covering the nipple.

Rigid feeding schedules are not advisable for the infant. If he is allowed to set up his own pace, he will eventually work out a fairly regular demand schedule of increasing duration per feeding and the process can be accomplished with little frustration on his or his mother's part.

If the mother has difficulty breast feeding her infant, it is wise for her to contact a member of the La Leche League International, Inc. This organization, largely composed of mothers who have nursed their own infants, has local chapters throughout the world.

Manual Expression of Milk. The technique of emptying the breasts when the infant has not done so is as follows:

Grasp the breast with the thumb above and the index finger below the outer edge of the areola. Press the thumb toward the fingers at the base of the nipple with firm, deep pressure. Support the breast with the other fingers. Use a forward stripping movement. Repeat this about 30 times a minute until the breasts are empty; the process usually takes from ten to 15 minutes. If the milk is to be used for the infant (e.g., if the mother will be away at the next feeding period), it can be kept in a sterile container under refrigeration.

Although the use of a hand breast pump or an electric pump may sometimes be advised, these methods of expressing breast milk may be very traumatic to the breast tissue.

Wet Nursing and Breast Milk Stations. Wet nurses are rarely used today to provide breast milk for infants other than their own. If they are used, they should have serologic tests and roentgenograms to assure the absence of syphilis and tuberculosis.

Breast milk stations have largely replaced the use of wet nurses in our society. These stations are found in a few of the large cities, but the milk is expensive, and constant supervision of the contributing mothers is necessary to prevent the milk's dilution with cow's milk or water. It is best to have the mothers come to the station and express the milk with the electric breast pump.

Breast milk may be pasteurized and kept in sterile containers under refrigeration. It can be frozen and shipped to distant points where it may be thawed and prepared for use as directed by the physician.

Artificial Feeding

Artificial feeding is based on scientific principles of nutrition and sterilization. When breast feeding is not possible and adequate artificial feedings cannot be provided, the morbidity and mortality rates of infants tend to rise.

The following conditions may adversely affect the success of artificial feeding: contaminated cow's milk; a formula not suited to the infant's needs, in either composition or quantity; lack of

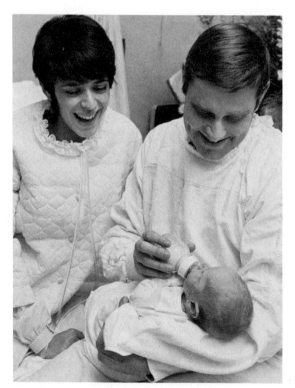

FIGURE 8–10. Bottle feeding. A close bond between father and son is beginning to be established. (From *Medical World News*, April 10, 1970.)

cleanliness in preparation of the formula and improper refrigeration of the 24-hour supply of feedings; haphazard and irregular feeding; and feeding entrusted to strangers, with implications of lack of interest and affection.

The importance of this last cause is seldom realized and is difficult to analyze. An infant becomes accustomed to one person's way and responds with restlessness on being fed in an unaccustomed way. Some persons believe that the mother responds more quickly to the infant's needs in regulating the flow of milk by tipping the bottle, bubbling him when he needs to expel air, and in general makes the procedure a more personal service adapted to her infant's needs.

REQUIREMENTS FOR ARTIFICIAL FEEDING

Low Bacterial Count of Milk. The fundamental requirement of a satisfactory artificial feeding mixture is that the milk, when taken from the cow, have a low bacterial count. Tuberculosis and undulant fever (brucellosis) can be acquired through milk from infected cows. Dairy herds are screened with the tuberculin test for tuberculosis and the Bang test for brucellosis.

The second requirement is that all milk handlers be free from diseases transmitted through milk, e.g., scarlet fever, streptococcal sore throat, typhoid fever, diphtheria, and tuberculosis.

A third requisite is cleanliness in the care of the cows and in the milking process. Most cities require strict inspection of the handling of commercial milk from the dairy to the retail store. The bacterial count and the fat content must conform to certain standards. The milk must be free from preservatives or any injurious substance. It must be pasteurized. Even this clean, pasteurized milk should be pasteurized again or boiled for use in an infant's formula.

Economy and Availability of Milk. For families of the low-income group it is necessary that an artificial feeding be inexpensive. This is one reason for the extensive use of sterile evaporated milk. It can be bought in small quantities, and if refrigeration is not available, a small tin can be opened for each feeding. What is not used for the infant can be used by the older children or by adults in their beverage.

Ease of Digestion of Milk. The average infant between four and six months of age can tolerate undiluted cow's milk. For infants under this age the milk is diluted with boiled water. Cow's milk in the infant's stomach forms large, tough curds which can be rendered more digestible by pasteurization, boiling, homogenization, evaporation, or the addition of an acid or alkali.

In these processes the curd tension is favorably altered.

Nutritional Requirements of Formula for Metabolism and Growth. An *adequate fluid intake* should be 2 to 3 ounces per pound of the expected body weight of the infant, allowance being made for loss of water in urine and stools, by evaporation from the skin and in expired air. The general rule is that a child of one year should take 1000 cc. a day, and an additional 100 cc. should be added for each year of life; e.g., a child of two years should take 1100 ml. of fluid per day.

The *protein requirement* for growth and for repair of tissue is 1.5 to 2 gm. per pound of body weight. One ounce of cow's milk provides 1 gm. of protein.

The *carbohydrate requirement* in the typical formula for the infant under five months is supplied in the form of Karo or cane sugar. One to 1½ ounces (30 to 45 gm.) is added to the formula. The addition of sugar brings the carbohydrate content of the formula to approximately that of breast milk. For other forms of carbohydrate suitable for use in infant formulas see page 176.

The *caloric requirement* for the infant under three months is approximately 50 calories per pound, and over four months approximately 45 calories per pound. In contrast, the average adult requirement is 20 calories per pound of body weight.

The *basal metabolic needs* are low during the neonatal period. Basal heat production rises rapidly, however, during the first year of life. The caloric requirements for basal metabolic needs are proportionately higher in infancy than at any other time of life. During the neonatal period about 80 calories per kg. of body weight per day are needed to satisfy the infant's nutritional requirements. This amount must be increased rapidly because, although basal metabolic needs do not change, the caloric requirements for growth and energy are much greater in the older infant. Soon a caloric intake of 100 to 130 calories per kg. (45 to 60 calories per pound) of body weight is needed; this requirement remains constant until the age of four months. Caloric needs vary with the infant's activity, his general well-being and his weight gain.

The *fat content* of the formula is not of great importance in the modification of cow's milk and is seldom mentioned in the calculation. Many of the proprietary milks, however, substitute varying proportions of olive, coconut, palm, or peanut oil for the butter fat.

Vitamins are usually lacking or in insufficient amount in the artificial feeding. Vitamin A, a fat-soluble vitamin, is needed for growth and for resistance to disease or infection. It, in conjunction with vitamin D, which prevents rickets (see p. 368), is derived from cod liver oil or some form of concentrate. The infant needs approximately 400 International Units of vitamin D each day. Vitamin B complex is needed for optimum health. Vitamin C prevents scurvy (see p. 368). The infant needs 25 to 50 mg. a day. Since vitamin C is easily destroyed in pasteurization of the milk, it must be provided from some other source. Breast-fed infants usually receive a sufficient amount in the mother's milk, though this depends upon her diet. Vitamin C may be supplied by giving the infant 2 ounces of orange juice daily, or ascorbic acid, 25 to 50 mg. a day. One problem that may result from the giving of orange juice is allergy.

Iron is essential in the infant's diet in order to prevent iron-deficiency anemia, which is currently a wide-spread problem. Proprietary formulas should be iron-fortified, and the infant, as he grows, should be given other foods to ensure an adequate iron intake.

In summary, the infant up to six months of age needs approximately 130 to 190 cc. of fluid per kg. (2 to 3 ounces per pound) of body weight per day. The total caloric, protein and fluid needs for the 24 hours of the day determine the composition of the formula. The number of feedings decreases as the infant grows older. At one month he will probably be taking five or six feedings. The amount given at each feeding increases as the intervals between feedings lengthen and the infant requires a greater total fluid intake.

Calculation of Formula. The following example may clarify the general statements made about an infant's daily nutritional need and fluid intake.

An infant one month of age weighing 8 pounds requires the following:

Fluid: 2 to 3 ounces per pound of body weight. Total fluid per day: 16 to 24 ounces

Whole cow's milk: 1½ to 2 ounces per pound of body weight. Total amount of milk: 12 to 16 ounces, *or*

Evaporated milk: 1 ounce per pound of body weight. Total amount of milk: 8 ounces

Water: A total of 24 ounces of fluid is required for the formula. Sufficient water is added to the milk to bring the amount of the mixture up to the required 24 ounces: e.g., 16 ounces with evaporated milk, 8 to 12 ounces with whole fresh cow's milk

Calories: 50 calories per pound of body weight. Total caloric requirement: 400 calories per day

Sugar: 1/10 ounce per pound per day

Volume per feeding: The infant's age in months plus 2 or 3; in this instance, 3 to 4 ounces of formula per feeding

Number of feedings: Total volume of feedings per day (24 ounces) given in 4-ounce feedings results in six feedings per day; given in 3-ounce feedings results in eight feedings per day. During the first six months up to 7 ounces may be given at a feeding. More than 8 ounces is rarely given at a feeding.

Schedule: Six feedings (every four hours) of 4 ounces each, or eight feedings (every three hours) of 3 ounces each.

An infant, regardless of his age, is seldom given more than 1 quart of whole milk or one can (13 fluid ounces) of evaporated milk during a 24-hour period because he receives solid food as he needs more nourishment.

TYPES OF MILK AND INGREDIENTS FOR ARTIFICIAL FEEDING

The caloric value of whole cow's milk is 20 calories per ounce.

Certified Milk. This is the purest form of raw milk. It contains less than 10,000 bacteria per cubic centimeter and no pathogens, even before pasteurization. It is produced under special hygienic conditions. All milk containers must be sterilized before use. The personnel who handle the milk must be inspected for evidence of disease which might be transmitted through milk. (Throat cultures are taken, and other tests are made.) Most certified milk sold today is also pasteurized.

Pasteurized Milk. In pasteurization raw milk is heated to 145° F. for 30 minutes. It is then cooled rapidly. In most cities pasteurization of commercial milk is required by law. Pasteurization kills pathogenic organisms, but does not sterilize the milk; it renders harmless *Salmonella typhosa,* tuberculosis bacilli, organisms causing diphtheria and those in the paratyphoid group, and hemolytic streptococci. Pasteurization destroys vitamin C, which is a heat-labile vitamin, and makes the curd in the infant's stomach smaller and softer. Pasteurized milk should be boiled for infant feeding purposes.

Vitamin D–Reinforced Milk. This is whole cow's milk to which has been added vitamin D, which prevents rickets. Milk from cows at pasture contains more vitamin D than that of cows which do not graze on fresh grass. The vitamin D content of milk may be increased by feeding the vitamin to the cow. In practice it is more satisfactory to add the vitamin directly to the milk. This is done in most large commercial dairies and in the production of evaporated milk. The procedure ensures the desired content of vitamin D in all the milk offered for sale.

Homogenized Milk. In homogenized milk the fat globules are broken down and distributed in a state of colloidal suspension throughout the milk. The curd is rendered softer and thus more digestible, and the flavor of the milk is improved. Digestion is thereby aided, since a larger surface area is offered by the smaller fat moieties for interaction with intestinal enzymes (lipase).

Evaporated Milk. This is a whole milk from which 60 per cent of the water has been removed. The caloric value is 44 calories (usually considered 40 calories) per ounce. There are 2 gm. of protein per ounce. It is sterile, relatively inexpensive, and available in all grocery shops, and can be stored in the home without refrigeration if the can is unopened. Evaporated milk is usually both irradiated and homogenized. It has a fine curd because of homogenization and because the casein has been altered in the evaporation process. To use as whole milk it is only necessary to dilute it with an equal quantity of water.

Condensed Milk. This is evaporated whole milk which contains 45 per cent sugar. The caloric value is approximately 100 calories per ounce. It should not be used for infant feedings since the sugar content is far too high. An infant fed on condensed milk is likely to be pale and fat, have flabby muscles and be subject to diarrhea due to fermentation of the excessive carbohydrate content of his feeding.

Dried Milk. In dried milk the water from skimmed milk has been completely evaporated. Dried milk contains various amounts of fat. It is valuable in the formulas of infants who cannot tolerate the amount of fat present in whole milk. Dried milk produces a fine curd, and any dilution desired can be easily made from the dry powder. It is packed in airtight cans and will keep for months without spoiling; for this reason it is useful in traveling with a baby and under conditions when fresh or evaporated milk is not available. In the drying process vitamin C is destroyed. One ounce by weight or 3½ packed level tablespoonfuls of dried milk mixed with 7 ounces of water gives a mixture having the composition of liquid milk. For infant feeding the powdered milk is mixed with enough cool water to make a paste; to this the desired amount of water is added gradually while the mixture is stirred to prevent the formation of lumps.

Carbohydrates. Carbohydrates are added to the formula to increase its caloric value and improve the flavor, and for their laxative effect. They contain, on the average, 120 calories per ounce. In order to dissolve the carbohydrate it is mixed with a warm fluid.

All types of carbohydrates must be broken down into monosaccharides in the intestinal tract before they can be utilized by the body. The carbohydrates commonly used in infant feedings include the following:

a. Dextrose or glucose. This is easily digested.
b. Sucrose or cane sugar, the most available and convenient form for use in the infant's formula, but with the disadvantage of being too sweet.
c. Lactose or milk sugar. Milk sugar is not sweet to the taste, is similar to the carbohydrate in breast milk and has a laxative value.
d. Dextri-Maltose, a relatively expensive form, but easily digested. This proprietary product consists of a mixture of maltose and dextrins. These are simplified by digestive processes prior to absorption.
e. Karo (corn) syrup, a cheap and easily digested carbohydrate. It should be kept in the refrigerator and carefully covered, since it is a good liquid culture medium for bacteria.
f. Starch, a polysaccharide. It is difficult for the infant to digest unless it is thoroughly cooked (cooking breaks down the starch molecules).

Prepared Infant Milk Products. These are made by commercial firms and have evaporated milk or dried milk as the base. The composition of the majority of prepared milks simulates breast milk; i.e., the protein content and mineral salts have been reduced; the fat has been modified by the substitution of vegetable fat for butterfat; and carbohydrate in the form of lactose or dextrin-maltose has been added. All these preparations contain added vitamin D, and many contain additional vitamins and iron. Other commercially prepared milks are available for infants requiring a modified diet such as one low in sodium or phenylalanine and for those allergic to a usual constituent of milk.

These preparations are relatively expensive, but have the advantages of convenience, sterility and compactness. The law requires the ingredients to be listed on the container. Usually only boiled water is added to the powdered preparation in order to prepare the formula. Some proprietary formulas are prepared in liquid form in disposable bottles and are ready for immediate use when opened.

PREPARATION OF THE FORMULA

The basic principles in the preparation of the infant's formula relate to cleanliness and accuracy. The formula must be clean and preferably sterile, since it can be a source of infection to the infant. In the milk laboratory of the hospital, personnel should wear gowns and caps, and many hospitals require that they also wear masks. In the home the formula is usually prepared in the kitchen. The mother should wear clean clothing and wash her hands thoroughly.

Equipment. All equipment and ingredients should be ready before preparation of the formula is begun. The ingredients are milk, sterile water and some form of carbohydrate.

BOTTLES. Enough 8-ounce feeding bottles should be provided for the entire 24 hours' feedings, and at least one extra bottle to replace any that might be broken. Wide-mouthed bottles are commonly used, since they are more easily and thoroughly cleaned with a brush and the nipple more nearly approaches the form of the mother's nipple. In the hospital each bottle is labeled clearly and accurately with either the infant's name or the type of formula the bottle contains. The formula in the individual feeding bottles should be kept in the refrigerator until feeding time.

NIPPLES. The newborn requires a firm nipple. A nipple which has become flabby from use and repeated sterilization makes sucking difficult. The aperture in the nipple should be a cross cut, i.e., two 4-mm. incisions in the shape of a cross. Some nipples on the market have this cross cut, but others have the traditional three small holes dispersed in the shape of a triangle. The holes may be enlarged to suit the needs of the infant. Factors determining the size of the holes are the infant's ability to suck (the immature and feeble infant may become exhausted if he has to pull vigorously in order to obtain the milk through tiny holes) and the consistency of the formula.

To enlarge the holes in the nipple, the blunt end of a darning needle is inserted into a cork. The point of the needle is held in a flame until red hot and is then used to puncture the nipple. Since the point is red hot, the rubber melts to form a round aperture. It is better to make three small holes in the shape of a triangle than to make a single hole. The nipple is then placed in cold water to harden the rubber. The flow should be tested before the nipple is used. When the bottle is tipped upside down, milk should drip slowly from the nipple at the rate of one drop per second.

BOTTLE CAPS. Since the nipple must be sterile when it enters the infant's mouth, airtight sterile bottle caps are used. These may be of glass or plastic and are cone-shaped, covering the nipple. They are used if the nipples are put on the bottles when the formula is made. If the sterile nipple is to be put on the bottle just before being given to the infant, a close-fitting cap may be used to cover the bottle top.

PREPARATION OF FORMULA. There are two general methods used in the preparation of formulas: the aseptic or standard method and the terminal heating method.

Aseptic or Standard Method. The equipment needed to prepare a formula by this method includes the following:

Teakettle or pan
Bottles, nipples, bottle caps
Measuring cup
Pitcher
Measuring tablespoon
Large pan for boiling equipment (covered)
Long-handled spoon
Table knife
Can opener
Funnel
Small pan for boiling nipples and bottle caps (covered)
Tongs
Bottle brush
Small jar with tight lid for storing nipples

The procedure for the preparation of the formula is as follows:

1. Wash all equipment in hot, soapy water, and rinse in hot, clear water. Wash the bottles, funnel, nipples, and bottle caps with the bottle brush. Squeeze water through the nipple holes to make certain they are open.

2. Place *all* equipment except rubber articles in a covered container and boil for ten minutes.

3. Place nipples and rubber caps, only rarely used, in a covered pan and boil for three minutes.

4. Place nipples in the small, sterile covered jar.

5. Boil water in the teakettle or pan for five minutes. Measure the required amount in the sterile measuring cup and pour into the sterile pitcher.

6. Measure the required amount of sugar or syrup in the measuring tablespoon. Level the contents with a table knife. Add the carbohydrate to the water in the pitcher and stir until dissolved.

7. If canned milk is used, scrub the top of the can with soap and rinse with hot water.

8. Measure the required amount of milk in the measuring cup and pour into the sugar-water mixture. Stir thoroughly with the long-handled spoon.

9. Pour the formula into the sterile bottles through the funnel. Cover the bottles with bottle caps.

10. Place the bottles in a pan of cool water in order to cool them quickly. The water should be as deep as the level of the milk in the bottles. Place the bottles in the refrigerator.

11. When it is time to feed the infant, remove one bottle from the refrigerator. Remove the cap. Remove one nipple from the jar and place it on the bottle. Replace the cover on the jar.

12. Place the bottle in a pan of warm water to take the chill off the formula, and feed it to the infant.

Terminal Heating Method. Terminal heating is now used in many hospitals and homes for all formulas which can tolerate the degree of heat necessary for this form of sterilization. This process produces a bacteriologically safe formula.

The formula is prepared with clean but not sterile technique and poured into thoroughly clean bottles. Nipples are put on the bottles, and caps are placed loosely over the nipples.

In the hospital the bottles are placed in racks and autoclaved for ten minutes at a temperature of 246°F. (119°C.) and 15 pounds' pressure.

For the home a sterilizer may be bought and the hospital technique adapted to its use. The formula should be sterilized for 25 minutes at 212°F. (100°C.). The lid of the sterilizer should not be removed until it is cool enough to handle with the bare hand. This is a rough gauge of the time required for the nipples to cool slowly. Under rapid cooling the holes in the nipples tend to become clogged by a thin coagulum which tends to form at the surface. Remove the bottles, tighten the caps, and place them in the refrigerator at a temperature of 40 to 45°F. (4.4 to 7.2°C.) until they are to be used.

In many hospitals a commercial formula service is being used instead of having the feedings prepared in a formula laboratory. Mothers can also purchase commercially prepared formulas for use in the home. These may come ready for use, or they may require dilution with sterile water and the use of sterile bottles and nipples. Some formulas may also be purchased in disposable containers with nipples attached. In the home such feedings save mothers time and effort in formula preparation, but they tend to be expensive.

TECHNIQUE OF BOTTLE FEEDING

The nurse or parent should first wash the hands thoroughly with soap and water. The bottle may be placed in a pan of water at a temperature of 120°F. (48.8°C.) for ten minutes or in an electric thermostat-controlled warmer. To test the temperature and the rate of flow of the milk, the nurse lets a few drops fall on the inner side of the wrist. Warming the feeding to body temperature is not really necessary, however, since infants who have been fed cool milk thrive well.

The nurse checks the name of the infant and that on the bottle before giving the infant his feeding. A mistake in the formula may be as dangerous as a mistake in the giving of medication. The nurse takes a bib and a diaper to the infant's crib and places the bottle on the bedside stand. The diaper is changed and the soiled one placed in a pedal-controlled can or on a piece of newspaper or paper towel at the foot of the crib.

After washing the hands again, the nurse picks up the infant, wrapped in a blanket if the room is chilly, and sits down in a chair, or preferably a rocking chair, holding the infant with his head supported in the bend of the arm. If for any reason the infant cannot be held in the lap, the nurse should sit beside the crib, elevate his head and hold his bottle. The mother may hold the infant in her arms to feed him while she rests in bed during the postpartum period.

A bottle should never be propped on a pad.

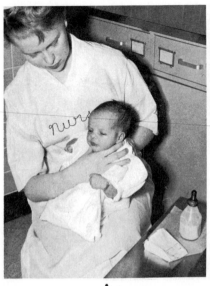
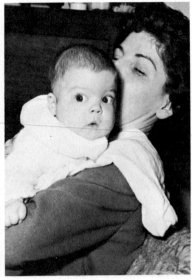

FIGURE 8–11. Bubbling the baby. A, The newborn can be bubbled most satisfactorily in the sitting position while gently leaning over the nurse's arm. This procedure is less likely to contaminate the newborn than if he is held over the shoulder. (Davis and Rubin: *DeLee's Obstetrics for Nurses.* 17th ed.) B, The infant can also be bubbled by holding him firmly against the shoulder, supporting his back and head. His back may be patted or rubbed gently in order to help him relax.

A **B**

Propping a bottle may be the severest form of unintentional maternal neglect. An infant is apt to lose his hold on the nipple and be unable to get it in his mouth again; there is also danger that the flow of milk will be too rapid and that the infant might choke. The bottle should be slanted so that the nipple is always filled with fluid; otherwise the infant will suck in air. He may need to be bubbled frequently, and always at the close of the feeding, usually in ten to 20 minutes. Indications that the infant may need to be bubbled because of his feeling of fullness include his stopping sucking, falling asleep, and having noisy respirations, especially on expiration. After this he should be placed on his right side or prone in his crib. In either of these positions the formula can most easily drain through the pylorus into the intestinal tract.

Any milk left in the bottle should be discarded. The bottle and the nipple are rinsed in cold water. If the infant is in isolation, all equipment should be boiled before being returned to the milk laboratory. The nurse should return to the infant after a few minutes to see whether he has regurgitated or vomited part of his feeding.

The feeding should be charted: the time when given, the amount taken and whether any was regurgitated or vomited. Words which may aid the nurse in charting are eructate, bubble, ruminate, regurgitate, and vomit. *Eructate* means to belch. *Bubble* has almost the same meaning, but implies that air is expelled while the nurse is holding the infant upright or is patting or rubbing him on the back. *Rumination* means voluntary or habitual regurgitation of formula into the mouth after it has been swallowed. Such milk may be swallowed again or spit out. An infant who spits out milk may lose a considerable amount of feeding. *Regurgitate* means to express—"spill over" as it were—a small amount of formula. *Vomiting* means bringing up an appreciable amount of the feeding. If the infant is sick, vomiting may be projectile.

DISCHARGE FROM THE NURSERY

Many pediatricians now recommend that prior to discharge from the nursery all newborn infants be tested for phenylketonuria, galactosemia, fructosemia and cystic fibrosis. The blood test for phenylketonuria should not be performed until the infant has been on milk feedings for 24 hours. Any infants who have questionable phenylalanine levels should be retested in four to six weeks. As to disorders involving galactose and fructose, the infants should be given feedings with these substances before urine tests are carried out. A strip or stick method of screening meconium for the presence of cystic fibrosis is used for the purpose of diagnosing the disease early. Infants born into families in which these or other inherited metabolic diseases are known should be carefully evaluated.

CARE AT HOME

Emotional Aspects of Care

After the newborn has been discharged from the hospital his care is primarily the responsibility of the mother. The mother must be lenient with herself at this time, realizing that if she becomes overburdened by her household duties, her care of the infant will not be beneficial for him. At such times she will need some kindly support or temporary relief from the responsibilities of managing her home, by either the father or another member of the family.

An infant in the low-income group is likely to receive as much loving care as one in the high-income group, but he may be cared for by many family members or neighbors, a number of whom may be children who will be awkward in their handling of him. This is in contrast to the more concentrated love and attention which the infant in the middle or upper class receives from a few relatives and friends who are "allowed" to hold him. This difference has an important effect on the emotional development of the child.

The overall responsibility of the mother for her child is well accepted in our society by all social groups. Not as frequently mentioned, however, is the task of the infant to respond to the mother, at first by smiling, and to communicate his needs to her, whether hunger, thirst, or need for contact. Thus the neonate's relation with his mother is truly an interaction. The newborn responds to the mother's stimulation with activities which orient him to his mother. His activities furnish her with cues that then influence her behavior toward him. If the mother sensitively responds to the infant's cues, satisfactory socialization begins. If she does not, a disturbed relation may be begun.

As mentioned previously, it is important that the father and the older siblings, if any, be involved in the infant's care. In this way the care of the new member does indeed become a family-centered cooperative venture.

The parents may decide to continue in the discussion group to which they belonged during the prenatal period or to find another type of parent education group. Members of such groups besides sharing information also help to reduce parental anxieties and fears concerning the care of the new family member.

Physical Aspects of Care

Aspects of the infant's care which the mother may possibly want to discuss with the nurse include shelter, room furnishing, bathing, clothing, elimination, sleeping, weighing, taking the temperature, and feeding, as well as follow-up care.

SHELTER

The nurse does not usually know to what kind of home a newborn infant will be taken on discharge from the hospital. The physical environment of the home of those in the low-income group is likely to be unhygienic, owing to poor neighborhood sanitation, to overcrowding and to parental attitudes toward health. In experiences in community or public health nursing the student will see many homes in poor neighborhoods and will be aware of the adaptations in child care which must be made under such conditions.

Here we can consider only an ideal home in a good neighborhood. It is important that the sewer and water systems be adequate and the house well built, with equipment for comfort and safety. The infant should have a room of his own. The floor covering and walls should be easy to keep clean; light colors are preferable. Heating and ventilation should be adequate. For the young infant it is wise to regulate the temperature during the day at 70 to 75° F. (21.1 to 23.8° C.) and at night 60 to 65° F. (15.5 to 18.3° C.); for the older child the temperature should be 68 to 70° F. (20.0 to 21.1° C.) during the day and 50° F. (10.0° C.) at night. There should be no drafts; ventilation can be secured by any of the devices for maintaining fresh air or indirectly from another room. The humidity should be 55 per cent. In winter any device providing evaporation of water will raise the humidity, such as a humidifier, a receptacle full of water placed on the radiator, or one of the patented devices which fit the radiator or can be attached to central heating. If moisture forms on the inside of a window on a cold day, the humidity in the room is adequate.

ROOM FURNISHINGS

The furnishings should be simple, durable, and easily cleaned. Paint in old homes or on old cribs may be a source of lead poisoning if the infant bites the painted surface or puts broken bits of paint-covered plaster from the wall in his mouth.

The infant should have a bed of his own. It is a needless expense to buy a bassinet, which is soon outgrown. A better plan is to buy a crib suitable for a child of four or five years. Many accidents have occurred because an infant has either fallen from the crib or become trapped between the side slats or the mattress and the frame. The mattress should fit snugly in the crib frame. The bars of the crib should be close together, no more than 2⅜ inches apart, and the side gates high enough to prevent his climbing over. When lowered, the drop rail must be at least nine inches above the mattress support. The latch should be out of his reach and accident-proof.

The mattress should be firm, but not hard, with a cover of waterproof material large enough to tuck in at the sides and ends or cover both sides of the mattress. A quilted pad large enough to cover the entire mattress is needed, as well as sheets long and wide enough to tuck 12 inches under the mattress at the sides, foot and top. The blankets should be of cotton or wool or a mixture of both. A sleeping bag is good if the infant tends to kick off the covers and the room cannot be kept sufficiently warm. He should not have a pillow until he is old enough to be propped up against it in a corner of his crib. A little infant may turn on his abdomen with the danger of suffocating as his face presses against the pillow.

It is convenient to have a small chest of drawers for the infant's clothing and personal equipment. As a preschool child he can use the chest and can be taught to put away his own things. There should be chairs for adults, one of them a low rocking chair. When the infant is old enough to sit up, he should have a small chair of his own, low enough for his feet to touch the floor, or the supporting foot rest if it is a high chair. Some high chairs can be lowered so that the infant is on a level with a small table. If the infant is to be left alone, it is safer to have the lower chair. There should also be a shelf for toys and a play pen raised off the floor.

The infant needs his own bathtub or bathinette. Plastic tubs are light, durable and smooth for the infant's skin. He will need a diaper pail, preferably of the pedal-controlled type, with a closely fitting cover, and later on a toilet seat or training chair. There should be a gate at the door of the nursery, or at the top of the stairs to prevent his falling if the family lives in a two-story house.

BATHING

The infant is bathed once a day and may be sponged off several times a day during warm weather. The temperature of the room should be 75 to 80° F. (23.8 to 26.6° C.). Either a bathinette or tub is used. If a tub is used, a bath towel is placed over the bottom to prevent sliding. The temperature of the water should be 100 to 105° F. (37.7 to 40.5° C.) for the newborn or small infant; for the normal healthy infant it can soon be reduced to 95° F. (35° C.). The mother tests the temperature with her elbow or a bath thermometer. Soft towels and a wash cloth are needed.

There should be a bath tray containing the following articles:

Jar of cotton swabs or cotton balls
Dish for soap (soap should be white and unscented)
Bottle or jar of baby oil or lotion if approved by the physician
Pin holder
Hair brush and comb
Orange wood stick
Paper bag for waste
Powder (if the mother wants to use it. Cornstarch powder is cheaper than most other powders and is suitable for use on the infant's skin; however, no powder should be used routinely.)
Bland ointment (A and D ointment is effective when necessary on an excoriated diaper area.)

The mother should be taught that there is no set procedure to be followed in bathing the infant, but certain principles must be remembered.

The scalp should be washed when bathing the infant. The football hold should be used (see p. 363). Mothers caring for their first babies may be fearful of washing over the "soft spot," or anterior fontanel. *Cradle cap*, a greasy crust or scale formation on the scalp, often occurs. Treatment of this seborrheic condition is by application of oil or a bland ointment at night and a scalp shampoo in the morning. This treatment should be repeated until the crust is removed. Commercial preparations may be used for this purpose and are successful if the directions are followed carefully.

The eyes, nose and ears require special attention to prevent injury. The creases of the body must be carefully cleansed and wiped thoroughly. The genitalia and the buttocks are bathed after each stool and, if the infant has a tendency to be chafed, after urinating.

The mother should be given complete directions on the care of the umbilicus before the infant is discharged from the hospital. Usually exposure of the cord to the air promotes rapid healing. There may be a slight bloody discharge from the navel; however, the umbilicus will heal in a few days after separation of the cord. Until the area is completely healed she should not give the infant a tub bath without permission from her physician. Before the infant is discharged the mother may give a demonstration to the nurse to ensure that she will not be anxious about her ability to care for the infant at home.

CLOTHING

Infants today wear very little clothing. Houses are usually comfortably warm in winter, and the less the infant wears in summer, the more comfortable he is. Children outgrow their clothing rapidly. All articles of infants' clothing should be soft and nonirritating, simple in design, comfortable, loose for activity, washable, suitable for the weather, easy to put on, absorbent, fire-retardant, safe — e.g., no ties around the neck which, if

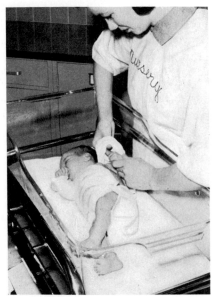

FIGURE 8–12. The simplest way to dress the infant is to put the entire hand through the sleeve, grasp the infant's hand and pull it through gently. (Davis and Rubin: *DeLee's Obstetrics for Nurses.* 17th ed.)

caught in any way, might choke the infant and in any case are uncomfortable—and tailored with safe fastenings to avoid the danger of loose or awkward buttons.

To dress the infant, if the cotton knit shirt is of the slipover type, it should be gathered in the hands so that it is easily pulled over the infant's head. The double-breasted shirt which ties is more popular, for it is easier to put on, gives double warmth across the chest and does not tear easily. To put the infant's arm through the sleeve, the nurse or mother should put her fingers through the end of the sleeve and put the infant's hand through the armhole. She can then take his fingers in hers and gently pull his hand through the sleeve. The diaper is put on like a pair of pants and pinned at either side to the shirt. The shirt is less likely to tear if it is turned up and the diaper is pinned through the two thicknesses. Turning it up also keeps it clean and dry when the infant voids or has a stool. The diaper should also be pinned securely around the leg openings to prevent spillage of feces. Many mothers today use disposable diapers, some even pinless, or the services of a commercial diaper service.

Stockings or socks as a rule are used only if the infant's feet are cold, and should be large enough to allow the infant to move his toes without being cramped. If long stockings are used, they are pinned to the diaper, above the knee on the outside of the leg. They are likely to become wet whenever the infant voids. Socks are pretty, but tend to come off when the infant kicks.

Bibs are used when the infant is fed. The young infant needs no other clothes, but as he grows older he should be provided with nightgowns, overalls, or dresses, sun suits, and outdoor clothes for all weather.

ELIMINATION

The breast-fed infant has several stools a day which are soft and rather spongy and may contain a little mucus. They are not likely to chafe him. Their odor is rather aromatic. The stools of the infant fed on cow's milk and cane sugar are yellow and more solid than those of the breast-fed infant. One or more stools a day is normal.

SLEEP

The newborn infant sleeps or appears to be sleeping practically all the time he is not feeding. His sleep is light, and there are frequent spontaneous movements of the face and body. He stretches and puckers up his face. When he is only a few weeks old, his sleeping periods are longer and more quiet, but he is also awake and alert for longer periods. This trend continues as he grows out of early infancy.

WEIGHT

Mothers should learn in the hospital how to weigh their infants if they have or intend to have scales at home. Safety factors should be emphasized. The mother should keep one hand over the infant at all times when she is weighing him. She should place the head end of the scale near, but not touching, the wall so that he may not slide out from that end. She should hold her hand close enough to his body to prevent his sliding down and over the other end of the scale.

In the home weekly weighings are sufficient. If they are attempted daily, mothers tend to worry about minor fluctuations. *Scales are not absolutely necessary,* for the infant can be weighed when taken for his check-up to the physician's office or the Child Health Conference (see p. 374). The average infant will gain from 7 to 8 ounces (210 to 240 gm.) each week. Some infants, however, gain 5 to 12 ounces (150 to 360 gm.) a week. If the gain is more or less than this, the mother should notify the physician.

TEMPERATURE

Although mothers should be taught how to take the infant's temperature, this should not be considered part of the daily care. The temperature should be taken only when the mother believes that it is not normal.

FEEDING

The feeding of the infant should be considered part of the routine activities of daily living in which all the members of the family are engaged. If everyone in the home is to be subordinated to the infant, he is likely to become a disturbing factor. This consciously or unconsciously creates a feeling that he is privileged and influences the emotional relations of parents and siblings toward him and indirectly toward each other. All plans for his care, from the first day in the hospital on, should be made with reference to what is best for him in the family situation.

Feeding time should be pleasant for both the infant and the family. The infant learns to like the one who feeds and cuddles him. The average infant at six weeks of age will smile at his mother when she picks him up and smiles at him. In time he is conditioned to smile because smiling always brings more cuddling and expressions of love from his mother. This is his way of wanting to please her, and it lays the foundation for willingness to do what she wants (obedience), so essential to the willing acceptance of discipline, which in turn leads to self-discipline.

While the mother is in the hospital the nurse should give her (1) a recipe for the formula, (2) a set of instructions and (3) a demonstration of formula preparation. The mother may be taught either the aseptic technique or the terminal heating method, or both. Teaching may be supplemented by the use of booklets; these illustrate the steps by which formulas can be prepared by either method.

FOLLOW-UP CARE

After discharge the infant should be under continuing medical care.

The mother who has a private physician will put her baby under his care. The infant of a mother who is a clinic patient is routinely referred by either the social service department of the hospital or the head nurse (or supervisor) of the obstetrical unit to the Child Health Conference in the district in which he lives. The public health agency will be notified of his discharge from the hospital, and a community or public health nurse will visit in the home to instruct the mother in the adaptation of all she has learned to the home situation. The nurse will check on the equipment for the infant's care and demonstrate his bath and the making of his formula. If further guidance or help which he or she cannot give is needed, the parents may be referred to The Family Service Society or equivalent agency.

TEACHING AIDS AND OTHER INFORMATION*

American Academy of Pediatrics

Comments on Health Legislation, Medical Research, and New Nursery Design.
Hexachlorophene and Skin Care of Newborn Infants.
Hospital Care of Newborn Infants.
Neurotoxicity from Hexachlorophene.
Vitamin K Supplementation for Infants.

The American Journal of Nursing Company

Care of the Well Child.
Techniques of Infant Feeding.

La Leche League International, Inc.

How the Nurse Can Help the Breastfeeding Mother.
When You Breastfeed Your Baby.
Why Breastfeed Your Baby?
Why Nurse Your Baby?

Public Affairs Committee

Carson, R.: Your New Baby.
Riker, A. P.: Breastfeeding.

Ross Laboratories

Barness, L. A.: On Developmental Nutrition: Fat, 1972.

Drash, A.: On Developmental Nutrition: Carbohydrate and Energy Metabolism, 1976.
Fomon, S. J.: On Developmental Nutrition: Protein and Amino Acids, 1972.
Goldbloom, R. B.: On Developmental Nutrition: The Fat-Soluble Vitamins, 1973.
Greene, H. L.: On Developmental Nutrition: Carbohydrate Absorption, 1976.
Hambidge, M., and O'Brien, D.: On Developmental Nutrition: Trace Metals, 1973.
Iatrogenic Problems in Neonatal Intensive Care, 1976.
Iron Nutrition in Infancy: Current Status, 1974.
Iron Nutrition in Infancy, 1970.
Kretchmer, N.: On Developmental Nutrition: Developmental Biochemistry, 1973.
Narins, D. M. C., and Weil, W. B.: On Developmental Nutrition: Calories, 1972.
Pearson, H. A.: On Developmental Nutrition: Iron, 1972.
Regionalization of Perinatal Care, 1974.
Reynolds, J. W.: On Developmental Nutrition: Water, 1974.
The Endocrine Milieu of Pregnancy, Puerperium and Childhood, 1974.

---

*Complete addresses are given in the Appendix.

Tsang, R. C.: On Developmental Nutrition: Calcium and Phosphorus, 1975.

Winick, M. (Ed.): Year One: Nutrition, Growth, Health, 1975.

United States Government

Breast Feeding Your Baby, Revised 1970.
El Cuidado de Su Bebe (Infant Care), 1975.
Infant Care, 1973.

REFERENCES

Books

Abramson, H. (Ed.): *Resuscitation of the Newborn Infant.* 3rd ed. St. Louis, The C. V. Mosby Company, 1973.

American Academy of Pediatrics: *Standards and Recommendations for Hospital Care of Newborn Infants.* 5th ed. Evanston, Ill., American Academy of Pediatrics, 1971.

American Hospital Association Committee on Infections Within Hospitals: *Infection Control in the Hospital.* 3rd ed. Chicago, American Hospital Association, 1974.

Arena, J. M.: *Poisoning: Toxicology-Symptoms-Treatments.* 3rd ed. Springfield, Ill., Charles C Thomas, 1974.

Burton, B. T.: *Human Nutrition.* 3rd ed. New York, McGraw-Hill Book Company, 1976.

Curley, A., et al.: *Hexachlorophene; A Possible Toxin for Infants Via Absorption Through the Skin.* The American Pediatric Society, Inc., and the Society for Pediatric Research Combined Program and Abstracts. Atlantic City, N.J., April 28–May 1, 1971.

Fomon, S. J. (Ed.): *Infant Nutrition.* 2nd ed. Philadelphia, W. B. Saunders Company, 1974.

Jelliffe, D. B., and Jelliffe, E. F. P.: *Human Milk in the Modern World.* St. Louis, The C. V. Mosby Company, 1976.

Klaus, M. H., and Kennell, J. H.: *Maternal-Infant Bonding: The Impact of Early Separation or Loss on Family Development.* St. Louis, The C. V. Mosby Company, 1976.

Moore, M. L.: *The Newborn and the Nurse.* Philadelphia, W. B. Saunders Company, 1972.

Pearlman, R.: *Feeding Your Baby; The Safe and Healthy Way.* New York, Random House, 1971.

Robinson, C. H., and Lawler, M. R.: *Normal and Therapeutic Nutrition.* 14th ed. New York, Macmillan Company, 1972.

Periodicals

Amsel, P. L.: The Need to Wean—As Much For Mother As For Baby? *RN,* 39:52, May 1976.

Beer, A. E., and Billingham, R. E.: Immunologic Benefits and Hazards of Milk in Maternal-Perinatal Relationship. *Ann. Intern. Med.,* 83:865, December 1975.

Brack, D. C.: Social Forces, Feminism, and Breastfeeding. *Nursing Outlook,* 23:556, September 1975.

Brackbill, Y., Douthitt, T. C., and West, H.: Psychophysiologic Effects in the Neonate of Prone Versus Supine Placement. *J. Pediatr.,* 82:82, January 1973.

Brown, M. S., and Hurlock, J. T.: Preparation of the Breast for Breastfeeding. *Nursing Research,* 24:448, November-December 1975.

Clark, L.: Introducing Mother and Baby. *Am. J. Nursing,* 74:1483, August 1974.

Estok, P. J.: What do Nurses Know About Breastfeeding Problems? *JOGN Nurs.,* 2:36, November-December 1973.

Gaensbauer, T. J., and Emde, R. N.: Wakefulness and Feeding in Human Newborns. *Arch. Gen. Psychiatry,* 28:894, June 1973.

Goldsmith, H. S.: Milk-Rejection Sign of Breast Cancer. *Nursing Digest,* 4:37, January-February 1976.

Gowdy, J. M., and Ulsamer, A. G.: Hexachlorophene Lesions in Newborn Infants. *Am. J. Dis. Child.,* 130:247, March 1976.

Greenberg, M., and Morris, N.: Engrossment: The Newborn's Impact Upon the Father. *American Journal of Orthopsychiatry,* 44:520, July 1974.

Herrmann, J., and Light, I. J.: Infection Control in the Newborn Nursery. *Nursing Clin. N. Am.,* 6:55, March 1971.

The Hexachlorophene Controversy. *RN,* 35:27, March 1972.

Johnson, N. W.: Breast-Feeding at One Hour Age. *The American Journal of Maternal-Child Nursing,* 1:12, January-February 1976.

Klaus, M. H., et al.: Maternal Attachment: Importance of the First Post-Partum Days. *N. Engl. J. Med.,* 286:480, March 2, 1972.

Knafl, K.: Conflicting Perspectives on Breast Feeding. *Am. J. Nursing,* 74:1848, October 1974.

Lopez, A. P., and Howell, Sr. J.: Is This Culture Necessary? *JOGN Nurs.,* 2:45, January-February 1973.

Lutz, L., and Perlstein, P. H.: Temperature Control in Newborn Babies. *Nursing Clin. N. Am.,* 6:15, March 1971.

Meng, K. Y., and Soo, B.: Breastfeeding in the Lower Socio-Economic Group. *Nurs. J. Singapore,* 15:6, May 1975.

Nishida, H., and Risemberg, H. M.: Silver Nitrate Ophthalmic Solution and Chemical Conjunctivitis. *Pediatrics,* 56:368, September 1975.

O'Brien, T. E.: Excretion of Drugs in Human Milk. *Nursing Digest,* 3:23, July-August 1975.

Olds, S. W.: Breast-feeding Is Nature's Way of Saying Mother Knows Best. *Today's Health,* 54:47, March 1976.

Phillips, C. R. N.: Neonatal Heat Loss in Heated Cribs vs. Mothers' Arms. *Nursing Digest,* 4:49, January-February 1976.

Poznanski, A. K., Kanellitsas, C., Roloff, D. W., and Borer, R. C.: Radiation Exposure to Personnel in a Neonatal Nursery. *Pediatrics,* 54:139, August 1974.

Rice, R. H., and Seacome, M.: Attitudes of a Group of Mothers to Breast Feeding. Parts I and II. *Midwife Health Visit,* 11:149, May 1975; 179, June 1975.

Rubin, R.: Maternity Nursing Stops Too Soon. *Am. J. Nursing,* 75:1680, October 1975.

Salk, L.: The Role of the Heartbeat in the Relations Between Mother and Infant. *Sci. Am.,* 228:24, May 1973.

Shaw, N. R.: Teaching Young Mothers Their Role. *Nursing Outlook,* 22:695, November 1974.

Taggart, M. E.: A Practical Guide to Successful Breast-Feeding. *The Canadian Nurse,* 72:25, March 1976.

Théberge-Rousselet, D.: Babies at Risk? *The Canadian Nurse,* 72:34, March 1976.

Théberge-Rousselet, D.: Freezing Breast Milk at Home. *The Canadian Nurse,* 72:31, March 1976.

Yanover, M. J., Jones, D., and Miller, M. D.: Perinatal Care of Low-risk Mothers and Infants. *N. Engl. J. Med.,* 294:702, March 25, 1976.

Yu, V. Y. H.: Effect of Body Position on Gastric Emptying in the Neonate. *Arch. Dis. Child,* 50:500, July 1975.

AUDIOVISUAL MEDIA*

American College of Nurse-Midwifery

Breast Feeding: A Family Experience
10 minutes, sound, color.
Portrays simplicity, beauty and ease of nursing.

Management of Breast Feeding
15 minutes, sound, black and white.
Portrays two mothers getting started on breast feeding.

Preparation of the Breast for Breast Feeding
10 minutes, sound, color.
This film is intended as an aid to teaching one technique of breast preparation to parent educators and expectant parents. For those educators who have no facilities for private instructions, it will, of course, fill a void.

The American Journal of Nursing Company

Maternity Nursing Class
44 minute classes, 16mm film or videotape, audio-tape cassettes, sound, color or black and white.

Hospital Care of the Newborn
Demonstrates care of the newborn in the delivery room and through the neonatal period. Includes legal responsibilities, with emphasis on identification procedures. Shows rooming-in arrangements and discusses parent education.

Postpartum Care—Hospital to Home
Demonstrates how the nurse may meet the teaching needs of families during the postpartum period, with emphasis on the discharge procedure, including explanation of community resources.

Respiratory Distress in Children
12 minutes, color.
This film is limited to illustrations of signs of respiratory distress in children, without reference to cause or treatment. The film contrasts examples of children with healthy breathing patterns to examples of infants experiencing respiratory distress.

Resuscitation of the Newborn
25 minutes, color.
The essential principles involved in the resuscitation of infants who do not breathe or whose respiration is impaired at birth. Procedures and equipment shown in actual resuscitations and through animated drawings.

Charles Press–Prentice-Hall, Inc.

Nursing Skills and Techniques Series
2–5 minutes, Super-8mm filmloop, color, guide.

Delivery Room Care: Newborn Part I
Equipment necessary for care of newborn shown, plus actual care.

Delivery Room Care: Newborn Part II
Continued care of the newborn in delivery room.

Nursery: Bathing Newborn I, Part I
Preparation for bathing newborn in nursery plus pertinent observations and charting.

Nursery: Bathing Newborn I, Part II
Continuation of procedure for bathing newborn in the nursery.

Nursery: Bathing Newborn I, Part III
Final steps of procedure for bathing newborn in nursery.

Nursery: Bathing Newborn II, Part I
Equipment and procedure for daily care of infant in hospital.

Nursery: Bathing Newborn II, Part II
Continued daily care of infant in hospital.

Nursery: Bathing Newborn II, Part III
Continued daily care of infant in hospital.

Nursery: Discharge of Infant, Part I
Procedure for discharging newborn from the hospital.

Nursery: Discharge of Infant, Part II
Completion of procedure for discharge of infant from hospital.

Health Sciences Communication Center, Case Western Reserve University

Breast Feeding: Prenatal and Postpartal Preparation
16mm film or videocassette.
This presentation was designed to guide nurses and physicians in instructing expectant and new mothers in the preparation and care of their breasts for breast feeding.

W. B. Saunders Company

Pediatric Conference with Sydney Gellis
Early Feeding of the Newborn
First Feeding

Trainex Corporation

Bathing the Baby
35mm filmstrip, audio-tape cassettes, 33 1/3 LP, color.
Provides the mother with instructions on how to sponge-bathe and tub-bathe her baby. Emphasis is placed on bathing and care of baby's face, scalp, and navel and genital areas. Various types of diapers are shown, and instruction is given on how to make different diaper folds with regard to baby's sex and physical size.

Bottle Feeding
35mm filmstrip, audio-tape cassettes, 33 1/3 LP, color.
Informs and instructs a mother on formula preparation and the feeding of her baby. It explains what baby is fed, and his feeding schedule while in the hospital. Formula preparation in the home, along with the equipment required, is shown, with emphasis on equipment and formula sterilization.

Infant Care—Breast Feeding
35mm filmstrip, audio-tape cassettes, 33 1/3 LP, color.
An illustrated presentation shows how to position the infant for feeding and how to help the infant find the breast. Discusses the importance of using alternate breasts and explains how to relax.

Introduction to Infant Care
35mm filmstrip, audio-tape cassettes, 33 1/3 LP, color.
This program shows how to generate self-confidence in the new mother. Provides information on: feeding, bathing, skin care, safety precautions, taking the rectal temperature, care of diapers, and home environment adjustments; also included is information on self-care for the mother.

Skin Care and Bathing Preparation
35mm filmstrip, audio-tape cassettes, 33 1/3 LP, color.
Instructs a mother on the care of her baby's umbilical cord stub and circumcision, and the trimming of baby's fingernails and toenails. Some forms of skin irritation (rashes) are mentioned, and the mother is instructed on how to care for them. The program enumerates the equipment required to bathe a baby, and describes how the mother should prepare herself prior to giving her baby his bath.

---

*Complete addresses are given in the Appendix.

Chapter Nine

THE DYSMATURE INFANT— PREMATURITY AND POSTMATURITY

The term *dysmaturity* refers to a clinical syndrome in which the levels of growth and development evidenced by the newborn either exceed or fall short of those normally seen at birth. *Premature* infants may be included in this syndrome; however, they are usually set apart and discussed separately. Premature infants are those delivered before 37 weeks from the first day of the last menstrual period; thus they have a shortened gestational period. *Low birth weight* infants are those who weigh 2500 gm. or less at birth, owing to either a shortened gestational period or a less than expected growth rate, or both. These infants of low birth weight are sometimes categorized as small-for-gestational-age (SGA) or small-for-dates (SFD) infants. Prematurity and low birth weight usually occur together, both carrying a high rate of morbidity and mortality. For this reason the conditions will be discussed together in this text under the diagnosis of prematurity. *Postmature* infants, those born after a prolonged gestation, show attainments in growth and development that surpass those seen in the term infant (see p. 210).

Dysmature infants must be observed carefully during the first few days of life; however, they may progress more quickly in their development than those of similar weights at birth.

PREMATURITY

Newborns born prematurely or those having a low birth weight account for the highest mortality rate among infants in the first year of life. This is probably the reason for the increasing amounts of research done during the last few decades on the causes of prematurity and the needs of these infants.

Approximately 10 per cent of all live births are premature. The standard of prematurity should be the number of days of gestation, but this standard correlates with the weight, length and activity of the newborn. Because weight is often indicative of prematurity and physiologic immaturity, a premature or a low birth weight infant is considered to be one who weighs 2500 gm. (5 pounds 8 ounces) or less at birth. The length from crown to heel is likely to be close to 18.5 inches (47 cm.). His behavior shows his immaturity: he lacks the normal reflexes and a general ability to carry on vital functions.

INCIDENCE AND CAUSES OF PREMATURITY

In many cases the causes of prematurity and low birth weight are not known, partly because the incidence is highest among the low socioeconomic groups. Prospective mothers in such groups are least likely to have adequate prenatal care. Many of these women are first seen by an obstetrician when they are in labor.

Multiple births are a frequent cause of prematurity; few triplets are carried to term. The relation between the use of contraceptives and multiple births may be important in the occurrence of prematurity. Toxemia of pregnancy is an im-

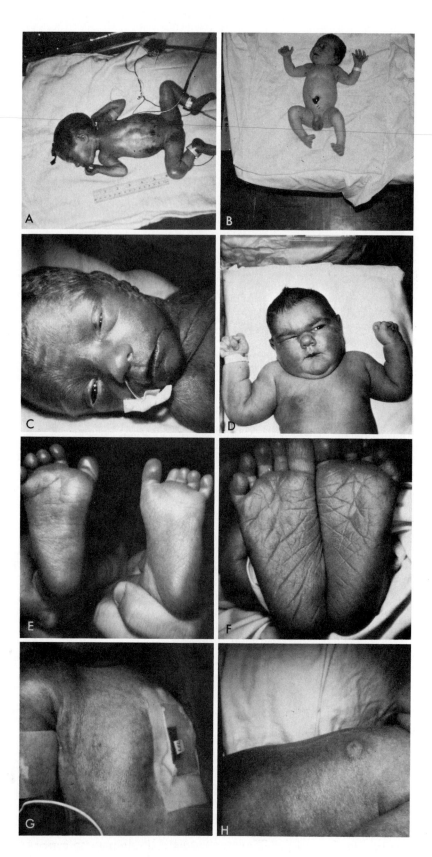

FIGURE 9–1. External criteria for estimating gestational age. General appearance: *A*, Premature infant lies frog-legged with elbows, wrists, knees, and ankles touching bed; inactive, few spontaneous movements, head turned to one side. *B*, Term infant lies with arms and legs flexed; moves actively, head moves from side to side. Skin: *C*, In premature infant very transparent, gelatinous, shiny, superficial blood vessels apparent, abundant lanugo. *D*, Thick in term infant; flakes soon after birth, no lanugo, no superficial blood vessels visible. Feet: *E*, In premature infant creases not present or only cover part of the sole. *F*, Creases found over entire sole of term infant. Breast: *G*, In prematures little breast tissue and nipples just barely visible. *H*, In term infant breast tissue is 10 mm. in diameter.

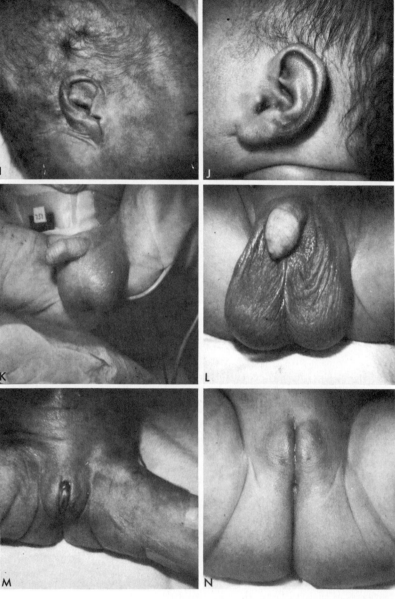

FIGURE 9-1 *Continued.* Scalp hair and ears: *I*, In premature, fine fuzzy hair; earlobe very pliable, with little cartilage. *J*, In term infant, distinct and identifiable individual scalp hairs; earlobe firm. Genitalia: *K*, Premature male has testicles high in scrotum or down at edges of canal; scrotum has few rugae, not very pigmented. *L*, Term male has pendulous scrotum, pigmented, and rugated testicles well descended. *M*, In premature female, labia major widely separated by protruding labia minor and clitoris. *N*, In term female, labia majora most prominent covering structure. (From Myers, M. S.: *RN*, 38:23, January 1975.)

portant cause, particularly among women not under observation of a physician. Antepartum hemorrhage is likely to occur in two important complications of pregnancy: premature separation of the placenta (abruptio placentae) and placenta praevia. Both conditions may contribute to premature birth of the infant. Premature rupture of the membranes invariably causes premature birth.

Among maternal conditions related to premature or high-risk delivery are those of noninfectious origin, e.g., cardiac disease, hypertension, underweight, overweight, diabetes mellitus, and severe sensitization to the Rh blood factor; those of infectious origin, whether acute or chronic,

and those due to heavy smoking, drinking, or drug taking during pregnancy. Problem pregnancies may also occur when the mother is under 17 years or over 35 years of age, has a family history of inherited disorders, has a structural abnormality of the pelvis, or has reported a history of previous miscarriage, low birthweight, or premature infants.

Fetal abnormalities or injury to the mother or fetus, or both, may make it impossible for the infant to be carried to term. Overwork and inadequate diet or chronic maternal malnutrition are important factors in the incidence of premature births. They are seldom the immediate cause of a premature delivery but predispose to poor health, if not chronic or acute illness, which interferes with carrying the fetus to term. With further long-range research perhaps more contributory factors to prematurity will be found.

PREVENTION OF PREMATURITY

The great preventive measure to reduce the number of premature births is adequate prenatal care for all prospective mothers. The incidence of prematurity could be substantially decreased if high-risk pregnancies could be diagnosed and monitored in time. The incidence of prematurity and low birthweight are increasing because of the growing number of teenagers who become pregnant, many of whom are not physically mature enough to meet the demands of pregnancy (see p. 884). Maternal and child health programs—federal, state, and local—have provided good obstetrical care for thousands of women who otherwise would have lacked even a minimum of medical supervision during the prenatal period. Maternal care is provided to protect the infant as well as the mother, since *the longer the fetus can be retained* in utero, *the better are its chances for survival.*

Characteristics of Premature Infants

PHYSICAL CHARACTERISTICS

The premature infant that we see in the incubator is at the same stage of development as the fetus of the same gestational age. The age of viability is commonly said to be seven months. Many premature infants, then, will resemble the fetus of seven months' gestation. The premature infant is adapted to life *in utero.* His immaturity is evident as we look at him. He is small and limp. His skin is thin, wrinkled, and red; there is an excess of lanugo and little or no vernix caseosa. His head is relatively large, with prominent eyes, soft ears, and receding chin. The thorax is less firm than that of the full-term infant. The abdomen protrudes, and the genitalia are small. The extremities are thin, the muscles small. The fingernails and toenails are abnormally soft and short. The subcutaneous tissue is deficient, so he has a wizened appearance. Extremely small prematures may have a plump appearance because of edema due to a low total serum protein concentration. This is lost, however, in a few days. Engorgement of the breasts, normal in the full-term infant, is absent in the premature, since it is due to hormones from the mother which are passed to the fetus in the late months of gestation. The normal sucking, swallowing, and gag reflexes are absent in very immature infants.

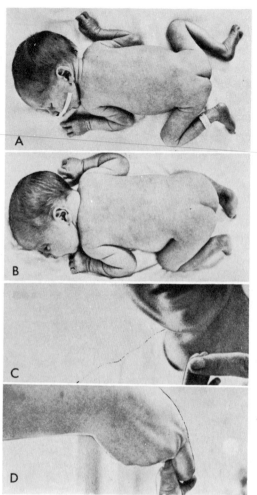

FIGURE 9–2. The contrast in neuromuscular development and muscle tone between the premature infant and the normal newborn. In the prone position. *A,* the premature lies with pelvis flat and legs splayed out sideways like a frog. *B,* The normal full-term infant lies with his limbs flexed, pelvis raised and knees drawn under the abdomen. In the grasp reflex. *C,* the premature infants grasps the finger weakly, but there is little muscle tensing. *D,* The normal newborn reinforces the grip when his arm is drawn upwards. (Courtesy of Mead Johnson and Company.)

PHYSIOLOGIC HANDICAPS

The nursing care of the premature infant, so far as it differs from that of the normal infant, is based on the physiologic handicaps of immaturity: poor control of body temperature, difficult respiration, inability to handle infections adequately, tendency to hemorrhage and anemia, tendency for rickets to develop, disturbances of nutrition, and impairment of renal function.

Poor Control of Body Temperature. What was said of the normal newborn's dependency on the temperature of his environment to maintain a normal body temperature (p. 160) is even more important in planning the care of the pre-

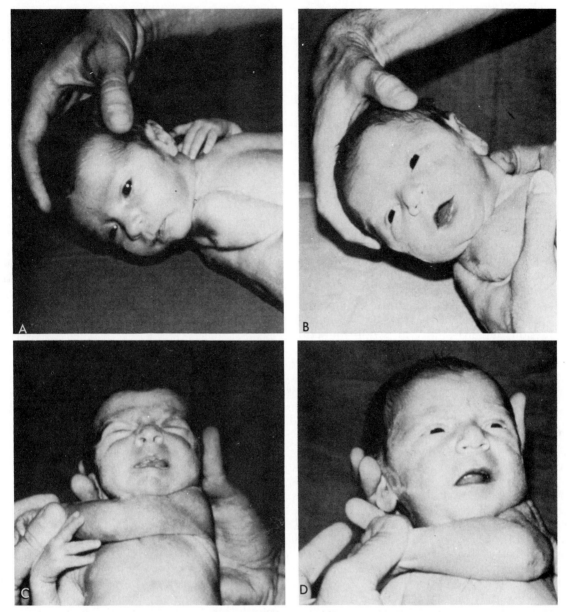

FIGURE 9–3. Estimation of muscle tone in newborn infants. A, "Owl" sign in premature infant. Head can be rotated past shoulder so that the child seems to be looking backward. In B, term infant's head is parallel with top of shoulder. C, "Scarf" sign in same infant as shown in A. Arm can be pulled over so far that the bend of the elbow lies well beyond the chin. In term infant, D, the elbow comes only under the chin. (Hodgman, *Hosp. Pract.*, May, 1969.)

mature infant. His nervous system is poorly developed, and the heat-regulating center in the brain is immature. The skin surface of the premature is great in proportion to his weight. He lacks the insulation of the subcutaneous fat layer, which is developed in the last month of gestation. His muscular development being poor, he is inactive. The metabolic rate is low. If the environment is too warm he becomes overheated, since his sweating mechanism is underdeveloped. Yet internal conditions which would cause a fever in a normal infant may be present in the premature without an elevation of tem-

perature (this often happens in the dehydrated premature or one with an infectious condition).

Difficult Respiration. Respirations are difficult and irregular in the premature infant. Since his lungs are immature, there is incomplete development of the alveoli and weakness of the thoracic cage and of the respiratory muscles. Gaseous exchange is retarded by the immature alveolar membrane. If mucus lodges in his throat or if a few drops of feeding enter the trachea, his gag and cough reflexes are too weak to clear the airway.

CYANOSIS. The premature's tendency to

cyanosis is evidence of inadequate oxygenation of his arterial blood. This may be due to increased intracranial pressure from birth trauma, obstruction of the respiratory tract, poor development of the respiratory muscles or some interference with the normal expansion of the lungs. Abdominal distention may interfere with the action of the diaphragm.

APNEA. Apnea is a condition of suspended respiration. It may result from excessive analgesics or anesthetics given the mother during labor. Expert care during delivery decreases the danger of birth trauma with resulting cyanosis. General immaturity of the nervous system and the respiratory tract is a cause of apnea which is inherent in the premature infant's condition and cannot be controlled by the obstetrician, although modern methods of resuscitation keep many such infants alive who would have died at birth.

Inability to Handle Infections Adequately. The premature infant is highly susceptible to infection, and his ability to handle infection of any sort is poor because he has poorly developed globulin synthesis, antibody formation and cellular defense. He does not react to infection with fever or an elevation of the white blood cell count. He lacks immune substances from his mother, which are transmitted to the fetus during the last months of gestation.

The immature infant has more avenues for access of infection than does the normal infant. His skin and mucous membranes are not as protective as the more mature skin and membranes of the full-term infant.

Tendency to Hemorrhage and Anemia. The blood vessels of the premature infant are incompletely developed and therefore more fragile, the supporting tissue lacks normal elasticity, and the plasma is hypoprothrombinemic. He lacks the normal supply of vitamin K. Anemia results from hemorrhage as with the normal infant, but the premature suffers more from loss of blood than does the normal infant because he lacks iron and other essential hematogenous factors which the fetus receives during the last months of gestation. His body growth is rapid and therefore requires a greater blood supply. He has an increased proportion of fetal hemoglobin. His red blood cells are easily destroyed, and even a slight loss of blood is of great consequence.

Tendency for Rickets to Develop. The premature infant lacks the calcium, phosphorus, and usually the vitamin D normally stored in the body of the full-term infant. Yet his potentially rapid rate of growth requires an ample supply of these minerals, and vitamin D is needed for their utilization. He also lacks the ability to ab-

sorb fat-soluble vitamins given in his feedings. Hence the premature is more likely to acquire rickets than is the normal infant.

Disturbances of Nutrition. This subject is discussed on page 195.

Impairment of Renal Function. The incomplete development of the kidneys of the premature causes difficulty in concentration of urine, and a proportionately large amount of fluid is lost. He has an unstable acid-base and electrolyte balance.

Care and Treatment of the Premature Infant

Differences in the nursing care of the premature infant from that of the full-term infant are based on the anatomic and physiologic characteristics of prematurity.

CARE IMMEDIATELY AFTER BIRTH

Warmth. The infant may be placed in a bubble plastic wrap or in a warm incubator provided with the necessary facilities for increasing environmental oxygen and humidity. Research has shown that premature as well as normal infants survive best when their body heat loss is reduced (see p. 192).

Initiation of Respirations. The airway should be cleared. Mucus may be removed from the nose and throat by gentle suction. A mucus trap may be used with a small soft catheter. The infant is placed in a level position or with his head down; this position increases the natural drainage of secretions (see p. 160).

If the infant has hypoxia, he may be given artificial respiration with a mechanical device providing measured positive pressure. If no mechanical device is available, *gentle* mouth-to-mouth insufflation by blowing "puffs" of air through several layers of gauze may be used. Air enriched with oxygen may be given to the infant if an oxygen tube is placed in the operator's mouth. Other more vigorous measures may cause the infant to gasp once or twice, but are not helpful in establishing respiration.

Oxygen Administration. Oxygen should be in readiness if respirations are not established in the first few seconds of life, and later if the infant shows signs of cyanosis. Immediately after birth he may be placed in an atmosphere having an oxygen content of 30 to 40 per cent.

Medications. The nurse should know the drugs commonly used in treating conditions usual in premature infants, and such drugs should be in readiness in case of emergency.

Epinephrine is given intramuscularly as a cardiovascular stimulant, and caffeine and sodium benzoate are given intramuscularly for respiratory stimulation. To reduce the tendency to bleeding, vitamin K may be given. The recommended dose of 1.0 mg. of vitamin K_1 is safe and effective. Forms of vitamin K_1 used include Menadione, Synkavite, Konakion, and Aquamephyton. Excessive doses are to be avoided, since the drug may cause increased bilirubinemia. Nalorphine hydrochloride (Nalline) should be given intravenously into the umbilical cord to counteract the respiratory depression due to morphine, codeine, or other opiates given the mother before delivery and transmitted to the infant via the placenta. If the physician knows that the infant is premature, the mother will probably not receive analgesia.

CARE IN THE NURSERY

The premature infant may be cared for in a premature nursery or in a special area set aside in a newborn intensive care unit (see p. 75). Some large hospitals, in accordance with regional planning, have several such units: an intensive care level for the most critically ill, an intermediate care level for those who have begun to thrive, and a level for normal infants preparing for discharge. There may also be an admission or isolation area nearby. In some places, transport incubators, emergency ambulance type mobile intensive care nurseries, and helicopters have become available for the transportation of critically ill infants. Many hospitals that do not specialize in the care of high-risk newborns must transfer them to regional intensive care nurseries. The nurse's role after the call has been received from the outlying hospital is to assess the kind of preparation that must be done for the individual newborn. The team of a physician and nurse goes out in the transport vehicle to evaluate the condition of the infant and to administer care en route to the receiving hospital. In any such unit all essential diagnostic and therapeutic equipment should be available *immediately* to each infant at any time.

In an intensive care unit, near each newborn should be equipment for oxygen, compressed air, and suction among others, and outlets for respirators, monitoring devices, and infusion pumps. Also readily available should be cardiopulmonary monitoring and resuscitation devices. Apnea monitors should be available to prevent brain damage and mortality in premature infants who suddenly stop breathing, but the best apnea monitor is still the nurse. In such

a unit nurses must be available who can handle both infants and machines in any emergency.

In smaller hospitals having units for newborns an attempt should be made to provide prompt care similar to that given in a larger setting.

Environment. In order to simulate certain features of the intrauterine environment, preterm infants may be placed on waterbeds, gently rocked, and exposed to auditory stimulation such as a recording of a mother's voice and her heartbeat. This minimizes the change from the environment of the mother's uterus to that of the nursery. No nurses may enter the premature nursery except those assigned to it. There is usually an isolation nursery for prematures brought to the hospital from other hospitals or from the home.

The infant should be taken from the delivery room to the nursery in a heated carrier. A portable oxygen tank should be available when transporting the infant. The nursery should be isolated from all other units to ensure protection from infection. It should preferably be air conditioned. The humidity of the nursery should not be below 55 or above 65 per cent, the temperature not below 77 or above 90° F. (25 to 32.2° C.). Each infant should have his own incubator or crib.

Good nursing care is essential to the preservation of the premature, and the survival rate is highest where nursing care is adequate in both quantity and quality. Such care must be constant. Any omission lessens the infant's chance for survival. Nurses caring for premature infants must know the principles on which care of the premature is based and must be skilled in their adaptation to the needs of the individual infant. They must be able to judge his needs at any time and be devoted to providing the best possible care. In no other area of pediatric nursing is the ability to observe and record accurately all symptoms of greater importance. Observations which the nurse should make on the premature infant include quality of respirations, color, sucking ability, activity, cry, and change in his condition such as increased retractions and degree of cyanosis.

Handling the Premature. The nurse should handle a small premature no more than is absolutely necessary and remove him as few times from his incubator or crib as possible. Minimal skillful, gentle handling lessens the danger of infection and conserves the infant's strength.

The nurse should accomplish as much as possible in every contact with the infant. Nursing care should be planned around the feeding time. This minimizes the danger of infection, does not interfere with his rest more than is necessary, and tends to keep the concentration of oxygen at the prescribed level in the incubator.

Research has shown, however, that the premature should have close contact with a maternal figure and adequate sensory stimulation *as soon as possible* in order to prevent developmental variations. Touching is indeed a therapeutic technique in the care of infants. In order to establish an early parent-child bond, the mother and father should be included in giving the infant care.

MAINTENANCE OF BODY TEMPERATURE

The premature infant is unable to maintain a stable body temperature. Even minor deviations from the optimum environmental temperature cause a corresponding change in his body temperature. In caring for the premature the danger of his being cold is always stressed. A warm nursery and the use of incubators (see Fig. 9–5) make it possible to provide the required environmental heat to maintain each infant's body temperature at 96 to 98° F. (35.5 to 36.5° C.). Ideally, the infant's body temperature should be 98° F., but stability of temperature is more important than maintenance of exactly 98° F. Overheating is as bad for the infant as being cold. The ideal temperature and humidity of the nursery prevent loss of water through the skin and excessive loss through breathing.

Incubators are indicated for infants of 3 pounds (1360 grams) or less. If for any reason a premature is placed in the general nursery, the incubator will probably be used until he weighs well over 3 pounds, and even longer if he cannot maintain his temperature, has difficulty in breathing or becomes cyanotic. One great advantage of the incubator is that it can be regulated to meet the needs of the individual infant. In general, the temperature in the incubator should not be over 90° F. (32.2° C.); it may be raised or lowered, according to whether the infant requires more or less heat.

Since the objective of applying external heat is to maintain the infant's temperature within a normal range, it is necessary to take his body temperature in order to determine the amount of external heat required. It may be necessary to take the temperature every hour until it is stabilized. The temperature should be taken when the infant is first brought to the nursery. This is done rectally, thereby simultaneously testing for the presence of anal occlusion (see p. 247).

Preparation and Use of Incubators. Types of incubators include the Armstrong, the Isolette and the heated crib among others. Each varies from the other in some detail of operation, and the nurse must study the operating instructions provided by the manufacturer.

In the selection of an incubator the points on which it is to be evaluated are (1) easy maintenance of heat and humidity, (2) ease in administration of oxygen, (3) transparent top for easy visibility, and (4) safety alarms to indicate overheating or lack of circulating air.

The incubator should be prepared before the infant arrives. The regulator is set at approximately 90° F. (32.2° C.). Thereafter it is adjusted so that the infant's temperature is maintained between 96 and 98° F. (35.5 to 36.5° C.). When the infant is cared for in the Isolette, not only can the temperature of the incubator be regulated by the nurse, but also, if an Infant Servo Control

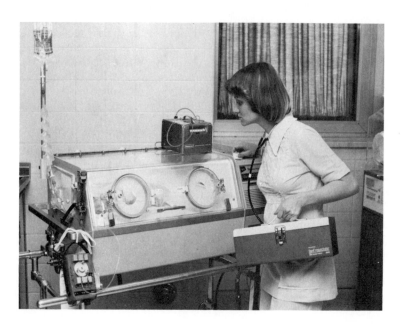

FIGURE 9–4. Transport incubator. The infant can be safely moved within the hospital or to the hospital from another location. Note the intravenous "Holter" pump for continuous infusion, oxygen analyzer, temperature control. The baby in the incubator is wrapped in bubble plastic with a nasogastric tube in place. The nurse holds a case containing emergency equipment. (From Johnson, M.: *The Canadian Nurse*, 72:20, May 1976. Reprinted with permission.)

Power Unit is attached, the infant himself can act as the Isolette's thermostat. A highly accurate temperature-sensing thermistor is taped directly to the skin of the infant's abdomen. When the infant's abdominal skin temperature changes, the Isolette's heater is turned on or off and the infant's body temperature is stabilized at the desired control point.

The water chamber is filled with sterile distilled water so that the humidity can be increased if necessary. In some instances no increase in humidity is provided. The bed is adjusted as ordered so that the infant's head is level with or slightly lower than his body. The oxygen flow is adjusted and tested every five minutes for concentration, to determine whether it is what the physician ordered. After the concentration has been stabilized it should be rechecked every four hours and the results recorded on the patient's chart. Prematures should be kept in 30 to 40 per cent oxygen only as long as they have symptoms of respiratory distress or cyanosis. The infant may be weighed in the incubator daily or according to the physician's order, depending on his size and condition.

One problem to which insufficient attention has been paid is the noise level in the incubator. This may be a perinatal risk factor with regard to later hearing impairment of the child.

If an incubator is not available, other methods of applying heat must be provided. The most commonly used is the hot-water bottle, especially in rural areas. The procedure for the use of hot-water bottles has been discussed previously (see p. 160).

Maintenance of respirations

The respirations of the premature may be rapid, shallow and irregular. The abdominal muscles are used, and there may be some periods of apnea. Gentle suction may be needed to clear the respiratory tract of mucus and other fluid. Stomach lavage may be ordered if the secretions are excessive.

A vaporizer should be used to produce the high humidity necessary for premature infants or those born by cesarean section. This is adjusted to produce a humidity within the incubator of 55 per cent or higher. If the respiratory difficulty is relieved, the vaporizer may be discontinued after 24 to 36 hours. Routine nebulized water is not necessary and may predispose to skin infections and sepsis. (High humidity may be obtained in the home through the use of humidifiers, steam kettles, inhalators, or wet towels placed over a radiator. The towels are kept wet by immersing one end in a pan of water.)

The infant should be on his side in the incubator in order to get the maximum amount of air into his lungs. If he is inactive, his position should be changed every one to three hours. If artificial respiration is necessary, it should be given very gently (see p. 202).

When the oxygen concentration in the incubator is above 40 per cent, there is danger of development of retrolental fibroplasia (see p. 200). Several methods may be used to limit the concentration of oxygen to the percentage ordered by the physician. The oxygen flow can be adjusted until analysis shows that the desired concentration has been established. A mixture of 40 per cent oxygen and 60 per cent nitrogen can be used in the incubator; by this means the infant cannot receive more than 40 per cent oxygen. An oxygen-diluting meter can be used to regulate the concentration of oxygen. This device mixes the air of the room with pure oxygen and can be set to produce any concentration ordered by the physician. It is not, however, a substitute for oxygen analysis (see Fig. 9–7), but keeps the

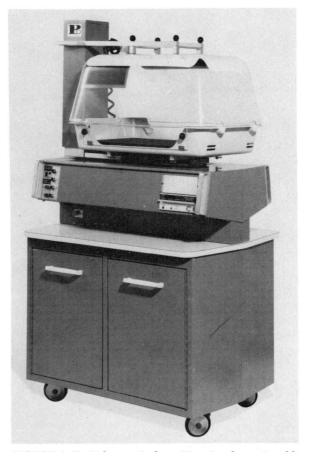

FIGURE 9–5. Infa-care Radiant Heat Incubator. In addition to providing the efficiency of radiant heat for infant warmth, this system contains physiologic monitoring modules for temperature, ECG/heart rate, respiration rate, and oxygen concentration. (Courtesy of Puritan-Bennett Corporation.)

ADVANTAGES AND DISADVANTAGES OF CPAP DELIVERY SYSTEMS

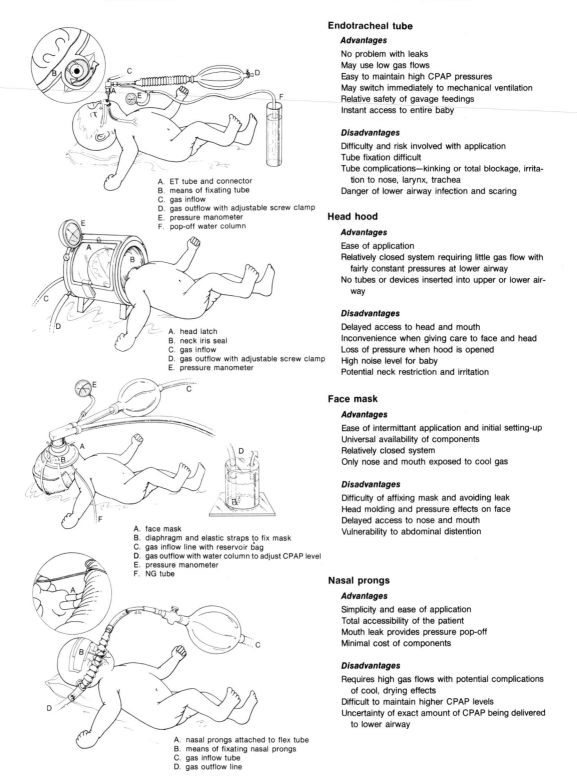

A. ET tube and connector
B. means of fixating tube
C. gas inflow
D. gas outflow with adjustable screw clamp
E. pressure manometer
F. pop-off water column

A. head latch
B. neck iris seal
C. gas inflow
D. gas outflow with adjustable screw clamp
E. pressure manometer

A. face mask
B. diaphragm and elastic straps to fix mask
C. gas inflow line with reservoir bag
D. gas outflow with water column to adjust CPAP level
E. pressure manometer
F. NG tube

A. nasal prongs attached to flex tube
B. means of fixating nasal prongs
C. gas inflow tube
D. gas outflow line

Endotracheal tube

Advantages

No problem with leaks
May use low gas flows
Easy to maintain high CPAP pressures
May switch immediately to mechanical ventilation
Relative safety of gavage feedings
Instant access to entire baby

Disadvantages

Difficulty and risk involved with application
Tube fixation difficult
Tube complications—kinking or total blockage, irritation to nose, larynx, trachea
Danger of lower airway infection and scaring

Head hood

Advantages

Ease of application
Relatively closed system requiring little gas flow with fairly constant pressures at lower airway
No tubes or devices inserted into upper or lower airway

Disadvantages

Delayed access to head and mouth
Inconvenience when giving care to face and head
Loss of pressure when hood is opened
High noise level for baby
Potential neck restriction and irritation

Face mask

Advantages

Ease of intermittant application and initial setting-up
Universal availability of components
Relatively closed system
Only nose and mouth exposed to cool gas

Disadvantages

Difficulty of affixing mask and avoiding leak
Head molding and pressure effects on face
Delayed access to nose and mouth
Vulnerability to abdominal distention

Nasal prongs

Advantages

Simplicity and ease of application
Total accessibility of the patient
Mouth leak provides pressure pop-off
Minimal cost of components

Disadvantages

Requires high gas flows with potential complications of cool, drying effects
Difficult to maintain higher CPAP levels
Uncertainty of exact amount of CPAP being delivered to lower airway

FIGURE 9–6. Advantages and disadvantages of CPAP delivery systems. (From Affonso, D., and Harris, T.: *Am. J. Nursing,* 76:570, April 1976. © April, 1976, The American Journal of Nursing Co. Reproduced from the *American Journal of Nursing* with permission.)

range of concentration within limits. Oxygen should be given at as low a level as possible in order to afford relief for the infant and should be discontinued as soon as possible.

Charting Oxygen Intake. Each infant's chart should contain a separate oxygen record, which should include (1) the physician's written order for oxygen and its method of administration, (2) the duration of administration, (3) the oxygen concentration, and (4) the infant's response to the concentration and to its duration. The extent of time during which the infant received oxygen must be determined accurately (all interruption in therapy required when caring for the infant must be noted). The oxygen concentration should be analyzed at four-hour intervals, or more frequently if necessary, and charted. The analyzer should be checked periodically against the concentration of oxygen in the air (20.9 per cent oxygen at sea level) and by sampling pure oxygen. If the analyzer provides a correct reading at these extremes, intermediate readings should be reliable. The infant's response, including changes in his color, respirations, pulse, and degree of activity, should be carefully observed and accurately charted.

Research is currently being done on an effective body-surface oximeter that continuously monitors arterial oxygen saturation and sounds an alarm if the saturation is above or below normal limits.

NUTRITION

The problem of nutrition in the premature infant is complicated by his difficulty in sucking and in swallowing. Often these reflexes are absent, and he makes no response to stimulation of his lips by a nipple or medicine dropper; food placed in his mouth either runs out or causes

him to choke. If he is able to take the feeding or is fed by gavage, the small capacity of his stomach often results in distention and vomiting, which may cause respiratory embarrassment. The gastric acidity is low, and the capacity for absorption of fat is not that of the normal full-term infant. His entire digestive enzyme system is incompletely developed, and he may be unable to handle satisfactorily any kind of feeding, even breast milk.

The problem is accentuated by his need for a nutritional intake higher than that of the normal infant, whose weight at birth allows for the initial loss which normally occurs until feeding is established. The premature needs 60 to 80 calories and 3 to 4 gm. of protein per pound of body weight, plus an adequate carbohydrate and liquid intake. Since his ability to absorb fat is poor, skimmed milk rather than whole milk is generally used as the basis for his formula. Premature infants have a need for an increased intake of vitamin C in order to metabolize phenylalanine and tyrosine properly, vitamin D because of the loss of fat-soluble vitamins and calcium in their stools, and iron to prevent iron deficiency anemia.

Premature infants must be fed carefully. In the past such an infant was seldom given an oral feeding during the first 18 to 24 hours because it was believed that his inactivity, his low rate of heat production if his body heat was conserved, and his edema at birth reduced the need for electrolytes, calories and water. More recently it has been found that early feeding of saline or glucose solutions tends to reduce the occurrence of hyperbilirubinemia and hypoglycemia. If problems exist which prevent oral feeding, fluids, electrolytes, and calories may be given intravenously.

The initial feeding may be as little as 2 to 4 ml.

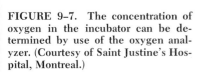

FIGURE 9–7. The concentration of oxygen in the incubator can be determined by use of the oxygen analyzer. (Courtesy of Saint Justine's Hospital, Montreal.)

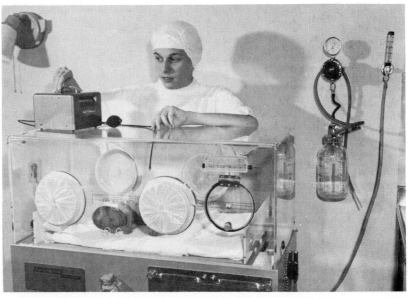

and may consist solely of a 5 per cent sugar solution. Feedings are slowly increased, and both fat and protein are added to the carbohydrate given in the first few days.

There is no set standard for his feeding; it must be adapted to his individual needs. In general he does not tolerate cow's milk unless the fat and protein content has been altered. If possible, he should be given breast milk, though it may be necessary to dilute it with water. The mother may be able to provide breast milk. If so, it should be expressed manually and given to the infant. The supply is thereby maintained, and the infant may be put on the breast when he is able to suck and swallow adequately.

Mention has been made of breast milk stations where human milk can be bought (see p. 172). Such milk is expensive, however, and it may be difficult to secure a steady supply. Often mothers on the obstetrical unit who have an overabundance of milk will donate the excess to the premature infants in the nursery.

The formula for the premature should be high in protein, low in fat, and of average carbohydrate content. Proprietary or prepared milks which resemble breast milk in composition are often used.

Methods of Feeding. The method of feeding is extremely important, since there is danger that the infant may aspirate a little of the milk and also since no formula is of advantage unless it is taken and retained. The infant takes so little milk at a feeding that it is generally ordered in cubic centimeters or milliliters rather than ounces. The selection of the proper nipple for the size and strength of the premature is important. The warmed feedings are given slowly in small amounts and at frequent intervals. The infant is bubbled frequently. He should never be forced to take the feeding. Underfeeding is less harmful than overfeeding. When feeding a premature in an incubator, he should be held in a semisitting position and placed on his right side when he is finished. He should not be permitted to suck longer than 20 minutes at a feeding because he may become too fatigued.

A fixed schedule or an occasional missed feeding may be indicated for weak infants or those whose condition is complicated by vomiting, convulsions, cyanosis, or hemorrhage. For an older premature who is gaining weight, a flexible schedule is advantageous.

TOTAL INTRAVENOUS ALIMENTATION. When feeding by mouth is impossible for an extended period of time, total intravenous alimentation may be necessary (see p. 436). By this method sufficient fluid, electrolytes, calories, and vitamins may be given to sustain growth. This

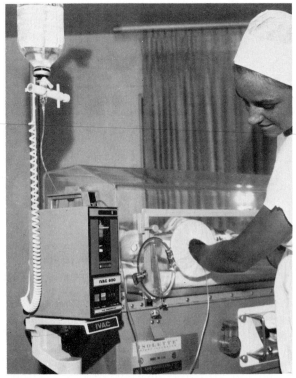

FIGURE 9–8. I.V. volume pump, which provides precise control of fluid and drug infusions down to 1 ml. per hour. (Courtesy of the IVAC Corporation.)

method of feeding is not without danger. Complications of intravenous alimentation include sepsis, thrombosis, dislodgment of the catheter, and metabolic complications. Continuous chemical and physiologic monitoring of infants receiving intravenous alimentation is essential to prevent these complications.

GAVAGE. The infant who is unable to suck or swallow or who becomes fatigued with the effort of nursing or is apt to become cyanotic after feeding by bottle or medicine dropper should be fed by gavage. An indwelling catheter may be used for the infant who cannot suck or swallow. If necessary, mummy restraint may be used (see p. 412). Research has shown that gavage feedings cause physiologic cardiorespiratory changes in the infant.

For gavage feeding the following equipment is needed: (1) a sterile plastic catheter, no. 5 to 8 French, with a rounded end, (2) the barrel of a glass syringe (sterile), (3) medicine glasses (sterile), (4) sterile water, (5) the warmed formula.

The method of *gavage feeding with an indwelling catheter* (generally inserted by the physician) is as follows:

1. Measure the distance from the bridge of the

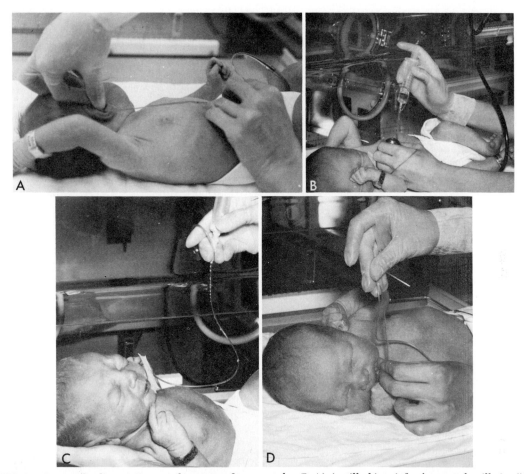

FIGURE 9-9. Gavage feeding. A, Proper placement of gavage tube. B, Air instilled into infant's stomach will give "growling stomach" sound on auscultation and indicate proper tube placement. Air is then withdrawn. C, Infant is then placed in a slightly elevated position to aid flow of fluid by gravity. Graduated reservoir above infant's head, used to give feeding, is raised and lowered to alter rate. D, Tube is flushed with 1 or 2 ml. of water after feeding, pinched tightly, and then withdrawn. Sterile gloves are sometimes worn to handle distal end of tube to reduce chances of contamination. (Chinn, P. L., Am. J. Nurs. 71(10), 1971.)

nose to the lower end of the sternum, and place a mark on the catheter.

2. Lubricate the tube with water. Do not use oil, because of the danger of aspiration with subsequent lipoid pneumonia.

3. Insert the catheter through a nostril until the mark is reached.

4. Check for placement of the catheter in the stomach by placing the free end under sterile water in one of the three medicine glasses. If many bubbles rise and then cease, the catheter is in the stomach and the infant is relieved of air which might cause him to vomit during or after the feeding. Bubbles rising periodically, however, are caused by air expelled with each respiration, an indication that the catheter is in the trachea. The infant is then likely to choke and become cyanotic. The tube should be withdrawn at once and reinserted.

Another method to determine the location of the catheter in larger infants and children is by gently aspirating a small amount of stomach contents. This may not be possible in a premature who receives extremely small amounts at each feeding. Only slight

suction should be used because of the danger of traumatizing tissue at the end of the catheter. Actually, when gavaging a premature infant, it is relatively difficult to enter the trachea with a gavage tube; however, these tests should be done in order to prevent any possible error.

An additional method to determine the location of the catheter in larger infants and children is by the injection of a small amount of air into the catheter and listening with a stethoscope for its entrance into the stomach. This method should not generally be used for prematures because of the possibility of distention of the infant's stomach with air unless it is withdrawn.

5. When it is certain that the tube is in the stomach, it is taped to the infant's cheek.

6. The barrel of the syringe is connected to the catheter by means of a no. 20 needle, which acts as an adaptor.

7. The syringe is held 6 to 8 inches above the infant and the milk poured very slowly into the syringe barrel. No air should precede the milk, and no pressure is used. The milk flows into the infant's stomach by gravity.

8. After the feeding a small amount of sterile water is poured into the syringe to wash out the milk and prevent clogging of the catheter. In a very small infant the amount of sterile water to be used may be ordered by the physician, since overdistention of the stomach may result in vomiting.

9. When the syringe is empty, the catheter may or may not be occluded, depending on the physician's order. Some physicians believe that the tube should be left open, but elevated above the infant's body. If vomiting occurs, the tube acts as a safety valve so that the possibility of aspiration of vomitus is minimized. If the catheter is to be changed, it must be compressed while being withdrawn. This prevents milk from dripping into the pharynx and causing the infant to gag or aspirate it.

10. Place the infant on his right side with a blanket rolled behind him for support.

11. The catheter should be changed at least every four days. The use of an indwelling catheter for the purpose of gavage may cause local irritation of the upper gastrointestinal tract.

An indwelling catheter is usually thought to be a better procedure to use with small infants than the catheter which is inserted for each feeding; however, a judgment as to the advisability of using each method must be made for the individual premature infant.

Gavage feeding without an indwelling catheter differs in several respects from the foregoing procedure. A soft small catheter is passed through the mouth toward the back of the throat. Its location must be tested carefully. The catheter is held in place with the hand near the infant's mouth. The catheter is withdrawn after the feeding and during withdrawal is compressed firmly. Before withdrawal it is a good plan to run sterile water through the catheter at once to clear it of milk, and to avoid drippings which might be aspirated.

Gavage feedings without an indwelling catheter are done to decrease the irritation that an indwelling catheter may cause. Nurses in many critical care nurseries are responsible for carrying out this procedure.

Gastrostomies have been done as a method of feeding premature infants; however, their value has not been established.

FEEDING WITH A MEDICINE DROPPER. This method is used for small prematures who have a good swallowing reflex, but cannot suck with sufficient strength to draw the milk through the nipple or cannot swallow rhythmically as they suck. The tip of the medicine dropper is protected with a bit of soft tubing pulled well over the end of the glass dropper. The soft rubing is less irritating than glass to the delicate mucous membranes of the mouth, and also less dangerous should the tip break. The feeding is

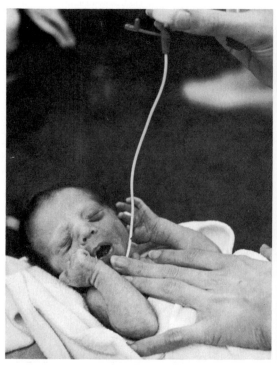

A

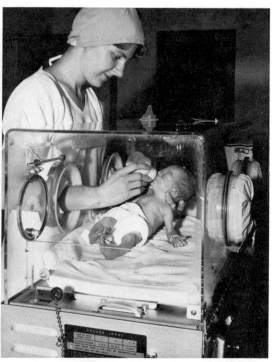

B

FIGURE 9–10. Feeding behavior in infants. *A*, Hand-mouth gestures and capacity to mouth feeding tube indicate that this premature infant will soon take feeding from nipple instead of tube. *B*, Infant contentedly takes feeding from nipple. (O'Grady, R. S., *Am. J. Nurs.* 71(4), 1971. Photographs: *A*, by Dominick; *B*, by Armstrong-Roberts.)

given a few drops at a time, with time allowed for the infant to swallow before the bulb is again compressed. If the infant becomes exhausted by this method, he should be fed by gavage until he is stronger.

The use of the Breck feeder, by which fluid is forced into the infant's mouth, is not safe since aspiration of the fluid into the lungs is a real possibility.

BOTTLE FEEDING. Bottle feeding is used with more mature prematures or those with an unusually strong sucking reflex (and adequate ability in swallowing) for their stage of development. There are special nipples on the market for small prematures. If these are not available, a regular nipple which is soft but not flabby may be used. The holes in the nipple should not be so small that the exertion of sucking tires the infant, nor too large, for he might not be able to swallow the milk which fills his mouth as he sucks and as a result might gag or aspirate it. Furthermore, the infant who drains the milk too easily is deprived of the natural satisfaction which sucking brings. The bottle should be held during the entire feeding. Infants large and strong enough to be fed from a bottle also need the closeness and cuddling a mother gives when feeding her child.

MEDICATIONS

Only those medications necessary for growth and health are considered here.

The premature infant's vitamin requirements are greater than those of the full-term infant, since his antenatal storage of vitamins is incomplete, his growth rate is greater, and the milk given him is small in amount and has been boiled (if he is not breast-fed), thereby reducing the vitamin C content. Defective fat absorption reduces the utilization of such fat-soluble vitamins as he receives in his formula. In general he requires 50 mg. a day of vitamin C (this is started as soon as he receives a formula) and 1000 units a day of vitamin D, which is given him within two weeks after birth.

Iron must be added to his intake by about six weeks of age, but may be given earlier with the hope that he can utilize it if his hemoglobin level is under 8 gm. or if he has lost blood. Iron should be included in proprietary infant formulas given to prematures.

PREVENTION OF INFECTION

Gastrointestinal Infections. Infections of the gastrointestinal tract are common in premature infants and are most likely to be caused by contaminated feeding equipment.

Skin Infections. Infections can find entrance through slight trauma to the skin. Some skin infections are transmitted by contact; such infections are likely to be transmitted from infant to infant, if equipment is shared in common or if the nurses fail to wash their hands thoroughly after care of each infant. Skin infections may also be contracted from linen not sterilized before use.

BATHING THE INFANT. The incidence of staphylococcal epidemics in nurseries can be reduced through the use of hexachlorophene in soap or solution form. Recent research has shown, however, that hexachlorophene can be absorbed through the skin (see p. 163) and may cause brain damage. For this reason soap solution without hexachlorophene may be used according to the policy of the agency (unless the physician specifically orders that hexachlorophene be used if infection is present). In bathing the premature the nurse should wet the hands, take one teaspoonful of soap solution and work it into a lather. The lather should be applied over all the baby's body, cleansing the diaper area last. The nurse should be careful not to get any into the infant's eyes. The lather should then be removed with sterile cotton and water and the infant patted dry with a soft towel.

Respiratory Infections. Organisms that cause respiratory infections are likely to be carried to an infant by the personnel who care for him. The staff caring for prematures should keep their hands clean by washing thoroughly, and should wear gowns and possibly caps. In some hospitals masks are also required, but in others are considered unnecessary, except when the nurse is doing sterile procedures. A mask should never be used for the purpose of allowing a person having a respiratory infection to enter the nursery.

Organisms causing respiratory infections may be carried by the air from infant to infant. For these reasons each infant should be in strict isolation, and any infant showing signs of a respiratory infection should be removed from the nursery.

In the majority of hospitals airborne organisms are prevented from drifting into the premature nursery, when the door is opened, by an antechamber between the main hall and the nursery.

General Suggestions for Prevention of Infection. No nurse should ever touch a premature without thoroughly cleaning the fingernails and washing the hands and arms to the elbow with ample soap, if this is the policy of the agency, and running water. Rings and watches must never be worn in the nursery.

Each infant should have his own equipment.

All other equipment used for the infants and for their examination should be kept in the nursery, and traffic there should be at a minimum.

Supplies such as linens, blankets, and cotton should be sterile when brought into the nursery and as far as possible sterile when used in the care of the infants. The outer wrapping of all such equipment should be removed before being brought to the nursery, in an area set aside for the purpose.

Nurses caring for a premature infant who exhibits evidence of infection must not care for the well prematures in the nursery.

There should be no dry dusting or sweeping in the nursery. A damp mopping should be done daily with a clean mop, hot water, and a cleansing powder. The daily dusting should be done with a damp cloth.

Treatment of Infections. The premature infant has an unpredictable response to many antibiotics. Doses of medication suitable for full-term infants can cause untoward reactions in a premature who cannot detoxify or excrete them at a rate expected for his size. More research must be done to determine effective yet safe dosages for these infants in order to prevent deaths from toxic levels of drugs.

Diseases of the Premature Infant

The ability to observe and describe symptoms so that the physician has an accurate and reliable account of an infant's symptoms and behavior is one of the chief distinguishing characteristics of the professional nurse. *Important among the observations which a nurse should make of the premature infant are (1) nature of the cry, respirations, color, activity, condition of the skin and umbilicus, and bladder and bowel function; (2) stability of body temperature under slight variations of external environmental conditions; (3) response to feedings in relation to the method used, the swallowing and sucking reflexes, the amount taken and retained, and the activity of the infant during feeding; (4) symptoms of unfavorable response to the environment; (5) symptoms of illness, knowledge of which is necessary to the physician's diagnosis and treatment, especially of serious conditions likely to occur in the premature.*

Retrolental fibroplasia

Incidence. Retrolental fibroplasia is the chief cause of neonatal blindness and has replaced ophthalmia neonatorum as the most common cause of blindness in children. The condition was diagnosed and the cause discovered within the last several decades. The condition is peculiar to infants under 1500 gm. in weight and of gestational age of six to seven months, thus it occurs in the smaller, less mature infants more frequently than in the larger and more fully developed prematures. The condition involves both eyes and may produce complete or almost complete blindness. The effects are not immediately apparent, but can be detected by the physician when the infant is several weeks or months of age.

Etiology. The cause of this condition is related to the pO$_2$ of the premature infant's blood rather than to the specific atmospheric concentration of oxygen in his environment. The normal oxygen tension of the blood is about 100 mm. Hg. If the infant breathes 40 per cent oxygen, the blood oxygen tension is usually 140 to 150 mm. When the infant receives oxygen and responds well, the partial pressures of oxygen in the arterial blood should be monitored and kept at or below 100 mm. The oxygen acts upon the primitive vasculature of the eyes. A high concentration of oxygen causes spasm of the retinal vessels; this leads to exudation of blood and serum through the walls of these vessels.

Pathology. The retinal veins dilate and become tortuous. There is hemorrhage with exudate into the retina, and finally separation of the retina from the inner surface of the eye occurs. Some of these changes may regress, but in other instances they continue until the retina detaches and floats forward in the eye. Eventually the retina may become atrophic, a completely detached and useless fibrotic mass (Fig. 9–11). Some light perception may be present, but the child has no useful vision. Glaucoma may occur in the late stage of the disease, and corneal opacities may result.

Diagnosis. Routine ophthalmoscopic examinations of premature infants should be made so that the condition may be detected early. Such examinations should be begun in the nursery.

Prevention. Oxygen therapy should be given only when an infant is in immediate need of oxygen, and then only in the lowest concentration which will satisfy his need. The concentration should never exceed 40 per cent unless it is needed as a lifesaving measure. Even in this situation oxygen should be discontinued as soon as possible. Physicians order oxygen by concentration rather than by rate of flow. The nurse must check the oxygen concentration in the incubator and adjust the flow so that it does not exceed 40 per cent unless ordered. This requires that an accurate oxygen analyzer be part of the standard equipment of every nursery (see Fig. 9–7).

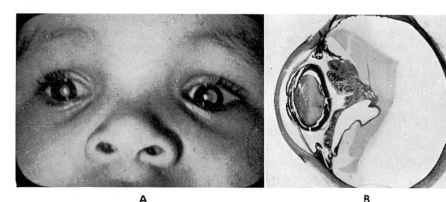

FIGURE 9–11. Retrolental fibroplasia. *A,* Photograph of eyes of an infant to show the complete white opacification of the tissues behind the pupil. This is the end-stage of retrolental fibroplasia. *B,* Sagittal section of an eye removed from this child. One sees the entire retina detached and pulled forward toward the lens and a band of scar tissue encircling the posterior aspect of the lens. The whole disorganized mass makes up the retrolental eschar. (From the collection of Dr. Arnall Patz, Baltimore.)

Frequent analysis of oxygen concentration is necessary even if oxygen-limiting devices are used on the incubator.

If the infant's condition is such that he should have a higher oxygen concentration, the exact concentration should be ordered by the physician and not given on the judgment of the nurse, except in dire emergency (the pediatric staff may be asked for routine orders to cover such emergencies). Frequent determinations of blood gases must be done on infants receiving oxygen concentrations over 40 per cent.

There is no obvious contraindication to the use of oxygen therapy in infants over 5 pounds, but such infants seldom need it, since their respiratory and circulatory systems are more completely developed.

RESPIRATORY CONDITIONS

Respiratory distress in the newborn may be due to a number of causes, but for a better understanding of the nursing problems of these infants two main groups of pathologic conditions which seriously interfere with normal respiration will be considered. (1) Failure of the respiratory center of the central nervous system may be due to anoxia, intracranial hemorrhage, anomaly, trauma, or narcosis. (2) The second group includes peripheral respiratory difficulty (alveolar exchange of oxygen and carbon dioxide) due to atelectasis, respiratory distress syndrome, pneumonia, or aspiration pneumonia. Conditions not discussed in this chapter are treated elsewhere (see Index).

ANOXIA OF THE NEWBORN

Types, Incidence, and Etiology. Anoxia of the newborn is a condition in which his organs, especially the brain, receive much less oxygen than they need for optimum functioning. Anoxia is not a clinical entity in itself. Some of its causes are known, but others have not yet been identified. Anoxia is an important cause of perinatal death or lasting damage to the tissue of the central nervous system. Cerebral palsy may result or mental retardation be evident later in life.

Fetal anoxia may be due to any cause which limits the oxygen supplied by way of the maternal and fetal circulations from reaching the brain of the fetus. Causes include systemic conditions of the mother such as poor oxygenation of the blood due to cardiac failure or low blood pressure. Anoxia may also be caused by conditions of the uterus and the placenta which impede the maternal-fetal circulation or by physical obstruction to adequate circulation due to a knot or kink in the umbilical cord.

Postnatal anoxia may be due to any cause which limits the supply of oxygen or renders the cells unable to use the oxygen available. This is the case, for example, if an overdose of barbiturates has been given. During severe shock, oxygen is not sent to the cells in adequate amounts. Even obstruction of the air passages by mucus may drastically diminish the supply of oxygen reaching the brain. Lasting causes of anoxia include severe anemia due to hemorrhage or hemolytic disease, poorly oxygenated blood due to a cyanotic type of congenital heart disease, or inadequate pulmonary ventilation due to malformation of the lungs.

Clinical Manifestations. It is extremely important that the nurse know the signs of both fetal anoxia and anoxia in the newborn. Fetal anoxia is evidenced by an increase in activity of the fetus followed by diminution. The fetal heart beat slows and weakens. When fetal anoxia is present, the infant is delivered immediately in order to save his life.

Symptoms of anoxia in the newborn include signs of yellow, meconium-stained amniotic fluid and yellowish vernix caseosa, pallor or cyanosis (even duskiness of the skin), lack of muscle tone, and variable heart beat.

Treatment. The treatment depends upon the stage of the anoxia and the cause of the condition. Mechanical techniques include mouth-to-mouth insufflation, administration of oxygen by moderate pressure (20 to 30 cm. of water for less than 0.2 second) or through an intratracheal catheter, and the use of "seesaw" respirators. Artificial respiration is of no value unless some expansion of the lungs has taken place. Nalorphine hydrochloride (Nalline) may be given intravenously to reverse respiratory depression due to narcotics given to the mother.

The method of mouth-to-mouth *artificial respiration* for infants and small children advocated by the American Red Cross is as follows:

Clear the child's mouth of any foreign matter.

Place the child on his back, and use the middle finger of each hand to lift the lower jaw from beneath and behind so that it juts out. Hold the jaw in that position with one hand. Place your mouth over the child's mouth and nose, making a reasonably leakproof seal, and breathe into the child smoothly and steadily until you observe the chest rise. As you start this action, move your free hand to the child's abdomen, between the navel and the ribs. Apply continuous moderate pressure to the abdomen to prevent the stomach from filling with air. When the lungs are inflated, remove your lips from the child's mouth and nose and allow the lungs to empty. Repeat this cycle, keeping one hand beneath the jaw and the other hand pressing on the stomach at all times.

Inflation of the lungs with oxygen or air can also be accomplished by the use of well fitting bag-mask devices. The lungs should be inflated rapidly (at a rate normal for the age of the child) between each three to four cardiac compressions.

If cardiac resuscitation is necessary in small infants, cardiac output can be effectively produced by applying firm pressure over the middle third of the sternum. In larger infants and small children the pressure must be applied with the heel of the right hand over the sternum, opposite the fourth interspace. The pressure is applied for large children by placing the heel of the left hand over the right hand in order to provide strength from both arms and shoulders. In all instances the vertebral column must be firmly supported. In infants the usual rate is 100 compressions per minute, in children about 80 per minute.

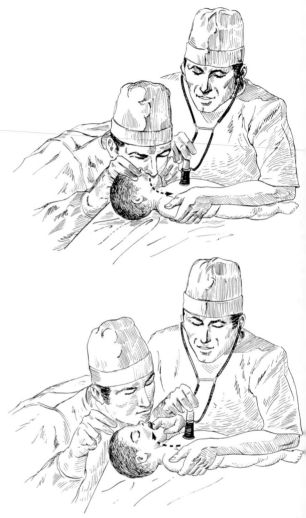

FIGURE 9–12. Mouth-to-mouth insufflation. *A*, Air is breathed into the infant's lungs. *B*, The lungs are allowed to empty. The stethoscope is placed over the abdomen in order to determine whether air is being forced into the stomach.

Nurses should develop skill in carrying out the procedures of artificial respiration and external cardiac massage.

Infants with respiratory distress should be wrapped in a warm blanket or placed in an incubator. Aspiration to remove mucus from the throat is a routine procedure.

Responsibilities of the nurse are the same as for the newborn having atelectasis (see below).

Prevention. Preventive measures applying to the management of labor include reduction of analgesia and anesthesia and administration of oxygen during the second stage of labor. Preventive measures applying to the care of the infant include maintenance of an open airway, administration of oxygen as needed, provision of skin stimulation, and keeping the infant warm.

ATELECTASIS

The lungs are collapsed in fetal life, and the fetus receives oxygen through the maternal circulation. After birth, with the infant's first breath, the lungs normally expand to a variable degree. It may be days or weeks before full expansion takes place.

Atelectasis—collapse or imperfect expansion of lung tissue which carries air—is found in greater or less degree in almost all infants dying soon after delivery. The condition may be either primary or secondary. In *primary* atelectasis the alveoli fail to expand initially. This is common in premature infants and in full-term infants who have suffered brain injury. In *secondary* atelectasis the alveoli collapse after they have once been expanded by air; this may occur when the infant has pulmonary disease.

Clinical Manifestations. The symptoms are irregular, rapid, shallow respirations accompanied by a respiratory grunt and flaring of the nostrils. The skin is mottled. Cyanosis may be persistent or intermittent; it decreases if the infant cries or is given oxygen. There are intercostal and suprasternal retractions. Fine rales may be heard. On auscultation of the chest poor respiratory exchange is evident. X-ray films reveal increased density which may be present throughout both lungs.

Treatment. By bronchoscopy the physician determines whether any obstruction is present and removes it if possible. Oxygen may be given so that the open areas of the lungs will have a sufficient supply. The environmental humidity is raised in order that secretions may be liquefied. Caffeine and sodium benzoate may be given intramuscularly. The infant's skin may be stimulated in order to induce crying. His position may be changed every hour or two to provide opportunity for collapsed areas to expand. Antibiotics are given for persistent atelectasis in order to prevent secondary infections. The fundamental treatment is directed toward the underlying condition.

Course, Prognosis, and Prevention. The *course* is difficult to predict. Even with early diagnosis and treatment the *prognosis* is poor and death not infrequent. *Prevention* of atelectasis in the infant includes prenatal care of the mother. Premature labor or a difficult delivery in which intracranial hemorrhage occurs is the cause in many cases. Fetal or neonatal anoxia is evidently a predisposing factor, as are pneumonia and respiratory distress syndrome.

Responsibilities of the Nurse. The nurse should keep in mind the infants who are likely to have atelectasis, such as those who were born prematurely or by cesarean section, those whose mothers had problems during pregnancy, and those who have had intracranial injury or are sick from pneumonia or other respiratory conditions. The nurse must observe these infants closely to detect the first symptoms of distress and also to give an accurate description of their condition to the physician. These infants should be kept warm, preferably in incubators where oxygen can easily be given and the humidity raised. It may be necessary to aspirate the upper respiratory tract if the infant's nose and throat appear to be clogged with mucus. The physician may also order aspiration of the gastric contents in order to prevent aspiration of vomitus should vomiting occur. The infant must be fed slowly and with great care, and the physician may order gavage feedings. All possible measures to prevent abdominal distention must be taken.

The nursing care should be planned so that the infant is disturbed as little as possible; there is more than the usual need for gentle handling. Every precaution should be taken to prevent infection, since even a simple respiratory infection may prove fatal.

IDIOPATHIC RESPIRATORY DISTRESS SYNDROME (PULMONARY HYALINE MEMBRANE DISEASE)

Incidence. This condition is found in about 50 per cent of premature infants who die within a few days after birth. It seldom occurs in full-term infants, but may develop in infants whose mothers have diabetes or in infants delivered by cesarean section.

Etiology. In the normal fetus the majority of the venous blood goes from the venous to the arterial circulation by way of the ductus arteriosus and the foramen ovale without passing through the lungs. When breathing begins, the high vascular resistance present in the fetal lung is reduced and pulmonary blood flow is increased.

In hyaline membrane disease pulmonary vascular resistance remains high. Pressure on the venous side of the circulation causes blood to be shunted to the arterial side without going through the lungs. Respiratory distress and cyanosis result. Carbon dioxide tension rises and the pH of the blood drops.

Resuscitation efforts frequently result in chilling the newborn because of his lack of insulating body fat, small energy reserve, and low thermal stability. The combined effect of the increased carbon dioxide tension, the lowered pH of the blood, and chilling results in vasoconstriction of the pulmonary arterioles leading to hypoperfusion of the lungs and shunting of blood past the lungs. Atelectasis may also add to the problem.

The respiratory distress syndrome may also be explained etiologically as due to an overactivity of the sympathetic nervous system in response to the stress of hypoxia and hypercapnia leading to the typical symptoms of this condition.

A surface-tension-reducing film of lipoprotein, surfactin, is normally present in the alveoli. If there is a deficiency of this substance due to an inhibiting substance derived from inhaled amniotic fluid or from damaged pulmonary tissue, the lungs will not be able to function and the respiratory distress syndrome or hyaline membrane disease will result.

Pathology. The lungs are liver-like in consistency and a deep purplish-red in color. Atelectasis is present, and the alveoli and respiratory bronchioles are lined with membranes. Amniotic substances, pneumonia, hemorrhage, and interstitial emphysema may be present.

Clinical Manifestations. Many of these infants required resuscitation at birth. Clinical manifestations of the respiratory distress syndrome include rapid, shallow respirations up to 60 or more per minute within two hours after birth, intercostal retractions, a respiratory grunt, cyanosis, and increasing evidence of air hunger and fatigue due to increased respiratory efforts.

Course and Prognosis. Death may occur in a few hours. In milder forms of the condition the symptoms increase for three days, and then improvement begins. If recovery occurs, the prognosis is usually good. The mortality rate is increased among infants born before term.

Prevention. Factors in the prevention of the respiratory distress syndrome include the prevention of prematurity, optimum care of the diabetic mother, and the avoidance of cesarean sections if at all possible. Other preventive measures include the avoidance of maternal hypoxia, systemic hypotension, and acidemia; reduction of the newborn's pulmonary vasoconstriction; reduction of intervals of diminished umbilical blood flow; and avoidance of chilling and hypoxia.

Treatment, Complications, and Responsibilities of the Nurse. Since the basic problem is inadequate pulmonary exchange of oxygen and carbon dioxide leading to metabolic acidosis, treatment consists in avoiding chilling the infant and in the administration of oxygen and a buffer. Intravenous feedings including a buffer solution, calories, and fluid may be given to prevent fatigue from oral feedings. Mechanical assistance in breathing may be necessary and can best be carried out in an intensive care nursery (see p. 75).

The abdominal skin temperature of the infant should be kept between 96.8 and 98.6° F. (36 and 37° C.). Temperature control can be maintained by means of special thermoregulating equipment controlled by a thermistor taped to the skin of the abdomen. If no such equipment is available, an incubator should be used and the temperature kept between 89.6 and 93.2° F. (32 and 34° C.) with a relative humidity of 80 to 90 per cent. When special thermoregulating equipment is used, a relative humidity of 30 to 60 per cent is adequate. If proper humidification is available, nebulized water mist is usually not necessary and may be dangerous if too much water is inhaled.

The oxygen and carbon dioxide tension and the pH of arterial and capillary blood must be monitored periodically. Arterial oxygen tension, carbon dioxide tension and pH may be measured in blood drawn from the temporal artery or from an indwelling plastic catheter in one of the umbilical arteries threaded to just above the bifurcation of the aorta. Care must be taken that the infant does not suffer anemia due to the frequent withdrawal of blood. If anemia does develop, replacement of blood may be necessary. The umbilical arterial catheter may also be utilized for the administration of drugs and fluids.

When the infant is receiving oxygen, periodic measurements of the level of oxygen in the inspired air must be made in order to prevent retrolental fibroplasia (see p. 200). The oxygen tension of the infant's arterial blood should be between 60 and 100 mm. Hg when assisted ventilation is used.

Assisted ventilation may be provided through the intermittent use of a mask and bag resuscitator at intervals adapted to the needs of the individual newborn. A patient-cycled positive-pressure respirator with an endotracheal tube in place, a head hood, a face mask, or nasal prongs may also be used (see Fig. 9–6). Such devices may cause trauma or oxygen toxicity to the lungs.

Continuous positive airway pressure (CPAP) through the tube is useful during spontaneous respirations to increase positive end-expiratory pressure. It provides a means of reducing atelectasis, increasing lung volume, and improving arterial oxygenation in newborns having respiratory distress syndrome. *Continuous negative pressure* (CNP) reduces the air pressure surrounding the lung and thorax. CNP and oxygen are more therapeutic than increasing oxygen alone in improving oxygenation. *Positive end-expiratory pressure* (PEEP) or *continuous positive pressure ventilation* (CPPV) also increases end-expiratory transpulmonary pressure during artificial ventilation.

Monitoring of aortic blood pressure and central venous pressure may give a guide in managing the shock which may occur soon after the birth of a premature infant.

Some physicians order antibiotic therapy for these infants because of the possibility of infection, particularly pneumonia.

A serious complication resulting from nasotracheal intubation is cardiac arrest while intubating or suctioning. Other local complications may occur and can be reduced through the use of polyvinyl endotracheal tubes that do not contain tin, which is toxic to cells, the use of the smallest tube that is practical, the reduction in the amount of vigorous moving, suctioning or changing of the tube, and avoidance of infection by extreme cleanliness of equipment and personnel. If an anesthetic gas mask is used, care must be taken that the infant's eyes and skin are not injured because of pressure.

Serious complications may occur as a result of catheterization of the umbilical artery. These include reflex arterial spasm, blockage of a smaller artery leading to gangrene of the area supplied by the vessel, hemorrhage, and thrombi. An umbilical arterial or venous catheter should be removed as soon as possible.

Intensive care of infants having hyaline membrane disease as well as other high-risk newborn infants reduces their mortality. Optimum working relations between members of the medical and nursing teams are essential.

OTHER CONDITIONS

NECROTIZING ENTEROCOLITIS

Necrotizing or ischemic enterocolitis is a very serious, life-threatening, idiopathic condition diagnosed with increasing frequency in premature infants. This illness had previously been termed perforation of the ileum and colon, colitis, or "functional ileus."

Symptoms of necrotizing enterocolitis include retention of gastric contents, distention of the abdomen, vomiting of blood-streaked bile, and possibly diarrhea. Primarily, the ileum and colon are involved pathologically, being dilated, necrotic with superficial ulcerations, and submucosal hemorrhages. Perforation occurs commonly.

Necrotizing enterocolitis may occur because of decreased blood flow to the bowel, a complication of a severe infection or of an exchange transfusion. It has also been shown to occur in newborns who are fed an artificial formula and not breast milk. Mothers who are unable to breast feed their infants may be able to obtain a supply of breast milk from other mothers or from a breast milk bank (see p. 172).

On x-ray examination the small intestine shows multiple dilated and separated loops with air-fluid levels in the upright position, intramural gas, air in the peritoneum, and gas in the portal vein.

Treatment includes giving nothing by mouth but involves intravenous alimentation and hydration, blood transfusions, gastric suction, and antibiotic therapy. Arterial oxygenation must be maintained. If the intestine perforates or there is evidence of peritonitis, surgery is necessary. The gangrenous or perforated portions of the bowel are removed.

Responsibilities of the Nurse. The alert nurse may be the first to observe early symptoms of necrotizing enterocolitis, which include lethargy, temperature instability, bilious vomiting, abdominal distention, bloody stools, and apnea leading to hypoxia. The nurse's role in the care of such an infant is the nursing care given to any acutely ill newborn plus measurement of the degree of abdominal distention, checking for bowel signs, and reporting of signs of distress. Since the bowel is so fragile, the nurse should avoid lifting the infant to prevent pressure on the abdominal wall. For this reason also diapers should not be placed on the infant. Since diarrhea is a symptom of this illness, the rectal and adjacent areas should be kept clean and dry to avoid irritation to the skin. Ointments having a zinc oxide base may be used on the skin, especially when the diarrhea is watery.

If surgery becomes necessary, immediate postoperative care includes stabilizing all body systems and caring for the ileostomy or colostomy in order to maintain skin integrity (see Fig. 9–13). Karaya powder may be sprinkled around the stoma for this purpose. Later, when oral feedings are begun, careful feeding techniques must be utilized. Reestablishment of intestinal continuity may be done when the infant can tolerate oral feedings and his general health has improved.

The nurse is responsible for listening to the shocked parents when they are told of the diagnosis and for providing realistic information concerning the infant's condition. As soon as possible the parents are encouraged to assist in caring for their infant, socializing, and providing love for him. When the infant is moved to the intermediate nursery from the intensive care nursery, the parents have concrete evidence of improvement in the infant's condition. Following discharge the infant will need long-term special care, especially if he has an ostomy. Although the parents learned the care of the infant from the nurse while he was in the nursery, they may receive additional support in caring for their infant from parents who also have had an infant with this condition.

VOMITING

The most common causes of vomiting are overfeeding or too rapid feeding. The prevention, therefore, is reduction of the intake and slow feeding. If the infant's condition permits his being held for his feeding, he may be bubbled several times during the feeding and before he is put back in his incubator. Abdominal distention not only causes vomiting but also hinders respiration because of elevation of the diaphragm. Congenital malformation of the esophagus hampers the swallowing of milk, and that taken into the mouth is ejected. Increased intracranial pressure is a serious cause of vomiting, which may be projectile.

The nurse should chart not only the amount, color and nature of the feeding vomited but also the conditions under which vomiting occurred. This will aid the physician in his diagnosis and may also indicate defective feeding technique on the part of the nurse which could be corrected.

DIARRHEA

A premature infant normally has four or five stools a day. Increased frequency or loose stools are serious in the premature, since he needs all the nutriment of his feeding for metabolism and growth; also he cannot easily tolerate excessive fluid loss. Because of the low tolerance of his gastrointestinal tract for fat, the fat content of his feeding may be the cause of the diarrhea, or overfeeding may be responsible.

Diarrhea in infancy may occur with either an enteral or parenteral infection. The physician should be notified at once and the infant placed on strict isolation so that the infection—if that is the cause of the diarrhea—is not transmitted to other infants in the nursery. Vomiting often accompanies diarrhea and should be carefully observed and charted, since these observations will help the physician in making his diagnosis and planning therapy. Diarrhea can cause death of the premature infant quickly, and therefore immediate therapy is necessary.

DEHYDRATION

Dehydration is more important in infancy than in childhood and even more serious in the premature than in the normal infant. In the premature, dehydration is certain to follow an inadequate fluid intake. It has already been noted that diarrhea and vomiting cause dehydration.

JAUNDICE

Jaundice in the premature, as in the full-term infant, may be physiologic, that is, due to bilirubinemia in the early postnatal period. The current treatment of *physiologic jaundice* or *hyperbilirubinemia* is phototherapy or the use of lamps which are positioned over the infant's bassinet or incubator (see p. 240). Since there is no full explanation of the way in which such light effects bilirubin metabolism, nor of any adverse immediate or long-term effects to the infant, this method of treatment is used in the therapy of specific babies, not as a preventive measure routinely.

The infant who is to receive phototherapy is completely undressed and placed in either his Isolette or bassinet. His eyes are closed and immediately covered to prevent corneal damage and ulceration. Eye shields may be made or purchased for this purpose. The infant may be removed from the light and have his eye shields removed for feeding. Because the amount of light used in this treatment produces heat, the newborn's temperature should be taken every four hours in order to check for any elevation of temperature. The newborn may have loose, bright green stools, may have a rash, and may show alterations in his pattern of activity as a result of this treatment. After phototherapy has been discontinued, rebound elevations of bilirubin concentration may occur.

Physiologic jaundice is of no great importance, but jaundice which persists or becomes excessive is indicative of some serious condition, such as erythroblastosis fetalis, congenital anomaly or obstruction of the bile ducts, congenital toxoplasmosis, cytomegalic inclusion disease, syphilis, or septicemia. The nursing care is that of the condition causing the jaundice.

PALLOR

Pallor accompanies shock and hemorrhage. It is often seen in infants who fail to breathe at birth and may be a symptom of intracranial injury.

CONVULSIONS

One reason why premature infants should be under constant observation is the danger of convulsions. The accompanying anoxia and stress threaten his welfare. A description of the convulsion may assist the physician to arrive at a diagnosis and correct the cause if correction is possible. A convulsion may be a symptom of intracranial hemorrhage or of a congenital cerebral defect, or may be the result of prolonged anoxia. It may be caused by hypoglycemia or hypocalcemia or an overwhelming bacteremia.

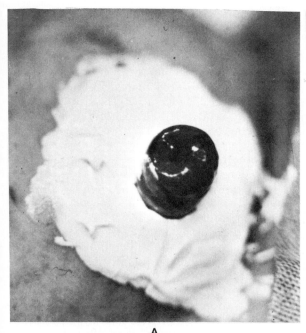

A

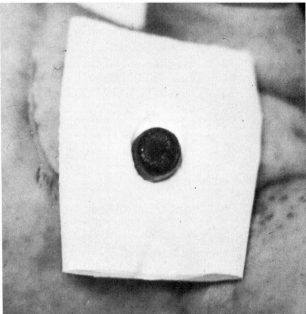

B

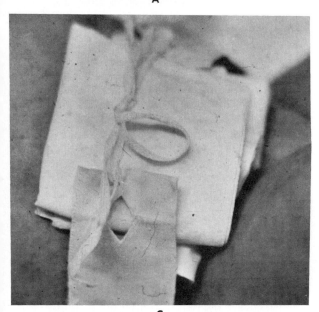

C

FIGURE 9–13. Dressing to prevent skin breakdown in the infant who has a stoma. *A*, To form a water-repellent layer, zinc oxide ointment is applied to the skin starting at the edge of the stoma and working outward. *B*, Next a facial tissue, folded four times and cut to fit around the stoma, is placed over the zinc oxide ointment to absorb the drainage from the stoma before it reaches the skin. *C*, Another folded tissue, which acts as a nonirritating absorbent pad, is placed directly over the stoma, and the whole dressing is secured with Montgomery straps. (From Bishop, W. S., and Head, J. J.: *The American Journal of Maternal Child Nursing*, 1:315, September–October, 1976.)

INFECTIONS OF THE NEWBORN

See Chapter 11.

Prognosis in Prematurity

The premature's chances of survival are much less than those of the full-term infant. About half of all deaths in the first month of life occur in infants classified as prematures. The smaller the infant, the less are his chances of survival. About half of the deaths in the premature group occur on the first day of life.

Causes of Death. Immaturity itself is the fundamental cause of the high death rate among premature infants. Only a small number of those who weigh less than 1000 gm. survive. Respiratory failure is responsible for many deaths. Birth injury such as intracranial hemorrhage with resulting damage to brain tissue may cause immediate death. Congenital malformations may make vital physiologic functions impossible. Infection, as already noted, is far more likely to be fatal to the premature than to the full-term infant, since the premature can neither combat the infection nor withstand its systemic effects. Also, the cause of the prematurity, if known, may affect the ultimate prognosis.

Factors Favoring Survival. Favorable prognostic signs in the premature are a birth weight of more than 1500 gm., good muscle tone and normal respiratory activity. If the infant is not cyanotic and exhibits an active response to stimulation, his immediate condition is likely to be good. When the gag and swallowing reflexes are present, he will be able to take his feedings with less danger of aspirating fluid. The importance of stabilization of body temperature has been shown. Absence of other serious conditions is additionally hopeful.

Parental Problems Due to Prematurity

The birth of a premature infant presents a crisis for the family. Usually, unless the mother has expected a multiple birth and knows that the infants may be premature, she has no warning and is therefore not prepared for the event and more anxious than the mother of a full-term infant. After a fast trip to the hospital following the onset of labor, she is usually treated with some degree of apprehension and is rushed to the delivery room to give birth to her infant without anesthesia. If a cesarean section becomes necessary, the mother may have anesthesia and therefore not be aware of her infant's birth.

The mother may or may not see her infant before he is placed in the incubator. If she does see him, his unattractive appearance may startle her. Both mother and father should be prepared for the appearance of their premature prior to

seeing him. They should be assured of the method used to identify their infant so that no mistakes can be made at the time of discharge from the hospital.

Although the parents may have many questions after the birth, physicians and nurses often avoid answering them directly because they do not want to arouse either false hope or despair. The parents may sense the air of suspense concerning the infant's condition, with resulting anxiety and fear. Furthermore, when the mother is ready for discharge, she must leave her frail infant in the nursery until he weighs 5 or 5½ pounds. This may mean separation from the parents for weeks or months.

Nurses must be aware of certain behavior that suggests future parent-child relationship disturbance: parents who are unable to express feelings of fear, anxiety, or guilt, even to each other, who do not try to secure information about the infant and when they do, misinterpret it, or who are unable to accept help from family, friends, or community services even when offered.

As with other crisis situations, parents should be helped to confront their problem realistically instead of trying to pretend that it does not exist. Ways to help such parents include the physician's discussing frankly the infant's condition with them, having both parents speak of their fears for the infant, and having nurses who understand the degree of guilt and anxiety such parents feel. The nurses who care for the mother should be informed about the infant's progress or condition and help the parents to understand

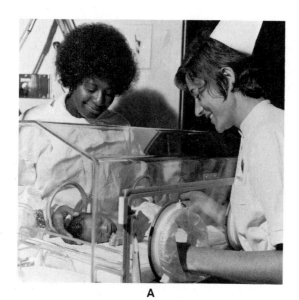

A

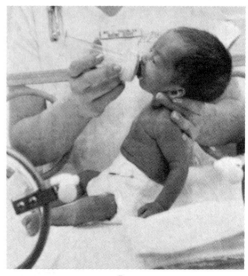

B

FIGURE 9–14. The premature is almost ready for discharge. *A*, The mother gradually gains confidence in caring for her premature child. *B*, A photograph of the premature baby is taken for the siblings. If it might be too threatening because of the infant's appearance or the equipment in use, a standard picture, such as this, is shown to them. (*A*, from Warrick, L. H., *Am. J. Nurs.*, 71:11, 1971. *B*, Photograph courtesy of Ross Laboratories.)

the routines of premature care. Also, friends can function in a beneficial way if they are willing to help with necessary tasks and if, instead of sending the usual "get well" cards, they send wishes that indicate their concern for the infant's survival.

The mother who is told realistically what chances for life her infant has may not be comforted, nor is she necessarily made less anxious, but she is probably less frightened about the future than the mother who is afraid to ask the question, "Will my baby live?"

Many mothers of premature infants try to blame someone or something for this unfortunate event, even though the real cause of the prematurity may not be known. An individual mother may blame an older child because he asked to be lifted up, her husband because he did not carry the groceries or the laundry for her, or the physician or the nurse for some imagined failure in therapy. The process of blaming is one way to avoid facing the truth and does not contribute to coming out of this crisis strengthened.

If the infant dies, the nurse should expect responses of grief and loss because the parents may actually mourn the loss of the healthy infant they anticipated (see p. 106). The parents should be helped to mourn and not merely be told that they should forget about him and have another child. Unfortunately such advice has been too freely given.

Every effort should be made to have the parents see their infant early, after assessing and validating their desire to do so, in order to preserve the parent-child relationship despite this separation. The role of the nurse in this situation is to have both parents feel comfortable in caring for their infant: to touch or talk to him through the portholes of the incubator, to rock him in a rocking chair, and to feed or give him other care when possible. Contact with their newborn helps to prevent the parents' developing a feeling of estrangement later on. Any feelings of guilt, anger, or rejection may interfere with their ability to care for their child.

Parents need encouragement in learning to handle a small, delicate infant when they visit him in the nursery, although by the time he is discharged he is almost the size of a normal newborn. In many hospitals areas are set aside where parents can attend demonstrations of the care of the infant, including bathing, dressing, methods of formula preparation and feeding techniques. As they practice these techniques, they gain confidence in their own abilities and have less anxiety over the infant's care.

The nurse should also emphasize the protective care of the infant in the home environment, stressing principles of safety and hygiene throughout all the teaching. Anticipatory counseling about the infant's probable growth and development even though the physician will also follow the child's growth in the future should be given.

If the mother is a clinic patient whose infant will be followed up by a community or public health nurse and will attend the Child Health Conference, she should meet the nurse who will visit her home and should be made familiar with the help which will be given her. The public health nurse should visit the home before the infant's discharge to evaluate the setting and to make suggestions as to how conditions may be improved for the infant's welfare. The nurse should make suggestions as to his physical environment, including the equipment needed in his care, and should evaluate the mother's feelings about the infant.

The public health nurse should also visit the family after the infant's discharge from the hospital in order to give necessary guidance and assistance. After discharge the public health nurse or the clinic nurse is responsible for assessing family interaction and parenting behavior toward the infant, as well as screening to determine whether the infant is developing as expected.

Mothers in the middle class have probably read a great deal about premature infants and may have studied their characteristics and care in classes on child development. These mothers understand the theory of premature care, but need help in putting it into practice. Since they are not likely to be clinic patients and to receive the routine help of a public health nurse, they are in even greater need of an opportunity to care for the infant while he is still in the hospital.

Mothers of premature infants often worry for fear that the infant will not develop normally and will be mentally retarded, frail, and small. This is not wholly so, and the nurse may tell the mother that studies of children born prematurely show that by and large they develop more rapidly than infants born at term, and that if age were dated from the time of conception rather than from birth, prematures are frequently on a par with infants born at term. Any lag in development of the premature in comparison with term infants tends to decrease with age and at the end of several years to become indistinguishable.

In early infancy the premature may appear backward in motor control, less so in sensory acuity, but still not up to the level of the normal infant. Prematurity does not influence intelligence, but emotional and social behavior is likely to be less mature than in children born at term. Some premature infants tend to develop undesirable behavior patterns. They may be overdependent and are likely to be negativistic. This is largely due to the overprotective attitude of his parents in infancy and to later pressure upon him to catch up with other children of his age. He is confused by the change of attitude and finds it difficult to adjust to the new demands made upon him.

Probably helping the mother to feel secure in her ability to care for the premature is the most important factor in forming good mother-child relations. If such a relation exists, a mother is not afraid to correct the child. She should let the child experience the minimal frustrations that occur in daily life and develop early independence.

PLACENTAL DYSFUNCTION SYNDROME

Incidence and Etiology. About 80 per cent of infants having placental dysfunction syndrome are premature infants or those born of elderly primigravida or toxemic mothers or those mothers with small or poorly attached placentas. The other 20 per cent of infants having this syndrome are postmature. In this condition the placenta does not function adequately in the nutritional and oxygen exchange between mother and fetus. As a result the fetus does not grow properly.

Clinical Manifestations. Evidences of fetal distress appear as a result of oxygen lack *in utero*. The vernix, umbilical cord, skin, and nails absorb bile pigment from the released meconium. In mild degrees the nails and vernix are stained green. In more severe forms they are stained bright yellow. In infants who do not live, lanugo hairs and evidences of meconium can be found in the finer branches of the bronchial tree, probably due to the vigorous respiratory efforts of the fetus resulting from hypoxia.

Treatment and **nursing care** of these infants center on their respiratory difficulties.

Prognosis. If the newborn lives for the first 48 hours, his chances for survival are good.

POSTMATURITY

The infant who remains in the uterus from one to three weeks or more after the expected date of delivery, in other words, beyond 43 weeks or 300 days of gestation, is classified as *postmature*. Postmaturity is difficult to diagnose because it is based on the questionable date of the mother's last menstrual period. About 5 per cent of newborn infants are born postmaturely. Recent research suggests that the causative factor of postmaturity may be a relative adrenocortical insufficiency.

Characteristics of Postmature Infants. The postmature infant has the behavior and appearance of an infant from one to three weeks of age. He is more mature, mentally alert and thinner (owing to recent weight loss) than the normal newborn infant. His nails and scalp hair are longer than those of a full-term infant, and he has no lanugo or vernix caseosa on his skin. His skin may be peeling and appear to have the consistency of parchment. These infants generally do not exceed 23 inches (57.5 cm.) in length.

Very large infants, such as those of diabetic mothers, are not products of prolonged gestation, but are the result of an abnormally rapid rate of growth before term.

Treatment. Labor may be induced before the cervix is soft, but such treatment may pose a greater risk than postmaturity. Cesarean section may be done on older women having their first infants, especially if the fetus shows signs of distress.

Prognosis. Among infants born three or more weeks after the expected date the mortality rate is likely to be two to three times greater than that among infants born at term.

TEACHING AIDS AND OTHER INFORMATION*

American Foundation for the Blind, Inc.

Chase, J. B.: Retrolental Fibroplasia and Autistic Symptomatology: An Investigation Into Some Relationships Among Neonatal, Environmental, Developmental and Affective Variables in Blind Prematures, 1972.

Froyd, H. E.: Counseling Families of Severely Visually Handicapped Children.

Johnson & Johnson

Klaus, M. H., Leger, T., and Trause, M. A. (Eds.): Maternal Attachment and Mothering Disorders: A Round Table, 1975.

*Complete addresses are given in the Appendix.

The National Easter Seal Society

Allied Health Approaches to Program Planning for Infants at Risk, 1974.
Battle, C. U., and Ackerman, N.: Early Identification and Intervention Programs for Infants with Developmental Delay and Their Families, 1973.

Public Affairs Committee

Brody, J. E., and Engquist, R.: Women and Smoking.

Ross Laboratories

Barness, L. A.: On Developmental Nutrition: Fat, 1972.
Iatrogenic Problems in Neonatal Intensive Care, 1976.
Necrotizing Enterocolitis in the Newborn Infant, 1975.

Perinatology—Neonatology—Pediatric Nutrition—Currents, 1976.
Your Premature Infant.

United States Government

A Study of Infant Mortality from Linked Records by Birth Weight, Period of Gestation, and Other Variables, United States, 1972.
Projects for Intensive Care: New Hope for the Newborn, 1975.
Respiratory Diseases: Task Force Report on Problems, Research Approaches, Needs, 1973.
Trends in "Prematurity," United States 1950-1967, 1972.
Your Premature Baby.
Projects for Intensive Infant Care—U. S., 1974.

REFERENCES

Books

Abramson, H. (Ed.): *Resuscitation of the Newborn Infant and Related Emergency Procedures in the Perinatal Center Special Care Nursery.* 3rd ed. St. Louis, The C. V. Mosby Company, 1973.
Aladjem, S., and Brown, A. K. (Eds.): *Clinical Perinatology.* St. Louis, The C. V. Mosby Company, 1974.
Avery, M. E., and Fletcher, B. D.: *The Lung and Its Disorders in the Newborn Infant.* 3rd ed. Philadelphia, W. B. Saunders Company, 1974.
Avery, G. B. (Ed.): *Neonatology: Pathophysiology and Management of the Newborn.* Philadelphia, J. B. Lippincott Company, 1975.
Behrman, R. E. (Ed.): *Neonatology: Diseases of the Fetus and Infant.* St. Louis, The C. V. Mosby Company, 1973.
Catzel, P.: *A Short Textbook of Paediatrics.* Philadelphia, J. B. Lippincott Company, 1976.
Cockburn, F., and Drillien, C. M. (Eds.): *Neonatal Medicine.* Philadelphia, J. B. Lippincott Company, 1975.
Feldman, S., and Ellis, H.: *Principles of Resuscitation.* 2nd ed. Philadelphia, J. B. Lippincott Company, 1975.
Harper, R. G., and Yoon, J. J.: Handbook of Neonatology. Chicago, Year Book Medical Publishers, Inc., 1974.
Klaus, M. H., and Fanaroff, A. A.: *Care of the High-Risk Neonate.* Philadelphia, W. B. Saunders Company, 1973.
Korones, S. B.: *High Risk Newborn Infants: The Basis for Intensive Care.* 2nd ed. St. Louis, The C. V. Mosby Company, 1976.
Lubchenco, L. O.: *The Infant of Low Birth Weight.* Philadelphia, W. B. Saunders Company, 1976.
MacGillivray, I., Corney, G., and Nylander, P. P. S.: *Human Multiple Reproduction.* Philadelphia, W. B. Saunders Company, 1975.
Scarpelli, E. M., and Auld, P. A. M. (Eds.): *Pulmonary Physiology of the Fetus, Newborn and Child.* Philadelphia, Lea & Febiger, 1975.
Winters, R. W., and Hasselmeyer, E. G. (Eds.): *Intravenous Nutrition in High-Risk Infants.* New York, John Wiley & Sons, Inc., 1975.

Periodicals

Affonso, D., and Harris, T.: CPAP... Continuous Positive Airway Pressure. *Am. J. Nursing,* 76:570, April 1976.
Ahlström, H., Jonson, B., and Svenningsen, N. W.: Continuous Positive Airways Pressure Treatment by a Face Chamber in Idiopathic Respiratory Distress Syndrome. *Arch. Dis. Child,* 51:13, January 1976.
Anderson, G. C.: A Preliminary Report: Severe Respiratory Distress in Transitional Newborn Lambs with Recovery Following Nonnutritive Sucking. *J. Nurse Midwife,* 20:20, Summer 1975.

Auld, P. A. M.: Resuscitation of the Newborn Infant. *Am. J. Nursing,* 74:68, January 1974.
Bishop, W. S., and Head, J. J.: Care of the Infant with a Stoma. *The American Journal of Maternal-Child Nursing,* 1:315, September–October 1976.
Blennow, G., Svenningsen, N. W., and Almquist, B.: Noise Levels in Infant Incubators (Adverse Effects?). *Pediatrics,* 53:29, January 1974.
Bliss, V. J.: Nursing Care for Infants with Neonatal Necrotizing Enterocolitis. *The American Journal of Maternal-Child Nursing,* 1:37, January-February 1976.
Boros, S. J., and Reynolds, J. W.: Hyaline Membrane Disease Treated with Early Nasal End-Expiratory Pressure: One Year's Experience. *Pediatrics,* 56:218, August 1975.
Brown, E. G., Krouskop, R. W., McDonnell, F. E., and Sweet, A. Y.: Blood Volume and Blood Pressure in Infants with Respiratory Distress. Part 2. *J. Pediatr.,* 87:1133, December 1975.
Chamorro, I. L., Davis, M. L., Green, D., and Kramer, M.: Development of an Instrument to Measure Premature Infant Behavior and Caretaker Activities: Time-Sampling Methodology. *Nursing Research,* 22:300, July-August 1973.
Colle, E., et al.: Insulin Responses During Catch-Up Growth of Infants Who Were Small for Gestational Age. *Pediatrics,* 57:363, March 1976.
Cranley, M. S.: When a High-Risk Infant is Born. *Am. J. Nursing,* 75:1696, October, 1975.
Deonna, T., Payot, M., Probst, A., and Prod'hom, L. S.: Neonatal Intracranial Hemorrhage in Premature Infants. *Pediatrics,* 56:1056, December 1975.
Dinwiddie, R., et al.: Quality of Survival After Artificial Ventilation of the Newborn. *Arch. Dis. Child,* 49:703, September 1974.
DuBois, D. R.: Indications of an Unhealthy Relationship Between Parents and Premature Infant. *Nursing Digest,* 4:56, Fall 1976.
Gabriel, M., Albani, M., and Schulte, F. J.: Apneic Spells and Sleep States in Preterm Infants. *Pediatrics,* 57:142, January 1976.
Galet, S., and Schulman, H. M.: The Postnatal Hypotransferrinemia of Early Preterm Newborn Infants. *Pediatr. Res.,* 10:118, February 1976.
Galloway, K. G.: The Uncertainty and Stress of High-Risk Pregnancy. *The American Journal of Maternal-Child Nursing,* 1:294, September-October 1976.
Johnson, M., and Gash, J.: Transport of Neonates—A Matter of Prevention. *The Canadian Nurse,* 72:19, May 1976.
Jung, A. L., and Thomas, G. K.: Stricture of the Nasal Vestibule: A Complication of Nasotracheal Intubation in Newborn Infants. *J. Pediatr.,* 85:412, September 1974.
Korner, A. F., Kraemer, H. C., Haffner, E., and Cosper, L.

M.: Effects of Waterbed Flotation on Premature Infants: A Pilot Study. *Pediatrics*, 56:361, September 1975.

Kramer, L. I., and Pierpont, M. E.: Rocking Waterbeds and Auditory Stimuli to Enhance Growth of Preterm Infants. *J. Pediatr.*, 88:297, February 1976.

Miller, H. C., and Hassanein, K.: Maternal Factors in Fetally Malnourished Black Newborn Infants. *Am. J. Obstet. Gynecol.*, 118:62, January 1, 1974.

Mockrin, L. D., and Bancalari, E. H.: Early Versus Delayed Initiation of Continuous Negative Pressure in Infants with Hyaline Membrane Disease. *J. Pediatr.*, 87:596, October 1975.

Myers, M. S.: Mature or Immature: Assessing Gestational Age. *RN*, 38:22, January 1975.

Nwosu, U. C., Wallach, E. E., Boggs, T. R., and Bongiovanni, A. M.: Possible Adrenocortical Insufficiency in Postmature Neonates. *Am. J. Obstet. Gynecol.*, 122:969, August 15, 1975.

Omer, M. I. A., Robson, E., and Neligan, G. A.: Can Initial Resuscitation of Preterm Babies Reduce the Death Rate From Hyaline Membrane Disease? *Arch. Dis. Child*, 49:219, March 1974.

Ostrea, E. M., and Schuman, H.: The Role of the Pediatric Nurse Practitioner in a Neonatal Unit. *Nursing Digest*, 4:8, March-April 1976.

Rubin, R. A., Rosenblatt, C., and Balow, B.: Psychological and Educational Sequelae of Prematurity. *Pediatrics*, 52:352, September 1973.

Stern, L.: The Use and Misuse of Oxygen in the Newborn Infant. *Nursing Clin. N. Amer.*, 20:447, May 1973.

Stocks, J., and Godfrey, S.: The Role of Artificial Ventilation, Oxygen, and CPAP in the Pathogenesis of Lung Damage in Neonates: Assessment by Serial Measurements of Lung Function. *Pediatrics*, 57:352, March 1976.

Van Caillie, M., and Powell, G. K.: Nasoduodenal Versus Nasogastric Feeding in the Very Low Birthweight Infant. *Pediatrics*, 56:1065, December 1975.

Wittner, D.: Life or Death. *Today's Health*, 52:48, March 1974.

Yashiro, K., Adams, F. H., Emmanouilides, G. C., and Mickey, M. R.: Preliminary Studies on the Thermal Environment of Low-Birth-Weight Infants. *J. Pediatr.*, 82:991, June 1973.

Zaslow, S.: New Touches in Caring for Preemies. *RN*, 39:31, February 1976.

AUDIOVISUAL MEDIA*

The American Journal of Nursing Company

Maternity Nursing Class

15 44 minute classes, 16mm film or videotape, audio-tape cassettes, sound, color or black and white.

Premature Infant—The causes of prematurity are discussed. Shows care of an infant at premature center and demonstrates nursing care of the premature infant in Isolette. Explains the causes of premature mortality; stresses implications for nursing care.

Resuscitation of the Newborn

25 minutes, color.

The essential principles involved in the resuscitation of infants who do not breathe, or whose respiration is impaired at birth. Procedures and equipment shown in actual resuscitations and through animated drawings.

American Lung Association

Smoking Can Affect the Two of You.

Poster—colors, 8½ x 11.

Startling but touching drawing of unborn child still in the womb.

Charles Press–Prentice-Hall, Inc.

Pediatrics: Newborn Respiratory Tract

25 35mm slides, 11 overhead transparencies, guide.

A step-by-step comparison of the newborn and adult respiratory tracts for nurses, respiratory therapists, and advanced students of pulmonary anatomy.

Health Sciences Communication Center, Case Western Reserve University

The Neurological Evaluation of the Maturity of Newborn Infants

32 minutes, 16mm film or videocassette, sound, color.

This program has been designed for teaching the Tison method of neonatal neurological examination. The demonstration includes the examination of a full term newborn infant, and four neonates ranging in gestational age from 30 to 38 weeks. The Amiel-Tison charts are sent with each film.

The Use of Nasal CPAP

21 minutes, 16mm film or videocassette, sound, color.

This film describes the detailed technique for administering nasal continuous positive airway pressure to the infant with respiratory distress syndrome, reviews the background and indications for CPAP, and discusses general basic treatment of the infant with RDS.

McGraw-Hill Book Company

The Normal Premature Infant

Ritz, A. and Dickason, E.

16mm film, Super-8mm filmloop, sound, color, guide.

Characteristics of the Premature Infant

Preparing for Admission of the Premature Infant

Daily Care of the Premature Infant

Gavage Feeding of the Premature Infant

Administering Medications to the Premature Infant

Intravenous Therapy for the Premature Infant

Educating the Parents of the Premature Infant

W. B. Saunders Company

Current Topics in Obstetrics and Gynecology

Director: Tyson, J. E.

Audio-cassette periodicals, approximately 1 hour in length.

A Perinatal Intensive Care Unit, Effer, S. B.

Pediatric Conferences with Sydney Gellis

Audio-cassette periodicals, approximately 1 hour in length.

Early Discharge from Hospital of Low Birth Weight Infants, Berg, R.

Fetal Development and Respiratory Distress, Gluck, L.

Treatment of Convulsions, Rabe, E. F.

Trainex Corporation

Cardiopulmonary Resuscitation of the Newborn

35mm filmstrip, audio-tape cassettes, 33 1/3 LP, color.

The major portion of the program is a comprehensive explanation of cardiopulmonary resuscitation, presented within the framework of an actual emergency filmed in a pediatrics intensive care unit. The scope of the material includes: indications for resuscitation; procedures for intubation and ventilation, external cardiac massage, and treatment of acidosis with bicarbonate; three adverse conditions that are often factors underlying cardiopulmonary arrest; and administration of medications for cardiac stimulation.

Gavage
35mm filmstrip, audio-tape cassettes, 33 1/3 LP, color.

This program focuses on the step-by-step procedure for two methods of gavage by gravity drainage: the funnel method, and variations in the procedure when a feeding bag is employed. Basic principles of administering medications through a nasogastric tube are also presented. Common problems and reactions of the patient to tube feeding are stressed, along with appropriate nursing intervention to enlist the patient's cooperation, assess his response, and avoid complication.

Management of Newborn Emergencies
Two 35mm filmstrip, audio-tape cassettes, 33 1/3 LP, color.

Both filmstrips feature actual case studies depicting clinical evaluations, diagnoses, medications, and procedures required to stabilize the stricken infant.

Respiratory Distress Syndrome in the Newborn
35mm filmstrip, audio-tape cassettes, 33 1/3 LP, color.

This program reviews the etiology and pathophysiology of respiratory distress syndrome in the newborn and details treatment and care of an infant with severe RDS. Included are comprehensive descriptions of signs and symptoms, the procedures for umbilical artery catheterization and oropharyngeal intubation of an infant, respiratory therapy and other supportive measures, and prevention of complications.

*Complete addresses are given in the Appendix.

Chapter Ten

THE IMPORTANCE OF HEREDITY AND ENVIRONMENT IN DISEASES OF CHILDREN

Whether a newborn or older child is healthy or has a hereditary or a congenital disease or anomaly depends on many factors, which can be grouped under the main headings of *heredity* and *environment*. These are discussed broadly in Chapter 2; however, the student must have a more specific knowledge of their influence in order to understand the causes of many of the diseases of children. This chapter is therefore a brief review of the theory of genetics and embryology learned earlier in the student's educational experience.

HEREDITY

The term *heredity* means the transmission of potential traits from the parents to their children. The life of each child begins with a ferti-

lized egg or *zygote* composed of cytoplasm and a nucleus. Within the nucleus there are genes on the chromosomes. Many defects found in children can be traced to abnormalities of the chromosomes and genes; however, even if the components of the zygote are normal, a child may have abnormalities due to an injurious *environment in utero*.

Chromosomes are threadlike structures which carry the genes. In the human being each sperm and each egg carries a set of 23 chromosomes, 22 of which are somatic chromosomes, numbered from 1 to 22 in order of decreasing size, plus one sex chromosome. After the egg and the sperm have united at conception, the fertilized egg contains 44 autosomes (22 pairs) and two sex chromosomes. These chromosomes can be identified under the microscope by their shape. Each chromosome in the egg can be matched with one in the sperm cell except for those that determine the sex of the individual. These consist of two large X chromosomes in the female and one large X and a smaller Y chromosome in the male.

Although male cells differ from normal female cells in their complement of sex chromosomes, they also show a visible difference in the interphase cells. A mass of chromatin in the nuclei of some cells, namely nerve cells, epithelial cells, and polymorphonuclear leukocytes, is called the sex chromatin or *Barr body*. The Barr body is found in the tissues of females and only rarely in males. The most convenient way to study this sex chromatin is by an examination of the epithelium of the buccal mucosa by doing a buccal smear.

The *karyotype* shows the chromosome constitution of the normal human somatic cell or a photographic representation of the human chromosomes arranged in pairs or groups in the order of descending size or position of the centromere or constricted area which joins the two chromatids of any metaphase chromosome.

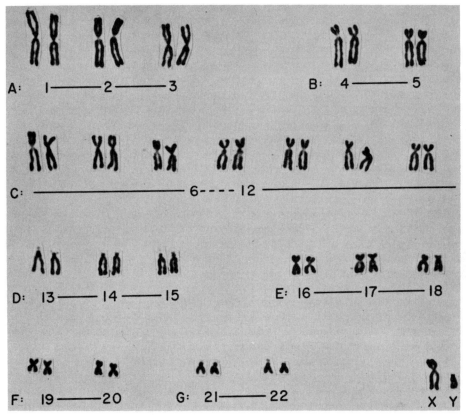

FIGURE 10–1. The cell most often used in study of the mitotic chromosome is the small lymphocyte of peripheral blood. After 72 to 96 hours in a nutrient medium, cell growth is stopped in metaphase. A hypotonic solution is then applied to swell and separate the chromosomes. They are then stained, photographed, cut out, and arranged into seven groups according to chromosome length and centromere position (position at which arms meet). This orderly arrangement is called a karyotype. Shown here is a normal male karyotype. (From Wright, S. W.: in W. E. Nelson, V. C. Vaughan, and R. J. McKay (Eds.): *Textbook of Pediatrics*, 9th ed.)

Some persons have two populations of cells with different karyotypes derived from a single zygote. The alterations in the karyotypes are either numerical or structural. These persons are known as *chromosomal mosaics.* Clinically they may show findings intermediate between the normal and abnormal constitutions represented by the two groups of cells.

Chromosomes are composed of nucleic acid and protein. Chemically speaking, the genes within the chromosome are composed of nucleic acid, of the type known as deoxyribonucleic acid (DNA). *DNA* is now generally accepted as being the storehouse of genetic information. Some evidence seems to indicate that genes, the units of heredity, are actually segments of DNA and that possibly many thousands of genes exist in each DNA molecule. The structure of a DNA molecule is like a rope ladder which has been twisted around itself or is in the form of a double helix.

The genetic code is contained in DNA, which is in the chromosomes of the cell nucleus. Polypeptide synthesis takes place in the cyto-plasm, in association with small cytoplasmic organelles called ribosomes. The link between the DNA in the nucleus and the polypeptide in the cytoplasm is *RNA.* A molecule of RNA is similar to a molecule of DNA except that it is single-stranded, and contains ribose instead of deoxyribose and uracil (U) instead of thymine. There are three types of RNA: messenger RNA, which transmits genetic information from the DNA molecule to the cytoplasm; transfer RNA, acting as an adaptor which brings amino acids into place in the growing polypeptide chain; and ribosomal RNA, serving a nonspecific function in connection with the ribosomes.

Deoxyribonucleic acid plays an important role in determining hereditary characteristics. Each gene carries instruction about a particular trait or characteristic of the organism. Like the chromosomes, the genes are also paired. Genes at the same locus on a pair of homologous chromosomes are alleles (alternate forms of a gene). When both members of a pair of alleles are identical, the individual is *homozygous* (a homozygote); when two different alleles are present, the individual is *heterozygous* (a heterozygote or carrier). If different instructions are carried by a gene pair, the resulting trait can be determined by only one member of the pair. The gene that is the determinant is called *dominant*, and the one not expressed is the *recessive*.

In order to diagnose *autosomal dominant inheritance* in a family a trait must appear in every generation; i.e., the trait is passed by the affected parent to half his children. In any specific family the ratio of affected to normal children may not be exactly 1:1; however, on the average, half of the children will have the trait. Unaffected parents cannot transmit the trait to their children. This sort of inheritance is not sex-linked.

Examples of pathologic conditions discussed in this text which may be inherited as dominant traits include osteogenesis imperfecta, sicklemia, and thalassemia minor.

In a family having an *autosomal recessive inheritance* a trait appears only in the children, not in the parents or other relatives in a family. An autosomal recessive trait appears in a person who receives the recessive gene from both parents and thus is homozygous for it. In such a family of four children produced by two carrier parents, one child will be homozygous normal, two heterozygous normal, and one homozygous abnormal.

A carrier of a recessive gene can have affected children only if he or she marries a carrier. The risk that a carrier will marry another carrier is higher if he marries a close relative than if he marries outside his own family. Laws exist in the United States for the prohibition of marriage between relatives; however, they vary as to their definitions of types of familial relationships. The reason for these laws is to prevent like genes from coming together at the time of conception. This sort of inheritance is not sex-linked.

Pathologic conditions which may show autosomal recessive inheritance include Tay-Sachs disease, mucoviscidosis, galactosemia, phenylketonuria, sickle cell anemia, and thalassemia major. These clinical conditions may also result from genes which have undergone mutation.

Mutation causing abnormal gene development is a process which is not completely understood. *Mutation* means a fundamental change in the structure of a gene which results in the transmission of a trait different from that normally carried by the gene. Research has been done on high-energy radiation as one cause of mutations. Such radiation can come from cosmic rays, radium, x-rays, and isotopes. We do not know exactly how much radiation a human being can be exposed to safely. Heat and some chemicals have also been found to be mutagenic agents.

Mutations can change the genetic constitution of the child so that body function is changed. These have been termed *inborn errors of metabolism*. Such mutations produce biochemical disorders (resulting from a deficiency of an essential body chemical), which are evidenced in anomalies of metabolism. Many structures of the body can be affected. In some conditions only a single known enzyme is affected. In other conditions the defect has not yet been identified, so that it is classified by the deficiency of some normal product which should be present or by the

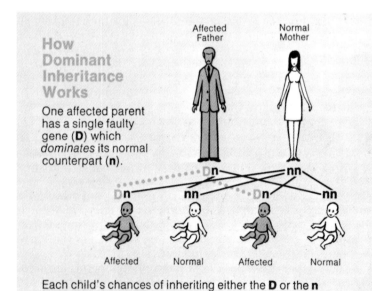

How
Dominant
Inheritance
Works

One affected parent has a single faulty gene (**D**) which *dominates* its normal counterpart (**n**).

Affected
Father

Normal
Mother

Dn   nn

Dn   nn   Dn   nn

Affected   Normal   Affected   Normal

Each child's chances of inheriting either the **D** or the **n** from the affected parent are 50%.

FIGURE 10–2. Inheritance of an autosomal dominant condition. (Courtesy of the National Foundation—March of Dimes, White Plains, N.Y.)

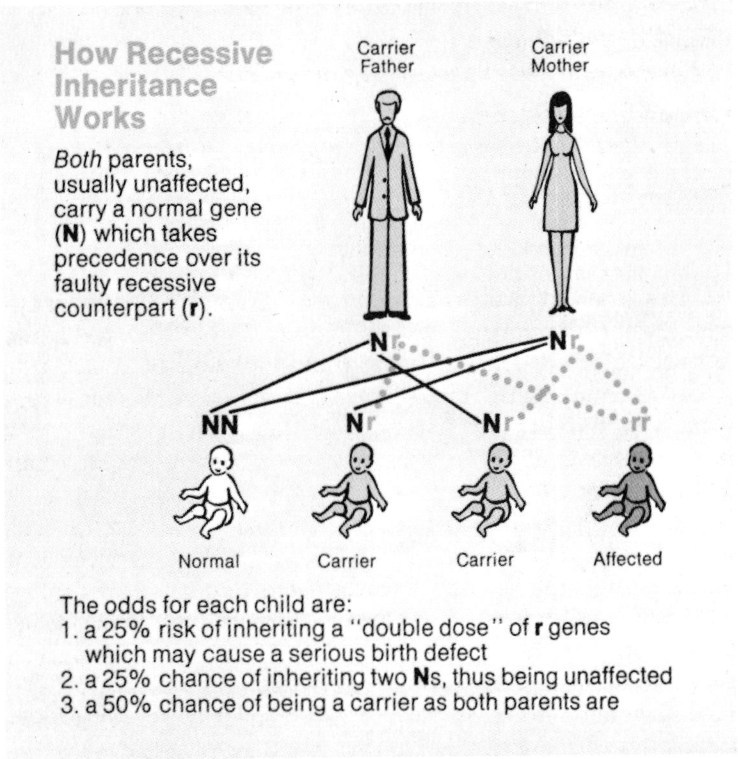

FIGURE 10-3. Inheritance of an autosomal recessive condition. (Courtesy of The National Foundation—March of Dimes, White Plains, N.Y.)

abnormal product which accumulates in the body.

Inborn errors of metabolism do not produce symptoms which can be recognized at birth. Examples of such conditions are agammaglobulinemia (a manifestation of a defect in plasma protein metabolism—immunoproteins) and phenylketonuria (a manifestation of a defect in metabolism and transport of an amino acid—phenylalanine). These conditions will be discussed in Chapter 15.

Certain characteristics such as color blindness and certain diseases such as hemophilia are sex-linked. As was mentioned above, in males the sex chromosomes are unequal in size, the X chromosome being large and the Y chromosome small. The X chromosome carries many genes. The Y chromosome is concerned only with maleness. The X chromosome of the male therefore has genes which are not matched with those of the Y chromosome. If a gene located in the X chromosome of the male is not normal, it can become evident even if it is recessive. Thus the trait is passed through an affected male to all his carrier daughters and on to half their sons. Fathers never transmit the trait directly to their sons. This is the reason why certain hereditary pathologic traits such as that for hemophilia A may be seen in the males of the family and only rarely in the females.

Some genes lead to congenital defects which are incompatible with life. These defects may cause death *in utero* or soon after birth.

Recently anomalies have been associated with abnormal size and configuration of chromosomes and abnormal chromosome counts rather than with alterations of specific genes. Normally before fertilization both ovum and sperm undergo a reduction division by which the cell separates into two parts, each one normally containing one member of each chromosome pair (haploid). Sometimes during cell formation two chromosomes fail to separate at cell division. The nucleus of one daughter cell has one more and the other one less than the normal number of chromosomes. This process is termed *nondisjunction*. If a defective haploid ovum is fertilized by a normal haploid sperm, or vice versa, the result is a new organism having either an excessive number of chromosomes (47) or a deficient number (45). When the chromosomal number is reduced to 45 by the absence of one of the sex chromosomes, the well-known gonadal dysgenesis or Turner's syndrome may occur. There is apparently no cause for most cases of nondisjunction; however, they seem to occur more often in the cells of older parents.

When an extra representative of any chromosome is present (*trisomy*), a number of abnormal traits characteristic of that chromosome will appear. When this germ cell unites with a normal one at the time of fertilization, the embryo that

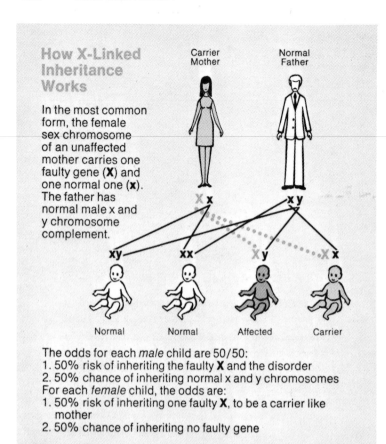

FIGURE 10–4. Inheritance of an X-linked condition. (Courtesy of The National Foundation–March of Dimes, White Plains, N.Y.)

results will have an abnormal chromosome count. If the embryo survives, it will have various congenital defects. Probably the best known example of trisomy is Down's syndrome (mongolism), in which there are usually 47 chromosomes, with an extra chromosome number 21. This condition may be called trisomy 21. A few children have this chromosomal material arranged not as a separate chromosome, but as a *translocation* of the long arm of the twenty-first chromosome onto either a chromosome of the D group (13–15) or another chromosome of the G group (21–22). (See Figures 12–23 and 12–24, page 308.)

Other conditions besides Down's syndrome are caused by chromosomal abnormalities. These are trisomy 18 (E-group syndrome) and the D group trisomy. Trisomy 18 is a syndrome of multiple congenital malformations, including those of the ears, hands, feet, and heart. These children are also mentally retarded and fail to thrive. Trisomy for a chromosome in the D group is less common and produces anomalies which are more severe than those in trisomy 18.

Partial trisomy or deletion of a portion of the short arm of a B (no. 5) group chromosome produces the group of anomalies called the cri

du chat syndrome because of the resemblance of the infant's cry to the mewing of a cat. These newborns have poor sucking reflexes and peculiarly formed faces. They fail to thrive physically and undergo severe mental retardation. (For further discussion of the care of the mentally retarded child, see page 696.)

With further research in this area more chromosomal defects are being found associated with clinical abnormalities.

ENVIRONMENT

The geneticist is intensely interested in the environment of the embryo and the fetus because it is difficult to distinguish between the influences of heredity and those of environment. Prenatal development takes place within the shelter of the uterus; however, various influences—infectious, endocrine, mechanical, nutritional, irradiation, and chemical agents—may affect the growing organism. The development of organ systems in the human fetus may be seen in Table 10–2 and Figure 10–5. When studying the congenital anomalies of the newborn, the student should learn to determine the ability of

TABLE 10–1. SOME HUMAN CHROMOSOMAL ABNORMALITIES

NAME	GENETIC FEATURES	CLINICAL ASPECTS
Turner's syndrome (gonadal dysgenesis)	XO	Short stature, streak ovary, juvenile female genitalia, poorly developed breasts
Klinefelter's syndrome	XXY	Gynecomastia, small testes
Triple X females	XXX	Two "Barr bodies" present, fairly normal females but secondary sex characteristics may be poorly developed
Down's syndrome	Trisomy 21	Epicanthal folds, protruding tongue, hypotonia, mental retardation
Trisomy 18	Trisomy 18	Mental retardation, multiple congenital malformations
D trisomy	Trisomy 15	Mental retardation, severe multiple anomalies, cleft palate, polydactyly, central nervous system defects, eye defects
Translocation mongolism	15/21, 21/22, or 21/21 translocation	Mongolism, clinically similar to trisomy 21
Philadelphia chromosome	Deletion of one arm of chromosome 21	Chronic granulocytic leukemia
Oral facial digital syndrome	Translocation of part of chromosome 6 to 1	Defects of upper lip, palate, and mouth, stubby toes with short nails
Cri du chat syndrome	Deletion of short arm of chromosome 15	Mental retardation, facial anomalies

From Page, E. W., Villee, C. A., and Villee, D. B.: *Human Reproduction.* 2nd ed., Philadelphia, W. B. Saunders Co., 1976.

each organ to function when the anomaly occurred.

The organism is most vulnerable to injury during the first trimester (*embryonic period*) of pregnancy, when the principal organ systems of the body are forming. During the *fetal period*, or the last six months of pregnancy, when the fetus is growing, injury may occur, but major anomalies do not result.

Infections such as rubella and toxoplasmosis among others may cause congenital anomalies in the embryo during the first trimester of pregnancy. Although rubella is usually a mild disease, the virus may penetrate the placental barrier and damage the developing embryonic tissue. It is important, therefore, that each woman should develop immunity to this disease before childbearing age. If the disease is not acquired naturally, rubella vaccine should be given to children of school age. Susceptible women should be given the vaccine when it is certain that they are not pregnant, i.e., immediately after the menstrual period. For legal reasons, some physicians have such women sign a statement that they are not pregnant at the time. Researchers are attempting to determine how long women should avoid conception following immunization. If a woman is not immune and contracts rubella in the first eight weeks of her pregnancy, the chance of her having a grossly defective infant is one in three or four. Problems associated with congenital rubella include car-

diac lesions, microcephaly, brain damage, eye disorders, and deafness.

Infections occurring later in the prenatal period produce clinical manifestations similar to those which would be seen after birth. The spirochete causing syphilis can infect a fetus before it is born. The mother should be adequately treated with penicillin before the birth of her child. Abnormal endocrine factors, such as exist in the diabetic mother, may influence the development of the embryo. Mechanical injury due to pressure from outside the mother's body may result in the death of the embryo or fetus. Positional defects due to pressure from the uterus or a portion of his own body may deform the jaw, face or legs of the growing organism.

The mother's nutritional state is important, since the fetus requires adequate nutrition. Without it, either death *in utero* or deformity may result. Experience with infants born in concentration camps and in areas where the level of living is down to little more than the maintenance level has shown the deleterious influence of poor maternal nutrition upon the fetus. Nevertheless the fetus tends to be nourished at the expense of the mother's body.

Irradiation of a pregnant woman's abdomen may cause malformations of the embryo, especially if it is done very early in the course of pregnancy. X-ray examination of the abdomen of any woman of childbearing age should be done

Text continued on page 224.

TABLE 10–2. DEVELOPMENT OF ORGAN SYSTEMS IN THE HUMAN FETUS

TIME (WKS)	RESPIRATORY TRACT	ERYTHROPOIETIC SYSTEM	LYMPHORETICULAR SYSTEM	KIDNEY	NERVOUS SYSTEM	GASTROINTESTINAL TRACT
2		Erythropoiesis begins. Primitive erythroid cell lines				
3	Lung buds present	"Blood islands" in yolk sac				Liver anlage seen
4	Right and left primary bronchi				Fore-, mid- and hind-brain present	Hepatic buds and ducts
5	Five main bronchi (3 right, 2 left)		Granulocytes appear	Metanephros begins to develop	Brain now has five regions. First reflex arc	Hepatic lobes recognizable
6		Definitive erythropoiesis in yolk sac and liver. Erythrocytes have Hb	IgG levels = 10% of adult values			
7	Dichotomous branching continues. Glands form and airway is lined with ciliated columnar epithelium (continues through twelfth week)		Lymphocytes seen in thymus	Nephrogenesis begins	Cerebral hemispheres develop	Gastric pits present
8		End of synthesis of primitive erythroid cells			Cerebellar rudiments begin. First recordable electrical activity	
10		Liver = major site of erythropoiesis, but gradually regresses	IgM synthesis detectable	Pelvis and calyces form. A.F. = 30 ml.	Medulla exerts some control over spinal cord	Glycogen and bilirubin synthesis begins in liver. Intestine capable of peristalsis and of absorbing glucose
12		Erythropoiesis in spleen begins	Fetal liver and G.I. tract can synthesize IgG	Glomeruli and prox. convol. tubules. Urine formed	Cerebral hemispheres cover diencephalon	Parietal cells and later chief cells
14		Begin gradual transition from Hb_F to Hb_A		Loop of Henle functional but short. 20% of nephrons mature	Some mesencephalic control	Bilirubin found in A.F. Liver can synthesize fatty acids

From Page, E. W., Villee, C. A., and Villee, D. B.: *Human Reproduction*, 2nd ed. Philadelphia, W. B. Saunders Co., 1976.

TIME (WKS)	RESPIRATORY TRACT	ERYTHROPOIETIC SYSTEM	LYMPHORETICULAR SYSTEM	KIDNEY	NERVOUS SYSTEM	GASTROINTESTINAL TRACT
16	Alveolar epithelial cells flatten			30% of nephrons mature		Mucus formed by epithelial cells of stomach
18			IgG synthesized by spleen			
20	Capillaries around potential air sacs proliferate	Erythropoiesis in bone marrow begins	Lymphoid tissue appears in spleen	350,000 nephrons. A.F. vol. = 350 ml.	Myelinization in brain-stem	
24	Alveolar cells start to make surfactant		IgG levels rise rapidly, reaching maternal values			
26					Beginning of alertness and neurovegetative behavior. Hypotonia. Rooting and incomplete Moro reflex	
28	Lungs capable of breathing air	Erythropoiesis in spleen ends; bone marrow becomes major site				
30					More muscle tone in legs and trunk. Pupillary light reflex. Moro reflex	
32		Erythropoietin formed				
35					Flexed limbs; firm grasp. Spont. orientation to light. Crossed ext. reflex incomplete	
40			Cord blood: IgM = 10% of adult, IgA = little or none. IgG = maternal origin primarily	A.F. vol = ca. 1000 ml. 830,000 nephrons	Myelinization reaches level of hemispheres. Crossed ext. reflex complete. Hypertonic upper and lower limbs	

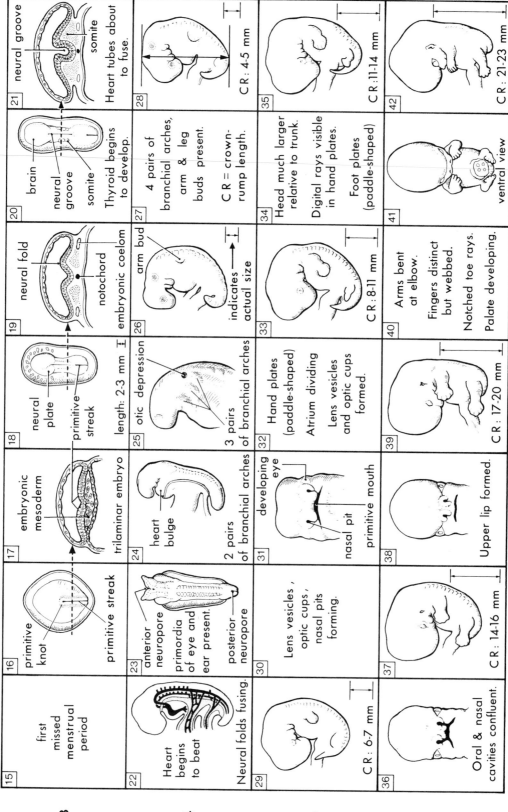

FIGURE 10-5. Maturation of a follicle containing a developing ovum (egg), ovulation and the menstrual cycle. Development begins at fertilization, about 14 days after the onset of the last menstruation. Cleavage of the zygote in the uterine tube, implantation of the blastocyst and early development of the embryo are also shown. (From Moore, K. L.: *Before We Are Born*, Revised Reprint. Philadelphia, W. B. Saunders Co., 1977.)

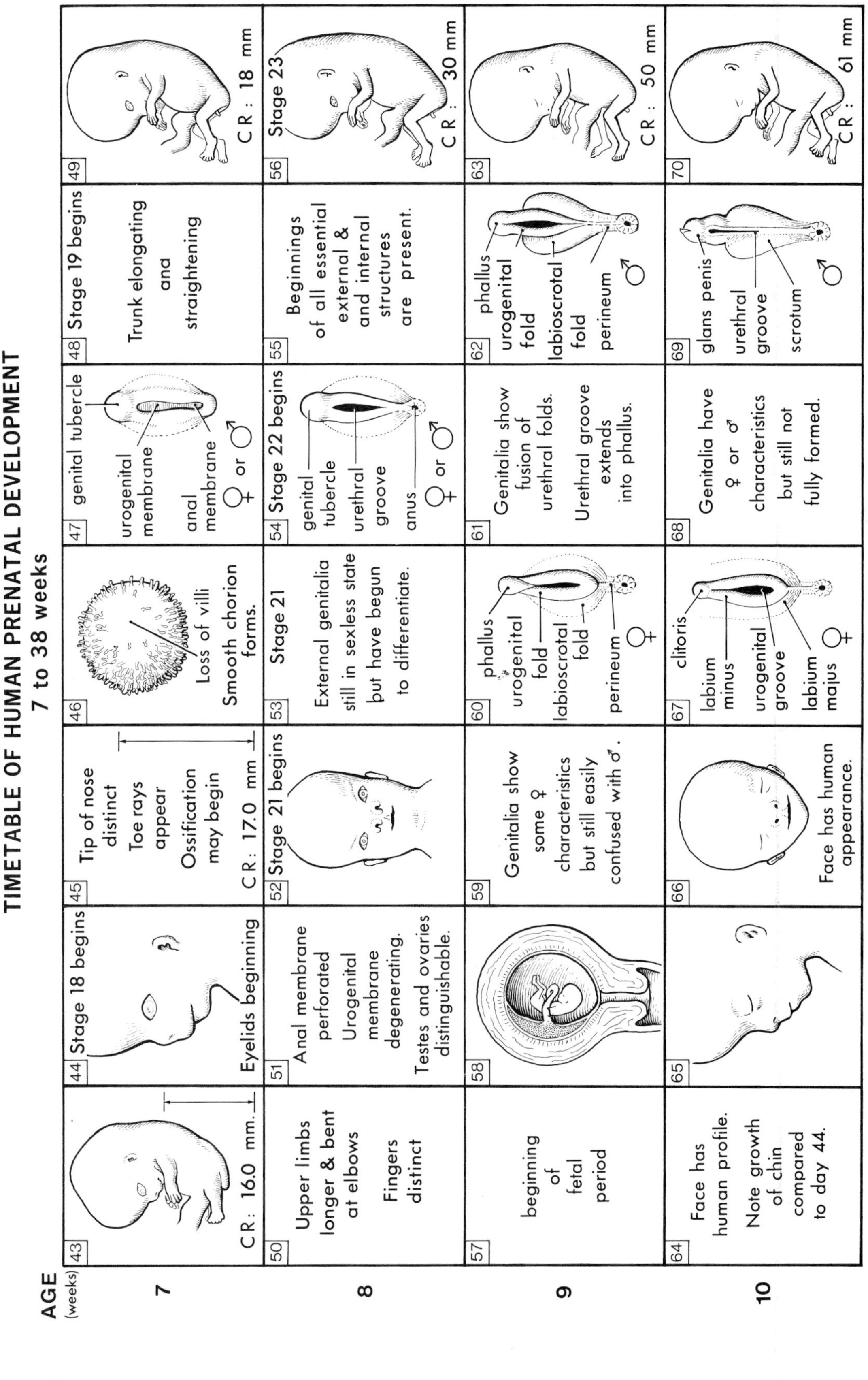

FIGURE 10–5 *Continued.*

only during the first two weeks after a regular menstrual period. Research is being done on the effect on the children of irradiation of fathers near the time of conception.

Injury to the fetus from the use of chemicals by the mother has had wide publicity. Drugs found to be teratogenic include thalidomide, which causes defects of the limbs mainly, but may also cause deformities of the heart, kidneys, and blood vessels. During the 1950's and 1960's women were given stilbestrol or related drugs during pregnancy to prevent miscarriages. As a result, many instances of vaginal and cervical adenocarcinoma have been found in their female children after the onset of puberty. There is also a possibility that the male children of these mothers face the problem of sterility.

There is some question also as to whether LSD and other hallucinogenic drugs may cause abnormalities. Current research shows that potentially all drugs can cross the placenta, but many variables determine whether a drug has a teratogenic or a depressant effect on the fetus. The nurse should caution all pregnant women to take *no* medications except those prescribed for her by her physician.

Recent research has raised the question concerning whether drugs taken by the father during the time of conception may also cause birth defects in the child. Further study must be done

TABLE 10–3. *MATERNAL MEDICATIONS WHICH MAY ADVERSELY AFFECT THE FETUS AND NEWBORN INFANT*

DRUG	EFFECT ON FETUS	DEPENDABILITY OF EVIDENCE
Adrenal corticosteroids	Cleft palate	Suggestive
Amphetamines	Congenital heart disease, transposition of the great vessels	Conclusive
Aminopterin	Abortion, malformations	Conclusive
Azathioprine	Abortion	Suggestive
Busulfan (Myleran)	Stunted growth, corneal opacities, cleft palate, hypoplasia of ovaries, thyroid and parathyroids	Doubtful
Chlorambucil	Renal agenesis	Suggestive
Chloroquine	Deafness	Doubtful
Chlorothiazide	Thrombocytopenia	Conclusive
Cigarette smoking	Low birth weight for gestational age	Suggestive
Cyclophosphamide	Multiple malformations	Suggestive
Dicumarol	Fetal bleeding and death, hypoplastic nasal structures	Conclusive
Insulin shock	Death	Conclusive
Lysergic acid diethylamide (LSD) or impurities in commercial preparations	Skeletal defects	Doubtful
	Chromosome damage	Suggestive
Meclizine (Bonine)	Congenital malformations	Doubtful
Mepivacaine	Bradycardia, death	Conclusive
6-Mercaptopurine	Abortion	Suggestive
Methimazole	Goiter	Conclusive
Methyltestosterone	Masculinization of female fetus	Conclusive
17-Alpha-ethinyl-19-nortestosterone (Norlutin)	Masculinization of female fetus	Conclusive
Phenmetrazine (Preludin)	Defect of diaphragm	Doubtful
Potassium iodide	Goiter	Conclusive
Progesterone 17-Alpha-ethinyl testosterone (Progestoral)	Masculinization of female fetus	Suggestive
	Masculinization of female fetus	Conclusive
Propylthiouracil	Goiter	Conclusive
Quinine	Abortion, thrombocytopenia	Conclusive
	Deafness	Doubtful
Radioactive iodine (^{131}I)	Destruction of fetal thyroid	Conclusive
Stilbestrol	Masculinization of female fetus	Suggestive
	Vaginal adenocarcinoma in adolescence	Conclusive
Streptomycin	Deafness	Suggestive
Tetracycline	Retarded skeletal growth	Suggestive
	Pigmentation of teeth, hypoplasia of enamel	Conclusive
	Cataract, limb malformations	Doubtful
Thalidomide	Phocomelia, other malformations	Conclusive
Trimethadione and Paramethadione	Abortion, multiple malformations, mental retardation	Conclusive
Tolbutamide	Congenital malformations	Doubtful
Vitamin D	Supravalvular aortic stenosis, hypercalcemia	Doubtful

From Vaughan, V. C., III, and McKay, R. J.: *Nelson Textbook of Pediatrics,* 10th ed., Philadelphia, W. B. Saunders Co., 1975.

TABLE 10-4. MATERNAL MEDICATIONS WHICH MAY ADVERSELY AFFECT THE NEWBORN INFANT

DRUG	EFFECT ON NEWBORN
Anesthetic agents (volatile)	Central nervous system depression
Adrenal corticosteroids	Adrenocortical failure
Ammonium chloride	Acidosis (clinically inapparent)
Caudal anesthesia with mepivacaine (accidental introduction of anesthetic into scalp of baby)	Bradypnea, apnea, bradycardia, convulsions
CNS depressants (narcotics, barbiturates, tranquilizers) during labor	Central nervous system depression
Cephalothin	Positive direct Coombs test reaction
Coumarin derivatives	High perinatal mortality
Hexamethonium bromide	Paralytic ileus
Intravenous fluids during labor, e.g. salt-free solutions	Electrolyte disturbances Hyponatremia
Lysergic acid diethylamide (LSD) or impurities in commercial preparations	Convulsions (?) Chromosome damage (?)
Morphine and its derivatives (addiction)	Withdrawal symptoms (poor feeding, vomiting, diarrhea, restlessness, yawning and stretching, dyspnea and cyanosis, fever and sweating, pallor, tremors, convulsions)
Naphthalene	Hemolytic anemia (in glucose-6-phosphate dehydrogenase [G-6-PD]-deficient infants)
Nitrofurantoin	Hemolytic anemia (in G-6-PD-deficient infants)
Primaquine	Hemolytic anemia (in G-6-PD-deficient infants)
Reserpine	Drowsiness, nasal congestion
Sulfonamides (long-acting)	Interfere with protein binding of bilirubin: kernicterus at low levels of serum bilirubin
Thiazides	Neonatal thrombocytopenia
Vitamin K (excessive amounts)	Hyperbilirubinemia

From Vaughan, V. C., III, and McKay, R. J.: *Nelson Textbook of Pediatrics*, 10th ed., Philadelphia, W. B. Saunders Co., 1975.

to determine the answer to this important question.

In summary, it may be stated that most congenital deformities are the result of the interaction between genetic and environmental factors, and that often more than one anomaly may occur in the same fetus. There may be abnormal development of any part of the body or any organ.

HEREDITARY AND CONGENITAL DISEASES AND ANOMALIES

It has been noted that *hereditary diseases* and a tendency to certain diseases are fixed at the time of conception. In contrast, *congenital disease* is acquired while the infant is *in utero*. Congenital disease, then, is subject to preventive medicine. Prenatal care of the prospective mother is not only for her sake, but also for the health of the fetus.

Congenital deformities or anomalies are extremely important, since many of them permanently disable a child. The influence of anomalies upon the child's personality cannot be disregarded; many of them limit his social life and activities of daily living.

Congenital anomalies are structural anomalies present at birth. They may be obvious on examination of the newborn, or they may be defects of histologic structure.

One reason why more deaths occur in the first month than during the remaining months of the first year of life is that many congenital abnormalities are compatible with intrauterine life, but not with extrauterine life. Approximately 15 per cent of deaths in the neonatal period are caused by such gross malformations.

Only about 20 per cent of recognizable birth defects are hereditary in origin. Another 20 per cent are apparently caused by environmental

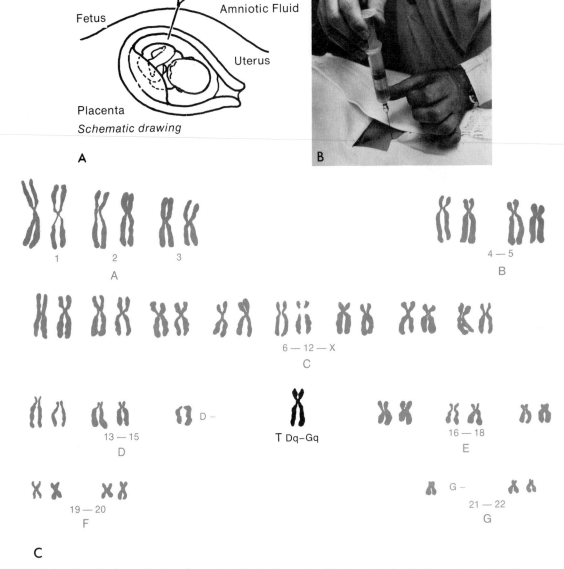

FETUS IN UTERUS

Abdominal Wall

Fetus

Amniotic Fluid

Uterus

Placenta

Schematic drawing

A

B

C

FIGURE 10–6. Steps in determination of genetic defect in fetus. *A* and *B*, Amniotic fluid is drawn by needle. After processing the mother's karyotype (*C*) shows a defective number 15 chromosome, with a number 21 chromosome attached to it, and the probability of a mongoloid baby.

Legend continued on the opposite page

factors such as drugs, venereal disease, viral infections, radiation, or malnutrition of the mother. The majority of birth defects, about 60 per cent, are due to the interaction of hereditary and environmental factors.

Fetology, an exciting new word in medicine, is the concept that the unborn child is a treatable patient. In recent years the term *intrauterine diagnosis* has been used to indicate diagnostic procedures for identifying disease in the fetus. These procedures may be used as a basis for treatment of the fetus *in utero* or for medical ter-mination of pregnancy. One such procedure is *amniocentesis,* or withdrawal of amniotic fluid during pregnancy for the purpose of examination for antibodies, Rh antigens, nonhemin iron, and erythropoietin and bilirubinoid pigment, as well as for the purposes of determining the sex of the baby in the case of a possible sex-linked inheritance and for diagnosing Down's syndrome or Tay-Sachs disease. If the diagnosis of erythroblastosis fetalis is made, treatment may be given or the time of delivery may be planned early.

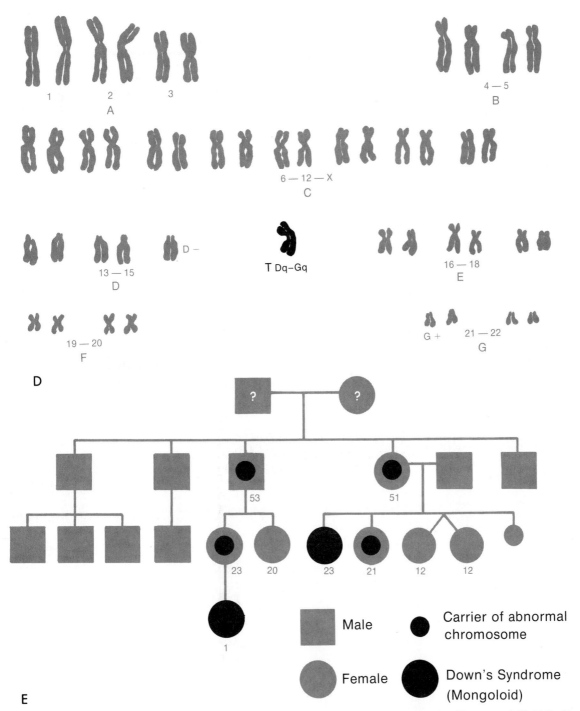

FIGURE 10–6 Continued. *D*, Fetal karyotype indicates that baby if not aborted would indeed be mongoloid. *E*, Pedigree indicates how mother inherited chromosome abnormality. (*B*, courtesy of National Institutes of Health. *C*, *D*, and *E*, courtesy of Laird Jackson, M.D.)

Amniography, by which contrast medium is introduced into the amniotic fluid, may show on roentgen examination the soft tissue outline of the fetus, whether the fetus has atresia of the gastrointestinal tract following his swallowing of the amniotic fluid, or whether the fetus is dead.

Roentgenologic examination of the fetus may be used late in pregnancy for the purpose of detecting skeletal abnormalities.

Amnioscopy does not require puncture of the uterus. Instead, an instrument may be passed through the vagina into the cervical canal. Sam-

Text continues on page 231

TABLE 10–5. DIAGNOSIS OF HEREDITARY METABOLIC DISORDERS BEFORE BIRTH BY AMNIOCENTESIS*

DISORDER	INHERITANCE	CLINICAL MANIFESTATIONS	ACCUMULATED PRODUCTS	DEFICIENT ENZYME ACTIVITY	PRENATAL DIAGNOSIS POSSIBLE
Disorders of lipid metabolism					
Fabry's disease	X*	Purple skin papules; renal failure; cardiac and ocular involvement	Ceramidetrihexoside	Ceramidetrihexoside galactosidase	?*
Gaucher's disease	A*	Infantile and adult forms; hepatosplenomegaly, erosion of long bones, neurologic involvement, anemia and thrombocytopenia	Glucocerebroside	Glucocerebrosidase	+*
G_{M1} gangliosidosis (generalized gangliosidosis)	A	Mental retardation from birth, unusual facies, hepatosplenomegaly and skeletal changes	G_{M1} ganglioside and ceramide tetrahexoside visceral mucopolysaccharide of keratan sulfate type and a sialomucopolysaccharide	β-galactosidase A, B and C; B and C only	+
G_{M2} gangliosidosis (Tay-Sachs disease)	A	Onset at age 5 to 6 months, degenerative neurologic disorder with cherry-red spot within macula, progressing from normal state to apathy, hypotonia, profound psychomotor retardation and death	G_{M2} ganglioside and its asialo derivative	Hexosaminidase A	++*
				Hexosaminidase A and B	+
Metachromatic leukodystrophy	A	At least two forms: degenerative neurologic disease progressing from normal state to weakness, ataxia, hypotonia, mental retardation and paralysis; excessive sulfatide in urine	Sulfatide	Arylsulfatase A (sulfatidase)	++
Niemann-Pick disease	A	Four types: hepatosplenomegaly; variable skeletal and neurologic involvement	Sphingomyelin	Sphingomyelinase	++
Refsum's disease	A	Cerebellar ataxia, peripheral polyneuropathy, retinitis pigmentosa, and other cardiac, skin, neurologic and skeletal changes	Phytanic acid	Phytanic acid α-hydroxylase	+
Mucopolysaccharidoses					
Hurler's syndrome	A	Gargoyle-like facies, early clouding of cornea, early psychomotor retardation, increased linear growth in first year; then decline to become dwarfed, hepatosplenomegaly, kyphosis, joint stiffness, excessive dermatan sulfate and heparitin sulfate in urine	Dermatan sulfate and heparitin sulfate	Specific β-galactosidase	++
Hunter's syndrome	X*	Gargoyle-like facies less obvious and seen later than in Hurler's syndrome, clear cornea, psychomotor retardation, increased linear growth in first year; declines later, hepatosplenomegaly, joint stiffness, excessive dermatan sulfate and heparitin sulfate in urine	Dermatan sulfate and heparitin sulfate	Unknown	?

Disease		Clinical features	Substance	Enzyme	
Maroteaux-Lamy syndrome	A	Severe skeletal changes, cloudy cornea, normal intellect; excessive dermatan sulfate in urine	Unknown	Unknown	?
Morquio's syndrome	A	Severe skeletal changes, with dwarfism, cloudy corneas, aortic regurgitation, intellect usually within normal range, excessive keratan sulfate in urine	Unknown	Unknown	?
Sanfilippo syndrome	A	Severe mental retardation, joint stiffness, excessive heparitin sulfate in urine	Unknown	Unknown	?
Scheie's syndrome	A	Coarse facies, stiff joints; usually normal intellect, aortic regurgitation, excessive dermatan sulfate in urine	Unknown	Unknown	?
Amino acid and related disorders					
Argininosuccinic aciduria	A	Mental retardation, trichorrhexis nodosa, ammonia intoxication	Argininosuccinic acid	Argininosuccinase	+
Citrullinemia	A	Ammonia intoxication, mental retardation	Citrulline	Argininosuccinic acid synthetase	?
Cystinosis	A	Failure to thrive, rickets, glycosuria, aminoaciduria, cystine deposition in tissue	Cystine	Unknown	+
Homocystinuria	A	Dislocated lenses, skeletal abnormalities, vascular thrombosis, mental retardation	Methionine and homocystine	Cystathionine synthase	+
Hyperammonemia Type II	A	Ammonia intoxication, mental retardation	Ammonia	Ornithine carbamyl-transferase	+
Hyperlysinemia	A	Mental retardation, muscular asthenia (may be normal)	Lysine	Lysine-ketoglutarate reductase	+
Hypervalinemia	A	Mental retardation, failure to thrive	Valine	Valine transaminase	?
Ketotic hyperglycinemia	A	Ketoacidosis, protein intolerance, developmental retardation	Glycine	Propionyl CoA carboxylase	?
Maple syrup urine disease Severe infantile	A	Ketoacidosis, neurologic abnormality, mental retardation, early death	Valine, leucine, isoleucine, and their keto acids	Branched-chain keto acid decarboxylase	++
Intermittent	A	Ketoacidosis, neurologic abnormality, mental retardation, early death	As above	As above	+
Methylmalonic aciduria	A	Acidosis, lethargy, failure to thrive, early death	Methylmalonic acid, glycine, homocystine, and cystathionine	Methylmalonyl CoA isomerase or vitamin B_{12} coenzyme (decreased carbon dioxide production from propionate)	++
Ornithine–α-ketoacid transaminase deficiency	A	Liver disease, renal tubular defect, mental retardation	Ornithine	Ornithine-α-keto acid transaminase	
Disorders of carbohydrate metabolism					
Fucosidosis	A	Severe progressive cerebral degeneration, intense spasticity, thick skin and excessive sweating, increased salinity of sweat	Fucose containing heteropolysaccharide	α-fucosidase	+
Glycogen-storage disease (Type II)	A	Failure to thrive, hypotonia, hepatomegaly, cardiomegaly	Glycogen storage	α-1,4-glucosidase	++

(Table continued on the following page)

TABLE 10–5. DIAGNOSIS OF HEREDITARY METABOLIC DISORDERS BEFORE BIRTH BY AMNIOCENTESIS* (Continued)

DISORDER	INHERITANCE	CLINICAL MANIFESTATIONS	ACCUMULATED PRODUCTS	DEFICIENT ENZYME ACTIVITY	PRENATAL DIAGNOSIS POSSIBLE
Glycogen-storage disease (Type III)	A	Hepatomegaly, cardiomegaly, hypoglycemia	Abnormally structured glycogen	Amylo-1,6-glucosidase	+
Glycogen-storage disease (Type IV)	A	Familial cirrhosis with splenomegaly	Abnormally structured glycogen	Branching enzyme	+
Galactosemia	A	Cirrhosis, cataracts, mental retardation and failure to thrive	Galactose	Galactose-1-P-uridyl transferase	+
Mannosidosis	A	Gargoyle-like facies, psychomotor retardation, accelerated growth in infancy, hypotonia, mild hepatosplenomegaly	Mannose and glucosamine containing heteropolysaccharide	α-mannosidase	+
Pyruvate decarboxylase deficiency	A	Intermittent cerebellar ataxia and choreoathetosis, with elevated urinary alanine	Pyruvic acid, alanine and lactate	Pyruvate decarboxylase	?
Glucose-6-PO_4 dehydrogenase deficiency	A	Hemolytic anemia		G-6-PO_4 dehydrogenase	+
Miscellaneous disorders					
Acatalasemia	A	Recurrent anaerobic infections of gums and oral tissue	Unknown	Catalase	?
Adrenogenital syndrome	A	Virilization or pseudohermaphroditism, adrenal insufficiency with salt loss, hypertensive cardiovascular disease, pregnanetriol and 17-ketosteroids in urine		C21, C11 or C17 steroid hydroxylase	++
Chediak-Higashi syndrome	A	Photophobia, decreased pigmentation of skin, hair and eyes, increased susceptibility to infections	Cellular inclusions	Unknown	?
Congenital erythropoietic porphyria	A	Photosensitive dermatitis, anemia, splenomegaly, hypertrichosis, massive porphyrinuria	Uroporphyrin 1 and coproporphyrin I in tissues	Cosynthetase	?
Cystic fibrosis	A	Recurrent pulmonary infection, malabsorption, failure to thrive, increased sodium chloride in sweat	Mucopolysaccharide storage or increased production in cultured fibroblasts	β-glucuronidase deficiency in skin components	?
I-cell disease	A	Gargoyle-like facies, dwarfism from birth, gingival hyperplasia, psychomotor retardation	Acid mucopolysaccharide and glycolipids	Reduced β-glucuronidase and excessive acid phosphatase	?
Lesch-Nyhan syndrome	X	Self-mutilation, choreoathetosis, spasticity, mental retardation	Uric acid	Hypoxanthine-guanine phosphoribosyltransferase	++
Lysosomal acid phosphatase deficiency	A	Failure to thrive, progressive neuromuscular involvement, hypoglycemia, seizures and hepatomegaly	Unknown	Lysosomal acid phosphatase	++
Marfan's syndrome	D	Connective-tissue disorder with skeletal, cardiovascular and ocular signs	Hyaluronic acid in cultured fibroblasts	Unknown	?
Orotic aciduria	A	Infantile megaloblastic anemia, orotic acid in urine	Unknown	Orotidylic pyrophosphorylase and decarboxylase	?
Xeroderma pigmentosum	A	Photosensitive dermatitis, skin cancers	Unknown	DNA "repair enzyme"	+

*A, autosomal recessive; D, autosomal dominant; X, sex-linked recessive; ++, prenatal diagnosis made; +, prenatal diagnosis possible; ?, prenatal diagnosis questionable.

From Page, E. W., Villee, C. A., and Villee, D. B.: *Human Reproduction*, 2nd ed. Philadelphia. W. B. Saunders Co. 1976.

ples of blood may be taken through the amnioscope from the presenting part of the fetus in order to carry out microanalysis to determine the pH and oxygen and carbon dioxide tensions of the blood. If the fetus is acidotic, the question arises as to whether immediate delivery is indicated. Amnioscopy may also be utilized for direct intrauterine visualization and photography and for determining the appearance of the amniotic fluid. If the fluid is dark, it is stained with meconium. This is an indication of fetal distress and thus an indication for immediate delivery.

Fetal electrocardiography has been used to monitor the fetal heart rate. This diagnostic method traces the progress of the fetus during gestation, labor, and delivery. It is particularly valuable during labor contractions when fetal heart tones are not easily detected by auscultation.

Ultrasonography, an important recent advance in diagnostic medicine, has a growing use in obstetrics. The ultrasonoscope sends an ultrasonic beam into body tissues, and echo waves return as a picture of the scanned area on the oscilloscope or receiver. Ultrasonography can be used to make a positive diagnosis of pregnancy as early as the sixth week. The growth of the fetus and the localization and size of the placenta can also be determined. Abnormalities which may have an effect on the fetus can thus be determined early.

Still another area of research concerns the effect of chemicals such as alcohol, drugs, even aspirin, on the fetus and the potentially deleterious effect of LSD in "psychedelic" doses on the fetus if taken early in the course of pregnancy. It is essential that the mother should not self-medicate at any time during the period of gestation.

Research continues to be done on methods to protect the newborn from defects. These measures include among others the use of vaccines to prevent rubella (German measles) and to prevent Rh disease (see p. 241).

Although treatment of some conditions of the fetus has been successful, such as intrauterine transfusions for those having erythroblastosis fetalis, much more research must be done before the prevention and treatment of many diseases and malformations can be accomplished. Research is also being done to determine the need for a national birth defects surveillance system in order to prevent the tragedy which occurred during the thalidomide episode when thousands of infants were born with serious defects (see p. 325).

PARENTS' AND NURSES' REACTIONS TO AN IMPERFECT INFANT, AND HOW THE NURSE CAN HELP THE PARENTS WITH THIS PROBLEM

Parental education should include the possibility of giving birth to an imperfect infant. In a class with other prospective parents, husbands and wives together can consider this possibility objectively. If their first knowledge on the subject comes when their child is born with a disease or an anomaly, it is difficult for them to maintain an objective point of view. Men and women of marriageable age should know that prevention begins with conception, i.e., impregnation of the ovum by a spermatozoon, neither of which carries genes causing hereditary abnormality. Once the ovum has been impregnated, medical care is no longer centered on the unfortunate combination of disease- or abnormality-bearing genes which might have been avoided, but rather on the developing fetus.

Parents have an aversion to the idea of something inherent in themselves which has been or could be transmitted to their children. Primitive people were not alone in their belief that a congenital malformation or illness was punishment for wrongdoing. Even modern parents, when told that their child has a congenital anomaly, will many times respond with some such statement as, "What did I do wrong during my pregnancy?" "What did my husband do wrong in the past?" "What have we ever done to others to deserve this?" "What great sin did we commit that our child has to suffer so much?"

When a defect is discovered in a newborn infant, the physician is responsible for telling the parents the sad news. After the parents have been told that an imperfect infant has been born, it is only natural that they evidence disappointment, grief, and despair. The perfect infant they had anticipated was born an imperfect human being. *Parents need help at this time to resolve their grief over the healthy perfect infant they had imagined they would have. They also need help in accepting the fact that their imperfectly formed infant exists and in establishing a warm relationship with their child.*

In the instance of discovery of a defect in a newborn, the parents need to be helped to stay with their responsibility. They need help in making necessary decisions, such as when operation is necessary immediately after birth. As a matter of fact, although exceptions may be made, depending on the individual mother, father, and physician, the mother should be helped to see her infant and care for him if possible so that the period of separation of mother and child is minimized. Some physicians believe that a mother should be protected from seeing her malformed infant for several days after his birth. In this situation, if the child dies, the mother will have to mourn for him on the basis of fantasy and not reality.

Most parents feel some degree of guilt and blame others or feel self-blame for their infant's condition. If the mother can be helped to see that an abnormal condition in her infant is not her fault, nor that of her husband, and that the physician is not to blame, she is more likely to accept the condition realistically and adjust to the infant's needs.

When parents continue to assume their responsibilities to satisfy their needs to be mothers and fathers, nurses should encourage them, because this is how they learn to know their child as a person. If the parents are truly involved, their despair or guilt may turn toward more adequate problem-solving.

When a hereditary disease is discovered later in the child's life it must be discussed in an honest, matter-of-fact manner. The nurse should have some knowledge of what has been discussed in order to support and assist the parents in the most appropriate way.

After the immediate action on the problem the members of the health team, including the nurse, must help the parents to face the situation realistically so that they do not go shopping around for a magical cure. The parents must be helped to plan for therapy, if anything can be done about the problem, to capitalize on the child's assets, and to become familiar with the patterns of growth and development of such children. In order to help the parents in this way, the nurse should know what therapy can be carried out in the various kinds of malformations and conditions, and their eventual prognoses.

The nurse should help the mother discuss her feelings about her ill infant, whether of guilt, embarrassment, anger, or fear but should not probe for information. If the mother wishes to talk, the nurse should demonstrate nonverbal and verbal acceptance and understanding by showing support and warmth.

After the mother's discharge and prior to the infant's discharge from the hospital, especially if the mother has been unable to accept his problem, the public health nurse may encourage her to return to the nursery to see her infant. If such a mother can then express her feelings, she may be better able to mother her baby in spite of what the future may hold.

The nurse can help parents create positive yet realistic attitudes toward their defective child. They must be helped to rid themselves of guilt feelings in order to prevent their treating the child too permissively. If they do not help him toward whatever degree of maturity and independence he is capable of, they will fail in their responsibility of preparing him for life.

Also, if their guilt feelings are intense, parents may so focus their attention on the defective child that the normal children in the family are not given the emotional care they need for healthy development. It may also be true that the mother focuses so much attention on the child that the father feels neglected. Often even the needs of the mother for her own recovery and care may be overlooked as the focus is shifted to her infant and his progress.

The attitude which parents develop toward their imperfect child will in many ways be the attitude his siblings, peers, relatives, and other members of the community will develop toward him. If a misfortune is accepted as a part of life, the manner of life may have to be changed accordingly, but in most situations the child can still learn to enjoy his areas of normality to the fullest as an individual and as a community member.

Since some malformed infants require prolonged care and training, the nurse should be cognizant of the care facilities and the financial resources available in the community and state which can assist such parents and their children and the ways these children can be referred to such sources of help.

Nurses can share information with parents concerning the national and local organizations that can provide help for their handicapped children and the location of groups of parents who also have children with birth defects. Parents benefit from meeting with such parents who have had to search for answers to problems they will face in the future.

Much of the information in Chapter 5 concerning the manner by which a nurse can comfort and further assist the parents when their child is dying can be utilized when a child is born with a hereditary or congenital disease or anomaly.

The nurse who cares for an imperfect infant faces several challenges. The physical aspects of the infant's care may be complex. Specific care is discussed in later chapters in this text.

The nurse, like the parents, may be emotionally disturbed by the infant who has a hereditary or congenital disease or anomaly. Before being able to support the family the nurse must be aware of personal feelings concerning the situation. These involve attitudes toward both the affected infant and his parents. The nurse's attitudes may also be complicated by imagining that the infant is the nurse's own child.

If the student has difficulty in handling per-

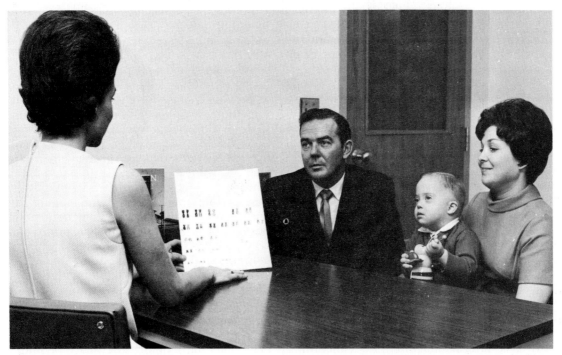

FIGURE 10–7. Genetic counseling is done with parents of a child having Down's syndrome. (Courtesy of The National Foundation—March of Dimes.)

sonal feelings comfortably, the guidance of the instructor should be sought so that a positive, helping relationship with the parents and a less stressful personal experience for herself in providing care for the child can be achieved.

Great strides have been made in genetics, not all of which can be included in this text. The inexperienced nurse or student is referred to the references at the end of this chapter for further explanation of specific areas of interest.

GENETIC COUNSELING AND THE RESPONSIBILITIES OF THE NURSE

The process of genetic counseling includes providing information concerning hereditary and congenital disorders to individuals, couples, or families who know that they have a potential problem, being themselves affected or having a relative with such a disorder. This may mean that an individual who recently discovered a defect that had not been diagnosed before may seek guidance. A couple who is not yet married but is closely related to each other or know of a medical problem with a possible genetic base existing in one or both of the families may seek help in deciding not to marry, to marry and take the risk of having affected children, or to marry and plan to adopt children. Such a decision is a major one for the individuals involved. A family that has had a child having a congenital defect or one who

is delayed in physical or mental development may seek guidance concerning the wisdom of having future children. An individual may also seek counseling if he or she has been exposed to a substance that could cause defects in a child. Some of these substances have been discussed previously (see p. 224).

The degree of disturbance felt by parents after the birth of a child who is not perfect may depend on the relationship of the family members prior to the birth, how they have reacted to other crisis situations, and whether or not they have been able to verbalize their feelings to each other or to others; the presence of other normal or abnormal children in the family; and their hopes for the newest family member. On the basis of these factors, some parents react deeply to a child born with a minor deviation from normal, while others are able to work through their grief over a serious defect with relative equanimity. The members of the helping professions who guide and support such parents have an important role to play in alleviating much of their distress.

The members of the genetic counseling team— the family or referring physician, the geneticist, the nurse, and other concerned members of the helping professions—may influence greatly not only the individuals mentioned here but also their children. The lives of the affected and apparently normal siblings may be changed through learning more about the chances of their having normal families in the future.

Before such discussions can take place and the decisions can be made, members of the team must have a detailed and accurate medical history of the persons involved as well as a family pedigree or family tree. Some families are embarrassed when discussing a possible genetic problem they have been trying to hide for years. A carefully taken family history is an important aid in genetic counseling and may be the responsibility of the nurse. Each family member, beginning with the child or the individual seeking help and going back to the grandparents and beyond when possible, should be included in this history, which leads to the outlining of a family pedigree.

The nurse can function within a multidisciplinary setting in genetic counseling as a visitor to the home of the individuals to observe other family members and collect pictures that might indicate others in the family having the problem. The nurse, in addition to being a data collector, can also give information to clients concerning the genetic clinic or its team members. The nurse can also assume the role of family advocate, helping each individual to obtain the best guidance possible.

Depending upon the size of the genetic team and his or her own experiences and educational background, the nurse may assist with counseling or may do actual counseling alone. An important part of genetic counseling is helping parents who already have an affected child to learn about the genetic problem they have and help them to accept the impact of such information by acquiring new coping mechanisms for handling the crisis.

Following the birth of a child having a physical or mental anomaly, the parents face increased responsibilities and important decisions that will affect them the rest of their lives. They must decide whether to have more children of their own or whether to adopt children in the future. Such clients need psychologic support in helping them to plan for the years ahead. Genetic counseling in this situation provides the guidance to avoid unhappiness later.

If the parents have already conceived another child who is in danger of having a genetic defect, the physician should be informed early so that a prenatal diagnosis, possibly through amniocentesis, could be made and a decision made about the wisdom of continuing the pregnancy.

In genetic counseling of a family both parents should be present at the discussions to prevent possible misinterpretations from occurring. The conferences should be scheduled in a private room without the presence of the affected child, who might be traumatized by the emotional tone of the discussions. If the nurse is doing the counseling, important points made in the meetings are summarized and shared with the parents to provide a basis for later discussions. Memory difficulties may occur in any crisis situation and such sharing helps to clarify any misinterpretations that may arise. The parents may wish to include their teenage offspring, if there are any, in these conferences so that they too may know what may lie ahead for them.

Sometimes parents or clients cannot think of questions to ask the nurse or genetic counselor during these conferences because the decisions they face are too overwhelming. The nurse can help them formulate questions by expressing gentle concern and making tactful inquiries. Throughout the counseling process the nurse must maintain an objective viewpoint and provide the emotional support which is so needed.

To reduce feelings of parental guilt and shame the nurse can explain that many people, if not all, have hidden genetic defects, but that most of them marry persons with a different set of affected genes and therefore do not have affected children. The probability of their having another affected child should also be explained. The matter of risk is difficult for parents to understand and should be repeatedly discussed until it is understood.

Throughout the genetic counseling process the nurse can function as a liaison person between the individual or family and the members of the genetic team. The nurse may assist not only with planning diagnostic examinations in conjunction with other team members, but also may be the one responsible for transmitting the results. The nurse may visit in the home to help clarify decisions already made or refer the individual or family to a community resource for follow-up care. If a child in the family is affected, the nurse may provide guidance to resources for further care of the child. The nurse may also provide guidance to the parents concerning ways of meeting other parents who have had a child like theirs.

Finally, the nurse who is aware of the importance of genetic counseling will be ever alert for opportunities to refer potential clients to known sources of help for genetic problems.

Genetic counseling will play a large part in the efforts of preventive medicine in the future. The nurse as a member of the health team will have an increasingly important role as a member of this multidisciplinary team.

THE COLLABORATIVE PROJECT

Leading medical centers in the United States, in cooperation with the Public Health Service's National Institute of Neurologic Diseases and Stroke are carrying out what is known as the *Collaborative Perinatal Research Project.* The purpose of this Collaborative Project is to try to determine the roles played by heredity, environment, psychologic aspects, sickness, or accident of the mother, and other factors occurring before, during, or after birth in contributing to neurologic, mental, and congenital deficits of children. Many thousands of mothers and their children are being studied in the project. Wide use is being made of physicians, nurses, allied health personnel, including social workers and nutritionists, and aides and assistants of various kinds. These mothers are examined, observed, and interviewed at routine intervals. The results are recorded along with data concerning pregnancy, labor, and delivery, and the growth and development of the child from birth through school age.

Results of this project to date have proved helpful in reducing the mortality rate among the study infants and have contributed to other areas of research.

TEACHING AIDS AND OTHER INFORMATION*

American Academy of Pediatrics

Counseling Opportunities in Human Reproduction.
Screening of Newborn Infants for Metabolic Disease.

Consumer Product Information

The Right to Be Well-Born, 1975.

Maternity Center Association

A Survey of Recent Medical Advances in Maternity Care, 1974.

Mead Johnson & Company

Galactosemia in Infancy: A Review of the Problem and Its Dietary Management, 1976.

National Association for Retarded Citizens

Facts on Mental Retardation, Revised 1973.
It Can Happen to Anyone.
Kelsey, F. O.: Drugs and Pregnancy.
Schimke, R. N.: Inheritance and Mental Retardation.
Your Head Is Your Own Thing.
Zellweger, H.: Genetic Counseling in Clinical Medicine.

The National Foundation–March of Dimes

Birth Defects: The Tragedy and the Hope.
Fast Facts About Sickle Cell Anemia.
Genetic Counseling.
It's Possible: Birth Defects Prevention.

Preventing Birth Defects Caused by Rubella.
Questions and Answers on Birth Defects.
Tay-Sachs Disease & Birth Defects Prevention.

Planned Parenthood Federation of America, Inc.

I've Been Tested for Sickle-Cell Anemia. Have You?

United States Government

Antenatal Diagnosis and Down's Syndrome, 1974.
Drugs and Pregnancy, 1974.
Early Diagnosis of Human Genetic Defects, 1971.
Genetic Screening for Inborn Errors of Metabolism, 1975.
Lin-Fu, J. S.: Prevention of Hemolytic Disease of the Fetus and Newborn Due to Rh Isoimmunization, 1975.
Mental Retardation Publications, 1971.
Phenylketonuria, An Inherited Metabolic Disorder Associated With Mental Retardation, 1972.
Russell, F. F. (Ed.): Identification and Management of Selected Developmental Disabilities; A Guide for Nurses, 1975.
Sickle Cell Screening and Education Clinics, 1975.
So, I Have the Sickle Cell Trait…, 1972.
The Maternity and Infant Care Projects: Reducing Risks for Mothers and Babies, 1975.
What Are the Facts About Genetic Disease, 1976.

*Complete addresses are given in the Appendix.

REFERENCES

Books

Arey, L. B.: *Developmental Anatomy: A Textbook and Laboratory Manual of Embryology.* 7th ed. Philadelphia, W. B. Saunders Company, 1974.
Beck, F., Moffat, D. B., and Lloyd, J. B.: *Human Embryology and Genetics.* Philadelphia, J. B. Lippincott Company, 1973.
Corliss, C. E.: *Patten's Human Embryology: Elements of Clinical Development.* New York, McGraw-Hill Company, 1976.
Fraser, F. C., and Nora, J. J.: *Genetics of Man.* Philadelphia, Lea & Febiger, 1975.
Fraser, G. R., and Mayo, O.: *Textbook of Human Genetics.* Philadelphia, J. B. Lippincott Company, 1975.

Gardner, L. I. (Ed.): *Endocrine and Genetic Diseases of Childhood and Adolescence.* 2nd ed. Philadelphia, W. B. Saunders Company, 1975.
Kelley, V. C. (Ed.): *Metabolic, Endocrine and Genetic Disorders of Children.* New York, Harper & Row Publishers, 1974.
Konigsmark, B. W., and Gorlin, R. J.: *Genetic and Metabolic Deafness.* Philadelphia, W. B. Saunders Company, 1976.
Milunsky, A.: *Prevention of Genetic Disease and Mental Retardation.* Philadelpha, W. B. Saunders Company, 1975.
Moore, K. L.: *Before We Are Born: Basic Embryology and Birth Defects.* Philadelphia, W. B. Saunders Company, 1974.

Murphy, E. A., and Chase, G. A.: *Principles of Genetic Counseling*. Chicago, Year Book Medical Publishers, Inc., 1975.

Nathan, D. G., and Oski, F. A.: *Hematology of Infancy and Childhood*. Philadelphia, W. B. Saunders Company, 1974.

Niswander, K. R. and Gordon, M.: *The Collaborative Perinatal Study: The Women and Their Pregnancies*. Philadelphia, W. B. Saunders Company, 1972.

Nora, J. J., and Fraser, F. C.: *Medical Genetics: Principles and Practice*. Philadelphia, Lea & Febiger, 1974.

Pai, A. C.: *Foundations of Genetics: A Science for Society*. New York, McGraw-Hill Company, 1974.

Rothwell, N. V.: *Understanding Genetics*. Baltimore, Williams & Wilkins Company, 1975.

Smith, D. W.: *Recognizable Patterns of Human Malformation: Genetic, Embryologic and Clinical Aspects*. 2nd ed. Philadelphia, W. B. Saunders Company, 1976.

Sucheston, M. E., and Cannon, M. S.: *Congenital Malformations: Case Studies in Developmental Anatomy*. Philadelphia, F. A. Davis Company, 1973.

Thompson, J. S., and Thompson, M. W.: *Genetics in Medicine*. 2nd ed. Philadelphia, W. B. Saunders Company, 1973.

Valentine, G. H.: *The Chromosome Disorders: An Introduction for Clinicians*. 3rd ed. Philadelphia, J. B. Lippincott Company, 1975.

Whaley, L. F.: *Understanding Inherited Disorders*. St. Louis, The C. V. Mosby Company, 1974.

Williams, R. A. (Ed.): *Texbook of Black-Related Diseases*. New York, McGraw-Hill Company, 1975.

Periodicals

Aase, J. M.: Environmental Causes of Birth Defects. *Nursing Digest*, 4:12, September-October 1976.

Chan, W. H., Paul, R. H., and Toews, J.: Intrapartum Fetal Monitoring. Maternal and Fetal Morbidity and Perinatal Mortality. *Obstet. Gynecol.*, 41:7, January 1973.

Cibils, L. A.: Clinical Significance of Fetal Heart Rate Patterns During Labor. II. Late Decelerations. *Am. J. Obstet. Gynecol.*, 123:473, November 1, 1975.

Collins, E., and Turner, G.: Maternal Effects of Regular Salicylate Ingestion in Pregnancy. *Lancet*, 2:335, August 23, 1975.

DiPalma, J. R.: Drug Therapy Today: The Growing New Field of Pharmacogenetics. *RN*, 37:109, September 1974.

Donley, D. L.: The Immune System: Nursing the Patient Who Is Immunosuppressed. *Am. J. Nursing*, 76:1619, October 1976.

Dorrance, D. L., Janiger, O., and Teplitz, R. L.: Effect of Peyote on Human Chromosomes. Cytogenetic Study of the Huichol Indians of Northern Mexico. *JAMA*, 234:299, October 20, 1975.

Galloway, K. G.: Placental Evaluation Studies: The Procedures, Their Purposes, and the Nursing Care Involved. *The American Journal of Maternal-Child Nursing*, 1:300, September-October, 1976.

Gelfand, E. W., Biggar, W. D., and Orange, R. P.: Immune Deficiency: Evaluation, Diagnosis, and Therapy. *Pediatr. Clin. N. Am.*, 21:745, November 1974.

Golbus, M. S., Conte, F. A., Schneider, E. L., and Epstein, C. J.: Intrauterine Diagnosis of Genetic Defects: Results, Problems, and Follow-up of One Hundred Cases in a Prenatal Genetic Detection Center. *Am. J. Obstet. Gynecol.*, 118:897, April 1, 1974.

Hardgrove, C., and Warrick, L. H.: How Shall We Tell The Children. *Am. J. Nursing.*, 74:448, March, 1974.

Harmetz, A.: Medical Breakthrough: Curing A Deadly Defect *Before* The Baby is Born. *Today's Health*, 52:14, December 1974.

Herbst, A. L., et al.: Clear-Cell Adenocarcinoma of the Genital Tract in Young Females. *New Eng. J. Med.*, 287:1259, December 1972.

Holtzman, N. A., Meek, A. G., and Mellits, E. D.: Neonatal Screening for Phenylketonuria. I. Effectiveness. *J.A.M.A.*, 229:667, August 5, 1974.

Isler, C.: Infection: Constant Threat to Perinatal Life. *RN*, 38:23, August 1975.

Jackson, P. L.: Chronic Grief. *Am. J. Nursing*, 74:1288, July 1974.

Lambert, L.: Genetic Screening: Learning What You Never Wanted to Know. *Today's Health*, 54:28, March 1976.

Nadler, H. L.: Prenatal Diagnosis of Inborn Defects: A Status Report. *Nursing Digest*, 4:63, Fall 1976.

Newton, M.: Will Our Baby Be 'Normal'? *Family Health/Today's Health*, 8:18, July 1976.

Nysather, J. O., Katz, A. E., and Lenth, J. L.: The Immune System: Its Development and Functions. *Am. J. Nursing*, 76:1614, October 1976.

Osborn, F.: The Emergence of a Valid Eugenics. *Nursing Digest*, 2:89, January 1974.

Osoff, A.: Caring for the Child with Familial Dysautonomia. *Am. J. Nursing*, 75:1158, July 1975.

Riccardi, V. M.: Health Care and Disease Prevention Through Genetic Counseling: A Regional Approach. *Am. J. Public Health*, 66:268, March 1976.

Robinson, J. C., and Forbes, W. F.: The Role of Carbon Monoxide in Cigarette Smoking. *Arch. Environ. Health*, 30:425, September 1975.

Rodman, M. J.: Drug Therapy Today: The Pregnant Patient: Treating Her Without Harming the Baby. *RN*, 38:61, February 1975.

Rosenfeld, A.: Thymosin: Breaking the Immune Barrier. *Nursing Digest*, 3:48, September-October 1975.

Rudd, N. L., and Youson, B. M.: Dilemma. *The Canadian Nurse*, 72:51, August, 1976.

Russin, A. W., O'Gureck, J. E., and Roux, J. F.: Electronic Monitoring of the Fetus. *Am. J. Nursing*, 74:1294, July 1974.

Sahin, S. T.: The Multifaceted Role of the Nurse As Genetic Counselor. *The American Journal of Maternal-Child Nursing*, 1:211, July-August 1976.

Seitz, P. M., and Warrick, L. H.: Perinatal Death: The Grieving Mother. *Am. J. Nursing*, 74:2028, November 1974.

Silva, M. C.: Science, Ethics, and Nursing. *Am. J. Nursing*, 74:2004, November 1974.

Speidel, B. D., and Meadow, S. R.: Maternal Epilepsy and Abnormalities of the Fetus and Newborn. *Lancet*, 2:839, October 21, 1972.

Stenchever, M. A., Kunysz, T. J., and Allen, M. A.: Chromosome Breakage in Users of Marihuana. *Am. J. Obstet. Gynecol.*, 118:106, January 1974.

Turner, J. H. et al.: Fetal and Maternal Risks Associated With Intrauterine Transfusion Procedures. *Am. J. Obstet. Gynecol.*, 123:251, October 1, 1975.

Zahourek, R., and Jensen, J. S.: Grieving and the Loss of the Newborn. *Am. J. Nursing*, 73:836, May 1973.

AUDIOVISUAL MEDIA*

The American Journal of Nursing Company

Growth and Development—Birth Through Adolescence
  Heredity and Behavior
  Participating Instructor: Ginsburgh, B., 44 minutes, black and white.
  Development and its dependency upon heredity and environment are discussed.

Maternity Nursing Class
  Chromosomal Aberrations
  Participating Instructor: Levitsky, J. M., 44 minutes, 16mm film or videotape, sound, guide.
  A geneticist discusses normal chromosomal development and abnormalities. Emphasizes supportive role of nurse during chromosomal studies and traumatic postpartum period.

Churchill Films

Have a Healthy Baby
  16 minutes, 16mm, sound, color.
  Uses animation to show human development from conception to birth. Warns how damage may occur.

Harper & Row Publishers

The Biological Aspects of Sexuality
  Allen, J. M., 35mm slides, 22 minutes each, audio-tape cassette, sound, color, guide.

The Nature of Human Sexuality
  Pervasive nature of sexuality; reproductive phase of the life cycle; physiologic significance of puberty; sexual anatomy; sex inheritance mechanisms; genetics of sex determination; mechanisms of sex differentiation in vertebrates; duality of sexual anatomy as evidenced by differentiation of external genitalia.

Human Development
  Development of the fetus from conception to birth (drawings and photographs); the first trimester as a demonstration of concepts relating to the developmental process; the nature and process of birth.

Accidents of Development
  The public health aspects of developmental abnormalities; genetic factors in congenital defects; amniocentesis as a diagnostic tool; rubella, radiation, thalidomide, and hormonal factors as examples of environmentally caused defects; high sensitivity of the embryo to damage during the first trimester.

Mechanisms of Differentiation
  How characteristic differences in body parts develop; early phases of development, including cell movement; aspects of new cell interactions related to the induction of new cell types (differentiation); importance of cellular environments in altering cell response; regulation of differentiation explained through experiments; the possibility of programming retrieval of genetic information.

Germ Cell Formation and Fertilization
  The biology of germ cell production in male and female; the process of egg and sperm cell formation from primordial germ cell to mature gamete; importance of meiosis in sperm and egg formation; physiology of fertilization; twinning; Down's and Turner's syndromes as examples of developmental accidents related to chromosome distribution errors.

W. B. Saunders Company

A Color Atlas of Human Embryology
  Editor: O'Rahilly, R., 294 35mm slides, or 4 microfiche color, booklet.
  All views are from the *Carnegie Embryological Collection.* Many of the specimens have never before been reproduced; others have not heretofore been seen in color.

Current Topics in Obstetrics and Gynecology
  Director: Tyson, J. E.
  Audio-cassette periodicals, approximately 1 hour in length.
  Diagnosis of Intrauterine Birth Defects, Kaback, M. M.
  Fetal Monitoring and Labor, Friedman, E. A. and Freeman, R. K.

Human Embryology
  Moore, K. L., 129 black and white 35mm slides, 21 full-color 35mm slides, contents card.
  These slides portray the timetable of development for the human fetus. Most illustrations are diagrammatic, complete with legends. Congenital malformations are displayed in actual clinical photographs.

Pediatric Conferences with Sydney Gellis.
  Audio-cassette periodicals, approximately 1 hour in length.
  Diagnosis of Fetal Disease, Milunsky, A.
  Hurler's Disease, Gellis, S.
  Indications for Karyotyping, Feingold, M.
  The XYY Karyotype, Gardner, L. I.

Trainex Corporation

Baby Cries
  Audio-tape cassette.
  An interview with Dr. Murray Feingold, specialist in diagnosis of congenital abnormalities, correlating detailed case histories with his personal tape collection of infant cries.

Fetal Development
  35mm filmstrip, audio-tape cassette, 33⅓ LP, color.
  Detailed, full-color artwork is used to explain the process of fetal development: implantation; formation of the placenta and fetal membrane; development of each of the major systems of the body; and the growth, maturation, and further refinements that occur in the fetus after the eighth week.

Syndromes in Pediatrics
  35mm filmstrip, audio-tape cassette, 33⅓ LP, color.
  Discusses some pediatric syndromes encountered on occasion by nurses. Inasmuch as many of the syndromes presented are genetic disorders, a succinct review of basic genetics is included.

V.C.I. Studios, CBS

Prescription for Living
  Life Begins at 40—Weeks
  30 minutes, videotape, sound, color.
  Development of human embryo from conception to birth.

Yale University School of Medicine

Development of the Human Gastrointestinal Tract
  15 minutes, 16mm, sound, color.
  Shows, by animation, the development of the human gastrointestinal tract in the fetal stage.

---

*Complete addresses are given in the Appendix.

Chapter Eleven

CONDITIONS OF THE NEWBORN REQUIRING IMMEDIATE OR SHORT-TERM CARE

What was said in Chapter 6 (see p. 124) and Chapter 9 (see p. 209) concerning the psychologic need of the newborn for contact with his parents and of his parents' need for contact with him is true also when the infant must stay in the hospital for short- or long-term treatment after the discharge of his mother. Not only is it important for parents to touch and talk to their infant, but it is also important for them to assist with his care if at all possible. Helping the parents develop a strong attachment to their infant and the infant attain feelings of warmth and security from the parents, so vital to normal development, are the responsibilities of the nurse.

In order to provide care to the newborn infant the nurse must understand the various illnesses he may have. These include congenital diseases, congenital anomalies, birth injuries, respiratory conditions, infections, and addiction. For the sake of clarity, the conditions included in each of these classifications will be divided into those which require immediate or short-term care, discussed in the present chapter, and those which require long-term care, discussed in Chapter 12.

CONGENITAL DISEASES

Hemolytic Disease of the Newborn (Erythroblastosis Fetalis)

Hemolytic disease of the fetus or newborn includes a number of hemolytic processes.

Etiology. Hemolytic disease is due to the development of an isohemagglutinin in the maternal serum, the result of incompatibility of parental genetic factors. Antibodies traverse the placenta and produce agglutination of the infant's red blood cells. The two most important hemolytic diseases are due to isoimmunization to (1) the Rh factor and to (2) A or B substances.

HEMOLYTIC DISEASE DUE TO RH INCOMPATIBILITY

There are three blood combinations which are always compatible, i.e., when the Rh factors of the blood of each parent are such that an infant-mother sensitization cannot arise. These are (1) when both parents are positive, (2) when both are negative, and (3) when the mother is Rh-positive and the father is Rh-negative. Erythroblastosis fetalis occurs when the mother is Rh-negative and the father—and therefore the fetus also—Rh-positive. About 15 per cent of the white population are Rh-negative and 85 per cent positive. Very few Asian or black women are Rh-negative.

Etiology. Erythroblastosis fetalis does not always occur in the infant born of an Rh-incom-

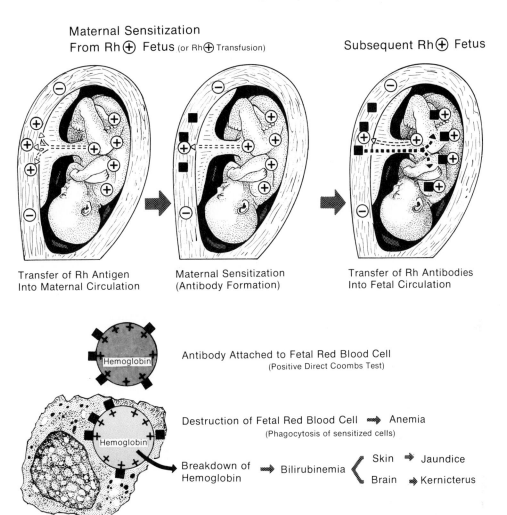

Key: ⊕ Rh Positive ⊖ Rh Negative ■ Rh Antibody

Maternal Sensitization
From Rh ⊕ Fetus (or Rh ⊕ Transfusion)

Subsequent Rh ⊕ Fetus

Transfer of Rh Antigen
Into Maternal Circulation

Maternal Sensitization
(Antibody Formation)

Transfer of Rh Antibodies
Into Fetal Circulation

Antibody Attached to Fetal Red Blood Cell
(Positive Direct Coombs Test)

Destruction of Fetal Red Blood Cell ➡ Anemia
(Phagocytosis of sensitized cells)

Breakdown of ➡ Bilirubinemia ⟨ Skin ➡ Jaundice
Hemoglobin   Brain ➡ Kernicterus

FIGURE 11–1. Etiology of erythroblastosis fetalis (hemolytic disease of the newborn). (Drawing after Ross Laboratories.)

patible mating, because of the vagaries of maternal sensitization, paternal heterozygosity, and small families. The first child is less apt to be affected than are later ones. The reason for this is that the mother who produces antibodies easily will begin to do so in response to the stimulus of the first fetus. The titer is further stimulated by succeeding pregnancies.

Rh isoimmunization evidently results from a relatively large transplacental hemorrhage at delivery or, probably more often, from sometimes undetectable bleeding which occurs at any time during pregnancy. All Rh-negative women are at risk because even when their postpartum blood specimens contain no Rh-positive fetal erythrocytes, Rh immunization can still take place. Sensitization may also result if the mother has had a transfusion or an injection of Rh-positive blood cells. These anti-Rh agglutinins are carried from the mother's blood across the placenta into the

blood stream of the fetus and destroy the fetal erythrocytes by their specific reaction with the Rh-positive cells.

Clinical Manifestations. The vernix caseosa is often yellowish; in some cases there may be severe edema (*hydrops fetalis*). Jaundice appears on the first day, and there is progressive anemia due to the severe hemolysis. Enlargement of the liver and the spleen is common. In severe cases the central nervous system may be affected, as evidenced by opisthotonos, spasticity, abnormal Moro reflex, inactivity, and anorexia present from the third to fifth day after birth. Under such circumstances kernicterus (jaundice of the basal ganglia) may be present.

Laboratory Findings. The mother's blood is found to be Rh-negative and the infant's Rh-positive. The Coombs test result on the infant is positive. His blood picture shows anemia with an increased number of nucleated red blood cells. The indirect serum bilirubin level is increased. The anti-Rh titer of the mother's blood is elevated.

In order to determine how ill an infant of an Rh-negative mother is, the physician can do an amniocentesis by injecting a needle into a pregnant uterus and withdrawing from the amniotic sac a few drops of amber fluid. A spectrophotometric analysis of the bilirubin concentration of this amniotic fluid can determine the diagnosis or degree of illness of the fetus. Therapy is aimed at inducing birth early and carrying out an exchange transfusion.

Course. In severe hemolytic disease the infant may be born dead or may die within the first few days of life. On the other hand, with prompt therapy complete recovery is the rule.

Kernicterus sometimes follows severe hemolytic disease of the newborn. The symptoms may appear within the first week of life or months later. The more important symptoms are noted above. Such sequelae, it is believed, can be avoided through the use of exchange transfusions when the serum bilirubin threatens to rise above a critical level of 20 mg. per 100 ml. If the infant survives, there may be central nervous system damage.

Treatment. If the newborn is only mildly affected, phototherapy (see p. 206) may be used; however, frequent determinations of the indirect bilirubin level and other blood studies must be made. The more severely affected infant should receive an exchange transfusion with fresh Rh-negative blood which is compatible with the mother's serum by the indirect Coombs test. This should be done as soon as possible after delivery and repeated later if necessary.

EXCHANGE TRANSFUSION. A polyethylene catheter is inserted into the umbilical or other large vein. Small amounts (approximately 10 to 20 ml. at a time) of the newborn's blood are withdrawn and equal amounts of Rh-negative blood injected. This process is continued until most of the newborn's blood has been replaced; approximately 500 ml. of blood are generally used in this procedure. Antibiotics are given after transfusion to prevent infection.

During this procedure the infant must be kept warm. The blood used for the transfusion must be kept at 98.6° F. (37° C.). During the transfusion one person should be responsible for monitoring the pulse and respirations, observing the infant's general condition, including his color, suctioning him if necessary, and recording the venous pressure as well as the amount of blood injected and withdrawn. After the procedure the infant must be observed for hemorrhage from the transfusion site as well as for his general condition.

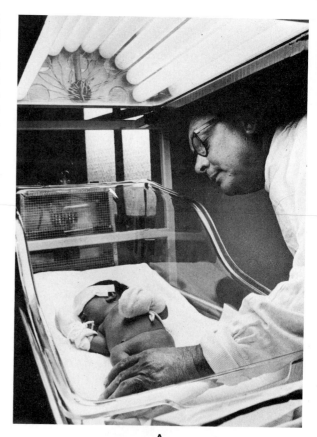

A

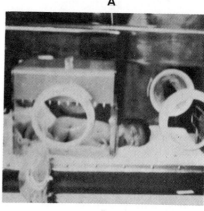

B

FIGURE 11–2. The light used in phototherapy reduces the infant's serum bilirubin level and consequently the icterus. A, The infant should wear an eye shield to protect his eyes from the fluorescent light. (From S. Nocella: *Medical World News*, June 13, 1969.) B, A phototherapy device concentrates maximum radiant energy on the infant, with no light spillage. The infant's head is excluded from radiation. A neon light source is used rather than a conventional fluorescent unit. (Courtesy of Medi-Spec Corporation.)

If the infant is too young for an emergency delivery and an exchange transfusion is indicated, the physician can administer an intrauterine transfusion into the abdomen of the unborn child. The position of the needle in the abdomen of the fetus is checked by x-ray to determine its location. Since transfused blood survives only temporarily, repeated transfusions may be necessary.

The degree of anxiety which the mother feels during the intrauterine transfusion may be great. The nurses caring for the patient must share her hope that the fetus will survive and strive to support her confidence in her physician. Many pregnant women complain of backache during the procedure because they must lie on a hard x-ray table. Comfort measures such as backrubs to reduce the strain should be carried out. Waiting for the birth of the infant produces further anxiety in the mother. The nurse must be supportive until the infant is actually born and the outcome of the procedure is known.

Prevention. Prevention begins in the prenatal period. All pregnant women should have their blood typed. Any woman who is Rh-negative should have her antibody titer ascertained after the thirty-sixth week. Thus in the event of a rising titer a tentative diagnosis can be made even before the birth of the child. If the newborn infant is Rh-positive, if the Coombs test result is positive, and if the infant exhibits a rapidly rising bilirubin level, treatment is indicated.

Physicians are currently giving RhoGAM, special anti-Rh immunoglobulin, intramuscularly to Rh-negative mothers within three days after delivering their first Rh-incompatible infant so that they will not develop the antibodies that will destroy Rh-positive blood. This vaccine is a highly concentrated solution of Rh antibodies obtained from Rh-negative persons who have been sensitized to the Rh factor. Later, when the blood of these mothers is tested, it is found to lack anti-Rh-positive antibodies. Each mother is thus passively protected against incompatibility with a future Rh-positive fetus. Unfortunately the vaccine is expensive and is not effective on Rh-negative mothers who have already developed their own active antibodies by having given birth to an Rh-positive infant.

HEMOLYTIC DISEASE DUE TO ABO INCOMPATIBILITY

Etiology. The etiologic process is the same as in Rh incompatibility. Clinical manifestations of hemolytic disease are more commonly due to ABO incompatibility than to Rh incompatibility. In ABO incompatibility the difficulty is caused by the presence of the blood group A or B factors.

Hemolytic disease due to A or B incompatibility is not usually anticipated unless there is a history of this problem among previous children in the family.

Course. A or B isoimmune disease of the newborn is usually mild and may even pass unnoticed. It should be treated, however, if signs are well developed.

Clinical Manifestations. Mild jaundice appears during the first 36 hours of life. On physical examination the physician may find enlargement of both the liver and the spleen. Central nervous system complications are rare. There is little or no edema.

Treatment. The majority of affected infants need no treatment, but an exchange transfusion (using group O blood of appropriate Rh type) may be needed if the infant's serum bilirubin level approaches 20 mg. per 100 ml. Treatment is aimed at the prevention of kernicterus.

Responsibilities of the Nurse in Hemolytic Disease of the Newborn. Skillful nursing is needed. An incubator to maintain the infant's temperature should be in readiness, as well as oxygen in case he becomes cyanotic. Preparation for exchange transfusion should be made when it is known that the birth of a possible erythroblastotic infant is expected or as soon as possible after it has been proved that the infant needs an exchange transfusion. His condition must be closely watched during and after treatment, and special attention must be paid to respirations, pulse, temperature, and evidence of increasing lethargy. At all times the nurse should watch for and report to the physician the following symptoms: increasing jaundice, pigmentation of urine, edema, cyanosis, convulsions, and changes in any of the vital signs. The nurse should change the lethargic infant's position frequently to prevent atelectasis and infection. If kernicterus is present, however, the infant should be handled as little as possible, since movement is likely to result in increased spasms. Because the infant is weak and may have difficulty in sucking, a soft nipple with a large hole should be given him, or he should be fed with a medicine dropper. These infants may be breastfed, since it is doubtful whether agglutinins in the breast milk would affect their circulating erythrocytes to a great extent.

Hemorrhagic Disease of the Newborn

Etiology. This disease is due to a deficiency of prothrombin resulting from either immaturity of the liver or a deficiency of vitamin K. Vitamin K, which is ordinarily elaborated by bacterial action within the intestinal tract during later life, is lacking in the sterile newborn. It is essential to the formation of prothrombin by the liver.

Clinical Manifestations. There is bleeding from the skin, retina, conjunctiva, mucous membranes, umbilical wound, or viscera. The infant may have tar-colored stools, owing to blood in the fecal matter, or hematemesis (vomiting of bright red blood). Such bleeding may occur with or without trauma and is most likely to appear between the second and fifth days of life, when the available prothrombin is at the lowest level (see Physiologic Hypoprothrombinemia, p. 145).

Laboratory Findings. The prothrombin time is prolonged; the coagulation time may be normal or prolonged.

Treatment. Vitamin K_1 is given intramuscularly once or repeated as necessary. The effect is much slower, however, than if the vitamin is given intravenously. A transfusion of fresh, matched whole blood may be given.

Prevention. The mother may be given synthetic water-soluble vitamin K intravenously, intramuscularly or orally before the beginning of labor is expected. This will help to correct maternal hypoprothrombinemia due to poor diet and thus may help to raise the prothrombin level of the infant at the time of birth. Direct administration of vitamin K_1 to the full-term infant is more effective than administration to the mother before delivery. Vitamin K_1 may be given intramuscularly to the infant immediately after birth. Large doses of vitamin K do not increase the therapeutic effect.

Responsibilities of the Nurse. The nursing care is that of the normal or premature newborn, with special care in handling to avoid the slightest danger of trauma and resulting bleeding. The nurse must observe these infants even more carefully than others for evidence of bleeding from the umbilical wound or gastrointestinal tract.

CONGENITAL ANOMALIES

Emergency Surgery and the Newborn

Several of the congenital anomalies seen in newborns can be corrected by surgery immediately or soon after birth. The normal newborn is an excellent surgical risk during the first 48 hours of life, but the mortality rate rises rapidly when the infant is more than 72 hours old. After this period several factors make operation more dangerous. The most important of these factors are (1) changes in fluid and electrolyte balance, (2) the normal breakdown of the red blood cells, and (3) the lessening of the infant's physiologic reserve, i.e., all the elements necessary for carrying on the vital functions, which he received through the placenta while still *in utero*.

TRANSPORTATION OF THE NEWBORN TO THE HOSPITAL

Newborns delivered in the home or in a hospital in which surgery is not done on this young age group must be transferred to a hospital or medical center where adequate personnel and facilities for therapy are available. All too often the infant is simply wrapped in a blanket and transferred in a vehicle in which no emergency equipment is available.

The newborn should be transferred in an ambulance or other safe means of transportation which has a portable incubator (see p. 191) with oxygen available in order to maintain his body temperature and the oxygen level in his blood. Equipment for suctioning should also be available in case of the need for removal of secretions.

The person responsible for the transfer of the newborn should be medically oriented and aware of the observations to be made and the appropriate treatment to be given in an emergency. For instance, the nurse or other skilled attendant should prevent the torsion of an omphalocele and prevent the aspiration of fluid by suctioning the esophagus or stomach when a diagnosis of esophageal atresia or intestinal obstruction has been made. Other observations and methods of therapy will be discussed under the various appropriate diagnoses in this chapter.

PREPARATION FOR SURGERY

On arrival at the hospital or medical center the newborn requiring immediate surgery should be cared for in an area where emergency equipment and experienced personnel are available such as in a newborn intensive care unit (see pp. 75 and 191). The nurse should make certain that equipment for determining levels of blood gases, for endotracheal intubation, for assisted respiration, and for other emergency procedures is available. A catheter placed in the radial artery to obtain arterial blood for blood gas determinations is essential to determine the need for the use of a ventilator.

The same care exerted when transporting the infant from hospital to hospital should be taken when transporting him from his crib or incubator to the x-ray department or operating room.

Preoperative preparation gives diminishing returns if it is prolonged. Opaque material should not be used in establishing the diagnosis of atresia of the esophagus or upper intestinal

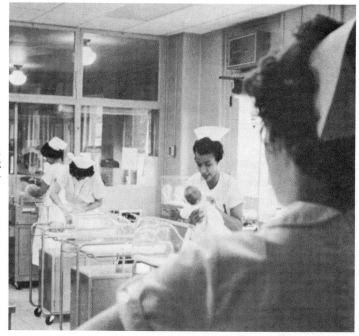

FIGURE 11–3. Nursery for newborn surgical patients. Each infant requires intensive nursing care. (Courtesy Children's Hospital of Philadelphia.)

obstruction because of the possibility of aspiration of fluid into the lungs with resulting pneumonia. Blood chemistry studies, if done at all, should be done by microtechniques to prevent depletion of blood volume. The newborn should be handled as little as possible. He should be hydrated, but surgery should not be postponed beyond the second day of life.

Extremely small doses of preoperative medication will prevent secretions from accumulating in the respiratory tract, and emptying the stomach of gastric contents will prevent vomiting with the danger of aspiration of vomitus. An environment with a high oxygen content is required so that the infant may not become exhausted by his efforts to have a sufficient intake.

To be successful, surgery of the newborn requires early diagnosis, minimal preparation and an expert team, including a surgeon, a pediatrician, a radiologist, and an anesthesiologist who are experienced in working with infants, and nurses who are thoroughly accustomed to nursing the newborn who undergoes operation.

PHYSIOLOGIC PROBLEMS IN SURGERY OF THE NEWBORN

There are many problems in surgery of the newborn which make it a specialty for surgeons and nurses alike. The newborn does not show gradually increasing signs of loss of blood as do older children and adults. Because of the elasticity of his blood vessels, the infant may show no danger signs until he suddenly goes into shock. Then he is pulseless, and the blood pressure is low and the skin mottled. Because of this characteristic response of the newborn undergoing operation, hemorrhage must be anticipated and blood given before his condition is serious. It is difficult to give the correct amount of blood

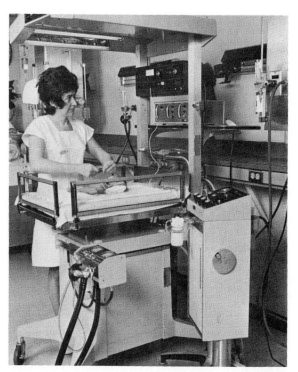

FIGURE 11–4. The Ohio Neonatal Intensive Care Center includes equipment for warmth, resuscitation, aspiration, and inhalation therapy. (Courtesy of Ohio Medical Products.)

when he is in shock, since too much fluid given then may cause pulmonary edema.

Other problems include an unstable weight status, diminution of certain aspects of renal function, labile control of body temperature, and a response to a lack of oxygen by increased respirations which, if allowed to continue, may result in exhaustion and death.

RESPONSIBILITIES OF THE NURSE IN THE CARE OF THE NEWBORN AFTER SURGERY

Infants have a remarkable resilience; on the other hand, they lack the physiologic reserve which older children have. If all goes well, an infant's recovery is rapid, but if complications arise, a state of emergency may develop with little warning.

Since the condition of the newborn postoperatively may change rapidly, the nurse must check his condition frequently, especially his temperature, the quality of his respirations and color, and the presence of bleeding, among other observations, and assume the responsibility for carrying out lifesaving procedures in the absence of the physician.

The most crucial period after surgery of the newborn is the first postoperative hour. He must be assisted to maintain his body temperature between 97 and 99° F. (36.1 and 37.2° C.) by the use of an incubator, to recover from anesthesia, and to maintain the patency of his small airway by positioning of his head and by suctioning of secretions from his nasopharynx. High humidity is usually maintained in the incubator in order to dilute secretions in the nasopharynx and to compensate for fluid lost because of a rapid respiratory rate. Oxygen is also usually given to newborns postoperatively in approximately 40 per cent concentration; however, higher concentrations may be given as necessary.

The newborn may die quickly from exhaustion unless his nursing care is planned to protect him from unnecessary external stimuli. Such care as the changing of dressings, the administration of medications and the taking of vital signs should be planned to be done together so that the infant does not have to be disturbed repeatedly.

The newborn postsurgical patient may be placed on a waterbed, if ordered by the physician, and should be turned from side to side without disturbing him more than necessary; however, he should be prevented from assuming any position which would constrict his diaphragmatic movements on respiration. The nurse should also observe the newborn carefully to prevent constriction of any dressings which might hinder respirations.

Fluid balance is maintained initially by the intravenous route. Intravenous solutions, electrolyte solutions and medications are given very slowly. Intravenous fluids are ordered in drops per minute as well as in cubic centimeters per hour in order to prevent too much fluid being given too rapidly. (See page 409 for further discussion of intravenous therapy.) When it is necessary to bypass the gastrointestinal tract completely, the method of total parenteral nutrition or *hyperalimentation (parenteral alimentation)* may be used.

The site of the needle insertion or of the cutdown should be inspected frequently for leakage. The infant should be weighed within his incubator if possible in order to determine whether adequate or more than adequate fluid is being given.

The nurse is responsible for observing gastrostomy or chest tubes, catheters, and intravenous tubing to determine their adequate functioning. If the newborn is fed by gastrostomy tube, it should never be clamped for fear of regurgitation through the esophagus and aspiration into the lungs, and for the purpose of relieving gaseous distention. After feedings the end of the tube should be elevated approximately 6 inches, or at a height determined by the physician, so that, should the stomach contract, the contents could be easily expelled. Depending on the procedure used in the hospital, the gastrostomy tube should be irrigated with a small amount of saline solution prior to feedings. (See page 196 for the procedure of feeding by gavage.)

When oral feedings are begun, a small amount of glucose water may be given. The nurse must observe the infant carefully to determine whether he has adequate sucking and swallowing reflexes. If suctioning is indicated, it should be done promptly.

Since the newborn has an inadequate cough reflex and thus cannot clear the nasopharynx, the danger of vomiting with aspiration into the lungs is ever present. In order to prevent this, constant suction drainage from his stomach may be established, or his head may be placed lower than his body and turned to the side so that secretions and vomitus can drain from his mouth. If aspiration does occur, endotracheal suctioning must be instituted promptly.

As the newborn shows progress he is gradually removed from his incubator and given decreasing concentrations of oxygen until he can live comfortably and safely in a bassinet in the stable temperature of the newborn unit.

The emotional support which the parents of a malformed newborn need has already been discussed on page 231. The inexperienced nurse should review this subject in order to obtain a more complete view of total family care.

The care of the postoperative newborn is an exceedingly important area of pediatric nursing. The details of nursing care of infants having various conditions will be discussed when the conditions are described.

Conditions Which May Require Surgical Correction

CONGENITAL LARYNGEAL STRIDOR

Noisy respiration—a crowing sound on inspiration—is a condition which may be due to a number of factors. The physician will determine the cause of the stridor, and the treatment is based upon his findings. No therapy may be required, or immediate treatment may be necessary if the child is to survive. The nursing care will be based upon the plan of treatment outlined by the physician.

Etiology. Laryngeal stridor lasting after the first few days of life is due to some abnormal condition in or around the larynx which may be located by laryngoscopy (Fig. 11–5). The most common cause is flabbiness of the epiglottis and the supraglottic aperture. Other causes include epiglottal redundancy, relaxation of the laryngeal wall, absence of the rings of the trachea, deformity of the vocal cords, or a web which partially occludes the larynx. In the older infant or child, stridor may be caused by laryngeal infection (see p. 539), tetany (p. 442), or a foreign body in the larynx (p. 404).

Clinical Manifestations, Diagnosis, and Treatment. The main diagnostic symptom is noisy breathing, often with a crowing sound on inspiration. This is most noticeable when the infant cries, and is present at birth or shortly thereafter. This symptom may be accompanied by mild or severe intercostal and supraclavicular retractions. The infant may become cyanotic and dyspneic.

Treatment is based on correction of the underlying cause. For mild stridor there is no specific therapy, but for severe stridor operation may be necessary. If the infant appears unable to take in sufficient oxygen on inspiration, an emergency tracheotomy (see p. 541) may be done. Such an operation may be only a step toward further corrective surgery. For deformity of the larynx, laryngoplasty may be necessary.

Course and Prognosis. If the condition is uncorrected, constant retractions of the thorax may cause deformity, since the bones readily bend under pressure. If the infant has difficulty in nursing, he may not take sufficient nourishment, and malnutrition may result. Naturally a respiratory infection increases the difficulty and may cause a mild chronic condition to become severe.

The mild, simple form of congenital laryngeal stridor usually subsides by the time the infant is six to 18 months old. The child does not become cyanotic, and he shows no symptoms other than

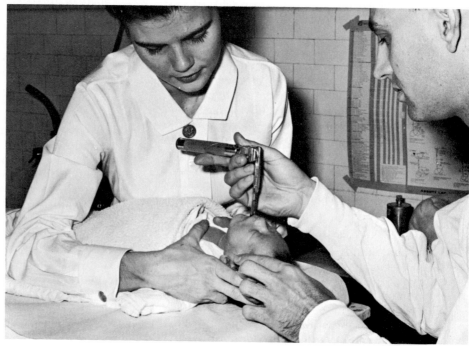

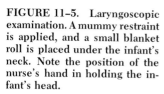

FIGURE 11–5. Laryngoscopic examination. A mummy restraint is applied, and a small blanket roll is placed under the infant's neck. Note the position of the nurse's hand in holding the infant's head.

his noisy breathing. But the *prognosis* in congenital stridor due to some malformation of the larynx will depend upon the cause.

Responsibilities of the Nurse. Feeding may be a problem, since any interference in breathing makes sucking difficult. The infant will have to be fed slowly, stopping frequently for him to breathe unimpeded by nursing. The respiratory process is more imperative than his desire for food, and so he will stop to breathe without the hindrance of sucking. This does not mean that his hunger is satisfied. The nurse should wait a few moments and then offer him the nipple again. If he appears to have difficulty in swallowing the milk, the nurse should remove the nipple from his mouth at once. A small nipple will probably give the best results. The size of the hole in the nipple should be carefully chosen to give the rate of flow which the infant finds easiest to handle. All infants, of course, should be held when fed and never left with the bottle propped on a pad, but with these infants it is imperative that they be held in the correct position and the bottle supported at the proper angle.

The mother should have ample opportunity to become accustomed to the infant's noisy breathing before she leaves the hospital; otherwise she has no standard by which to judge whether his condition becomes worse. The difficulty in breathing is likely to increase if a respiratory infection develops or if the infant aspirates a little of his feeding or in some other way undergoes an added strain on his already inadequate breathing. The mother should give the infant his bottle with the nurse beside her to show her the proper technique. The nurse should call her attention to the infant's reaction to too rapid feeding or failure to withdraw the nipple from his mouth if he appears unable to take the milk. If he is a breastfed infant, the mother will have had ample opportunity to learn the technique of feeding him before she takes him home.

Since a respiratory infection increases the infant's breathing problem, it is important that he be kept from every source of respiratory infection. He should be kept warm, dry, and away from drafts at all times. Raising the humidity in his environment is helpful.

CHOANAL ATRESIA

Choanal atresia is a congenital obstruction of the posterior nares at the entrance to the nasopharynx. The obstruction is usually caused by a membrane, but in rare cases by a bony growth. The condition may be unilateral or bilateral.

Clinical Manifestations, Diagnosis, and Treatment. The *symptoms* of bilateral obstruction are mouth-breathing and difficulty in taking his feedings. Mouth-breathing is difficult for the infant to do, especially when he is trying to suck at the same time. There may be dyspnea because he cannot obtain enough oxygen. If the obstruction is unilateral, the infant may do well unless infection occurs and persists on the side opposite the obstruction.

The *diagnosis* is confirmed by passing a sound, probe or soft catheter up the nostril until it meets the obstruction.

Bilateral atresia should be relieved *as early as possible*, since it is one cause of asphyxia of the newborn. By using a nasoscope the physician is able to pierce the obstruction if it is membranous. A bony obstruction requires extensive operation. Unilateral choanal atresia need not be corrected until the infant is in optimum condition.

Responsibilities of the Nurse. There is little in the nursing care of these infants which is specifically directed toward relief of their condition. The nostrils should be kept clean. Feeding the infant is difficult, since he has trouble in breathing and sucking at the same time, and since there is danger of aspiration of the formula. This is the reason for early treatment if the condition is bilateral. The precautions and techniques are similar to those outlined in the nursing care of the infant with congenital laryngeal stridor.

Conditions Incompatible with Life, but Amenable to Surgical Correction

There are several congenital anomalies of the gastrointestinal tract which, though incompatible with life, may be corrected by surgical treatment. These anomalies are imperforate anus, atresia of the esophagus, omphalocele, diaphragmatic hernia, and intestinal obstruction. These lesions are often associated with other congenital anomalies and are also seen in premature infants. Early diagnosis and treatment are essential in saving life. Operation immediately after birth is indicated when the infant has a diaphragmatic hernia or a large omphalocele.

The difficulties of surgery of the gastrointestinal tract in the newborn increase hour by hour. The infant swallows air, and the gastrointestinal tract becomes distended. He becomes progressively more exhausted because of his increased respiratory rate and is less able to withstand operation. Providing adequate nutrition is a problem that has become less difficult with the development of techniques of parenteral alimentation (see p. 436, Chapter 15).

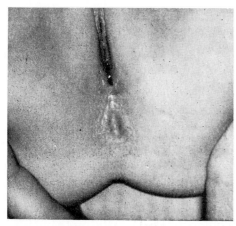

FIGURE 11–6. Photograph of imperforate anus, type III (Fig. 11–7 C). (From P. Hanley and M. O. Hines, in *Christopher's Minor Surgery.* 8th ed., edited by Ochsner and DeBakey.)

Three procedures were outlined under Examination of Internal Organs (p. 146) which nurses may carry out to determine the presence of anomalies which require immediate treatment. The nurse should report the findings to the physician, who would then check the symptoms and determine the treatment to be given.

In addition, the nurse should observe an infant closely for four important signs which indicate the possibility of a lesion incompatible with life. These signs are *cyanosis, vomiting, absence of stools, and abdominal distention.*

Cyanosis is indicative of many conditions. Those we are concerned with here are diaphragmatic hernia and atresia of the esophagus. *Vomiting* of bile-stained material is a sign of intestinal obstruction. An infant with a diaphragmatic hernia may have repetitive vomiting. In atresia of the esophagus there is immediate vomiting of the glucose solution, given if there is any question of the presence of an abnormal condition. *Absence of stools* is the characteristic sign of any form of intestinal obstruction, as is *abdominal distention.* Although these four signs may be seen in the normal newborn, they should be reported promptly to the physician in order to lead to early diagnosis and treatment of conditions incompatible with life, but amenable to surgical correction.

IMPERFORATE ANUS

Incidence and Etiology. This is the most common congenital anomaly of the newborn which is incompatible with life. In the eighth week of embryonic life the membrane which separates the rectum from the anus normally is absorbed, and thus a continuous canal is formed whose outlet is the anus. If this membrane is not absorbed and union does not take place, an imperforate anus results. A fistula between the rectum and the vagina, perineum, or fourchet in the female, or the urinary tract, scrotum, or perineum in the male, is likely to be formed when the infant has an imperforate anus.

Diagnosis. The diagnosis is made when (1) no anal opening is found on cursory examination of the infant in the delivery room; (2) the physician or nurse cannot insert a small finger or thermometer into the infant's rectum; (3) there is no meconium stool; and (4) later abdominal distention occurs. In the presence of these signs the distance between the closed end of the rectum and the anal dimple is ascertained by x-ray examination. The infant cries, and the air which he swallows goes only to the closed end of the rectum. In order to force air down through the bowel, the infant is held upside down or on his side with his knees pushed against the abdomen. An opaque object is placed at the anal dimple, and the roentgenogram thus shows the distance of the rectum from the anus.

Obstruction in a male infant must be relieved at once, for the stool cannot be passed, but an emergency is not so likely in a female, since a fistula probably exists into the vagina, perineum, or fourchet. The outlet of the fistula is easily found on inspection. The urine should be watched for flecks of meconium.

Treatment. The surgical procedure depends upon the type of anomaly. The anal defect may be such that the opening is covered by a thin membrane through which meconium can be

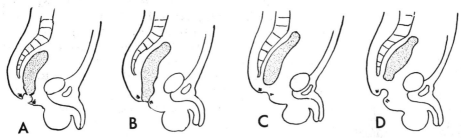

FIGURE 11–7. Diagrammatic illustration of 4 types of congenital anorectal malformation. (From P. Hanley and M. O. Hines, in *Christopher's Minor Surgery.* 8th ed., edited by Ochsner and DeBakey.)

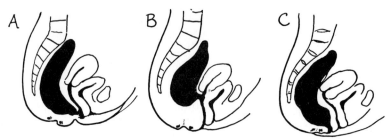

FIGURE 11–8. Schematic representation of imperforate anus, type III (Fig. 11–7 *C*), with associated fistula in the female. *A*, Low rectovaginal. *B*, High rectovaginal. *C*, Rectoperineal. (From P. Hanley and M. O. Hines, in *Christopher's Minor Surgery*. 8th ed., edited by Ochsner and DeBakey.)

seen. In this case the physician is able to perforate the membrane with a blunt instrument, and no further treatment is required. If the distance between the anal dimple and the blind end of the colon is not more than 1.5 cm., correction is made through the perineum, but if the distance is greater than 1.5 cm., a colostomy is performed while awaiting definitive operation, or the colon is brought down through the anal dimple by an abdominal-perineal procedure. If the anus is normal, but the closed end of the rectum ends in a blind pouch a few centimeters from the sphincter, the condition, called *atresia of the rectum,* must be surgically corrected as would any other colonic obstruction.

Responsibilities of the Nurse. One of the most important characteristics of the professional nurse is the ability for intelligent interpretation of meaningful observations. The detection of imperforate anus is a case in point. In the appraisal in the nursery the nurse should observe the newborn for the indications of imperforate anus mentioned previously and report promptly those found.

After the diagnosis of occlusion has been made the physician may order gastric suction. If operation is to be done, there may be no specific preoperative preparation. Postoperatively, if the operation has involved only the anal area, that site should be kept dry and clean. A diaper should not be used. When a stool is expelled, it should be cleaned away immediately. The infant should have nothing inserted into his rectum. No tension should be placed on the perineal sutures. Since the newborn when placed on his abdomen pulls his legs up under him, putting tension on the perineal area, he should be positioned on either side and turned frequently.

If a colostomy has been made, the skin around the wound must be kept clean. The infant's skin is more readily irritated than that of the older child or adult, and cleanliness is very important. Aluminum paste or zinc oxide ointment is used to protect the skin. If the skin breaks down, karaya gum powder may be sprinkled liberally on the area. The paste which is formed should be allowed to adhere to the skin for several days. When it comes off, the skin beneath is healed. The adhesive straps with ties which hold the colostomy dressing in place should be adjusted so that they remain clean and so that the dressing may be easily changed. An abdominal binder or a folded diaper (pinned around the abdomen) may be used instead of adhesive tape to prevent breakdown of the skin. If the mother is going to care for her infant at home before the colostomy is closed, she should be taught the correct procedure so that her anxiety can be reduced (see Fig. 9–13).

If surgery for this condition is not successful, the child may become a rectal cripple unable to control the seepage of feces from his rectum. This condition, depending on its severity, causes social problems as he grows older in that he may not be acceptable to his peer group who have been successfully bowel-trained.

ATRESIA OF THE ESOPHAGUS

Incidence, Pathology, Clinical Manifestations, and Diagnosis. Among the obstructive anomalies of the gastrointestinal tract in the newborn, this condition ranks second (imperforate anus holding first place). The esophagus, instead of being an open tube from the throat to the stomach is closed at some point. A fistula is common between the trachea and the esophagus. In ap-

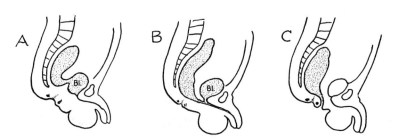

FIGURE 11–9. Diagrammatic representation of imperforate anus, type III (Fig. 11–7 *C*), with associated fistula in the male. *A*, Rectovesical. *B*, Rectourethral. *C*, Rectoperineal. (From P. Hanley and M. O. Hines, in *Christopher's Minor Surgery*, 8th ed., edited by Ochsner and DeBakey.)

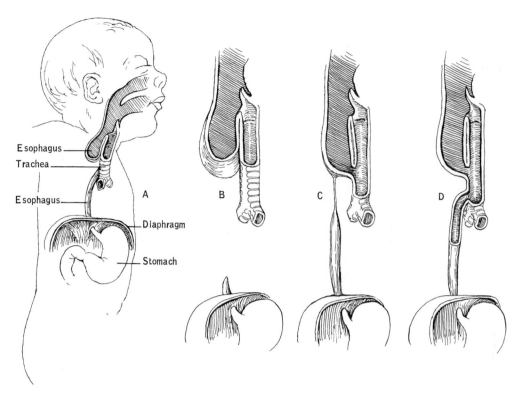

FIGURE 11–10. Atresia of the esophagus. *A*, Most common form. The upper esophagus ends in a blind pouch. The lower esophagus communicates with the trachea. *B*, The upper esophagus ends in a blind pouch. The lower segment does not communicate with the trachea. *C*, The upper esophagus ends in the trachea. A cordlike connection with the lower esophagus may or may not be present. *D*, Both upper and lower portions of the esophagus connect with the trachea.

proximately 80 per cent of these newborns the esophageal atresia is proximal and the tracheo-esophageal fistula is distal.

The presence of maternal polyhydramnios should provide a clue that the newborn has atresia of the esophagus. The fetus normally swallows amniotic fluid; however, with an obstruction of the gastrointestinal tract, especially atresia of the esophagus, he cannot do so.

At birth the infant has excessive mucus in the nasopharynx and therefore is cyanotic. When the mucus is withdrawn by aspiration and oxygen is given, the difficulty in breathing subsides, and the infant acquires the normal pink of the newborn. But as the secretions in the nasopharynx accumulate, he again becomes cyanotic. Nurses who care for newborns either in the delivery room or in the nursery should recognize this typical behavior and report the presence of excess mucus *immediately!* If this condition is suspected, the infant should not be fed until he is thoroughly examined and the patency of the esophagus determined.

If a small soft catheter cannot be passed through the infant's nose and down the esophagus, it is probably blocked by the area of atresia. An x-ray film shows the tip of the catheter coiled

back upon itself in a dilated esophageal pouch. *No radiopaque substance should be instilled into the esophagus because of the danger of the infant's aspirating it.* If the infant has a tracheoesophageal fistula, the roentgenogram will show air in the gastrointestinal tract.

If the newborn's condition is not recognized and he is fed, the nurse will note that the first mouthful goes down, but since the fluid can go no farther than the atretic area, the second is immediately expelled through the nose as well as the mouth. The infant chokes, sneezes, coughs and shows his discomfort by generalized movement. He is likely to aspirate some of the feeding, and pneumonia results. If he has a distal tracheoesophageal fistula, the stomach contents may be vomited into the tracheobronchial tree.

Treatment. Immediate operation is necessary. Depending upon the type of atresia, the following operations are performed: *(a)* An end-to-end anastomosis of the upper and lower segments of the esophagus is done and the fistula ligated. *(b)* If there is no lower portion of the esophagus or if the distance between the lower and upper esophageal pouches is too great for anastomosis, a cervical esophagostomy is performed, a gastrostomy is done for feeding pur-

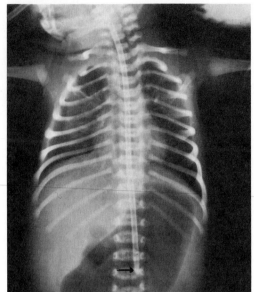

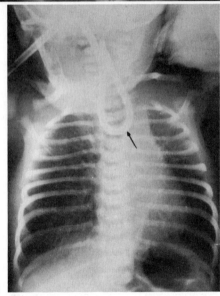

FIGURE 11–11. Atresia of the esophagus. *A,* Newborn with catheter passed through normal esophagus into stomach. *B,* Newborn with esophageal atresia, showing catheter coiled back in blocked esophagus. (Courtesy of Radiology Dept., Children's Hospital of Philadelphia.)

poses, and a colon transplant is done about a year later.

In some premature infants and in infants having severe pneumonia a double-lumen polyethylene catheter is passed into the esophagus and attached to a pump so that the drainage can be collected. The catheter is attached to the nose with adhesive tape. A gastrostomy is then made, and the infant is fed through a tube inserted into the stomach. An end-to-end anastomosis is carried out when the infant has gained weight and has been cured of his pneumonia. If an end-to-end anastomosis is not possible, an operation is performed in which either the right or transverse portion of the colon is brought into the chest to join the upper normal portion of the esophagus with the stomach. If a stricture occurs at the site of the anastomosis, it can be dilated later. The chance of survival depends upon the age, weight and general condition of the infant and upon whether other anomalies are present.

Responsibilities of the Nurse. It is advisable to place the infant in an incubator where he can be kept warm and is protected from infection. He should also be in an environment of high humidity, since this will tend to liquefy the thick mucous secretions which accumulate in the trachea. The nurse should observe the infant's respirations constantly to determine the need for aspiration of secretions. The physician will perform tracheal aspirations if necessary, but the nurse may do nasopharyngeal aspirations. Tracheotomy may be necessary if respiratory difficulty persists (see p. 541).

After operation the infant needs the individual attention of a nurse because frequent suctioning is necessary. He must be stimulated to cry and turned so that his lungs expand fully. Whenever a chest tube is in place, the nurse must remember to move the attached drainage bag or bottle when the infant is moved so as not to cause tension on the tube. The bag or bottle, of course, must never be raised. The tubing should not be disconnected, compressed or kinked. If clots of blood appear in the tube, the tube should be milked away from the infant. The nurse should have nearby two rubber-tipped hemostats in the event that there is a break in the system. The chest tube can be clamped immediately to prevent pneumothorax. The fluid level should be marked on the bag or bottle and checked frequently, depending on the amount of drainage.

If a gastrostomy has been done, feedings are begun several hours after operation. The feeding may be given by slow drip (by gravity) from an infusion bottle or by gastrostomy tube, according to the following procedure.

GASTROSTOMY FEEDING AND CARE. The equipment for feeding includes a tray on which are the warm formula, a sterile funnel or Asepto syringe, and a sterile pacifier.

Attach the funnel or syringe to the gastrostomy tube and fill with the formula before the clamp is removed. This will prevent air from being forced into the stomach. The funnel or syringe is then elevated to allow the fluid to run *slowly* into the stomach. Force should never be used. Since up to this time the stomach has not received food, distention by introducing air or feeding too rapidly must be avoided.

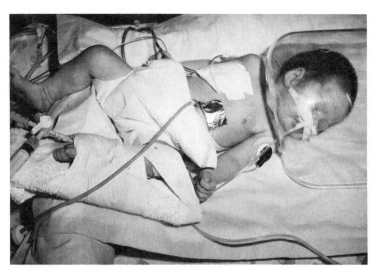

FIGURE 11–12. Intensive care for this infant after surgery for esophageal atresia includes oxygen by hood; chest drainage; constant temperature and ECG monitoring; hyperalimentation through an I.V. cutdown in her foot; and gastric drainage by N.G. double-lumen tube connected to continuous suction and gastrostomy tube to straight drainage. (C. D. Nalepka: © December 1975 The American Journal of Nursing Co. Reproduced from the *American Journal of Nursing*, Vol. 75, No. 12, with permission.)

Some physicians prefer that for infants under one year the gastrostomy tube remain open for variable periods of time, depending on the order, but elevated above the infant's body. If vomiting then occurs, the tube provides a safety valve.

The infant fed through a gastrostomy tube should be given the opportunity to satisfy his need for sucking. He is given a sterile pacifier to suck on while the milk is running into the stomach through the gastrostomy tube. Sucking on the nipple provides him with normal sucking pleasure, exercise for his jaw muscles, and relaxation while being fed. This facilitates the flow of milk. During and after the feeding the infant should be held in the nurse's arms if possible so that he learns to associate feeding with the comfort of being cuddled.

The care of the skin around the gastrostomy is exceedingly important. This area must be kept clean and protected with aluminum paste or zinc oxide ointment. To prevent displacing the tube when the dressings are changed, the inner side of the adhesive strap which holds the dressing in place should be covered with a second strip so that the part of the tape which extends over the dressing will not stick to it. The adhesive straps can then be tied together over the dressing.

The use of antibiotics will depend on the type of organism cultured from the cut end of the tracheo-esophageal fistula. As in other conditions involving the gastrointestinal tract, blood or plasma is given as necessary, and fluids are administered parenterally. There should be a minimum of salt content in these fluids so that the tissues do not become edematous. Depending on the infant's condition, feedings may be given by mouth, or through a tube into the esophagus or through a gastrostomy. Feeding by mouth should be done as soon as it is safe to do

so, for fluid passing through the esophagus lessens the danger of a stricture which will require dilation.

If the infant has a cervical esophagostomy, some physicians order "sham" feedings of strained foods after the age of two months. Even though the infant cannot digest this food, he can become used to various tastes and textures as he grows. The skin opening must be protected from secretions and kept scrupulously clean so that it does not become infected.

The psychologic needs of these infants for sucking and warmth and comfort from body contact must be met so far as is possible by both the parents and the nurse. They are in the hospital for a relatively long time and might easily become emotionally starved, though physically well cared for.

Because these infants need specialized care for long periods of time, parents may welcome referral to an appropriate community or state agency both for financial assistance and for the emotional support of the nurses from such an agency.

OMPHALOCELE

Incidence and Diagnosis. An omphalocele is a herniation of abdominal viscera at the point where the umbilical cord connects with the abdomen. The defect occurs from the sixth to the tenth week of intrauterine life. The sac which covers the hernia is composed of transparent avascular membrane.

The *diagnosis* is made by inspection. Although the omphalocele is easily seen, it is sometimes so small that it appears to be part of the normal umbilical cord.

Clinical Manifestations, Treatment, and Prognosis. On examination of a large omphalocele the mass of abdominal viscera seems to be

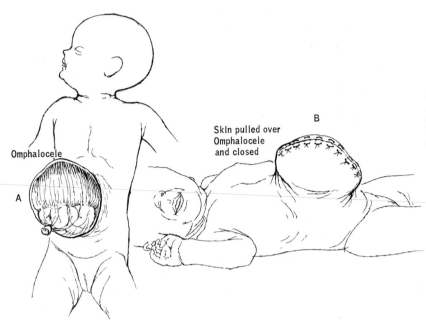

FIGURE 11-13. Omphalocele. A, An omphalocele is a herniation of the abdominal viscera at the umbilicus. B, The skin is closed over the omphalocele.

greater than the size of the abdominal cavity into which the viscera must be placed.

The *treatment* is by covering the defect with sterile saline dressings and immediate operation—replacement of viscera into the abdomen and closure of the abdominal wall—before the bowel is expanded by swallowed air and before the sac dries or is contaminated by bacteria. Even if it is protected by a sterile dressing, the sac may become infected by airborne bacteria. The operation may be done in one or two stages.

Currently the surgical treatment of a large omphalocele involves the use of a silastic bag.

The bag is sutured to the fascia or full thickness of abdominal wall and forms a pouch over the exposed abdominal contents. The bag is suspended from the top of the incubator. Every few days pressure is exerted on the pouch, thus forcing the organs into the abdominal cavity and stretching the abdominal wall over the defect. The defect can then be sutured closed. Mersilene or a similar synthetic material may be used instead of silastic.

With tremendously large omphaloceles some surgeons postpone operation and instead paint the area with a 2 per cent aqueous solution of

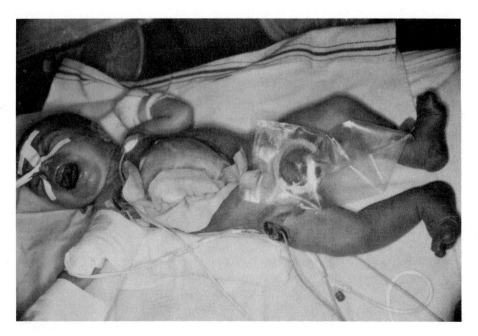

FIGURE 11-14. Newborn with omphalocele is being treated through the use of a silastic bag. Note that this seriously ill infant is being fed intravenously, has a nasogastric tube in place, and has a plastic receptacle attached to his genitalia to collect his urine. (Courtesy of Dr. C. Everett Koop, Children's Hospital of Philadelphia.)

Merthiolate applied 2 or 3 times daily, which produces an eschar that eventually converts the omphalocele into a large ventral hernia.

Because of these newer techniques of treatment, the mortality rate for this defect has been reduced in recent years; however, it still remains relatively high if other anomalies are present also.

DIAPHRAGMATIC HERNIA

Incidence, Pathology, Clinical Manifestations, and Diagnosis. Although this condition is reported today more frequently than it was in the past, this may be due not to an increase in the number of infants born with the anomaly, but rather to earlier and more accurate diagnosis.

A diaphragmatic hernia is more common on the left side. The lesion ranges from a slight to an extensive protrusion of the abdominal viscera through an opening in the diaphragm into the thoracic cavity.

The *symptoms* form a characteristic clinical picture, and the diagnosis can often be made in the delivery room if the lesion is extensive. On the other hand, in less severe states no symptoms may appear until later. The symptoms are severe respiratory difficulty, often with resulting cyanosis; a relatively large chest; failure of the affected side of the chest to expand as does the unaffected side; and a relatively small abdomen. When the herniated bowel fills with gas, all these symptoms increase in severity. Obviously

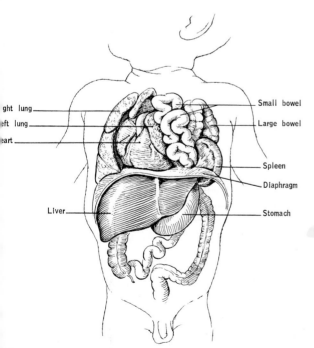

FIGURE 11–15. Diaphragmatic hernia. The abdominal viscera have herniated into the thorax. The thoracic viscera have been displaced and compressed.

Labels on figure: Right lung, Left lung, Heart, Liver, Small bowel, Large bowel, Spleen, Diaphragm, Stomach

no breath sounds are heard in the side of the defect when the lung is collapsed by abdominal viscera.

The *diagnosis* is made by physical examination and confirmed by roentgenograms of the chest. These show air from the intestinal tract in that part of the bowel which has protruded into the hernia and is pressing against the organs of the chest.

Treatment, Prognosis, and Responsibilities of the Nurse. Immediate operation is indicated. Gastric suction is used to remove secretions and swallowed air from the stomach and the intestinal tract. The infant should have his head elevated to reduce the pressure of the abdominal organs on his diaphragm. He may be placed on the affected side so that the unaffected lung can expand to its fullest potential. The operation consists in replacing the abdominal viscera in the abdominal cavity and in repair of the diaphragmatic defect. The lung on the affected side will then fill with air, and normal breathing will occur. If operation is not done immediately, the *prognosis* is very poor: the infant will probably die within the first month of life.

Postoperative *nursing care* is extremely important. Gastric suction is used to prevent abdominal distention immediately after operation. Transfusions of plasma or whole blood are given when necessary, and fluids are given intravenously until the infant can take them by mouth without abdominal distention. Feedings may be given by gavage on the second or third postoperative day. When fed by gavage, the infant is not so likely to swallow air as he is when sucking.

INTESTINAL OBSTRUCTION

Etiology. Intestinal obstruction in the newborn may result from a number of conditions—congenital atresia or stenosis of the intestine, malrotation of the colon with volvulus of the midgut, internal hernias, peritoneal bands, meconium ileus, or Hirschsprung's disease (p. 455).

CONGENITAL ATRESIA AND STENOSIS OF THE INTESTINE. Atresia, an absence of a lumen, in a portion of the intestinal tract is caused by an intrauterine interference with the blood supply due to a vascular accident, intussusception (see p. 422) or volvulus (see below). In stenosis there is partial occlusion of the gastrointestinal tract. There are three types of atresia: a diaphragmlike block of the lumen, a blind end which is not continuous with a distal segment, and segments of bowel connected with cordlike connections.

MALROTATION OF THE COLON WITH VOLVULUS. During the tenth week of embryonic development the emerging ileocecal structure normally rotates so that the cecum lies in the lower right quadrant of the abdomen and is fixed there by the mesentery. If this process does not occur, the colon may remain in the right upper quadrant. Here an abnormal membrane may obstruct the duodenum. This obstructing band is one of the most significant findings in malrotation. A more serious complication is volvulus of the midgut, which happens because of lack of mesenteric attachment. The freely mobile loops of small intestine twist on themselves, produce obstruction and may go on to necrosis from lack of blood supply.

INTERNAL HERNIAS AND OBSTRUCTION CAUSED BY PERITONEAL BANDS. Internal hernias are caused by a loop of bowel slipping out of the normal position and becoming caught in a defective area of the mesentery or becoming compressed between bands of the peritoneum. In either case intestinal obstruction occurs.

MECONIUM ILEUS. This condition occurs in 5 to 10 per cent of infants born with cystic fibrosis (see p. 444). The infant lacks the enzymes normally supplied by the pancreas and discharged into the intestinal tract. While the infant is still *in utero* this deficiency causes the meconium to be more sticky than is normal. It is of a putty-like consistency which causes it to adhere to the mucosa of the intestinal wall, and obstruction results. Solutions containing proteolytic enzymes may be used to irrigate the intestine during surgery and postoperatively if necessary. Other symptoms of cystic fibrosis can be expected to appear later in infancy.

Clinical Manifestations. The three main symptoms of intestinal obstruction are (1) absence of stools. If the infant has no stool within four hours after birth, examination for the presence of meconium may be made by inserting a gloved finger into the anus. If no indication of meconium is found, a colonic irrigation with not more than 10 ml. of physiologic saline solution may be ordered. (2) Vomitus stained with bile is diagnostic of intestinal obstruction, though obstruction may produce nonbile-stained vomitus as well. In general, whether the vomitus is bile-stained or not depends on the location of the obstruction. The vomitus will contain bile if the obstruction is below the ampulla of Vater. (3) Abdominal distention is a symptom of intestinal obstruction, though it may be physiologic in a normal child until meconium is passed. All infants have these symptoms to a degree, but the presence of two of these manifestations should suggest investigation.

The higher the obstruction, the earlier the symptoms appear, and the earlier can the diagnosis be made and treatment instituted. For this reason the lowest mortality rate is among infants with high obstruction.

Diagnosis. The decisive factor in the diagnosis is the roentgenogram, which shows the presence or absence of obstruction.

Treatment. The treatment is surgical. The majority of operations performed upon the newborn are for intestinal obstruction. The mortality rate is relatively high, but lowest among those cases in which the diagnosis is made early and relief is obtained before the infant's condition has degenerated.

Responsibilities of the Nurse. It is the nurse who is most likely to observe the main symptoms of intestinal obstruction in the newborn infant. The nurse observes readily whatever has meaning for him or her. That is why the pathology and etiology of this condition have been given in somewhat extensive detail.

BIRTH INJURIES

This is an inclusive term embracing both avoidable and unavoidable trauma at birth and also permanent damage occurring soon after birth.

INTRACRANIAL HEMORRHAGE

Etiology, Incidence, and Diagnosis. Trauma to the cranium is especially apt to occur when the infant's head is large in proportion to the size of the mother's pelvic outlet, when labor is prolonged and during a breech presentation or a precipitate delivery. It may also be seen in newborns with hemorrhagic disease. The two common types of hemorrhage are *subdural* and *subarachnoid*. Hemorrhage may extend into the ventricles or the brain substance itself.

Intracranial hemorrhage is the most common and severe type of birth injury. It occurs more frequently in premature than in full-term infants.

Diagnosis is based on a history of difficult delivery and an increase in cerebrospinal fluid pressure. The presence of a few blood cells in the cerebrospinal fluid is not of particular diagnostic value, because a minute amount of bleeding into the fluid may be normal in the newborn.

Clinical Manifestations, Treatment, Prevention, and Prognosis. Intracranial hemorrhage may be evident at birth or may be diagnosed later in an infant apparently normal at birth. The nurse may observe somnolence or limpness in the infant, or irritability and restlessness. Opisthotonos may be present, the Moro reflex absent, muscular twitchings and convulsions may occur, and the cry may be high-pitched and shrill. Cardiac and respiratory functions may be abnormal with resulting pallor and cyanosis. The temperature may be even less stable than that of the normal newborn. The fontanels may bulge if the increase in intracranial pressure is great. Paralysis may appear in a few days.

The results of *treatment* may be quite satisfactory. The infant needs warmth and rest and may be placed in an incubator where oxygen is available if needed. His head should be elevated. Hemorrhage may be controlled by the administration of vitamin K. The physician may order a sedative such as phenobarbital to control the convulsions. Prophylactic antibiotics are given. If a subdural hematoma is present, it is generally treated as described on page 475.

As with many other birth injuries, better obstetrical care is the best *preventive.*

In the majority of cases the *prognosis* is good, and the child may completely recover. Other infants may show mental retardation or a tendency to convulsions or may be handicapped by cerebral palsy. Those who do not survive usually die within the first few days after delivery.

Responsibilities of the Nurse. These infants are generally placed in incubators. Since the sucking and swallowing reflexes are weak or absent, the infant must be fed with great care. If he vomits after feedings, he should be placed on his abdomen or on his right side with a rolled blanket at his back, unless the physician has ordered that this is not to be done. In this position, drainage from the stomach to the duodenum is favored, and vomiting may be decreased. The infant must be observed for increased intracranial pressure and for convulsions (see p. 473).

Medications such as sedatives, vitamins or prophylactic antibiotics may be given orally or by injection. The nurse may assist the physician with treatments such as lumbar punctures (see p. 294) or aspiration of a subdural hemorrhage.

Peripheral Nerve Injuries

BRACHIAL PLEXUS PALSY (ERB-DUCHENNE PARALYSIS)

Etiology and Clinical Manifestation. Brachial plexus palsy is a paralysis of the upper arm. The cause is trauma involving the fifth and sixth cervical spinal nerves or their trunks. The injury results from pulling the infant's shoulder away from the head during delivery. The arm on the affected side is adducted, extended and internally rotated with pronation of the forearm. The hands and fingers are not affected. The arm cannot voluntarily be abducted from the

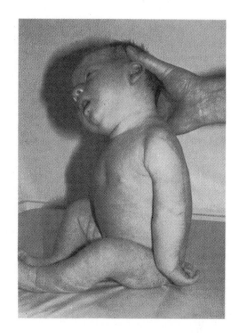

A

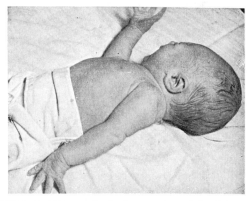

B

FIGURE 11–16. Brachial plexus palsy of the left arm. A, Erb-Duchenne paralysis in four-week-old infant weighing 4100 gm. at birth. The arm is hanging down in a typical position, with adduction, internal rotation and pronation. (From Moll, H. *Atlas of Pediatric Diseases.* Philadelphia, W. B. Saunders Co., 1976.) B, Asymmetric response to Moro reflex. (R. J. McKay, Jr., and C. A. Smith in W. E. Nelson: *Textbook of Pediatrics.* 8th ed.)

shoulder or externally rotated, and the forearm cannot be supinated. The Moro reflex is absent on the affected side, and there may be sensory loss on the lateral portion of the arm.

Treatment. The arm should be immobilized in a position of maximal relaxation, i.e., abducted and rotated externally with the elbow flexed. Later an airplane splint may be used to keep the arm in this position. To prevent contraction deformity, the physiotherapist may manipulate and massage the arm gently. In persistent cases neuroplasty may be necessary.

Responsibilities of the Nurse. The arm is to be immobilized as the physician may order. In

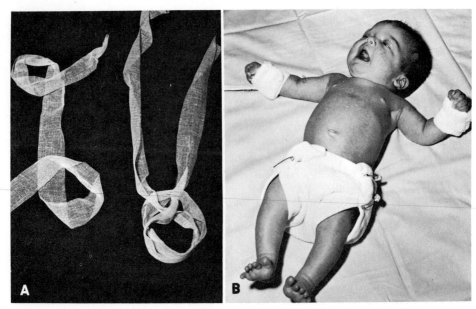

FIGURE 11–17.   Clove hitch restraint. *A*, In the middle of a strip of gauze make a figure of 8. Place one loop over the other. *B*, Place the restraint over the wadding wrapped around the wrist (or ankles). Pull the gauze restraint securely, but not tightly enough to cut off the circulation. The response of this infant, namely crying, is the typical response to restraint. When the clove hitch restraint is used on an infant having brachial plexus palsy, the affected arm should be elevated and the ends of the gauze tied to the head of the crib.

general a clove hitch restraint is used. The equipment needed for this is (1) a strip of gauze bandage 2 inches wide and 1½ yards long, and (2) cotton wadding covered with gauze, cut to 2 inches wide and long enough to encircle the infant's wrist.

To apply the restraint, spread the gauze strip out on the bed with one end toward the nearer side of the bed. In the middle of the strip make a figure of eight, as shown in Figure 11–17. Place the gauze wadding around the infant's wrist. Place circles of restraint around the padding on the wrist. Pull the ends of the gauze to the bedsprings at the head of the bed so that the arm is elevated to the proper angle. Care must be exercised to prevent cutting off the circulation and yet have the bandage tight enough not to slip over the infant's hand.

The fingers and the hand should be observed for coldness or discoloration and the skin under the restraint for signs of irritation. These infants need even more love and affection than the normal infant does because of their immobilization.

Prognosis.   The prognosis usually cannot be determined for several months. If the paralysis is due to edema and hemorrhage around nerve fibers with no laceration, the prognosis is good. If laceration of the nerve has occurred, operation must usually be considered.

FACIAL NERVE PARALYSIS

Etiology, Clinical Manifestations, and Prognosis.   Facial nerve paralysis results from pres-

sure over the facial nerve in front of the ear. This pressure may have occurred during labor or may have been due to the use of forceps during delivery. The paralysis is generally unilateral. When the infant cries, movement is observed on only one side of his face. The mouth is drawn to that side. The eye on the affected side is partially open. If the nerve is only injured by pressure, recovery can be expected in a few weeks; if the nerve is torn, however, neuroplasty may be required.

Responsibilities of the Nurse.   The nurse

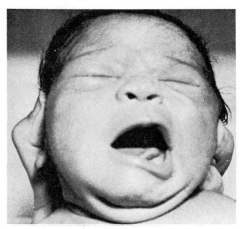

FIGURE 11–18.   Right facial nerve paralysis in infant delivered without forceps. (Davis and Rubin: *DeLee's Obstetrics for Nurses.* 17th ed.)

must be patient when feeding the infant, since sucking may be difficult for him. The physician will order care of the exposed eye. If a shield is applied, it may be necessary to restrain the infant's arms so that he does not pull it off. He can be held and cuddled like a normal infant.

Injuries to Bones

Etiology and Types of Fractures. Although the newborn's bones bend easily on pressure, as when traction is applied during delivery, a fracture may occur. Fractures occur mainly in the skull, clavicle, or long bones.

Fractures of the skull are of two types: *(a)* linear fractures, the more common type, do not produce symptoms and require no treatment; *(b)* depressed fractures appear as a dent in the infant's head. Treatment is by early operation, which prevents injury to the cortex due to prolonged pressure.

Fracture of the clavicle is the most common fracture of the newborn. It may occur when delivery of the shoulder is difficult. The infant fails to raise his arm on the affected side, and the Moro reflex is possible only with elevation of the unaffected arm. The infant may be able to raise his arm, however, if the fracture is of the greenstick type, which is common in infants and little children. The prognosis in either type of fracture is excellent. Treatment is by immobilization of the arm and the shoulder on the affected side.

Fractures of the long bones of the arms or legs, unless of the greenstick type, prevent the infant from moving the limb. The treatment of a fracture of the humerus is strapping the arm to the chest and later placing it in an airplane splint or shell cast. For a fracture of the femur the leg is placed in Buck's extension (see p. 565). Splints are used for immobilizing other bones of the extremities. Excessive callus formation is likely to accompany rapid healing.

Responsibilities of the Nurse. Nursing care of these infants includes maintenance of good body alignment, splint or cast care (see p. 322), and prevention of pressure areas. Care has to be adapted to the position in which they must lie or the part of the body which is immobilized. Demonstrations of affection for the infant must also be adapted to his condition. The infant in traction cannot be fed at the breast, but his mother's milk may be expressed and given him. In this way the supply of breast milk will be maintained, because the infant is likely to have a longer hospital stay than is customary.

INJURY TO THE STERNOCLEIDOMASTOID MUSCLE

Etiology, Pathology, and Treatment. About two weeks after birth, or even earlier, a small, firm mass may be noted in the midportion of the sternocleidomastoid muscle. This may be caused by a small hematoma resulting from injury or may be a fibromatous malformation in the muscle itself. The injury generally, but not always, results in *torticollis* (wryneck), a condi-

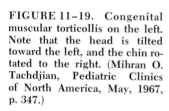

FIGURE 11–19. Congenital muscular torticollis on the left. Note that the head is tilted toward the left, and the chin rotated to the right. (Mihran O. Tachdjian, Pediatric Clinics of North America, May, 1967, p. 347.)

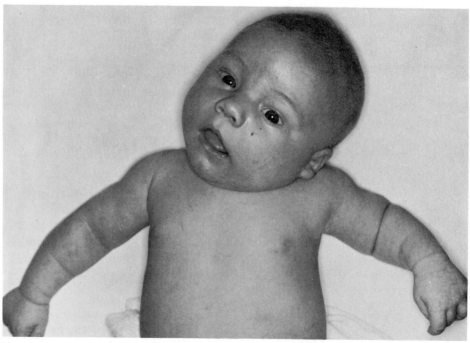

tion in which the head inclines to one side. The majority of these problems resolve under treatment before the infant is one year old.

Treatment lies in gently extending the neck so that the face is in the opposite direction. The mother can be taught to turn the infant's head to the normal position and flex the neck toward the unaffected side. This may be done as often as 25 times twice or three times a day. If the condition is present when the child is two years old, operation may be required.

Responsibilities of the Nurse. Nursing care must be adapted to the limitation of movement of the infant. The nurse should talk to the infant and should cuddle him before and after the exercise.

RESPIRATORY CONDITIONS

PNEUMONIA

Incidence and Pathology. Pneumonia is responsible for approximately 10 per cent of neonatal deaths. The disease may accompany an infection which is not of the respiratory tract. Pneumonia in the newborn and the older infant is usually bronchopneumonic rather than lobar.

Etiology. Organisms which may cause pneumonia in the infant are not the same as those responsible for the disease in older children and adults. In the newborn, pneumonia may be due to bacteria or viruses. The chief causative agents in pneumonia occurring within the first few weeks of life are coliform organisms, enterococci, Klebsiella, Pseudomonas, Proteus, Salmonella, and Staphylococcus.

The causes of pneumonia in the newborn are connected with the birth process as well as with contact with infection after birth. During delivery, infection may come from aspiration of infected amniotic fluid or vaginal secretions. Infection may be carried to the respiratory tract by way of the blood stream. After birth the infectious organism is most commonly acquired through contact with the mother or with a nurse who has a cold. Although slight respiratory infections in the newborn do not always result in pneumonia, the danger is so great that no one with even a simple cold should care for him. Skin infections caused by a staphylococcus are also a cause of pneumonia in the newborn, whose resistance to any kind of infection is low.

Clinical Manifestations. The first sign of pneumonia in the newborn is rapid respiration, which may reach 80 per minute, more than the nurse can count with accuracy. Respiratory distress is evident in flaring of the nostrils. The infant appears listless, is pale or cyanotic, and has a temperature higher or lower than normal.

He is likely to refuse his feedings and suffers from abdominal distention.

Treatment. In general the plan of treatment includes chemotherapeutic agents against the common organisms causing pneumonia in infancy. Bacitracin or an antistaphylococcal synthetic penicillin may be used in the treatment of staphylococcal infections. If the exact causative organism can be isolated through laboratory tests, treatment can be made more specific. Oxygen is routinely used to relieve the respiratory distress.

ASPIRATION PNEUMONIA

The first *symptom* of aspiration pneumonia is generally an attack of coughing or, since the cough reflex of the newborn is imperfect, of choking. The usual symptoms of pneumonia are likely to follow within a short time. *Prevention* lies in careful feeding of infants and is therefore the responsibility of the mother and the nurse.

One advantage of breast feeding is that aspiration is not too likely. The newborn has not learned the technique of correlating sucking and swallowing. If the flow of milk is too rapid for him to swallow, he can pull away from the breast more readily than from a bottle held in a nurse's hand. The size of the hole in the nipple is important, and the nurse should be sensitive to the infant's need to swallow what he has in his mouth before more flows in.

If the infant chokes on the feeding and is in immediate danger, the emergency measure is to suspend him by his feet. This permits aspirated milk to drain from the lungs. (For artificial respiration see page 202.) After feeding, the infant should not be placed on his back, but on his right side or abdomen so that if he vomits, the material will drain from the mouth.

Treatments which disturb the infant emotionally or physiologically, e.g. puncture of the jugular or femoral veins, should be done two hours or more after feedings.

INFECTIONS

Immunity in the Newborn, Infant, and Child

When the infant is born he comes into contact with antigens foreign to him, for example bacteria, viruses, fungi, and protozoa, as well as other agents taken in orally or inhaled from the surrounding air. *The most important function of the immune system is to prevent the occurrence of illness as a result of such contact.*

Immunology is undergoing a period of very

rapid and exciting growth. Recently, observations concerning the structure of the immune system have significantly changed the course of immunologic research. One of these discoveries is that the immune system is divided into two parts: the one composed of lymphocytes that produce antibodies is known as the B-cell system; the other, known as the T-cell system, is composed of lymphocytes whose responsibility it is to ward off viral infections, recognize and reject foreign tissues, and protect against cancer. B-cells are lymphocytes that are not influenced by the thymus. T-cells are lymphocytes that have migrated to the tissues via the thymus or are otherwise influenced by the thymus. Together, B- and T- lymphocytes have an important role to play in antibody production, cellular immunity, and immunologic memory. Research continues on the nature of these B- and T-cells.

It is not the intent of this text to review the theory of immunology, but rather to make application of it to the care of newborns, infants, and children. A discussion of immunology may be found in recent textbooks on anatomy and physiology that the student may review if lacking knowledge in this area.

During the first trimester of fetal life immunologic competence is probably lacking. After this period the fetal lymphoid system is gradually populated with immunologically competent cells. During the last six months of gestation, the fetus can develop delayed hypersensitivity and can form plasma cells that are capable of synthesizing specific immunoglobulins usually of the IgM and IgA classes. If more than 20 mg/dl of IgM globulin is present in cord blood, it is suggestive of prenatal infection. There is a transfer of maternal IgG to the fetus through the placenta, but the levels of IgM and IgA are low.

During the postnatal period the development of the immunologic system is dependent on the experience of the growing child. If an infant is raised in a germ-free environment, he will have small lymph nodes, few plasma cells, and very low rates of immunoglobulin synthesis. If an infant is raised in a normal environment, he will respond to antigenic stimuli from the organisms with which he comes in contact as well as from the vaccines he receives (see p. 381). If the infant's immunologic system is normal, there will be a progressive hyperplasia of the follicles and a gradual appearance of plasma cells in lymphoid tissue in the body. This results in enlargement of the tonsils (see p. 649) and lymph nodes from their miniature size at birth. As the child has contact with other immunologic substances, immunoglobulin synthesis increases. During adolescence, adult levels of immunoglobulins are produced.

The passive immunity obtained from the maternally derived IgG antibodies is gradually lost. The duration of the young infant's immunity to a particular infection depends on the level of that particular antibody in the mother's plasma during pregnancy. It also depends upon the amount of antibody required to protect the infant from that particular kind of infection. Protection against measles may last through the second half of the first year, but protection against pyogenic bacterial infections may last only one or two months. This passive immunity of the infant may interfere with his response to active immunization. In other words, measles vaccine should not be given under ordinary circumstances before the infant is one year old. Maternal diphtheria antitoxin may reduce the infant's response to diphtheria toxoid; however, since multiple injections of DPT are given (see p. 379) the infant does become immune.

The reason newborn infants are so susceptible to infections due to the gram-negative enteric bacilli such as *Escherichia coli* is probably the fact that bactericidal antibodies to this group of organisms are IgM globulins. These are not transferred to the fetus from the mother. Breast-fed infants receive high concentrations of all immunoglobulins, especially IgA, from the mother. This ingested concentration of antibodies from colostrum and breast milk may provide local gastrointestinal immunity against organisms entering the body via the oral route.

Cell membranes and skin offer the child some protection against infection, but many invaders may gain access to the body through natural or traumatic openings or by making their own portals of entry. Many organisms that invade the body live in a parasitic relationship with their host, either in a benign fashion, causing little problem, or in a destructive fashion, damaging the host severely. The immune system is a way by which the host can be protected against such external dangers.

When the immune system is impaired, every microbe has a chance to become a pathogen, and even common pathogens may become more virulent. In addition, when an individual is immunologically depressed, the incidence of cancer rises in comparison with that in the general population. Certain congenital anomalies, disease states, malnutrition syndromes, and other causes such as surgery, radiation, chemotherapy, and drug abuse may cause immunologic depression.

Many parents have complained to physicians and nurses that their child has "poor resistance to infection." The cause of such a complaint must be comprehensively investigated since there are many possible causes for poor resistance. The parents may be unreasonable in their expectations concerning the health of their child, believing that he should have as few infections as they have. The environment in which the child lives may be overcrowded, leading to cross infections from siblings and others. If the child has persistent infections in one site such as in an ear, this indicates an anatomic or physiologic defect. If he has frequent infections in different sites, the question of a general immunologic deficiency such as agammaglobulinemia must be investigated.

If there is a congenital absence of the thymus gland or stem cells, the precursors of B- and T-lymphocytes, the affected infant will be unable to live a long normal life. Since the immune system cannot develop without B- and T- lymphocytes, the infant will acquire severe bacterial, viral, or fungal infections. If protective isolation is not provided for such an infant, he will probably die soon after birth. A child may possibly be raised in complete protective isolation to prevent infection, but he is likely to have serious emotional effects because of his lack of physical contact with others.

The condition of agammaglobulinemia (Bruton's disease) is due to a lack in the lymph nodes and spleen of the normal follicular structure. Because of the complete absence of B-cells with a normal number of T-cells, a part of the antibody pool is lost (see p. 468).

Malnutrition, the result of poor food intake or poor absorption of essential nutrients, decreases the ability of the body to form circulating antibodies against certain bacterial and viral antigens (see p. 435). If there is a defect in antibody structure and production and diminished phagocytosis by leukocytes, the child is susceptible to bacterial, viral, or fungal infections.

The younger the child the more likely he is to develop immunologic depression. The premature infant cannot develop his own antibodies and must, therefore, depend on the passive immunity obtained from maternal antibodies. As the child grows toward adolescence, he is less susceptible to infections unless he has a deficiency of gamma globulin. Active immunity does not develop spontaneously. It develops gradually as the child is repeatedly exposed to an antigen.

An overwhelming systemic infection, particularly viral, can depress the immune system. The nutrients available are being used to manufacture one type of antibody, resulting in no nutrients to manufacture another type. The child who can respond to one infection, such as influenza, may therefore not be able to recover from a secondary infection such as pneumonia (see p. 546).

Children who are severely burned (see p. 556) also may become immunologically depressed. Such a child has lost his defense by means of an intact skin. Infections may be caused by the invasion of microorganisms normally present on the skin or in the environment. Also, the loss of serum through the burned surfaces reduces the body's supply of gamma globulin, leading to a reduction of antibodies.

Major surgery in children decreases immunologic competence, thus leading to infection. Several reasons have been given for this immunosuppression. The stress related to surgery stimulates the adrenal cortex to release cortisol. Although a little cortisol can help prevent infection, a large amount is lympholytic. Immunosuppression following surgery may also be due to the interruption in nutrition. If essential nutrients are not given, the healing process is retarded and the antibody production is slowed.

Emotional stress also stimulates the adrenal cortex in children. While mild stress increases resistance to disease, high stress levels reduce resistance (see Asthma, p. 689).

Allergy (see p. 688) is a specifically altered state produced by the immunologic response of the individual to an initial contact with a foreign substance or an infectious agent. It is an inherited tendency of certain children to overrespond to a variety of foreign substances when they come in contact with the skin, mucous surfaces, or vascular endothelium.

In this and future chapters conditions such as infections and allergic responses are discussed.

Organisms Causing Infection Before Birth

Certain infections may be passed from the mother to the child either before or during birth. These include ophthalmia neonatorum, thrush, congenital syphilis, toxoplasmosis, and cytomegalic inclusion disease.

OPHTHALMIA NEONATORUM (GONORRHEAL CONJUNCTIVITIS)

Etiology. The causative organism, *Neisseria gonorrhoeae* (a gram-negative, coffee bean-shaped diplococcus), is found in a smear or culture taken from the purulent exudate from the eye.

The newborn acquires the infection during the birth process by direct contact with infected material in the vagina of the mother. As the incidence of gonorrhea among adults increases, the incidence of gonorrheal conjunctivitis may also increase. The condition is to be reported to the Board of Health as a contagious disease.

Clinical Manifestations. The onset is usually within two or three days after birth, but symptoms may appear earlier. There is redness and swelling of the lids and a profuse, purulent discharge.

Complications. The common complication is corneal ulceration with resulting opacity and partial or complete loss of vision. The extent of the handicap depends on the duration and severity of the untreated condition.

Treatment. Penicillin is the preferred drug, but erythromycin, a tetracycline, or chloramphenicol may be administered topically and systemically. The infant is kept in strict isolation. Symptomatic therapy consists in removing the discharge thoroughly with irrigations, usually of physiologic saline solution.

Prognosis. Excellent results are obtained with treatment of the infant. An epidemiologic follow-up should be done on the mother.

Responsibilities of the Nurse. It is difficult to instill drops into the eyes of a newborn infant at the time of delivery. The nurse must be absolutely sure that the drops are instilled within the eyelids. The medication may cause a slight irritation and redness of the eyes and the lids for a few days.

If the infant develops ophthalmia neonatorum, his arms must be restrained so that he does not rub his eyes. If only one eye is affected, a shield is placed over the other one to protect it from infection. The purulent discharge is removed by frequent irrigations. When irrigations are done, the infant should be restrained in mummy fashion (see p. 413), and a second nurse should steady his head. As in all eye irrigations, the fluid should be warmed to body temperature, and the flow should be directed from the inner canthus outward. Extreme care must be taken that no drops of the return flow splash into the nurse's eyes.

Prevention. The prophylactic measure is to keep the mother free of infection. If the mother does not come under the care of a physician until the time of delivery, however, instillation of silver nitrate or penicillin safeguards the infant. State laws require prophylactic treatment of all infants at birth even though there is no reason to believe that a particular newborn is infected (see p. 157).

THRUSH (ORAL MONILIASIS)

Etiology and Mode of Transmission. The causative agent of this infection is *Candida (Monilia) albicans*. The organism is normally present in the vagina of the mother, and is a saprophyte in the mouth of older children and adults. Thrush is a fungus infection; the spores grow on the delicate tissue of the buccal mucosa, producing mycelia. The infant may become infected from improperly sterilized nipples or the unclean hands or breast of his mother. Antibiotic therapy may cause changes in the flora of the mouth which may also predispose to thrush.

Clinical Manifestations. The mouth of the infant who has thrush contains white patches which resemble milk curds. They are different from milk curds, however, in that they are difficult to remove from the mucous membrane and, when removed, leave a bleeding area. These pearly-white, elevated lesions, which occur on the tongue margin, inside the lips and cheeks and on the hard palate, are painless. If the infection is localized in the mouth, the systemic symptoms tend to be mild, although the infant has anorexia. Esophagogastritis or pneumonitis may develop, however, as a result of invasion by the infective organism. (Color Plate 1–6.)

Treatment, Responsibilities of the Nurse, and Prognosis. Nystatin or 1 per cent aqueous solution of gentian violet is effective in the *treatment* of these lesions and may be applied locally with a soft swab. Care should be taken to place the solution on the lesions gently so that it is widely distributed before it is swallowed. Gentian violet may be irritating if it is swallowed. If the infant is placed face downward after it has been applied, the drug will drain from the infant's mouth.

If the physician orders gentian violet therapy, the mother should be warned of the purple discoloration of the infant's skin and also of the fact that the drug stains bed linen and clothing. These stains can be removed with sodium bicarbonate paste.

To prevent the spread of thrush, the infant should have his own feeding equipment, which should be sterilized after use. If the nipple irritates his mouth, a medicine dropper may be used.

Preventive *nursing* is based on absolute cleanliness of all articles which enter the infant's mouth, including the nipples used in feeding him. Applicators used in the infant's mouth should be sterile. An older infant's toys and pacifiers must be clean.

The nurse should inspect the mouth of each infant receiving antibiotic therapy at least once daily in order to note the presence of thrush early.

The *prognosis* in general is good, recovery taking place in three or four days. If the infant is malnourished or chronically ill, the underlying disturbance should be corrected.

Congenital syphilis (lues)

Etiology and Description. The causative agent of syphilis is a spirochete, *Treponema pallidum.* Congenital syphilis and childhood syphilis will be considered here.

Congenital syphilis and acquired syphilis have been greatly reduced in incidence throughout most of the United States; however, their incidence has begun to rise again in the past few years. The mode of transmission to the fetus is by direct inoculation into the blood stream through the placenta during the latter half of pregnancy. Thus the disease is beyond the primary stage when the infant is born.

Clinical Manifestations. Although a variety of other conditions have symptoms similar to those of syphilis, a typical combination of symptoms points to the diagnosis of syphilis. The symptoms may be divided into two groups: those which appear early and those which appear later in the course of the disease.

Early Symptoms. The more severe the infection, the earlier will the symptoms be apparent; in general they appear before the sixth week. Characteristic symptoms are as follows: (1) a persistent rhinitis, which has been given the name of "snuffles." This is a profuse mucopurulent nasal discharge, which may be blood-tinged and is irritating to the upper lip. The lip may become excoriated from the discharge. (2) There is a rash, heaviest over the back, buttocks, and thighs, and involving the palms and soles. (3) There may be bleeding ulcerations and moist lesions of the mucous membranes of the mouth, lips, anus, and genitalia. (4) The infant is anemic. (5) There may be osteochondritis or periostitis, or both, of the bones. (6) Pseudoparalysis or pathologic fractures may be present. (7) The liver and the spleen are enlarged. (8) There may be chorioretinitis with later atrophy of the optic nerve (see Color Plate 2–8).

Later Symptoms. Later clinical manifestations are as follows: (1) destruction of the bones of the nose, so-called saddle nose, in which the nose dips slightly beyond the bridge and rises again toward the tip; (2) a periostitis of the tibiae in which these bones develop a sharp forward curve, a condition called saber shins. (3) The deciduous teeth are normal, but the central incisors of the permanent teeth are peg-shaped with a characteristic Gothic-shaped notch, so-called Hutchinson's teeth (Fig. 11–20). (4) The lesions of early syphilis around the mouth and nose become linear fissures which form radiating scars on healing (rhagades). (5) Interstitial keratitis may develop when the child is 6 to 12 years old. Photophobia, lacrimation,

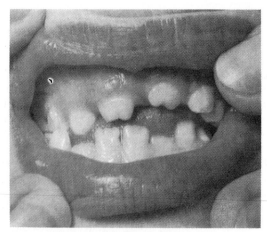

FIGURE 11–20. Hutchinson's teeth. The upper central incisors of the second dentition show characteristic peg shape and central notching; the adjacent teeth are also deformed. Such dentition is diagnostic of congenital syphilis, especially when associated with diffuse interstitial keratitis and deafness (Hutchinson's triad). (From Kimmig, J., and Jänner, M.: *Frieboes Schönfeld Color Atlas of Dermatology.* Stuttgart, Georg Thieme Verlag, 1966.)

general discomfort, and impairment of vision are symptoms of this condition. (6) Neurosyphilis, manifestations of which may appear at any time from one to ten years of age. The symptoms are hemiplegia, spastic paralysis, and mental retardation. The child is slow in talking and is irritable and restless.

Diagnosis. The diagnosis is confirmed by serologic tests. A Wassermann reaction may be determined at any time, or blood may be obtained from the cord at delivery. Blood tests, however, are less accurate in providing proof of the presence of syphilis in the newborn than later in life. When the infant is six months of age, positive serologic results are more indicative of a syphilitic infection. A second test should be done, however, before the diagnosis is confirmed even at this age if no other manifestations of the disease are evident. Scrapings from moist lesions may show *Treponema pallidum* (darkfield examination is done on the scrapings).

Prognosis. Prompt treatment of early congenital syphilis will usually result in a cure and in normal growth and development. Although late congenital syphilis may be cured, the pathologic changes will remain for life.

Prevention. A serologic test is required in most parts of the United States before marriage or during pregnancy. This is probably the greatest preventive measure against congenital syphilis. Case finding in adults is furthered by the requirement of physical examinations in many kinds of work and in the armed services. The availability of prenatal care during pregnancy has increased the opportunity for early treatment of syphilis if a woman is found to have the disease. Cure may then be effected before the infant is born. Even later treatment may prevent syphilis in the infant or mitigate his condition.

Treatment. For early syphilis any of the penicillins may be given by injection. If the patient is sensitive to penicillin, erythromycin or tetracycline may be given. Follow-up serologic tests should be done on both the infant and the mother.

Responsibilities of the Nurse. Basic to the nursing care is the danger of transmission of the disease. Although the organism dies rapidly on exposure, it may be transmitted by direct or indirect contact. The organisms are found in the skin lesions and the nasal discharge of the host and invade the body of another through a break in the mucous membranes or skin. In many hospitals, nurses caring for infectious syphilitic infants are required to wear rubber gloves and a gown. During the infectious period no pins should be used in the infant's clothing because of the possibility of the nurse being injured with a contaminated pin. Diapers should be tied in place temporarily. After a few days of treatment the infant is probably no longer infectious.

Feeding is made difficult by the presence of snuffles. The nose should be cleansed of discharge before the bottle or breast is offered. The upper lip should be kept clean, and cold cream should be applied to prevent excoriation from the irritating nasal discharge. Careful handling of the infant is necessary, for bone lesions cause him pain on movement. If the nurse is caring for an older child who shows signs of photophobia due to interstitial keratitis, darkening the room increases his comfort; if he is old enough, he may wear dark glasses.

Congenital syphilis represents a failure in finding a syphilitic infection in an antepartal patient; therefore community or public health nurses stress the need of prenatal care, including serologic examinations, treatment if necessary, and follow-up study on infants on whom treatment has been started.

TOXOPLASMOSIS

Incidence, Etiology, and Transmission. This is an uncommon disease of the central nervous system. The causative organism is the *Toxoplasma gondii,* which is considered to be a protozoon.

This organism crosses the placenta only when the pregnant woman has a primary infection. It is not possible, therefore, for a woman to have more than one infant having this condition. The severe infantile form occurs when the fetus acquires the infection *in utero* because of his general immunologic immaturity. As a consequence, the infection remains active longer in the neonate, permitting parasitization of the brain and eye. Frank encephalitis with hydrocephalus may develop. The fetus may be prematurely born, stillborn, or born at term. The disease may also be acquired after birth.

Clinical Manifestations, Prognosis, and Treatment. Evidence of chorioretinitis (inflammation of the choroid and of the retina) may be detected in the eyegrounds. Cerebral calcifications may be present. Hydrocephalus (see p. 301) or microcephalia (see p. 308) may occur. Psychomotor retardation and convulsions are also symptoms. During the acute stage, symptoms of encephalitis may appear. The organism may be isolated from cerebrospinal fluid or from other tissues of the body.

In the infantile form the *prognosis* is poor. Although active congenital toxoplasmosis may cause death in days or weeks, the illness may regress, leaving one or more of the various disabilities mentioned above.

Pyrimethamine (Daraprim), which is a folic acid antagonist, and a sulfonamide in combined *treatment* give promising results. When these drugs are used, frequent leukocyte counts must be made, since both may produce leukopenia.

Responsibilities of the Nurse. The nursing care is based on the relief of symptoms. The child is made as comfortable as possible. The nurse should keep in mind both the symptoms and the possible complications so that an accurate account may be given to the physician.

Prevention. Since individuals acquire toxoplasmosis either by eating poorly cooked meat that is infected or by exposure to infected cats or cat litter pans, the nurse should counsel pregnant women to avoid these sources of infection. If exposure to such sources is necessary, disposable rubber gloves should be worn. Serologic testing of all pregnant women for evidence of *Toxoplasma* infection should be done. If seroconversion or rise in titer occurs in the first trimester, a decision must be made regarding continuation of the pregnancy.

CYTOMEGALIC INCLUSION DISEASE (SALIVARY GLAND VIRUS DISEASE)

Incidence, Etiology, and Transmission. This condition is a generalized illness caused by a salivary gland virus. The occurrence of symptoms with this disease is unusual, although salivary gland virus may cause symptomatic human infection. Transplacental transmission occurs, resulting in infection of the newborn.

Clinical Manifestations, Prognosis, and Treatment. *Symptoms* may be mild with recovery, or severe, leading to a rapidly fatal disease. In severely affected infants, hepatosplenomegaly, purpura, jaundice, and signs of central nervous system involvement may be present. The child may have convulsions, microcephalia, hydrocephalus, and chorioretinitis. If the infant survives, permanent neurologic sequelae such as mental retardation occur. Clinically, this condition resembles toxoplasmosis. The only *treatment* known at present is to support the patient and to keep him as comfortable as possible.

HERPES SIMPLEX

Etiology, Incidence, Types, and Transmission. *Herpesvirus hominis (HVH) is a DNA-containing virus* and occurs commonly in man. It can produce generalized systemic disease or specific clinical manifestations in the skin, the mucous membranes, the central nervous system, the eye, and the genital tract of both sexes.

There are two types of infection. The primary infection occurs when the host has an initial infection with the virus. This may result in a subclinical infection, local superficial lesions, or a systemic reaction. In neonates and infants who are malnourished, a severe systemic infection may occur without previous localized lesions. In infants who survive, circulating antibodies develop. Recurrent infections may occur even though the individual has antibodies as a result of a reactivation of a latent infection. These lesions are localized and are not accompanied by a systemic infection.

There are two *types* of herpesvirus: type 1 and type 2. In the newborn the infection is usually caused by type 2 virus as a result of contamination from the infected genitalia of the mother during the process of birth. Type 1 virus may also infect the neonate, perhaps owing to transplacentally or postnatally acquired infection.

The *incidence* of herpetic disease is not known, since the infection may be mild, with localized involvement of the eye or skin and a low-grade fever, or severe, leading to systemic disease and death.

Herpesvirus may be a cause of congenital malformations similar to those of cytomegalic inclusion disease. Further research is necessary for confirmation of this observation.

Clinical Manifestations, Treatment, Responsibilities of the Nurse, and Prognosis. The *clinical manifestations* of herpesvirus infection occur between the fifth and ninth days after birth in a previously well neonate. Infants having a severe infection feed poorly and appear to have a widespread infection like septicemia with manifestations of elevation of temperature, hypothermia, jaundice, vomiting, dyspnea, listlessness, or convulsions. The liver and spleen are enlarged, and myocarditis may develop leading to circulatory collapse. In infants infected with herpesvirus, a terminal infection with *Pseudomonas aeruginosa* may occur. If the disease is severe or if the central nervous system is involved as in encephalitis, the prognosis is poor. In half the surviving infants severe sequelae may be present.

With mild infection, local vesicular lesions may or may not be present on the skin and mucous membranes, or a conjunctivitis may be diagnosed. Some infants may recover if they have only a mild infection.

Treatment and *nursing care* are symptomatic, supporting the neonate and keeping him as comfortable as is possible. Gamma globulin may be tried in an attempt to replace the missing antibodies of the neonate. If the mother has known genital herpes, a cesarean section may be done to prevent infection from the vagina. If the fetus had already been infected transplacentally or if the membranes had been ruptured for a prolonged period, a cesarean section would not prevent the disease.

No new drugs have been proved therapeutic for this disease.

Neonates whose mothers have a herpesvirus infection are usually isolated to prevent spread of the disease to other newborns in the nursery.

Prevention. During the prenatal period nurses should help mothers understand the importance of their not having sexual contact with an infected male, especially during the last trimester of pregnancy.

Organisms Causing Infection After Birth

Any pathogenic bacteria or virus may cause infection in the newborn. The chief organisms affecting the newborn are coliform organisms and *Staphylococcus aureus;* others include enterococci, Klebsiella, Pseudomonas, Salmonella, and Proteus.

Types of Infections. The most common types of infections occurring in the nursery are septicemia, pneumonia, and skin and umbilical infections. Diarrhea is still a common infection, although its incidence has been reduced in this country.

Clinical Manifestations and Treatment. It is extremely difficult for the nurse to recognize infection in the newborn, since his reactions to it may be so general that infection is not suspected. This is one reason why the nurse should report anything slightly abnormal even in an apparently normal newborn. The pediatrician makes the diagnosis by appraising the significance of every factor in the total clinical picture.

Signs indicative of something wrong with an infant include cyanosis, convulsions, listlessness, anorexia, vomiting, jaundice, and diarrhea. Fever may or may not be an indication of infection, since it may be the result of keeping the infant too warm. Absence of fever has little diagnostic significance, since the newborn may not react to even a massive infection with an elevation of temperature. The difficulties in making a diagnosis of infection are even greater in the premature than in the normal newborn. Laboratory studies and x-ray examination may be necessary.

If a specific infecting organism is found, *treatment* is mainly by administration of the appropriate chemotherapeutic agent; if a specific organism is unknown, an agent effective against a number of organisms is given.

INFECTIONS CAUSED BY ESCHERICHIA COLI

Escherichia coli is the most common cause of serious infection of the newborn and is capable of producing a number of pathologic conditions, among them septicemia, pneumonia, meningitis, and diarrhea. Neomycin is commonly used for intestinal infections; kanamycin, for systemic infections.

INFECTIONS CAUSED BY STAPHYLOCOCCUS AUREUS

Etiology, Onset, Types, and Modes of Entry. *Staphylococcus aureus* is a gram-positive organism which under the microscope appears in clumps. It is second only to *Escherichia coli* as a cause of infection in the newborn. Unfortunately the incidence of this type of infection in newborn nurseries is increasing. Many strains of the organism appear to be resistant to the majority of known chemotherapeutic agents.

The initial infection usually occurs while the infant is in the hospital, but may appear weeks or months later. This is one of the many reasons why all infants should be under the care of a private physician or be visited by a community or public health nurse and taken regularly to a Child Health Conference or clinic. An infection of this type acquired while the infant is in the nursery is likely to spread to other infants even though the customary isolation technique has been followed.

If the infant is breast-fed, the mother may acquire mastitis due to infection of the nipple from the organisms in his mouth. An infant may also infect other members of the family if he is discharged before the infection has been recognized and treated.

The primary infection with *Staphylococcus aureus* is commonly but not always of the skin. It may be an infection of the nasopharynx or of the cord stump carried from one infant to another. Pneumonia, septicemia, or enteritis may represent infection with *Staphylococcus aureus*. Osteomyelitis or meningitis may be a complication of septicemia. A leaking meningocele or a circumcision wound may also be the site of an infection.

SOURCES OF INFECTION IN THE NURSERY. Pathogens may be brought into the nursery by the nurses caring for the infants or by other personnel. The mother also is a possible source of infection to her child. Infection is spread readily from one infant to others.

Treatment and Prevention. Systemic *therapy* requires giving an antibiotic effective against the specific organism infecting the infant. The drugs include methicillin, oxacillin, nafcillin, or other antibiotics. Indiscriminate use of prophylactic antibiotics should not be condoned, because this will only result in the emergence of more resistant strains of bacteria. Skin lesions in general are treated by bathing the infant with a soap or a detergent containing hexachlorophene, if this is ordered by the physician. Bacitracin ointment may be applied to the skin lesions, but in some cases it may be necessary to drain the lesions surgically.

Prevention is as important as treatment. No one with a skin infection should enter the nursery or the rooms occupied by the mothers. A mother who becomes infected should be isolated, and her child, if there is any reason to believe that his contact with her may have caused him to become infected, should be isolated from other infants in the nursery.

Every infant in the nursery should have his individual equipment, and all personnel should wash their hands thoroughly after caring for each infant. Personnel should be aware also that the anterior nares are the main reservoir in carriers of *Staphylococcus aureus*. (See page 166 for the advisability of wearing masks when caring for infants.) The nursery must not be overcrowded, for then it is almost impossible to maintain isolation technique.

If an epidemic starts, certain measures are routine. New patients are isolated. Rigid isolation technique is enforced. Another nursery should be opened for newborns delivered after the epidemic started and therefore not exposed to the infection in the contaminated nursery. Contaminated equipment should be thoroughly scrubbed with soap and water and sterilized if possible. The floor and walls should be cleaned and aired, curtains and furnishings washed. Nose and throat cultures should be taken of all nurses and other personnel who have cared for the infants in the infected nursery. It is imperative that each nursery have its own staff of nurses. As a preventive measure, an antibiotic effective against the particular strain of staphylococcus responsible for the original epidemic may be given to each infant in the clean nursery from his admission until discharge.

If these drastic measures are carried out for three weeks, the epidemic will probably come to an end. Such an epidemic is one of the most serious which may occur in a nursery for newborns.

IMPETIGO OF THE NEWBORN

Etiology, Incidence, and Transmission. (Color Plate 1–6). The causative organism may be staphylococci or streptococci. These organisms invade the superficial layers of the skin. The condition occurs more readily in the newborn than in older children and adults because their resistance is lower. Impetigo may be carried from one infant to another in the nursery.

Clinical Manifestations, Treatment, Prognosis, and Responsibilities of the Nurse. The first symptomatic lesions are erythematous papules. Then superficial vesicles containing fluid appear. The covering of these vesicles is loose and wrinkled. The fluid soon becomes purulent, and an area of erythema develops around each vesicle. The pustule ruptures, and crusts may develop, although this is more common in older children than in the newborn. The lesions usually occur on moist surfaces or body creases, and last from one to two weeks. Constitutional symptoms are rare.

Treatment consists in removing the epidermis with alcohol sponges and exposing the denuded areas to sunlight if possible. Affected areas may also be treated by washing with soap containing hexachlorophene, if this is ordered by the physician. Bacitracin or neomycin ointment may be applied locally. Systemic antibiotic therapy may be necessary.

Impetigo of the newborn was formerly a dangerous infection which led to sepsis and pemphigus, but today, with antibiotic treatment, the *prognosis* is good. Superficial lesions heal without scarring, although more extensive, deeper lesions may leave scars. Strict isolation technique should prevent the occurrence of impetigo in the nursery.

FURUNCULOSIS

Etiology, Incidence, Pathology, and Clinical Manifestations. Staphylococci are, in general, the pathogenic organisms which cause furunculosis. Although the condition may occur at any time during childhood, it is most frequent and most dangerous in malnourished newborn infants. Furuncles are most likely to occur on the head, but may appear on the back or the back of the extremities.

Furunculosis is an infection of the sebaceous glands or hair follicles. The furuncle soon develops into a red, pointed or rounded lump. In a few days it softens, and a core is formed. When a number of such lesions are present, the condition is called *furunculosis*. The infant seldom shows systemic symptoms. In extreme cases, however, anorexia and toxemia may occur.

Treatment. Antibiotic therapy depends upon the specific organism causing the condition. This can be found through an epidemiologic survey of nursery personnel or the family. A neomycin-bacitracin ointment may be applied in the nostrils, under the fingernails and around the perianal area to help prevent spread of the infection. The infant should be bathed daily, using soap containing hexachlorophene, if this is ordered by the physician, or a similar antiseptic to prevent spread of the infection. Hot compresses may be ordered to further maturation of the furuncle and, after it has opened spontaneously or been incised, to further drainage.

The diet should be low in carbohydrate and high in vitamin content. A sufficient fluid intake is necessary, and the electrolyte balance must be maintained.

Responsibilities of the Nurse. Aseptic nursing technique in the nursery is the best prevention against furunculosis. Particularly in hot weather the infant's position should be changed so that all surfaces of the skin are exposed in rotation to the air.

If furunculosis develops in an infant in the nursery, he should be removed and placed in isolation. With the first sign of the lesion the area should be cleansed with care. If the lesion is on the scalp, the area around the furuncle should be shaved. The nurse will carry out the physician's orders for treatment. The infant must not be allowed to rub the area; arm restraints (see Fig. 12–2) should be applied if necessary. The nurse should be careful not to become infected; the slightest scratch or abrasion on the hand may easily be a point of entrance for the organism.

EPIDEMIC DIARRHEA

Etiology, Incidence, and Transmission. In the newborn no single organism has been identified which is invariably the cause of epidemic diarrhea, though severe epidemics have been caused by virulent strains of *E. coli* bacilli or by viruses producing respiratory infections in adults. Diarrhea is a highly contagious disease easily carried from one infant to another. An infant who acquires the condition should be taken from the nursery and isolated elsewhere.

An infant may contract the disease through a contaminated formula or from the hands of his mother or nurse who themselves carry the organism, but are without clinical symptoms, since they have the adult's resistance to the infection. The importance of this source of infection is seldom realized. It is impossible to sterilize human hands completely, and even careful washing may not eliminate the risk of carrying the pathogenic organism to the infant.

Clinical Manifestations, Treatment, and Course. The main *symptom* is frequent watery stools, which are likely to be expelled with considerable force. The infant has abdominal distention; he may refuse his feedings or, if he takes them, vomit. As a rule there is elevation of the temperature. The weight loss is largely due to loss of fluid, which may be extremely rapid. Loss of fluids results in electrolyte imbalance and dehydration. Acidosis may result.

The *treatment* is similar to that given older infants with diarrhea (see p. 409). The obstetric unit should be closed unless all new cases can be cared for in other quarters by nurses who have not been in contact with the infants suffering from this infectious condition. If the cause of the infection is the enteropathic strain of the colon bacillus, neomycin may be ordered and given orally. Fluids and electrolytes are given parenterally to supplement or replace the oral intake.

The disease must be reported to the health authorities because of its infectiousness. The *course* is severe, and the mortality rate may be as high as 25 to 40 per cent of affected infants.

Responsibilities of the Nurse. Nursing care is both preventive and supportive. Rules and regulations safeguarding infants from all sources of infection are an administrative responsibility, but conscientious application of these regulations in the direct care of infants is the function of the nurse. It is the nurse who will see the first loose stool and note the presence of mucus in it, observe the infant's refusal of part or all of his feeding—probably vomiting what he has taken—and note his rise in temperature. The pathologic organism must be isolated in the laboratory examination of a stool specimen before the diagnosis of infectious diarrhea is made, but measures to protect the other infants in the nursery must be taken as soon as infection is suspected. In the majority of hospitals the nurse has a standing order to place an infected infant in isolation even before the physician has made a diagnosis and given written orders to do so.

The probable treatment which the physician will order has been outlined. All but the parenteral administration of fluids is carried out by the nurse. Few infants having medical conditions require such constant attention as those suffering from epidemic diarrhea.

Prevention of excoriated buttocks is an immediate problem in the nursing care. The diaper must be changed frequently. If the room is warm enough, it is advisable not to diaper the infant, but rather to place a pad made of folded diapers under his buttocks and leave him uncovered.

In some hospitals the diapers from an infected infant are soaked in a disinfectant before being sent to the laundry, or they may be placed in a container marked for special care in the laundry.

For additional care of infants with diarrhea, see page 411.

UMBILICAL INFECTION

Etiology, Clinical Manifestations, Complications, Treatment, Prevention, and Responsibilities of the Nurse. Umbilical infection is usually due to *Escherichia coli* or staphylococci, but may be due to other pyogenic organisms. The *symptoms* are redness and moisture of the stump of the cord. These symptoms may be slight or severe, but in no case should they be disregarded. In severe cases there may be a characteristically foul odor from the stump. The condition may clear up without systemic effects. But if the causative organism is one of the pus-producing type, septicemia may develop. Infection by the tetanus bacillus is less common, but produces a higher mortality rate (see p. 268).

Treatment consists in the administration of a broad-spectrum antibiotic immediately. Cultures with antibiotic sensitivities should be obtained. Some physicians may order hexachlorophene baths and the application of triple dye to the umbilical area. If an abscess forms, incision and drainage become necessary.

Prevention of the infection is discussed on pages 156 and 165.

This is another condition in which close, intelligent observation of the newborn by the nurse is of the utmost importance. The responsibility for noting the first signs of infection rests with the nurse.

Early recognition and treatment may prevent serious, if not fatal, systemic complications. As with any infection, the infant should be isolated and, preferably, removed from the nursery.

SEPSIS NEONATORUM

Etiology, Clinical Manifestations, and Treatment. Sepsis neonatorum may be caused by any pathogenic organism which has entered the blood stream. The portal of entry may be through the skin, mucous membranes, respiratory or gastrointestinal tract, umbilicus, or circumcision or other wound. The infection may occur prenatally, during delivery or postnatally.

The *symptoms* and signs may appear suddenly after an insidious onset, the infant at first appearing only restless or listless with anorexia and poor weight gain. Later there is evidence of dehydration and emaciation. There may be vomiting and diarrhea. The infant's temperature and white blood cell count may be elevated, depressed or normal. Convulsions may or may not be present. Signs of jaundice may appear. On examination the spleen and the liver may be found enlarged. The majority of these symptoms are so variable that the diagnosis is made upon the general picture and the laboratory findings, particularly the blood culture and nasopharyngeal culture.

Immediate *treatment* consists in administration of large doses of broad-spectrum antibiotics. After the laboratory blood examination has proved the specific organism causing the septic condition the specific antibiotic is given. Symptomatic therapy is carried out from the onset of the disease. The infant is isolated. He may be placed in an incubator so that he can be more easily observed and so that the temperature, humidity, and oxygen administration can be regulated accurately. Fluids may be administered parenterally, and a blood transfusion may be necessary. Oxygen is given as the need arises.

Prognosis and Course. If the condition is recognized early and treatment is instituted at once, the mortality rate is low. The probability of death increases as the untreated condition becomes more severe. The nidus of the infection should be sought; it may be in the meninges, the perineum or elsewhere. The organism in the blood stream may cause secondary infection in almost any part of the body. If meningitis develops, convulsions may ensue. If the infant survives, hydrocephalus may result. Characteristic signs of damage to brain cells may be evident as the child grows older (mental retardation).

Prevention and Responsibilities of the Nurse. *Prevention* lies in aseptic technique during delivery and in the technique which has already been outlined for the prevention of infection among infants in the nursery. Personnel caring for newborn infants must be exceptionally conscientious in reporting any infection, however slight, in their own bodies. In a modern hospital where good technique prevails it is probable that bacteria in the nose and throat of some member of the hospital personnel who comes in close contact with the infants are the greatest potential source of danger to them.

The preventive *nursing care* which has already been described in relation to infectious conditions applies in the care of infants suffering from sepsis neonatorum. Again, accurate observation and prompt reporting are of tremendous importance. From the discussion of signs and symptoms it is evident that the condition at the onset may easily be considered only a minor ailment and may go untreated until grave symptoms develop and the probability of complete cure is slight.

TETANUS NEONATORUM

Etiology, Incidence, and Incubation Period. The causative organism is the tetanus bacillus (*Clostridium tetani*), an anaerobic, spore-forming, gram-positive bacillus. Entrance into the blood stream of the newborn is through the umbilical wound. Tetanus is most unlikely to occur in a well regulated hospital, since the natural environment of the organism is in the soil. In children and adults the organism enters the blood stream through a deep puncture of the skin and underlying tissue. Since infants and children today receive antitetanus injections with the other types of early immunization, the incidence of tetanus among them is low.

Tetanus cannot be transmitted through contact; it must enter the body through a break in the skin. It develops only where it is not exposed to the air. Isolation of the infant is not necessary, but may be carried out to protect the child from other infections.

Tetanus of the newborn is extremely rare in the United States, but occurs in other countries where the hands of the attendant at delivery (untrained midwife, neighbor or one of the family) are contaminated and a contaminated knife is used to cut the cord.

The *incubation period* is five days to several weeks. The shorter the period of incubation, the greater is the probability of a fatal outcome. In the average hospital in the United States an infant is not in the nursery more than five days, and if the condition were to occur, it would probably be after the infant had been sent home. Again we see the need of follow-up of all infants who are not under the care of a private physician.

Clinical Manifestations. The symptoms

which accompany tetanus neonatorum are produced by the toxic effects on the nervous system of the exotoxin of the tetanus bacillus. The infant is irritable and restless; he cannot open his mouth or suck because of *trismus*, or tetanic spasm of the muscles of the jaw, and has great difficulty in swallowing. The facial expression is drawn and anxious. A symptom of diagnostic importance is stiffness of the neck. Painful muscular contractions or convulsions recur periodically. *Opisthotonos*, with the head drawn back and the back arched, occurs as a result of contraction of the strongest muscles in the body. As a result of spasms of the facial muscles a fixed expression, or *risus sardonicus*, may be seen. Tactile or auditory stimuli may induce convulsions. The temperature may be elevated, rising to 104°F. (40°C). The white blood cell count is 8000 to 12,000, and there is a slight increase in the cerebrospinal fluid pressure.

Treatment, Prevention, and Responsibilities of the Nurse. Adequate *treatment* and nursing care cannot be given unless a nurse is with the child at all times. Tetanus antitoxin is given to neutralize the free toxin in the body and around the site of the infection. Before administration of the antitoxin the infant's sensitivity to horse serum should be tested in order to prevent a serum reaction.

Measures to control convulsions are essential. Sufficient doses of sedatives are given to keep the infant relaxed and semiconscious. The level of sedation should be kept constant. Stimulation or unnecessary handling should be reduced to a minimum.

Nursing care should be planned around the periods when medication or necessary treatment is given. Secretions in the nasopharynx should be aspirated. Oxygen and carbon dioxide may be ordered to stimulate respirations. The equipment for tracheotomy should be ready for immediate use if needed. (For care of a child having a tracheotomy see page 541.) Since the infant is heavily sedated and unable to suck or swallow, it is necessary to feed him by gavage. Fluids will probably be administered parenterally. An intake and output chart must be kept.

Prevention of tetanus neonatorum lies in the use of sterile instruments to cut the cord and adequate care of the cord during the neonatal period. For prevention of tetanus in the infant, see page 379.

Prognosis. The prognosis is very poor, the mortality rate being up to 50 per cent of the cases. Death is usually due to respiratory failure, exhaustion or a complicating aspiration pneumonia. If the infant survives, however, recovery is complete.

ADDICTION — NARCOTIC DRUGS

Etiology, Incidence, and Clinical Manifestations. As the incidence of addiction to drugs such as morphine, heroin, and methadone has increased among the adult population, so has it also increased among infants born to addicted mothers (see p. 169).

Clinical manifestations of drug addiction in the newborn usually appear within 24 to 72 hours after birth, but may not appear until the newborn is ten days old. The symptoms include central nervous system irritability evidenced by tremors, an incomplete Moro reflex, and hyperirritable, distraught behavior with an increased need for sucking. The cry of the addicted infant is piercing, similar to that of the infant having central nervous system damage. He may also have excessive mucus, diarrhea, and vomiting and may show more than the usual weight loss after birth. Since these manifestations are commonly seen with other problems in the newborn, the mothers of these infants should be observed for scarring of the extremities due to needle punctures, cellulitis, thrombophlebitis, and withdrawal symptoms.

In order to make an accurate diagnosis, specimens of blood and urine from the newborn should be collected soon after birth because the narcotic metabolites disappear rapidly.

Treatment and Responsibilities of the Nurse. The drugs most commonly used for the treatment of addicted newborns are phenobarbital and chlorpromazine. Paregoric may be used to control diarrhea. These infants should be handled as little as possible because of their extreme hyperirritability. The use of parenteral

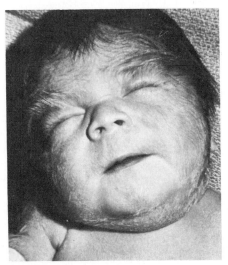

FIGURE 11–21. Fetal alcohol syndrome. One-year-old affected child of a chronic alcoholic woman at his birth. (From Smith, D. W.: *Recognizable Patterns of Human Malformation*, 2nd ed. Philadelphia, W. B. Saunders Co., 1976.)

fluids may be necessary to correct dehydration and electrolyte imbalance.

FETAL ALCOHOL SYNDROME

Etiology, Incidence, and Clinical Manifestations. The "fetal alcohol syndrome" may occur in the neonate of a mother who has chronic alcoholism. It is not known how much alcohol may be necessary to bring about adverse effects to the developing fetus or whether there is a particularly critical time in fetal growth when exposure to alcohol in the mother's blood stream may influence the fetus. Perinatal mortality occurs much more frequently in these infants than in those of nonalcoholic mothers.

In the survivors, lowered intelligence, a borderline-to-moderate degree of mental retardation, is the most frequent problem. These newborns are shorter in length, lower in weight, and have a smaller head circumference than normal newborns. Their growth is slow after birth. They may also have various types of deformities: congenital heart disease, joint defects, and underdeveloped cheekbones.

When the mother is intoxicated, the blood alcohol levels are high enough so that alcohol is carried across the placenta. These babies at birth may experience symptoms of alcohol withdrawal just as adult alcoholics do.

It is true that the other factors that may contribute to the lack of development of these infants at birth include heavy smoking and an inadequate diet, problems which may exist together with alcoholism.

Prognosis. The frequency of adverse outcome in the chronic alcoholic woman who is pregnant is so great that a decision must be made concerning the continuation of pregnancy. Women who drink alcohol excessively should not become pregnant until they have their problem under control. The organization Alcoholics Anonymous may help them to achieve this goal (see Chapter 27).

TEACHING AIDS AND OTHER INFORMATION*

American Academy of Pediatrics

Infectious Diseases (Red Book).
Venereal Disease and the Pediatrician.

Johnson & Johnson

Narcotic Addiction in the Newborn.

The National Foundation — March of Dimes

Are You His/Her Type?
Birth Defects — Causes, Incidence, Prevention, Treatment.
Birth Defects: The Tragedy and the Hope.
It's Possible: Birth Defects Prevention.
Preventing Birth Defects Caused by Rubella and Rh Blood Disease.

National Society for the Prevention of Blindness, Inc.

Control of Ophthalmia Neonatorum — A Position Statement.

Ross Laboratories

Common Orthopedic Conditions in Childhood, 1973.
Iatrogenic Problems in Neonatal Intensive Care, 1976.
Regionalization of Perinatal Care, 1974.

United States Government

Lin-Fu, J.S.: Prevention of Hemolytic Disease of the Fetus and Newborn Due to Rh Isoimmunization, 1975.
Promoting Community Health, 1975.
Russell, F.F. (Ed.): Identification and Management of Selected Developmental Disabilities: A Guide for Nurses, 1975.

----

*Complete addresses are given in the Appendix.

REFERENCES

Books

Abramson, H. (Ed.): *Resuscitation of the Newborn Infant.* 3rd ed. St. Louis, The C. V. Mosby Company, 1973.
American Hospital Association: *Infection Control in the Hospital.* 3rd ed. Chicago, American Hospital Association, 1974.
Arey, L. B.: *Developmental Anatomy: A Textbook and Laboratory Manual of Embryology.* 7th ed. Philadelphia, W. B. Saunders Company, 1974.
Avery, G. B. (Ed.): *Neonatology: Pathophysiology and Management of the Newborn.* Philadelphia, J. B. Lippincott Company, 1975.
Babson, S. G., Benson, R. C., Pernoll, M. L., and Benda, G. I.: *Management of High-Risk Pregnancy and Intensive Care of the Neonate.* 3rd ed. St. Louis, The C. V. Mosby Company, 1975.

Balinsky, B. I.: *An Introduction to Embryology.* 4th ed. Philadelphia, W. B. Saunders Company, 1975.
Behrman, R. E. (Ed.): *Neonatology: Diseases of the Fetus and Infant.* St. Louis, The C. V. Mosby Company, 1973.
Cockburn, F., and Drillien, C. M. (Eds.): *Neonatal Medicine.* Philadelphia, J. B. Lippincott Company, 1975.
Corliss, C. E.: *Patten's Human Embryology: Elements of Clinical Development.* New York, McGraw-Hill Book Company, 1976.
Fochtman, D., and Raffensperger, J. G. (Eds.): *Principles of Nursing Care for the Pediatric Surgery Patient.* 2nd ed. Boston, Little, Brown & Company, 1976.
Frobisher, M., and Fuerst, R.: *Microbiology in Health and Disease.* 13th ed. Philadelphia, W. B. Saunders Company, 1973.

Gasser, R. F.: *Atlas of Human Embryos.* New York, Harper & Row Publishers, Inc., 1975.

Gellis, S. S., and Kagan, B. M. (Eds.): *Current Pediatric Therapy 7.* Philadelphia, W. B. Saunders Company, 1976.

Gold, E. R., and Butler, N. R.: *ABO Hemolytic Disease of The Newborn.* Chicago, Year Book Medical Publishers, Inc., 1972.

Hanshaw, J. B., and Dudgeon, J. A.: *Viral Diseases of the Fetus and Newborn.* Philadelphia, W. B. Saunders Company, 1977.

Korones, S. B.: *High Risk Newborn Infants: The Basis For Intensive Nursing Care.* 2nd ed. St. Louis, The C. V. Mosby Company, 1976.

Langman, J.: *Medical Embryology: Human Development— Normal and Abnormal.* 3rd ed. Baltimore, Williams & Wilkins Company, 1975.

Moffet, H. L.: *Pediatric Infectious Diseases.* Philadelphia, J. B. Lippincott Company, 1975.

Moore, K. L.: *Before We Are Born: Basic Embryology and Birth Defects.* Philadelphia, W. B. Saunders, 1974.

Raffensperger, J. G., and Fochtmann, D.: *Pediatric Surgery for Nurses.* 2nd ed. Boston, Little, Brown & Company, 1976.

Remington, J. S., and Klein, J. O. (Eds.): *Infection of Fetus and Newborn Infant.* Philadelphia, W. B. Saunders Company, 1976.

Schaffer, A. J., and Avery, M. E.: *Diseases of the Newborn.* 4th ed. Philadelphia, W. B. Saunders Company, 1977.

Smith, C. A., and Nelson, N. M. (Eds.): *The Physiology of the Newborn Infant.* 4th ed. Springfield, Ill. Charles C Thomas, 1975.

Smith, D. W.: *Recognizable Patterns of Human Malformation: Genetic, Embryologic and Clinical Aspects.* 2nd ed. Philadelphia, W. B. Saunders Company, 1976.

Stevenson, R. E.: *The Fetus and Newly Born Infant: Influences of the Prenatal Environment.* St. Louis, The C. V. Mosby Company, 1973.

Vaughan, V. C. III, and McKay, R. J. (Eds.): *Nelson Textbook of Pediatrics.* 10th ed. Philadelphia, W. B. Saunders Company, 1975.

Periodicals

Amarose, A. P., and Norusis, M. J.: Cytogenetics of Methadone-Managed and Heroin-Addicted Pregnant Women and Their Newborn Infants. *Am. J. Obstet. Gynecol.,* 124:635, March 15, 1976.

Barnard, M. U.: Supportive Nursing Care for the Mother and Newborn Who Are Separated from Each Other. *The American Journal of Maternal-Child Nursing,* 1:107, March-April 1976.

Bonta, B. W., and Warshaw, J. B.: Importance of Radiant Flux in the Treatment of Hyperbilirubinemia: Failure of Overhead Phototherapy Units in Intensive Care Units. *Pediatrics,* 57:503, April 1976.

Brown, M. S.: Syphilis and Gonorrhea: An Update for Nurses in Ambulatory Settings. *Nursing '76,* 6:71, January 1976.

Cozzi, F., and Wilkinson, A. W.: Low Birthweight Babies With Esophageal Atresia or Tracheoesophageal Fistula. *Arch. Dis. Child.,* 50:791, October 1975.

David, L.: The Tiniest Patients: How Do You Operate on a Baby no Larger than Your Two Hands? *Family Health/Today's Health,* 8:30, June 1976.

Faden, H. S., Burke, J. P., Glasgow, L. A., and Everett, J. R.: Nursery Outbreak of Scalded Skin Syndrome. *Am. J. Dis. Child,* 130:265, March 1976.

Finnegan, L. P., and Macnew, B. A.: Care of the Addicted Infant. *Am. J. Nursing,* 74:685, April 1974.

Francis, D. P., et al. Nosocomial and Maternally Acquired Herpesvirus Hominis Infections. A Report of Four Fatal Cases in Neonates. *Am. J. Dis. Child,* 129:889, August 1975.

Griscelli, C., Desmonts, G., Geny, B., and Frommel, D.: Congenital Toxoplasmosis: Fetal Synthesis of Oligoclonal Immunoglobulin G in Intrauterine Infection. *J. Pediatr.* 83:20, July 1973.

Handsfield, H. H.: Gonococcal Orogastric Contamination in the Newborn. *Medical Aspects of Human Sexuality,* 8:32, February 1974.

Harper, R. G., et al.: The Effect of a Methadone Treatment Program Upon Pregnant Heroin Addicts and Their Newborn Infants. *Pediatrics,* 54:300, September 1974.

Hecht, M.: Children of Alcoholics. *Am. J. Nursing,* 73:1764, October 1973.

Hyperbilirubinaemia and Bacterial Infection in the Newborn. *Arch Dis. Child,* 50:652, August 1975.

Jones, K. L., Smith, D. W., Streissguth, A. P., and Myrianthopoulos, N. C.: Outcome in Offspring of Chronic Alcoholic Women. *Lancet* 1:1076, June 1, 1974.

Kibrick, S., and Loria, R. M.: Rubella and Cytomegalovirus: Current Concepts of Congenital and Acquired Infection. *Pediat. Clin. N. Amer.,* 21:513, May 1974.

Kimball, A. C., Kean, B. H., and Fuchs, F.: Toxoplasmosis: Risk Variations in New York City Obstetric Patients. *Am. J. Obstet. Gynecol.,* 119:208, May 15, 1974.

Kron, R. E., Litt, M., Phoenix, M. D., and Finnegan, L. P.: Neonatal Narcotic Abstinence: Effects of Pharmacotherapeutic Agents and Maternal Drug Usage on Nutritive Sucking Behavior. *J. Pediatr.,* 88:637, April 1976.

Marx, J. L.: Cytomegalovirus: A Major Cause of Birth Defects. *Science* 190:1184, December 19, 1975.

Moncrieff, M. W., and Dunn, J.: Phototherapy for Hyperbilirubinaemia in Very Low Birthweight Infants. *Arch. Dis. Child,* 51:124, February 1976.

Nalepka, C. D.: The Oxygen Hood for Newborns in Respiratory Distress. *Am. J. Nursing,* 75:2185, December 1975.

Ostrea, E. M., Chavez, C. J., and Strauss, M. E.: A Study of Factors That Influence the Severity of Neonatal Narcotic Withdrawal. *J. Pediatr.,* 88:642, April 1976.

Pattison, K.: Drug Addicted Mother & Child. *Nursing '73,* 3:46, February 1973.

Rementeria, J. L., Janakammal, S., and Hollander, M.: Multiple Births in Drug-Addicted Women. *Am. J. Obstet. Gynecol.,* 122:958, August 15, 1975.

Rudoy, R. C.; and Nelson, J. D.: Breast Abscess During the Neonatal Period. *Am. J. Dis. Child,* 129:1031, September 1975.

Sardemann, H., Madsen, K. S., and Friis-Hansen, B.: Follow-Up of Children of Drug-Addicted Mothers. *Arch. Dis. Child,* 51:131, February 1976.

Shafer, N.: Toxoplasmosis. *N.Y. State J. Med.,* 75:1049, June 1975.

Stimmel, B., and Adamsons, K.: Narcotic Dependency in Pregnancy. *J.A.M.A.,* 235:1121, March 15, 1976.

Tan, K. L.: Comparison of the Effectiveness of Phototherapy and Exchange Transfusion in the Management of Nonhemolytic Neonatal Hyperbilirubinemia. *J. Pediatr.,* 87:609, October 1975.

Venereal Disease Control Advisory Committee: Syphilis: USPHS Guide to Treatment. *Medical Aspects of Human Sexuality,* 10:106, August 1976.

Weissberg, E. D., Smith, A. L., and Smith, D. H.: Clinical Features of Neonatal Osteomyelitis. *Pediatrics,* 53:505, April 1974.

AUDIOVISUAL MEDIA*

The American Journal of Nursing Company

Maternity Nursing Class
  Hemolytic Diseases of the Newborn
  44 minutes, 16mm film or videotape, guide.
  Physician discusses erythroblastosis fetalis and antigenic blood group incompatibilities, their effects on the fetus, prenatal management including amniocentesis, and the treatment of the neonate.

CIBA and Wayne State University

Abdomen in Infants and Children
  Platou, R. V., 32 minutes.
  This film shows the technique of examining infants and children for more than 20 diseases and conditions including hernia, intestinal atresia, pyloric stenosis, intussusception, appendicitis, and Wilms' tumor.

W. B. Saunders Company

Current Topics in Obstetrics and Gynecology
  Director: Tyson, J. E.
  Emergency Management of Disorders of the Newborn, Haller, J. A.

Pediatric Conferences with Sydney Gellis
  Cytomegalovirus Infections, Hanshaw, J. B.
  Herpes Simplex Infections, Nahmias, A. J.
  Identification of the Newborn at Risk of Infection, Cochran, W.
  Narcotic Addiction in the Newborn, Wasserman, E.
  Phototherapy for Hyperbilirubinemia of the Newborn, Lucey, J. F.
  Staphylococcal Infections, Melish, M. E.

Viral Infections in Childhood
  Sussman, S. J.
  4 35mm filmstrips, 2 audio-tape cassettes, color, booklet.
  This presentation emphasizes the important visual component in diagnosis and management of viral diseases and includes an in-depth verbal discussion of the infection and its clinical implications. Essential aspects of differential diagnosis and management of pediatric viral infections are included: skin eruptions, various exudates, swelling, upper respiratory tract inflammations, signs on radiographs, and other visual manifestations.

Trainex Corporation

Pediatric Dermatology
  35mm filmstrip, audio-tape cassette, 33 ⅓ LP, color.
  Provides an introduction to common skin manifestations and diseases of infants and children. Clinical photographs of characteristic skin eruptions are accompanied by a narration that discusses etiology, incidence and progression of the condition. Included are such disorders as those manifested in the newborn, inherited disorders, papulosquamous diseases, and infections and infestations of the skin.

Pediatric Surgery for Congenital Defects
  35mm filmstrip, audio-tape cassettes, 33 ⅓ LP, color.
  Defects and corresponding surgical management and techniques presented include hypertrophy of tongue, cystic hygromas, mandibular cysts, sacrococcygeal teratomas, omphalocele, gastroschisis, imperforated anus, bowel atresias, meconium ileus, ischemic necrosis of the bowel, colon perforation, Hirschsprung's disease, congenital webs, Meckel's diverticulum, and intussusception. Full-color photographs of the defects and corrective surgical techniques, diagnostic X-rays, descriptive narration.

Respiratory Problems in the Newborn
  35mm filmstrip, audio-tape cassettes, 33 ⅓ LP, color.
  Discusses and illustrates conditions that result in respiratory problems in the newborn: respiratory distress syndrome, meconium aspiration, chylothorax, pulmonary hemorrhage, and transient tachypnea. Describes clinical signs of respiratory problems in the newborn and discusses methods of diagnosis and treatment, oxygen therapy, and complications resulting from O_2 toxicity.

---

*Complete addresses are given in the Appendix.

Chapter Twelve

CONGENITAL DEFORMITIES

Several congenital anomalies require care over a period of weeks, months, or years. Long-term conditions such as inborn errors of metabolism, which are not usually diagnosed during the first few days of life, will be discussed in later chapters. For many of the anomalies discussed in this chapter, surgery early in life is the treatment of choice. The risk to life must be considered in relation to the probable advantage to the child of operation. It is difficult for parents to be objective in making the decision for or against surgical treatment. Before operation is undertaken the parents should be convinced that their decision is right, that the probable benefit justifies the risk. Then, if the child should die, they do not blame themselves for permitting the operation.

Surgical correction may be necessary later. The treatment and nursing care of some of these children will be discussed in this chapter.

CONDITIONS OF THE NEWBORN REQUIRING LONG-TERM CARE

Skin Lesions

NEVI

Nevi in the newborn are of two types: *(a)* the vascular group, due to hyperplasia of blood or lymph vessels; and *(b)* nonvascular nevi, caused by an overgrowth of connective or epidermal tissue. In either type the defect probably originates in the germ plasm. The hereditary factor is apparently important.

Nevus Vasculosus. The nevus vasculosus, commonly called a birthmark, is composed entirely of blood vessels. These marks are likely to be flat and to appear on the back of the head. No treatment is required, since the majority disappear spontaneously.

The *nevus flammeus* or so-called *port-wine mark* is a flat, irregularly shaped mark often found on the side of the face. It is light pink in the newborn, but later becomes deep purple. It is due to a malformation of superficial capillaries and does not respond too well to local treatment. A small or faint lesion which appears to be similar to these marks on the face may appear on the nape of the neck, bridge of the nose or on the eyelids. These lesions, unlike those of the face, disappear without treatment.

The so-called *strawberry mark* is the most common of the vascular nevi. It is a slightly raised, bright red to deep purple nevus which may disappear spontaneously, although the growth pattern of these marks may be variable during the first six to eight months of life.

A *cavernous hemangioma* is formed by large sinus-like blood vessels. These lesions are cystic, deep-lying vascular anomalies that are blue or purple. In rare instances when the cavernous hemangioma grows widely and is deforming the face, anemia may develop because of the vol-

273

ume of blood within the tumor. Fresh blood or platelet-rich transfusions may be necessary. Prednisone may be used to produce regression in cavernous hemangioma. Complete excision of the entire vascular defect may be indicated.

Pigmented Nevi. These lesions vary in size and color from harmless freckles to dark hairy nevi. Although such lesions are rarely malignant, the child should be kept from irritating the area. Although nevi do not grow rapidly, they develop in proportion to the child's growth and therefore become increasingly more difficult to remove. If they are large, dark, and on the face, they may cause both parents and child the emotional trauma likely to accompany any conspicuous disfigurement.

TREATMENT. The most satisfactory treatment of pigmented nevi is by surgical excision, including a portion of the nearby normal skin. Nevi on parts of the body where constant irritation of the skin occurs must be observed at regular intervals and removed if changes in size or nature occur. Operation must be done if they appear to be growing at a disproportionately greater rate than the body skin. If only the cosmetic effect is the concern of the physician and the parents, the time for removal makes little difference. In general, however, it is advisable that operation be done during the first year of life or in the early school years.

Gastrointestinal System

CLEFT LIP AND CLEFT PALATE

Etiology, Pathology, and Incidence. The terms "cleft lip" and "cleft palate" describe the condition. The cause is a failure of union of the embryonic structures of the face. Fusion of the maxillary and premaxillary processes normally occurs between the fifth and eighth weeks of intrauterine life. The palatal processes fuse about one month later. Failure of fusion results in the typical cleft lip and cleft palate.

This partial or complete nonunion may involve more than the palatal bone and the upper lip. It may affect the maxilla, premaxilla, and tissues of the soft palate and uvula. All these defects or any combination of them may occur. The abnormality appears to run in families and therefore to be influenced by heredity, but other factors may be involved. The condition is often one of several anomalies in the infant.

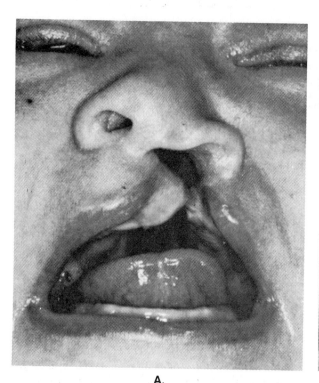
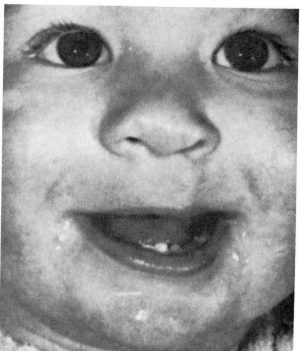

A.   **B.**

FIGURE 12–1.   Correction produced by the combination of preoperative orthodontic treatment and operation. *A*, The typical deformity of a unilateral complete cleft. The midline is deviated away from the cleft and the premaxilla is tilted. The alar cartilage is concavoconvex. *B*, After treatment the midline of the nose and the shape of the cartilage have been corrected. (From Davis, J. A., and Dobbing, J. (Eds.): *Scientific Foundations of Paediatrics.* Philadelphia, W. B. Saunders Co., 1974.)

The *incidence* of cleft lip or cleft palate is about 1 in 800 of the population.

Psychologic Trauma. To learn that their newborn infant suffers this abnormality is a great shock to the parents—less so, however, if some relative on either side of the family lines has had a successful repair of the same condition. A sympathetic, tactful nurse can do a great deal to relieve their distress. The nurse may show them "before and after operation" pictures of infants who had this deformity. These pictures may relieve parents of some of their anxiety about the appearance of their own infant. Immediate evaluation should be done by a plastic surgeon. The surgeon's discussion of therapy with the parents may also help them in their adjustment to their newborn's malformation.

CLEFT LIP

Incidence and Pathology. Cleft lip is one of the most frequently occurring congenital anomalies. It is more common in males than in females.

The defect is due to incomplete fusion of the central processes with one or both of the external processes from which the area around the upper jaw, lip, and nose is formed. If the fissure is unilateral, it is generally below the center of one of the nostrils; if bilateral, beneath both nostrils. The extent of the defect varies from a slight indentation to an open cleft. The incomplete cleft may be little more than a notching of the vermilion border of the lip, but on the other hand may extend to the nostril. The complete cleft usually involves the alveolus to some degree, and the ala (the flap of flesh forming the side of the nostril) is displaced toward the side. The floor of the nares and even the gum in which the upper teeth are set may also be deformed.

Treatment and Prognosis. Plastic surgery should be done for the child's comfort as well as the cosmetic effect. The psychologic effect upon the parents, even if they try to be objective in their attitude toward the child's deformity, is likely to hinder the usual face-to-face cuddling which infants normally receive. If they show him to friends, he may not receive the warm greeting which adults generally give to perfect, healthy infants and which the infant needs to develop his trust in others.

Some plastic surgeons will do the surgical repair as soon as the infant begins to gain weight and is free from infection or before one to two months of age. Early repair prevents trauma and difficulty for the parents, since friends and relatives are not disturbed by seeing the newborn.

In the mild, incomplete type of cleft lip the child is not hampered by the deformity.

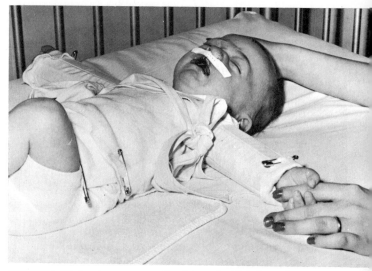

FIGURE 12–2. Appearance of a 2-month-old infant after repair of a cleft lip. A Band-aid is used to hold the suture line together. Elbow restraints prevent the infant from rubbing his face. The mother remained with this child throughout his hospitalization.

With complete cleft lip, repair should be made as soon as the child's condition permits, since the deformity interferes with feeding. The infant also becomes accustomed to breathing through his mouth, with the result that the mucous membrane becomes dry and cracked, and infection is more likely. In the rapidly growing structure of the infant's face the cleft prevents normal development.

The *prognosis,* when repair is made by a competent plastic surgeon, is good. Postoperatively a Band-aid may be used to hold the suture line together. In many hospitals a *Logan bar* (a wire bow placed over the wound with each end taped to the cheek on which it rests) is used to prevent stretching of the wound postoperatively when the infant cries.

Responsibilities of the Nurse Preoperatively. While the infant is at home the nurse should encourage the mother to treat him as if he were a normal infant. He should not be overprotected and certainly never rejected. If the operation is to be postponed, the mother should not keep him from relatives and friends. She must realize, however, that the first impression of a child so disfigured is startling, and allow others to become accustomed to his appearance before expecting from them the normal reaction to an infant.

The mother should be told that the infant's difficulty in feeding is due to the fact that he cannot create a vacuum in his mouth and so is unable to suck. A soft nipple with a relatively large hole, a special type of nipple or a rubber-tipped medicine dropper may be used to feed him, although in extreme cases gavage may be necessary. The mother can be taught whatever procedure is appropriate for her child. If a soft nipple is used, the infant should be assisted in sucking with a biting type of movement. In feeding with the dropper the rubber tip should be put on the top and to the side of the tongue and as far back in the mouth as is practical. He should be bubbled frequently, for he swallows more air than the infant nursing from the breast or the bottle.

Some physicians believe that the infant's hands should be restrained when he is not being held if he shows any tendency to irritate the cleft lip. With a small infant it is usually sufficient to pull the sleeves of the shirt down over the hands and to pin the edge of each sleeve to the diaper. Because of his need for sucking pleasure, some physicians recommend the use of a pacifier by such infants. The older infant's hands may be restrained by using the clove hitch restraint (see p. 256), or elbow restraints, only if absolutely necessary.

Because of mouth-breathing the lips are dry, and it is important to prevent cracks or fissures through which infection may enter. The area should be kept clean, and water should be given after feedings to rinse out the mouth. The mother or nurse should also watch for signs of aspiration, respiratory distress, or gastrointestinal disturbance. Every precaution should be taken to protect him from infection. The routine care of an infant must be taught the mother, since the infant will be at home until he is old enough for operation.

Responsibilities of the Nurse Postoperatively. The infant will require close observation to keep the airway open. He is accustomed to mouth-breathing, which may be difficult postoperatively. The nurse should report to the physician if the tissues of the tongue or mouth or the lining of the nostrils is swollen from surgery. A laryngoscope, endotracheal tube, and suction apparatus should be ready for use if necessary.

The solution to be used for cleansing the nostril and the incision is ordered by the physician. The nurse cleanses the suture line frequently and with great care. The lip should be patted, not wiped. In some hospitals suture line care consists of applying sterile cotton-tipped applicators soaked in hydrogen peroxide to the incision to cleanse it. Mineral oil may be applied following the gentle cleansing to prevent crusting. If a crust forms, a scar is likely to result; if a suture is pulled or sloughs out, the suture line will not be even.

The infant receives the routine nursing care needed by all infants; he should be kept comfortable, warm, and dry. He should be kept from crying, for even with the Band-aid or Logan bar, crying puts some strain on the suture line. His mother should be encouraged to stay and comfort the infant so that he will not cry. He can be held and carried about. The infant may be given clear liquids for several days.

If a medicine dropper is used, it is inserted in the corner of the mouth so as not to touch the area about the suture line. He is fed slowly and in a sitting position. He is bubbled frequently both for relief of air which he has swallowed and for its general comforting effect. Water is given to cleanse the mouth of milk after the feeding. As with any infant, water should be given between feedings.

If the hands must be restrained to prevent the infant from rubbing his face, normal movement is prevented. To improve the circulation and make the infant more comfortable, the arms can be released, first one and then the other. Since the infant cannot suck, he is held and cuddled frequently to provide emotional satisfaction. The infant should never be placed upon his abdomen, or even upon his side if there is a likelihood that he may roll over on his face. In the lateral position he is less likely to aspirate mucus or regurgitated milk. His position should be changed frequently to lessen the danger of hypostatic pneumonia. If it is impossible to support him on his side, or if his position is changed and he lies upon his back, he may be held in the desired position by bands about the wrists fastened with the clove hitch restraint (see p. 256).

The adhesive anchoring a Band-aid or Logan bar should be kept clean and dry and be replaced if it loosens.

After approximately two weeks, when the lip is completely healed, bottle or breast feeding may be resumed. Only an infant with an incomplete cleft can nurse, and therefore few of these infants are breast-fed satisfactorily. For a breast-fed infant, however, the mother should express her milk before and during the postoperative period when the infant is unable to suck.

CLEFT PALATE

Incidence, Etiology, Pathology, and Clinical Manifestations. Unlike cleft lip, which occurs more frequently among boys than among girls, cleft palate is more common in girls. Although it is often associated with cleft lip, the two anomalies are not always simultaneously present. Cleft palate is more serious than cleft lip. It interferes more with the infant's feeding and breathing and is far more difficult to repair. There seems to be an increased incidence of associated congenital malformations, intellectual impairment, and hearing impairment in infants with cleft palate.

The fissure may involve only the soft palate or

may extend into the nose and also the hard palate. The cleft is in the midline of the soft palate and on one or both sides of the hard palate, and of course is longitudinal. The cleft forms a passageway between the nasopharynx and the nose. This passageway causes part of the difficulty in feeding and is a factor in susceptibility to infection.

The infant is unable to suck well, and even if he tries to suck, part of the feeding may be expelled through the nose.

As soon as the child has enough teeth to hold a dental speech appliance in place, one can be made to fit the deformity. If the cleft is not repaired before the child learns to talk, and if a dental speech appliance is not used, the guttural tone produced by the deformity may become habitual and persist after repair of the cleft has made normal speech possible.

Instructions to the Parents on Discharge of the Infant from the Nursery. As with the infant with cleft lip, the parents of a child with cleft palate are apt to either overprotect him or emotionally reject him. While he is still in the nursery the parents should be taught how to care for him, and he should become accustomed to their feeding him.

The *nutritional problem* is immediate. An adequate fluid intake is necessary to prevent dehydration. The parents should be taught how to feed the infant with a soft nipple having holes large enough to permit the milk to drop into the infant's mouth without sucking, or with a special nipple with a flange that covers the defect in the cleft palate so that the infant can suck. The infant may also be fed with a medicine dropper. Some physicians recommend the use of a Brecht feeder; however, there is a danger in using it because the feeding may be expressed too rapidly into his mouth and the infant may choke. Gavage should be used as a last resort. The infant should be held in an upright position in order to facilitate swallowing the feeding without regurgitation through the nose or without aspirating it. He should be bubbled frequently. Later on, perhaps when several months old, he may be fed with a spoon or may learn to take his milk from a cup.

The infant's mouth is easily infected. Some physicians believe that until he is old enough to cooperate, his arms must be restrained to prevent him from sucking his fingers or otherwise irritating the cleft. Other physicians and those interested in early childhood development believe that if the infant can be observed frequently, restraints should not be used, since they prevent him from exploring his world and his own body. If the infant is not permitted to explore and discover himself, he will have missed a sensory stage which is almost impossible to make up later. The mouth should be kept clean at all times, and for this purpose the physician may order a mild antiseptic. Feedings should be followed by a little water to rinse out the mouth.

Unless these infants are under the care of a private physician, it is essential that they be taken to a cleft palate clinic or a pediatric clinic at regular intervals in order to determine the proper time for operation. Repair may be attempted when the infant is as young as six months or two years old, or may be postponed until later, depending on the wisdom of taking advantage of the changes which occur with palatal growth. The optimum time for operation depends upon the condition of the individual child. If correction of the defect is not made before the child has learned to talk, he may retain his guttural speech.

Total Program of Care or Habilitation. The care and habilitation of the child with cleft palate may require many years of medical, dental, surgical, and speech treatment. The personnel involved act as a team, functioning better as a group so that the parents are not confused by the ally. The *cleft palate team* includes the pediatrician, plastic surgeon, dentist, prosthetic dentist, orthodontist, otolaryngologist, audiologist, medical social worker, nurse in the hospital, speech pathologist, psychologist or psychiatrist or both, and the public health or community nurse. The child's physician may act as coordinator of the group so that the parents are not confused by the apparent complexity of the treatment. The parents may need guidance from each of the team members at various times as treatment progresses. Cleft palate teams such as these are usually centered in the clinics of large medical centers.

If the parents cannot afford this care, the child is treated at one of the large medical centers connected with the state program for crippled children or at a children's hospital under private auspices. In either case he is treated without cost to his parents, or for whatever fee they are able to pay.

Dealing with the anxieties of the parents is one of the main functions of the cleft palate team, and specifically of the nurses in the newborn nursery, the nurses in the home or clinic, and the nurses in the hospital when the child is admitted for surgery. The parents should be reassured that all possible therapy will be given the child. They must also be told that improvement will take time and will require their full cooperation. The parents must be helped to accept the child with his disfigurement and to help him to adjust to his deformity. The physical defect can be corrected more successfully than can hampering personality traits which may develop if he believes that others turn away from him because of his cleft palate.

Surgical Correction. The child should be placed under the care of the cleft palate team as early as possible so that changes occurring with growth can be observed and plans can be made for long-term needs.

Operation is delayed because the surgeon wants to take advantage of changes in the palate which occur with growth. The time for operation varies because of differences in the size, degree and shape of the deformity. The surgeon tries to correct the defect so that there is optimum union of the cleft in the palate, without injury to the developing maxilla, and so that intelligible speech will be possible.

If operation is postponed until the child is learning to speak—about the third year—a dental speech appliance can be fitted so that the child can speak clearly enough for others to understand him. If the deformity is too severe and surgical repair is not possible, a *prosthetic speech appliance* is used as an important means of speech habilitation. Such appliances must be replaced periodically as the child grows.

Surgical Management and Responsibilities of the Nurse. *Preoperative care* is minimal. Any infection is a contraindication to operation. The nurse must watch the child closely and report any evidence of infection. The clotting and bleeding times should be determined preoperatively. Feedings are given until six to eight hours before operation if the child is in good nutritional condition, with good fluid and electrolyte balance.

Postoperative care is extremely important. Special nursing care is essential immediately after operation to keep the mouth clean and free from irritation. Antibiotics are ordered only if infection is suspected. Directly after the operation the child is placed on his abdomen and may have the foot of his bed slightly elevated to prevent aspiration of drainage material. His head is turned to one side. The nurse should watch closely for signs of an occluded airway and for hemorrhage. If necessary, the child is placed in a position favorable to postural drainage.

The physician may order aspiration of the nasopharynx to reduce the possibility of development of pneumonitis or atelectasis. It must be done very gently. Many physicians, however, prefer that no suction be used.

The nurse should tell the child not to rub the site with his tongue, in words he can understand, such as, "Don't put your tongue on the part of your mouth which feels sore." Restraint may be necessary to keep the child from putting his fingers or even toys in his mouth. If the child is not old enough to cooperate, his arms must be securely restrained with elbow restraints. The restraints should be placed over the shirt, with the shirt sleeves turned back and pinned in position. The restraints should be removed periodically and passive exercise given.

The nurse may be asked to assist the physician in giving parenteral fluid therapy.

The diet is limited to clear sterile or other fluids as ordered by the physician. Milk is usually not permitted immediately after the operation because of the danger of curds forming along the suture line. The child's mouth should be rinsed or cleansed with sterile water after each feeding.

The diet is fluid or semifluid for ten days to two weeks after operation. For the following two weeks a soft diet is given, and after that a regular diet.

As far as possible all strain on the sutures must be prevented. The first postoperative feeding is given with a rubber-tipped medicine dropper, with the physician's permission, or from a paper cup or the side of a spoon. A straw is not used, for he should not suck.

If possible, crying should be prevented even though he is usually irritable postoperatively and may have an elevation of temperature. The child should be kept dry and as comfortable as possible. Quiet diversion such as showing him pictures in his favorite picture book and reading the accompanying story will help to keep him from crying. The physician may order sedatives to be given.

Instructions to the Parents on Discharge of the Child. The parents must be cautioned to prevent injury to the palate. Since the area may be without sensation, the child may show no sign of pain if the healing area is scraped with some hard object such as a spoon. It may be necessary for the child to wear arm cuffs constantly except when he is bathed or when his parents give him passive exercise and allow him to move his arms freely. At such times they must guard against his putting his hand into his mouth.* Sucking and blowing movements bring a strain upon the wound. If the parents see that he is amusing himself in this way, they should play with him and divert his attention with a toy.

Upper respiratory tract infection increases his discomfort. He should be kept from infection by

---

*The mother can make arm cuffs out of rolled cardboard and tie them in place with string. Care must be taken that the restraints do not rub the skin in the axilla.

isolating him from anyone who has a sore throat or a cold.

Complications. These children may have recurring attacks of otitis media (see page 399) with resulting loss of hearing. The mother should report any indications of otitis to the physician. Excessive dental decay may accompany cleft palate. The mother should be taught the correct method of brushing the child's teeth so that she can keep them clean when the physician says that it is safe for her to use a brush. Later she will teach the child the correct technique. The mother should also be told of the need for dental supervision of the child. The teeth must receive special attention if an appliance is to be fitted. If displacement of the maxillary arches and malposition of the teeth occur, orthodontic correction may be necessary.

Prognosis. The prognosis is fair, but depends upon the extent of the deformity at birth. A speech defect may still exist after surgical correction of the palatal defect or after insertion of a speech appliance. Speech therapy should be given if the defect persists.

Circulatory System

HYPOGLYCEMIA

Incidence, Etiology, Clinical Manifestations, Treatment, and Prognosis. In recent years not only infants of diabetic mothers but also infants of nondiabetic mothers have been diagnosed as having hypoglycemia. This condition is seen mostly in male infants whose mothers had toxemia. The overall incidence of hypoglycemia is 2 to 3 per 1000 live births. It is higher among

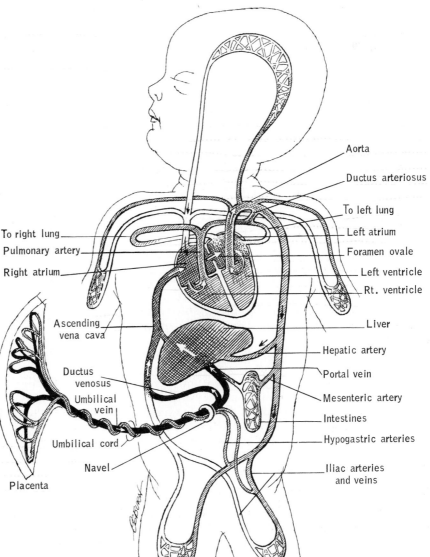

FIGURE 12–3. Diagrammatic illustration of fetal circulation. The degree of oxygen saturation is indicated by the blackness of the vessels.

Aorta

Ductus arteriosus

To left lung

Left atrium

Foramen ovale

Left ventricle

Rt. ventricle

To right lung

Pulmonary artery

Right atrium

Ascending vena cava

Liver

Hepatic artery

Portal vein

Mesenteric artery

Intestines

Hypogastric arteries

Ductus venosus

Umbilical vein

Umbilical cord

Navel

Iliac arteries and veins

Placenta

newborns of low birth weight for gestational age than among normal newborns.

The *cause* of this type of hypoglycemia is thought to be the infant's having inadequate stores of glycogen in the liver before birth, and a very sensitive insulin release mechanism after birth. This may be due to a rare inborn error of enzyme synthesis.

Clinical manifestations may be seen soon after birth and during infancy. These include tremors, convulsions, listlessness, periods of respiratory distress and cyanosis, abnormal cry, and feeding difficulties.

Treatment includes giving glucose solution intravenously until the blood glucose level has been stabilized. ACTH may also be given in an attempt to maintain the blood glucose level within normal range. This condition may recur during infancy.

The *prognosis* for life is good; however, these infants may be impaired intellectually as a result of this condition, because the brain, except under unusual conditions, is able to utilize only glucose.

CONGENITAL HEART DISEASE

Changes Occurring in the Circulatory System at Birth. With the severing of the umbilical cord and expansion of the lungs there is increased pressure from the incoming blood in the left side of the heart. This eventually causes the foramen ovale to close. In fetal life much of the pulmonary arterial blood passed through the ductus arteriosus to the aorta, because the pressure was greater on the right side, owing to pulmonary resistance to blood flow. At birth the muscles in the wall of the ductus arteriosus constrict, although complete closure may not occur until the second or third month of life. The heart has less work after than before birth, since placental circulation has been replaced by that of extrauterine life.

Etiology, Incidence, Diagnosis, and Types of Cardiac Defects. The heart is completely developed in the first eight weeks of intrauterine life. One or several anomalies may result from maldevelopment of the heart or great blood vessels leading to and from the heart, with the result that the infant is born with congenital heart disease. Such defects may be hereditary, e.g., those caused by defects inherent in the genes or germ plasm. They may be caused by vitamin deficiency or viral infection such as rubella (German measles) occurring during the first trimester of pregnancy. Fetal intracardiac disease is possible. After birth there may be failure of obliteration of the ductus arteriosus or foramen ovale. The teratogenic effects of radiation and drugs are well known. The thalidomide syndrome may include congenital heart disease as one of its manifestations. Newborn infants of mothers on anticonvulsant therapy may also have this condition.

Cardiovascular malformations occur in about 8 per 1000 births. They cause about half the deaths due to congenital defects in the first year of life.

The *diagnosis* is based on the health history of the mother during pregnancy and on the characteristics of congenital heart disease in the infant. Early diagnosis is essential so that treatment, if possible, can be given. The nurse can play an important role in early diagnosis by observing all newborn infants. Observations should include the infant's vital signs, especially the rate and nature of his pulse (tachycardia) and respirations (dyspnea), his skin color (cyanosis), his weight gain or loss, his feeding behavior, his cry, and his general level of activity. The nurse should also observe newborns for excessive perspiration which may lead to miliaria (see p. 163) and for abnormal fatigue and irritability. The signs and symptoms of congenital heart disease include abnormal murmurs, and in later months or years generalized poor development and clubbing of the fingers and toes.

The diagnosis is confirmed when radiographic examination shows divergence of the heart from its normal position and contour. Such an examination repeated at intervals of several months may reflect continued changes in the structure of the heart as the infant's body develops. Examination with barium given by mouth may show indentation of the esophagus by the aorta and other vessels.

By *electrocardiography* variations in the normal electrical potentials of the different parts of the heart can be noted. The electrocardiogram shows the condition of the muscular structure of the heart.

For *angiocardiography* the child is usually anesthetized, and radiopaque material is injected into a peripheral vein; its course through the heart chambers appears on a succession of x-ray pictures taken at rapid intervals. Abnormal communications between the chambers of the heart are also evident. *Selective angiocardiography* is being used more than venous angiocardiography because it is a more satisfactory method of determining specific heart defects. The radiopaque catheter is moved into the heart chambers themselves, and the contrast material is injected into specific areas. The structure of the heart can thus be more clearly seen by roentgenogram.

Cine-angiocardiography is the process by which motion pictures are taken of successive images seen on the fluoroscopic screen. Because of improved techniques angiocardiography and cine-angiocardiography are now considered by many to be part of the cardiac catheterization technique.

Cardiac catheterization is done under either general or local anesthesia. If local anesthesia is used, the infant should be under heavy sedation. The physician who catheterizes the heart must be supported by a well trained team of assistants accustomed to working with him. A small radiopaque catheter is inserted into a large vein of an arm or leg and pushed into the right atrium. With the tip of the catheter the physician can examine the heart minutely for anomalies of structure, often found in the right ventricle and the pulmonary artery. He is able to determine the blood pressure within the heart itself, and samples of blood can be taken to determine the exact degree of oxygenation. After cardiac catheterization the nurse should observe the child for hemorrhage from the site of insertion of the catheter, for his color, for the rate and regularity of the vital signs, and especially for the presence of peripheral pulses, reporting any irregularities. This procedure is not without risk; hence the nurse should be careful how reassurance is given to parents of a very ill child who is having this study done. Parents should also understand that this is a diagnostic test and not a corrective surgical procedure.

Echocardiography is a noninvasive procedure that works like sonar to produce an accurate picture of the inside of an infant's heart. For certain infants, use of the echocardiograph may eliminate the need for further diagnostic tests.

Congenital defects in cardiac structure may be classified in two groups: (1) *acyanotic* heart disease, in which the infant is not cyanotic, and (2) *cyanotic* heart disease, in which the infant shows varying degrees of cyanosis.

A detailed approach to the treatment and care of children having congenital cardiac disease will be discussed under the condition tetralogy of Fallot.

ACYANOTIC TYPES OF CONGENITAL HEART DISEASE

In acyanotic congenital heart disease either there is no abnormal communication between the pulmonary and systemic circulations or, if such a connection is present, the pressure forces the blood from the arterial to the venous side. The peripheral blood is therefore oxygenated as in a normal infant, and cyanosis does not result. If the anomaly is such that venous blood eventually mixes with arterial blood when the heart weakens, cyanosis may result.

COARCTATION OF THE AORTA

Types, Clinical Manifestations, and Diagnosis. There are two types of coarctation. In the *infantile* or *preductal* type there is a constriction between the subclavian artery and the ductus (Fig. 12–4). This condition can be corrected by surgery. The *postductal* type consists of a constriction at or distal to the ductus arteriosus. The symptoms in this type depend upon the degree of coarctation. Blood pressure is higher than normal in the upper part of the body, resulting in headache, dizziness, epistaxis, and later cerebrovascular accidents. Blood pressure in the legs is relatively low, resulting in absence or diminution of of femoral pulses.

The *diagnosis* is based on the reversal of normal blood pressure relations in the arms and legs and is confirmed by x-ray study. In older children, roentgenograms may show enlargement of the heart which was not evident during routine examination of the newborn, together with notching of the ribs due to enlarged collateral vessels.

Treatment and Prognosis. Surgical repair consists in cutting out the narrowed portion of the aorta, with anastomosis of the ends. In some cases a graft of transplanted aorta is inserted where the narrowing is so extensive that removal with anastomosis is not practical.

If the infant's condition is such that the physician believes that he can live until he has reached the preferred age for correction, operation is postponed until the child is from 8 to 15 years old. Operation should be performed at this age rather than during early childhood because the segment used as a graft will not grow as does the aorta. The shorter the time after operation before maximum growth of the child is reached, the less is the danger from difference in the rate of growth between the graft and the main structure of the aorta.

The *prognosis* is dependent upon the success of surgery. If the operation is successful, life expectancy should be normal.

AORTIC STENOSIS

In this condition blood cannot pass freely from the left ventricle to the systemic circulation because of stenosis of the aorta. The degree of constriction varies from so mild that the child is asymptomatic to so severe that it causes dizziness and can lead to sudden death. This normally can be surgically corrected (using the open-heart technique) by dividing the stenotic valves of the aorta or dilating the constricting aortic ring.

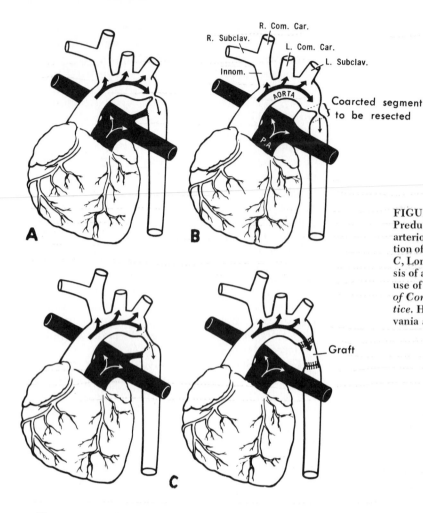

FIGURE 12–4. Coarctation of the aorta. *A*, Preductal coarctation of the aorta with the ductus arteriosus open or closed. *B*, Postductal coarctation of the aorta with the ductus arteriosus closed. *C*, Longer areas of constriction, where anastomosis of aortic segments is not feasible, require the use of a graft to bridge the gap. (From *Diagnosis of Congenital Cardiac Defects in General Practice.* Heart Association of Southeastern Pennsylvania and American Heart Association.)

PATENT DUCTUS ARTERIOSUS

Etiology, Incidence, and Clinical Manifestations. The ductus arteriosus (Fig. 12–5) normally closes shortly after birth. If the ductus remains open, blood under pressure from the aorta is shunted into the pulmonary artery, since the blood pressure in that vessel is less than in the systemic circulation. As a result, oxygenated blood recirculates through the pulmonary circulation. This may lead to increased vascular pressure in the pulmonary tree and diminished blood flow in the aorta.

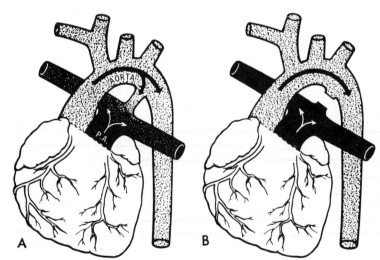

FIGURE 12–5. Patent ductus arteriosus. *A*, Relation of ductus arteriosus to great vessels. *B*, Ductus arteriosus transected (as shown here) or ligated. (From *Diagnosis of Congenital Cardiac Defects in General Practice.* Heart Association of Southeastern Pennsylvania and American Heart Association.)

Patent ductus arteriosus is one of the most common cardiac anomalies. It is frequently the only cardiovascular anomaly, but may occur in conjunction with other cardiac defects. It is almost twice as frequent in female infants as in male infants.

The symptoms of patent ductus arteriosus in the infant are usually so slight that the condition is not discovered at the initial examination, but is found during a routine examination later. As the child grows older and is more active, the characteristic symptoms appear. He is likely to show progressively greater dyspnea on exertion. Examination may reveal a malfunctioning left ventricle or congestive heart failure (see p. 292). Progression of the lesion is due to the strain upon the heart of pumping blood which passes a second time through the pulmonary circulation while at the same time supplying adequate systemic circulation for an active infant or child. It is easy to prevent overexertion in an infant, but far more difficult to limit the activities of a growing child without overprotecting him and building up the very qualities which may make a handicapped child disliked by his playmates.

If the ductus is large and much blood from the aorta is shunted into the pulmonary circulation, there may be retardation in growth.

Physical signs include increased pulse pressure, sometimes felt when taking the radial pulse. Signs of a large pulse pressure, including water-hammer pulsations and arterial Corrigan pulsations in the neck, are produced. After exertion the low diastolic pressure may fall further. A cardiac thrill in the second left interspace is usually present; this may radiate over a larger area of the chest. There is the classic machinery murmur, continuous from systole into diastole. The electrocardiogram usually shows no abnormality, but roentgenograms show a vigorously pulsating pulmonary artery and increased pulmonary vascularity. The heart may be normal in size, but is more likely to be enlarged.

Diagnosis, Treatment, and Prognosis. The diagnosis is made on the clinical symptoms and signs of a machinery murmur of the heart and a low diastolic blood pressure. Cardiac catheterization (see p. 281) shows a normal or increased pressure, roentgenograms show the shadow of the pulmonary artery to be larger than normal, and angiocardiography shows the ductus arteriosus.

The treatment is surgical, by division and ligation of the ductus, preferably when the child is about three years of age. If necessary, however, operation may be done earlier if the child is in serious difficulty. After the repair the heart becomes normal in size, murmurs disappear, and there is a general improvement in the child's condition.

With modern surgery done by a skilled specialist, the prognosis is excellent. The surgical mortality rate in the uncomplicated condition during childhood is extremely low. Without repair subacute bacterial endocarditis or cardiac failure may develop as the child leads the less sheltered and more strenuous life of the school-age group.

DEXTROCARDIA

In this condition the heart is in the right side of the chest. This may occur with or without reversal of the other organs (situs inversus). Although the heart may be normal, associated anomalies often complicate the condition. Treatment then depends on the underlying defect. If no other anomalies are present, no treatment is necessary, and the prognosis is excellent.

DOUBLE AORTIC ARCH

Infants and children with this defect may have respiratory symptoms or dysphagia, or both. These symptoms, beginning in the first year of life, arise from compression by the branches of the aorta on the trachea or esophagus, or both. This is due to the persistence of embryologic vascular precursors of the aorta and stem branches. The infant, in an effort to find relief, will hold his head in an extended position. The diagnosis is made on x-ray examination, which shows constriction of the esophagus by the aorta. Constriction or deviation of the trachea can also be seen. The treatment is surgical, and the prognosis is excellent.

INTERATRIAL SEPTAL DEFECT

This is one of the more common congenital anomalies. The incidence is higher among girls than among boys. There is a communication between the left and right atria. Since oxygenated blood in the left atrium is under the higher pressure, it is forced through the defect in the separating wall into the right atrium. Such an arterial-venous shunt does not produce cyanosis. If, however, the right atrial pressure becomes increased as a result of pulmonary stenosis or pulmonary hypertension, venous blood may be shunted across the patent foramen ovale and into the left atrium, with resultant cyanosis. Once the blood flow has reversed, surgical repair is difficult. When cardiac failure occurs, cyanosis is also evident.

The diagnosis is made on the basis of the roentgenogram and the electrocardiogram. The heart is enlarged, and there is congestion of the pulmonary circulation. On auscultation a loud murmur is heard in the area of the pulmonary artery.

The *treatment* is surgical repair of the defect. The edges of the opening are pulled together and sutured, or the opening is occluded by a plastic patch placed over the aperture. This operation may be done with the aid of the heart-lung machine. The size and location of this defect are important. Some patients do not require surgical correction and can live normal lives.

INTERVENTRICULAR SEPTAL DEFECT

This anomaly consists of an opening between the right and left ventricles. The condition may be slight or severe.

In the *mild form* the defect is low or in the muscular portion of the septum and is so slight that only a small amount of oxygenated blood passes from the left to the right ventricle. It is a common congenital defect. The heart is seldom enlarged, and the only clinical finding is a murmur accompanying the heart beat. The treatment is by surgical closure of the opening. Since the ventricle must be entered, the heart-lung machine must be used in order to enable the surgeon to reach the defect. In this condition subacute bacterial endocarditis may develop at the site.

In the *severe form* there is a large opening in the upper or membranous portion of the septum, and oxygenated blood in greater amount passes from the left to the right ventricle. The result may be pulmonary hypertension. The symptoms include cardiac failure, a tendency to pneumonia, and retarded growth. The diagnosis is made from the roentgenogram and the electrocardiogram. The treatment is by surgical closure of the defect. The heart is opened, and the edges of the septal opening are drawn together, or a plastic sponge patch is placed over the opening. This kind of operation involves the use of a cardiac bypass by means of the heart-lung machine. Without operation the prognosis is poor.

If pulmonary hypertension with a ventricular septal defect becomes so severe that the predominant shunting of blood is reversed, the child is cyanotic and the condition is inoperable. This phenomenon is known as the *Eisenmenger complex*. A technique currently used to prevent the development of the Eisenmenger complex is banding of the pulmonary artery. This is usually done on the infant with a ventricular septal defect prior to the development of irreversible pulmonary hypertension. A piece of Teflon tape is sutured circumferentially around the pulmonary artery to decrease the pulmonary blood flow.

PULMONIC STENOSIS

Although these constrictions may exist in newborn infants, symptoms may not be present for several years. Cardiac failure may occur, and the prognosis is generally poor. Treatment is surgical, by valvulotomy or mechanical dilatation of the passage through which blood must pass from the heart into the respective vessels.

CYANOTIC TYPES OF CONGENITAL HEART DISEASE

The common cause of the congenital cyanotic types of heart disease is a communication between the pulmonary and systemic circulations through which venous (unoxygenated) blood enters the systemic circulatory system. Cyanosis may be seen at birth or may not be apparent until later, commonly during the first year of life; it tends to increase as the child grows older.

Polycythemia (an increase in the number of red blood cells per milliliter of blood) results from the need of the tissues of the body for an adequate supply of oxygen. The symptoms vary in degree with the extent and nature of the anomaly. In general, there is clubbing of the fingers and toes, retarded growth, and shortness of breath on exertion. If the blood, thickened by an abnormal concentration of red blood cells, clots in the blood vessels, further complications result. It is important to give adequate fluids to these infants to reduce the possibility of clot formation.

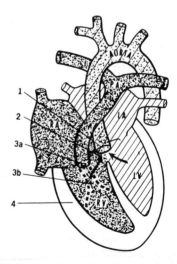

FIGURE 12–6. Tetralogy of Fallot. Anomalies include (*1*) overriding aorta, (*2*) high ventricular septal defect, (*3a*) valvular pulmonary stenosis, and (*3b*) infundibular pulmonary stenosis, and (*4*) hypertrophy of right ventricle. (From *Diagnosis of Congenital Cardiac Defects in General Practice.* Heart Association of Southeastern Pennsylvania and American Heart Association.)

TETRALOGY OF FALLOT

Incidence and Pathology. This is the most common type of cyanotic congenital heart disease which is compatible with continued existence into childhood. Pathologically, there are four associated anomalies: (1) funnel-like or valvular pulmonic stenosis, (2) interventricular septal defect, (3) dextroposition of the aorta, and (4) hypertrophy of the right ventricle.

Pulmonary stenosis restricts the flow of blood from the heart to the lungs; the right ventricle hypertrophies and facilitates venoarterial shunting. Dextroposition of the aorta also leads to venoarterial shunting. Since cyanosis is dependent upon the absolute concentration of reduced hemoglobin in the capillary circulation, it is evident that in the systemic circulation, containing a rich admixture of venous blood from the start, this value is almost invariably surpassed, and cyanosis is thus clinically manifest.

Clinical Manifestations and Diagnosis. The arterial blood is not normally saturated with oxygen, and as a result the skin is not the natural pink, but has a bluish tint. The fingers and toes become clubbed and have a purplish hue, since the capillaries are distended with poorly oxygenated blood. The condition worsens during even the first year of life. The body's reaction to the inadequate supply of oxygen is an increased production of red blood cells (polycythemia). The child's general condition is poor. Growth is retarded; exercise causes severe dyspnea. In order to relieve the strain of standing, he favors the *squatting position.* This behavior has diagnostic value.

Anoxic "blue" spells or *paroxysmal dyspneic attacks* may occur during the first 24 months of life and last for a few minutes to hours. During the spell the infant becomes more cyanotic, dyspneic, and restless. He gasps for breath and may have a weak or a loud cry. Short episodes may be followed by sleep, but prolonged spells may lead to unconsciousness, convulsions, hemiparesis, or death. These spells may occur with no warning, although they may follow feeding, an emotional upset, or defecation. These infants have hypoxia and metabolic acidosis.

Treatment of these paroxysmal dyspneic attacks includes placing the child on his abdomen in the knee-chest position, releasing restrictive clothing, administering oxygen, and giving morphine. In severe attacks sodium bicarbonate may be administered intravenously to return the pH of the blood to normal. Since acidosis may recur, repeated measurements of the blood pH should be done.

Although the child may be of normal intelligence, the poor supply of oxygen to the brain

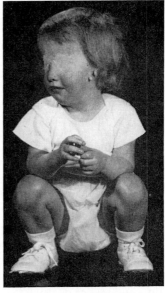

FIGURE 12–7. Tetralogy of Fallot. Child squatting. (Nadas: *Pediatric Cardiology.* 2nd ed.)

is likely to produce mental retardation, syncope, or convulsions. The child is apt to be emotionally unstable, irritable, and overdependent upon others. His parents, concerned over his physical condition, are likely to avoid discipline to prevent frustration, since they do not want him to become excited or cry. The child realizes that if he cries he will get his way.

The *diagnosis,* based on the symptoms, is confirmed by radiographic examination of the heart, which shows the enlarged chamber on the right side, the decrease in size of the pulmonary artery, and reduced blood flow through the lungs. The unusual shape of the heart has led to its being called the wooden shoe or *boot-shaped heart (coeur en sabot).* The child should be allowed to handle the diagnostic equipment before examination so that the procedures will be less frightening to him. If he is to take barium, the addition of chocolate to the mixture may make it look and taste like the chocolate milk to which he is accustomed. Laboratory findings show the decreased oxygen saturation of the blood, and exercise tolerance tests prove the child's tendency to extreme dyspnea.

Instructions to the Parents. On the parents rest the responsibility for giving the child good care until the time when operation is to be performed.

The parents may become anxious about the possibility of attacks of paroxysmal dyspnea occurring after they have taken the infant home. To reduce anxiety about his care they should spend time with him in the hospital learning how to feed him, how to conserve his energy in a normal routine, and how to provide care during an attack. The nurse at this time can identify specific problems and can plan with the parents how these problems can be resolved. The nurse can also assist in planning follow-up care after the infant has gone home.

Both physical and mental hygiene must be considered. Provision for normal growth and development is essential, but requires constant good judgment so that the child is neither overprotected nor allowed an independence in which he overtaxes his weakened heart. This program is easy to carry out while the infant is still so young that he accepts parental plans for all his activities of daily living.

During this period the infant becomes accustomed to limitation of activities without overdependence on others. He also learns to trust others to give him the help he needs. Overfatigue should be avoided, and certainly he should never be urged to exertion beyond his tolerance. It may be difficult for the entire family and those adults he contacts outside the family circle to carry out such a regimen with a young child whose handicap is not visible, but it is in this period that the foundation for a strong, happy personality is made.

The child should never acquire the feeling of undue importance which is apt to develop in one who feels that his heart condition makes him a special child who must always have his own way and be given first consideration. The influence upon the other children in the family must be considered. Although his needs may be more important than their pleasures, his pleasure is not to be gained at the expense of their constant inconvenience. He should lead as normal a life as is compatible with his welfare, but learn to accept frustration and the inevitable restrictions which his condition imposes on his activity and social relations. He cannot do all that other children do.

The physician will discuss with the parents the influence of cyanosis upon the child's intelligence. If he is retarded, the parents are apt to attribute the retardation entirely to his physical condition, forgetting that low intelligence may be due to a number of factors. To lead as normal a life as is compatible with his condition is the best way to realize to the full his potential mental capacity. The experiences which develop the normal child, but in which he cannot participate, should be replaced by experiences of comparable learning value. His toys should be light and easily handled. He should learn that a ball rolls, though he may not be able to creep after it for any length of time. He may not creep up a flight of stairs, but he may go up one or two steps. He should be carried about more than the average child is and should be allowed to handle everything within the nursery. Picture books are valuable. He can pat-a-cake to slow music. Overexcitement is as taxing for him as overactivity. As he grows older he must learn not to compete in games requiring agility and strength. As a rule, competitive games are too exciting for these children. Even the very little child can learn that fun does not necessarily come through getting ahead of someone else.

If the parents prove able to give good care and to observe signs of a worsening in his condition, he may not need frequent visits to the physician. But if they are unable to judge his condition and to give him the care he requires, he should be seen regularly by the family physician or pediatrician. If he has been referred from the hospital to the children's clinic, he should be under the observation of the pediatrician there and should be visited by the community or public health nurse. He should be seen by his physician before even minor surgery is done. The danger is not only from the anesthetic—often minor surgery would not require the use of an anesthetic—but also from the possibility of infection. Prophylactic antibiotic medication may be indicated.

Treatment, Responsibilities of the Nurse, and Prognosis. The *treatment* is surgical, and may be corrective or merely palliative. Palliative surgery does not correct the deformity. Without operation the life expectancy of the child is almost always shortened. Operation is postponed as a rule until the child is three years of age or even older, but if his condition is critical, operation may be done upon the infant.

PREOPERATIVE CARE AND TREATMENT. The inexperienced nurse, after learning the detailed care of children having one type of congenital cardiac anomaly, should be able to transfer this knowledge to the care of children having other kinds of cardiac surgery.

SURGICAL CORRECTION. One of several types of surgical correction may be done on children having tetralogy of Fallot. In closed-heart surgery (palliative surgery) there are the Blalock-Taussig operation, the Potts operation, and the Brock procedure.

Closed-Heart (Palliative) Surgery. In the *Blalock-Taussig operation* a branch of the aorta is anastomosed to the pulmonary artery. In children under two years the innominate artery is used; in children over two years the subclavian artery is preferred. The result of this operation is that a connection is made between a systemic artery and the pulmonary artery, thus increasing

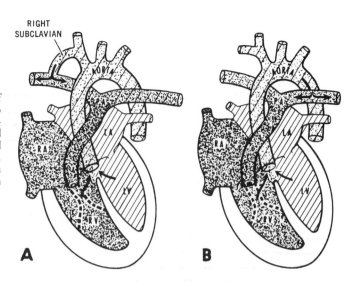

FIGURE 12–8. Tetralogy of Fallot. *A*, Volume of blood to lungs increased by joining right subclavian to right pulmonary artery (end-to-side anastomosis – Blalock procedure). *B*, Volume of blood to lungs increased by creating stoma between left pulmonary artery and aorta (side-to-side anastomosis – Potts procedure). (From *Diagnosis of Congenital Cardiac Defects in General Practice.* Heart Association of Southeastern Pennsylvania and American Heart Association.)

the blood flow to the lungs, improving exercise tolerance, and reducing cyanosis.

In the *Potts operation* a direct connection is made between the aorta and the pulmonary artery. The same results are achieved as with the Blalock-Taussig operation.

Neither of these operations is corrective. The operative risk with anastomotic procedures is low. Although the immediate clinical improvement is good, some incapacity may remain.

The *Brock procedure* is a direct operation for the pulmonary stenosis and is done through a right ventricular approach. This operation increases the flow of blood to the lungs, but does not correct the ventricular septal defect.

Open-Heart (Corrective) Surgery. Techniques developed to permit open-heart surgery include the following: (1) hypothermia. Hypothermia may be induced by the use of water-cooled mattresses of varied sizes, ice bags, or gastric lavage with iced liquid. The degree of cooling is dependent on the surgeon; however, maximum benefit with minimal danger can be achieved when the child's temperature is reduced to between 86 and 90° F. (30 to 32.2° C.). Some surgeons may request temperatures lower than these. Vigorous shivering must be prevented if this therapy is to be effective. The use of hypothermia is not without danger, and therefore the child so treated must be watched carefully by a team of experts for complications. In hypothermia the body temperature is lowered so that the metabolic rate is reduced. Reduction of the metabolic rate decreases the need for oxygen in the tissues of the body and so lessens the danger of anoxia. (2) Heart-lung machine. The heart-lung machine is interposed in the circulation, allowing blood flow to bypass the heart and lungs. Gaseous exchange occurs within the apparatus. The venous blood passes through two

catheters in the venae cavae to the machine, and the oxygenated blood is returned to the large arteries for systemic distribution. Since the machine carries on the functions of the heart and lungs, the surgeon is able to open the bloodless heart and repair the defective structures.

Open-heart surgery would seem to be best for the child having tetralogy of Fallot, since it affords relief of the pulmonary stenosis and closure of the ventricular septal defect. The operative risk is higher than that of the anastomotic

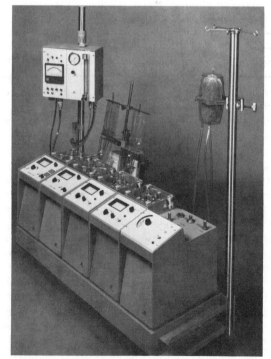

FIGURE 12–9. Modular pump and oxygenator. (Courtesy of Artificial Organs Division, Travenol Laboratories, Inc.)

procedures. The results are spectacular, however, in successful cases.

During these operations a thoracotomy tube is usually inserted into the pleural space and attached to a gravity suction bottle placed lower than the chest. The pleural space is thus kept free from drainage. If the fluid were permitted to remain in the chest, the lungs would not be able to expand completely, and the fluid might become infected, resulting in empyema. The fluid in the tube oscillates with respiration, indicating that there is an airtight seal at the site where the thoracotomy tube is inserted.

Emotional Preparation for Surgery. Not only should the parents explain the procedure of admission to the hospital to the child, but they should also have explained to him in simple language the nature of his illness and the treatment to be done. If the child has siblings, they should also understand the child's condition so that they do not become jealous of the extra attention which of necessity he must receive.

The child admitted for cardiac surgery is usually somewhat insecure and unstable in spite of the preparation he may have had. He has probably observed the anxiety of his parents over his physical health, and he in turn becomes anxious about his own welfare. Since the majority of parents, realizing that crying by a child who has a cyanotic type of cardiac defect results in frightening cyanosis, they have minimized frustration for him so that he has not been able to learn to stand the usual frustrations of childhood. In addition, he has to minimize his physical activity, not only by not playing actively with other children, but also by becoming overdependent on his parents for meeting the normal physical needs which other preschool children handle themselves. Although some children will revolt in the face of such restrictions and exercise to the limit of their tolerance, most of them submit because of the attention they receive. These children may lack self-confidence, may feel inferior to their peers, and may withdraw from other children, yet may be demanding and aggressive with their parents and other adults.

In order to plan care for the child, the nurse through discussion with the parents should determine how much preparation for his operation the child has actually had, what experiences he has had in the past which would prepare him for this experience, and how he usually relates to adults other than his parents. On the basis of this information the nurse should be able to determine an approach to make the child feel more secure.

The parents usually regard surgery with an ambivalent attitude: of exaggerated fear because of the relative newness of cardiac surgery and of hope for the child's recovery. The parents need someone with whom they can discuss their hopes and fears and from whom they can get easily understood answers to their questions.

Both the child and his parents need emotional preparation for the tests and operation which the child is to undergo. Any diagnostic procedures which may be done, such as the exercise tolerance test, roentgen examination and fluoroscopic examination, oxygen saturation tests, electrocardiography, cardiac catheterization, and angiocardiography, should be explained when appropriate. The child and his parents may be taken to the operating suite and to the intensive care unit so that they will become familiar with the physical setting, the brightness of the lights, and the increased activities as well as the appearance of the gowned and masked personnel. Details of the operation such as how the anesthetic will be given, where the incision will be, and what sort of tubes will be inserted can be discussed in a nonthreatening manner. The purposes of therapy should be discussed. The equipment to be used should be shown *gradually,* such as that used for the administration of parenteral fluids, tracheal suctioning, drainage apparatus, intermittent positive-pressure apparatus, oxygen tent, and the inevitable injections. The child should be placed temporarily in the oxygen tent in order to accustom him to the experience. He should also be taught how to use the intermittent positive-pressure respirator if this is to be used postoperatively. This machine is frightening to many children because of the gust of air it emits and because the face mask makes them fear that they will suffocate when it is used. Suggestions for gaining the child's cooperation include a demonstration of the use of the mask by the nurse, and making a game of the treatment by pretending that the mask is of the same kind as astronauts use. Prior to operation the child should also be oriented to other aspects of the nursing care which he will receive: the taking of vital signs, taking of fluids, necessity for turning, coughing, and deep breathing. If the child understands that he can tell the nurse how he feels about the care he receives, he will be free to express his emotions easily postoperatively. The nurse should stress the fact that the child and his parents may forget some of the aspects of the care described. Then when they do forget something postoperatively, they know that the nurse expected this to happen, and they feel confident in asking for assistance.

Throughout this preparatory phase the nurse should make every effort to assure both parents and child that a nurse will be with the child constantly so that he will not be alone. The nurse, through an accepting manner, can also convey the fact that emotions which either parents or child feel should be expressed, whether of fear, anger, or dependency, and that they will be accepted. Regression, which is a usual response to stress, should also be recognized and accepted.

The nurse at this time can also help the parents to understand that their child will need a great deal of attention and that activity around his bed is not an indication that his condition has become worse.

Physical Preparation for Surgery. Since many children are not in optimum physical condition preoperatively, adequate diet and fluid intake, rest, and controlled exercise are needed. Adequate hydration is especially needed if the child has a compensatory polycythemia (see p. 284). If cardiac failure is present, absolute rest, digitalis, diuretics, and oxygen therapy may be needed (see p. 292). Antibiotics are given prophylactically before operation. The child must be protected from patients and personnel having infections. Fluids are given parenterally before and during the operation to prevent dehydration.

The child's skin is shaved and prepared on the evening before operation. A cleansing enema may be ordered. Sedation is given so that he may get as much rest as possible. He is weighed on the same scale that will be used to weigh him after the operation. By comparing the difference in weights it can be determined whether the child received too much or too little parenteral fluid during the operation. The child should be permitted to take his favorite toy or security object with him to the operating room.

The nurse who cares for the child preoperatively should care for him postoperatively so that changes in his condition can be easily noted and the child may feel secure. During operation the nurse must give the parents support by answering their questions and preparing them for the child's appearance after operation so that their anxiety may be reduced. It may be wise to show the parents a child who has had the same operation their child will have so that they are not overwhelmed by his appearance.

During the operation the nurse should also check on the equipment needed for the child's care, including a cardiac arrest tray, and make certain that it is assembled in readiness for his return. Immediately postoperatively the nurse should become familiar with the operative procedure which was done, the medications and parenteral fluids which he received, and the orders which were written for his postoperative care.

Postoperative Care. On admission to the intensive care unit or recovery room the child is given oxygen immediately. Each catheter in his chest must be carefully checked and attached to the suction machine. The vital signs must be taken, and if there is any indication for the use of a cardioscope, it is attached to the patient. The heart rate and rhythm and the electrocardiogram can thus be observed constantly. The administration of intravenous fluids must be checked and regulated carefully, perhaps using a special regulating pump if one is available. If a tracheotomy has been done, the child should receive the care described on page 541.

When the child reawakens from his anesthesia, he should be told that his operation is over. The child may be confused, restless, drowsy, and in obvious pain. A narcotic may be given on the physician's order. The child may be unaware of his environment and the medical and nursing personnel around him, and be concerned only with himself and his pain.

The vital signs are taken each hour, or more often if necessary. The nurse must take the temperature rectally, since the cool atmosphere (68 to 72° F. or 20 to 22.2° C.) in the oxygen tent may affect an oral reading. If fever is present, rectal administration of aspirin, tepid water sponges, ice bags to the groin and axillae, an ice-water mattress or a hypothermia blanket may be ordered. Fever must be reduced, since this increases both the rate of blood flow through the body and the metabolic rate.

The nurse should check the rate and depth of respirations and note whether chest expansion on both sides is equal. If the child has noisy or rapid breathing indicating an accumulation of mucus in his respiratory passages, the nurse should use suction to remove the secretions. The nurse should also note the difference in rate, quality, rhythm, and volume between the radial and pedal pulses. The blood pressure should be taken with the other signs. If the pulse rate becomes irregular and the blood pressure drops, the physician should be notified immediately, because these signs may indicate impending cardiac arrest. If the pulse and respiratory rates rise, if the blood pressure drops, and if the child is very thirsty, the physician should also be notified, because these are signs of hemorrhage. The cardiac monitor in use in many institutions is of great value in the care of these patients. The color of the child's nailbeds and skin and the condition of his skin, whether moist, dry, cool, or warm, should also be observed and recorded. If cyanosis and respiratory embarrassment are severe, a tracheotomy may be necessary (see p. 541) if it was not done previously.

Intravenous fluid therapy is given by cutdown

in the child's arm or leg. The administration of fluids must be carefully recorded (see p. 412) so that they are not given too rapidly. It must be remembered that a change in the child's position or from a resting to a crying state may change the rate of flow. The nurse must also check on whether the tubing is kinked or obstructed in any way and whether fluids are infiltrating into the tissues.

Fluid intake by mouth is usually limited during the postoperative period in order to prevent added strain on the heart due to overloading the circulation. A Levin tube may be inserted to prevent gastric dilatation. Mouth care and frequent rinsing of the mouth with water will alleviate some of the thirst the child experiences. Since both the parents and the child may be disturbed by this limitation of fluids, the nurse should assure them that thirst is a normal reaction and explain the reasons why unlimited fluids may not be given.

If the child is unable to void within eight to 12 hours after operation, a Foley catheter may be inserted. The specific gravity, color, and amount of urine should be recorded.

Immediately after operation the one or two chest catheters are connected to underwater suction. These tubes remove fluid which has collected in the pleural cavity. By observation of the drainage, bleeding can be readily detected. If the physician so orders, the tubes are "milked" in the direction of the drainage bottles to assure that they are patent and free of blood clots, and to facilitate drainage. Some physicians "milk" the tubes toward the patient in order to avoid pulling a clot into the tube and causing obstruction. The nurse must check to see that the tubing is not kinked and the connections with glass connectors are tight, that the tubing is long enough to permit the child to move, that there is no rapid increase in the amount of drainage, and that the fluid in the tube fluctuates with each respiration. *The nurse must remember that the drainage bottle and the water bottle must remain below the bed level,* i.e., below the bottom level of the child's thorax. To ensure that they are not elevated, they should be attached to the floor or placed in a holder which cannot be moved easily. Chest drainage must be observed accurately for color, amount, and consistency. The time is marked on the vertical tape on the side of the drainage bottle every hour so that the amount of drainage can be easily seen.

The nurse must realize that if air leaks into the pleural cavity, a pneumothorax may occur with restlessness, apprehension, cyanosis, sudden sharp chest pain around the area of insertion of the catheter, tachycardia, and dyspnea. If these signs and symptoms occur, the nurse should clamp the chest catheters as close as possible to the child's chest and immediately call the physician.

Postoperatively chest x-rays are taken so that the lungs can be visualized. Because the oxygen is turned off while the x-ray picture is being taken, the child may become very apprehensive. His vital signs should be taken, and he should be reassured of his progress.

Although the child was oriented preoperatively to the necessity for coughing and deep breathing, he may have difficulty cooperating postoperatively when such activity produces pain. The nurse can help him by supporting his chest, especially over the incision area, with both hands. The child should be praised for any effort he makes to cooperate. Since coughing is important in order to prevent retention of secretions and atelectasis and to promote lung expansion, the physician should be notified if the child cannot cooperate.

The use of the intermittent positive-pressure respirator may be helpful in encouraging the child to cough. The nurse should observe his color, respiratory and pulse rates, and his general response during this treatment. The nurse should remember that coughing is very painful and tiring for the postoperative cardiac patient. Therefore, if a narcotic is ordered, it should be given prior to this therapy. Either hot or cold steam vapor may be used to prevent drying of mucus in the respiratory tract with resulting greater ease in expectoration.

The child's position should be changed every hour to promote good circulation and ventilation of the lungs, and to maintain good range of motion of the extremities. The child's body should be adequately supported with pillows if he cannot maintain his position. As soon as possible the child should be encouraged to help move himself. After moving the child, some increase in drainage from the chest tube may be noted.

The nurse should make the following additional observations: the absence of pedal pulses, or presence of cyanosis or coldness of the legs indicating a possible embolus in an artery, distention of the veins in the neck, nausea, abdominal distention, or bleeding or infection of the incision or the intravenous site. Any twitching of the extremities, signs of congestive heart failure (see p. 292), petechiae, or complaints of dizziness, restlessness, or headache should be reported. The nurse is responsible also for assisting the physician in the removal of the chest tubes, and, if one was used, the pacemaker wire from the heart muscle.

Rest is of primary importance; therefore the

nurse should plan the child's care so that the patient has as much rest as possible. Narcotics or sedation should be given as prescribed; however, careful nursing care can relieve the child's fear and thus lessen his need for medication. Depending on the severity of the surgical procedure, the child may be permitted out of bed in a wheelchair within a few days after the chest tubes have been removed.

As mentioned previously, the child who has had cardiac surgery may regress to an infantile state. He may cry, become more demanding, or require more physical contact than he did before the operation. The nurse, recognizing his need, provides care suitable for an infant in order to help the child rebuild his sense of trust in others. The nurse must, as the child's condition improves, help him once again gain control of his situation, to regain the autonomy he has temporarily lost. As convalescence progresses the child feels increasingly well and is ready to assume more responsibility for his own care and to play with other children.

Before the child is discharged from the hospital the physician, parents, social worker, community or public health nurse, and the hospital nurse must work out together a plan of care for the child. The child is usually more active, aggressive, and independent than he was preoperatively. These changes may frighten the parents because they fear that he will overexert himself. Also the mother may have difficulty in giving up the pleasure she gained from caring for a sick dependent child prior to surgery. The nurse can help them by pointing out his obvious enjoyment of new activities and his new freedom from dyspnea and fatigue. The mother must be helped to find satisfactions to replace those of caring for an ill child.

Complications and Prognosis. The *prognosis* is generally good after operation and depends on the quality of the surgical correction. If complete correction is achieved by the open-heart technique, the prognosis is excellent.

PULMONIC STENOSIS WITH PATENT FORAMEN OVALE

In this condition venous blood from the right atrium is shunted to the left atrium with resulting cyanosis. Clinically, the condition may simulate the tetralogy of Fallot. Treatment is by surgical valvulotomy of the stenosed pulmonary valve with or without closure of the septal defect. The prognosis after repair is good.

TRANSPOSITION OF THE GREAT VESSELS

Incidence and Pathology. The incidence of this condition is almost as great as that of tetral-ogy of Fallot. In this anomaly the aorta has its origin in the right ventricle, and the pulmonary artery has its origin in the left ventricle. Hence the aorta carries unoxygenated blood to the systemic circulation, and the pulmonary circuit carries oxygenated blood back to the lungs. An infant can survive initially only if an associated defect such as an atrial or ventricular septal defect or a patent ductus arteriosus is present.

Clinical Manifestations and Diagnosis. An infant born with transposition of the great vessels may not be too cyanotic at birth because of the patent ductus arteriosus, but may become extremely cyanotic soon after birth. Such an infant is likely to be dyspneic and unable to suck. Later growth is severely retarded, and there is clubbing of the fingers and toes. The *diagnosis* is made by cardiac catheterization and related roentgenograms. Laboratory findings include an elevated hematocrit value and polycythemia.

Treatment and Prognosis. As a result of recent research into the treatment of this condition, more infants live today than ever before. Palliative *treatment* is aimed at achieving adequate mixing of oxygenated and unoxygenated blood. This can be accomplished by removing the atrial septum and can enable the infant to survive until corrective surgery can be done.

One palliative nonsurgical technique currently used is the Rashkind-Miller procedure. This involves passing a double-lumen cardiac catheter via the femoral vein to the right atrium and across the foramen ovale into the left atrium. One lumen runs through to the end of the catheter, and the second runs to a balloon just behind the tip of the catheter. When in the left atrium, the balloon is inflated with a dilute solution of radiopaque contrast material so that proper size can be determined. When the balloon is pulled back to the right atrium, it leaves a septal defect, allowing the unoxygenated and oxygenated blood to mix. This procedure is repeated until the filled balloon can be drawn without resistance from the left to the right atrium. After this procedure the infant's color improves, and heart failure, if present, disappears.

If a child having a ventricular septal defect develops pulmonary hypertension, a pulmonary artery banding may be necessary to prevent irreversible damage.

The second and corrective stage of this therapy is done when the child is between 18 months and three or four years of age with the aid of the cardiopulmonary bypass machine. This complex Mustard procedure is one by which total correction of the transposition can be obtained. An intra-atrial baffle of pericardium is made that directs systemic venous blood to the left ventricle and pulmonary venous blood to the right ventricle. Through this procedure the systemic venous blood is pumped by the left ventricle to the lungs. The pulmonary venous blood is pumped by the right ventricle to the aorta. Any existing ventricular septal defect or patent ductus arteriosus is closed. If present, the banding is removed from the pulmonary artery.

The *prognosis* of infants having transposition of the great vessels has been greatly improved since the discovery of these procedures. If the condition is recognized early enough, most children can be ultimately cured.

Responsibilities of the Nurse. The nurse caring for the newborn in the nursery should recognize the infant having this condition, although cyanosis may not be too severe because of the patent ductus arteriosus. The nurse should, however, recognize the increasing dyspnea and the infant's inability to suck. These newborns have increased secretions, though not as profuse as the child having atresia of the esophagus. The sooner newborns having this condition have their palliative operation, the better are their chances for life. It is therefore extremely important for the nurse to report observations as soon as they are made.

There are other rare cardiac anomalies, nearly all of which are surgically correctible at present.

Congestive Heart Failure

A heart that has been under physiologic strain or is actually damaged is said to be compensated when it has adjusted to its handicap. If it cannot adjust, i.e., does not maintain an adequate circulation, it is said to be decompensated or in failure.

Clinical Manifestations. The nurse should be aware of the fact that infants, like adults, having severe cardiac problems may suffer congestive heart failure suddenly, or it may be predictable. The first indication of this problem occurs when the mother or nurse notices that the infant does not feed as well as he did. He may tire easily when he sucks, but cries soon after the feeding. If permitted to rest after every ounce or two of formula, he may have a sufficient intake of nutrients. If he does not, he may fail to gain weight.

Other indications of congestive heart failure may be a weak cry, cyanotic or pale color, edema, rapid heart beat, and rapid respirations which may be accompanied by an expiratory grunt or wheeze, suprasternal retractions, and flaring of the alae nasi. On x-ray films the heart may appear enlarged.

The signs and symptoms of congestive heart failure in older children are similar to those in adults. These include anorexia, fatigue, dyspnea, cough, cyanosis, abdominal pain, enlarged liver, and dependent edema. Cardiomegaly is present.

Treatment and Responsibilities of the Nurse. *Therapy* for an infant or a child having congestive heart failure includes the use of digitalis, diuretics if edema is present, and oxygen. The aldosterone antagonist spironolactone (Aldactone) may be used in the management of heart failure to supplement diuretic therapy.

Treatment begins with digitalization. The types of digitalis used most frequently are digoxin and digitoxin for slow digitalization and lanatoside C (Cedilanid) for rapid digitalization. Digoxin is used because it is available in liquid form and is easy to control. It is important when giving digitalis preparations to check carefully the dose to be administered. The dose is estimated according to body weight and is adjusted according to the child's response. The use of maintenance doses of digitalis is necessary unless the cause for the failure is completely corrected. If it is continued, the amount given must be adjusted upward as the child gains weight. Toxicity may occur and is especially to be feared, since there are few warning symptoms other than bradycardia, anorexia, vomiting or diarrhea prior to ventricular fibrillation, or heart block itself occurs. Treatment consists in stopping the medication until signs of toxicity are gone and then resuming the drug, if necessary at a lower dosage.

The infant or child in congestive heart failure needs more rest than normal. He should have small frequent feedings higher than average in calories. Some physicians recommend for the infant the use of a pacifier to keep him happy and content.

An infant having this condition is most comfortable in a sitting position when held over his mother's or nurse's shoulder. A special cardiac chair (see Fig. 12–10) may be utilized especially to advantage if the infant has rapid labored respirations.

When pulmonary edema is present, any superimposed infection should be treated appropriately. Salt may need to be restricted in the diet in order to prevent the retention of excess fluid. A low-salt formula such as Lonalac may be ordered. A salt substitute may be used to make the diet more palatable. As the child recovers he may be graduated to a moderately low sodium preparation. Morphine sulfate may be given for its beneficial effect in pulmonary edema.

Further observations the nurse should make,

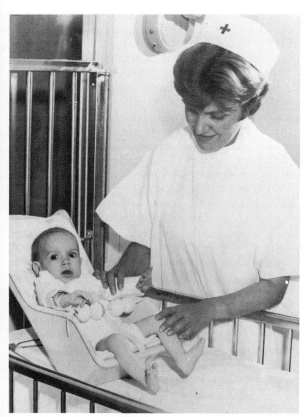

FIGURE 12–10.   Children, particularly babies with pulmonary congestion, seem more comfortable in the sitting position. (Courtesy of Saint Justine's Hospital, Montreal, Canada.)

in addition to edema and other signs and symptoms, include the daily weight of the infant or child, and the amount of intake and output of fluids.

Any condition complicating congestive heart failure such as infection, anemia, or electrolyte imbalance should be promptly treated.

Before the child is discharged from the hospital the parents not only must be taught the kinds and amounts of medication to be given and the side effects to be observed, and the type of diet and possibly low-salt foods which are available, but must also be aware of observations they should make such as for edema, and illnesses to prevent such as infection. The decision as to whether the parents of a child who is being discharged from the hospital on digoxin should be taught to take the apical pulse at home or whether only the physician or nurse should carry out this procedure depends on the individual parents, and whether it would increase their anxiety to such an extent that it would reflect on the total care given the child. The physician and the nurse should also help to plan for the continued care of their child.

SUMMARY OF THE RESPONSIBILITIES OF THE NURSE IN CONGENITAL HEART DISEASE

The nursing care of infants and children with congenital anomalies of the cardiovascular system is extremely important. What is done for the child is, of course, dependent upon the treatment outlined by the physician and involves difficult procedures and nursing skills.

The nurse should become familiar with the parents' reaction to being told that their child has a congenital cardiac condition, and should learn how to reassure them without minimizing the danger of the defective heart. The nurse should teach the parents how to care for the child in the interval between his leaving the newborn nursery and his re-entrance into the hospital for operation. What has been said about the care of the child with the tetralogy of Fallot may also be applied to other types of congenital heart disease.

In summary, the general objectives of nursing care for the child having congenital heart disease include prevention of physical and emotional fatigue, provision of adequate fluid and nutritional intake, prevention of infection, and helping the parents and their child to cope with the problems that arise before and after cardiac surgery.

GENETIC COUNSELING

As mentioned before, the incidence of congenital heart disease is 8 per 1000 newborns. The incidence in live-born siblings of affected children is between 14 and 22 per 1000. It can be explained to parents that if they have one child with congenital heart disease, the recurrence rate is about two per cent. The incidence of cardiovascular malformation in children of parents who have been treated for congenital heart disease is only 3 per cent.

Diagnostic Examinations for Neurologic Conditions

There are several congenital anomalies that can occur in the central nervous system as well as those injuries, tumors, or other conditions that occur as the child matures (see p. 473 and p. 791). Parents are understandably anxious concerning their child's condition when such abnormalities exist. Not only do they need as much reassurance and support as possible, but they also need explanations concerning the diagnostic examinations required.

Generalizations concerning parent education were discussed previously in this text (see p.

90). The student should remember that preparation of the parents and child, if he is old enough to understand verbal explanations, includes an accurate description of what is going to happen: the purpose of the procedure, the preparation required, the equipment to be used, whether there is a need for sedation or parenteral fluids, how much discomfort there will probably be, and the care of the child after the procedure is completed. As a result of such explanation, the need for hospitalization or outpatient care is simple to explain.

During the procedure the nurse observes the child carefully and gives verbal and nonverbal assurance to him. After the procedure the nurse continues to observe the child for any reaction that may occur. The nurse and the parents can help the child express his feelings about the procedure either verbally or through play.

Diagnostic procedures done for conditions involving the central nervous system include the following:

Lumbar puncture is done to determine the level of intracranial pressure, to reduce intracranial pressure, to identify hemorrhage in the central system, to do a culture and sensitivity, or to test for the cell count, globulins, protein, or sugar in the cerebral spinal fluid. This procedure is not done on a child having a space-occupying lesion that produces increased intracranial pressure, in the presence of an untreated clotting defect, or through a skin site that is infected.

Prior to this procedure, local anesthesia may be given at the injection site. An infant may be given a pacifier to suck or an older child may need to be sedated.

The nurse's most important responsibility in assisting with the procedure is firm restraint of the patient in such a way that his back is rounded and parallel with the side of the treatment table in order to open the lumbar space. In the neonate the sitting position may be preferable. To restrain an older infant or young child in the lateral recumbent position, the nurse may place one hand behind his neck or one arm around his neck and grasp his legs, while placing the other arm around the buttocks and grasping his hands. By putting pressure on the neck and legs the nurse can bend the child's body as necessary. An older child can be restrained with a sheet folded lengthwise and applied in a figure of eight around the neck and under the buttocks in the same way as can an uncooperative adult.

In this procedure a needle is inserted into the lumbar area (L 3-4 is the preferred site) of the subarachnoid space. A manometer is attached to the needle to determine the cerebrospinal fluid pressure. A Queckenstedt test is performed. The cerebrospinal fluid is collected in tubes that are accurately labeled and numbered.

After this procedure the child is kept flat in bed until rested. This procedure may be done on an outpatient basis or when the child is hospitalized.

Subdural tap or ventricular tap is performed for diagnosing subdural effusions or hematoma, to diagnose ventricular hemorrhage, to obtain a culture or an analysis of the cerebrospinal fluid, to relieve increased intracranial pressure, or to instill medication. If the child has unexplained excessive head growth, a bulging anterior fontanel, and a positive transillumination of the skull, a subdural tap is performed.

The hair is shaved over the injection site (with the permission of the parents) and strict aseptic precautions are observed throughout the procedure. The nurse's additional responsibilities in assisting with a tap are to apply a mummy restraint to an infant or small uncooperative child if necessary and to hold his head securely in the correct position.

The needle is inserted into the subdural space or the ventricle through the open anterior fontanel or during a craniotomy. The tubes of fluid are numbered in the order they are collected and labeled. They are taped to the foot of the child's crib or elsewhere in his unit. Following the procedure the child should be kept flat in bed and observed for changes in intracranial pressure or leakage of cerebrospinal fluid from the site where the needle was inserted. With the physician's approval the child may be placed in a semi-erect position in an infant seat to reduce prolonged leakage from the puncture site.

The child is usually hospitalized for this procedure.

Electroencephalography (EEG) examines the electrical activity of the cerebral cortex to determine nonfunctioning areas or areas producing seizures. During the maturation process brain waves slowly become more regular and increase in frequency. This procedure may also be done to follow the progress of a child after a central nervous system infection or a head injury.

The parents and the child may be informed that multiple electrodes will be attached to various areas of the head with adhesive and readings taken when the child is awake, asleep, and hyperventilating. The hair should be clean so that the oil will not interfere with the electrode readings. No stimulants or depressants may be given on the day the EEG is to be done. Medications are given as ordered. After the examination the electrode paste may be washed from the hair and the patient encouraged to rest.

An electroencephalogram may be done on either an inpatient or an outpatient basis.

Skull series or x-rays are done to study the bony framework of the skull for identifying fractures, intracranial calcifications, separation of the cranial sutures due to elevated cerebral spinal fluid pressure, or developmental disorders such as premature (craniosynostosis, see p. 479) or postmature closing of the fontanels. If old fractures are present, the diagnosis of battered child syndrome (see p. 481) must be ruled out.

This study involves taking x-rays of the head. The parents and child are informed that while the study is not painful, the x-ray equipment may be frightening. Any foreign objects such as glasses or barettes are removed from the head, face, or mouth.

This diagnostic procedure may be done on an outpatient basis.

Brain scan is performed to identify certain focal brain lesions. Test material tends to accumulate where the blood-brain barrier is defective as in tumors or surrounding brain abscesses. With subdural hematoma and encephalitis, positive uptake of material is also seen.

Parents and child are told that a radioactive material will be given intravenously and that radioactivity will be counted over the skull after a fixed time interval.

This test may be done on an outpatient basis.

Pneumoencephalography is done by injecting air or oxygen into the subarachnoid space from a lumbar or cisternal site. The child is heavily sedated or anesthetized, and the procedure is done with the child in a sitting position. X-rays of the head are taken. The purpose of this procedure is to identify structural abnormalities of the brain: the size, shape, symmetry, and position of the ventricular system and subarachnoid spaces, in order to determine the presence of tumor, mass, or abnormality of the brain and meninges. The child is permitted nothing by mouth for the number of hours ordered prior to this procedure.

After the pneumoencephalogram the child is kept flat in bed and is observed for indications of a headache, irritability, fever, vomiting, and increased meningeal irritation or increased intracranial pressure. The vital signs are taken frequently, and fluids are given as ordered.

The pneumoencephalogram is done while the child is hospitalized.

Ventriculography is performed to visualize the ventricles of the brain to determine the presence of a lesion, mass, or hydrocephalus. General anesthesia is given, and air is injected into the ventricles. X-rays are taken during and after the procedure. The child is permitted nothing orally prior to this procedure. Medications are ordered by the physician.

After the procedure the child is kept at rest flat in bed. Vital signs are taken, and medication is given for headache as ordered. The child should be observed for changes in intracranial pressure following this procedure. Fluids are encouraged to replace the cerebrospinal fluid that was withdrawn during the procedure.

Hospitalization is necessary for this procedure.

Myelography visualizes the subarachnoid space of the spinal cord in order to identify any interference in the flow of cerebrospinal fluid: any tumor, dislocation, fracture, or foreign body that may be present. Before the procedure the child is given nothing by mouth and is sedated as ordered. After an iodinized contrast medium or air is injected into the subarachnoid space by way of a lumbar or cisternal puncture, x-rays are taken. After successful x-ray of the child, the foreign material is removed.

When the test is completed the child is kept flat and at rest in bed in a comfortable position. Observations are made for any alterations in intracranial pressure and for temperature deviations from normal. The child is encouraged to increase his fluid intake.

Hospitalization is preferred for this procedure.

Cerebral angiography is carried out to identify a tumor or other lesion, a cerebral vascular anomaly, or a hemorrhage.

Before the procedure the child is given nothing by mouth as ordered and is given general anesthesia. A radiopaque substance is injected into an artery, usually the femoral, or a vein, possibly by surgically exposing the vessel to be injected, or into a dural sinus. After the x-rays are taken the procedure is completed.

The child should be kept comfortable and observed for complications such as changes in intracranial pressure, decreased level of consciousness, seizures, transient hemiplegia, loss of vision, petechiae, or a thrombus or hemorrhage at the site of injection.

The child should be hospitalized as an inpatient.

Computerized axial tomography (CAT) works on the same principle as conventional radiology, but with much greater precision. Film is not used with CAT. Electronic tubes called photomultipliers that are much more sensitive to changes in the intensity of tissue than the usual x-ray are utilized. The CAT can determine differences of density of tissue of less than 1 per cent. The child lies on a couch, and the portion of the head to be studied is placed between the scanner sending out the x-ray beam and the photomultiplier, which picks it up. The device is rotated slowly 180 degrees around the child's head, with readings taken at each degree. A picture of the tissue appears on the television screen. A photograph is taken of the picture for a permanent record that can be interpreted by the physician. This is a rapidly performed procedure. The child receives radiation exposure no greater than from conventional x-ray devices. The CAT scan is expensive to perform, but is still cheaper than the more complicated and dangerous methods of angiography and pneumoencephalography, which require hospitalization and in some cases exploratory surgery for diagnosis.

Benign conditions that can be diagnosed through the use of CAT scans are abscesses, cysts, arteriovenous malformations, subdural hematomas, and aneurysms. Malignant lesions can be localized. The physician can determine with this diagnostic tool whether a substance visualized is air, cerebrospinal fluid, brain tissue, blood, bone, or calcifications.

There is no preparation of the child for this procedure in terms of altered diet or medication. While an explanation should be given to both parents and child that this procedure is painless and safe, the child especially must understand the necessity for immobility while this test is done. Because he must lie perfectly still, a young child often requires sedation prior to the procedure.

The CAT scan may be done on an inpatient or an outpatient basis.

Central Nervous System

SPINA BIFIDA

Incidence and Types. Spina bifida is a malformation of the spine in which the posterior portion of the laminae of the vertebrae fails to close. It may occur in almost any area of the spine but is most common in the lumbosacral region. It is the most common developmental defect of the central nervous system, occurring in about one out of 1000 newborn infants.

Three types are discussed: (1) spina bifida occulta, in which the spinal cord and meinges are normal, the defect being only of the vertebrae; (2) meningocele, in which the meninges protrude through the opening in the spinal canal; and (3) meningomyelocele, in which both the spinal cord and the meninges protrude through the defect in the bony rings of the spinal canal. Meningomyelocele is the most serious type.

SPINA BIFIDA OCCULTA

Clinical Manifestations, Diagnosis, and Treatment. The majority of patients have no symp-

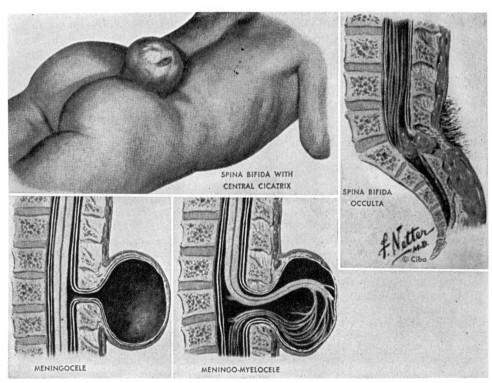

SPINA BIFIDA WITH CENTRAL CICATRIX

SPINA BIFIDA OCCULTA

MENINGOCELE

MENINGO-MYELOCELE

FIGURE 12–11. Diagrammatic representation of types of spina bifida, meningocele and meningomyelocele. (Copyright, The Ciba Collection of Medical Illustrations, by Frank H. Netter, M.D.)

toms. Some may have a dimple in the skin or a growth of hair over the malformed vertebra. If the condition is suspected from these signs or upon physical examination, a roentgenogram will rule out or confirm the diagnosis. There is no need for treatment unless neurologic symptoms indicate that the defect is greater than was thought. If there is a possibility that the spinal cord may be involved in the defect, surgical treatment is indicated.

MENINGOCELE

Clinical Manifestation, Diagnosis, Treatment, and Prognosis. On examination the newborn infant is found to have a defect in the spinal column large enough for the meninges to protrude through the opening. The defect is usually in the center line. There is generally no evidence of weakness of the legs, for the infant stretches and kicks in a normal manner, or of lack of sphincter control, though this is difficult to ascertain in the newborn.

The *prognosis* is excellent. Surgical correction is done on these defects. Hydrocephalus may be an associated finding or may be aggravated after operation for a meningocele (see p. 301).

MENINGOMYELOCELE

Clinical Manifestations, Diagnosis, Treatment, and Prognosis. In this condition an imperfectly developed segment of the spinal cord, as well as the meninges, protrudes through the spina bifida. The round, fluctuating bulge resembles that of the meningocele and is usually located in the lumbosacral region. There may be a minimal weakness to a complete flaccid paralysis of the legs and absence of sensation in the feet. The feet may be clubbed. Bowel and bladder functioning require careful evaluation.

The objectives of *treatment* and nursing care are to prevent infection of the sac and to help preserve whatever function is present orthopedically and urologically.

Operation removes a cosmetically unacceptable deformity, prevents infection, and in many instances improves the neurologic deficit, since traction is removed from the nerve pathways. Currently, correction is done as early as possible, preferably in the first 24 to 48 hours of life. The reason for this early correction is that some newborns appear to have a degree of motor ability in the legs at birth which decreases soon after birth. Early operation is advocated therefore to prevent further deterioration of neural tissue. If the defect is extensive, there may not be enough skin to cover it. Skin flaps may be made first and the infant returned to the operating room later to have the defect covered. When

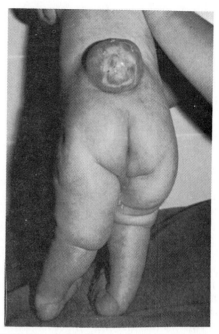

FIGURE 12–12. Epithelialized lumbosacral meningomyelocele in a three-month-old twin. Paralyses of the legs, bilateral neurogenic clubfeet, and permanent dripping of urine are evident. Among nine siblings, there is another case of meningomyelocele. (From Moll, H.: *Atlas of Pediatric Diseases.* Philadelphia, W. B. Saunders Co., 1976.)

skin flap rotations are made, skin grafts are necessary to cover the areas from which the skin was taken.

Usually clinically silent, the *Arnold-Chiari syndrome* is a congenital malformation of the occipitocervical region, with displacement of the cerebellar tonsils and adjacent structures into a funnel-shaped enlargement of the upper cervical canal and swelling and displacement of the medulla against the upper portion of the spinal cord. The defect originates between the sixteenth and twentieth weeks of fetal life. This syndrome may occur in children having lumbosacral spina bifida with meningomyelocele. The medulla and part of the cerebellum are pulled into the foramen magnum because the cord is attached at the site of the defect in the spine. The result may be an acute obstruction to the flow of cerebrospinal fluid; hence hydrocephalus may follow repair of a meningomyelocele.

The *symptoms* are the result of complete or partial block of the flow of cerebrospinal fluid. In infants clinical manifestations include a running nose (sometimes confused with an upper respiratory tract infection) and crowing respirations. The nurse must observe these manifestations because immediate relief of pressure is indicated. The nurse may also be requested to measure the occipital-frontal head circumference daily to determine the rapidity of enlargement of the skull. In older children, manifestations include stiff neck, headache, and dizziness. When the child is old enough to walk or talk, his gait is unsteady, and his speech impaired.

Surgery is the only known *treatment* for the Arnold-Chiari syndrome. (See p. 303 for the surgical procedures used in the treatment of hydrocephalus.)

RESPONSIBILITIES OF THE NURSE IN MENINGOCELE AND MENINGOMYELOCELE

Responsibilities of the Nurse Preoperatively. Until the operation is performed, the newborn should be kept flat on his abdomen with a single layer of sterile petrolatum gauze or a Telfa pad over the lesion. No diaper should be applied. The object of care is to prevent breaking the meningocele sac; therefore no pressure is to be put upon it.

Prompt surgical closure of the skin defect, preferably within 24 to 48 hours after birth, is done to prevent meningeal irritation. If for some reason the neurosurgeon prefers to wait to operate on the lesion, preoperative nursing care is that of a normal infant so far as it can be given while protecting the sac from pressure, injury, or infection. To decrease the danger of infection of the area from urine and feces, the genitalia and buttocks must be kept scrupulously clean. The infant should not be diapered if the meningocele is in the lower portion of the spine. The infant is placed in bed, and a meningocele apron is applied. This is done by taping an oblong piece of plastic sheeting below the defect. The larger portion of the piece of plastic should be in the direction of the child's head. Either Scotch tape or masking tape should be used to hold it in place. The piece of plastic should then be folded back on itself and taped again to the skin so that it covers the buttocks and shields the defect from feces. It is customary in some hospitals to place the infant on a Bradford frame with the cover divided so that urine and stool may pass between the sections of the frame.

USE OF A BRADFORD FRAME. The frame is covered as follows:

Canvas covers the head and foot areas of the frame, and foam rubber is placed between the covers. The open area between the covered head and foot sections of the frame is provided for the purpose of drainage of urine and feces away from the body. The covers are stretched tightly over the frame to prevent sagging from the weight of the infant's body. Plastic covers are placed over the top and bottom sections of the divided canvas frame cover. A sheet is put tightly over each section of the frame. The frame is then placed on blocks to elevate it slightly from the bed.

Since the infant is incontinent, sheets of plastic are draped over the top and bottom edges of the opening in the frame cover to permit urine and feces to drain into a bedpan placed below the opening. Folded diapers are placed over the plastic and under the infant so that the plastic does not irritate the skin.

Parents can be taught to construct a Bradford frame for use in the home. A plastic-covered mattress can be shaped appropriately and placed on the frame.

Fixation in the correct position is important. Ankle restraints, using a clove hitch restraint, are applied. The child is not to be placed on his back, since such position would cause pressure on the sac. If the surgeon permits, the child should be supported in the side position with a rolled blanket or pillow behind the head and the buttocks. The pillow or blanket behind the but-

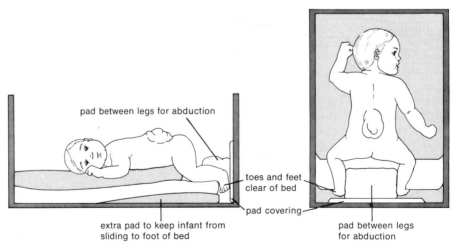

FIGURE 12–13. Positioning of infants with myelomeningocele. The infant is positioned so that there is minimal pressure on the defect and on the feet and toes. This is managed by placing a pad between the legs. To prevent the infant from slipping to the end of the bed, an extra pad is placed beneath the mattress.

tocks must be protected from fecal staining by a plastic cover. If the infant is unable to move his legs, foam rubber pads covered with soft cloth may be placed between the legs to prevent pressure on the skin of the knees and ankles. The infant's position should be checked and changed slightly at least every hour.

To prevent deformity of the feet when the infant is placed on his abdomen, the ankles should be supported with foam rubber pads so that the toes do not rest upon the bed. To prevent injury from rubbing the skin of the elbows, face, and knees, a mild ointment such as A & D ointment or zinc oxide may be used. To prevent chafing of the knees, ankles, toes, and sides of the heels, should the infant move his legs back and forth on the sheet, it is a good plan to use long stockings, but since he has no diaper to which they may be pinned, it is difficult to keep them on his legs.

To change the frame covers or bed, the child may be placed on his abdomen or side in a baby carriage. If the physician permits, the nurse, aide, or mother may hold the child to prevent complications arising from constant lying on the mattress or frame.

Antibiotics may be used if infection is suspected.

In addition to the danger of infection of the sac, the bladder of an infant having a meningomyelocele may also become infected. According to the urologist's evaluation, the infant's bladder may need to be Crédéd if the sphincter is tight and urine is retained. The nurse, or the parents when the child is at home, is responsible for emptying the infant's bladder every two hours during the day and once at night. Pressure should be applied firmly but gently, beginning in the umbilical area and slowly progressing under the symphysis pubis and toward the anus. The parents should be helped to learn this procedure as early as possible. They should practice under supervision until feeling secure. As the child grows, his urine may be expressed less frequently. If he has normal intelligence, by the time he is three or four years of age he should be able to assume part of the responsibility for doing this procedure himself. If evidence of urinary infection occurs, cultures should be done to determine the appropriate antibiotic to be used.

The infant may be transferred directly from the nursery to the pediatric unit. If he is taken home before his readmission to the hospital for operation, his parents will care for him. They can make a substitute for the Bradford frame, and cover it as described above. They can carry out the essential features of nursing care and

will have more time to hold the infant than do hospital personnel. Both parents should be shown how to hold him without causing pressure upon the sac.

The infant should be held for his feedings, if the physician permits. He may be held in the normal feeding position with the nurse's elbow rotated to avoid touching the sac. If the sac is large, he can be held on the shoulder, his mother's or the nurse's hands supporting him above and below the sac, while a second person, standing behind, holds the bottle to his mouth. He cannot be bubbled like the normal infant, but the feeding should be stopped and the nipple withdrawn from his mouth several times during the feeding so that he may rest and air be expelled. If the lesion is in the lumbosacral area, he may be gently rubbed between the shoulders; this has a soothing effect and may aid in expulsion of air. These infants can also be fed lying on their side on the nurse's or mother's lap.

Contamination of the sac can be prevented by covering it with sterile gauze or a sterile towel when the infant is removed from bed.

If the physician believes that the infant should not be removed from the frame or bed for feeding, the restraints may be loosened and the infant turned slightly on the side. The nurse or mother should elevate his head with one hand when feeding him. The mother or nurse can offer substitute pleasure for that of being held for his feeding, such as stroking his skin or singing to him.

One of the most essential functions of the nurse is observation and accurate reporting of the behavior of these infants, as well as of signs and symptoms directly connected with their condition. The nurse records activity of the legs and the degree of continence, whether there is constant or intermittent dribbling, noting whether there is retention of urine or fecal impaction. All the vital signs should be taken and recorded with extreme care.

Responsibilities of the Nurse Postoperatively. The goal of surgical treatment is closure of the surface defect while preserving all functioning nervous tissue.

The nurse is responsible for observing and reporting all signs and symptoms of the infant's condition. Temperature, pulse, and respiration must be noted frequently. Symptoms of shock must be anticipated and an incubator be in readiness for use. If an incubator is not available, a heat cradle may be placed over the infant. Since he may have respiratory difficulty, oxygen should be kept near his bed. Abdominal distention caused by paralytic ileus or distention of the bladder follows most spinal cord surgery and should be reported immediately.

The physician may request that the circumference of the infant's head be measured frequently in order to determine whether hydrocephalus follows repair of the meningomyelocele.

The surgical dressing should be kept clean and dry by the use of a meningocele apron.

Casts applied to the child's legs should be positioned properly and handled carefully (see p. 323).

Nutrition is important. Postoperatively, some surgeons prefer to have the infant fed in as natural a position as possible, while others prefer to have him fed in bed until the operative site is completely healed. If the infant is fed in the prone position in bed, his head should be slightly elevated either with the nurse's hand or by elevating the top end of the frame if one is used. The nipple should be withdrawn several times during the feeding to allow the infant to rest and to facilitate expulsion of air. Gavage feeding may be necessary (see p. 196).

All the foregoing suggestions for postoperative care are subject, of course, to the physician's orders.

Postoperative Habilitation. Orthopedic and urologic physicians should be consulted during the infant's first admission for evaluation. *Habilitation* of the child is necessary after operation. Functional improvement of the legs and bowel and bladder function will require a long time and diligent care. Habilitation emphasizes constructive use of the normal parts of the body and minimizes the disabilities, making the child as self-helpful as possible in the activities of daily living. It also implies anticipation on the part of the nurse or mother of the child's need for various observations and experiences in living in order to prevent sensory deprivation and to expand his world. Although the child is to be taught activities which render him less dependent on others, he must also learn to accept help which normal children do not need. The adult must make an attempt to help the child keep up with the appropriate growth and development sequence for his age.

The parents will need help to learn and to carry out the following aspects of care of the child. Incontinence after infancy creates social problems. It may be helpful for the nurse to review with the parents the process of toilet training a normal child (see p. 495). The child should be taken to the toilet at the time he usually has a bowel movement. A suppository may be used until he establishes regularity. The child may need a special diet to avoid constipation. If he can achieve regularity of stool, he will

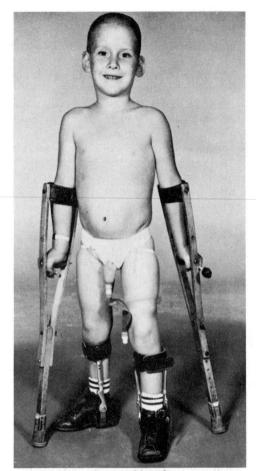

FIGURE 12–14. Hill Pediatric Male Urinal (Davol).

be more socially acceptable. Regularity of urination is of even more importance. Mechanical means for making pressure on the urethra may be used to prevent incontinence. If he cannot urinate, his bladder will need to be emptied by the Credé method (i.e., pressed upon periodically to expel urine), as it was prior to operation. A child of three or four years can be taught to Credé his own bladder by blowing up a party balloon as he bends over and presses on his bladder. His parents and later the school nurse or teacher can then do Credé for residual urine. A distended bladder must be prevented, since it is more subject to infection. Reflux from a distended bladder may result in hydroureter and hydronephrosis with resulting kidney damage. For all these reasons a schedule of toileting should be instituted.

Follow-up care by a urologist is necessary. Some urologists have attempted by surgical means to form a substitute bladder by transplanting the ureters into the sigmoid colon. Unfortunately, ascending infection often followed this procedure. Another procedure, the uretero-ileal cutaneous ureterostomy (an ileal loop), involves isolating a section of ileum and anastomosing the remaining portions. One end of the isolated segment of ileum is closed and the other end brought to the surface of the abdomen. The ureters are transplanted into this substitute bladder. An ileostomy bag, if fitted carefully over the stoma, receives the urine and prevents leakage. The advantage of this procedure is that it prevents the child from soiling his clothing.

Although his legs may be totally or partially paralyzed, the infant can be taken about in a stroller and later can learn to use a wheelchair and possibly to walk with braces and crutches. If the physician prefers to use braces on the child, currently the belief is that heavy bracing should be used first, gradually reducing their weight as the child grows. The parents will need to be taught the methods of putting on the braces, of providing skin care beneath them, and the care of the braces themselves. The parents can be taught by the nurse or physiotherapist to exercise the child's legs appropriately and how to help him to use his crutches properly, if these are ordered.

Care must be taken to prevent obesity or malnutrition and secondary contractions or other deformities. Any infection that occurs should be promptly treated with antibiotics. If the child is normal mentally, he can become a socially useful member of society.

These children have varied and complex problems. The importance of coordination of the medical and health services required for the total care of these children must be stressed. The nurse is many times in a position to assist with the coordination of such services on a long-term basis in conjunction with other community agencies such as schools.

ENCEPHALOCELE

An encephalocele is a protrusion of brain substance through a congenital defect in the skull. It occurs through a failure of the bones of the fetal skull to unite in the normal manner. It is commonly found in the midline and in the occipital or parietal area, although it may also be found in the frontal bone, the orbit of the eye or in the nose.

Clinical Manifestations, Diagnosis, Treatment, Prognosis, and Responsibilities of the Nurse. The *symptoms* depend upon the degree of involvement of the nervous tissue and upon the location of the defect. The diagnostic evidence is a sac or hernia into which the meninges, cerebrospinal fluid, or cerebral tissue has entered. Roentgenograms show the defect in the skull. Early surgical repair is indicated.

The *prognosis* depends upon the extent and location of the encephalocele. If it ruptures, there is danger of meningitis.

The *nursing care* is that of a normal infant, plus relief of symptoms and extreme caution in handling him. It is essential that no pressure be brought upon the sac and that it be not injured in any way. The infant should also be observed for normal developmental milestones.

HYDROCEPHALUS

Hydrocephalus is due to inadequate absorption of cerebrospinal fluid, with a corresponding increase of fluid under pressure within the intracranial cavity, or to obstruction within the ventricular system. To understand this process it would be well to review the formation, flow, and absorption of cerebrospinal fluid (see Fig. 12–16).

Cerebrospinal fluid is formed by the choroid plexus of the four ventricles and by filtration from capillaries. It passes from the lateral ventricles by way of the foramina of Monro into the

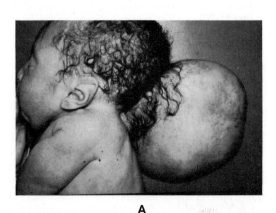

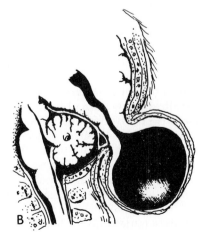

A **B**

FIGURE 12–15.   Encephalocele. *A,* Occipital encephalocele. (Courtesy Luis Schut, M.D.) *B,* Diagrammatic representation. (After Netter.)

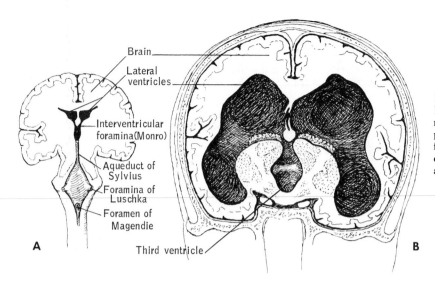

Brain
Lateral
ventricles
Interventricular
foramina(Monro)
Aqueduct of
Sylvius
Foramina of
Luschka
Foramen of
Magendie
Third ventricle

A   B

FIGURE 12–16. Noncommunicating hydrocephalus. *A*, Diagrammatic representation of brain showing sites of possible obstruction of cerebrospinal fluid. *B*, Diagrammatic representation of brain showing dilatation of lateral and third ventricles of brain.

third ventricle. From the third ventricle it flows through the aqueduct of Sylvius into the fourth ventricle, and then into the cisterna of the subarachnoid space by way of the foramina of Luschka and the foramen of Magendie. From there it passes under the base of the brain and up over the convexity into the cortical sulci until it is finally absorbed into the venous sinuses by way of the arachnoid villi. It flows along the tissue spaces of the sheaths of all the cranial and spinal nerves and is taken up by the vascular system. Normally the amount absorbed equals that secreted.

Etiology. Obstruction in the flow of cerebrospinal fluid may be due to one of several causes. There may be congenital maldevelopment of the ventricular foramina, neoplasm may be present, or a fibrous residue of meningitis may occlude the reabsorptive surfaces. Hemorrhage from trauma may cause hydrocephalus in the young infant.

The accumulation of fluid in the ventricles generally enlarges the infant's skull, since the sutures are not closed, and the bones are soft and yielding under pressure. The cranial enlargement tends to decrease the pressure upon the brain.

Treatment should be started as soon as the clinical manifestations are observed, before damage to the brain itself occurs. Several shunting procedures are now in use: e.g., ventriculovenostomy (shunting from the ventricle through the internal jugular vein to the right atrium of the heart), ventriculoperitoneostomy, ventriculoureterostomy, and lumbar subarachnoid peritoneostomy.

The **prognosis** is dependent to a great extent on the promptness of treatment and the kind of operation performed.

COMMUNICATING HYDROCEPHALUS

Etiology. In communicating hydrocephalus there is a normal communication between the ventricles and the subarachnoid space at the base of the brain. There may, however, be adhesions between the meninges at the base of the brain, meningeal hemorrhage, or a congenital defect in the brain, which prevents the absorption of cerebrospinal fluid. Hydrocephalus may occur after a successful operation for meningocele (see p. 297).

Clinical Manifestations, Diagnosis, and Treatment. The obvious *symptom* is an increase in size of the infant's head because of an excessive amount of cerebrospinal fluid. The fluid which is not absorbed in the subarachnoid space accumulates, compressing the brain and distending the cranial cavity. The sutures fail to close, and the bones of the skull become thin.

There is an excess of spinal fluid outside the brain. The convolutions of the brain are flattened and atrophied. Usually, however, the presence of the fluid does not enlarge the head as much as in noncommunicating hydrocephalus, because of the brain atrophy, which increases the space that the fluid may fill without enlargement of the skull. The fontanels are tense and widened. The child tends to be irritable and to have anorexia.

The *diagnosis* is confirmed by puncture of the fontanels, and ventriculography may be used.

The *treatment* is surgical. Sometimes spontaneously a balance may rarely occur in the young child between the secretion of fluid and its absorption. Operation, however, should be performed as early as possible to prevent damage to the brain. Since the difficulty is mostly mechanical, corrective measures are aimed at forming an outlet for the surplus fluid.

Noncommunicating Hydrocephalus

Etiology and Pathology. In noncommunicating hydrocephalus, which is more important than the communicating type, there is a block between the ventricular and subarachnoid systems. Such a block may be partial or complete. It may have begun in the latter months of intrauterine life. Mechanical causes include tumor, hemorrhages, or anomalous development of the pathway. A mechanical block may result from absence of an aqueduct or stenosis or obstruction by exudate or a blood clot. The foramina of Magendie and Luschka may be occluded.

Fluid distends the ventricles. There is a gradual thinning of the brain substance, which is compressed between the distended ventricles and the expanding skull. The bones of the cranium become thin, the fontanels large, and the sutures separated.

Clinical Manifestations and Diagnosis. In the congenital type of noncommunicating hydrocephalus the infant may die *in utero,* or a cesarean section may be done to deliver the child.

After birth an increase in size of the head is noticeable. The fontanels widen instead of narrowing and are tense. Irritability, anorexia, and vomiting occur. The infant becomes increasingly helpless and less able to raise his head. The neck muscles are underdeveloped from lack of use. Affect and normal responses may be diminished. Nystagmus or convergent strabismus may be present. There is possibly some interference with sight. The eyes seem to be pushed downward and protrude slightly. The sclerae are visible above the iris, since the upper lids are retracted by the taut skin over the bulging forehead. The scalp is shiny, and the veins are dilated.

The muscle tone of the extremities is frequently abnormal. As the child's condition deteriorates, his body becomes emaciated, often weighing less than the head. The cry is high-pitched and shrill. Convulsions may occur. These infants have little resistance to infection; therefore the administration of antibiotics may be necessary.

If no contraindications exist, operation is done to prevent further enlargement of the head and to facilitate nursing care of a child with massive enlargement.

Symptoms in hydrocephalus due to infection, e.g., that resulting from meningeal inflammation, develop slowly or are clinically unrecognized. The bones yield to pressure as in the congenital type. The course is progressive.

Diagnostic tests are done to indicate the site of the obstruction. The head circumference is measured daily around its widest diameter to compare its growth with that of the normal child. By ventricular puncture the presence of excess fluid and the approximate thickness of the cortex are determined. *Ventriculograms* or *pneumoencephalograms* using small amounts of air are helpful in establishing a diagnosis.

Treatment and Prognosis. Since the causes of noncommunicating hydrocephalus are mechanical, *treatment* must be surgical.

Modern surgery bypasses the point of obstruction by attempting to shunt the cerebrospinal fluid to another area where it will be absorbed and finally excreted. After a shunting procedure, x-rays are taken to determine whether placement of the shunt is correct.

Probably the most common treatment now in use is a shunt from one lateral ventricle into the circulating blood by way of the internal jugular vein to the right atrium of the heart or the superior vena cava just proximal to it. A Pudenz or Holter valve prevents blood from flowing back into the ventricles, but allows the cerebrospinal fluid, when under pressure, to enter the circulation. Several complications can follow this procedure, such as thrombosis of the jugular vein, obstruction of the valve, or sepsis. The tube must be replaced at intervals with the further possibility of infection.

In the ventriculoperitoneal shunt a tube is run from the ventricle to the peritoneum. An omentectomy is done to prevent blocking of the end of the tube.

In spinal ureterostomy the effectiveness of the tube is not influenced by the child's growth, but when a ventriculoureterostomy is done, longer tubes must be inserted as the child grows. This

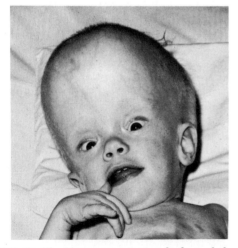

FIGURE 12–17. Noncommunicating hydrocephalus. The infant is helpless and lethargic. Strabismus is present. The "sunset sign" of the eyes is obvious. The scalp veins are dilated. A covered pad of sponge rubber is kept under the infant's head. A blanket roll is kept under his shoulders.

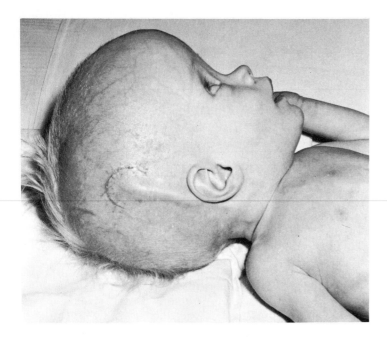

FIGURE 12-18. A hydrocephalic infant on whom was done a ventriculoperitoneal shunt. Note the presence of the tube as it emerges from the skull and passes under the skin of the scalp and the chest.

is why the ventriculoureterostomy is not done more frequently in addition to the fact that in both spinal ureterostomy and ventriculoureterostomy it is necessary to remove one kidney in order to insert the tube into the ureter.

A problem in the management of children having a ureterostomy is the loss of great quantities of salt in the fluid passed through the shunt. Massive sodium depletion may result. Infection reaching the cerebrospinal fluid from the bladder by way of the shunt is combated by the use of antibiotics.

In the Torkildsen operation (ventriculocisternostomy) a tube is run from the lateral ventricle to the cisterna magna.

The *prognosis* in the past was poor, but with

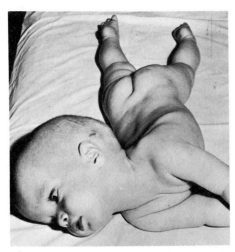

FIGURE 12-19. Opisthotonos resulting from meningitis in a hydrocephalic infant.

newer surgical techniques excellent results have been obtained. If the brain is not seriously malformed at the time of operation, mental function may not be impaired. Motor function is retarded if the child cannot lift his head and move as a child would normally do. In many cases there is neurologic impairment. Death may occur from extreme malnutrition or intercurrent infection.

Responsibilities of the Nurse. The hydrocephalic infant may be admitted to the hospital for diagnosis before operation is undertaken. The nursing care will include assisting with a number of tests. The basic care of the child admitted for diagnosis is that of the child admitted for operation.

PREOPERATIVE CARE. With early diagnosis of the enlarging head, treatment is given before nursing care becomes difficult. The nurse is responsible for observing the degree of irritability and changing vital signs and should report such changes promptly. The nurse must also provide care for the child who exhibits the manifestations of anorexia and vomiting.

The child may be unable to raise or even move his head, brain damage may have delayed his mental development, and malnutrition may have resulted from inadequate food intake and frequent vomiting.

The infant must be kept clean and dry, especially in the area around the creases of the neck where perspiration and vomitus may collect.

To maintain nutrition, the feeding schedule should be arranged to avoid vomiting; i.e., the intervals between feeding should be those ordered by the physician, and all necessary care should be given *before* a feeding to avoid moving the infant after he has been fed. He should be held for his feedings. Since the head is heavy, the nurse should rest one arm upon a pillow or pad placed over the arm of the chair, or upon the mattress of the crib if it is low enough to do so. If the head is very large, the infant cannot be bubbled. The bottle should be taken from his lips several times during the feeding, and his head and shoulders be slightly elevated (if the physician permits) while he is gently rubbed between the shoulders. When he is returned to his crib, he should be placed on his side to prevent aspiration of vomitus.

The infant's position should be changed frequently to prevent hypostatic pneumonia and to lessen the danger of pressure areas. These lesions are likely to appear on the head and ears unless every precaution is taken to prevent them. A pad of lamb's wool or sponge rubber may be placed under his head or a water pillow may be used. A full-length sponge rubber mattress or an alternating pressure mattress is excellent. If pressure areas develop, great care must be taken to prevent infection, which, in the infant's debilitated condition, might result in septicemia.

When the child is lifted from his crib, his head must be carefully supported in order to prevent trauma. In changing his position in bed, the weight of the head should be borne in the palm of the nurse's hand, thereby freeing the other hand to move the body. It is essential that head and body be rotated together, bringing no strain upon the neck. To lift the infant, the nurse leans over the crib, places an arm under his head and adjusts his head against the nurse's chest. The infant is then raised, with the nurse's other arm supporting his body, as with a normal infant.

If a lumbar puncture is to be done for diagnostic purposes, the nurse gives the usual assistance to the physician (see p. 294).

For the nurse's responsibilities in assisting with a ventricular tap, see p. 294.

The parents should have constant contact with the neurosurgeon. All diagnostic procedures should be explained to them, and they should be encouraged to help with the infant's care while he is in the hospital.

POSTOPERATIVE CARE. The temperature, pulse and respiration should be noted every 15 minutes until the infant is reactive; blood pressure readings, if ordered, are taken at the same time (a small blood pressure cuff is needed; see p. 92). Signs of increased intracranial pressure are irritability, bulging of the fontanel, lethargy, vomiting, elevated systolic blood pressure, widened pulse pressure, slowing or a change in the pulse and respiration rates, or change in body temperature.

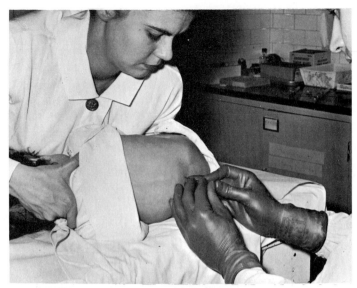

FIGURE 12–20. Restraint of a child for a lumbar puncture. The nurse places one hand behind the child's neck and the other under his buttocks. By resting her body gently on the infant's body and by applying pressure on the neck and legs, she can thus round his back and keep it parallel with the side of the treatment table.

Recording of the vital signs may be ordered hourly for several days. If the temperature is elevated, sponging with tepid water, and aspirin may be ordered, and the infant should be clothed only in his diaper.

Fluids are given intravenously slowly in quantities proportionate to weight until the infant can be fed orally. If they are given too rapidly there is danger of circulatory overload and cardiac falure.

Mucus from the nose and throat should be aspirated whenever necessary to prevent difficulty in breathing and the danger of aspiration of mucus. As in the care of every hydrocephalic infant, there is danger of pressure areas developing on parts of the scalp which support the weight of the head. Cotton may be placed behind the ears, and over the ears under the head dressing. The child should be turned at least every two hours.

The elevation of the infant's head and his general position depend upon the amount of fluid draining through the tube used to shunt fluid from the ventricular system to another site—atrium, peritoneal cavity, or ureter. The nurse and parents should know the kind of apparatus that has been inserted. The nurse should also know the location of the pump in the valve so that it can be pressed through the skin surface as ordered. The nurse should record observations of bulging or tenseness of the fontanel. The physician will direct the elevation of the head and shoulders and the general position of the infant to increase or decrease the rate of drainage. If the fontanel becomes depressed too rapidly, a subdural hematoma may develop. If the anterior fontanel is depressed, the infant should be placed flat in bed with the head slightly lower than the body. When the tenseness of the anterior fontanel is normal, his head should be slightly elevated or flat.

If a spinal ureterostomy or ventriculoureterostomy has been done, a 24-hour urine specimen must be collected to determine the amount of fluid and electrolytes being excreted from the body.

The infant may be placed in a mobile metabolic crib (see Fig. 12–21). Accurate urine collections may be obtained by the use of this device from children from birth to two years of age. The infant lies on a nonirritant, nonwettable nylon mesh hammock, which is held taut between stainless steel rods. This "bed" is suspended in a transparent box made of heavy-duty acrylic plastic. The front of the box is hinged to allow easy access to the infant. The top of the box is open to allow for ventilation. The urine from the child passes through the mesh to a collecting bottle below. The stools, unless of a diarrheal consistency, remain on the nylon mesh. The infant requires no restraint when urine is collected in this manner.

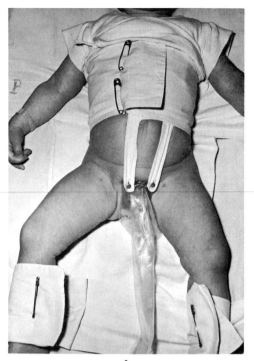

A

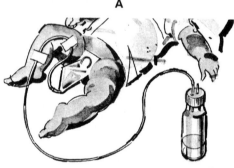

B

FIGURE 12–22. Procedure to be used for the collection of a 24-hour urine specimen from an infant girl. *A*, A specimen halter to which is snapped a plastic ring and tubing is used. The other end of the plastic tubing is placed in the drainage bottle attached to the bottom of the infant's crib. The abdominal and extremity restraints are used to restrain the infant adequately. *B*, A different type of equipment used for collecting the 24-hour urine specimen. (*B*, Sterilon Corporation.)

A device similar to the one used for the collection of a single specimen of urine (see p. 96) can be used for the continuous collection of urine if it is attached to a container at the foot of the bed.

The infant is restrained on the back by abdominal and ankle restraints. Such restraints (Fig. 12–22) are made of double-thickness muslin with ties at both ends to tie on the springs of the bed. The abdominal restraint has a flap of double-thickness muslin stitched to its center. This flap may be pinned around the infant's abdomen. The ankle or extremity restraint has two smaller flaps sewn to it. These flaps may be pinned securely around the ankles or wrists. If this restraint is too large, a tuck can be pinned in the center (Fig. 12–22).

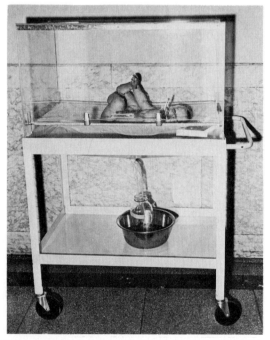

FIGURE 12–21. The mobile metabolic crib. (Courtesy of Lester Baker, M.D., and Charles W. Thomas Plastics, Inc., 4540 Worth Street, Phila., Pa.)

The head of the crib should be slightly elevated, if the infant's condition permits, to prevent a backflow of urine. The genitalia should be cleansed frequently to prevent excoriation. The restraints should be removed frequently, and passive exercise should be given to the legs and arms if the child cannot move himself. The nurse should not leave him until the restraints are again in position.

The physician usually orders sodium chloride to replace the amount lost through a ureteral shunt.

If a peritoneostomy (ventriculoperitoneal shunt) has been performed, the infant immediately postoperatively is given nothing by mouth. Abdominal distention is handled with a nasogastric tube which may be connected to mechanical suction. Irrigation of the tube may be necessary. The drainage is measured, and the amount and color are charted.

The infant's mouth becomes dry, and mouth care is required four times a day. As soon as the child can tolerate them, clear fluids are given orally. The milk formula is introduced gradually, and later solid foods, suitable to the age of the infant, are given. A high protein diet should be offered.

The nurse should closely observe and report to the physician any of the following: signs of infection, tenseness of the anterior fontanel (an indication of inadequate drainage of the cerebrospinal fluid), vomiting (an indication of increased intracranial pressure or intolerance of diet), signs of dehydration such as loss of skin turgor, convulsions (duration, where initiated, all parts of the body involved, and the kind of movements), the vital signs, coldness or clamminess of the infant's body, pallor or mottled condition of the skin, the state of consciousness, movements or signs of paralysis, the kind of drainage from the incision, and the degree of restlessness and irritability of the child.

A child having hydrocephalus may return to the hospital with an infected shunt. This is common cause for children with this disease. Treatment consists of surgical removal of the indwelling shunt and placement of an external constant ventricular drainage system. Cerebrospinal fluid cultures are taken, and the physician administers the appropriate antibiotics through the external shunting system.

The nurse's main responsibility is to observe the drainage system and to make certain that the fluid is fluctuating and draining. Any cessation of drainage indicates a blockage in the system and requires immediate action. Increased intracranial pressure may result if the system is not patent. The nurse must observe for any leakage or kinks in the tubing. Fluid should be measured every eight hours. Sodium replacement depends on the amount of fluid drainage.

When the infection has cleared, the child is returned to surgery and a new shunt is put into place.

A child with hydrocephalus is often hospitalized to lengthen the shunt because he has outgrown the original one. Preparation for hospitalization is indicated, since these admissions are usually elective. The clinic nurse or the nurse working in the pediatric neurology practice of a large hospital may be responsible for preparing the child for hospitalization.

Successful shunting must be maintained throughout the life of the child. Careful medical supervision is necessary to detect early evidence of shunt malfunctioning. If the shunt in an older child malfunctions, the intracranial pressure may increase rapidly, with symptoms of vomiting, headache, stupor, and ultimately coma. Other evidence of shunt malfunctioning includes failure in school, drowsiness, and deterioration of gait. For early detection of a decline in mental ability, intelligence testing may be of value.

Teaching the Parents Before Discharge of the Infant. The importance of the parents' understanding the care for their infant, and important conditions they should watch for and report to the physician, cannot be overestimated. Parents should be instructed in a way which will not increase anxiety. They may be told of the success other parents have had in caring for infants such as theirs. This will help them to gain confidence in their ability to give the infant the care he needs. To understand the operation which was performed is a basis for understanding the reason for the care taught and for following instructions exactly. They should understand the signs of increased intracranial pressure and of dehydration and their importance. With the surgeon's guidance the nurse may suggest exercises to the parents that will help to strengthen the infant's muscles so that he will learn to lift his head.

If the parents cared for the child before operation, they are probably skillful in handling him, but must learn to pump the shunt, if the surgeon advises this, and be aware of the problems which may arise in relation to the shunt. They should know the danger signals of too rapid drainage and should watch for them.

If the child is completely helpless and cannot move his body, there is always danger of pressure areas not only on the head but also on the body. In hot weather the danger of such lesions is increased. Methods of prevention such as passive exercises, frequent turning, and cleanliness can be taught to the parents. The infant should lead as normal a life as possible. He should be given toys, and should be taken about in a baby carriage or stroller whenever possible.

MICROCEPHALIA (MICROCEPHALY)

Etiology, Clinical Manifestations, and Treatment. Microcephalia is a relatively uncommon congenital anomaly. It is accompanied by mental retardation. It is easily recognized at birth by the smallness of the skull. Growth of the skull is largely dependent upon development of the brain. Arrested brain growth is the cause of microcephalia and may be due to hereditary factors, toxoplasmosis, German measles during pregnancy, or irradiation of the mother during the second or third month of pregnancy.

The *symptoms* are the small skull (less in volume and in circumference than normal in relation to the body build of the infant) and severe mental retardation.

There is no *treatment* for this condition. Habilitation should be attempted to whatever extent is possible.

DOWN'S SYNDROME (MONGOLISM)

Incidence, Etiology, Clinical Manifestations, Treatment, and Prognosis. This condition occurs most frequently in the Caucasian race, although it sometimes appears among blacks. The *incidence* is the same among all socioeconomic classes and both sexes.

The *cause* has only recently been discovered. There are three known causes of mongolism, all of which are associated with chromosomal abnormalities (see p. 218). The most common chromosomal abnormality in mongolism is trisomy of chromosome 21. This occurs once in every 600 births. The total chromosome count, instead of the normal forty-six, is forty-seven. This type of mongolism is rarely familial, but usually occurs

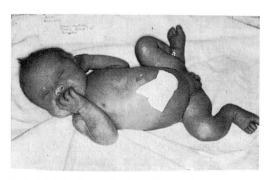

FIGURE 12–24. Over-all view of mongoloid infant made on the second day of life. General hypotonia is suggested by the relaxed appearance in what appears to be an awkward position. (Schaffer and Avery: *Diseases of the Newborn.* 4th ed.)

in children born to older women. The other causes of Down's syndrome—translocation of chromosome material or mosaicism—are rare.

The *signs* may be recognized at birth, but not all need to be present in order for the diagnosis to be made. The infant's physiognomy resembles that of an Oriental. The head is relatively small, the occiput flat and the face round. The eyes are set close together and slant slightly upward. The palpebral fissures (the openings between the eyelids) are narrow. Brushfield's spots are present on the iris of each eye. The nose is flat, and the tongue protrudes. These children breathe through the mouth and may drool. Eruption of the teeth is delayed. The hands are short and thick, the little finger is curved, and the creases of the palms and the prints of the feet are unlike those of a normal infant. There is a wide space between the first and second toes. The muscles are underdeveloped, the joints loose, and the child can assume unusual positions. Growth and development are slow; mental development seldom reaches beyond that of the average child of five to seven years of age. Associated anomalies are frequent, among them

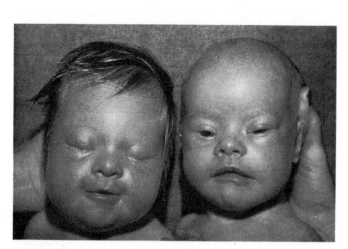

FIGURE 12–23. Mongoloid facies in two newborns with trisomy 21. (From Moll, H.: *Atlas of Pediatric Diseases.* Philadelphia, W. B. Saunders Co., 1976.)

TABLE 12–1. *MAJOR CLINICAL FEATURES OF THE THREE MOST COMMON AUTOSOMAL TRISOMIES*

CHARACTERISTIC FEATURES	21-TRISOMY	18-TRISOMY	13-TRISOMY
General	Mental retardation; hypotonia	Mental retardation; hypertonia; failure to thrive; preponderance of females; low birth weight	Mental retardation; failure to thrive; capillary hemangiomas; increased nuclear projections in neutrophils; persistent fetal hemoglobin; seizures
Craniofacies	Flat occiput; oblique palpebral fissures; epicanthic folds; speckled irides (Brushfield spots); protruding tongue; prominent, malformed ears; flat nasal bridge	Prominent occiput; small features; micrognathia; low-set, malformed ears	Microcephaly; cleft lip ± palate; midline scalp defects; microphthalmia, colobomata; low-set malformed ears; apparent deafness
Thorax	Congenital heart disease, mainly septal defects, especially of the endocardial cushion	Congenital heart disease, mainly V.S.D. and P.D.A.;* short sternum	Congenital heart disease, mainly septal defects, P.D.A.
Abdomen and pelvis	Decreased acetabular and iliac angles; small penis; cryptorchidism	Horseshoe kidney; small pelvis; cryptorchidism; limited hip abduction; inguinal or umbilical hernia	Polycystic kidneys; bicornuate uterus; cryptorchidism
Hands and feet	Simian crease; short, broad hands; hypoplasia of middle phalanx of 5th finger; gap between 1st and 2nd toes	Flexion deformity of fingers; short, dorsiflexed big toes; rockerbottom feet or equinovarus	Polydactyly; hyperconvex fingernails; simian crease
Other features observed with significant frequency	High-arched palate; strabismus; broad, short neck; small teeth; furrowed tongue; intestinal atresia; imperforate anus	Cleft lip ± palate; ocular anomalies; simian crease; hypoplasia of fingernails; widely spaced nipples; webbed neck; single umbilical artery	Flexion deformity of fingers; single umbilical artery; shallow supraorbital ridges; micrognathia; retroflexible thumb; rockerbottom feet

*V.S.D.=ventricular septal defect; P.D.A.=patent ductus arteriosus.

From Vaughan, V. C., III, and McKay, R. J.: *Nelson Textbook of Pediatrics.* 10th ed. Philadelphia, W. B. Saunders Co., 1975, p. 305.

congenital deformities of the heart, including atrial septal defect, ventricular septal defect, and patent ductus arteriosus. Chronic myelogenous leukemia has been found to be about 20 times as frequent in the mongoloid population as in the normal population.

Such children need continuous health care and supervison. They have little resistance to infection and may die early of an intercurrent infection. Modern drug therapy has prolonged their life expectancy to some extent.

Although there is no *treatment* for the condi-

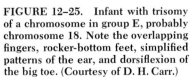

FIGURE 12–25. Infant with trisomy of a chromosome in group E, probably chromosome 18. Note the overlapping fingers, rocker-bottom feet, simplified patterns of the ear, and dorsiflexion of the big toe. (Courtesy of D. H. Carr.)

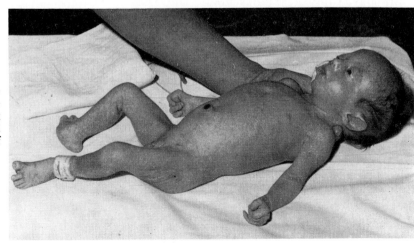

tion, habilitation is important. These children may or may not be difficult to train. They respond to training by copying techniques shown to them repeatedly in a consistent manner. In adolescence vocational training may be considered. Some communities have organized classes so that these children can be trained to the limit of their abilities.

It is difficult for the parents to accept the child's condition. This is especially true if he is the only child of older parents. If the infant is the child of young parents, they may be afraid to have other children. In any event the parents need help from professional persons in understanding the child's limitations and in planning his life to make the most of his capacities and to give him a happy childhood.

Many community resources are available to help the parents of children having Down's syndrome to meet the short- and long-term problems presented by these children. The nurse should be cognizant of the specific resources available for them in the community in which they live.

For further discussion of the care of the mentally retarded child, see page 696.

Genitourinary System

Some malformations of the genitourinary system are present and are diagnosed at birth. Others may not be diagnosed immediately. The nurse in the nursery and later the parents at home are responsible for observing the amount and color of urine, the pattern of the infant's voiding, the strength of the urinary stream, and indications of infection such as an elevation of temperature. Any deviation from normal should be reported to the physician.

OBSTRUCTION OF THE URINARY TRACT

Etiology, Clinical Manifestations, and Diagnosis. Obstruction to the flow of urine is important because of the back pressure produced above the level of the obstruction. The back pressure of accumulated urine causes the tract to become distended proximal to the point of obstruction. This may lead to stasis, hydroureter, hydronephrosis, possible infection, and death due to renal insufficiency.

The *symptoms* are obstruction while voiding, dribbling, bladder distention, or the presence of an abdominal mass. Infection of the urinary tract results in fever, chills, pyuria, and convulsions. If there is eventual loss of kidney function with uremia, death results.

A number of tests are used to determine the location of the obstruction. It may be in the upper or lower urinary tract, above the bladder, or below it. The symptoms are not always indicative of the site of the obstruction.

Diagnostic tests include catheterization immediately after voiding to determine the amount of residual urine. Intravenous urography is used to visualize the urinary tract and to measure renal excretory function. Cystoscopic examination and retrograde pyelography may be performed. The blood urea nitrogen level and phenolsulfonphthalein excretion rate may be determined to measure renal function.

OBSTRUCTION OF THE LOWER URINARY TRACT

Pathology and Clinical Manifestations. Causes of lower urinary tract obstructions include urethral valves (filamentous valves that obstruct urinary flow are most commonly found in boys), urethral diaphragm or congenital narrowing of the urethra, obstruction of the neck of the bladder (the most common site of obstruction), severe phimosis (obstructive phimosis is rare), neuromuscular dysfunction such as is found in association with cord injury and meningomyelocele, and meatal stricture.

All these obstructions result in dilatation and hypertrophy of the bladder. Residual urine is constantly present. The ureters dilate and become tortuous from the back pressure of urine which cannot pass into the distended bladder. Later the renal pelves enlarge from pressure of urine which cannot pass down into the distended ureters. Destruction of kidney tissue inevitably results.

The *signs* and *symptoms* are abnormalities of urination, a palpable, distended bladder and possibly distended ureters and kidneys. Infection of the urinary tract may be frequent.

OBSTRUCTION OF THE UPPER URINARY TRACT

Upper urinary tract obstructions are usually unilateral. The bladder is not involved. There is no problem of urination unless an infection occurs. Anomalies involving the ureters are the most common anomalies of the urinary tract.

The following *types* occur: obstruction or stricture of a ureter, congenital absence of one ureter, duplication of the ureter of one kidney, pressure of an aberrant blood vessel which blocks drainage through the ureter, neoplasm, calculi, or an inflammatory stricture. The most common stricture or obstruction of the ureter occurs at the pelvic-ureteral or the vesicoureteral region.

Clinical Manifestations. Often there are no symptoms, or there may be vague symptoms such as failure to grow normally, hypertension, fever, bacteriuria, pyuria, or a mass in the abdomen.

Treatment and Nursing Care of Upper and Lower Obstructions. Preliminary drainage by a cystostomy or an indwelling catheter may be done prior to surgery. Irrigation of the bladder with an antibacterial agent may prevent infection from these procedures. If the obstruction can be relieved by surgical means, operation is attempted in spite of the reduced renal function (see p. 312 for surgical treatment of exstrophy of the bladder). Accurate intake and output records are needed. The nurse should exercise care to prevent contamination of the catheters utilized for urinary drainage. Acute or chronic infections should be eradicated with appropriate chemotherapeutic medications.

Course and Prognosis. Untreated obstruction results in renal insufficiency. Little can be done for chronic renal insufficiency, manifested by progressive renal dysfunction. Death results from renal failure. If operation can remove the obstruction, improvement may result, and the child may live for many years.

PATENT URACHUS

Etiology and Pathology. Patent urachus is due to persistence of the embryonic connection of the umbilicus with the bladder. Occasionally the urachus may persist, and urine is discharged through the umbilicus after birth. Often there is also an obstruction of the urinary tract below the bladder. Many times there is only a cyst at the upper end of the tract, extraperitoneally under the umbilicus.

Clinical Manifestations and Treatment. When the entire urachus is present, urine dribbles from the umbilical region. When a urachal cyst is present, there is a deep midline swelling below the umbilicus.

If the urachus is patent, the tract should be obliterated surgically. Urachal cysts should be removed before they become infected. If they do become infected, they should be drained surgically before removal. Appropriate antibiotics are given for infection.

CONGENITAL CYSTIC (POLYCYSTIC) KIDNEYS

Etiology, Pathology, Clinical Manifestations, and Treatment. The *cause* is unknown. The infantile form is probably transmitted as a mendelian recessive trait. The renal tissue is filled with cysts of varying sizes. The kidneys are enlarged, and at operation or autopsy have a spongy appearance. The renal pelves and calices are distorted because of the amount of surrounding tissue. The condition is rarely unilateral.

Other anomalies may also occur, e.g., hydrocephalus, polydactylism, or cardiac malformations.

The *clinical findings* depend upon the location of the cysts. On palpation both kidneys (less frequently only one) are found to be enlarged. There is increasing renal insufficiency and, as a result, hypertension and signs of congestive cardiac failure. There may be severe growth retardation. Laboratory findings show recurrent bacteriuria, hematuria, proteinuria, and elevated blood nonprotein nitrogen levels. X-ray films (urograms) show enlargement of the kidney and deformity of the calices and pelves.

There is no specific *treatment*. Supportive and palliative measures may be used to combat renal acidosis and insufficiency. Surgical drainage of large cysts may be done when they interfere with renal function.

The *prognosis* depends upon the type and severity of the interference with function. In severe types the infant dies *in utero*. Among infants living at birth renal function decreases over the years. In less severe cases, although the first symptom may appear in childhood, the condition may not become too evident until adult life.

WILMS' TUMOR (NEPHROBLASTOMA)

Incidence, Clinical Manifestations, and Diagnosis. Wilms' tumor is a highly malignant embryonal adenosarcoma of the kidney. It develops from abnormal tissue in the embryo, beginning to grow before or after the infant is born. It is one of the most frequent neoplasms occurring during infancy or the toddler age. It is commonly unilateral, but may be bilateral.

There are seldom *symptoms* other than a mass in the abdomen which is usually discovered by the physician in a routine examination of the child, or by the parent while bathing him or changing his diaper.

After the diagnosis has been made the physician and the parents must be careful not to palpate the infant's abdomen, since handling might favor metastasis. The tumor extends through the kidney capsule or renal vein and then spreads to other areas of the body by way of the circulatory system. The late symptoms are anemia and cachexia.

The *diagnosis* is confirmed by intravenous pyelography, which shows the distortion and displacement of the pelvis of the kidney.

Prognosis, Treatment, and Responsibilities of the Nurse. The condition without treatment is always fatal. In general, the *prognosis* is better for infants under one year of age than for older children because the mass has been detected early. With adequate treatment there is a high rate of cure with early diagnosis. The tumor metastasizes to regional lymph nodes. It also produces pulmonary metastases via the renal vein and venous circulation to the right side of the heart and thence through the pulmonary artery to the lungs.

The *treatment* is surgical extirpation with possible x-ray irradiation before and/or after surgery. Operation should be done immediately after the diagnosis has been made. Actinomycin D (dactinomycin) and vincristine are given preoperatively and postoperatively to a child having Wilms' tumor.

The *nursing care* is that of the normal infant, with special attention to nutrition. The specific danger in preoperative care is manipulating the abdominal wall inadvertently, as in bathing the infant or when fondling him, and thereby increasing the danger of metastasis. The parents should be cautioned against this, and in the hospital a sign should be placed on the infant's crib or on his abdomen—"Do not palpate abdomen."

Newborns who have malignancies require nursing care that takes into consideration their physical, intellectual, and emotional needs. They require good skin care, especially when either irradiation or chemotherapy is given. The skin is kept clean and dry; if it becomes irritated, a bland ointment may be applied.

Personal feelings about children having malignancies should be recognized by the nurse and accepted in order to be more effective in attempting to help parents with their feelings. A diagnosis of a malignancy in a child produces high levels of anxiety in parents. With the improvement of therapy in Wilms' tumor, the outcome is no longer as bleak as it once was. The student should review the material in Chapter 5 concerning the nurse and the terminally ill child.

EXSTROPHY OF THE BLADDER

Pathology and Clinical Manifestations. Complete exstrophy is an extensive anomaly. The lower urinary tract—i.e., the entire bladder to the external urethral meatus—is exposed and may be without ventral covering. The defect in the male infant may be accompanied by a short penis, epispadias, undescended testes, or an inguinal hernia. In the female infant the clitoris may be cleft, the labia separated, and the vagina absent. In either sex the rectus muscles below the umbilicus are separated, and the pubic rami are not joined.

In complete exstrophy the posterior bladder lining is exposed and appears bright red through the fissure in the abdominal wall. The condition is more common in boys than in girls.

The defect is obvious at birth. Urine seeps onto the abdominal wall from the abnormal ureteral outlets. This causes a constant odor of urine and excoriation of the surrounding skin. There may be ulceration of the mucosa of the bladder. The separation of the pubic rami causes a waddling gait when the child learns to walk.

Treatment, Complications, and Prognosis. If the exstrophy is not complete, the abdominal and bladder walls may be closed by plastic surgery. Even complete exstrophy including the external genitalia has been corrected by plastic surgery with excellent results. The child then voids normally.

If continence is not obtained after surgery on the bladder neck, urinary diversion by a sigmoid or ileal conduit is done soon thereafter. Reflux of urine into the ureters occurs in more than three quarters of closed bladders because of an abnormal vesical wall and the position of ureteral entrance. An antireflux operation may be necessary in order to prevent an ascending infection and to allow for a continence procedure on the bladder neck. Chronic ureteral reflux may lead to pyelonephritis, due to chronic urinary tract infection, or to hydronephrosis, due to increased pressure in the renal pelvis from the refluxing

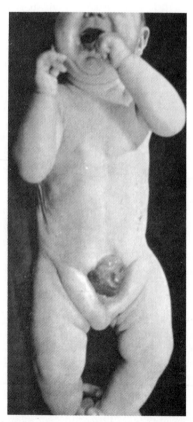

FIGURE 12–26. Exstrophy of the bladder. Five-month-old infant with exstrophy of the bladder and bilateral indirect inguinal hernias. The association of these 2 conditions is common. (Gross: *The Surgery of Infancy and Childhood.*)

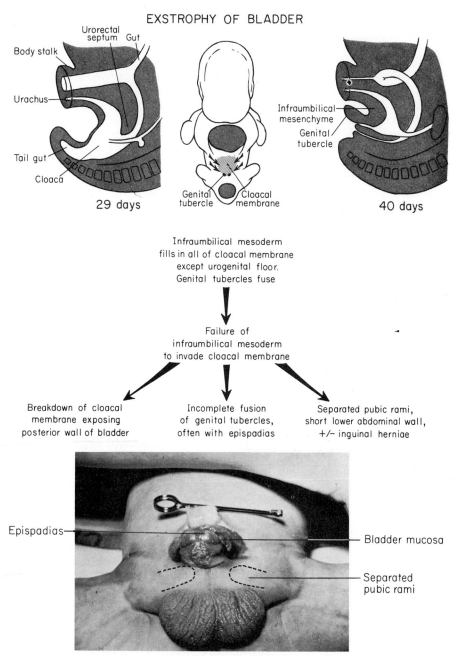

FIGURE 12–27. The fetal development of exstrophy of the bladder. (From Smith, D. W.: *Recognizable Patterns of Human Malformation*, 2nd ed. Philadelphia, W. B. Saunders Co., 1976.)

urine. When there is upper urinary tract damage from hydronephrosis or pyelonephritis, urinary diversion is indicated.

A type of urinary diversion may be carried out between 12 and 18 months of age when the functional status of the anal sphincter can be assessed. A ureterosigmoidostomy with an antireflux ureteral anastomosis is done to free the child from any external urinary appliance. Urine is then passed with stool from the anus. When the child is old enough to have control of his bowel movements, he learns to retain the urine in the colon by tightening the sphincter muscle. He is given antibiotics to combat infection.

A procedure used frequently is ureteral reimplantation of the ureters. Normally, the ureters enter the bladder at an oblique angle. They are surrounded by bladder muscle and terminate at the ureteral orifice on the bladder mucosa. When the bladder contracts, as in voiding, the increased pressure results in collapse of the intravesical portion of the ureter, preventing backflow. The urine is expelled through the urethra.

If the vesicoureteral valve is incompetent, compression of the ureter by the muscle of the bladder is not possible, and reflux occurs. Ureteral reimplantation may be required to prevent damage to the kidney. The objective of surgery is to straighten the affected ureters and to position a long enough segment of ureter within the bladder or its wall so that intravesical pressure during voiding compresses the ureters and prevents reflux.

The waddling gait is improved by a brace, which corrects the deformity of the pelvic girdle, or by surgery.

The *prognosis* depends upon the injury done to the kidneys by the back pressure of urine for which there is no adequate outlet, and upon whether the child has suffered severe or chronic infection of the urinary tract. Even if there is no infection of the kidney, children having a ureterosigmoidostomy may have a chronic disturbance of the body chemistry, since the bowel surface may absorb secretory products from the urine when the ureters are transplanted.

Parent Teaching Before Discharge of the Infant from the Nursery. It is important that the parents be taught the general care of these infants. Good hygiene is necessary so that the infants may be in optimum condition to withstand an infection of the skin or kidney and, later, surgical correction of the anomaly. The nurse should understand the parents' distress over the child's condition and appreciate that his care may be a task which they cannot immediately undertake. The nurse's acceptance of the child's condition is as important in teaching the parent as are the procedures in the care of the anomaly.

The mother may not have sufficient self-control to cleanse the area around the exposed bladder until she has become accustomed to the sight of the defect. If she is to be taught before she leaves the obstetrical unit, she should be fully recovered from parturition. If she is not ready for his care, it would be better to keep him in the hospital for a few days and have the public health or community nurse instruct her after he has been sent home. The mother should learn to keep the bladder area very clean and to apply sterile petrolatum gauze over it in order to prevent infection and possible ulceration. A bland ointment may be applied around the bladder area in order to protect the skin from draining urine. The diaper should be changed frequently for the infant's comfort and to prevent the odor of urine, which will embarrass the parents when they show him to friends. Stool should be removed immediately so that it does not contaminate the bladder mucosa. The in-

fant's clothing should be light so as to avoid pressure on the exposed bladder.

Responsibilities of the Nurse. *Preoperative* nursing care includes the care outlined above to be taught the parents. If the infant is not a newborn in the nursery, but an older infant admitted to the pediatric unit for tests or operation, the parents may be able to give good hints on his care. This will ensure the continuity of care which makes the transition from home to hospital less disturbing for the infant. If operation is to be done when the child is old enough to understand that he is to undergo surgery, he should be emotionally prepared for the experience. The parents must be psychologically ready for operation before it is undertaken. It is helpful to both the parents and the child to allow the parents to help with his care in the children's unit.

If a urine specimen is needed, it is collected from the opening in the bladder with a medicine dropper, or the child may be held over an emesis basin in such a position as to allow urine to drip into the basin.

Postoperative care is that of any surgical patient. The dressings must be kept clean and dry. If the ureters have been transplanted into the sigmoid colon and if the child is old enough to establish control of the anal sphincter muscle, he should be taught to hold the muscle tight to prevent seepage of urine. There will be some soiling of his clothes while he is acquiring this control. He should never be made to feel ashamed of "accidents." Control will be acquired more readily if he is not too anxious about his condition.

If a ureteral reimplantation has been done, the main goal of the nurse caring for the child is maintaining the patency of the urinary drainage system. The nurse must regularly measure and record the amount, color, and consistency of urine, including the presence of clots, mucus, or other material. Adequate hydration, orally or parenterally, must be assured to produce sufficient urine to flush the bladder and help dislodge clots. The child is usually kept flat in bed to prevent kinking of the drainage tubing that might obstruct urinary flow. Many young children feel uncomfortable when they do not have their underpants on, so loose pants that do not obstruct the catheters may be worn.

Parents need few instructions before discharge of their child if they have been involved in his care during hospitalization. Adequate fluid intake should be continued, and an antibiotic may be ordered to prevent infection. If the child has a fever, hematuria, or purulent drainage from the incision, the physician should be notified.

HYPOSPADIAS

Etiology, Treatment, and Prognosis. Hypospadias is a congenital malformation in which the urethra, in the male, opens on the lower surface of the penis just behind the glans, in the body of the penis or on the perineum; rarely, in the female, the urethra opens into the vagina. This condition occurs in about 1 in 125 male infants. First-degree relatives of children having hypospadias are five to ten times more likely to have hypospadias than others in the general population. In the male, associated congenital *chordee* is a cordlike anomaly that extends from the scrotum up the penis and pulls it downward in an arc. Urination with the penis in the normal elevated position is impossible.

Treatment to correct the chordee is by surgery at about two years of age. If the hypospadias is slight, no treatment may be given, since only severe forms interfere with procreation. If it is severe, the anomaly should be repaired before the child is of school age so he will not be embarrassed when voiding before his peers. Surgery may be done in one or more stages, depending on the defect. Newborns having hypospadias should not be circumcised, since the foreskin is used in the repair.

Responsibilities of the Nurse. In the newborn nursery it is important for nurses to observe the voiding pattern of all infants. If an infant cannot void normally, a meatotomy may be done. When surgery is performed on the hypospadias, a perineal urethrotomy, a Foley catheter, or a suprapubic tube is used to remove urine from the operative area. If the incision is kept dry and trauma to the area is prevented, the repair should be successful.

Since preschool children have a fear of body mutilation, the timing of surgery is important, especially to their self-image. The psychologic preparation of the child and his parents is important also because the surgery may be done in one or more stages.

EPISPADIAS

In this anomaly the urethra opens upon the dorsal surface of the penis. The urethra may lie just behind the glans or, in conjunction with exstrophy of the bladder, extend the whole length of the penis.

The treatment is surgical. The emotional and psychologic problems involved are the same as those in hypospadias.

Intersexuality

Parents feel guilty about the birth of a child whose sex is not easily determined. Intersexuality is an extremely disturbing anomaly, although its influence on physical health is slight. If there is any question about the sex of the child because of the lack of distinctive genitalia, the newborn should have an exploratory examination to determine the gonadal sex, as well as chromosomal studies (see p. 214). This should be done before the parents announce the child's sex to their friends and information for the birth certificate is given. If the parents wish to name the infant before absolute determination of sex is made, they can use names such as "Lee" or "Vern." The social role of the boy is different from that of the girl; clothing, activities, and the pronominal references of speech all set off one sex from the other. It is psychologically harmful to both parents and the child if the infant believed to be of one sex is later found to be of the other. All psychologic identifications have been made in terms of the sex originally determined by the physician.

Parents, and the child when he is old enough, need to understand the anatomic problems involved and the treatment which should be given. The treatment, depending upon the causes of the problem, may be surgical or medical. They need support from professional people who consider the problem objectively, without the morbid curiosity and pity which friends and relatives may show. A child with such a problem needs help at school in adjustment to his peer group. It is advisable to have the child under the supervision of the guidance clinic. Parents, even the most understanding ones, cannot judge the depth of such a child's emotional problems.

Three types of intersexuality will be discussed: pseudohermaphroditism in the female, pseudohermaphroditism in the male, and hermaphroditism.

PSEUDOHERMAPHRODITISM IN THE FEMALE (CONGENITAL ADRENAL HYPERPLASIA)

Etiology, Clinical Manifestations, Diagnosis, and Treatment. Female pseudohermaphroditism is the most common problem in intersexuality or sexual differentiation. It is due to an inability to synthesize hydrocortisone from its precursors. The deficiency of hydrocortisone results eventually in adrenocortical hyperplasia and overproduction of androgens. Increased androgenic—i.e., producing male characteristics—steroid secretion by the fetal adrenal cortex causes masculinization of the external genitalia in the female infant. Recently more cases have been seen in infants born of mothers treated with steroids during pregnancy than have occurred spontaneously.

The *clinical findings* are enlargement of the phallus or clitoris, fusion of the labia resembling

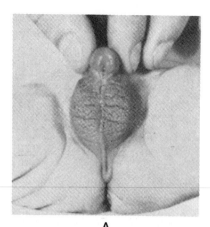

A

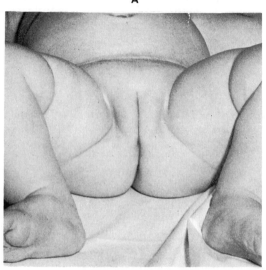

B

FIGURE 12–28. Pseudohermaphroditism. *A*, Female pseudohermaphrodite having untreated adrenal hyperplasia. This infant had normal female sex chromosomes, but was designated a male at birth. (J. McFarlane, *Am. J. Nursing*, 76:1290, August 1976.) *B*, Pseudohermaphroditism in the male. View of torso of one-month-old infant showing normal female configuration. A swelling can be seen in the right inguinal region. At operation this proved to be a testis which had herniated into the inguinal canal. The external genitalia appear to be made up of completely normal female labia, clitoris, vulva, and vagina. Skin biopsy revealed the male chromosomal pattern. At laparotomy no female internal organs were found. (Gaspar, Kimber, and Berkaw, in A.M.A. *J. Dis. Child*, Vol. 91, with the permission of the authors.)

a bifid scrotum, and hypospadias. Such infants have a cervix and a uterus and the female chromosomal pattern.

The *diagnosis* may be made by exploration and biopsy of the gonads during the neonatal period, by assay of steroid excretion products in the urine, and by chromosomal studies (see p. 214).

In spite of the anomalous external genitalia, these children should be reared as girls. If the child is given hydrocortisone, the production of corticotropin will be inhibited and the production of androgens reduced. Infants who do not have adrenal hyperplasia require no treatment other than corrective plastic surgery. Correction should be undertaken between the ages of 18 months and four years.

If the diagnosis is made in infancy and plastic surgery is performed in the toddler or preschool age, the *prognosis* is very good.

PSEUDOHERMAPHRODITISM IN THE MALE

Etiology and Treatment. There are several types of this condition, but all such infants are chromosomal males. One type is caused by gonadal dysgenesis. These are infants whose testes were damaged early in fetal life, resulting in feminization of the fetus. Another type is characterized by normal female external genitalia, but testes, not ovaries, internally. In this type the testes should be removed and the child reared as a girl. At the usual time for puberty the child should be given estrogens to compensate for those normally produced by the ovaries of the female. In still another type the genitalia are predominantly masculine or ambiguous. Such children masculinize at puberty. Any structures not of the male sex should be removed surgically.

TRUE HERMAPHRODITISM

True hermaphroditism is rare. The clinical findings show both ovarian and testicular tissue in the same infant. The chromosomal sex may be male or female. True hermaphroditism must be excluded in all infants showing intersexuality except those with congenital adrenal hyperplasia. The treatment is the same as for male pseudohermaphroditism.

Diseases of Muscle

MUSCULAR DYSTROPHY

A group of disorders of genetic origin in which slow degeneration of muscle fibers occurs is known as the muscular dystrophies. Two of this group are discussed here: *congenital muscular dystrophy* and *pseudohypertrophic muscular dystrophy (Duchenne or childhood form)*. *Congenital muscular dystrophy* is an autosomal recessive disorder that causes weakness and hypotonia in infants. The problem originates *in utero*. Clinical manifestations include profound muscular atrophy, limitations of joint movements or contractures that may be evident at birth. Tendon reflexes may be absent. Respiratory muscles, including the diaphragm, may be involved. Before one year of age severely affected infants may die; those less affected will have a prolonged survival. Diagnosis can be made from muscle tissue biopsies, which show dystrophic changes and from a study of serum enzymes, especially CPK (creatine phosphokinase) at birth. At present, intrauterine diagnosis is not possible.

Pseudohypertrophic muscular dystrophy is the most common form of this disease, but it is still uncommon when compared with other illnesses in childhood. It classically occurs only in boys. Sex-linked inheritance is found in about one half of these children. Although the diagnosis is rarely made before age three years, there may be a history of slow motor development from birth. The infant may not sit, stand, or walk at the usual ages. A waddling gait, difficulty in running and climbing stairs, and hypertrophied calf muscles are usual findings. Other muscles such as the deltoid and the tongue may also be increased in size. The increase in muscle size is due to fatty infiltration, which does not provide strength. Walking on the toes and contracture of the heel cords are frequently seen and may cause this condition to be confused with cerebral palsy (see p. 578). The child has characteristic waddling, lordotic gait, and has difficulty in rising from the floor because of weak muscles of the pelvic girdle. When the moderately severely affected child is on the floor, Gowers' sign can be seen. Gowers' sign is evidenced by the child rolling to the prone position, kneeling, and raising himself by pushing with his hands against his shins, knees, and thighs in order to stand. As the child grows older, profound muscular atrophy occurs. By puberty walking is usually impossible and death occurs in three quarters of patients by the end of the second decade of life. Cardiac myopathy may be the cause of death. Mild or severe mental retardation may be present in the Duchenne form of muscular dystrophy.

Diagnosis is made by measurement of serum enzymes, especially CPK (creatine phosphokinase), by muscle biopsy, and by electromyography. Certain identification of female carriers of this disease is not possible.

Treatment, Genetic Counseling, and the Responsibilities of the Nurse. *Treatment* is not effective. *Genetic counseling* (see p. 233) is an important part of management, since one half of the male siblings of a child having muscular dystrophy are affected and one half of the females are carriers of the disease. The level of creatine phosphokinase is elevated in some known carriers, and in the preclinical and clinical states.

These children should remain ambulatory as long as possible. Although strenuous exercise is to be avoided because it may speed the breakdown of muscle fibers, long-term bedrest may hasten muscular atrophy. Lengthening the heel cords surgically may improve ambulation. Assisted ventilation and tracheotomy may become necessary if respiratory infection occurs.

The *responsibilities of the nurse* include supportive care of the child and understanding for the parents. Affected children should have regular examinations to note the progress of the disease. If the nurse is interested in the child and his care, the family will gain immeasurable solace. The nurse can encourage a reasonable amount of activity according to the child's ability. When weakness is severe, the nurse can teach the family how to do passive manipulation or range of motion of the joints in order to prevent contractures and restricted joint motion. Overzealous passive manipulation of muscles may injure the muscle fibers and hasten the restrictive process. When the child is no longer able to walk without falling, the nurse can help the family with the use of a wheelchair.

As the muscles of respiration become more involved, the possibility of lung infection increases. The nurse can help the family avoid these infections and secure early treatment if they occur.

If cardiac failure due to a myopathy of the heart muscle occurs, the nurse can help the family care for the child if he develops congestive heart failure (see p. 292).

MYASTHENIA GRAVIS

Etiology, Incidence, Types, Clinical Manifestations. Myasthenia gravis is not a common condition in infancy. When it does occur, early diagnosis and treatment are important. The *etiology* of the disease is not known; however, it may be due to an immunologic dysfunction because there is a high incidence of hyperplasia of the thymus. The weakness of muscles may also be due to a deficient action of acetylcholine on the motor end-plates of involved muscles, probably caused by a competitive (acetylcholine-inhibitory) block. There are three forms of myasthenia gravis syndrome: *transient neonatal myasthenia gravis, persistent neonatal myasthenia gravis,* and *juvenile myasthenia gravis.*

Transient neonatal myasthenia occurs in neonates whose mothers have the disease, perhaps with or without any symptoms. Such an infant is hypotonic, with weakness, poor sucking ability, difficulty in breathing, and ptosis (drooping eyelids). If these newborns are not treated, they may die in hours or days after birth, or they may improve to recovery within two weeks to a month.

Persistent neonatal myasthenia gravis occurs in neonates of mothers who do not have the disease. More than one child in a family may have the symptoms of the transient form noted already. This disease continues throughout life, with the eyelids and extraocular muscles most seriously affected.

Juvenile myasthenia gravis usually occurs after ten years of age. Treatment is the same as in the other two types. Girls are affected six times as often as boys. The most common clinical manifestations include ptosis and double vision. The facial and neck muscles and bulbar and intercostal muscles may also be affected. Weakness is exacerbated on repetitive movement. Myasthenia crisis, a life-threatening exacerbation, may occur during stress, such as emotional upheaval, severe infection, or surgical procedure. Diagnosis is made when there is a characteristic distribution of muscle weakness and when further weakness is evident, such as a sustained muscular contraction when the child is asked to gaze at the ceiling and develops ptosis.

Treatment, Responsibilities of the Nurse, and Prognosis. *Treatment* is by anticholinesterase compounds, which tend to reduce the weakness. The compounds used in treatment include intravenous or intramuscular edrophonium chloride (Tensilon), a short-acting drug used for testing as in diagnosing, or neostigmine (Prostigmin), a longer-acting drug. If the child develops evidence of excessive parasympathetic stimulation, such as salivation, bradycardia, abdominal cramps, vomiting, or diarrhea, atropine sulfate should be made available and given immediately. As the child improves, the parenteral anticholinesterase compound may be replaced by oral pyridostigmine bromide (Mestinon) or a less toxic drug, neostigmine bromide. As the child improves, the need for anticholinesterase medication will decrease. The drug should be discontinued when possible.

Further treatment and nursing care include intermittent assisted ventilation, tracheotomy, and suctioning if needed (see p. 541). Parenteral or nasogastric feeding is given as necessary. Thymectomy or corticosteroid therapy may be indicated in severe myasthenia. Antibiotics may be given if infection occurs.

The *prognosis* of myasthenia gravis in childhood is better than that in the adult form. Most affected children can lead lives that are nearly normal. About one quarter of these children have complete remissions.

Orthopedic Anomalies

As recently as 20 years ago children with minor orthopedic deformities were hospitalized for months. Today, with the recognition of the psychologic importance of the separation of the child from his family, such children are treated largely on an outpatient basis. They are admitted to the hospital only for application of a cast or for operation and are cared for at home between admissions. This places increased responsibility upon the nurse to help the parents understand the care of the child.

The nurse may be the first person to observe that the infant has an orthopedic deformity. It is the responsibility of the nurse to report this observation to the physician as early as possible. Long-term care of the infant should be discussed with the parents in order to gain their cooperation.

CLUBFOOT

Clubfoot is a foot which has been twisted out of shape or position *in utero* and cannot be moved to an overcorrected position. An infant may appear to have this deformity because of the fetal position of comfort *in utero*. Unlike true clubfoot, however, his foot can be moved to a correct or even overcorrected position and made normal by simple exercises. In such a case before the mother is given the infant to nurse or fondle, she should be told that the defect is only temporary.

Incidence, Etiology, Diagnosis, Pathology, and Types. True clubfoot is one of the most common orthopedic deformities. Several theories have been advanced to explain the *etiology*. The condition may be due to a defect in the ovum, a familial tendency, or arrested growth. It may be a paralytic deformity occurring in conjunction with meningomyelocele. Not all cases of clubfoot in older children are congenital in origin. The defect may have been caused by injury or poliomyelitis.

The *diagnosis* of the specific type of clubfoot (several types are recognized) depends upon the anomaly in the individual child. The *pathology* varies from slight changes in the structure of the foot to abnormalities in the bones of both the foot and the leg.

The two most common types of clubfoot are talipes equinovarus and talipes calcaneovalgus. Both types are usually bilateral. In *talipes equinovarus* the foot is fixed in plantar flexion and deviates medially; i.e., the heel is elevated. The child walks on the toes and outer border of the foot. More than 95 per cent of cases of congenital clubfoot are of this type. In *talipes calcaneovalgus* the foot is dorsiflexed and deviates laterally; i.e., the heel is turned outward, and the anterior part of the foot is elevated on the outer border. The child walks on the outwardly turned heel and the inner border of the foot.

Treatment and Responsibilities of the Nurse. *Treatment* should be started as soon as possible. Delay makes correction more difficult, since the bones and muscles of the leg develop abnormally, and the tendons will be shortened. In infancy, treatment is usually conservative. It may consist in manipulation, the application of a cast to hold the foot in a corrected position, or use of a wedged cast. The advantage of a wedged cast is that a position of greater correction can be achieved and that the cast need not be changed. A hungry infant is more cooperative when a cast is being applied if he can be fed during the procedure. A toddler is usually more cooperative if he is given a toy to distract his attention. Parents can assist with the application of a cast in this manner.

The young child should be prepared for the application of the cast before it is scheduled to be done. The child should be well aware of what is going to happen to him through the informed nurse's teaching. The child should know what the cast will look like: a simple way to

help him understand is to show him a model of the type of cast he will have on a doll. Actually having the child put a cast on a doll himself will help him feel more secure in his own treatment. He may enjoy taking such a doll to the plaster room with him. The nurse may be responsible for immobilizing and holding the child during cast application. A Denis Browne splint is often used for infants under one year of age. The appliance is made of two foot-plates attached to a crossbar. When the splint is fitted to the shoes, varying positions of angulation of the feet may be maintained by set screws. As the child kicks, he automatically moves his feet into a corrected position.

When the physician orders a Denis Browne splint, the nurse should discuss the care of the child using this appliance with the parents. The parents are told when and for how long the splint must be worn. The infant's feet may be attached to the splint with adhesive tape or slipped into well-fitting shoes attached to the splint. The nurse can assist parents in applying the splint, emphasizing that socks should be used to protect the feet. The parents must check the skin of the feet for reddened areas. Parents must also be taught how to tighten the shoes against the Denis Browne splint with a key if they become loose.

If conservative measures fail, correction to as

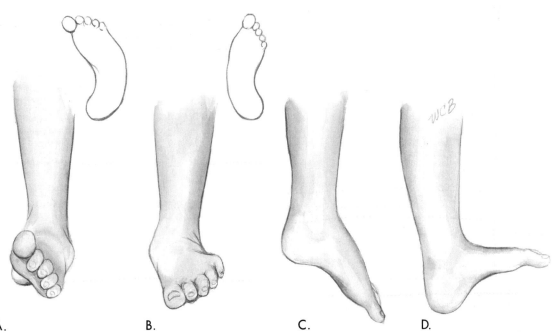

A.   B.   C.   D.

FIGURE 12–29. Club feet in a newborn child. If left untreated, the deformity will become increasingly severe. *A*, Varus; *B*, Valgus; *C*, Equinus; *D*, Calcaneus deformities. (M. O. Tachdjian, *Pediatric Orthopedics*.)

near normal position as possible may be done under anesthesia and a cast applied. Surgery on the tendons and bones may be done in early childhood, and the leg and foot placed in a cast.

Most of the nursing care of children having club foot is given by the mother at home. When the child is admitted to the hospital, the usual method of applying a cast is followed. A plaster of Paris bandage is closely fitted over stockinet or wadding extending from below the knee to the toes. In the Kite method of correction the cast is wedged. When the child returns to the pediatric unit after application of a cast, the nurse should observe for areas of pressure and should note the condition of the skin around the edges of the cast, the circulation in the toes as shown by color and temperature, the child's ability to move his toes, and any sign of discomfort. If pressure areas develop or if the circulation is impaired, the cast is split to relieve the pressure or is removed. The nurse may put adhesive petals around the edges of the cast to prevent the plaster from irritating the skin. A discussion of further care of a child in a cast can be found on page 323.

If manipulation is used to place the foot in a corrected position and a cast is applied, the child should remain in bed for 24 hours with the leg and the foot elevated on pillows or in a sling which supports the cast evenly. Elevation prevents swelling of the foot and leg and also constriction of the circulation.

If the child has undergone operation and a cast has been applied, upon his return to the pediatric unit the nurse must watch for evidence of impairment of circulation or sensation and bleeding, i.e., for discoloration of the cast over the wound, and report these observations to the physician. The nurse should circle the area of discoloration and write the time this was done on the cast. After operation it is necessary to change the cast about every three weeks in order to bring the foot gradually into normal

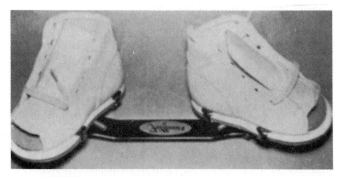

FIGURE 12–30. Denis Browne bar attached to shoes. Reverse shoes hold the infant's feet in position while sleeping. (Courtesy of F. James Funk, M.D.)

position and ensure permanent correction. When the cast is no longer needed, exercises and special orthopedic shoes may be required.

Instructions to the Parents. Before the infant is discharged from the nursery the nurse should discuss with the parents the necessity of taking the infant regularly to the clinic or to a private physician. Parents are naturally distressed at the discomfort of corrective measures. They may need encouragement to follow treatment through until all possible correction has been made and the surgeon has discharged the child. If the parents are to manipulate the foot, they should be taught by the physician and supervised in practice until they can do so correctly.

If the child is sent home from the pediatric unit in a cast, the mother and father should understand that after the position of the foot has been corrected, as shown by roentgenograms, the cast will be removed and the foot manipulated. If they have not already been taught how to do this, the physician will show them the procedure, and they should practice under his supervision or that of the nurse. The parents should be told that eventually the child will be fitted with shoes designed to correct a clubfoot and will learn to walk, but that it may be necessary for him to wear a splint on the leg and the foot at night.

After manipulation or surgery and the application of a cast (see care of a child in a cast, above) the mother and father should be told that it will be necessary to bring the child back to the surgeon for examination over a period of months. Often parents believe that operation will correct the condition without further ado.

If the family is unable to bear the expense of frequent changes of cast, special shoes, and possibly surgery, the parents should be referred to the medical social worker. Often an apparent lack of interest in returning for necessary treatment of the child may be due to financial difficulty in meeting the cost of his care.

Prognosis. The prognosis depends to a great extent upon the age of the child when treatment was begun. If the deformity is corrected in infancy, there is usually a good functional result, although exercises may have to be continued for years. The shape of the foot is not always normal in severely affected children.

DISLOCATION OF THE HIP (CONGENITAL HIP DYSPLASIA)

Etiology, Incidence, and Diagnosis. Congenital dislocations of the hip are believed to be due to lack of embryonic development of the joint. Although this seems to be true, the cause is not entirely clear. It has been suggested that heredity is a factor.

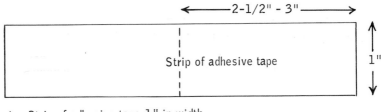

A. Strip of adhesive tape 1" in width.

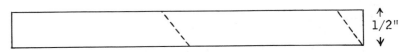

B. Strip of adhesive folded in half with the adhesive side out. Cuts are made as indicated by the broken lines approximately every 2-1/2" to 3" apart. Petals may be longer depending on the thickness of the cast.

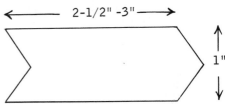

FIGURE 12–31. Method of applying adhesive petals around the edges of a cast to prevent the plaster from irritating the skin.

C. Completed petal. Petals are placed over the edge of the cast as shown in the figure below.

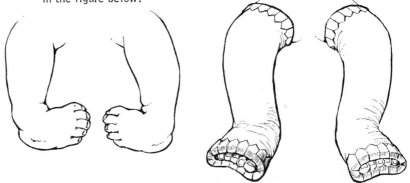

D. Bilateral talipes equinovarus before and after application of the plaster casts. Adhesive-petals have been placed around the ends of the casts.

Newborn infants seldom have a complete dislocation of the hip. Rather, the head of the femur does not lie entirely within the shallow acetabulum. When the child begins to walk, weight bearing may convert this condition to a true dislocation.

The anomaly is more frequent among girls than among boys, the ratio being seven to one.

This is one of the congenital anomalies which should be discovered in the neonate; however, if it is not, it may be found during the regular monthly examinations which every infant should have.

The initial *diagnosis* is based upon the following symptoms. The first and most reliable sign is limitation in abduction of the leg on the affected side. When the infant is lying on his back with knees and hips flexed, the normal hip joint permits the femur to be abducted until the knee almost touches the table at an angle of 90 degrees. With dislocation, abduction on the affected side is limited to no more than 45 degrees.

Pathology, Clinical Manifestations of Complete Dislocation, and Treatment. The early sign of dislocation of the hip is a shallow and extremely oblique acetabulum. The head of the femur on the affected side tends to be smaller than normal, and the ossification centers are delayed in appearance. Evidence of true dislocation is found on the roentgenogram, which shows lateral and upward dislocation of the head of the femur in relation to the acetabulum.

Signs and symptoms of complete dislocation are shortening of the leg and asymmetry of the gluteal skin folds, limited ability to abduct the leg and, when the child begins to walk, a charac-

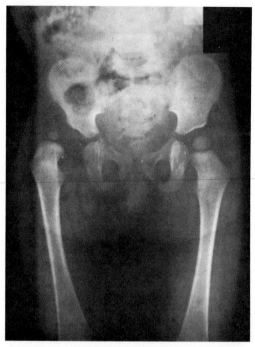

FIGURE 12–32. Untreated congenital dislocation of the right hip, demonstrating superior and lateral displacement of the underdeveloped femoral head and capital epiphysis, underdevelopment of the acetabulum, and an increase in the slope of the acetabular roof. (From Vaughan, V. C., III, and McKay, R. J. (Eds.): *Nelson Textbook of Pediatrics*, 10th ed. Philadelphia, W. B. Saunders Co., 1975.)

teristic limp. *Ortolani's sign* is present when a "click" can be felt by the examiner as the femoral head moves with Barlow's maneuver into and out of the acetabulum. *Trendelenburg's sign* is present: lowering of the normal hip when the child is placed upon the affected leg and raises the normal leg.

If the dislocation is bilateral, the gait will be waddling and lordosis will be evident. The child is likely to be late in walking.

Treatment should be started as soon as the diagnosis is made. Delay prolongs treatment and may result in conversion of a partial to a complete dislocation. The objective of treatment is to place the head of the femur within the acetabulum and by constant pressure to enlarge and deepen the socket with ultimate correction of the dislocation. This is achieved in the young infant by placing rolled cotton diapers or a pillow between his thighs, thereby keeping the knees in a froglike position. The pillow should be protected by a plastic covering over the infant's diaper or under the cotton pillow cover. The Frejka pillow splint is a more elegant modification and is easier to maintain in position. Initially Bryant traction may be ordered by some physicians to achieve abduction (see p. 565). With the older child a stiff, shell-like cast may be used which spreads his legs apart and forces the head of the femur into the acetabulum. Complete casts are not used during the first few months of life, but, when applied, will be maintained for six to nine months.

If operation is performed, an open reduction of the dislocation or repair of the defect in the acetabular shelf is done. A cast is applied after operation to hold the head of the femur in the corrected position, i.e., fitted into the socket of the acetabulum.

Responsibilities of the Nurse. The nurse is responsible for observing all newborns for abnormalities. Suspicion should be aroused by observation of asymmetric creases and limitation of abduction of the hip. When a child learns to walk, the nurse should observe him for a waddling gait and a positive Trendelenburg's sign.

If a Frejka pillow splint is ordered, the nurse must explain the purpose of the splint and demonstrate its application to the parents. They should be informed when the splint is to be worn and for what period of time it can be removed for physical care of the infant. The hips should be abducted during the application and removal of the splint. Clothing worn under the splint protects the child's skin from irritation. Sufficient pillow covers provided with the Frejka splint allow laundering. If exercises are ordered for the infant, these are also explained to the parents.

In general a child is admitted to the hospital for application of a hip spica cast. If a cast is used, it encircles the waist and extends down to the toes. The cast holds the leg in an abducted position. In bilateral and unilateral dislocation both legs are abducted and held in position by the cast.

When the child returns to the unit after having his cast applied he should be placed on a mattress covered with water-repellent material. Boards should be placed under the mattress to prevent it from sagging. The child's head should be slightly higher than his feet so that urine and stool will not soil the cast. This can be accomplished by supporting the child's head, back, and each leg with plastic-covered pillows. If the pillows are arranged properly, the heels will not rest on the mattress, and the upper part of his body will be higher than the buttocks. Another purpose of placing the child on plastic-covered pillows is to avoid pressure on the cast or denting it as it dries. The nurse, in moving or turning the child, should do so with the palms of the hands rather than the fingertips for the same reason. Depressions made in the cast may lead to pressure areas on the skin, and such irritation may lead to infection beneath the cast. Drying of the cast may be facilitated by the use of a hair dryer type of apparatus; however, this is not usually necessary.

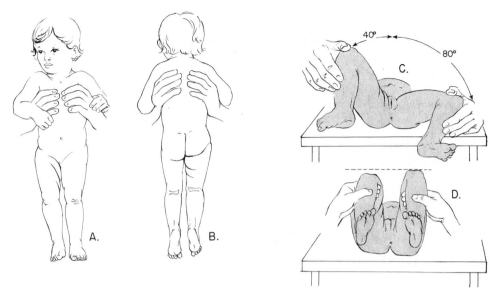

FIGURE 12–33. Physical findings in congenital dislocation of right hip. *A, B,* Asymmetry of the thigh folds, popliteal and gluteal creases with apparent shortening of the extremity on the right. *C,* Limited abduction of the right hip, *D,* Galeazzi's sign—apparent shortening of the femur as shown by the difference of the knee levels with the hips and knees flexed at right angles and the child lying on a firm table. (Courtesy of M. O. Tachdjian: *Pediatric Orthopedics.* Philadelphia, W. B. Saunders Co., 1972.)

After application of the cast, a child who is not toilet-trained may be placed on a Bradford frame (see p. 298). This helps to keep the cast clean. If ponies or blocks are used under the head of the frame, they should be placed under the child's shoulders, never directly under the head. Lower blocks should balance the ponies, and the corners of the frame should be tied to the bed to prevent its slipping. Pillows should be placed at the sides of the frame to support the child's arms. A restraining jacket and ankle restraints are used to maintain the child's position and to prevent his falling.

If the child is old enough to be continent, in order to prevent soiling the cast when a bedpan is used, a piece of plastic is tucked under the front and back edges of the opening around the buttocks and genitalia. The fracture bedpan is then slipped beneath the buttocks with the ends of the plastic strips hanging into the pan. For urination unaccompanied by stool, a male or female urinal is more convenient and comfortable than the bedpan.

The cast may be painted with white shoe polish or shellac according to the procedure adopted by the hospital. The skin around the edge of the cast is in danger of becoming excoriated. To prevent this the edges should be smoothed or lined with a waterproof material (see p. 321). "Petals" of waterproof adhesive tape, moleskin, or pieces of polyethylene plastic drapes or other substance are placed around the openings of the cast to protect the plaster and

the stockinet lining from soiling and to prevent bits of plaster from cracking off and slipping under the cast.

The perineum should be kept clean. The nurse should wash the skin under the edge of the cast whenever necessary and dry it *thoroughly.* Neither oil nor powder should be used on the skin under the cast. The opening around the buttocks and genitalia is covered with plastic material taped in place. If a diaper is necessary, it should be small and changed as soon as it is soiled.

The nurse should watch closely for signs of impaired circulation such as pallor, discoloration, or cyanosis of the skin, impaired movement, loss of sensation, edema, or temperature change in the toes. If the nurse presses on the child's toenail, normally the nail will blanch, but the color returns. Delay in the return of color indicates poor circulation. The nurse should also watch for evidence of discomfort. These indications of poor circulation are generally caused by pressure of a cast which fits too closely over some area of the extremity.

If operation has been done, the nurse watches for bleeding, and if there is evidence of hemorrhage, reports it to the physician.

Children are mischievous and are likely to slip small particles of food or anything else under the edge of the cast. It requires close observation to prevent a child from doing this, but prevention is essential, since such particles may cause irritation and possibly infection. The nurse should have frequent physical contact with the child, giving him toys too large to be pushed under his cast. The nurse should also investigate the area under the cast to make certain that no excoriations or foreign material is present. When the cast is to remain in place for a long time, the parents are instructed to "smell" the cast each day. A musty or unusual odor may indicate infection.

A hospital for acutely ill patients may have a special unit for convalescent and chronically ill children. If the child cannot be sent home, he may be placed here. Every effort should be made to give children who are not sent home as normal a life as is possible in an institution. Many of the suggestions outlined below for parents to follow are applicable to the care of the institutionalized child. Carts built for crippled children, adult wheelchairs with the back dropped and the foot raised level with the seat, or kiddie cars may be provided for children able to use them.

Guidance of the Parents After the Child's Discharge from the Hospital. Children with long-continued disabilities can be helped to lead as normal a life as possible. They should be given the means to help themselves in habilitation in all daily life activities. A large plaster cast which holds the legs in frog position is unsightly and difficult to fit into clothing, furniture, or equipment made for normal children. Practical ideas in use in many convalescent units will help the parents care for the child. Wide flaring pants extending down to the ankles may be used to cover the cast. These are made of attractive material and worn with a jacket of the same or a contrasting color. In such an outfit the child feels dressed up.

A homemade substitute serves the same purpose as the Bradford frame. It will resemble a sling in which the child's legs can extend over the edges. The canvas sling is suspended from a wooden frame. Another appliance which can be used is a stroller made of wood with openings for the legs on either side. The base must be large so that the stroller does not tip. Casters put at the corners should be large enough to permit pushing the stroller easily.

A wooden cart is often used in hospitals and convalescent units. It resembles a long wooden box mounted on a chassis which has large wheels at the top and small wheels, which pivot,

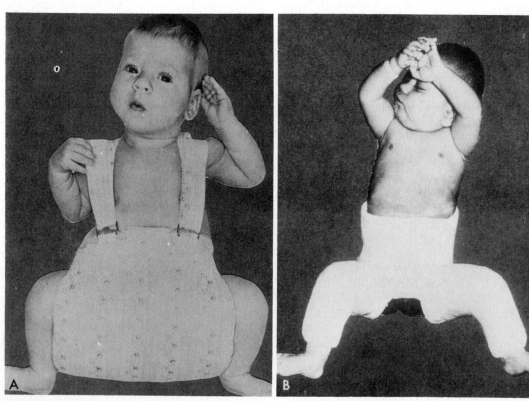

FIGURE 12–34. *A,* With a Frejka pillow splint, shown here on a 3-month-old child, the hips are not rigidly immobilized and yet are maintained in a stable position. This type of splint is particularly useful for newborn infants. *B,* With a hip spica cast the hips are in more than 90° flexion but only slight abduction. A subcutaneous adductor tenotomy has been done, and there is virtually no compression of the cartilage between the immature femoral head and the acetabulum. (Dr. R. B. Salter: *Modern Medicine,* November 17, 1969, p. 205.)

at the bottom. The cart can be pushed like a baby carriage, and the child can turn the cart so that he can look this way or that by revolving the large wheels. The cart will hold a Bradford frame the width of the child's body, but support must be provided for the legs, which extend over the side of the cart. If the child has control of urination and defecation, he may be laid upon the mattress in the cart rather than upon a Bradford frame.

Any appliance made by the parents or any technique used in his care should be checked by the physician to ensure the child's safety and to protect the cast from cracking.

If the parents take the child home before the cast is completely dry, they must be taught how to inspect the cast for cracks, dents, or breaks, how to observe the extremity and skin around the edges of the cast for signs of infection and pressure, and how to keep the cast clean.

These are long-drawn-out cases, and the final result is uncertain. All that has been said previously about the psychologic management of handicapped children should be applied in the care of these children, whether at home, in a convalescent unit, or in a hospital. Since the child will be readmitted to the hospital many times during the course of treatment, a good working relation between nurses and parents is essential or, in the clinic situation, among the parents, hospital and public health or community nurses, and social service worker.

OSTEOGENESIS IMPERFECTA

Etiology, Incidence, Diagnosis, and Clinical Manifestations. Osteogenesis imperfecta is a systemic disease due to a defect in the mesenchyme and its derivatives, a disorder that affects especially bones and ligaments. The congenital form of osteogenesis imperfecta is rare. It is an inherited disease and is characterized by ribbon-like bone shadows with numerous fractures. Fractures may occur *in utero* or during the process of birth. Minor trauma just from a change of position can result in relatively painless fractures of the bones. Many of these children are dwarfed because of multiple fractures of the long bones and compression fractures of the vertebral bodies. Children with this condition have blue scleras, poor dentition, hypermobility of the joints due to flaccid ligaments, and deafness.

Treatment and Responsibilities of the Nurse. Orthopedic management may help these children, but the condition cannot be cured. They should be kept in a state of good nutrition, and handled gently in order to prevent further fractures. Traction and immobilization may be used.

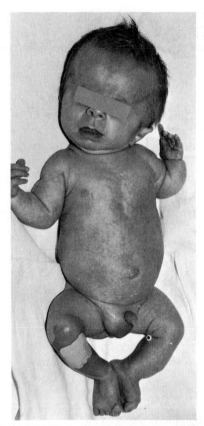

FIGURE 12–35. Osteogenesis imperfecta. Two-month-old infant, length 19 inches, with blue sclerae, inguinal hernia and hepatosplenomegaly. (From Smith, D. W.: *Recognizable Patterns of Human Malformation*, 2nd ed. Philadelphia, W. B. Saunders Co., 1976.)

Parents and child need help in coping with the difficult limitations that severely restrict the kind of physical activity that is such a large part of a child's world. Parents may need continuing support after the child is discharged from the hospital.

DEVELOPMENTAL ANOMALIES OF THE EXTREMITIES

Congenital anomalies of the extremities vary in severity from a slight defect of one extremity to an absence of a functional limb. *Polydactyly,* the presence of more than the ordinary number of digits, may be inherited as a dominant trait. *Syndactyly,* a partial or complete fusion of fingers or toes, may involve only skin, or the bones themselves may be fused. These conditions can usually be corrected by surgery.

In more severely affected infants there may be an absence of a part or all of any of the four limbs. Within the past several years such deformities became publicized because of the effect of the drug thalidomide on the embryo. The habilitation of such children is complex, involving skeletal, neuromuscular, psychologic, social,

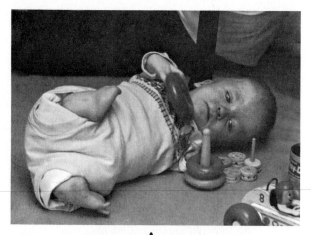

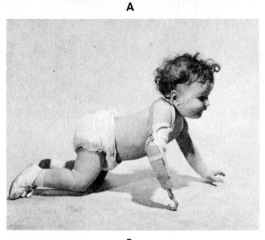

FIGURE 12–36. *A,* Born with only portions of all extremities, this young child attempts to play with his toy. (Courtesy of The National Foundation–March of Dimes.)

B, An infant with a passive hook, below-elbow prosthesis which enables him to crawl in essentially normal fashion. He may thus maintain a more normal progression of the milestones of motor development. (From Blakeslee: *The Limb Deficient Child,* University of California Press, p. 242.)

and intellectual factors. Successful treatment of such a child involves the whole medical team, including pediatrician, orthopedist, psychiatrist, psychologist, prosthetist, social worker, occupational therapist, physiotherapist, nurses, and other professional persons as needed. The parents and the child himself are of great importance in therapy if the objectives of habilitation are to be achieved.

In order for this comprehensive therapy to be successful, these children must be well motivated to learn how to use the usual prosthetic devices or the newer externally powered prostheses necessary for them to achieve independence.

If the parents see other children with amputations who are adjusted to their prostheses, they will be more likely to accept such treatment for their own child. How a parent reacts to the prosthesis often determines to a large degree how useful it will be, since the child generally adopts the attitude of his parents.

The accepted method of treatment today is to fit the child *early* with a functioning prosthesis, because this leads to more normal development and less atrophy of the parts of limbs present, and to greater patient and parent acceptance of the prosthesis. The nurse must learn how to help each patient manipulate his own prosthetic devices, since there are too many types of prostheses to be discussed here.

A congenital limb deficiency has a profound effect on the life of the afflicted child and his parents. Even professional persons may have to control their reactions to a seriously deformed child. The parents of such newborns must be told the truth about their child as soon as possible after birth even though this is a difficult thing to do. Because medical and nursing personnel may not invite further communication about such anomalies, the parents may, in addition to their feelings of guilt, feel rejected, hopeless, and helpless.

The parents and the child should be accepted by the medical team and helped to verbalize their feelings about their disappointment. They should be told about the use of prosthetic devices early so that they are realistic in their hopes for the child. With support and guidance the parents ultimately should be able to discuss the disability realistically, to accept the child's need for both independence and dependence, and to free themselves from self-blame so that they can help the child to accept his difference from other children. When the child asks about his deformity, the parents should give a simple, truthful answer such as, "You were born like that." Later he will need more detailed answers to his questions and further help with his problems. If the parents receive help with their own problems, they will be in a better position to help their child through his difficulties. If the parents' attitude toward the deformity is one of acceptance that it exists, but that it does not bar the child from living, the child and his friends will adopt this attitude also.

Special clinics have been established throughout the country for children having developmental anomalies of their extremities; however, not all states have them. The goal of every clinic for children having amputations is the same: to fit and train the child as early in his life as possible.

CLINICAL SITUATIONS

Mr. and Mrs. Jamison had moved into a moderately low-income housing area a short time before their first child, Joan, was born. Mr. Jamison planned to attend college while his 19-year-old wife looked forward to caring for her infant. Since Mrs. Jamison knew few people in her new community and had no previous experience with children, the public health nurse was asked to visit Mrs. Jamison and her five-day-old infant on their first day home from the hospital. Mrs. Jamison asked several questions.

1. "I have read about 'demand feedings' for babies. Why are these important?"
   a. "The more often you feed Joan, the better her nutritional status will be."
   b. "If you give Joan feedings every four hours, she will quickly learn correct eating habits."
   c. "If you feed Joan when she is hungry, you will be meeting her individual needs."
   d. "If you feed Joan frequently, you will not have to adhere to a rigid schedule and to plan your other household responsibilities around it."

2. "I am concerned because Joan's breasts are swollen a little even though the doctor said this was normal. What could I do about this?"
   a. "All newborn girls have breast changes to a degree. It is nothing to worry about."
   b. "Be certain to ask your doctor again about these changes. They may be important."
   c. "Some newborn infants respond in this way because of hormone activity originating from the mother. No treatment is necessary."
   d. "Fortunately few infants have this congenital condition. Be certain that you express the secretion from the breasts so that the swelling is reduced."

3. "Sometimes when I feed Joan her bottle, she has 'air on her stomach' and vomits a little formula when I place her in her crib. How can I prevent this?"
   a. "Do not give her all the formula the doctor recommended, because she is obviously eating too much."
   b. "Bubble her frequently during her feeding and especially after she has finished eating. Then place her in bed on her right side."
   c. "Bubble her frequently during her feeding and especially after she has finished eating. Then place her in bed on her left side."
   d. "Bubble her frequently during her feeding and prop her against a pillow in the corner of her crib so that it will be mechanically more difficult for her to vomit."

4. The nurse should know in discussing infant feeding with mothers that breast milk in comparison with cow's milk per volume contains
   a. More carbohydrate, less protein.
   b. More carbohydrate, more fat.
   c. More carbohydrate, more protein.
   d. More calories per ounce.

5. When the nurse was examining Joan, she realized that the infant should be referred to the physician if she had the following manifestations:

   a. Positive rooting reflex and positive sucking reflex.
   b. Positive grasping reflex and negative Chvostek's sign.
   c. Negative startle reflex and negative tonic neck reflex.
   d. Positive tonic neck reflex and positive swallowing reflex.

6. The nurse tested Joan's Moro reflex. A normal baby would respond by
   a. Sudden, generalized, symmetrical movement with the arms thrown outward in an embrace position and the legs drawn up together.
   b. Rapid movement of the arm and leg on the side where the nurse stimulated her.
   c. Slow, generalized, random activity of the whole body followed by a rigid positioning of the extremities.
   d. Rapid movement of all the extremities, but with no fixed pattern.

Mr. and Mrs. Basito had a five-year-old daughter, Dolores, when Juan was born prematurely in the emergency room of their local hospital. Since both parents had to work because of financial problems, Mrs. Basito had not taken time to visit the clinic for prenatal care. At birth Juan weighed 4 pounds 1 ounce. He was admitted to the pediatic unit and placed in an incubator.

7. The nurse regulated the temperature in the incubator on the basis of
   a. The environmental temperature of the unit.
   b. The temperature of the infant's extremities.
   c. The set temperature of 88° F. (31° C.) for all prematures.
   d. The infant's body temperature.

8. Juan had a period of apnea about three hours after delivery. The nurse, in order to stimulate his respirations since no mechanical resuscitator had been brought to his unit,
   a. Held him by his ankles with his head down and spanked him.
   b. Plunged the infant alternately into a bath basin of warm, then a basin of cool water.
   c. Carefully suctioned the infant, then gently carried out mouth-to-mouth insufflation.
   d. Gently suctioned the infant, then applied rhythmic pressure to his chest.

9. Oxygen was ordered for Juan in the usual concentration. The nurse should realize that in order to prevent retrolental fibroplasia it is important to
   a. Maintain a constant level of oxygen concentration less than 40 per cent in the incubator.
   b. Give at least 70 per cent oxygen to prevent this condition.
   c. Open the arm holes of the incubator in order to mix the oxygen with room air to prevent too high a concentration.
   d. Use an oxygen analyzer once a day to check the concentration of oxygen in the incubator.

10. A few hours after delivery Juan's skin began to be increasingly jaundiced. His bilirubin level was found to be near the critical level. A diagnosis of erythroblastosis fetalis was made. The nurse should realize that

   a. His mother was Rh-positive, his father Rh-negative.

   b. Both parents were Rh-negative.

   c. Both parents were Rh-positive.

   d. His mother was Rh-negative, his father Rh-positive.

11. An important reason why one or more exchange transfusions are done on an infant having erythroblastosis fetalis is to prevent

   a. Hemorrhagic disease of the newborn.

   b. Kernicterus.

   c. Ophthalmia neonatorum.

   d. Toxoplasmosis.

12. When Mrs. Basito was discharged from the hospital, she came to the pediatric unit to visit her son. She became emotionally disturbed when she saw the nurse feeding Juan by gavage even though the physician had told her he was doing well. The nurse could explain the reason for this procedure and reassure her by saying

   a. "I am feeding Juan this way in order to prevent infecting his mouth with a rubber nipple, since he has very little resistance to infection."

   b. "Although Juan is gaining weight well, we do not want to tire him by having him suck on a nipple."

   c. "Juan is more likely to vomit and inhale his formula if we feed him by nipple."

   d. "I am very busy. This is the quickest way I can feed Juan and be certain that he gets all his formula."

13. When Juan weighed 6 pounds, the physician discharged him from the hospital. Before discharge the nurse demonstrated the physical care he would need at home. In view of the total family situation, which comment by the mother should alert the nurse to the mother's need for further guidance?

   a. "Dolores, his sister, is so anxious to help me take care of the baby."

   b. "Poor Juan. I have caused him so much trouble. I will never let anything happen to him again."

   c. "He is such a beautiful baby! All my neighbors will want him when they see him."

   d. "My husband wanted a son so much. He has prayed each night that he would live."

Tommy Walker, who had a unilateral cleft lip, was admitted to the pediatric unit from the newborn nursery because his mother was emotionally unable to care for him at home. Mrs. Walker had previously had two infants who died at birth. Both she and her husband were distraught over Tommy's obvious defect.

14. The nurse could best help Tommy's parents adjust to their situation on admission by

   a. Placing him in a crib where other parents and children could not see him.

   b. Explaining that Tommy's deformity is really mild in comparison with others on the unit.

   c. Agreeing with the parents that Tommy's deformity is difficult to accept.

   d. Treating Tommy as a normal infant and at the same time accepting the parents' feelings of disappointment.

15. After operation on the cleft lip Tommy's parents were delighted with the results. On his tenth postoperative day his mother asked for permission to hold her baby and to try to feed him. The nurse explained that

   a. The mother could hold Tommy on her lap and feed him with a rubber-tipped medicine dropper if she did not touch the area around the suture line.

   b. Tommy should lie flat in bed during his feeding because of the possibility of injury to his lip.

   c. Only nurses were permitted to feed babies while they were hospitalized.

   d. Tommy would have to be fed by gavage for at least a few more days and that the mother would have to wait until the baby was discharged to care for him.

16. Tommy's mother asked several questions about the skin of a newborn infant. The nurse should realize that only one of the following characteristics is found in all normal infants

   a. Mongolian spots.

   b. Miliaria.

   c. Intertrigo.

   d. Good turgor.

17. Since Tommy was Mrs. Walker's first living infant, she asked the nurse several questions about his care after discharge from the hospital. She asked, "Should Tommy's mouth be wiped out each morning when I bathe him?"

   a. "Yes, in order to clean away milk curds."

   b. "No, you will probably gag the baby and cause vomiting."

   c. "Yes, cleanse the mouth with a cotton swab moistened with boric acid solution in order to prevent thrush."

   d. "No, a baby's mouth should not be cleansed except by rinsing after feedings with boiled water."

18. "How can diaper rash be prevented?"

   a. "Powder the buttocks thoroughly, particularly in the creases, when you change Tommy's diaper."

   b. "Wash his buttocks with a mild soap and water and dry thoroughly whenever you change his diaper."

   c. "Wipe the buttocks with a dry swab and oil well when he is soiled."

   d. "When you change his diaper, wipe the buttocks with oil and powder in the creases well."

GUIDES FOR FURTHER STUDY

1. Make a list of questions asked by mothers of newborns who have been admitted to the pediatric unit for treatment of congenital anomalies. Discuss your answers to these specific questions in seminar.

2. List the specific differences between fetal and postnatal circulation. If expected changes do not occur at or after birth, which congenital heart lesion would result? What clinical manifestations of these conditions could you observe?

3. Observe a group of normal newborns for common traits and for individual differences in relation to sleep, i.e., bodily movements, facial grimaces, sucking activity, and reactions to hunger. Discuss your observations in seminar.

4. Discuss in seminar differences in practices of various religious and cultural groups in relation to the care of newborns.

5. Help an individual mother plan a 24-hour program of care for a normal newborn infant. What difficulties are encountered?

6. A newborn having a meningomyelocele is being discharged from the nursery. He will be admitted to the pediatric unit of another hospital in two weeks for operation. Help the mother plan a program of care for this infant at home. During your discussion note the mother's attitude toward this infant. What could you do or recommend in addition to helping her plan for his physical care that would assist her in adjusting emotionally to this situation?

7. How do you imagine you would feel if you discovered that you were Rh-negative? What thoughts would you have and what medical supervision and treatment would you expect for yourself and your future family?

8. A high school friend of yours has confided to you that she is planning marriage. She knows that her first cousin was diagnosed as having Down's syndrome when he was born. She is concerned about the possibility that she may have a mentally retarded child also. What guidance could you give your friend in order to reduce her anxiety?

TEACHING AIDS AND OTHER INFORMATION*

American Academy of Pediatrics

The Pediatrician and the Child with Mental Retardation.

The American Cancer Society, Inc.

Cancer Source Book for Nurses.
Nursing Problems of Children with Cancer.

American Heart Association

If Your Child Has a Congenital Heart Defect.
Innocent Heart Murmurs in Children.

Mead Johnson & Company

Berkowitz, S.: Steps in Habilitation—For the Cleft Lip and Palate Child, 1971.
Berkowitz, S.: The Road to Normalcy—For the Cleft Lip and Palate Child, 1971.

Muscular Dystrophy Associations of America, Inc.

Chart of Differential Diagnostic Characteristics of the Primary Diseases Affecting the Neuromuscular Unit.
Patient and Community Services Program.

National Association for Retarded Citizens

Beck, H. L.: The Advantages of a Multi-Purpose Clinic for the Mentally Retarded.
Dybwad, G.: The Mentally Handicapped Child Under Five.
Facts on Mental Retardation, Revised 1973.
Feeding Mentally Retarded Children.
Hunt, J. M. V.: How Children Develop Intellectually.
Into the Light of Learning.
Mather, J.: Make the Most of Your Baby.
Perske, R. A.: New Directions for Parents of Persons Who Are Retarded.

Pitt, D.: Your Down's Syndrome Child.
Schreiber, M., Feeley, M., and O'Neill, J.: Siblings of the Retarded.
Stabler, E. M.: Primer for Parents of a Mentally Retarded Child.
Stimson, C. W.: Understanding the Mongoloid Child.
Waskowitz, C. H.: The Parents of Retarded Children Speak for Themselves.

National Kidney Foundation

How Can Urinary Tract Obstruction Affect You?

United States Government

Antenatal Diagnosis and Down's Syndrome, 1974.
Children Served in Mental Retardation Clinics—Fiscal Years 1970–1972, 1973.
Congenital Malformations Surveillance, 1975.
Facts About Mongolism for Women Over 35, 1974.
International MCH Projects: Research to Improve Health Services for Mothers and Children, 1975.
Muscular Dystrophy: Hope Through Research, Revised 1968.
Research to Improve Health Services for Mothers and Children, 1974.
Services for Crippled Children, Reprinted 1975.
Studies in Handicapping Conditions: Research to Improve Health Services for Mothers and Children, 1975.
The Child with a Missing Arm or Leg, Reprinted 1970.

*Complete addresses are given in the Appendix.

REFERENCES

Books

Ferguson, A. B. (Ed.): *Orthopaedic Surgery in Infancy and Childhood.* 4th ed. Baltimore, Williams & Wilkins Company, 1975.
Fink, B. W.: *Congenital Heart Disease.* Chicago, Year Book Medical Publishers, Inc., 1975.

Grossman, W. (Ed.): *Cardiac Catheterization and Angiography.* Philadelphia, Lea & Febiger, 1974.
Hallman, G. L., and Cooley, D. A.: *Surgical Treatment of Congenital Heart Disease,* 2nd ed. Philadelphia, Lea & Febiger, 1975.

Kelikian, H.: *Congenital Deformities of the Hand and Forearm.* Philadelphia, W. B. Saunders Company, 1974.

Koch, R., and De La Cruz, F. F. (Eds.): *Down's Syndrome (Mongolism): Research Prevention and Management.* New York, Brunner/Mazel Publishing Company, 1975.

Milunsky, A.: *Prevention of Genetic Disease and Mental Retardation.* Philadelphia, W. B. Saunders Company, 1975.

Moller, J. H.: *Essentials of Pediatric Cardiology.* Philadelphia, F. A. Davis Company, 1973.

Moschella, S. L., Pillsbury, D. M., and Hurley, H. J., Jr.: *Dermatology.* Philadelphia, W. B. Saunders Company, 1975.

Mustarde, J. C. (Ed.): *Plastic Surgery in Infancy and Childhood.* Philadelphia, W. B. Saunders Company, 1971.

Pochedly, C., and Miller, D. (Eds.): *Wilms' Tumor.* New York, John Wiley & Sons, Inc., 1976.

Royer, P., Habib, R., Mathieu, H., and Broyer, M.: *Pediatric Nephrology.* Philadelphia, W. B. Saunders Company, 1974.

Rudolph, A. M.: *Congenital Diseases of the Heart.* Chicago, Year Book Medical Publishers, Inc., 1974.

Smith, D. W., and Wilson, A. C.: *The Child with Down's Syndrome (Mongolism): For Persons Concerned With His Education and Care.* Philadelphia, W. B. Saunders Company, 1973.

Smith, J. F.: *Pediatric Neuropathology.* New York, McGraw-Hill Book Company, 1974.

Strong, W. B., Levy, M., Tompkins, D., and Adams, M. J.: *An Introduction to Pediatric Cardiology.* Springfield, Ill., Charles C Thomas, 1975.

Sutow, W. W., Vietti, T., and Fernbach, D. J. (Eds.): *Clinical Pediatric Oncology.* St. Louis, The C. V. Mosby Company, 1973.

van Niekerk, W. A.: *True Hermaphroditism.* New York, Harper & Row, 1974.

Vince, D. J.: *Essentials of Pediatric Cardiology.* Philadelphia, J. B. Lippincott Company, 1974.

Weinberg, S., and Shapiro, L.: *Color Atlas of Pediatric Dermatology.* New York, McGraw-Hill Book Company, 1974.

Wells, C. G.: *Cleft Palate and its Associated Speech Disorders.* New York, McGraw-Hill Book Company, 1971.

Young, B. W.: *Lower Urinary Tract Obstruction in Childhood.* Philadelphia, Lea & Febiger, 1972.

Periodicals

Aisenberg, R. B., Wolff, P. H., Rosenthal, A., and Nadas, A.: Psychological Impact of Cardiac Catheterization. *Pediatrics,* 51:1051, June 1973.

Beck, M.: Attitudes of Parents of Pediatric Heart Patients Toward Patient Care Units. *Nursing Research,* 22:334, July-August 1973.

Bliss, V. J.: Sharing Another's Death. *Nursing '76,* 6:30, April 1976.

Braney, M. L.: The Child with Hydrocephalus. *Am. J. Nursing,* 73:828, May 1973.

Condon, M. R.: The Cardiac Child: What His Parents Need to Know. *Nursing '73,* 3:60, October 1973.

Clarkson, P. M., and Orgill, A. A.: Continuous Murmurs in Infants of Low Birth Weight. *J. Pediatr.,* 84:208, February 1974.

Cogswell, J. J., Hatch, D. J., Kerr, A. A., and Taylor, B.: Effects of Continuous Positive Airway Pressure on Lung Mechanics of Babies After Operation for Congenital Heart Disease. *Arch. Dis. Child,* 50:799, October 1975.

Culp, O. S.: Anomalies of Male Genitalia. *Medical Aspects of Human Sexuality,* 8:126, September 1974.

Donahoe, P. K., and Hendren, W. H.: Evaluation of the Newborn with Ambiguous Genitalia. *Pediat. Clin. N. Am.,* 23:361, May 1976.

Donley, D. L.: The Immune System: Nursing the Patient Who Is Immunosuppressed. *Am. J. Nursing,* 76:1619, October 1976.

Durand, B.: A Clinical Nursing Study: Failure to Thrive in a Child With Down's Syndrome. *Nursing Research,* 24:272, July-August 1975.

Erickson, M. P.: Talking With Fathers of Young Children With Down's Syndrome. *Children Today,* 3:22, November-December 1974.

Gayton, W. F., and Walker, L.: Down Syndrome: Informing the Parents. *Am. J. Dis. Child,* 127:510, April 1974.

Golden, D. A., and Davis, J. G.: Counseling Parents After the Birth of an Infant With Down's Syndrome. *Children Today,* 3:7, March-April 1974.

Gomez, M. R., and Reese, D. F.: Computed Tomography of the Head in Infants and Children. *Pediat. Clin. N. Am.,* 23:473, August 1976.

Hilt, N. E.: Care of the Child in a Hip Spica Cast. *RN,* 39:27, April 1976.

Jenkin, R. D. T.: The Treatment of Wilms' Tumor. *Pediat. Clin. N. Am.,* 23:147, February 1976.

Lavoie, D., Lierman, C. J., Fletcher, A. B., and Corbett, D.: Spina Bifida: Immediate Concerns.... Long-Term Goals. *Nursing '73,* 3:43, October 1973.

McElroy, C.: Caring for the Untreated Infant. *The Canadian Nurse,* 71:26, December 1975.

McFarlane, J.: Congenital Adrenal Hyperplasia. *Am. J. Nursing,* 76:1290, August 1976.

Maguire, D. C.: Death by Chance, Death by Choice. *Nursing Digest,* 2:36, October 1974.

Miezio, P.: Care of the Child with Myelomeningocele: An Overview. *Nursing Digest,* 1:45, November 1973.

Nysather, J. O., Katz, A. E., and Lenth, J. L.: The Immune System: Its Development and Functions. *Am. J. Nursing,* 76:1614, October 1976.

Park, I. J.: Vaginal Anomalies. *Medical Aspects of Human Sexuality,* 7:88, December 1973.

Passo, S. D.: Positioning Infants with Myelomeningocele. *Am. J. Nursing,* 74:1658, September 1974.

Penfold, K. M.: Supporting Mother Love. *Am. J. Nursing,* 74:464, March 1974.

Posey, R. A.: Creative Nursing Care of Babies With Heart Disease. *Nursing '74,* 4:40, October 1974.

Potter, A. E.: Psychiatric Nursing: A Human Experience. *Nursing Forum,* 13:157, 1974.

Raimondi, A. J., and Soare, P.: Intellectual Development in Shunted Hydrocephalic Children. *Am. J. Dis. Child,* 127:664, May 1974.

Ralis, Z. A.: Traumatizing Effects of Breech Delivery on Infants With Spina Bifida. *J. Pediatr.,* 87:613, October 1975.

Rowe, R. D., and others: Long-Term Management of Heart Defects. *Pediat. Clin. N. Am.,* 21:841, November 1974.

Saxen, I.: Epidemiology of Cleft Lip and Palate. An Attempt to Rule Out Chance Correlations. *Br. J. Prev. Soc. Med.,* 29:103, June 1975.

Schanche, D. A.: Two Facial Handicaps That Can be Conquered. *Today's Health,* 52:52, November 1974.

Schantz, Sr. M. E.: A Time to be Born: The Story of Mark. *JOGN Nursing,* 5:50, May-June 1976.

Scott, C. I., and Thomas, G. H.: Genetic Disorders Associated with Mental Retardation: Clinical Aspects. *Pediat. Clin. N. Am.,* 20:121, February 1973.

Stark, G. D.: Drummond, M. B., Poneprasert, S., and Robarts, F. H.: Primary Ventriculo-Peritoneal Shunts in Treatment of Hydrocephalus Associated with Myelomeningocele. *Arch. Dis. Child,* 49:112, February 1974.

Strangway, A., Fowler, R., Cunningham, K., and Hamilton, J. R.: Diet and Growth in Congenital Heart Disease. *Pediatrics,* 57:75, January 1976.

Waechter, E. H.: Developmental Consequences of Congenital Abnormalities. *Nursing Forum,* 14:108, April-May-June 1975.

Watt, R. C.: Urinary Diversion. *Am. J. Nursing,* 74:1806, October 1974.

Wise, D. J.: Crisis Intervention Before Cardiac Surgery. *Am. J. Nursing,* 75:1316, August 1975.

AUDIOVISUAL MEDIA*

The American Cancer Society, Inc.

Meeting Highlights: The American Cancer Society's National Conference on Childhood Cancer
Album with 2 standard C-60 audio cassettes.
The participants discuss the progress being made in the diagnosis and treatment of childhood cancer. Topics include: environmental, immunologic, genetics, and familial factors involved; management of Wilms' tumor, neuroblastoma, and other abdominal tumors; role of surgery, chemotherapy, radiation therapy, and immunotherapy; diagnosis and treatment of brain tumors; radiation therapy of central nervous system tumors; treatment of Hodgkin's disease and lymphomas; etiology, diagnosis, and treatment of leukemia.

The American Journal of Nursing Company

Care of Patients with Neurologic Conditions
2 filmstrips, 2 audio-tape cassettes, study guides.
Volume I: Anatomy and Physiology; Pathophysiology; Routine Diagnostic Tests; Special Diagnostic Tests; Increased Intracranial Pressure. This volume presents the essential anatomy and physiology of the central nervous system and diagnostic tests of the central nervous system.

Pediatric-Mental Health Nursing
44 minutes, black and white.
The Mentally Retarded Child (Down's Syndrome), Instructor: Brodie, B.
Introduces a child with Down's syndrome and discusses with his parents his growth and development patterns and associated problems.

Pediatric Nursing Series
44 minutes each, 16mm film or videotape, sound, instructor's guide and student syllabus.

The Child with an Orthopedic Anomaly
Participating Instructor: Lee, J.
Three conditions are emphasized: clubfoot, dislocated hip, and scoliosis. Clinical manifestations, pathology, diagnosis, and treatment of all three are discussed. Emphasis is on nursing care, especially after surgery.

The Child with a Neurological Condition
Three distinct conditions are emphasized; subdural hematoma, hydrocephalus, and spina bifida. For these neurological problems pathology, etiology, clinical manifestations, diagnosis, treatment, and prognosis are discussed.

The Mentally Retarded Child
Participating Instructor: Vuillemot, L. D.
A description is given of the child with Down's syndrome. Growth and development patterns, with associated problems, are discussed in an interview with the parents.

The Child with a Heart Condition
Participating Instructor: Miller, R.
The roles of nurses and physicians are described in diagnosis, criteria for and discussion of diagnostic tests, explanation of surgical procedures for three common heart defects, and the problems of rearing a child who has a heart defect.

The Child Who Undergoes Open-Heart Surgery
The progress of a young boy admitted for surgery is followed. Preoperative tests and teaching, cardiac catheterization, immediate postoperative stages, and return of normal activity are included. The nurse's role in caring for the child is outlined.

Cleft Lip and Palate
Participating Instructor: Elliot, C.
Description of cleft lip and palate including embryogen-esis, etiology, variations, and surgical correction. The child's problems in communication, eating, and oral hygiene are discussed. An interview is shown between speech therapist Dr. Elliott, and a teenage girl who demonstrates palate prosthesis and speech.

Charles Press — Prentice-Hall, Inc.

Nursing Skills and Techniques Series
2–5 minutes, Super-8mm filmloop, color, guide.
Pediatric Restraints: Arm Cuff and Crib Net. Demonstration of two types of restraint commonly used in pediatrics.

CIBA

Open-Heart Surgery
Distributor: Association Films, Inc.
57½ minutes, 16mm film, black and white.
An operation for repair of an interatrial septal defect in an eight-year-old boy.

CIBA and Wayne State University

Gait and Musculoskeletal Disorders
Green, W.
34 minutes, film.
Stance and swing phases of normal gait are covered along with associated arm movements. Abnormal gait due to pain, structural defect, and muscular disorders are considered. Polio patients illustrate gluteus medius and gluteus maximus limp, foot drop, quadriceps weakness. Scissors gait of cerebral palsy, muscular dystrophy and dystonia musculorum is also shown. Hip considered last with congenital dislocation, degenerative disease of hip, and slipped femoral epiphysis.

Introduction to Speech Problems
Darley, F. L., and Van Riper, C.
27 minutes.
Twelve patients with problems of speech-sound mastery, stuttering, cleft palate, speech retardation, aphasia, and dysarthria are presented. They point out not only the problems involved in speech, but also what can be done to help through speech therapy, surgical procedures, and speech appliances.

The Face — Part II
Myers, J. D.
33 minutes.
The physical diagnostic signs as related to edema and color change are seen. The pathophysiological mechanism causing the diagnostic sign is described. Patients with congenital defects with typical facies such as trisomy, missing chromosomes, etc., are presented.

Film & Videotape Library, National Institute on Mental Retardation, Canada

Kindergarten
Produced by: Communications Resources Division of the National Institute on Mental Retardation.
20 minutes, videotape, black and white.
The integration of children with handicaps into regular childhood education programs in Canada, and the effects on the handicapped child, the other children, and the teachers. Depicts the experiences of a child with Down's syndrome who attends a normal kindergarten class, and points out that integration is beneficial to all concerned.

J. B. Lippincott Company

Cardiac Auscultation
8 of a total of 18, each of which is made up of a booklet, a film, an audiocassette, and a set of slides.

Auscultation and the Normal Heart
Atrial Septal Defect
Ventricular Septal Defect
Fallot's Tetralogy
Pulmonary Valve Stenosis
Coarctation of the Aorta
Persistent Ductus Arteriosus
Transposition of the Great Arteries

New York University Medical Center, Institute of Physical Medicine and Rehabilitation

Congenital Anomalies of the Extremities
86 minutes, sound.
Reviews the problems of a child born without an extremity or parts of extremities. Discusses prostheses, schooling, and adaptation to living.

W. B. Saunders Company

Pediatric Cardiology
Schmidt, R., and Khoury, G. H.
35mm filmstrip totaling 145 frames, two tape cassettes, color, booklet.
A combination of line drawings, photographs, and actual taped auscultatory findings assist recognition of both rare and common pediatric heart disorders. In two units: *Cardiac Examination of the Child,* covering all aspects of the initial encounter from history-taking to specific diagnostic techniques, and *Rheumatic Fever in Children,* a full discussion of the subject.

Pediatric Conferences with Sydney Gellis
Treatment of Hemangiomas, Gellis, S.

Trainex Corporation

Abnormal Sexual Development
35mm filmstrip, audio-tape cassette, 33 1/3 LP, color.
Color photographs depict the specific physical characteristics of these abnormalities. Actual case histories, diagnoses, and treatments are given for the various abnormalities. Abnormalities covered in the filmstrip include precocious development, intersexuality, and delayed or incomplete development. Examples of adrenal hyperplasia, virilizing tumors, and asymmetric gonadal dysgenesis are shown. The filmstrip also includes a portion on surgical correction of external genitalia.

Baby Cries
35mm filmstrip, audio-tape cassettes, 33 1/3 LP, color.
An interview with Dr. Murray Feingold, specialist in the diagnosis of congenital abnormalities, who correlates detailed case histories with his personal tape collection of infant cries.

Pediatric Abdominal Surgery
35mm filmstrip, audio-tape cassettes, 33 1/3 LP, color.
Surgical abdominal problems of infancy covered in this filmstrip program include hernias, ectopic testes, atresia of the vas, hydroceles, testicular tumors, hydrometrocolpos, ovarian masses, Wilms' tumors, neuroblastomas, hepatic lesions and tumors, hamartomas, omental cysts, splenic cysts, neurofibromas, fibrosarcomas, and rhabdomyosarcomas. Color photographs depict these pediatric abdominal abnormalities and illustrate surgical management and techniques used to correct them. Diagnostic x-rays are included.

°Complete addresses are given in the Appendix.

UNIT THREE

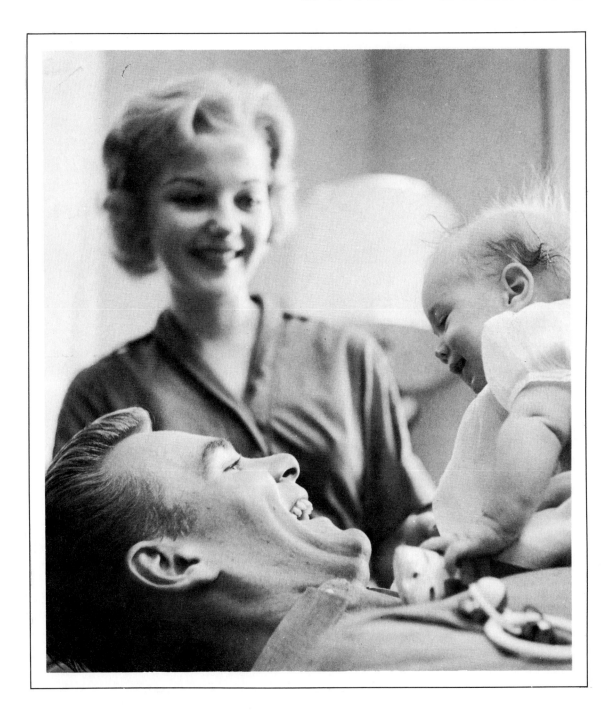

THE INFANT

TO MISS CHARLOTTE PULTENEY

Timely blossom, infant fair,
Fondling of a happy pair,
Every morn, and every night,
Their solicitous delight,
Sleeping, waking, still at ease,
Pleasing, without skill to please . . .

Ambrose Philips (1675?–1749)

Chapter Thirteen

An infant is someone who becomes a child and then an adolescent, passing through his parents' lives and disappearing into an adult, a full-fledged person, with a life and a future all his own. No one can slow this process at any point in time.

The care and development of the infant throughout the first year of life are considered in this unit. As with the newborn, his emotional and physical status and his needs in health and in sickness are discussed.

Just as growth and development occur in the child, so also must the process of development occur in his parents as they keep pace with his natural maturation. During the first year of an infant's life the parents must learn the cues, what the child is trying to tell them, and then act on their observations. They must learn to observe their infant's behavior and to act toward fulfilling his needs. Some parents unfortunately are not prepared to undergo the emotional development needed in relation to their child's development. These are the parents who particularly need help in understanding the usual steps in a child's development. Nurses many times can interpret this process to parents and thus alleviate much of their misunderstanding.

Parents also need help in becoming more flexible and adaptable in meeting their child's needs. Parents are influenced by the child each of them was in the past. It is not easy to change each parent's view of his or her own background experiences. Some parents retain within themselves the children they used to be and see things as though their past home situations still existed. At the same time they are also looking at the same events through an accumulation of adult experiences. Parents then see their children as they would a blurred photograph, using a camera which is out of focus. The phases through which a parent should progress as the child grows will be discussed in appropriate chapters throughout this text.

THE NORMAL INFANT: GROWTH, DEVELOPMENT AND CARE DURING THE FIRST YEAR

Stress must be placed on the fact that spontaneity and enjoyment of the infant by the adult are probably of greater significance than the specific procedures used in his care. If the parent or the nurse is particularly harassed and overburdened, care will not be beneficial for the infant. At such times some kindly support or temporary relief from the pressure may be necessary.

OVERVIEW OF THE INFANT'S EMOTIONAL DEVELOPMENT

The nurse should understand a child's developmental needs and should know how to respond to them so that he may continue to grow emotionally and physically while he is in the hospital as he would at home. This is particularly important with infants and young children because separation from their parents, in itself, produces problems with which they need help.

SENSE OF TRUST

As was stated earlier (see p. 44), different components of the healthy personality develop at various periods in the process of growing up. The first of these, and probably the most important, is the *sense of trust,* which normally develops in the first year of life. It is, of course, strengthened or weakened by experiences after that age, but the foundation is laid in infancy. If this sense of trust in others is not learned, the reverse, *a sense of mistrust,* is acquired. This tendency will be increasingly difficult to change as the infant enters childhood. A distrustful child is not friendly, and his attitude evokes a similar response in adults and other children.

During the first year the infant is completely dependent upon his mother or someone who is a temporary substitute for her such as his father, siblings, baby-sitters, or grandparents. His preference will probably be for his mother.

During the first six months the concept of mutual regulation between mother and infant, especially as it applies to feeding, must be established if the infant is to trust in his mother. The mother needs support from her husband and others in her environment in order to be able to provide the closeness to her infant which is essential to the development of trust.

The infant's earliest approach to life is *incorporative,* as shown in his wanting to put everything into his mouth, to make it a part of himself. If this need is satisfied, he has laid the foundation for *giving* as well as *receiving.*

Turning to his mother or her substitute for comfort and love is the first evidence of an infant's desire to *turn outward* for pleasure. His interest is no longer solely in physical sensations which he himself produces (sucking his fingers, sucking at the breast or on the nipple of his bottle, kicking, stretching, and the like) or which someone provides for him (the comfort of having his diaper changed or his warm bath). The growing infant learns very slowly that *people* give care which he enjoys and so learns to turn to them for relief of tensions.

The sense of trust does not develop independently of other aspects of growth. Initially it is based on consistently similar events such as the occurrence of hunger and the receiving of the proper feeding. If the feedings are not sufficient or are improperly given, the infant will begin to establish a sense of mistrust. Trust is an integral part of his total development. An infant learns to trust others through the relief of his basic needs; i.e., he learns to trust those who give him pleasant sensations. The young infant does not differentiate his body from that of others who handle him. He likes the warm feeding in his mouth, but does not differentiate his mother's hand upon the bottle from his own fingers. Later, when he has learned the limits of his body and knows in a vague way that he is a separate organism, he will respond to his mother's presence. *He has learned to associate her care and caresses with her.* He smiles and coos when he sees her, for he knows that something pleasant will happen to him. He has learned to trust his mother and has laid the foundation for trusting other people.

If, however, someone speaks to him in a harsh tone or is sudden and spasmodic in his movements, the infant is frightened. He has received his first lesson in *mistrusting* others. If this happens often, he is likely to grow uneasy and apprehensive. This may happen especially if the infant's parents are under considerable tension and anxiety in their marital relations. If such is the case, they may need marriage counseling or psychiatric care in order to prevent later severe mental illness characterized by mistrust in their child. *The sense of trust is indeed the cornerstone of a wholesome personality.*

Either a harmonious relationship of giving and getting is established or disruption occurs and other modes of behavior predominate in the infant, such as feeding difficulties and excessive crying. Instead of mutual satisfaction there is mutual frustration between mother and infant.

During the second six months the infant becomes capable of recognition of and response to others. He changes from a basically passive being to a more actively taking individual, watching his mother with his eyes, reaching out for her or crawling after her.

During this period the infant also learns to *bite.* The first teeth erupt between the fifth and seventh months, and he quickly learns to use them. Having experienced the world through food, the infant bites down on anything he draws into his mouth. He gradually becomes aware that if he clamps his mouth on the nipple it is taken away, or if he bites when teething it hurts him. The infant then learns that sometimes discomfort occurs when he trusts. He therefore has a conflict: to trust and possibly to be hurt or to mistrust. If the infant is basically trusting, he may maintain his urge and motivation to proceed to try new behaviors even though there are frustrations.

As he develops he becomes increasingly aware of himself as a separate organism. His mother, thinking that he is less dependent upon her, is likely to leave him more to himself while she resumes activities which she enjoyed before his birth. If she intends to resume employment outside the home, she wants to accustom the infant gradually to her absence. She leaves him alone while she does her housework. Although she has always done this, the infant while very young slept the greater part of the time, but now is awake and alone.

Toward the end of the first year a crisis develops around the adjustment which mother and infant make to their changed relations. The infant's successful adjustment depends less on the amount of time his mother now spends with him than on the *quality* of their relations during his first six months and while the crisis is being resolved. Another factor in his adjustment is the continuity of care from other members of the family, especially the father, which formerly supplemented that of his mother.

DEVELOPMENT OF SEXUALITY IN INFANCY

Sexual differences in human beings do not emerge suddenly when children reach puberty. Children are prepared for their sexual roles from birth to adulthood through a *process of socialization.*

There is a question about how much the behavioral differences between female and male persons are determined by genetic mechanisms (see p. 214) and how much by indoctrination. Learning is certainly important for feminine-masculine differentiation. The infant seems to induce its own gender role learning. The mother gets the original message about the newborn's sex from the genitalia at birth. She then creates a specific gender response early in the infant's life: the mother talks more to a female infant because the female infant is more responsive to words. This stimulates the mother to talk even more, so that the little girl develops an earlier and greater verbal aptitude than boys. Also, female infants apparently relate more intently to faces than males do. The infant girl thus molds the mother-infant relationship and the "pleasing cycle" between them. The mother also modifies the response cycle by responding further to gender cues by building certain hopes depending on the sex of the infant. The mother promotes, develops, or represses specific gender attitudes, thus contributing to later sex-specific conduct.

Sexual development follows biologic growth in the child. The young infant has practically undifferentiated sensuosity. Through touch he receives bodily delight from the total surface of his own skin and from proprioceptive sensations such as warmth, cuddling, caressing, and stroking. Later rolling, rocking, and squirming produce similar body sensations. The holding and cuddling of an infant play an important role in the subsequent sexual development of the individual. Male or female, both sexes want to be held and cuddled as adults and as adults will demonstrate love through this activity. Children who have been inadequately held and fondled will, as older children and adults, suffer from an affect-hunger for such attention.

Also, the source of bodily pleasure becomes concentrated in zones around the mucocutaneous junctions. These erotogenic zones displace one another in sequence as the child matures. Initially, the infant's erotogenic zone is the *mouth.* Activities such as sucking at the breast, drinking, and eating are pleasurable stimuli, as are sucking a pacifier and fingersucking. Orgasm-like responses can occur as a result of vigorous and excessive mouth stimulation in infancy.

The quality of the physical intimacy during breast-feeding, bathing, and other bodily contact between mother and child reflects the feelings of the mother concerning intimacy itself. Each contact with the child is an opportunity for him to experience the pleasures of intimacy. Tenderly handled, an infant acquires good feelings about himself and his body. If the mother is afraid of being close to another person, the child, even the infant, will sense the fear and feel it as rejection. When this occurs it will be reflected in every kind and degree of avoidance and mistrust of physical closeness. Mothers who observe obsessive cleanliness in caring for their infants often produce children who fear touching their own bodies. This prohibition interferes greatly with sexual awakening later in life.

Excluding anatomical defects and faulty biologic development, sexual health is dependent almost entirely on emotional factors.

NEEDS DURING THE FIRST YEAR

Although the infant's need to put everything into his mouth and later to bite was given priority among his essential needs because of its great psychologic importance, he has five other needs which must be met if he is to learn to trust the people about him: *feeding, sucking pleasure, warmth and comfort, both love and security, and sensory stimulation.*

NEED FOR FEEDING

The infant's world is small. He has no sense of time and lives entirely in the moment. The only rhythms he knows are those set up by his physiologic mechanism. He experiences hunger, which produces tension. He soon learns that people around him can satisfy this need and reduce his tension—make him comfortable—and that this is done with varying emotional attitudes on their part. This is a time for showing him love and affection.

An infant can receive the warmth and comfort from his mother when he is bottle-fed as when he is breast-fed if she holds him closely during feeding. Nurses are sometimes criticized for the professionally unemotional attitude they show when feeding hospitalized infants. This is unfortunate, since infants sense a lack of warmth and spontaneity. The mother's attitude or that of her substitute is expressed in voice, touch, and handling the infant while he is nursing. He associates this attitude with being fed and later on with food.

NEED FOR SUCKING PLEASURE

The infant's habit of putting fingers and toys into his mouth is closely allied to his pleasure in sucking. The need for sucking, however, is quite apart from the need for food. He thoroughly enjoys the act of sucking, and if he does not have the opportunity for it, tension results. Giving him something to suck on relieves the tension, and he promptly relaxes. Being put to the breast or held lovingly with the nipple of his bottle between his lips and the milk in his mouth is his first experience of love and comfort. The intensity of the sucking urge varies and is an example of individual differences in children.

During the second six months he may bite upon the nipple. If he is at the breast, this hurts his mother even if his teeth have not erupted. If the baby bites on the nipple while breast feeding, this can usually be corrected by the mother by using a breast shield for protection or removing the breast immediately. Thus he may learn not to bite. The mother may still, however, think of weaning him. If this is done and he is taught to drink from a cup before he has outgrown the need for sucking, he will suck upon anything else he can use for the purpose. If he wants to bite, he should be given a piece of toast or a suitable toy. The intensity of the urge to find satisfaction through sucking and biting gradually decreases as other gratifications become available.

NEED FOR WARMTH AND COMFORT

An infant enjoys the warmth and softness of his mother's body when held in her arms. He has a real hunger for this pleasant experience. He enjoys rhythmic rocking, being handled, and the comfort of having his position changed.

NEED FOR LOVE AND SECURITY

Just as the infant becomes hungry, is fed, and becomes relaxed, repeating the rhythm over and over, so he needs a rhythm of attention shown in bathing him, riding in the stroller, being played with, being cuddled close to his mother's body and being put to sleep. Throughout these activities of daily living he needs a feeling of security, of being wanted and loved. Infants are not consciously apprehensive about the future, but their daily care is the basis for either serenity or a tenseness which in an adult we would call apprehension or generalized anxiety.

NEED FOR SENSORY STIMULATION

The newborn infant first communicates with his environment through contact with his mother's body and the touch of other hands of persons who care. Later his perception of the world is based on his tactile and other sensory experiences. The infant also learns to communicate with himself by exploring his own body and thus gradually develops his own body image.

Research during the past several years has shown that sensory stimulation is necessary for the immature organism if the sensory organs and nerve fibers especially are to develop normally. Even the adult, if isolated from his environment for a prolonged period of time, will have disturbances of his thought processes, his problem solving ability and his perceptual ability. Infants and children are even more dependent on the environment than are adults for sensory stimulation.

Human beings learn to a varying degree throughout life. Research has been done recently in an attempt to identify critical periods when there is an optimum time for sensory experience to be of maximum value for learning. The desired learning, either quantitatively or qualitatively, may be reduced either before or after the time during which the stimulation of the environment has its most profound effects. Perhaps the critical period for any kind of learning is when the various motor, sensory, and psychologic capacities are combined with the motivation of the individual to learn.

Infants need to be stimulated by a change of environment, by a change in position, by contact with various textures of materials, by sights and sounds, and by human contact. If they do not receive such stimulation in their daily care, they will not grow and develop normally. The need for sensory stimulation can be met by a loving mother who takes her infant with her as she moves through her daily routine, who talks and sings to him as she cuddles him, and who gradu-

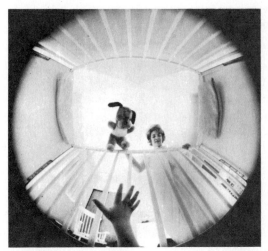

FIGURE 13-1. The infant's view from the center of his world. (Courtesy of Mr. Jack Tinney and *Baby Talk Magazine*, April 1967.)

ally introduces him to wider and more varied learning experiences and activities.

Methods of Meeting the Needs

Meeting the infant's needs is an interrelated process which begins immediately after birth. The infant's communication with the outside world is normally through his mother.

Breast feeding meets many needs simultaneously. The infant is held close to his mother and has the comfort of taking as little or as much as he wants. Many physicians believe that the breast can be given to comfort the infant even if he is not hungry.

If the infant is bottle-fed, he should be held in the same position as the infant at the breast. If the mother accepts the idea of a self-demand schedule (see p. 167), the infant will establish his own feeding rhythm. The holes in the nipple should be of such a size that two or more hours of sucking a day are required for him to take his entire feeding. *Bottles should never be propped*, because propping does not fulfill the basic needs of an infant and may produce a life-threatening situation if the infant chokes and aspirates his formula.

If his basic needs are met, an infant cannot be spoiled in early infancy. His mother should go to him if he is uncomfortable — wet, cold, or tired of lying in the same position. Spoiling does not result from his being kept comfortable, and he needs pleasant experiences in order to trust others.

When the infant has developed to the stage at which he identifies his mother and others who care for him as separate beings, he does not want to be left alone. He needs to have someone look into his room and speak to him frequently until he learns that temporary absence does not mean that the friends in whose presence he feels secure are permanently gone. If he has to endure long periods of separation, he may become chronically afraid that he will be left alone. (The family dog is a poor substitute for human companionship, but better than inanimate toys.) During this period the infant may become very shy and appear insecure and afraid of the world. Sympathetic adults must accept this lack of friendliness and, without forcing their attentions upon him, win his trust.

In early infancy the child cannot express his wants, and his mother must anticipate his needs. Later he will convey his wants through movements and sounds. Development of speech is primarily determined by his stage of mental growth and his need to communicate with others. But an important factor, often overlooked, is his mother's response to his coos and babbling. The smiling and cooing of the infant are enormously rewarding to the mother. If she responds by talking to him, showing her appreciation of his achievement in one way or another, he will continue to vocalize and will speak at an early age.

In summary, the infant will learn to adapt to his world by having his needs met initially. First of all he will cry to indicate his need for food. The mother will offer her breast or a bottle feeding to meet his need. If later the infant cries again, but the mother produces no feeding, the infant feels great discomfort because of his hunger and the fact that his crying produced no response. In turn the infant will evolve a new behavioral response. He will either suck his fingers and ultimately go to sleep or he will cry with rage. The infant thus learns to adapt to his world and in time to control his environment through a change in his behavior.

Although the very young infant needs maximum pleasure and minimum discomfort, the older infant needs small doses of anxiety to learn how to handle frustrations and be prepared for the usual problems every child must meet. If he has not been overprotected, everyday experiences are likely to provide all the frustration he requires to build up his ability to handle successfully the activities of daily living.

Frustration of Needs

If the child's need for food is not met, he may exhibit anxiety, shown by overeating or not eating enough.

Some infantile responses persist in adult life,

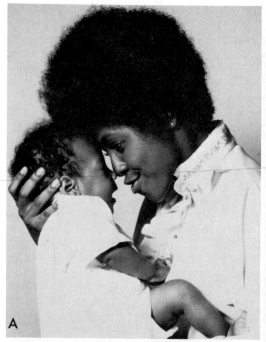

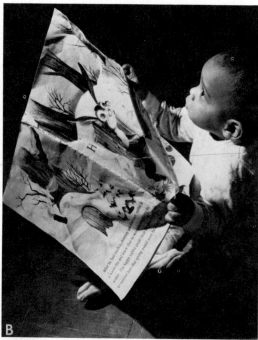

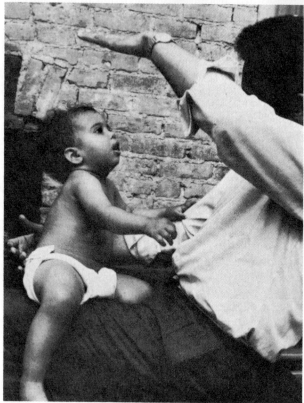

FIGURE 13–2. *A,* An adult can literally talk a baby into talking. Mother's words (and father's, of course, as well as those of any other person helping to care for a baby) are the "blueprint" for baby's words . . . a baby drinks in those "mother noises" as thirstily, eats them up as hungrily, as he does food. No baby is too young to talk to . . . to sing to . . . to laugh to . . . to sweet-talk to . . . and no day is too busy or too hectic for many such mother-baby (and father-baby!) "talks." *B,* Looking at pictures in an often-read-aloud picture book brings to mind the right word for the right thing . . . adds to a baby's "passive" vocabulary of words-understood before these become words-spoken. *C,* As more and more fathers join their wives in pregnancy classes, in the labor room (and often the delivery room), as they get an early jump on the getting-to-know-you via hospital rooming in, tender loving care from Dad becomes an invaluable part of a baby's world. (*A,* Paul Duckworth Photography. *B,* George W. Washington: *Baby Talk,* July, 1971. *C,* T. B. Brazelton: *Baby Talk,* 38:15, April 1973.)

but are modified by the culture of the group. Probably the adult fondness for biting into crisp food and for chewing gum is an infantile pleasure carried over into adult life.

If his need for love and security is not met, the child may doubt his own ability to influence his environment and become insecure in his personal world. He may not be able to take the next steps in personality development. If he does not learn to trust others, he does not merely remain neutral toward them, but rather is likely to be unable to make and hold friends, for he mistrusts them as he learned to mistrust those who cared for him in his early infancy.

If the infant does not receive sensory stimulation, he probably will not develop normally intellectually. He needs perceptual experience early in life in order to prevent growth failure and serious behavioral abnormalities.

When an infant is removed from his home as during hospitalization (see pp. 78 and 395), the members of the health and nursing teams must be aware that the needs of the parents, especially those of the mother, for emotional support are essential and must be met if they are to transmit a sense of security to their child. The mother needs to be able to participate in the care of her infant in some way. Since an infant's sense of trust needs to be developed and maintained, he needs as few persons as possible caring for him. He also needs sensory stimulation, but not overstimulation as may occur in an intensive care unit (see p. 75). The infant may also need a pacifier, not as a substitute for physical contact with his mother or her substitute, but as a means of satisfying his increased need for sucking pleasure.

OVERVIEW OF PHYSICAL AND MENTAL GROWTH AND DEVELOPMENT

PRINCIPLES OF GROWTH AND DEVELOPMENT

Chapter 2 dealt with the general principles of growth and development. These might be summarized as follows.

Development of the human organism is a *continuous process* which begins before birth, each stage being dependent upon the preceding

stages. A specific example of this would be the development of human dentition (Fig. 13–3).

An infant is usually born without teeth. Already, however, he has 20 deciduous (primary) teeth in his mandible and maxilla, some of which began to calcify *in utero*. Eruption of the primary teeth begins at approximately seven months postnatally (see Fig. 13–3). For some infants, teething brings no discomfort; for others it is a painful experience. Since the eruption of teeth is a physiologic process, the claim that teething causes directly a high fever, diarrhea, or other serious upset is not justified. If fever does occur, it is coincidental and may be related to the infant's increased exposure to infection, the loss of maternal antibodies, or the development of immunologic responses. A slight fever may also be related to the fact that his fluid intake may be decreased slightly, and if he does not eat well, he may have a slight electrolyte imbalance and sleep poorly.

The permanent teeth begin to form soon after birth. These erupt when the deciduous teeth are shed, usually about six or seven. The eruption of the last permanent teeth, the third molars, indicates the approximate time of cessation of growth.

The term *developmental sequence* means that these changes are specific, progressive, and orderly and lead eventually to maturity. All children progress through similar steps, but the age at which each child achieves these steps varies, since achievement depends upon his inherent maturational capacity interacting with his physical and social environment. It is especially important for nurses to observe *individual differences* in order to meet adequately the needs of each child.

The different areas of growth are *interrelated*.

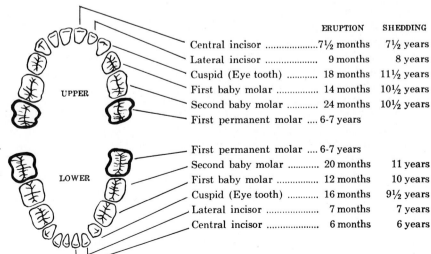

FIGURE 13–3. The development of human dentition is a continuous process from the fifth month *in utero* to maturity. (Courtesy of Niles Newton, Ph.D., and *Baby Talk Magazine*, November 1967.)

	ERUPTION	SHEDDING
UPPER		
Central incisor	7½ months	7½ years
Lateral incisor	9 months	8 years
Cuspid (Eye tooth)	18 months	11½ years
First baby molar	14 months	10½ years
Second baby molar	24 months	10½ years
First permanent molar	6-7 years	
LOWER		
First permanent molar	6-7 years	
Second baby molar	20 months	11 years
First baby molar	12 months	10 years
Cuspid (Eye tooth)	16 months	9½ years
Lateral incisor	7 months	7 years
Central incisor	6 months	6 years

All types of growth and development—physical, mental, emotional, social, spiritual, and sexual—proceed together and in various ways affect each other in the normal advance toward maturity.

Three principles should be stressed in motor development. (a) Muscular development is *cephalocaudal,** i.e., proceeding from the head to the feet. The result is that the child acquires the ability to control his neck muscles before those of his legs and feet. (b) The development of muscular control is also from *proximal to distal;* i.e., development begins near the body and progresses outward to the extremities. (c) The two preceding principles operate in conjunction with development from *general to specific* movement. Muscles controlling gross movements are in general the large muscles proximal to the body. The child uses the larger muscles of the upper arms and legs before he has control of the muscles of the hands and feet, fingers and toes. The infant waves his arms and kicks long before he is able to control the muscles of his fingers in handling anything. Children hold their toys, roll over and sit up before they are able to pick up a crumb as an adult would do.

Tests of motor ability are used as intelligence tests in the young infant, since a child of subnormal mentality is late in sitting, standing, walking, and achieving control of the arms and hands in any but gross movements. Such tests may not be valid, however, when used with infants having problems involving the central nervous system.

BASIC FACTORS IN DEVELOPMENT

Development results from two basic factors: maturation and learning.

Maturation refers to the inborn, genetically transmitted capacity for development. This capacity normally covers all areas of development.

Learning is the result of experience, experimentation, and training. The test of learning is whether it changes behavior. The ability to learn is highly dependent upon the inborn capacity for mental development. If the potential capacity for learning is poor, i.e., if the child has a low intelligence rating or quotient (I.Q.), he will find learning difficult. The child learns from experience that the floor is hard when he falls upon it and that strained fruit tastes good when he is given a spoonful. Later on he learns by ex-

*From *kephalos,* Greek for head, and *cauda,* Latin for tail, so called because of the location of the nerve cells of the central nervous system which control muscular activity. Tail is here the equivalent of the lower part of the spinal cord.

perimentation to open and close the door and the easiest way to creep up stairs.

When he has matured to a higher level, he will learn partially from the experience of others, both by observing them and by listening to what they tell him. He has learned that adults know much more than he does and that what they say—in earnest, not in jest—is true. When his mother tells him that the stove is hot and will burn his hand if he touches it, he believes her. If the child is of toddler age, he may still experiment by putting his hand on the hot stove because his mother's words of caution are in conflict with establishing his own independence. From a child who describes his stay in a hospital he learns what hospitalization may be like. When he goes to school, he will learn from the experience of men since man was first upon this earth.

Maturation and learning are interrelated. No learning takes place unless the child is mature enough to be able to understand, and change his behavior. If he is forced beyond his capacity to learn, unfavorable attitudes may be established which may later retard learning in that area. *The child who is not given opportunity to learn by experience and from others at the optimum time—that period in his development when he is best able to learn the particular task—is hindered in the learning process.* An adult in charge of a child for even a short period should consider his interest in learning, his perseverance in carrying out the activity over a period of time, and his progress.

For example, if a mother places her month-old infant in a sitting position in a corner of the crib, he will probably fall over because his muscles are not mature enough to support him in that position. He may be thoroughly frightened by the experience of having lost his balance and fallen. If, however, a mother observes her older infant repeatedly trying to pull himself to a sitting position even though he falls over many times, she should help him until he is able to sit without support. Thereby she will have aided him in his development by assisting him at the right time and in the right way.

In summary, the effectiveness of teaching or learning depends upon the child's maturity. His maturity, on the other hand, when tested by his behavior, will be greatly influenced by his opportunities to learn. The Denver Developmental Screening Test is a good tool for assessing the level of development in young children (see p. 31).

MENTAL DEVELOPMENT

Earlier in this text (see p. 42) the theory of development of Piaget was discussed. The stage concept was described in which development follows a sequence of stages over a period of time, with each stage having unique characteristics. When the child has attained a new level of functioning, he consolidates and progressively organizes it while at the same time beginning to learn a new level of functioning or stage. As an example, the infant may consolidate his sense of trust while at the same time progressing to the next stage, that of autonomy.

The order in which the child progresses through the various stages does not change, but the rate may differ, depending on his level of inherited intelligence and the influence of various factors in his environment. Although each stage is unique, the stages may blend with behavior seen in earlier stages. For example, when a preschool child who has been successfully toilet trained is under the stress of adjusting to a new sibling, he may revert to soiling himself, typical behavior for an infant.

The *sensorimotor stage* comprising six substages occurs during infancy and the first year of the toddler period, until the child is two years of age. In this period the child's behavior is related to immediate sensory experiences, objects and events that are present within his perceptual field. He has not yet achieved symbolism or mature object constancy. The infant's behavior does progress, however, from the biological reflexes present at birth through various accommodations to the environment until it becomes increasingly complex.

Four substages comprise the sensorimotor period during the first year; the other two substages will be discussed when a description of the intellectual development of the toddler is presented (see p. 506). A description of the first four substages follows.

Substage I (Birth to 1 month). The biologically given reflexes provide the bases for survival in the neonate (see p. 148). On the basis of experience during the first month of life the infant manifests *functional assimilation,* or he repeats reflexive actions such as sucking even though he is not hungry. *Generalized assimilation* occurs when the infant no longer sucks only the breast or bottle but other non-nutritive items such as his fist as well. *Recognitory assimilation* occurs when the hungry infant will not accept a substitute for the breast or bottle. He demonstrates primitive anticipation of his feeding even though it is only on a conditioned learning basis.

Substage II (1 to 4 months). The *primary circular reaction* occurs during substage II. What an infant learns during this time is related to his own body. While sucking his fist, the infant learns that sucking the thumb is much better. At first he brings his mouth to this thumb, later he brings the thumb to his mouth. The infant tries this many times until it is accomplished. When finally learned, this advances the infant because it introduces a new organized schema involving coordination of his movements and discrimination of one movement over another.

During this substage also the things the infant sees and hears belonging to the same experience become coordinated in his mind. This coordination of sensory experiences is the basis for the establishment of the permanent object, which will be discussed later.

Substage III (4 to 10 months). During substage III the *secondary circular reaction* occurs. This reaction involves events that are removed from the infant's body. Events that occur by accident in the environment are repeated by the infant. For instance, while holding a rattle, it accidentally makes a noise. The infant will try to repeat the action to make this noise by coordinating many schemas, finally reproducing the action consistently.

Primitive causality is implied in both primary and secondary circular reactions because the infant connects his participation with the effect it has produced. Primitive thought appears in the *abbreviated schema.* This, however, is not true thought because it occurs only in terms of action.

Development occurs further in establishing *object permanence* when the infant begins to search for an object that has disappeared; if he has dropped it he can anticipate where it is.

Substage IV (10 to 12 months). The secondary reactions the infant learned earlier are combined and extended to deal with new situations. When *coordination of secondary schemas* occurs, the actions of the infant are more flexible than his reactions were earlier.

Object constancy progresses during substage IV. For instance, if the mother hides his rattle, the infant will search for and find it. If the mother moved it from one place to another, however, the infant would still search for it in the place where it was last found.

The infant in this substage improves in his ability to imitate those around him.

In summary, during the *sensorimotor period* the infant learns through his sensations and his movements, and thus his learning is inseparable from his sensory and motor experiences. He also learns that objects continue to exist even when they are out of sight. The concept of object permanence is a prerequisite for the ability to think about things when they are not present and to be aware that one can control some aspects of one's environment. The infant also develops an early idea of goal-directed behavior and a primitive grasp of the connection between cause and effect. During the first year the infant does not learn to "think" per se. He cannot deal abstractly with things beyond the scope of his sensorimotor experience.

Just as emotional and physical development occur in stages, as seen in the accompanying tables and figures, so does intellectual development occur.

LIFE PERSPECTIVE

The infant has no life perspective of his own. He does not remember the past and cannot predict what will happen tomorrow. During the first year he can differentiate his mother and her substitute from strangers, but he cannot understand exactly what meaning they have in his life.

Levels and Achievements in Growth and Development

It is important for the student to review the overall principles of emotional and physical development in order to understand the specific growth levels and range of achievements typical of infants during their development month by month.

The behavior of infants as it changes with development has been the subject of much research. As was mentioned before, each achievement of a child may occur normally within a range of time. The age for specific achievements given in various tables in this book (see Table 13-1 and Figs. 13-4 through 13-16) is usually the average age of children in such a range. These schedules will probably not be typical of many infants whom the student knows, because they are *averages* and therefore do not necessarily apply to any one infant. Few infants are average for their age in all areas covered by these schedules. Furthermore, there are great individual differences among infants. These schedules will, however, provide a kind of yardstick with which the student can determine in a general way whether individual infants are developing according to the usual pattern.

PLAY

Purpose. Infants learn many things through play. In play they practice motor skills, acquire control of the body, and gain in general coordination of movements and specific coordination of hand-eye movements. Infants learn to relate to objects and to people, to express their feelings, and to work off frustrations through play. *Play, then, is all-important in the development of the child's personality;* it occupies almost all his waking hours.

Learning to play with things and to amuse himself with his own movements and the sounds he can make begins in infancy. Later on in childhood he learns to play with other children. This, it is said, lays the foundation for adult ability to work well with others.

TABLE 13-1. AVERAGE ACHIEVEMENT LEVELS OF INFANTS, 1 MONTH TO 1 YEAR

1 MONTH

Physical
  Weight: 8 pounds. Gains about 5 to 7 ounces weekly during first 6 months of life
  Height: Gains approximately 1 inch a month for the first 6 months
  Pulse: 120–150
  Respirations: 30–60
Motor Control (Figs. 13-4, 13-5)
  Head sags when supported. May lift head from time to time when he is held against his mother's shoulder
  Makes crawling movements when prone on a flat surface
  Lifts head intermittently, though unsteadily, when in prone position. Cervical curve begins to develop as the infant learns to hold his head erect
  Can turn his head to the side when prone
  Can push with feet against a hard surface to move himself forward
  Has "dance" reflex when held upright with feet touching the bed or examining table
  Shows a well developed tonic neck reflex (head turned to one side, the arm extended on the same side and the other arm flexed to his shoulder)
  Holds hands in fists. Does not reach with hands. Can grasp an object placed in his hand, but drops it immediately
Vision
  Stares indefinitely at his surroundings and apparently notices faces and bright objects, but only if they are in his line of vision. Activity diminishes when he regards a human face
  Can follow an object to the midline of vision
Vocalization and Socialization
  Utters small throaty sounds
  Smiles indefinitely
  Shows a vague and indirect regard of faces and bright objects
  Cries when hungry or uncomfortable

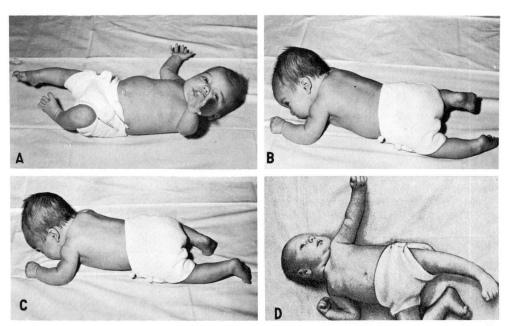

FIGURE 13–4. The one-month-old infant. *A*, Shows random, generalized activity in response to stimulation. *B*, Makes crawling movements when prone on a flat surface. Pushes with toes. Holds hands in fists. *C*, Lifts head from the bed a short distance. Can turn head to the side when prone. *D*, Has a well developed tonic neck reflex.

Although the general purposes of play are the same for all infants, each discovers how to use a particular toy or game for his own purposes. Thus *play is an individual matter.* Not all chil-

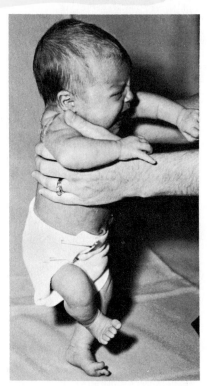

FIGURE 13–5. The one-month-old infant has a "dance" reflex when held upright with feet touching the bed or examining table.

dren learn in the same way from playing, because play is a result of each infant's or little child's need at the time. For this reason, play should be self-directed. Adults, through their interest in a child's development, are apt to overdirect his play activity. Some adults believe that they are "playing with" an infant when they toss him into the air and catch him or shake him roughly. Because of the weight of the infant's head and the relative weakness of his neck muscles, this action may cause brain damage. Nurses can help parents to understand the danger associated with this type of play.

Selection of Play Materials. The variety of toys generally listed as suitable for children of any age group is based on the assumption of normal growth and development. The nurse, knowing the characteristics of growth and development of each age level, will select from the toys suitable for the age group the ones best adapted to a particular child's needs, for he may be advanced or retarded for his age.

Selection is important, for toys have many functions, i.e., toys help children to learn different things in different ways. An essential factor in the selection of a toy is that it be safe for the child's use. This, in general, depends on his level of growth and development, but varies with his physical condition and other characteristics. Some children are more cautious than others. This may be due to slow or rapid development, but also to specific experiences from which a child has learned to be careful when

Text continued on page 357

TABLE 13–1. *AVERAGE ACHIEVEMENT LEVELS OF INFANTS, 1 MONTH TO 1 YEAR* (*Continued*)

2 MONTHS

Physical
 Posterior fontanel closed
Motor Control (Fig. 13–6).
 Can hold head erect in midposition. Can lift head and chest a short distance above bed or table when lying on his abdomen
 Tonic neck and Moro reflexes are fading
 Can turn from side to back
 Can hold a rattle for a brief time
Vision
 Can follow a moving light or object with his eyes
Vocalization and Socialization
 Shows a "social smile" in response to another's smile. This is the beginning of social behavior. It may not appear until the third month
 Has learned that by crying he will get attention. His crying becomes differentiated; the sound of his crying varies with the reason for crying, e.g. hunger, sleepiness or pain
 Pays attention to the speaking voice

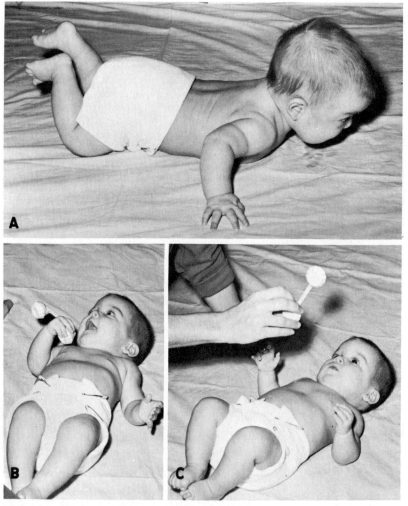

FIGURE 13–6. The 2-month-old infant. *A*, Can hold the head erect in midposition. Can lift the head and chest a short distance above the bed or table when lying on abdomen. *B*, Can hold a rattle for a brief period. *C*, Can follow a moving object with eyes.

TABLE 13–1. *AVERAGE ACHIEVEMENT LEVELS OF INFANTS, 1 MONTH TO 1 YEAR* (*Continued*)

3 MONTHS

Physical
  Weight: 12–13 pounds
Motor Control (Fig. 13–7).
  Holds his hands up in front of him and stares at them
  Plays with hands and fingers
  Reaches for shiny objects, but misses them
  Can carry hand or object to mouth at will
  Holds head erect and steady. Raises chest, usually supported on forearms
  Has lost the walking or dancing reflex
  Grasping reflex has weakened
  Sits, back rounded, knees flexed when supported
Vision
  Shows binocular coordination (vertical and horizontal vision) when an object is moved from right to left and up and
    down in front of his face
  Turns eyes to an object in his marginal field of vision
  Voluntarily winks at objects which threaten his eyes
Vocalization and Socialization
  Laughs aloud and shows pleasure in making sounds
  Cries less
  Smiles in response to mother's face

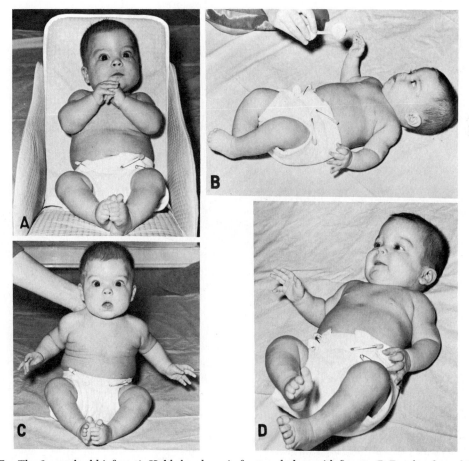

FIGURE 13–7.   The 3-month-old infant. *A*, Holds hands up in front and plays with fingers. *B*, Reaches for a shiny object, but misses it. *C*, Sits with support, back rounded, knees flexed. *D*, Smiles in response to mother's face and laughs aloud.

TABLE 13–1. *AVERAGE ACHIEVEMENT LEVELS OF INFANTS, 1 MONTH TO 1 YEAR (Continued)*

4 MONTHS

Physical
    Weight: Between 13 and 14 pounds
    Drools between 3 and 4 months of age. This indicates the appearance of saliva. He does not know how to swallow saliva, which therefore runs from his mouth
Motor Control (Fig. 13–8).
    Symmetrical body postures predominate
    Holds head steady when in sitting position
    Lifts head and shoulders at a 90-degree angle when on abdomen and looks around
    Tries to roll over. Can turn from back to side
    Thumb apposition in grasping occurs between third and fourth months
    Holds hands predominantly open. Activates arms at sight of proferred toy
    Sits with adequate support and enjoys being propped up
    Tonic neck reflex has disappeared
    Sustains portion of own weight
Vision
    Recognizes familiar objects
    Stares at rattle placed in his hand and takes it to his mouth
    Follows moving objects well. Even the most difficult types of eye movements are present
    Arms are activated on sight of dangling toy
Vocalization and Socialization
    Laughs aloud and smiles in response to smiles of others
    Initiates social play by smiling
    Vocalizes socially; i.e. he coos and gurgles when talked to
    He does not cry when scolded. He is very "talkative"
    "Talking" and crying follow each other quickly
    Shows evidence of wanting social attention and of increasing interest in other members of the family
    Enjoys having people with him

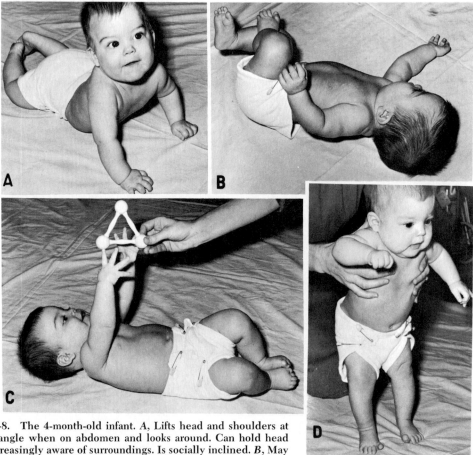

FIGURE 13–8. The 4-month-old infant. *A*, Lifts head and shoulders at a 90-degree angle when on abdomen and looks around. Can hold head steady. Is increasingly aware of surroundings. Is socially inclined. *B*, May roll from back to side. *C*, Grasps for a toy with whole hand. Has symmetrical body posture predominantly. Holds head in midline. Can open and close hands on rattle. Can coordinate hands and eyes sufficiently to reach and grasp on sight. *D*, Sustains part of own weight when held.

TABLE 13-1. *AVERAGE ACHIEVEMENT LEVELS OF INFANTS, 1 MONTH TO 1 YEAR (Continued)*

5 MONTHS

Physical
  Weight: Twice the birth weight (15–16 pounds)
Motor Control (Fig. 13–9).
  Sits with slight support. Holds back straight when pulled to sitting position
  Can use thumb in partial apposition to fingers more skillfully
  Can balance head well
  Reaches for objects which are beyond his grasp. Grasps objects independently of direct stimulation of the palm of the hand (partial grasp). Grasps with the whole hand. Accepts an object handed to him
  Has completely lost the Moro reflex
Vocalization and Socialization
  Vocalizes his displeasure when a desired object is taken from him

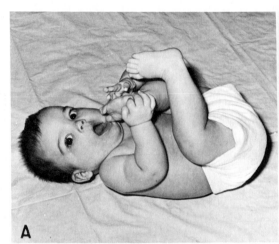 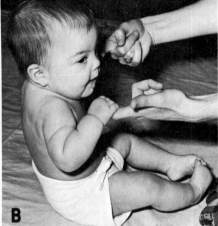

FIGURE 13-9. The 5-month-old infant. *A,* Reaches and grasps objects with the whole hand and carries them to mouth. *B,* Holds back straight when pulled to a sitting position. Continues to drool.

TABLE 13-1. *AVERAGE ACHIEVEMENT LEVELS OF INFANTS, 1 MONTH TO 1 YEAR (Continued)*

6 MONTHS

Physical
  Gains about 3 to 5 ounces weekly during the second 6 months of life
  Grows about ½ inch a month
  May be teething
Motor Control (Fig. 13–10).
  Sits momentarily without support if placed in a favorable leaning position
  Grasps with simultaneous flexion of fingers
  Retains transient hold on 2 blocks, one in either hand
  Pulls himself up to a sitting position
  Completely turns over from stomach to stomach with rest periods during the complete turn. This ability is important in protecting him from falling out of bed
  Springs up and down when sitting
  Bangs with object held in his hand, rattle or spoon
  Hitches. Hitching is locomotion backward when in a sitting position. Movement of the body is aided by use of his arms and hands. This ability is usually present by the sixth month
Vocalization and Socialization
  Babbles from the third to the eighth month
  Vocalizes several well defined syllables. Actively vocalizes pleasure with crowing or cooing. Babbling is not linked with specific objects, people or situations
  Cries easily on slight provocation (change of position or withdrawal of a toy)
  Thrashes arms and legs when frustrated
  Begins to recognize strangers (fifth to sixth month)

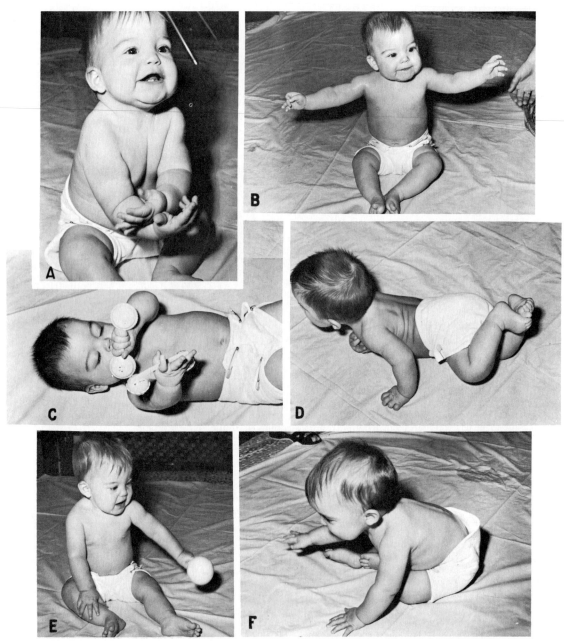

FIGURE 13–10. The 6-month-old infant. *A*, Has 2 lower central incisors. *B*, Sits momentarily without support. Holds arms out for balance. *C*, Retains transient hold on 2 objects. Grasps with flexion of fingers. *D*, Turns completely over. *E*, Bangs with a rattle held in hand. Balances well by leaning forward slightly on one or both hands. *F*, Can hitch. Moves backward in a sitting position by using arms and hands to push.

TABLE 13–1. *AVERAGE ACHIEVEMENT LEVELS OF INFANTS, 1 MONTH TO 1 YEAR* (Continued)

7 MONTHS

Motor Control (Fig. 13–11).
  When lying down, lifts head as if he were trying to sit up
  Sits briefly, leaning forward on his hands. Control of trunk is more advanced
  Plays with his feet and puts them in his mouth
  Bounces actively when held in a standing position
  Can approach a toy and grasp it with one hand
  Can transfer a toy from one hand to the other with varying degrees of success
  Rolls more easily from back to stomach
Vocalization and Socialization
  Vocalizes his eagerness
  Vocalizes "m-m-m" when crying
  Makes polysyllabic vowel sounds
  Emotional development, 7 to 8 months: Shows fear of strangers.
  Emotional instability shown by easy and quick changes from crying to laughing

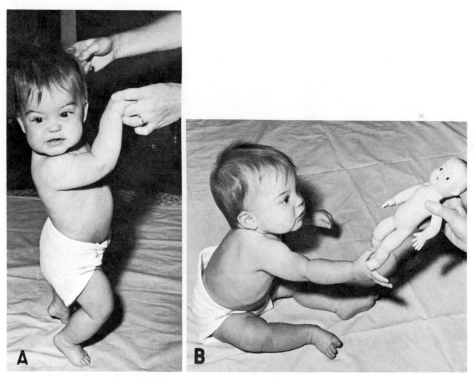

FIGURE 13–11. The 7-month-old infant. *A,* Bounces actively when held in standing position. Can support a larger portion of own weight for a longer time. *B,* Can approach a toy and grasp it with one hand.

TABLE 13–1. *AVERAGE ACHIEVEMENT LEVELS OF INFANTS, 1 MONTH TO 1 YEAR* (*Continued*)

8 MONTHS

Motor Control (Fig. 13–12)
  Sits alone steadily
  Complete thumb apposition
  Hand-eye coordination is perfected to the point that random reaching and grasping no longer persist
Vocalization and Socialization
  Greets strangers with coy or bashful behavior, turning away, hanging his head, crying or even screaming, and refuses to play with strangers or even accept toys from them
  Shows nervousness with strangers
  Emotional development: "Eight months' anxiety," to be distinguished from anaclitic depression (see p. 359), occurs between the sixth and eighth months as a result of the child's increased capacity for discriminating between friend and stranger
  Affection or love of family group appears
  Emotional instability still shown by easy changes from laughing to crying
  Stretches arm to loved adult as in invitation to come

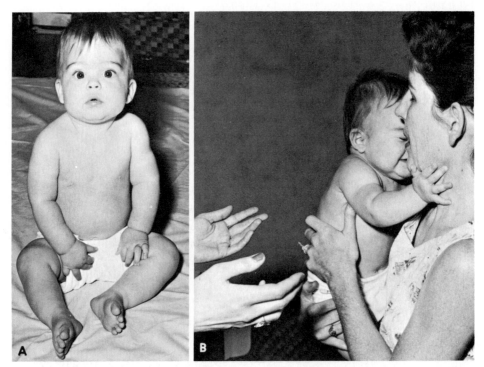

FIGURE 13–12. The 8-month-old infant. *A*, Sits alone steadily. Has increased interest in activity in environment. *B*, "Eight months' anxiety." Greets stranger by turning away and crying.

TABLE 13-1. *AVERAGE ACHIEVEMENT LEVELS OF INFANTS, 1 MONTH TO 1 YEAR (Continued)*

9 MONTHS

Motor Control (Fig. 13-13)

Shows good coordination and sits alone

Holds his bottle with good hand-mouth coordination. Can put the nipple in and out of his mouth at will

Preference for the use of one hand is marked

Crawls instead of hitching. Crawling may be seen as early as the fourth month; the average age is about nine months. In crawling the infant is prone, his abdomen touching the floor, his head and shoulders supported with the weight borne on the elbows. The body is pulled along by the movement of the arms while the legs drag. The leg movements may resemble swimming or kicking movements

Creeps. This is a more advanced type of locomotion than crawling. The trunk is carried above the floor, but parallel to it. The infant uses both his hands and knees in propelling himself forward. Not all infants follow this pattern of hitching, crawling and creeping. Different children stress different means of locomotion and may even skip a stage. (This is particularly likely if an infant is sick or for some other reason is unable to practice moving about)

Raises himself to a sitting position. Requires help to pull self to feet

Vocalization and Socialization

Shows the beginning of imitative expression. Sounds stand for things to him. Says "Da-da" or some such expression

Responds to adult anger. Cries when scolded

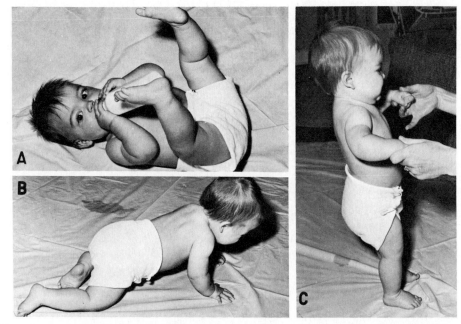

FIGURE 13-13.   The 9-month-old infant. *A,* Holds own bottle with good hand-mouth coordination. Can put the nipple in and out of mouth at will. *B,* Can creep. Carries trunk above the floor, but parallel to it. Uses both hands and knees in propelling self forward. *C,* Can pull self to feet if assisted.

TABLE 13–1. *AVERAGE ACHIEVEMENT LEVELS OF INFANTS, 1 MONTH TO 1 YEAR* (*Continued*)

10 MONTHS

Motor Control (Fig. 13–14)

 Sits steadily for an indefinite time. Does not enjoy lying down unless he is sleepy

 Makes early stepping movements when held

 Pulls himself to his feet, holding to the crib rail or similar support. (This is a good time to begin the use of the play pen or yard)

 Creeps and cruises about very well. (Cruising is walking sideways while holding on to a supporting object with both hands)

 Can pick up objects fairly well and pokes them with his fingers

 Feeds himself a cracker or some such food which he can hold in his hand

 Is able crudely to release a toy

 Can bring his hands together

Vocalization and Socialization

 Says one or two words and imitates an adult's inflection

 Pays attention to his name

 Plays simple games as bye-bye and pat-a-cake (motor control is such that he can bring his hands together) and peek-a-boo

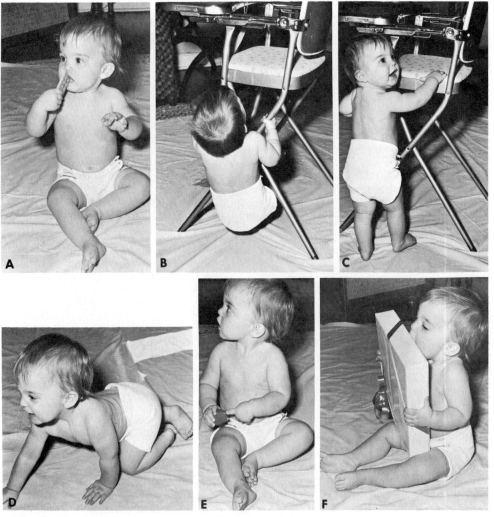

FIGURE 13–14. The 10-month-old infant. *A*, Sits steadily for an indefinite time. Feeds self a cracker. *B*, Pulls self to feet, holding on to legs of chair or similar support. *C*, Cruises or walks sideways around furniture while holding on to supporting object with both hands. *D*, Creeps well. *E*, Can pick up objects fairly well and pokes them with finger. *F*, Plays peek-a-boo over top of box.

TABLE 13–1. *AVERAGE ACHIEVEMENT LEVELS OF INFANTS, 1 MONTH TO 1 YEAR (Continued)*

11 MONTHS

Motor Control (Fig. 13–15)
  Stands erect with the help of his mother's hand or supporting himself by holding on to some object as the side of his play yard

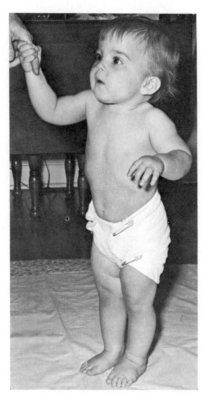

FIGURE 13–15.   The 11-month-old infant stands erect with the help of mother's hand.

TABLE 13–1. *AVERAGE ACHIEVEMENT LEVELS OF INFANTS, 1 MONTH TO 1 YEAR (Continued)*

12 MONTHS

Physical
  Weight: Three times his birth weight (21–22 pounds)
  Height: 29 inches
  Head and chest are equal in circumference
  Has 6 teeth
  Pulse: 100–140 per minute
  Respirations: 20–40 per minute
Motor Control (Fig. 13–16)
  Stands for a moment alone, or possibly longer
  Walks with help. Cruises, walking sideways around chairs or from chair to chair, holding on with one hand
  Lumbar curve and the compensating dorsal curve develop as he learns to walk
  Can sit down from standing position without help
  Holds a crayon adaptively to make a stroke and can mark on a piece of paper
  Can pick up small bits of food and transfer them to his mouth. Can drink from a cup and eat from a spoon, but requires help. He likes to eat with his fingers
  Cooperates in dressing; e.g. he can put his arm through a sleeve. Can take off his socks

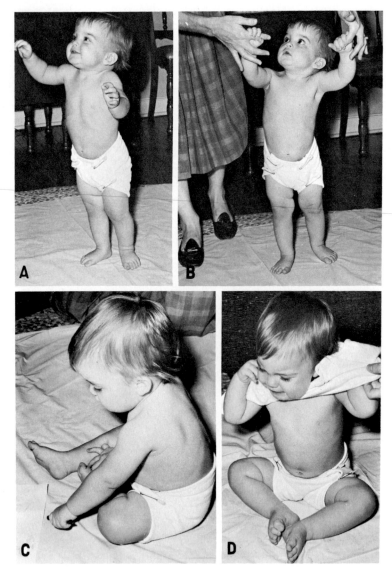

FIGURE 13–16.   The 12-month-old infant. *A*, Stands alone for a moment or possibly longer. *B*, Walks with help. *C*, Holds a crayon adaptively to make a stroke and can mark on a piece of paper. *D*, Cooperates in dressing. Puts arm through sleeve.

TABLE 13–1.   AVERAGE ACHIEVEMENT LEVELS OF INFANTS, 1 MONTH TO 1 YEAR (Continued)

Vocalization and Socialization

Can say 2 words besides "Mama" and "Dada"
Slow vocabulary growth, as a rule, owing to his interest in walking
Knows his own name
Uses expressive jargon. Communicates with himself and those around him
Inhibits simple acts on command. Recognizes the meaning of "No, no"
Shows jealousy, affection, anger and other emotions. He may cry for affection. He loves an audience, and will repeat a performance which brings a response. Crying is more often associated with irritation or frustration than it formerly was. Stiffens in resistance
Loves rhythms
Still egocentric, concerned only with himself

trying out a new use for toys. It is never safe to give toys designed for older children to infants. For instance, the small plastic parts which an older child uses in building a toy car would not be suitable for an infant, for he would put them into his mouth and might easily swallow or even aspirate them.

Toys should be washable, durable, easily handled, not too heavy, and smooth with rounded edges and no sharp points. Children enjoy gaily colored toys. If the toy is painted, it should be with nonlead paint. The size of the toy should be appropriate to the use the child will make of it. An infant's toy should be well constructed. For instance, a rattle should be one the infant cannot break when he bangs it against the rails of his crib. If it broke, he might pick up and swallow some of the pebbles it contained.

A toy should be one with many uses for the child, for developing motor abilities and for auditory and visual experiences. It is difficult to predict to what uses he may put it, and his creative ability should be encouraged. But safety factors must be considered.

Colorful mobiles may be hung across the crib, but should be changed frequently in order to vary the stimuli in the infant's line of vision. When he is learning to stand, such toys should be removed in order that he will have sufficient space in which to move and also to prevent his harming himself should he suddenly fall.

Blocks are meant for building, but the infant may throw them. For this reason they should be made of some relatively soft substance so that he can hurt neither himself nor another child. These he can place together, clap together, or toss as he happens to fancy. Cuddly toys can be used in many ways besides being cuddled at bedtime. They can be dropped, dragged along or sat upon. Many adults do not understand that the infant may use a toy for its express purpose and also for whatever other use he desires. They bring pressure upon the child to use a toy as an older child would do or even to watch them use it, withholding the toy if the child grasps for it.

Suggested toys include large wooden beads and spools strung on a cord or shoestring, rattles, soft toys (not fuzzy) of different shapes, balls, and large or small blocks.

Play Responses During Infancy. Toys to be used during the first year must be very simple. The infant's attention span is short.

BIRTH TO FIVE MONTHS. An early type of motor play is for exercise, but it is also thoroughly enjoyable to the infant. He reaches for objects and attempts to turn from back to side. He kicks, wiggles, and plays with his hands.

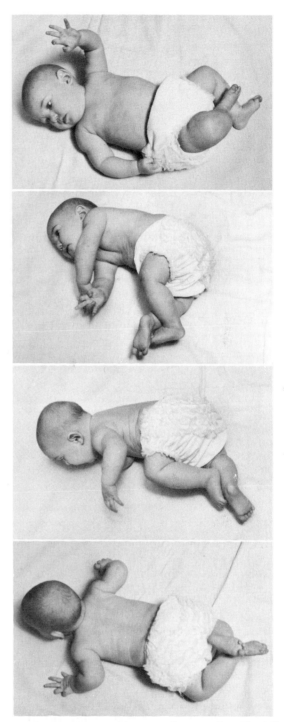

FIGURE 13–17. An early type of motor play. The infant turns well from back to abdomen. (Courtesy of Lew Merrim and *Baby Talk Magazine,* June 1967.)

FIVE TO EIGHT MONTHS. At this age the infant still finds pleasure in motor activity for its own sake. He plays with his feet, bounces his body, shakes his head, leans against objects when learning to sit, grasps at anything he can reach and moves on the floor or in his play yard by hitching. He usually plays contentedly by himself during the first six months. By seven months he enjoys company, but is still happy playing alone with his toys. He likes to explore his hands and feet and talks to himself. He enjoys his bath when free from the restraint of clothing and can move his body easily.

EIGHT TO TEN MONTHS. Motor activity is still the infant's chief source of play. He kicks his legs. Now that he can sit alone he likes to lean over the side of his carriage or the arm of his chair. He plays with his toes and rolls with ease. He crawls, creeps, or pulls himself into a sitting position and stretches to get toys which are out of his reach. He transfers a toy from one hand to the other and puts the toy into his mouth. He has learned where the toy goes when he drops it over the edge of the crib or the tray when he is sitting in his high chair, and looks down at it.

TEN TO ELEVEN MONTHS. The child still plays alone for relatively long periods, but lets the family know when he wants their company or the stimulus of having another toy. His play is becoming more highly developed. He plays in a sitting position, creeps about, pokes objects with his fingers, and enjoys pulling himself up to standing position.

TWELVE MONTHS. Now the child plays with several toys, picking them up and dropping them. He can grasp a ball and let it go, and will take or give a toy on request or gesture. He greatly enjoys walking with help.

EFFECTS OF SEPARATION FROM PARENTS

Factors in Development of the Child. *It may be said that the kind of person the infant will become depends in part upon the characteristics of his parents, their relations to each other, and the emotional atmosphere of the home in general. Their attitude toward the infant is of fundamental importance. He may receive from them a feeling of love and peace or anxiety and insecurity.*

Among the significant developments in psychiatry in recent years has been the increasing awareness that the kind of parental care given during infancy and early childhood is of great importance to the child's future mental and physical health.

During infancy and early childhood he should have an intimate, warm and continuous relationship with his mother or permanent mother-substitute in whom he finds happiness. In such a situation the basis for mental ill health characterized by excessive anxiety and feelings of guilt is not likely to develop.

As the infant grows he normally learns how to deal with his anxiety over his gradual separation from his mother. *Spoiling* of an infant may occur when the mother or her substitute does not give him opportunities to develop methods of dealing with this anxiety. The maternal figure is so afraid when the infant's behavior changes as he attempts to deal with his anxiety that she pacifies him constantly and does not leave him. The infant thus stays at his original level of development, since the adult fulfills his needs and gives him no encouragement to develop further.

Maternal Deprivation. *Maternal deprivation is the term used for an infant's lack of a warm relationship.* The condition occurs when the mother or her substitute cannot give loving care even though the infant lives with her, or when the child is removed from his mother's care, is hospitalized or institutionalized, or remains in the home while she is absent. Although maternal deprivation is emphasized here, if the father or his substitute has assumed the maternal role, the infant would be deprived if that individual were to be separated from him.

There are various degrees of deprivation. In a situation of *incomplete* or *partial deprivation* the infant or young child may show acute anxiety, at the same time experiencing an excessive need for love and affection. In *complete* or *total deprivation* the infant may become incapable of forming normal relations with others.

Since the infant learns to know his mother as a person when five or six months old and to recognize and fear strangers when seven to eight months old, he should have his mother or a permanent substitute to care for him and be near him during his first year.

Although deprivation during infancy is serious, the effects of deprivation differ according to whether it occurs in the first or the second half of the first year.

DEPRIVATION IN THE FIRST SIX MONTHS. Infants of this age have inadequate psychic and physical development to adjust to an impersonal sort of care given by a succession of kindly, competent persons who do not love them as they would their own infants. Infants deprived of maternal care by their own mothers or by an adequate mother-substitute lack all that goes with love and seldom receive sufficient stimulation to promote normal development. In foundling homes they become emotionally isolated from adults, and their activity is likely to be restricted. They generally show signs of retarded mental development, even if they receive the best possible physical care.

The result of such care in foundling homes is evident in the infant's behavior. The young infant may cry a great deal. He may not gain weight as he should, and his motor development is likely to be poor, since he is seldom handled or taken from his crib. Gradually he will refuse contact with adults. He will lose weight, and his sleep pattern will be altered. He will develop a rigid facial expression. He has poor resistance and is liable to contract infections readily. After a few months he will become completely passive and eventually appear retarded. He may make bizarre finger movements. The incidence of marasmus (see p. 435) and the death rate are relatively high among these children.

Prevention of maternal deprivation in foundling homes is almost impossible. Foster-home care should be provided in the earliest months of infancy, and the child should remain in the same home with his loving, permanent mother-substitute. If foster-home care is impossible, a permanent mother-substitute should be provided in the foundling home. She should be chosen from among the nursing personnel and should have a limited number of infants to care for so that she can give them individual attention. She must communicate to each child that he is loved and wanted.

An infant hospitalized because of a congenital deformity or illness may exhibit the same symptoms as the infant in a foundling home if warm, affectionate care and sensory stimulation are not provided. Such care is often more difficult to provide in a hospital than in a foundling home because of the constant change in the nursing personnel (both nursing students and auxiliary personnel) and also because the more acutely ill infants need more than their proportionate share of attention. An adequate, stable graduate nurse staff is essential on the pediatric unit if these children are to receive continuous loving care. There is a real need in each situation to determine whether the hospital is the best place for such an infant or whether the members of the health team can provide sufficient support and guidance to the parents so that the infant can be cared for at home.

DEPRIVATION DURING THE SECOND SIX MONTHS. This is the period when *anaclitic depression* occurs. It results from a change in the infant's life, from the warm relations with his mother and family to a situation in which he is one of a group of infants who do not receive continuous loving care from their mothers.

The result is that the infants become de-pressed, cry a great deal and look sad, and are withdrawn in their relations with adults caring for them. This is in decided contrast to their previous happy, outgoing behavior. They may refuse to eat and may lose weight. They will cling to a doll or a blanket brought from home. The last stage of detachment is evidenced by the children's delay in reponse to the parents when they visit them, by their establishing superficial positive relations with other adults, and by their increased autoerotic behavior. If deprivation continues more than three months, the constant crying subsides. The sad expression is replaced by a rigid facial expression. They may suffer anorexia and sleep disturbances. It may become difficult and eventually impossible for nurses to establish contact with them. If the child is restored to his parents within three months, recovery may be rapid. If deprivation continues, recovery becomes increasingly difficult and less likely to be complete.

In summary, after six to nine months of age reactions of infants to maternal deprivation can be classified into three time-sequence stages: protest (crying), despair (quiet and subdued behavior) and denial (even of the mother). After the mother reappears the child may continue to be withdrawn, to have altered sleeping or eating patterns, to cling to the mother and to be afraid of strangers. Although damage to the child due to maternal deprivation may be severe, recently some question has been raised about the effects of deprivation being irreversible in later years. Certainly not every deprived child has grown up to be a delinquent or an unloving adult or has had the serious personality problems formerly blamed on maternal deprivation early in life.

Although the probable results of extreme deprivation are those which have just been described, some infants who have lacked their mother's love for any number of reasons appear to suffer little permanent personality damage. The reasons for this are not clearly understood, but may depend upon the age of the child, length of separation, the care of the child by other adults during separation, and the stress of the illness itself. It must be remembered that each infant's environment is influenced by his characteristics. Though it should not be so, a pretty child who was friendly before separation from his mother is apt to evoke a warm response from those who care for him. His life is likely to be different from that of the child, who, on entrance to the institution, did not respond to the friendly advances of the personnel. The personnel of an institution are human and likely to be very different in their treatment of the likable and unlikable infants.

To fulfill the function of the profession, every nurse should provide the kind of warm, loving care which children need to prevent them from suffering the effects of maternal deprivation. The specific nursing practices, which may help to prevent the occurrence of maternal deprivation include frequent body contacts with the child, continuity in contact with the child of a few nursing personnel, genuine interest of these personnel in the child, provision for a variety of sensory stimuli for him, and finally the establishment of the nurse as a friend to the mother, a friend who can serve as a bridge between her and her child.

PREVENTION OF ANACLITIC DEPRESSION. After six months of age the normal infant takes the initiative and seeks adult contact. He needs sensory stimulation and room where he can investigate his environment. Above all, he needs the continuous warm affection of a mothering person who gives him individual attention. If these two requirements are fulfilled, he may continue to be an essentially normal infant; otherwise he will probably become depressed and unloving.

Foundlings and Adoptions. In the foregoing discussion the term "foundling home" was used. A *foundling* is an infant abandoned by its parents and found by others. Such infants in general are adopted, since the demand for infants eligible for adoption exceeds the supply. Although time must elapse between the finding of an infant and his legal adoption, he may be given temporarily to the future adoptive parents through a legally approved organization. Adoptive parents, as a rule, want to take the infant when he is only a few weeks old. Thus few foundlings, if they are normal infants, remain in institutions.

Homes for infants retain the word "foundling," since they were incorporated when in fact they did care for foundlings and because they still receive infants deserted by their parents and care for them until adopted. In general, the infants and children in these homes are illegitimate children whose mothers surrendered them to the institutions at birth and who are there only until adopted. Infants who are in a children's home for a long time are those whose parents are unable to care for them or are not considered by the court to be able to provide a suitable home for them. Such children generally come from homes where both the physical and the social conditions are poor, though the mothers might have had loving relations with the infants. It is these infants, rather than foundlings, who constitute the great problem of the institutionalized child.

Aid for dependent children under the Social Security Act has resulted in relatively few infants and children being institutionalized because of the death of one or both parents.

INFANT CARE

DAILY CARE

Every infant and every other member of the family—mother, father, and siblings—have their individual needs. The plan for the infant's care must take into consideration ways of adjusting all these common and conflicting needs. Parents should not feel that they must give up their whole lives for their infant. If they do, their care may ultimately lack spontaneity and warmth.

The natural rhythms of a normal infant and of the particular infant must be considered. These rhythms will change as he grows older. His pattern of sleeping and waking and his periods of playful exercise will alter. The parents have schedules which their activities require them to follow and with which the infant's schedule is interrelated. Both parents should plan to spend some time with the infant in the evening, and this requires a corresponding arrangement of his periods of sleep.

If the mother does her own housework and is not employed outside the home, she is able to spend considerable time with the baby at periods which best fit into her schedule. But if she works outside the home, it may be necessary to adapt his schedule to the hours when she is free to be with him. If there are siblings in the home, her activities must be adapted to their needs also. She and her husband should spend some time with the siblings without the infant being present to distract the parents' attention from the other children. This is important in the prevention of sibling jealousy of the infant (see p. 606) and in their acceptance of their status as older than he. Older siblings should realize that they are given prerogatives he does not receive, just as he receives attentions not given them.

As the infant shifts to having three meals a day with nourishment such as orange juice between meals, he may gradually be included in the family group at meal times.

Since an infant is not old enough to tell how he feels, his parents should watch for signs and symptoms of discomfort and illness. The infant's color is a good indication of his condition. His eyes should be clear and bright. When tired, he should fall asleep without fretting.

There is no set pattern of daily care for all infants, since their needs vary from month to month, and the family situation of each differs from that of the others.

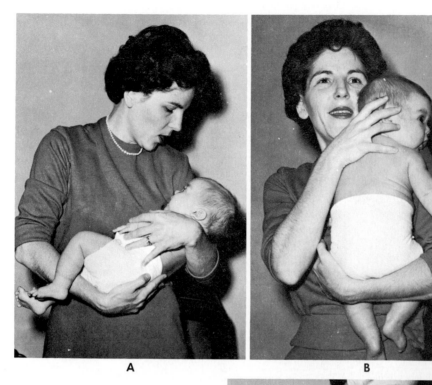

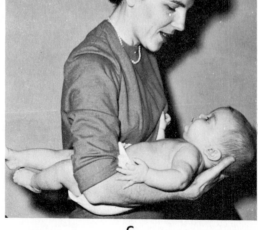

FIGURE 13–18. *A*, A modified cradle position. The young infant's head and back must be supported adequately. *B*, The infant may be held upright against the shoulder. The head must be supported until the infant is able to do so by himself. *C*, Football hold, side view.

CARRYING THE INFANT

The technique of carrying the infant is based on his anatomic structure and motor ability. His head is large in proportion to his body, and he is unable to hold his head erect without support until he is about three months old. The shoulders and back must be supported at first because of weakness. If these two facts are remembered, lifting and carrying the infant will be comfortable and safe for him and easy for the parent or nurse. Different techniques for carrying infants have been given descriptive titles, such as the *cradle technique* and the *football hold*. Each technique has its special use.

The *cradle technique* is commonly used in lifting,

turning, and carrying the infant. The nurse or parent grasps his feet with the right hand (keeping the index finger between the ankles in order not to press the ankle bones together), slides the left hand and arm under the infant's back, giving support to the buttocks, back, and head. The right hand is then brought up and under the buttocks, while moving the left arm and hand up to give greater support to the head, shoulders, and back. The infant is then raised so that he is cradled in the nurse's arms, his body against the chest.

If the nurse or parent holds him in an upright position, on the shoulder, the left forearm is under his buttocks, his body pressed against the chest and shoulder and his cheek resting slightly over the shoulder. Support for his back and head is given with the other hand. If for a moment the right hand must be used, as in opening a door, the body is bent

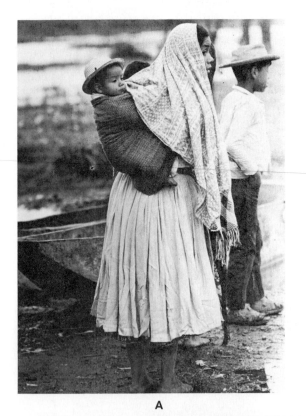

A

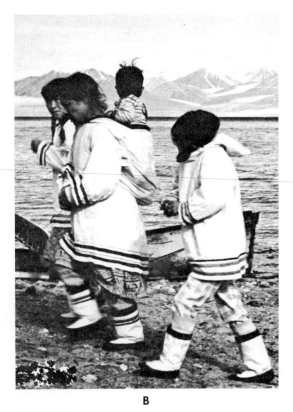

B

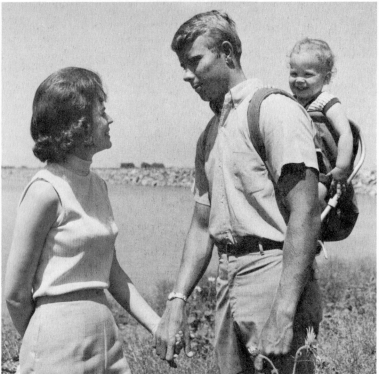

C

FIGURE 13–19. Examples of child care. A, A Mexican mother and child. The shawl-like rebozo spells security as well as transportation. (Courtesy of Peggo Cromer.) B, Children of the Arctic. (Courtesy of Canada's Health and Welfare, February, 1969.) C, When the infant can support his head well, he may be carried comfortably on his parent's back. (Courtesy of M. S. Hansson, Gerry Designs, Inc., Boulder, Colorado.)

backward so that the infant's body is pressed against that of the adult by gravity and he lies there without a sense of loss of support.

The *football hold* is useful in washing the infant's head over a basin or making the crib while holding the infant. His hips are supported in the bend of the nurse's or parent's arm, with the forearm and hand supporting his back and head. This frees the other hand and is therefore a convenient way of carrying an infant.

As the infant grows older and is able to support his head, the parents may take him with them outdoors in a sling (see Fig. 13–19). This mode of transportation of the infant permits the parents greater freedom for shopping or participating in outdoor activities.

BATHING

The purpose of the bath is not only cleanliness but also to give the infant a chance to exercise without clothing and, if he is put in a tub of water, to kick and splash. It is a time for parent or nurse to talk to him and play with him. It provides an opportunity to note his growth and development and to observe his body for evidence of rash or chafing (see p. 163).

The time for the bath can be whenever the parent or nurse finds it most convenient. It should have a regular place in the day's schedule of care. The modern father bathes the infant now and then in order to learn to know him better and to give him the same sense of being loved and cared for by his father that he has from his mother.

For the procedure of the bath, see page 180. The infant may have a sponge bath in bed or be bathed in a tub. A bathinette constructed for the purpose of infant bathing may be used if the parents can afford it. The tub cover has straps which buckle over the infant's chest so that the parent can change the infant's diaper and wash his buttocks without fear of his falling. When using this equipment, the parent may have difficulty in transferring the infant from the table to the tub. The equipment for bathing the infant should be conveniently near and everything required in readiness so that the parent will not have to leave him.

Safety factors must be kept in mind when bathing the infant; precautions to safeguard him and to avoid fear are necessary. An infant or little child should never be left alone in a tub of water even if he is old enough to sit up and hold on to the sides of the tub. It is not safe to give him a powder can to play with even if it appears to be empty, for he may inhale a little of the powder left in the bottom of the can if he shakes it vigorously.

It is important that the infant learn to like his bath. If he is immersed in the tub too quickly or does not feel that he is held securely, he may stiffen and appear startled. If this happens, he may acquire an adverse attitude toward his bath. The nurse or parent should place him in the tub very gently. His head and shoulders should be held on the forearm and the hand should grasp the opposite arm. He should not be soaped too liberally, since it is then difficult to retain a firm hold upon his body and limbs. He would be frightened if he were allowed to slip or if his face were covered with water.

CLOTHING

Clothing needed for the newborn and the infant was discussed on page 180. In general, when dressing the infant, the clothing should not be dragged over his face, but should be put on from the bottom up if at all possible.

Various kinds of sleeping garments are used for infants. Many mothers like to put a nightgown on the infant when he is old enough to kick the covers off. If the gown is open at the bottom and all down the back, the sides should be folded so that he does not lie upon the gown and wet it when he voids. If there is a drawstring through the hem and the gown is partially closed at the back, the drawstring can be tightened so that the gown covers his feet, but he must have room to kick unrestrainedly. As he grows older and becomes more active, he needs pajamas or sleepers with feet. The two-piece type saves laundry and time, since it is necessary to change only the half that is soiled.

A sleeping bag or garment made of blanket material like a loose, long, full-sleeved kimono with the bottom sewed up and closed with a zipper in front is useful for keeping the infant covered. It should be large enough for him to move freely within it. The neck should be loose so as not to bind him when he turns.

When the infant learns to creep or move around freely, his clothes should be loose in the crotch and armholes. Overalls will protect his legs when he creeps. They should be open in the crotch so that the diaper may be easily changed. Sunsuits are excellent in summer weather.

Shoes should be soft until the child walks. They are needed only to protect his feet when he crawls or creeps. If the floor covering is warm, smooth and clean, he should be allowed to go barefoot. Socks are worn with the shoes and should be at least ½ inch longer than his feet. Infants' feet grow quickly, and unless the socks are ample in size when bought, they will soon be too small.

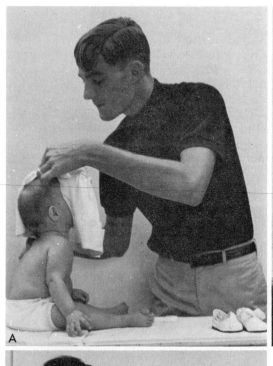

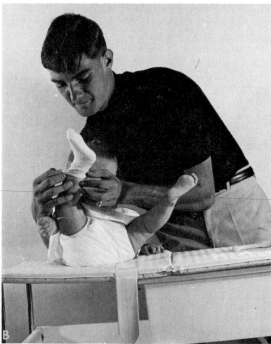

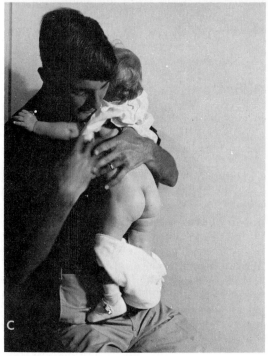

FIGURE 13–20. Father's care of his daughter not only helps him to know her better but also relieves mother of her responsibility for a short time. The father learns that dressing an infant is not always as easy as it appears. (Courtesy of Peggo Cromer: *Baby Talk*, August 1969, p. 7.)

FRESH AIR AND SUNSHINE

The infant should be outdoors as much as possible. He should be dressed according to the weather. Actual deep suntanning or sunburning of an infant should be avoided. Some pediatricians warn mothers not to intentionally expose babies to the sun until the second summer of life. The objective of sun baths is to acquire an even tan. While having his sun baths he should continue to take vitamin D (see p. 368).

EXERCISE

An infant gets exercise in a number of ways. He is active at bath time. Mere change of position is a form of exercise. When he is old enough to turn over—and later play in his play yard—his clothes should not restrict his movements. He should have toys which encourage activity.

SLEEP

The greater part of a young infant's time is spent in sleep. Currently research is being done on the amount of REM (rapid eye movement) sleep which an infant obtains as evidenced by his grimacing, sucking, and squirming activity during apparent sleep. The infant needs rest for his rapid growth, and his energy output. The amount of sleep he takes depends upon his needs, which vary from day to day. If he is given the opportunity, he will develop his own schedule.

The position in which an infant is placed for sleep is important (see p. 160, changing the position of the newborn). As soon as he can move his head from side to side to prevent his nose from being pressed against the surface on which he lies, it is safe to place him on either his back or his abdomen. The danger of sleeping on his back is that he may vomit and aspirate fluid. In general, lying on his side is preferred for comfort and safety.

Signs of increasing maturity in relation to sleep are a reduction in the total sleeping time and longer intervals between sleeping periods. Although each infant varies from any standard or norm, 15 to 18 hours of sleep a day is typical during the first few months of life. At three months the usual amount of sleep in a 24-hour period is about 15 to 16 hours. He will often sleep throughout the night. At six months the average amount of sleep is about 12 hours at night and 3 to 4 hours during the day. The number of naps and their length vary with the individual infant. At one year of age he sleeps about 14 hours out of the 24. At this age he is fearful of leaving his mother and of being deserted by her. A child of this age should have one or two naps a day.

Promotion of Sleep, and Care After Wakening. Overstimulation should be avoided before bedtime. The infant should be dry and comfortable. He should not be put to bed and immediately left alone in the dark. He may need to keep a favorite toy with him to hold so that he feels secure while he goes to sleep. Quieting activities should be provided, such as rocking him or singing to him.

The environment should be suited to his needs, one of which is a room of his own. Twilight is preferable to either a bright light or darkness. A soft light is often used to make the situation more familiar. The light should not shine directly in his eyes.

The temperature of the room should be such that the infant is neither chilled nor overheated.

A suitable temperature in the day would be 70 to 75° F. (21.1 to 23.8° C.) and at night 60 to 65° F. (15.5 to 18.3° C.). The room should be well ventilated, but there must be no drafts. Screens should be used to cut off unavoidable drafts, but blankets should not be hung over the sides of the crib, since they may fall on the infant and smother him.

The mattress should be firm and completely covered with heavy plastic material. A small piece of light plastic should not be used under the sheet. Should the infant pull the sheet from the bed, he might be covered with the plastic, which could cut off his supply of air. Pillows are not used, since there is danger of his burying his face in one or having it fall on his face and being suffocated. He should lie on a flat surface, since this is best for his bone development.

SAFETY MEASURES

Importance of Accident Prevention. Since accidents are a principal cause of death in infants and children of all ages, great emphasis should be placed on accident prevention. Nurses and parents must consider the child's interests and the hazards resulting from the activities into which his interests lead him. The protection and education needed by each sex and age group are then adapted to the prevention of accidents to which they are most liable. Health education during the prenatal period and while mothers are in the maternity unit should be constructive, not listing all possible dangers to which a child might be subjected, but emphasizing reasonable precautions against the hazards he is likely to encounter in the near future. Accident prevention education should be given slowly to parents and to children.

It may sound ridiculous to speak of teaching accident prevention to an infant. What is meant, of course, is merely that he becomes accustomed to the safety measures used in his care. He learns by observing his mother's actions what behavior of his displeases her, such as behavior which may lead to his harm. As he passes from the toddler into the preschool age simple explanations can be given. He should learn to exercise caution, because he may be hurt if he does not. A certain degree of fear of being hurt is normal and is the logical reason for caution. Health hazards tend to lessen as the child goes to school and later enters adolescence, but accident hazards increase. Accident prevention is taught in the schoolroom and on playgrounds. Accidents common to each age group will be mentioned in this text in their appropriate place.

Specific Safety Measures. Safety factors during the bath, in relation to toys or clothes and in the selection of furniture have already been discussed. The use of cotton-tipped swabs in cleaning the ears is to be avoided because if the infant moves during the procedure, severe injury to the ear with possible loss of hearing may result.

The sides of the crib should always be raised and secure when the infant is in it unattended. The crib should have narrow spaces between the rungs so that the infant's head, arms or legs cannot be caught between them. The infant's bed should not be placed near a radiator, since he may burn his hand if he touches it when reaching through the bars of his crib. It should also be out of range of windows with venetian blinds, since the infant may become fatally entangled in a dangling cord. Safety pins should always be closed and removed from the crib; they should never be stuck in the mattress or left in a receptacle or cake of soap (soap is sometimes used to lubricate the point of a safety pin so that it goes through the thick layers of diaper more readily).

Since an infant puts everything within reach into his mouth, small articles should not be left in his crib or close to his chair. Articles which frequently are aspirated are beads, coins, peanuts, and the like. With the increased use of adhesive fasteners on disposable diapers has come a new danger of the infant pulling the fastener off, putting it into his mouth and aspirating it.

Commonly regarded as a harmless way to soothe a crying infant, the pacifier may cause accidents. If the pacifier is tied around the infant's neck, the ribbon or string may catch on a protrusion on the crib and strangle the child. The infant may also suck the pacifier into his throat with resulting asphyxia. Parents should be taught to observe their infant closely if a pacifier is used.

Even an infant too young to roll may move himself upward by pushing with his feet. For this reason he should never be left unprotected on a bed or a stand. If the mother or nurse must reach for some equipment, she must keep one hand on the infant. An infant should not be left alone in a high chair even if he is strapped in place.

All toys and infant furniture should carry a guarantee that no paint containing lead (see p. 576) or other poisonous substance was used. The infant might ingest such substances when he licks and chews his toys or the bars of his play yard or crib.

Guard rails or gates at the top and bottom of steps will prevent serious falls when the infant begins to creep. When the infant is old enough to creep on the floor, all electrical outlets which he can reach should be covered. Tablecloths which hang over the edge of the table should not be used, since the toddler or even the infant who creeps about will pull on them. Anything on the table will be spilled or will fall on the child. An adult with a baby in arms should not walk on a slippery floor or where toys or other small articles have been left on the floor. It is difficult to regain balance after stumbling with an infant in one's arms.

Parents who take their infant with them in an automobile must be aware of the hazards involved. An infant seat which can be attached to the adult safety lap belt might prevent needless injury should an accident occur.

Infants living in highly populated metropolitan areas are many times the victims of rats. Rats attack infants especially when they are sleeping and may bite or chew the face, fingers, or toes. Prevention lies in the elimination of rats from the area.

INFANT FEEDING AND NUTRITION

Feeding of the newborn was discussed in Chapter 8. The infant will continue to feed from the breast or bottle until he is weaned. Recent research has shown that if a nursing infant refuses milk from one of his mother's breasts during feeding, the mother should be carefully and promptly examined for a malignancy in that breast.

Mothers who breast-feed their infants may want to give them experience in the use of a bottle, giving them water, a formula, or orange juice in this way. If an emergency arises and breast feeding must be discontinued, his acceptance of the bottle is helpful both to him and to those who care for him.

Many mothers do not understand the nutritional needs of infants. They want them to be well fed, but in the process permit social pressure or cultural customs to interfere with sound feeding habits. Some mothers believe that if a little food is good, more will be better, so they change their infant's formula as early as two weeks after birth. They prepare a more concentrated milk formula by either using heaped or packed scoops instead of level scoops of powder in preparing the formula. Some mothers also use fluid milk-like products such as a substitute for milk in the formulas. This "filled milk" is any milk, skim milk, or cream to which any fat or oil other than milk fat has been added. The nutrient quality of these filled milks may vary considerably. Filled milks are therefore not recommended for infant feeding. Some mothers also add cereal to the infant's diet soon after birth.

*TABLE 13–2. RECOMMENDED DAILY DIETARY ALLOWANCES FOR INFANTS
0 TO 12 MONTHS OF AGE*

	0–6 MONTHS WT.–6 KG. (14 POUNDS) HT.–60 CM. (24 INCHES)	6–12 MONTHS WT.–9 KG. (20 POUNDS) HT.–71 CM. (28 INCHES)
K calories	kg. × 117	kg. × 108
Protein	kg. × 2.2 g.	kg. × 2.0 g.
Fat-soluble vitamins		
Vitamin A activity	1400 I.U.	2000 I.U.
Vitamin D	400 I.U.	400 I.U.
Vitamin E activity	4 I.U.	5 I.U.
Water-soluble vitamins		
Ascorbic acid	35 mg.	35 mg.
Folacin[a]	50 μg	50 μg
Niacin[b]	5 mg.	8 mg.
Riboflavin	0.4 mg.	0.6 mg.
Thiamine	0.3 mg.	0.5 mg.
Vitamin B_6	0.3 mg.	0.4 mg.
Vitamin B_{12}	0.3 μg	0.3 μg
Minerals		
Calcium	360 mg.	540 mg.
Phosphorus	240 mg.	400 mg.
Iodine	35 μg	45 μg
Iron	10 mg.	15 mg.
Magnesium	60 mg.	70 mg.
Zinc	3 mg.	5 mg.

[a]The folacin allowances refer to dietary sources as determined by *Lactobacillus casei* assay. Pure forms of folacin may be effective in doses less than ¼ of the RDA.

[b]Although allowances are expressed as niacin, it is recognized that on the average 1 mg. of niacin is derived from each 60 mg. of dietary tryptophan.

From the Food and Nutrition Board, National Academy of Sciences–National Research Council: Recommended Daily Dietary Allowances (1974).

There are dangers of *hypernatremia* from taking concentrated milk feedings. Problems of *obesity* (some infants double their birth weight at three months of age) that may follow the very early introduction of cereals to the diet are due to the increased production of fat cells (see p. 440). Closer supervision of early infant feeding habits is indicated.

Table 13–2 gives the nutritional requirements of infants under one year of age.

ADDITION OF OTHER FOODS AND SUBSTANCES TO THE DIET

The age at which additional foods are added to the infant's diet depends on the physician and on the infant's mother. Some infants enjoy the addition of foods such as strained meats, fruits, vegetables and cereal before they are a month of age even though at first they may have difficulty swallowing them. Infants should in general be given solid foods before the age of three to four months in order to make their diets more nutritionally complete and to become accustomed at an early age to various tastes and textures of food. Infants under five to six months of age accept new foods easily, but after that age they may begin to resist new tastes and textures.

Specific substances to be added early are water, vitamin C, vitamin D, iron, and possibly fluoride.

Water. Newborn infants learn to drink water—boiled for safety—from a bottle. This is given them between feedings because they need more fluid than is supplied in either breast milk or their formula. The infant's thirst should determine the amount of water he takes. In the home the mother should prepare freshly boiled water daily. The water is put in 4-ounce sterile nursing bottles. When the infant is about five months old, some of the daily supply of boiled water should be kept in a sterile covered container and may be offered from a cup; this, however, is supplementary to the use of the bottle until he learns to drink from the cup. Some pediatricians believe that when the infant is about four months old he may be given unboiled water if the water supply in his community is considered safe.

Vitamins. The body requires vitamins in small amounts to guide various metabolic processes. The human being can ingest these in food and store them for future use; therefore a deprivation of vitamins does not produce symptoms immediately. Since infants grow rapidly, their vitamin requirements (see Table 13–2) are proportionately greater than those of adults and their stores are depleted more rapidly; hence *vitamin deficiency diseases* (see pp. 441 and 443) *are seen more frequently in infancy than during adult life.*

Because public education on the need for vitamins has been so effective, many infants as well as adults receive excessive amounts of these substances, leading not only to financial waste but more importantly to toxic effects. These effects in relation to vitamins C, D, and A will be discussed later.

VITAMIN C. Vitamin C, or ascorbic acid, is available in many fruits and vegetables, especially citrus fruits such as oranges, lemons, grapefruit, and limes. Fresh fruit juice is an excellent source of vitamin C, but frozen juice is an acceptable source if used soon after thawing. Tomato juice is also a good source of this vitamin. Exposure of these foods to air for long periods of time may reduce the amount of their vitamin C content.

The infant requires a minimum of 35 mg. of vitamin C daily to prevent scurvy. The addition of vitamin C is particularly important for the bottle-fed infant, since this vitamin is destroyed by heating the milk in the formula. Vitamin C is usually given also to breast-fed infants to assure an adequate supply (the mother's intake of this vitamin may be insufficient, in which case the infant will not receive enough to meet his needs).

The physician will order orange juice, tomato juice, or ascorbic acid in tablet form to satisfy the need of the infant for vitamin C, beginning by about two weeks of age.

To mothers of a low socioeconomic group and possibly to those of low intelligence it should be explained that orange-flavored drinks (orange soda and the like) usually contain no fresh orange juice and may contain ingredients harmful to the infant. It is also necessary to stress the need for cleanliness throughout the procedure of preparing and giving the orange juice.

Synthetic vitamin C is inexpensive. It is a nontoxic vitamin, even in overdosage. The amount not needed is excreted in the urine. A lack of vitamin C produces a condition known as scurvy (see p. 443).

VITAMIN D. Vitamin D can be produced by the human body in response to the action of ultraviolet light on the cholesterol in the skin (see p. 441). Since this source of vitamin D is not constant, especially in the temperate climates, adequate amounts should be given in the diet. Vitamin D can be found in some amounts in natural foods such as milk, butter, and egg yolks, but liver is a good source of supply. This vitamin can be produced artificially. It is a relatively stable vitamin, not as easily destroyed by heat as is vitamin C.

This vitamin is added to the diet when the infant is about two weeks old; in general, 400 International Units are required per day. Vitamin D helps the infant to make use of the calcium he receives in his milk; in this respect it is a substitute for sunshine or is needed in addition to sunshine. As was mentioned on page 175, vitamin D-reinforced whole milk or evaporated milk is available commercially. Many other preparations containing vitamin D are also available, such as cod liver oil and concentrates and other fish liver oil concentrates. The amount of these substances to be given to the infant depends on the physician's order. Vitamin D preparations vary so much in potency that the physician's order should be followed carefully.

The way in which a preparation containing vitamin D in fish oil is given is important. It is given cold. The mouth of the bottle should be wiped to remove all the old oil. No displeasure or disgust should be shown while giving this medication, since the infant will copy the attitude toward the oil from the adult who gives it. The infant's head should be elevated and the infant should be held in a sitting position when he is given the medication by dropper or spoon, in order to prevent aspiration (see p. 404). Preparations containing oil should never be given while the infant is crying.

The usual dosage of vitamin D concentrates is 5 to 10 drops a day.

Some vitamin D preparations can be given in milk, but the infant may not take all the milk and therefore will not ingest the full dose of the vitamin. It is not feasible to put any oily substance into the formula (1) because the oil adheres to the glass, and (2) since oil rises to the top when the feeding bottle is inverted, the infant sucks the oil through the nipple only at the close of the feeding.

Excessively high overdosage of vitamin D over a period of time may lead to abnormalities of calcium metabolism in the body, anorexia, and weight loss. A lack of vitamin D may lead to rickets (see p. 441).

OTHER VITAMINS. Although other vitamins are needed by the infant (see Table 13-2), he usually receives enough in his diet so that supplementation is not necessary. If the physician considers it necessary, multivitamin preparations may be ordered. Overdosage may, however, produce hypervitaminosis, such as is the case with vitamin D. An excessive amount of vitamin A over a period of time may result in anorexia, slow growth and poor weight gain. The infant may also have an enlarged liver, thickening of the cortex of the long bones, and itching of the skin. An excessive amount of other vitamins is usually not harmful.

Iron. The Committee on Nutrition of the American Academy of Pediatrics has emphasized the value of iron-fortified, proprietary milk formulas for the prevention of iron-deficiency anemia of infancy. The Committee recommends that mothers provide their infants with a source of dietary iron either by continuing an iron-fortified formula as long as an infant is bottle-fed and then as beverage milk until the infant is at least one year old by giving the infant iron-fortified whole milk or evaporated milk if it is available (see p. 174).

Although normal newborn infants have an extra supply of iron at birth, they need additional amounts to meet their requirements during growth, especially after the first few months of life, in order to prevent iron-deficiency anemia (see p. 460). In the usual infant diet one half or more of the total daily intake of iron is provided by iron-enriched cereals. For premature infants dietary iron is inadequate for their rapid growth, and supplemental iron should be given (p. 195).

Fluorides. The effect of fluoride in drinking water is to strengthen calcification of forming dental tissues and thus to make the enamel of the teeth more resistant to decay. In many cities the fluoride content of the water supplies is adjusted to adequate levels in order to improve the dental health of the children in the community. For infants who do not receive adequate fluorides in their drinking water the daily administration of a solution of fluoride or a vitamin preparation containing fluoride is recommended. As the child grows older the dosage should be increased, and the substance may be given in tablet form. A fluoride preparation can also be applied to erupted teeth to prevent cavity formation.

ADDITION OF SOLID FOODS

Foods Which Infants Like. The infant will take solid foods which he likes more readily than those which he dislikes. In general, infants like bland foods which are *slightly* sweet, sour, or salty. They do not like bitter foods or those strongly sour or salty. Some concern has been shown recently over the amount of sodium contained in commercially prepared infant foods and the possibility that this might lead to hypertension later. Sugar and starch that are added to commercially prepared infant foods encourage obesity. These substances are added to foods, presumably to make them more palatable to the mother, not necessarily to the infant. Consumer groups and various health professionals are striving to have the exact amount or percentages of ingredients, including salt, sugar, and starch

placed on the labels. Research continues on these matters.

The nutritional values of infant foods may be found in textbooks on nutrition.

An infant's preference for texture and consistency of food varies according to his age. Naturally the newborn infant likes only liquid food. An infant a few weeks old likes food which feels smooth (puréed food). When his teeth are coming through, he likes foods on which he can chew, such as teething biscuits, zwieback, or chopped foods. The shift from puréed to chopped foods should be a gradual one. Chopped foods ("junior foods") can be started from six to nine months, depending upon the infant's ability to chew.

Infants prefer food at moderate temperatures. An infant may be frightened by food too hot or too cold and may refuse it when it is offered him again.

Method of Introduction. The infant's reaction to his first solid food is to make sucking movements with his tongue which cause the food to be pushed out of his mouth. It must be remembered that the infant has to learn the method of smoothly transferring solid food from the front of the mouth to the pharynx. The nurse should explain to the young mother that this reaction is to be expected.

An infant's introduction to solid food should be a pleasant experience. The infant should be held securely in the same position as for taking his formula from the bottle, but his head and shoulders should be raised slightly more than in bottle feeding. A bib is necessary, since he will spit out the food and make his fingers sticky by putting them into his mouth. The food should be smooth and thin. Cereals should be diluted with the formula; fruit or a vegetable, with boiled water.

A small serving (1 teaspoonful) is all that an infant will take at first. A small spoon should be used. (Do not use a spoon with a curved handle; it is awkward in an adult's hand.) The food should be placed on the back of the infant's tongue, but no pressure should be exerted, since that would cause him to gag. New foods should be introduced one at a time, usually at an interval of several days in order to allow for the appearance of any allergic reaction which may occur. A new food should be offered before his formula or a food to which he is accustomed. The infant should not be hurried, coaxed or allowed to linger. Thirty minutes is long enough for a feeding. If he has not taken the food at the end of that time, the feeding should be discontinued and another attempt made the next day. Medication should not be mixed with the food unless the physician specifically orders that this be done.

Many parents and nurses become anxious when teaching an infant to take solid food. The feeder should be calm, patient, gentle, and pleasant in the approach to the infant. He is then more likely to take the food than if he is scolded or coaxed. He should never be held tightly in an effort to control his hands, nor be forced to eat. Such measures make him antagonistic to the feeding process. If the nurse or parent is giving the infant food that is personally distasteful, he or she should not show any evidence of this dislike. The infant is likely to imitate this reaction to the food. If he wants to touch the food, he should be allowed to do so. Touching is one of his methods of learning. His hands, of course, should be washed both before and after his feeding.

Just as physicians vary as to the time for starting solid foods, so they vary as to which food should be given first. Traditionally, cereal has been the first food given.

Cereal. Early administration of cereal was formerly advised because it contains iron. A young infant needs iron since he does not receive a sufficient quantity of it in breast milk or his formula. Currently proprietary enriched infant cereal contains more iron than most other puréed foods; therefore it is begun early.

Cereals which are ready-prepared for infant use may be given, or the infant's portion may be taken from that prepared for the family breakfast. Dry cereals, however, are not suitable for infants. Cereals especially prepared for infants are more finely divided and easily digested than those made for the family table. If the cereal cooked for the family is to be used for the infant, his serving should be cooked longer in order to break the starch or polysaccharide down to the simpler forms of carbohydrate—disaccharide or monosaccharide—which the infant can more readily digest. (It is best to use a double boiler to cook cereals so that the cereal does not stick to the bottom of the pan.) Cereals prepared for the infant should not be sweetened.

A variety of cereals should be given so that the infant may learn to accept a variety of tastes. Rice cereal may be given first; however, mixed cereals should not be given early because of the possibility of an allergic reaction to one of the ingredients. It is well to begin with a teaspoonful of cereal once a day. This may be increased gradually until at six or seven months he will take from 2 to 5 tablespoons a day.

As the infant grows older he may be given a baked or boiled potato in place of his cereal. The potato can be mashed with a fork and moistened with a little boiled milk or water.

Fruits. Fresh fruits (e.g., apples, peaches, apricots) should be stewed and put through a sieve. No sugar should be added. Banana can be given raw, mashed to a pulp with a spoon. The fruit should be thoroughly ripe. The giving of fruit should be started with 1 teaspoonful, and the amount gradually increased until the infant is getting 3 or 4 tablespoons a day. Several kinds of fruit should be tried so that he learns to like a variety.

Vegetables. As with fruit, the infant should be given only a teaspoonful at first, with an increase until he is taking 2 to 4 tablespoonfuls. The vegetables should be steamed or cooked in as little water as possible in order to retain their mineral and vitamin content. Vegetables, when first introduced, should be put through a sieve. The infant should be given green and yellow vegetables which have a bland taste and contain necessary vitamins. Later, when he is teething, he should be given coarsely mashed or chopped vegetables. Peas, carrots, or string beans may be included in the diet, and should be cooked until soft so that they can be readily chopped, mashed or crushed with a fork.

Eggs. Many physicians suggest that egg yolk be given the infant when he is from three to five months old. They also suggest that egg white not be given until toward the end of the first year, because infants may be allergic to egg albumen. Egg yolk contains iron and riboflavin as well as protein. It should be hard-cooked, mashed with a fork, and fed in small amounts until the infant has become accustomed to it and then gradually increased. It can be given alone or mixed with milk or cereal. When egg white is added to the diet, the egg may be boiled (hard or soft) or poached. Only small amounts of egg white should be given until it is evident that the infant is not allergic to the protein it contains; then the entire egg may be given.

Meat. Many physicians add strained meats to the diet early in the first year. Meat, like eggs and milk, provides protein. Meat especially prepared for infant feeding can be bought in small containers. It can also be prepared by scraping raw meat—liver or beef—with a knife; the scraped meat is then formed into a patty and cooked in a custard cup set in a pan of boiling water. When the meat is thoroughly cooked, the patty will be brown.

At first the infant is given only a teaspoonful of meat prepared in this way, but it is soon increased to 2 tablespoonfuls a day. Liver is especially valuable because of its high content of iron, vitamin A and vitamin B complex. Chicken and lamb are added to the diet later. The infant should not be given fatty meats because fat requires more time for digestion and is therefore less easily utilized. When he is able to chew, his meat may be finely ground rather than scraped.

Fish. Near the end of the first year, fish can be substituted for meat or egg several times a week. The fish should be boiled, baked, or steamed, but not fried, because of the increase in the fat content. The fish must be finely divided in order to be certain that it does not contain small particles of bones.

Bread. Dried bread or zwieback may be added to the diet when the infant is about six months old and his teeth are coming through the gums. If he is permitted to hold the bread, he will learn in an easy way to carry food to his mouth. This is the first step in acquiring the ability to feed himself. He will also get exercise for his jaws through chewing the dried bread.

Whole Milk. If the infant is not breast-fed, his formula may be discontinued by about three to five months, and he is given whole homogenized, pasteurized, boiled milk. Some pediatricians do not request the mother to boil the milk or the water she gives her infant if she lives in a community where the quality of the milk and water supplies is carefully controlled. Since he is receiving carbohydrate in his cereal and other foods, he does not need sugar added to the milk.

Desserts. Desserts are given in the latter part of the first year. Those suited to the infant's needs are fruits, gelatin, milk puddings, junkets, and custards.

HOME OR COMMERCIAL PREPARATION OF INFANTS' FOODS

Mothers may prepare infants' foods at home or buy ready-prepared foods; some may want to can food for his use.* Such foods must be thoroughly cooked without seasoning and strained for feeding the young infant. The advantages of homemade baby foods are that they are both safe and nutritious without any additives.

Mothers can buy precooked cereal. These powdered cereals can be made into a liquid or paste by the addition of boiled water or the infant's formula. Vegetables, fruits, meats, and egg yolk can also be obtained in puréed or chopped form for infant feeding. Mixed meat and vegeta-

ble dinners are available, but the infant should be observed for the possibility of an allergic reaction to one of the ingredients. These containers can be safely refrigerated for two or three days after being opened. It is good practice to remove from the container only one serving at a time. The remainder in the jar may be safely covered and refrigerated. The original container was sterilized in processing and is the safest receptacle for the food. The advantages of prepared infant foods are variety, convenience, year-round availability, uniform quality and consistency, and sterility.

DEVELOPMENT OF EATING HABITS

The mother is generally responsible if her child develops poor eating habits. If she makes the feeding period a happy one for him, feeding problems are not likely to develop. It is easier to make a good start in feeding than to correct a bad habit when the infant is older.

By *one month* the infant is able to take food from a spoon if it is offered to him. At *five to six months* the average infant begins to use his fingers in eating (finger-feeding), taking zwieback or dry, thin toast in his hand and learning to carry it to his mouth. At *eight to nine months* he has acquired the skill of holding a spoon and playing with it. At *nine months* the average infant can hold his own bottle and seems to prefer doing so. The *12-month-old* child drinks from a cup, although he may want his bottle at bedtime for the comfort of sucking. See p. 571 for a discussion of the bottle-mouth syndrome.

During the first year the infant's appetite will be good because of his increasing activity and rapid body growth. At the end of the first year his appetite will decrease because of his slower rate of growth and his corresponding decreased need for food. This is normal and should never be a signal for the mother or nurse to force him to eat or to become anxious lest he starve. Encouraging him to eat too much food at this time often results in feeding problems during the toddler period.

COLIC

Colic is most common during the first three or four months of life. By colic is meant paroxysmal intestinal cramps due to accumulation of excessive gas. This causes discomfort and pain. The infant may pass gas from the anus or belch it up from the stomach. In reaction to his pain the infant cries loudly, draws up his arms and legs and becomes red in the face. His abdomen feels hard to the mother's or nurse's hand.

Etiology, Treatment, and Prognosis. Colic may be caused by one or a combination of sev-

---

*Directions for canning fresh foods may be obtained from the United States Department of Agriculture, Washington, D.C., or from a state College of Agriculture.

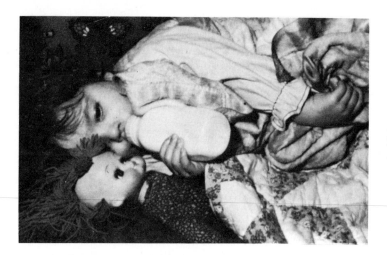

FIGURE 13–21. Bottle-mouth caries is a phenomenon seen in infants and young children who have had prolonged bottle feeding. (From Rabinowitz, M.: *Children Today* 3:18, March-April, 1974.)

eral factors, among them excessive air-swallowing, too rapid feeding, overfeeding, excessive intake of carbohydrate which fosters intestinal fermentation and thus gas production, and emotional tension in the infant.

The *treatment* is dependent on whatever is thought to be the cause of the condition and may include modification of the formula, careful infant feeding procedure with frequent bubbling of the infant, the use of a carminative such as peppermint water (a "home" remedy), the use of enemas, suppositories, or rectal tubes, the application of a hot-water bottle to the infant's abdomen or turning the infant on his abdomen to encourage the expulsion of flatus, the use of drugs such as antispasmodics, sedatives, or tranquilizers, or the use of a pacifier to calm the tense child.

This lengthy list of therapeutic measures provides evidence that no one treatment is successful in all infants having colic. Each mother with the help of the physician must therefore find the technique that works best for her infant. The nurse can often help the mother of an infant who has colic by listening to the problems caused by her infant's condition.

Colic is not a serious condition, and infants often gain weight in spite of the periods of pain.

WEANING

Psychologic Background. Weaning from the breast or bottle to drinking from a cup has a psychologic significance apart from pleasure in the new activity and from the mere motor ability to drink rather than to suck. It is the end of an infant's receiving his main pleasure from an object through the use of his mouth and sucking.

An infant usually indicates his readiness for advance in behavior when the old technique is no longer needed and its limitations frustrate him in his desire for new experiences and control of his environment. In his journey toward maturity he must experience a certain amount of frustration at his inability to control his physical and social environment, in order to be stimulated to try to achieve this control.

During the second half of the first year the infant both wants and needs more freedom to move about and to acquire increasing control of his body and knowledge of his environment. It is no longer necessary to hold him closely to communicate to him a feeling of love and protection. In fact, he is likely to resist such restraint. He now gains a feeling of trust in others through their smiling faces and through their words spoken in a tone of voice which he has always associated with pleasant experiences. He wants to leave his infant way of taking nourishment—sucking from the breast or bottle—and try to drink from a cup.

In all learning there is an optimum stage of development when a new activity is learned most readily. At this time opportunity for experimentation should be given the infant, under conditions which favor his success. He should not be hurried to drop the old pattern of behavior while learning the new. By six months or so he has learned that good things to eat come from dishes and cups and is ready to try milk from a cup when it is presented to him. He shows his readiness to drink from a cup by sitting up and reaching for it. He then looks to the adult for help in the technique of this new way of taking milk. If he fails to take it, the nurse or parent should wait a few weeks and then try again. The old and the new techniques will overlap.

Time for Weaning. The best time for weaning is generally in the second half of the first year. Although some infants learn to drink from a cup at five months, they seldom show pleasure in it and should not be forced to give up sucking pleasure until they are ready to do so.

The infant may be weaned from breast to formula or whole milk feedings, depending on the order of his physician, before six months of age if the mother's milk is diminishing in quantity or if it is necessary that she return to work outside the home. If some breast milk is available, this should also be given to the infant. The feeding should be given by bottle and not by cup, since a small infant needs the comfort of sucking.

Pregnancy and illness are other reasons for weaning before six months. It is a strain on a pregnant woman's physical strength to supply enough of the essential food elements for both the suckling and the fetus and at the same time meet her own physical needs. Chronic illness in the mother, such as cancer and diseases of the kidneys, heart, or blood, may necessitate weaning the infant. Severe, long-lasting infections in the mother are also a cause for weaning. Pulmonary tuberculosis in the mother is a contraindication to breast feeding, since the infant would be contaminated from such close contact with his mother.

Methods of Weaning. The infant should be weaned gradually so that he is less likely to be frustrated by the change from sucking to drinking.

As soon as he drinks well from the cup the number of breast or bottle feedings can be slowly reduced. Some breast-fed infants change to taking their milk from a bottle before learning to drink from a cup. It is an individual matter whether to use the bottle feeding as an intermediate step between breast feeding and drinking from a cup. It is a good plan to let the infant learn to like the taste of cow's milk before breast feeding is discontinued completely.

Weaning should never be undertaken when the infant is sick or hospitalized for any but a compelling reason, for he is already under a physical and emotional strain from his illness.

Reaction of the Infant to Weaning. When the complete process of weaning is too abrupt, the infant may show signs of discomfort (anxiety, sleeplessness, and irritability) and may cry a great deal. He is likely to suck his thumb excessively.

If the infant receives extra attention during and after the period of weaning, he will find many other pleasant experiences to compensate for the lost satisfaction of ingesting milk through sucking and will have little or no reaction to the weaning process.

Reaction of the Mother to Weaning. Earlier in this text the importance of early maternal attachment to the infant was discussed in relation to breast feeding (see p. 167). In addition, since breast stimulation alone evokes a range of reactions in women from little or no pleasure to orgasm, one should not be surprised that breast feeding may cause sexual arousal in some women. This is normal. Sudden cessation of nursing or even an unexpected interruption may thus cause a crisis not only for the child but for the mother as well. The ultimate need for the mother to wean the infant is real, but it must be by her choice and done gradually. If it is not done in this way, the mother may feel a great loss and become depressed. Anticipatory preparation for weaning is essential for the mother who breast-feeds her infant.

ELIMINATION

As different kinds of foods are added to the infant's diet, the color as well as the consistency of the stools will change. For example, if beets are given, the stools will have a reddish tinge. Gradually, as a variety of foods is taken in the daily diet, the stools will be formed, and their predominant color will be brown.

HEALTH PROTECTION

Participants in the 1970 White House Conference on Children and the Joint Commission on Mental Health of Children gave high priority to the recommendation of a nationwide network of comprehensive health services for children and youth. These services should take a broad view of the whole child in his environment and should be concerned with the maintenance of health or the prevention of illness as well as with its early treatment. To this end it has been necessary not only to develop new delivery systems but also to build on the strengths of programs already in existence (see Chap. 1).

Although there are some private ventures in prepaid group medical practice, health plans, and centers for handicapped children among others, the majority of ways comprehensive health services have been provided within the last ten years have been under the stimulus of the Federal government. These include the Children and Youth (C and Y) Program, which provides services for children from birth to 19 years in low-income families; Maternity and Infant Care (M and I) Program for high-risk mothers and infants to one year of age; Project

Head Start for preschool children; state crippled children's services; university-affiliated centers and community clinics for mentally retarded children; and neighborhood health centers, among others.

Even though these services have been available, the complete goal of comprehensive health services for our nation's children remains out of reach; only a fraction of the children needing service actually obtain it. Some of these children are cared for by private physicians or clinics with the help of the federal-state program of Medicaid. Obviously further planning will be necessary if each child is to receive the comprehensive preventive, diagnostic, and therapeutic care he needs.

A general movement is under way to decrease the fragmentation of existing health services. One aspect of the broader concern for comprehensive family health services is the concern about the need for comprehensive health services for children and youth. The value of the Child Health Conferences has already been proved, as evidenced by the reduction of morbidity and mortality rates among the children served. Children have been served by their screening programs for vision, hearing, and dental health as well as by their immunization programs.

Child Health Conference

PRIMARY CARE

One aspect of primary care, as discussed earlier, is that of distributive care, which is primarily designed *to maintain health and prevent disease* on a *continuing* basis. Distributive care is likely to occur in the community with *essentially well or ambulatory patients.*

Care of the infant in the Child Health Conference may be the first contact he has with the health care system other than during his mother's pregnancy, at birth, and during the postnatal period. The pediatric nurse or public health nurse or the pediatric nurse practitioner as a primary-care agent in the Child Health Conference not only works with the mother on the care of the child, but also continues to provide care for the individual infant and later to help him in self-care.

Although nurses have served this function for many years, pediatric nurse practitioners are increasingly seen in the community where services to children are provided: in private pediatric practices, in outpatient departments, in Child Health Conferences, and in Neighborhood Health Centers. They provide a major service to

essentially well infants and ambulatory children and adolescents. The pediatric nurse practitioner assumes the responsibility for children's health maintenance and thus frees the pediatrician to care for acutely ill children having medical or surgical conditions. The goal of both the nurse and the pediatric nurse practitioner is to be concerned with prevention as well as care and with anything that interferes with the physical or psychosocial well-being of this age group. They also function as health consumer advocates in providing the best family care possible for parents and their children.

The principal focus of care in this type of nursing is on the family rather than on specific illnesses or other problems. Families must be helped to utilize their own strengths when adapting to the stresses of family life or to crisis situations when they occur. The mother and father, and increasingly the child as he matures, are responsible for making their own decisions regarding their care. The nurse and the pediatric nurse practitioner, then, aid them in reaching this goal.

The Child Health Conference is part of a continuous program of health supervision which should start in the prenatal period and continue throughout childhood and into adult life. The family is studied in the Child Health Conference so that the personnel can help the family to make the most of their resources in the care of the individual child.

FAMILY APPROACH

Adjustments of general principles must be made for application to the individual family. It is essential that parents have an easy self-confidence in their ability to fulfill their parental roles. The physician, social worker, counselor, pediatric nurse practitioner, community or public health nurse must know the socioeconomic status and cultural background of the family when making recommendations, and should make no recommendation which the family will be unable to carry out.

It is difficult for many mothers to measure a child's development in terms of his capacities; they tend to compare growth, development, and abilities of one child with those of others. This is a matter in which the Child Health Conference is particularly useful, since it keeps a continuous record of the child's progress.

If the personnel of the Conference work as a team and show an intense interest in the children, the mothers will follow advice and instructions to the best of their ability. Not too much advice should be given at one time, since this might lead to confusion.

PURPOSES OF THE CHILD HEALTH CONFERENCE

Overall Purposes. The main purpose of the Child Health Conference is to provide health supervision for infants and young children who would not otherwise receive this service. Some children are not directly under the supervision of any physician; others may be taken to a private physician or to a clinic only when they are sick. The Child Health Conference does not displace the services of the private physician, but supplements them by giving a kind of service which some children would not otherwise receive.

A secondary purpose of the Conference is to educate parents in better ways of caring for children and to give them an understanding of growth and development.

The Conference personnel should strive to meet the mother's needs and to increase her confidence in providing care for her children. Personnel must not be autocratic or judgmental, but rather should be interested and understanding. Many parents as consumers are confused by the conflicting ideas of child-rearing gathered from relatives, friends, and magazine and newspaper articles. They should be helped to learn the best concepts of child care and feel secure in their ability to adapt these concepts to their particular needs and then put them into practice without doubts and misgivings.

Although direct teaching is one responsibility of the personnel, it is equally important that they accept the mother as she is. If she is suffering from anxiety or is fearful and possibly has feelings of guilt, the personnel should help her to understand the basis for these attitudes, so that the energy wasted in combating her frustration can be used in loving and working for the children.

Specific Purposes. The broad aims of the Conference are implemented through specific aims: (1) to help mothers understand the physical growth and emotional development of their children and to show them how serious problems can be averted if parents know what to expect of a child at various ages; (2) to recognize physical defects or illness through a complete examination and to inform parents of the sources in the community, such as a private physician or a clinic, where these conditions can be treated; (3) to provide protection against certain communicable diseases by immunization procedures; (4) to offer advice about specific nutrition of the child and to give general assistance with budgeting for the whole family diet; (5) to help es-

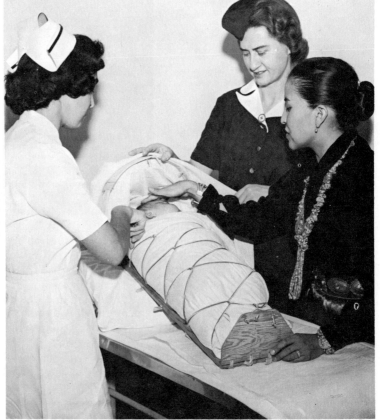

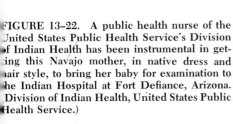

FIGURE 13–22. A public health nurse of the United States Public Health Service's Division of Indian Health has been instrumental in getting this Navajo mother, in native dress and hair style, to bring her baby for examination to the Indian Hospital at Fort Defiance, Arizona. Division of Indian Health, United States Public Health Service.)

TABLE 13–3. FLOW SHEET FOR HEALTH SUPERVISION: THE PROBLEM-ORIENTED MEDICAL RECORD

WELL CHILD FLOW SHEET   NAME: _____ DOB: _____

Age	Immunizations	HGB	U/A	P/R BP	Hearing	Vision	Guidance	Diet	Comments
1 mo.			PKU				Clothes, Travel, Infant Seat, Sleep, Thermometer, Father, Mother, Observation, Vitamins, Fluoride	Bottle in bed, Solids	
2 mos.	DPT TOPV			▼			Pain, Fever, ASA, Sibling Rivalry, Mother	Quant. Formula	
4 mos.	DPT TOPV			▼			Observation, Toys, URI, Foreign Objects, Car Seat, Discipline, Toilet Training	Milk, Vitamins, Solids	
6 mos.	DPT TOPV				▼		Crawler, Poisons, Ipecac, Strangers	Peanuts	
9 mos.	Tine ▼						Climber, Accidents, Temper Tantrums, Masturbation	Cup	
1 yr.	Measles Rubella			▼	▼	▼	Family play, Dental Care, Matches, Appetite	Candy	
1 1/2 yr.	DPT TOPV						Streets, Cars, Seat Belts	Soft Drinks	
2 yr.	Tine Mumps						Bed Wetting, Peers, Independence, Manners		
3 yr.		▼	▼	▼	▼	▼	Strangers		
4 yr.	Tine				▼		Water Safety		
5 yr.	DPT TOPV ▼			▼	▼	▼	School, Bike		
6 yr.	Tine			▼			Chores, Money		
7 yr.				▼					
8 yr.	Tine			▼			Drugs, Alcohol, Tobacco		
9 yr.	Rh HAI			▼			Menstruation, Sex		
10 yr.	Tine			▼			Guns, Rh		
11 yr.				▼		▼	Limits		
12 yr.	DT Tine			▼			Drugs, Alcohol, Tobacco, Sex		
13 yr.				▼			Freedom, Parents		
14 yr.	Tine			▼			Cars, Sex		
15 yr.				▼			Education		
16 yr.				▼			Future plans		
17 yr.	DT			▼			Marriage		
18 yr.	Tine			▼			Children		

▼ = mandatory

DEVELOPMENT

Milestone	Age
Smile	
Grasp & Reach	
Sit Alone	
Walk Alone	
Words	
Bowel Control	
Urine Control	

PREVIOUS IMMUNIZATIONS

DPT				
OPV				
Tetanus				
Smallpox				
Measles				
Rubella				
Mumps				
Tine				
Other				

Abbreviations: DOB=Date of Birth, Hgb= Hemoglobin, U/A=Urinalysis, P/R=Pulse/Respiratory rate, PKU=urine test for phenylketonuria, DPT=Diphtheria-Pertussis-Tetanus vaccine, TOPV=Trivalent oral poliomyelitis vaccine, ASA=aspirin, Tine=skin test for tuberculosis, Rh=Rh blood typing (girls), HAI=Hemagglutination inhibition test for rubella antibodies (girls), DT=Diphtheria-Tetanus toxoid.

From Vaughan, V. C., III, and McKay, R. J.: *Nelson Textbook of Pediatrics*, 10th ed. Philadelphia, W. B. Saunders Co., 1975.

tablish sound child-health team-mother relations and attitudes toward medical treatment; and (6) to provide assistance with behavior problems and to help the family in their total relations with the child.

The physician in some instances may refer a child to a social worker, psychologist, or psychiatrist. The nurse will help the mother to understand and accept the need for such service. This is best done by allowing the mother to express her fears and work through the problem with the emotional support of the nurse. The nurse should also help her to extend the constructive relations she has had with the Conference personnel to those in other professions who can provide the service the child needs.

Concomitant Outcomes. Records on the physical and developmental progress of children and on parental reactions to their roles are kept in the Child Health Conference. These records are of potential value in future care of the child. In some cities children are given physical examinations in the Conference, and the completed records of their health histories are sent with them when they go to school.

MOTHERS AND THE CHILD HEALTH CONFERENCE

A mother may learn of Child Health Conferences while receiving prenatal care or in the hospital after the birth of her child. Sometimes the public health nurse who delivers the birth certificate may inform the mother if she has not already been told of the availability of the Conference. Any nurse or pediatric nurse practitioner, whether working in a hospital, clinic, or public health service, should know of the facilities the community offers for child health supervision and should explain these to the mothers whose infants need such services. Any infant whose mother does not have a private physician should be taken to such a Conference.

Many mothers come to the Child Health Conference to find out whether they are doing a good job in bringing up a child. They want reassurance that their judgment is sound and that the child is responding normally to their care. Some mothers come because they feel discouraged and inadequate or want to be relieved of a sense of guilt. All come for information and to have their children examined and given the customary immunizations. Some come because their friends come, and they consider it a pleasant social gathering. Such mothers dress their children to be admired by other mothers and by the clinic personnel. Their attendance should not be discouraged, though obviously they need to take a more serious view of child care.

PERSONNEL

The minimal personnel required to meet the needs of the mother who brings her child to them includes the physician and at least one nurse or pediatric nurse practitioner. If there is a full staff, a social worker, a child guidance worker, a nutritionist, and a dental hygienist are available for consultation or treatment. The physician should be a pediatrician or should have had extensive experience with mothers and children. The nurse or pediatric nurse practitioner in charge of the Conference should have had public health experience and have worked successfully with children. In an ideal situation one or both parents and the child should see the physician and the nurse at each visit.

Functions of the Pediatric Nurse Practitioner or the Nurse in the Child Health Conference. In the general management of the Conference the atmosphere should be such as to reduce the strain on the mother and the child and to make them feel at ease. Each mother should be respected as a person and addressed by her proper name. If it is the mother's first visit, the nurse should explain each step of the routine to her. Facilities for privacy should be provided during the mother's conferences with the personnel. The nurse should introduce her to other mothers and talk with her before she sees the physician. The nurse screens patients and mothers on the basis of their different needs and problems. The nurse also observes them for signs of illness when they enter, in order to isolate any child whose condition may be infectious or to refer him immediately to the appropriate agency or the physician. It is desirable that the same nurse discuss with the mother the physician's recommendations after her conference with him.

The nurse should have adequate time for both individual and group teaching when an appointment system is used. Each child should be seen in order of his appointment. If a mother brings her child without an appointment, however, it is customary for the physician to see the child if he appears sick or if the mother is anxious about his condition. The appointment system is a good check on the regularity of the infant's visits to the clinic. Before the mother leaves, the date and time of the next appointment should be given her in writing and should be entered in the appointment book.

HOME VISITS. A visit to the home should be made after a child has been brought to the clinic, in order to observe the home environment, to teach the mother, and to inspect the child. Ideally, this visit is made by the nurse in charge of the clinic, but if this is not possible, the public health or community nurse makes the visit and sends a report to the clinic. During the home visit the nurse should observe the socioeconomic status, sanitary conditions, housing, and recreational facilities, which are important to both the infant's and the family's health. In the home the nurse can observe parent-child relations better than in the more or less formal atmosphere of the Child Health Conference.

THE NURSE AND VOLUNTEER WORKERS. The work of volunteers is valuable, for they help the nurses to serve as an important means of communication with the public. The nurse teaches the volunteers how to perform nonprofessional duties in the clinic.

Functions performed by volunteer workers in many clinics are as follows:

Check ventilation and light.
Assist in setting up the clinic.
Greet each mother and register the children.
Bring to the attention of the nurse the fact that a child does not appear well.
Begin the admission record.
Take the child's weight and height and record the findings on the chart.
Talk with the mother about educational material and interest her in it.
Supervise the play of the preschool children.
Assist with any additional duties.

ADMINISTRATION AND PROCEDURES

The Child Health Conference may be a voluntary organization with private support, or it may be a public service supported through public funds. Private physicians in the community are requested to support and to help plan and conduct the Conference.

If possible, the Conference should be held in a place convenient for the parents of the children who will be brought there. In large cities many are located in housing projects or health centers. In rural areas the Conference may travel by mobile health unit from community to community; some organization within the community to be visited makes all the necessary arrangements. These Conferences are highly successful and have done much to improve the health of children in rural areas.

The physical setup requires three or four rooms. One room is used as a reception or waiting room and should be large enough to accommodate the mothers and children without crowding. Posters and exhibits can be placed here. A small room is required for weighing and measuring the children. The physician's consultation room should be equipped for examining the child and should have a comfortable chair for the mother in which she can hold her infant while she talks to the physician. There should also be a separate room in which the mother and nurse or nutritionist may consult about any problems the mother may have.

If such space is not available, one or two rooms may be divided by screens so that the work of the clinic may be carried on. Ideally, room should be available for taking the child's history, for undressing and examining the child, for comfortable seating of mothers and children while waiting to be seen, and for play among older children. The play area should have small chairs and washable toys for the children. A volunteer worker may be available to supervise the children. The area where immunizations are given should be away from the room where the children and their mothers are waiting, so that they do not hear a child cry when he receives an injection.

SERVICES OF THE CONFERENCE

The pediatric nurse practitioner or a nurse in charge is responsible for the conduct of the clinic; one or more nurses may assist in this effort. The nursing personnel should strive to create an atmosphere of friendliness and dignity. The nurses should thoroughly understand the purposes of the Conference and the recommendations made by the physician for each child so that they may feel secure in conferences with the mothers. Nurses cannot impart a feeling of confidence in the clinic if they themselves are uncertain of the objectives and of the specific recommendations given by the physician for the individual child.

The services offered by the Child Health Conference include the following:

1. Keeping a complete health history of the child
2. Assessment of the child's physical and emotional status
3. Giving a complete physical examination
4. Recording the child's height and weight and taking his temperature
5. Anticipatory guidance, support, and counseling on behavior problems
6. Health education, promotion, and maintenance
7. Immunization according to the best medical advice
8. Nursing interpretation of the physician's advice
9. Referral to private or clinic physicians for illness or correction of physical defects or to a psychologist or psychiatrist for emotional problems
10. Keeping of accurate records through the use of problem-oriented health records (see p. 376)
11. Evaluation of the success or failure of care through peer-review techniques and the health-status audit.

Health History. A careful and complete history is of extreme importance in order to give the clinic personnel a picture of the whole child and to help them establish friendly relations with the mother. The history should not be taken hurriedly. The mother should have time to discuss her problems and those of her child or other family members who are constantly in contact with him. If the nurse takes the history, opportunities should be utilized for health teaching and explaining to the mother the purpose of the Conference, thereby preparing her for consultation with the physician.

Assessment of the Child's Physical and Emotional Status. Such appraisal is made by both the physician and the nurse of the Child Health Conference, as well as by the community or public health nurse who visits in the home. In planning care of the infant or child such factors as the history of transmissible defects or disease, the mother's condition during pregnancy, and the postnatal health history of the infant should be viewed in relation to the socioeconomic background of the family.

Physical Examination. Physical examination of an infant should be made as often as necessary, but the number of examinations given at various age levels and what is included in the examinations vary in different clinics. Such examinations even in infancy should include an evaluation of the infant's abilities to see and hear. Although the physician or the nurse may do the actual physical examination, they participate in a complementary way rather than duplicating the activity. For the manner of proceeding with a nursing assessment, the student can review pages 137 to 152.

Complete examination at each visit is not necessary. A thorough examination is made when the infant is first brought to the clinic and when he is 6 and 12 months old. After that once a year is considered sufficient. This is not, of course, a set rule. An infant should be examined whenever the physician thinks it is necessary. The need for a complete examination is determined by a limited examination made at each visit or by the mother's report of signs or symptoms of disease, abnormality or lack of normal development.

In general, a limited examination is directed toward finding abnormal conditions commonly connected with the stage of development reached by the infant, e.g., conditions of the feet, legs or back when he is learning to walk. The examination, even if limited, consists in noting the mother-child relations, the general growth and development, state of nutrition, general health and evidence of disease or abnormality.

A developmental screening tool can be utilized at the time of the physical assessment or on another visit.

A urine test for phenylketone bodies should also be done (see p. 466). The physical examination should precede immunization procedures, which are likely to make the infant cry and be uncooperative.

Height, Weight, and Temperature. Recording height and weight and taking temperatures are the nurse's responsibility, though these are often done by a volunteer. The undressed child should be observed for rashes or other signs of illness. Demonstrations can be made to the mothers of the procedures of weighing the infant and taking his temperature. As she observes the nurse, the mother learns how to utilize safety measures in handling the child and the importance of accuracy in taking these measurements.

Anticipatory Guidance, Support, and Counseling on Behavior Problems. These are the responsibility of both the physician and the nurse. The mother can be stimulated to ask questions by mentioning a few of the problems most likely to occur in infants the same age as hers. If the physician does not have time to give the mother all the attention she needs, the nurse-mother conference is commonly held before the mother leaves the clinic. The nurse should be thoroughly familiar with the physician's recommendations so as not to confuse the mother or alter the physician's plan of care by giving conflicting directions.

Health Education, Promotion, and Maintenance. All personnel of the Conference give guidance for feeding and general care of the child. The physician prescribes the formula and the addition of solid foods to the infant's diet. The nurse should help the mother to understand the recommendations given by the physician, and other suggestions for his care should be carefully explained. The nurse should be sure that the mother understands in detail *what* is to be done and *how* it is to be done.

The nurse must know enough of the home situation to be sure that the plan of infant care made by the clinic personnel is practical and will fit into the cultural complex of the family. If the plan does not meet these criteria, it should be remade; otherwise the service of the clinic is of little value. If the plan is not suitable, it is not likely to be carried out, or it may cause friction within the family which will adversely influence the mother-child relations.

Immunization. Prevention of disease is one of the most important goals in child care. During infancy and childhood preventive measures can be carried out against certain infectious diseases. Parents should be encouraged to keep their own records of immunization of their children, or the Child Health Conference record should be duplicated in the event the parents plan to move to another area.

Since infants learn rapidly to dislike the needles used in immunizations, one way to virtually eliminate the pain is by the use of an adhesive gauze patch medicated with a topical anesthetic and applied to the injection site about two hours before the time of injection.

DIPHTHERIA, PERTUSSIS, AND TETANUS. Active immunization against these three diseases can be accomplished at the same time through the administration of 0.5 ml. of combined alum-precipitated or aluminum hydroxide- or aluminum phosphate–adsorbed diphtheria and tetanus toxoids and pertussis vaccine, commonly known as D.P.T. A minimum of three intramuscular injections of this combined toxoid-vaccine mixture should be given at intervals of eight weeks, beginning at two months of age.

To reduce the possibility of occasional local or general reactions, the material should be given with a 1-inch needle inserted deeply into the midlateral thigh muscles. In older children it may be given in the deltoid muscles. When primary immunization is being given, inoculation should not be made more than once at a particular injection site. After the injections, reactions of irritability, fever, and swelling and redness at the site of injection may occur. In

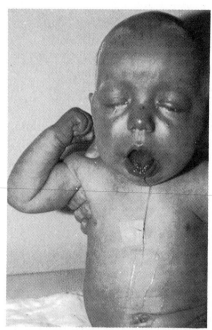

FIGURE 13–23. Four-month-old infant during a pertussis paroxysm: congestive, swollen face, lacrimation, and salivation. (From Moll, H.: *Atlas of Pediatric Diseases.* Philadelphia, W. B. Saunders Co., 1976.)

many Child Health Conferences the nurse may give advice to the mother about the care of the child who has such a reaction to an immunization. If these reactions persist, they should be reported to the physician.

Booster doses of D.P.T. should be given at 18 months and at four to six years. Pertussis vaccine is not necessary for children over this age, since the disease is most severe in infancy. Booster doses of adult type diphtheria-tetanus toxoids should be given at 14 to 16 years and every ten years thereafter.

An acutely ill child should not be given immunization materials. Pertussis vaccine should not be given to any infant or child who has a history of convulsions.

POLIOMYELITIS. Trivalent oral poliomyelitis virus vaccine should be given at two, four, six, and 18 months and between four and six years of age. This immunization is suitable for both breast-fed and bottle-fed infants.

MEASLES. At one year of age measles (rubeola) vaccine may be given in combination as measles-rubella or measles-mumps-rubella combined vaccines. This is especially important for children who, because of a chronic illness or institutionalization, might possibly suffer serious complications from the disease.

Vaccination against measles is delayed until one year of age because during the first year antibodies transmitted across the mother's placental circulation are still present in the infant. Since the purpose of the vaccination of live attenuated strain of measles virus is to produce a mild form of the disease, the passively transmitted maternal antibody may prevent adequate active immunity in the infant (see p. 152). A brief febrile disease may follow vaccination. Other complications generally do not occur. The virus does not spread from the vaccinated to the unvaccinated child.

Recent research has shown that because of the presence of passively transmitted maternal antibodies, which may persist in some 12-month-old infants and interfere with immunization, active

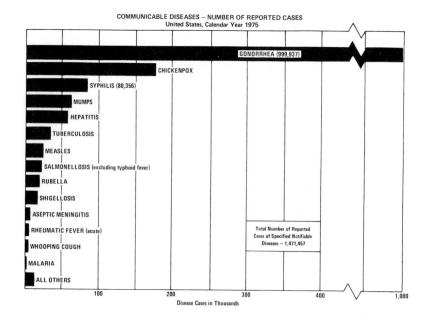

FIGURE 13–24. Reported cases of communicable diseases in the United States during the calendar year 1975. As the result of preventive health measures, such as immunization and improved sanitation, the incidence of many diseases associated with childhood has generally declined. (Courtesy of the Center for Disease Control, Atlanta, Ga.)

immunization using live, attenuated measles virus vaccine should be withheld until the child is 13 months of age or older. In the past, it was thought that waning antibody levels accounted for the lowered titer in actively immunized children. Now it is believed that vaccine failure in the infant of one year of age or younger was the cause. Recommendations have been made, therefore, that children should be immunized against measles between 13 and 15 months of age and that children who had been immunized before this age, be reimmunized when they reach the recommended age.*

The Advisory Committee on Immunization Practices (ACIP) of the United States Public Health Service and the Committee on Infectious Diseases of the American Academy of Pediatrics (AAP) now recommend that measles immunization be given at 15 months to infants living in areas where the disease is not prevalent. If a measles outbreak occurs, the vaccine may be given at any time after the age of six months, but a second inoculation should be given to these children at or after 15 months of age. This new recommendation concerning the age at which measles vaccine should be given applies also to combined measles-mumps-rubella vaccine and monovalent measles vaccine.

GERMAN MEASLES. German measles (rubella) vaccine is recommended for all children between the ages of one year and puberty. Priority is given to children in preschool and elementary school ages. This vaccine should be given to girls approaching puberty if they have not received it prior to this time and to seronegative women of childbearing age who are not pregnant and who can prevent pregnancy for two months after vaccination (see Table 20–1).

MUMPS. This vaccine should be given between the ages of one and 12 years. It is recommended for administration to young boys approaching puberty and for adult males who have not had mumps because of the danger of sterility following the disease. It may be given in combination with measles-rubella combined vaccines.

TUBERCULIN TEST. Tuberculin tests should be done on children at 12 months of age. The frequency of repeated tuberculin tests depends on the prevalence of tuberculosis and the risk of

*Yeager, A. S., et al.: Measles Immunization: Successes and Failures. *J.A.M.A.*, 237:347, January, 1977.

TABLE 13–4. RECOMMENDED SCHEDULE FOR ACTIVE IMMUNIZATION OF NORMAL INFANTS AND CHILDREN

2 mo	DTP[1]	TOPV[2]
4 mo	DTP	TOPV
6 mo	DTP	TOPV
1 yr	Measles[3]	Tuberculin Test[4]
	Rubella[3]	Mumps[3]
1½ yr	DTP	TOPV
4-6 yr	DTP	TOPV
14-16 yr	Td[5]	and thereafter every 10 years

[1] DTP – diphtheria and tetanus toxoids combined with pertussis vaccine.

[2] TOPV – trivalent oral polio virus vaccine. The above recommendation is suitable for breast-fed as well as bottle-fed infants.

[3] May be given at 1 year as Measles-Rubella or Measles-Mumps-Rubella combined vaccines.

[4] Frequency of repeated tuberculin tests depends on risk of exposure of the child and on the prevalence of tuberculosis in the population group.

[5] Td – combined tetanus and diphtheria toxoids (adult type) for those over six years of age in contrast to diphtheria and tetanus (DT) containing a larger amount of diphtheria antigen.

Tetanus toxoid at time of injury: For clean, minor wounds, no booster dose is needed by a fully immunized child unless more than 10 years have elapsed since the last dose.

For contaminated wounds, a booster dose should be given if more than 5 years have elapsed since the last dose.

Routine smallpox vaccination is no longer recommended.

From American Academy of Pediatrics.: Active Immunization Procedures. *Report of the Committee on Infectious Diseases.* 17th ed., 1974.

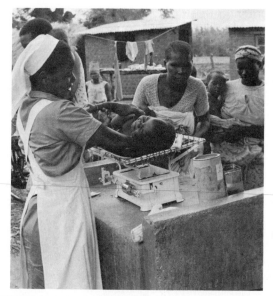

FIGURE 13-25. Student nurse weighs a baby at the clinic in Kalinde. Every governmental district in Malawi has a community development officer, who has received six months training at a government school and who contributes to the health and development of the people in his district. (Courtesy of Medical Mission Sisters, Phila.)

exposure of the individual child (see Table 13-4).

SMALLPOX. Routine smallpox vaccination is no longer recommended by the United States Public Health Service or the American Academy of Pediatrics. The risk of acquiring smallpox in the United States is so small that it does not justify routine primary vaccination of infants and children. This type of immunization has occasionally resulted in severe adverse reactions, some of which have been fatal. Those who travel where smallpox is endemic or where vaccination is required must be immunized.

OTHER IMMUNIZATIONS. If the parents plan to travel to other states or to foreign countries, further information about other immunizations which might be necessary can be obtained from health departments or the Public Health Service, Washington, D.C.

Nursing Interpretation of the Physician's Advice. This means more than a nurse interpreting what the physician has said; it means that the mother carries over into her nursing care the *medical advice* given by the physician, including preventive medicine and mental hygiene. Nurses often fail to realize that nursing has something to contribute to the child care program which medicine cannot give. Their recommendations to the mother are based on the physician's orders and on the body of knowledge which belongs to the profession of nursing.

Referral to Private or Clinic Physicians. Referral of an infant or child to a private or clinic physician for illness or correction of physical defects, or to a psychologist or psychiatrist for emotional problems, is certainly a necessary function of the clinic, for it is not prepared to handle such problems. Case finding and referral are two of the main functions of the Conference. The referral is sometimes made by the nurse under the physician's direction, or it can be made by the social workers with his approval.

Group Visits in Child Care Conferences. An innovative way to promote the health of infants and young children is through the use of group visits with mothers; that is, times usually set aside by the pediatric nurse practitioner or nurse when several mothers and their infants or children of the same age come together for a joint visit. During this time physical assessments are made on the infants. The findings on each are shared with his mother, and care instructions are given for any minor illness or problem. While one mother and infant are with the nurse, the other mothers become acquainted with each other.

Topics of general interest are postponed until discussion time. Such topics could include child rearing, nutrition, growth and development, or the individuality of infants. Mothers take the lead in these discussions, sharing their experiences with each other.

Group visits for each age group can be planned at regular intervals during the year. Visits with one mother and her infant or child can be alternated with group visits. Fathers are included in these visits whenever possible. In this way it is possible to spend more time with the parents and their child.

An individual mother in such a group may have a child-care problem she cannot solve, but one not serious enough to involve a professional. Such a mother can call a more experienced mother in her group for assistance or support in solving her problem.

PREPARATION FOR CARE OF INFANTS IN A MAJOR DISASTER

Parents, in addition to learning how to care for their infants and small children under normal circumstances, should also learn how to care for them under mass casualty conditions. Preparation for the care of children in advance of such a disaster might make the difference of life or death for them.

The main problem which would confront parents would be that of feeding the infants. If the infant is breast-fed, further breast feeding should be encouraged. Infants up to six months of age should be provided with 1 quart of fluid per day, such as milk, water, fruit juices or appropriate soft drinks (if nothing else is available). Infants up to one year of age should receive approximately 125 ml. of fluid per kilogram of body weight per day. For a period of 30 days vitamin and mineral supplements should be considered of no importance to a normal child. They should be added to the diet of the child, however, as soon as possible. For an artificially fed infant, bottles and nipples should be boiled before use, and the formula should be used as soon as it is prepared.

A two-week to two-month supply of uncontaminated water, dried or evaporated milk, sugar, cereal and other foods with which the child is familiar should be stored safely for emergency use for each child under the age of one year. Foods the child likes would be better accepted than those with which he is unfamiliar. Supplies of other necessary items such as diapers, pins, clothing, and feeding equipment should also be prestocked for emergency use.

Infants should be immunized according to the usual schedule so that they are protected as much as possible should an emergency occur. Immunization against typhoid and paratyphoid fevers would also be advisable. If diarrhea should occur, food should be withheld and oral electrolytes, if available, or boiled water should be substituted. Injuries to infants or small children should be treated as injuries to adults would be.

At the time of a major disaster infants and children should be kept under the care and supervision of their own parents whenever possible. From their parents they would get the love and security needed to prevent emotional disturbance during and after such a time of stress.

Although modern society denounces the primitive practice of allowing weak infants to die for the welfare of the group (see p. 3), this practice is reflected in our present-day concept of disaster nursing. Whether following an atomic or hydrogen bomb explosion or other catastrophic happening, preference in the care of survivors is given to those children and adults most likely to profit from care. The severely traumatized victims, many of them probably infants, who would need extensive therapy would be cared for when time and facilities permitted. In such an emergency would even our civilized society not be selecting those most able to survive in preference to the very young or those least likely to survive? It is obvious that our practices in times when we are not personally threatened change when our own lives are in danger.

SUMMARY OF THE CONTRIBUTIONS OF THE NURSE TO CHILD HEALTH

The nurse can contribute in many ways to improving the physical and mental health of infants and children. The nurse can contribute as an active member of the health and nursing teams, performing independent functions in various areas of expertise.

Observation of Children. The nurse is usually in a position to spend more time with children, whether in the home, clinic, hospital or other community agency, than are other members of the health team. The nurse is thus able to observe their levels of growth and development and their physical and emotional health, as well as their relations with their parents, siblings and peers.

The nurse will be perceptive and sensitive in the process of identifying and validating any immediate or long-term need, concern or problem and of responding to these by appropriate intervention. The nurse can help a child face the usual problems of growth and development, adjust to an illness, and cope with painful diagnostic or therapeutic procedures in the clinic or during a period of hospitalization (see p. 82). Specific ways nurses can contribute to the mental and physical health of the child are provided in this text.

Parental Education and Anticipatory Guidance. The role of the nurse in the expanding educational programs for families and children is of vital importance. The nurse can provide guidance not only in the formation of healthy parent-child relations but also in the areas of physical and emotional development of children and in their health care (see p. 50).

Parental education is of little value unless the parents are motivated to keep their child well. If they are indifferent to his health, and without motivation, they are not likely to put into practice what they are taught. Motivation is increased if teaching has reference to *their child* and is specific and not general.

Instructions should be simple and should cover the essential information. Excess information is apt to be confusing. Effectiveness of instruction is measured by whether the parents can answer questions posed by the nurse or the degree to which they make suggestions and think through their own problems. Self-direction is more effective than direction by others.

What and how much parents can be taught at any time depends on their social level (i.e., their living situation and their financial status), their intelligence level (how much knowledge they can absorb at any one time), and their past experience in child care.

Visual aids are valuable in clarifying the application of theory to the child in the home situation. Folders or pamphlets should be provided for the parents; they are most effective if given in answer to specific questions and reviewed with them.

The child's daily routine should be planned in sufficient detail to make it of practical value to the mother. Anticipatory guidance should be given in relation to the level of the child's growth and development. The feeding of the infant or child is extremely important and is a matter on which consumers receive a great deal of advice from miscellaneous sources.

The purpose and need for regular visits for health checks should be stressed, as parents are likely to feel that these are unnecessary if the child appears well. It is the mother, constantly with the child, who is in a position to observe the early signs of illness. It is imperative that she know these signs and realize the importance of reporting her observations and securing early treatment for the infant or child when he is ill.

Group instruction may be given to mothers on pertinent topics of common interest, such as the kind of clothing suitable to the weather and home conditions, routine immunizations carried out on all children, general principles of feeding, and the management of minor behavior problems.

Emotional Support of Parents. Parents many times need help in reducing their anxiety in relation to the care of their children. Not only can the nurse provide emotional support or first aid in an emergency by listening and helping them to express their feelings (see p. 83 for a discussion of interviewing), but can also guide those parents who need expert help to seek the services of a specialist. Before and during treatment by the physician or other specialist, the nurse can be supportive and clarify the ways by which other professionals can help in their particular situation.

Nurses can assist parents in their adjustment to problems involving their children, such as in the instance of the birth of an imperfect infant (see p. 231), acute or critical illness, prolonged illness, or death (see p. 109). Specific ways by which nurses can help parents are discussed throughout this book.

The Health and Nursing Teams. The professional nurse has responsibilities as a participating member of the health team and as a leader of the nursing team (see p. 79). In order to function effectively as a member of the health team, the nurse must know the responsibilities of the other members. To serve well as a leader of the nursing team, the nurse must know what can be expected from each member and how they as a group can work harmoniously toward a common goal. The ability to teach effectively is of vital importance in all aspects of the nurse's endeavors.

The Improvement of Child Health Care. Professional nurses are assuming increasing responsibilities for screening essentially normal children in Child Health Conferences and in other clinics. There is a great need to increase such facilities in order to reduce the morbidity and mortality rates of children. Nurses must use their influence to secure such services for as many children as possible. They may exert their influence as a body through their state nurses' associations and through united action in bringing pressure upon the city, county, and state legislatures and councils to provide more such services under public auspices. As individuals, nurses can help the public to know the value of such services. Nurses are assuming their professional and civic responsibilities by helping to procure care for all children not fully cared for by private physicians.

TEACHING AIDS AND OTHER INFORMATION*

Alexander Graham Bell Association for the Deaf

Can Your Baby Hear?

American Academy of Pediatrics

Childhood Diet and Coronary Heart Disease.
Disaster and Emergency Medical Services for Infants and Children.
Parents: Guidelines for Your Family's Health Insurance.
Personal Immunization Record Card.
Standard Health Examination Card.

American Dental Association

Fluoridation Facts.
Mothers Want to Help.

Schour, I., and Massler, M.: Development of the Human Dentition Chart.

American Lung Association

La Prueba de la Tuberculina.
The Tuberculin Skin Test.

Consumer Product Information

Crib Safety, 1974.
Safe Toy Tips, 1974.
Toys: Fun in the Making, 1973.

*Complete addresses are given in the Appendix.

Department of National Health and Welfare: Ottawa, Canada

Canadian Mother and Child.
Family Health Planning for Disaster.
Immunization—A Guide for International Travellers.

Johnson & Johnson

Klaus, M. H., Leger, T., and Trause, M. A. (Eds.): Maternal Attachment and Mothering Disorders: A Round Table, 1974.

Mead Johnson & Compnay

Good Infant Nutrition, 1976.
Nutrition...And the Critical First Year of Life, 1975.
Nutritional Aspects of Cow's Milk in Infant Feeding, 1976.
Overfeeding in Infancy: Causes and Implications, 1976.

National Association for Retarded Citizens

Murphy, L. B.: Spontaneous Ways of Learning in Young Children.

The National Foundation–March of Dimes

Family Medical Record.

Public Affairs Committee

Barman, A.: Motivation and Your Child.
Barman, A.: Your First Months with Your Baby.
Graves, J.: Right from the Start: The Importance of Early Immunization.

Ross Laboratories

Iron Nutrition in Infancy, 1974.
Perinatology—Neonatology—Pediatric Nutrition—Currents, 1976.
Smith, N. J.: On Developmental Nutrition: The Challenge of Obesity, 1972.
Year One: Nutrition, Growth, Health, 1975.

United States Government

Babies Look and Learn: A Guide for Parents, 1974.
Babies Touch, Taste, and Learn: A Guide for Parents, Reprinted 1973.
Child Development in the Home, 1974.
Cognitive Development in Young Children, 1976.
El Cuidado de Su Bebe (Infant Care), 1975.
Garfinkel, J., Chabot, M. J., and Pratt, M. W.: Infant, Maternal, and Childhood Mortality in the United States, 1968–1973, 1975.
Infant Care, 1973.
Learning Through Touch: A Guide for Parents, Reprinted 1974.
New Clues to Your Baby's Secret World, 1976.
Publications of the Office of Child Development, 1976.
The Maternity and Infant Care Projects: Reducing Risks for Mothers and Babies, 1975.
Your Baby's First Year, Reprinted 1975.

REFERENCES

Books

American Academy of Pediatrics: *Standards of Child Health Care.* Evanston, Ill., American Academy of Pediatrics, 1967.

American Academy of Pediatrics: *Report of the Committee on Infectious Diseases.* 17th ed. Evanston, Ill., American Academy of Pediatrics, 1974.

Babcock, D. E.: *Introduction to Growth, Development and Family Life.* Philadelphia, F. A. Davis Company, 1972.

Baer, M. J.: *Growth and Maturation; An Introduction to Physical Development.* Cambridge, Mass., Howard A. Doyle Publishing Company, 1973.

Brody, S., and Axelrad, S.: *Anxiety and Ego Formation in Infancy.* New York, International Universities Press, 1971.

Bullough, B., and Bullough, V. L.: *Poverty, Ethnic Identity, and Health Care.* New York, Appleton-Century-Crofts, 1972.

Caplan, F.: *The First Twelve Months of Life; Your Baby's Growth Month by Month.* New York, Grosset and Dunlap Publishers, 1973.

Cohn, H., and Tingle, J. E.: *Manual for Nurses in Family and Community Health.* Boston, Little, Brown & Company, 1974.

Comer, J., and Poussaint, A.: *Black Child Care.* New York, Simon & Schuster, 1975.

Dodson, F.: *How to Father.* Los Angeles, Nash Publishing Corporation, 1974.

Duvall, E. M.: *Family Development.* 4th ed. Philadelphia, J. B. Lippincott Company, 1971.

Emde, R. N., Gaensbauer, T. J., and Harmon, R. J.: *Emotional Expression in Infancy.* New York, International Universities Press, 1976.

Erickson, M. L.: *Assessment and Management of Developmental Changes in Children.* St. Louis, The C. V. Mosby Company, 1976.

Fomon, S. J.: *Infant Nutrition.* 2nd ed. Philadelphia, W. B. Saunders Company, 1974.

Frankenburg, W. K., and Camp, B. W.: *Pediatric Screening Test.* Springfield, Ill., Charles C Thomas, 1975.

Freedman, D. G.: *Human Infancy: An Evolutionary Perspective.* New York, Halsted Press, 1975.

Hobart, M. J.; and McConnell, I. (Eds.): *The Immune System: A Course on the Molecular and Cellular Basis of Immunity.* Philadelphia, J. B. Lippincott Company, 1975.

Hurlock, E. B.: *Developmental Psychology.* 4th ed. New York, McGraw-Hill Book Company, Inc., 1975.

Illingworth, R. S. (Ed.): *The Normal Child.* 6th ed. New York, Longman, 1975.

Jelliffe, D. B., and Jelliffe, E. F. P.: *Human Milk in the Modern World.* St. Louis, The C. V. Mosby Company, 1976.

Kaluger, G., and Kaluger, M. F.: *Human Development: The Span of Life.* St. Louis, The C. V. Mosby Company, 1974.

Knobloch, H., and Pasamanick, B. (Eds.): *Gesell & Amatruda's Developmental Diagnosis.* 3rd ed. New York, Harper & Row, 1974.

Leininger, M. (Ed.): *Transcultural Health Care: Issues and Conditions.* Philadelphia, F. A. Davis Company, 1976.

Lowrey, G. H.: *Growth and Development of Children.* 6th ed. Chicago, Year Book Medical Publishers, 1973.

Lynn, D. B.: *The Father: His Role in Child Development.* Monterey, Calif., Brooks/Cole Publishing Company, 1974.

Marcus, I. M., and Francis, J. J. (Eds.): *Masturbation: From Infancy to Senescence.* New York, International University Press, 1975.

McWilliams, M.: *Nutrition for the Growing Years.* 2nd ed. New York, John Wiley & Sons, 1975.

North, A. F. Jr.: *Infant Care.* New York, Arco Publishing Co., 1975.

Park, B. H., and Good, R. A.: *Principles of Modern Immunobiology: Basic and Clinical.* Philadelphia, Lea & Febiger, 1974.

Pomeranz, V. E.: *The First Five Years: A Relaxed Approach to Child Care.* New York, Doubleday and Co., 1973.

Recommended Dietary Allowances. 8th ed. Rev. Washington, D.C., National Academy of Sciences, National Research Council, 1974.

Uzgiris, I. C., and Hunt, J. M.: *Assessment in Infancy.* Urbana, Ill., The University of Illinois Press, 1975.

Valadian, I., and Porter, D.: *Child Growth and Development.* Boston, Little, Brown & Company, 1976.

Van der Linden, F., and Duterloo, H. S.: *Atlas on the Development of the Human Dentition.* New York, Harper & Row, 1976.

Visiting Nurse Association of New Haven, Ct.: *Child Health Conference—Nurses' Resource Manual.* New York, National League for Nursing, 1975.

Walters, C. E.: *Mother-Infant Interaction.* New York, Human Sciences Press, 1975.

Zachau-Christiansen, B., and Ross, E. M.: *Babies: Human Development During the First Year.* New York, John Wiley & Sons, 1975.

Zeitz, A. N.: *Postpartum As A Continuing Link in the Symbiotic Relationship of Parents and Child.* New York, Zanab Press, 1975.

Periodicals

Alley, R. D., and Heinz, W. C.: Attention Kids: This Holiday Story Won't Leave You With a Lump in Your Throat. *Today's Health,* 51:28, December 1973.

Are Baby Foods Good Enough For Babies? *Consumer Reports,* 40:528, September, 1975.

Bauernfeind, L.: Strengthening a Disorganized Family. *Am. J. Nursing,* 75:2198, December 1975.

Beardslee, C.: The Sleep of Infants and Young Children: A Review of the Literature. *Matern. Child Nurs. J.,* 5:5, April 1976.

Braden, C. J., and Price, J. L.: Encouraging Client Self-Discovery. *Am. J. Nursing,* 76:444, March 1976.

Brazelton, T. B.: Baby Care Teamwork...4...Tender Loving Care. *Baby Talk,* 38:12, April 1973.

Brown, M. S.: What You Should Know About Communicable Diseases and Their Immunizations: A Guide for Nurses in Ambulatory Settings, Part 1. *Nursing '75,* 5:70, September 1975.

Brown, M. S.: What You Should Know About Communicable Diseases and Their Immunization: A Guide for Nurses in Ambulatory Settings, Part 2. *Nursing '75,* 5:56, October 1975.

Brown, M. S.: What You Should Know About Communicable Diseases and Their Immunizations: A Guide for Nurses in Ambulatory Settings, Part 3. *Nursing '75,* 5:55, November 1975.

Bruner, J. S.: Child Development: Play is Serious Business. *Psychology Today,* 8:80, January 1975.

Burnip, R., et al.: Well-child Care by Pediatric Nurse Practitioners in a Large Group Practice. A Controlled Study in 1,152 Preschool Children. *Am. J. Dis. Child,* 130:51, January 1976.

Calderone, M. S.: Education in Human Sexuality for Health Professionals. *Nursing Digest,* 1:48, December 1973.

Clark, A. L.: Recognizing Discord Between Mother and Child and Changing it to Harmony. *The American Journal of Maternal Child Nursing,* 1:100, March-April 1976.

Clark, A. L., and Affonso, D. D.: Infant Behavior and Maternal Attachment: Two Sides to the Coin. *The American Journal of Maternal Child Nursing,* 1:93, March-April 1976.

Cohen, M.: A Warning to Conscientious Mothers. *Today's Health,* 52:22, February 1974.

Cooper, I.: Group Sessions for New Mothers. *Nursing Outlook,* 22:251, April 1974.

Cowell, C., Maslansky, E., Grossi, M., Dash, R., Kayman, S.,

and Archer, M.: Survey of Infant Feeding Practices. *Am. J. Pub. Health,* 63:138, February 1973.

Cranston, L.: Communicable Diseases and Immunizations. *The Canadian Nurse,* 72:34, January 1976.

Drye, R. C.: Sexual "Scripts": Behavior Patterns Established in Childhood are Revealed in Adult Psychosexual Roles. *Medical Aspects of Human Sexuality,* 9:32, October 1975.

Eoff, M. J. F., Meier, R. S., and Miller, C.: Temperature Measurement in Infants. *Nursing Research,* 23:457, November-December 1974.

Grantham, E.: Sore Bottoms in the Newborn. *Arch. Dis. Child,* 48:568, July 1973.

Greenberg, M., and Morris, N.: Engrossment: The Newborn's Impact Upon the Father. *Nursing Digest,* 4:19, January-February 1976.

Greenberg, R. A., et al.: Primary Child Health Care by Family Nurse Practitioners. *Pediatrics,* 53:900, June 1974.

John, J. T., Devarajan, L. V., Luther, L., and Vijayarathnam, P.: Effect of Breast-Feeding on Seroresponse of Infants to Oral Poliovirus Vaccination. *Pediatrics,* 57:47, January 1976.

Kitzman, H.: The Nature of Well Child Care. *Am. J. Nursing,* 75:1705, October 1975.

Kravitz, H., et al.: The Cotton-Tipped Swab: A Major Cause of Ear Injury and Hearing Loss. *J. N.Y. State Sch. Nurse Teach. Assoc.,* 6:33, June 1975.

Lindstrom, C. J.: No Shows: A Problem in Health Care. *Nursing Outlook,* 23:755, December 1975.

Mahler, H. T.: Smallpox: Point of No Return. *Bulletin of the Pan American Health Organization,* 9:48, 1975.

Maslansky, E., et al.: Survey of Infant Feeding Practices. *Am. J. Pub. Health,* 64:780, August 1974.

Mayer, J.: Charting a Course to Good Nutrition with Your Children. *Family Health/Today's Health,* 8:30, August 1976.

Miller, R.: Private Care in a Public Clinic: Typical Family Progress. *Am. J. Nursing,* 74:1644, September 1974.

Murray, A. D.: Maternal Employment Reconsidered: Effects on Infants. *Am. J. Orthopsychiatry,* 45:773, October 1975.

Neumann, C. G., and Alpaugh, M.: Birthweight Doubling Time: A Fresh Look. *Pediatrics,* 57:469, April 1976.

Nysather, J. O., Katz, A. E., and Lenth, J. L.: The Immune System: Its Development and Functions. *Am. J. Nursing,* 76:1614, October 1976.

Oates, R. K.: Infant-Feeding Practices. *Br. Med. J.,* 2:762, June 30, 1973.

Perkins, Sr. M. R.: Does Availability of Health Services Ensure Their Use. *Nursing Outlook,* 22:496, August 1974.

Rabinowitz, M.: Why Didn't Anyone Tell Me About Bottle Mouth Cavities? *Children Today,* 3:18, March-April 1974.

Safran, C.: What We're Finding Out About Sexual Stereotypes. *Today's Health,* 53:14, October 1975.

Shaw, N. R.: Teaching Young Mothers Their Role. *Nursing Outlook,* 22:695, November 1974.

Sirota, A. L.: Private Care in a Public Clinic. *Am. J. Nursing,* 74:1642, September 1974.

Skalka, P.: Solving the Mystery of the Decaying Teeth. *Today's Health,* 52:25, January 1974.

Slattery, J. S.: Nutrition for the Normal Healthy Infant. *The American Journal of Maternal Child Nursing,* 2:105, March-April 1977.

Thomstad, B., Cunningham, N., and Kaplan, B. H.: Changing the Rules of the Doctor-Nurse Game. *Nursing Outlook,* 23:422, July 1975.

Vaillancourt-Wagner, M.: Children's Value to Their Parents. *The Canadian Nurse,* 71:31, August 1975.

Yeager, A. S., et al.: Measles Immunization: Successes and Failures. *J.A.M.A.,* 237:347, January 1977.

AUDIOVISUAL MEDIA*

American Dental Association

Development of the Human Dentition Chart
Schour, I., and Massler, M.
14 7/8'' × 12'' chart, color, booklet.
Shows the development of both deciduous and permanent teeth.

The American Journal of Nursing Company

Growth and Development – Birth Through Adolescence
Series of 23 44 minute classes, black and white.
Class Instructor: Nicolay, R.C.

Overview
The study of children is introduced by discussion and demonstration of the continuity of development through the stages of infancy, toddlerhood, preschool years, middle years of childhood, and adolescence.

Unfolding Infant Behavior
The innate potential of infants is presented through examples of specific reflexive actions, cephalo-caudal sequences and the parallel development of language and physiological reactions such as crying and other sound productions and gestures.

Understanding Infant Behavior
Participating Instructor: Barger, P.
The infant's behavior as a reaction to his basic needs is described. Behavioral problems produced by parental expectancy, demands, and reactions regarding feeding procedures, masturbation, sleep, and toilet training are discussed.

Emerging Consciousness
Demonstrations are given of the development of the neonate's consciousness from the time when he is physiologically fused with his mother until he becomes an individual able to distinguish objects and himself.

The Infant and Society
Participating Instructors: Holliday, J., Vocalis, H. A., Aghi, M. V., and Ignatius, Sr. F.
Social and environmental factors involved in the socialization process of the infant are shown and discussed.

Emotional Development of the Infant
Participating Instructor: Donaldson, B.
The emergent patterns of emotion during the first years of life are demonstrated and discussed.

The First Two Weeks of Life
17 minutes, color.
Ideal for use in prenatal instruction classes for expectant parents, it is aimed specifically at reducing the levels of anxiety often felt by young couples about to have their first baby. The camera captures the completely spontaneous and unrehearsed excitement of childbirth and the parents' first moments with their new daughter. There is a visual cataloguing of the next two weeks of discovery and delight of the new parents.

Charles Press–Prentice-Hall, Inc.

Nursing Skills and Techniques Series
2–5 minutes, Super-8mm filmloop, color, guide.

Nursery: Infant to Mother Arm Carry, Part I
Procedure for arm carrying newborn who is breastfed to mother.

Nursery: Infant to Mother Arm Carry, Part II
Continued procedure for transporting a breastfed newborn to mother via arm carry.

Growth and Development: 1 Month, Part I
Observation of one-month-old infant: fontanels, reflexes, reactions, etc.

Growth and Development: 1 Month, Part II
Further observations of one-month-old infant.

Growth and Development: 3 Months
Observations of three-month-old infant: muscle tone, posture, reflexes, and reactions.

Growth and Development: 6 Months, Part I
Overview of six-month-old infant: movements, muscle tone, reactions.

Growth and Development: 6 Months, Part II
Further observations of a six-month-old infant: muscle tone, reflexes, reactions.

Growth and Development: 9 Months, Part I
Over-all appearance, abilities and characteristics of a nine-month-old infant.

Growth and Development: 9 Months, Part II
Further observations of nine-month-old infant and some reactions and interactions with mother.

Growth and Development: 1 Year
Observations of appearance, characteristics, abilities and reactions of a one-year-old.

Concept Media

Human Development: The First 2½ Years
7 programs of varied length, 35mm filmstrips/tape, sound, color, guide.
Pregnancy, Birth and the Newborn–27 minutes.
Physical Growth and Motor Development–18 minutes.
The Development of Understanding–23 minutes.
Styles of Interaction–22 minutes.
Emotional and Social Development: Part I–17 minutes.
Emotional and Social Development: Part II–17 minutes.
Language Development–21 minutes.
Explores the possible effects of various environments on babies' and children's emotional and social development.

Health Sciences Communication Center, Case Western Reserve University

Breast Feeding: Prenatal and Postpartal Preparation
16mm film or videocassette.
This presentation was designed as a guide in instructing expectant and new mothers in the preparation and care of their breasts for breast feeding.

J. B. Lippincott Company

Growth and Development: A Chronicle of Four Children
Thompson, J. K., and Juenker, D. M.
16mm film and Super-8mm film and/or videotape, sound, color.
This series of motion pictures demonstrates the range of normal variation in social, physical, and cognitive development during the first four years of life. Holistic in approach, the films focus on each child's social and emotional development, identification behavior, motor development, habitual responses, concepts of reality, and body structure and function.

McGraw-Hill Book Company

Infancy
19 minutes, 16mm film or videocassette, color.

The Child
Kagan, J., and Rabinovitch, M. S.

16mm films or videocassettes.
The Child, Part I: The First Two Months–29 minutes.
The Child, Part II: 2–14 Months–28 minutes.
The Child, Part III: 12–24 Months–29 minutes.

As these babies develop and grow, you are the silent participant in the countless events of their self-discovery. Each film lets you quietly observe them. The cameras unobtrusively direct your attention to the subtle nuances of behavior, highlighting a mercurial switch from tears to laughter. In natural settings alone and with parents, siblings.

National Communicable Disease Center

Stop Rubella
Producer: National Medical Audiovisual Center
14 minutes, 16mm, sound, color.
Urges parents to have their children inoculated against rubella. Traces development of the vaccine.

Ross Laboratories
Growth Charts
This collection of charts traces the physical and social development of children. Two separate sheets—one for boys, the other for girls—illustrate the normal patterns of adaptive social and physical development from birth to 56 weeks. Characteristic crying habits, smiling behavior, socializing tendencies, and self-concepts are described as they vary throughout the 56 weeks, as are physical attributes such as degree and type of hearing, and eye and hand control. A separate graph shows shifts in head circumference from birth to three years of age.

W. B. Saunders Company

Pediatric Conference with Sydney Gellis
Problems of Iron-Fortified Formulas, Oski, F.
Rubella Vaccine, Cooper, L. Z.

Trainex Corporation
Bathing the Baby
35mm filmstrip, audio-tape cassettes, 33 ⅓ LP, color.
Provides the mother with instructions on how to sponge-bathe and tub-bathe her baby. Emphasis is placed on bathing and care of baby's face, scalp, and navel and genital areas. Various types of diapers are shown, and instruction is given on how to make different diaper folds with regard to baby's sex and physical size.

Bottle Feeding
35mm filmstrip, audio-tape cassettes, 33⅓ LP, color.
Informs and instructs a mother on formula preparation and the feeding of her baby. It explains what baby is fed, and his feeding schedule while in the hospital. Equipment required for formula preparation is shown, with emphasis on equipment and formula sterilization. Instruction on baby feeding includes: formula temperature and flow, positioning of baby and bottle, burping, and the scheduling of feedings.

Growth and Development
35mm filmstrip, audio-tape cassettes, 33⅓ LP, color.
Provides parents with information on a number of growth patterns including head shape, sleep habits, teething, walking, and talking.

Health Care of the Normal Infant
35mm filmstrip, audio-tape cassettes, 33⅓ LP, color.
This program emphasizes for the mother of a newborn baby the importance of good health care early in the infant's life. It shows the special care the baby receives while in the hospital, and points out the importance of regular health care after the baby is taken home. In addition, the mother learns about routine immunization (baby shots), about fever, how to take baby's temperature by rectum, and about giving medication by mouth and by rectum (suppositories).

Immunizations
35mm filmstrip, audio-tape cassettes, 33⅓ LP, color.
Simply and succinctly explains the reasons for immunizations, and the important ones children should receive. Also explains reactions and how to treat them.

Infant Care—Breast Feeding
35mm filmstrip, audio-tape cassettes, 33⅓ LP, color.
An illustrated presentation shows how to position the infant for feeding and how to help the infant find the breast. Discusses the importance of using alternate breasts, and explains how to relax.

Intestinal Disturbances
35mm filmstrip, audio-tape cassettes, 33⅓ LP, color.
Advises parents about the causes of intestinal disturbances and how to treat colic, a "gassy" baby, constipation, and diarrhea.

Introduction to Infant Care
35mm filmstrip, audio-tape cassettes, 33⅓ LP, color.
This program shows how to generate self-confidence in the new mother. Provides information on: feeding, bathing, skin care, safety precautions, taking the rectal temperature, care of diapers, and home environment adjustments; also included is information on self-care for the mother.

Normal Patterns of Development
35mm filmstrip, audio-tape cassettes, 33⅓ LP, color.
Portrays the normal stages of growth and development during an infant's first year. Babies of various ages up to one year are used to illustrate the approximate stages at which the infant will begin new phases of development.

Preventive Dental Care
35mm filmstrip, audio-tape cassettes, 33⅓ LP, color.
Includes facts about normal and abnormal development of teeth. Explains the medical view of pacifiers and thumb-sucking.

Skin Care and Bathing Preparation
35mm filmstrip, audio-tape cassettes, 33⅓ LP, color.
Instructs a mother on the care of her baby's umbilical cord stub and circumcision, and the trimming of baby's fingernails and toenails. Some forms of skin irritations (rashes) are mentioned, and the mother is instructed on how to care for them. The program enumerates the equipment required to bathe a baby, and describes how the mother should prepare herself prior to giving her baby his bath.

Tuberculosis Skin Testing
35mm filmstrip, audio-tape cassettes, 33⅓ LP, color.
The nature of delayed hypersensitivity and of an induration, the differences between Old Tuberculin and Purified Protein Derivative, the Multiple Puncture Skin Test, and Mantoux Skin Test are illustrated and discussed. Giving, reading, and interpreting both the Mantoux Skin Test and the Multiple Puncture Skin Test are explained with emphasis on the patient's history during interpretation.

United States Government

Emotional Ties in Infancy
Producer: USPHS
12 minutes, 16mm film, optical sound, black and white.
Shows the importance of strong emotional ties between infant and adult by comparing four 8–10 month-old infants—a home-raised girl with strong attachment to her mother, a child in an institution who is equally attached to his nurse, an institutional baby who is indiscriminate in his attachment to any adult, and still another baby in an institution who has formed no attachment and who appears withdrawn and uninterested in his surroundings.

Learning to Learn in Infancy
 Producer: USDHEW
 30 minute, 16mm film, optical sound, black and white.
 Stresses the essential role of curiosity and exploration in learning, and points to the kinds of experience that cultivate and stimulate an eager approach to the world. It also points out the cumulative nature of learning—even in infancy the ability to absorb and use new experiences depends on a backlog or context of experience. Ways are suggested in which adults can help infants make approaches, differentiate between objects, and develop the earliest communication skills.

Person to Person in Infancy
 Producer: USDHEW
 22 minutes, 16mm film, optical sound, black and white.
 Stresses the importance of the human relationships between infant and adult, and shows that in group care as well as at home there can be a considerable range of warmth and adequacy of relationship. The impact of this relationship on the infant's readiness and eagerness for new experience is suggested.

Psychological Hazards in Infancy
 Producer: USDHEW
 22 minutes, 16mm film, optical sound, black and white.
 Presents how in group care and at home, the vital experiences and learnings of infancy may be hampered by inadequate stimulation, insufficient warm attention from adults, or inappropriate handling not geared to changing developmental needs. The film shows mild and severe psychological damage and suggests means of prevention.

Wayne State University

DENT: Directions for Education in Nursing Via Technology
 30-minute lessons, videotape and videocassette, 16mm film, color.
 Human Sexuality Series
  I. Infant-Pre-adolescent
  Sexual health care in the nursing process.

---

*Complete addresses are given in the Appendix.

Chapter Fourteen

CONDITIONS OF INFANTS REQUIRING IMMEDIATE OR SHORT-TERM CARE

infant with an elevated temperature may develop anorexia, vomiting, or diarrhea.

The young infant or child has a labile temperature-regulating mechanism. Temperature elevations are higher than in the adult patient in a similar situation. The infant can withstand a high fever better than the adult and after the temperature returns to normal may be ready for his usual activity, while an adult would be exhausted.

During an illness the infant may develop fluid imbalance due to the elevation of temperature, vomiting, or diarrhea. Nutrition may also suffer due to a lack of food intake during illness. In the infant this is especially apparent, since it occurs during a period of rapid growth. In addition to an inconsistent weight gain during illness, the lack of consistent growth may be evident on roentgenograms of the bones and the teeth in later years. The bones on x-ray may show dense transverse lines, which reflect a time of growth failure, and the teeth may show pitting and grooving of the enamel, which are due to the effects of disease at a time when the teeth were being formed.

Some acute illnesses of infancy and early childhood leave residual defects that are handicapping to the child. Certain infectious diseases are especially prone to cause permanent damage (see p. 658), whether physical or psychologic, with which the child must be helped.

Hospitalization during infancy is often a new experience for both parents and child. Since the parents are anxious, the infant also becomes anxious. The parents should be encouraged to verbalize fears about the child's welfare, thereby relieving some anxiety.

When an infant becomes ill for even a short time, his well-being, both physical and emotional, is threatened. This is especially true if he is hospitalized and deprived of his parents' love while he is in pain, restrained for treatment, or not permitted to suck.

ILLNESS IN INFANCY

Acute illness in the infant usually begins rapidly, with no warning. Before parents realize what is happening, the infant may suddenly change in his degree of interest in his surroundings and his level of activity. If an infection is present, his body temperature may rise quickly to 102° to 104°F. (38.8° to 40°C.) or higher. When the temperature rises the infant may have a convulsion. In the adult, chills occur in a similar situation. Parents may never have seen a child having a convulsion before and may therefore be very anxious concerning his welfare. An

390

Text continued on page 395

NURSING ADMISSION HISTORY   0–6 YEARS

DIAGNOSIS: _____

T_____ P_____ R_____ B.P. _____

HT. _____ WT. _____ ALLERGIES _____

PHYSICAL DESCRIPTION: _____

_____

_____

_____

_____

USE PLATE
OR PRINT

M.R. No. _____ DATE _____
PT. NAME _____
PARENT _____
ADDRESS _____
_____
DATE OF BIRTH _____ B.C. No. _____
M.A. No. _____
DIV. _____ CLIN. _____ A.P. DR. _____

Nickname _____ Age _____

Hist. From _____ Lang. _____

THE CHILDREN'S HOSPITAL MEDICAL CENTER, BOSTON, MASSACHUSETTS 02115

1. **FAMILY:** Household composition (i.e., parents, siblings, grandparents) _____

_____

Names and ages of siblings _____

_____

Primary caretaker for child _____

Does mother work ☐ YES ☐ NO If yes, who cares for child _____

How can parents usually be reached _____

Language spoken by parents _____

Any additional problems or changes in the family that might affect this child (i.e., births, deaths, illness, etc.) _____

_____

2. **EATING PATTERNS:**

☐ Bottle _____   ☐ Breast fed _____   ☐ Cup _____

Formula type _____ Frequency and amounts _____

Juices ☐ YES ☐ NO Types _____ Frequency and amounts _____

Solids ☐ YES ☐ NO ☐ Strained _____ ☐ Junior _____ ☐ Regular table food _____

Typical day's diet (including type of food, amounts, and time)

Breakfast @ _____	Lunch @ _____	Supper @ _____	Snacks @ _____
_____	_____	_____	_____
_____	_____	_____	_____
_____	_____	_____	_____
_____	_____	_____	_____
_____	_____	_____	_____

Approximate amount of milk per day _____

Any fluids or solids not tolerated _____

Special likes _____ Dislikes _____

If mother is presently introducing the use of the cup, how being done _____

Vitamins _____ Fluorides _____

Any additional feeding problems _____

_____

03595

FIGURE 14–1. Nursing admission history, 0 to 6 years. (Courtesy of Children's Hospital Medical Center, Boston, Mass.)

Illustration continued on following page

3. **SLEEPING:**

Naps _____ Time and length _____ a.m. _____ p.m.

Sleeps in ☐ Crib _____ ☐ Bed _____ ☐ Alone ☐ With _____

Bedtime rituals _____

Usual bedtime _____ Awakes at _____

Special needs related to sleep

Bottle ☐ YES ☐ NO   Pacifier ☐ YES ☐ NO   Fears _____

Special toy _____ Bed wetter ☐ YES ☐ NO   Climber ☐ YES ☐ NO

Needs to be taken to bathroom at _____

Any sleep problems ☐ YES ☐ NO   If yes, how handled _____

_____

4. **ELIMINATION:**

Number of bowel movements per day _____ Type _____

☐ Diapers   ☐ Pampers   ☐ Training pants   ☐ Toilet trained — Day ☐ YES ☐ NO   Night ☐ YES ☐ NO

☐ Uses potty chair   ☐ Toilet   ☐ Other _____

Taken to the bathroom at any particular time _____

Words for bowel movement _____ Urination _____

If being toilet trained now, how is mother doing this_____

_____

Any other problems regarding elimination ☐ YES ☐ NO   How handled _____

_____

5. **PERSONAL HYGIENE:**

☐ Dresses self   ☐ Bathes self   ☐ Brushes teeth by self   Usual bath time _____

Any fears of tub or water ☐ YES ☐ NO   How handled _____

6. **BEHAVIOR AND TEMPERAMENT:**

How would mother describe child's temperament (i.e., nervous, quiet, etc.) _____

_____

Fears ☐ YES ☐ NO   If yes, explain _____

Method of discipline used at home _____

What seems to comfort child when he is distressed _____

_____

Any behavior problems ☐ YES ☐ NO   How handled _____

7. **INTERPERSONAL COMMUNICATION:**

Talks well ☐ YES ☐ NO   If just learning, explain any special words_____

_____

If can't talk, how does child communicate needs _____

_____

How does he usually respond to strangers _____

FIGURE 14–1   *Continued.*

Is this his first time away from home □ YES □ NO If no, how has he reacted in the past _____

_____

Accustomed to baby sitters □ YES □ NO _____

8. **ACTIVITY AND RECREATION:**

Present motor ability (i.e., crawls, walks with help, etc.) _____

_____

□ Uses wheel chair   □ Crutches   □ Other _____

Type of toys and play activities enjoyed at home _____

Any special security toy _____ Brought with child □ YES □ NO

T.V. — favorite programs _____

Any special rules for watching T.V. _____

Plays mostly   □ Alone   □ With others

Are there any particular activities that could be done in bed that your child likes _____

Does he go to nursery school □ YES □ NO   Kindergarten □ YES □ NO   1st Grade □ YES □ NO

9. **PAST HEALTH CARE:**

Has child been hospitalized before □ YES □ NO When _____

Where _____ Why _____

How did he react while in the hospital _____

Any problems after discharge _____

Primary care received from _____

Any other health agencies involved (i.e., V.N.A.) _____

Has been or is presently involved with any CHMC facility (i.e., clinic, etc.) _____

_____

IMMUNIZATIONS

Circle the ones received: DPT   1   2   3   Booster   1   2

Polio   1   2   3   Booster   1   2

Measles   Mumps   Rubella

10. **ADJUSTMENT TO ILLNESS - PARENT AND CHILD:**

Why does child feel he has been hospitalized _____

Have you, or has anyone else, explained any possible procedures, etc., to the child □ YES □ NO By whom _____

Explain _____

How has your child reacted to his illness (i.e., behavior changes, irritable, etc.) _____

_____

Is there anything about his present or past illness which particularly upsets the child (i.e., fears injection, etc.) □ YES □ NO

_____

Does he take medicines at home □ YES □ NO What _____

How _____ Any problems _____

What medication has he had today _____

Does the child do any of his care himself (i.e., diabetic - gives own injection) _____

FIGURE 14–1 *Continued.*

Illustration continued on following page

PARENT

What is your understanding of your child's illness _____

_____

_____

How have you been involved in your child's care _____

_____

_____

How would you like to participate in your child's care in the hospital (i.e., feeding, etc.) _____

_____

_____

How much time will you be spending with your child in the hospital _____

_____

_____

Are there any aspects of your child's care that you already know you would like to be taught or have reviewed

_____

_____

What changes in your home routine have occurred due to the child's illness _____

_____

_____

11. **QUESTIONS ASKED BY PARENT AND/OR CHILD:**

_____

_____

_____

12. **ADDITIONAL OBSERVATIONS DURING INTERVIEW:**

_____

_____

_____

13. **INITIAL NURSING PROBLEMS FOR CARE PLAN:**

1. _____

2. _____

3. _____

4. _____

Comments _____

_____

_____

_____

Date: _____   Nurse Interviewer: _____

FIGURE 14-1 *Continued.*

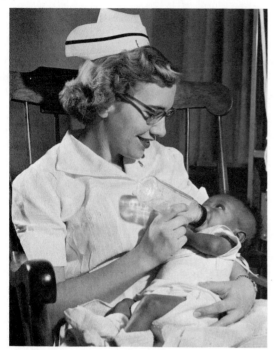

FIGURE 14–2. When feeding the hospitalized infant, the nurse gives him, in addition to food and sucking pleasure, warmth, comfort and a feeling of security. (National Institutes of Health Clinical Center photo.)

RESPIRATORY CONDITIONS

CONTROL OF RESPIRATION. Respiration is controlled by the respiratory center in the brain stem. Changes in carbon dioxide tension affect the respiratory center, which is stimulated by lack of oxygen. Certain drugs (anesthetic agents, opiates, barbiturates), brain injury, and hypothermia depress the respiratory center.

MUSCLES OF RESPIRATION. In normal breathing only the inspiratory muscles of respiration are used, mostly the diaphragm. When these muscles relax, expiration occurs. But when breathing is difficult, the intercostal, spinal extensor, and neck muscles are brought into use. In forced expiration, as in coughing, the abdominal muscles are used. If these are weak, the child will find it difficult to cough. The nurse can help the older child to cough by exerting manual pressure over the abdomen after he has taken a deep breath.

THE INFANT'S RESPIRATORY TRACT. Because the respiratory tract of the infant or little child is very small, any obstruction in the airway is extremely serious. Obstruction may be due to edema, mucus or an aspirated foreign body. If the obstruction is extensive and high in the respiratory tract, the whole lung is affected; if it is in the lower part of the tract, only tissue below the obstruction is involved.

Incidence. Respiratory disturbances as a group constitute one of the greatest problems in the care of children. The patient's age is important in the kind of disease from which he is likely to suffer and in its clinical picture.

Although respiratory infections are common in young children, it is difficult to identify them as separate clinical entities. The reason for this is that the tissues of the respiratory tract are continuous from the nose, pharynx and larynx to the tracheobronchial tree and also to the paranasal sinuses and the middle ear. Often an infection beginning in the upper respiratory tract will proceed downward to the lower tract.

Epidemiology. Infecting organisms are passed from person to person through the air. As the infant breathes, he draws into his lungs organisms carried on minute droplets of water or particles of dust. These organisms multiply rapidly in the mucous membranes, and the newly infected infant becomes a source of infection to others and of further infection to himself.

These pathogenic organisms die quickly in outdoor air, owing to the action of ultraviolet light from the sun and a temperature unfavorable to their growth. This is the reason why in summer, when infants and children are outdoors and houses are better ventilated, colds are few. In winter, when children are kept indoors, whether at home or at school, cross-contamination is apt to occur, and colds spread through the family, play group or class. Children during the first few years at school are likely to have more upper respiratory tract infections because they are more frequently exposed and have not built up resistance to infection as has the healthy older child. Infected preschool-age and school children thus become a source of infection for smaller siblings at home.

Etiology. Infection is the most common etiologic factor in respiratory conditions occurring after the neonatal period. The infant, however, may aspirate foreign bodies or irritating substances containing oil or zinc stearate.

Acute infection may be caused by viruses mostly or by some bacteria. The influenza virus has been recognized for many years as one of the organisms causing such infections. During recent years several other viruses have also been recognized, such as the adenoviruses, the Coxsackie viruses, the ECHO (enteric cytopathogenic human orphan) viruses, and the RS (respiratory syncytial) virus.

ACUTE NASOPHARYNGITIS (COMMON COLD)

This is the most common respiratory infection

in infants and children. The nasal accessory sinuses and the nasopharynx are involved. The difficulty in caring for children is that the infection spreads quickly, and serious complications may result. The clinical pattern in infants and small children is different from that in adults.

Etiology. The common cold is caused by a filterable virus or a group of viruses causing an acute catarrhal inflammation of the upper respiratory tract. Bacteria are the cause of the purulent, second stage of the cold; these may be pneumococci, hemolytic streptococci or staphylococci.

CONTRIBUTING FACTORS. Infants and children vary in their susceptibility to colds. Age, nutritional state, fatigue, degree of chilling of the body or emotional disturbance may influence the severity of a cold.

Immunity. Susceptibility to the common cold is universal. Children have little resistance to infection and therefore must be protected from exposure. Serious complications may re-

TABLE 14-1. PEDIATRIC MEDICATION GUIDELINES 1 TO 3 MONTHS

	Developmental Tasks and Behaviors	Nursing Implications
MOTOR	• Reaches randomly toward mouth; shows strong palmar grasp reflex.	• Infant's hands should be monitored or controlled to prevent spilling of medications.
	• Head drops or exhibits bobbing control.	• Head must be well supported.
FEEDING	• Sucks reflexively in response to tactile stimulation.	• Medication should be administered using this natural behavior: medication should be given via nipple. (See example.)
	• Corners of the mouth may not seal effectively and the tongue may be reflexively forced against the palate.	• Correct position of the nipple, if used, must be assured for adequate sucking.
	• Tongue movement may project food out of mouth.	• A syringe or dropper, if used, should be placed in the center back portion of the mouth. If placed along the gums, it must be toward the back of the mouth.
	• Sucking strength increases (3 mos.).	• Amount of medication presented must be controlled. Infant may choke or drool because he can take in more medication than he can control.
	• Stops taking fluids when full; progresses to fading of sucking reflex (3 mos.).	• Medication more easily given in small volumes and when infant is hungry.
INTERACTIVE	Basic Trust versus Mistrust Stage • Infant becomes socially responsible.	• Medication administration requires feeding behavior which establishes an easy, comfortable situation. This is part of the child's learning to form a trust relationship.

EXAMPLE: Jonathan, 2 months, has received 125 mg of ampicillin intravenously every 4 hours for 2 weeks and by mouth every 4 hours for 2 days. Irritable and febrile on admission, his status improves after the medication starts. He becomes alert and afebrile and orders for discharge are written. He is to continue the ampicillin for 5 more days and return to the clinic in 7 days.

Jonathan's mother is very nervous about "getting him to take medicine" at home. She explains that she herself "throws up" every time she tries to drink medicine.

The nurse helps mother prepare to give her son medication, which is available in a suspension. She teaches Jonathan's mother to draw the proper amount into a syringe and how to hold Jonathan in her lap so both her hands are free to hold the nipple and syringe. Then, touching the nipple to Jonathan's lips so his mouth opens and placing it well back in his mouth in a natural feeding position, the nurse drips the medicine into the nipple and follows it with some water to assure his getting full amount. For Jonathan this is like all feedings. Demonstrating this technique can help relieve the mother's fears and increase the likelihood of Jonathan's continued recovery as well.

From Ormond, E. A. R., and Caulfield, C.: *The American Journal of Maternal Child Nursing*, 1:320, September/October 1976.

TABLE 14–2. PEDIATRIC MEDICATION GUIDELINES 3 TO 12 MONTHS

	Developmental Tasks and Behaviors	Nursing Implications
MOTOR	• Advances from sitting well with support (3-4 mos.) to crawling (10 mos.). • Begins to develop fine motor hand control. • Advances from lying as placed (3 mos.) to standing with support (12 mos.).	• Safety precautions regarding where medications are placed and kept become extremely important. • Child who does not want to cooperate has ability to resist with his whole body.
FEEDING	Starting at 12-month-old level: • Smacks and pouts lips in act of shifting food in mouth and in swallowing. Lower lip active in eating. • Tongue may protrude during swallowing. • Learns to drink from cup. Generally has poor approximation of corners of the mouth when drinking. • Learns to finger-feed self. • Feeding behaviors become individualized.	• Child may spit out food and medicine he does not want. • Eating is inefficient, so medications may need to be retrieved and refed. A small medicine cup may be more effective than a spoon. • Feeding patterns and routines at home need to be considered.
INTERACTIVE	Basic Trust versus Mistrust and Oral Sensory Stages • Communication skills develop from random social responses (3 mos.) to making simple requests by gesturing (12 mos.). • Is sensitive and responsive to tactile stimulation. Begins developing responsiveness to other stimuli. • Recognizes immediate family and, very important, may exhibit intense separation anxiety.	• One must be alert for child's indicating his own needs (12 mos.). • Physical comforting will be most effective with child. Verbal comforting secondary. • Exhibits early memory. May recall negative experiences, precipitating negative response in another similar situation.

EXAMPLE: Herman, age 8 months, has had recurrent otitis media, and his mother has given him medications from a syringe since he was 2 months. Currently admitted with fever, dehydration, and otitis media, he has received ampicillin intravenously. Herman's condition improves and oral fluids and medications are initiated. Knowing he drinks from a cup, the nurse pours his ampicillin suspension (200 mg) into a medicine cup. In his room she holds Herman, talks with him in a relaxed manner, then puts the cup to his mouth.

After a brief pause, Herman begins crying and reaching for his bottle. Herman's mother arrives to visit and explains that at home she uses a syringe and he does not seem to mind taking medicine. Leaving Herman with his mother, the nurse gets a syringe for the remainder of the dose, and Herman's mother then gives him a bottle of juice to drink. Familiar activities are very important to Herman. Six hours later the same approach works for the nurse. She describes Herman's familiar routine in the Kardex before going off duty.

From Ormond, E. A. R., and Caulfield, C.: *The American Journal of Maternal Child Nursing*, 1:321, September/October 1976.

sult, particularly among infants in infants' homes, in a children's hospital, or in children's units of a general hospital.

Pathology. The initial lesion is an edema of the submucosa followed by infiltration with leukocytes. There are separation of epithelial cells and destruction of nasal epithelium.

Clinical Manifestations. The child is fretful, irritable and restless. He sneezes and has a nasal discharge which at first is thin and later purulent. The discharge may irritate the edge of the nostril and the upper lip.

Respiration is difficult, owing to congestion of the mucous membrane of the nostrils. The throat is sore, and the cervical lymph nodes are swollen. Gastrointestinal disturbances such as vomiting and diarrhea are common. Fever of 102 to 104° F. (38.8 to 40° C.) is prominent in patients up to two to three years of age. The temperature in older children is not likely to be over 102° F. (38.8° C.), and the school child and the adult may have little or no fever. Anorexia, cough, and general malaise are common. In the small infant obstruction of the nostrils may interfere with sucking, since he cannot breathe and swallow at the same time.

Differential Diagnosis. One of the problems in the diagnosis of the common cold in young children is that its onset resembles that of a number of infectious diseases, e.g., measles, pertussis, poliomyelitis, or congenital syphilis. The nasal discharge in allergic rhinitis may appear to be the first sign of nasopharyngitis; it does not progress to a purulent stage, however, as does a cold. Also, in allergy the nasal mucous membranes are pale, whereas in a cold they are inflamed.

Complications. Serious complications such as sinusitis, otitis media, mastoiditis, brain abscess (due to extension of infection from the mastoids), tracheitis, bronchitis, pneumonia, pleurisy, or empyema are more common in infancy than in childhood. These complications are caused by extension of the infection from the nose to the sinuses, ears, mastoids (and possibly to the brain), throat, larynx, bronchi, and lungs.

Treatment. The treatment is largely symptomatic. In the hospital the child is isolated. It is important to maintain his nutritional state with a suitable diet and adequate vitamins. The fluid intake is increased. The child is kept in bed during the febrile stage. Nasal congestion should be alleviated so that the infant may suck properly. Nose drops are used in an aqueous solution. Neo-Synephrine hydrochloride (0.25 per cent) or ephedrine (0.5 to 1 per cent) is frequently used to decrease the swelling of the mucous membrane and thus to permit drainage. Whatever the drug, in general one half to one quarter of the adult strength is used for infants and young children. Oily nose drops should *never* be used because of the danger of lipoid pneumonia (see p. 404). Medication such as aspirin reduces the temperature. The dose is generally figured as 60 mg. (1 grain) of aspirin per year of age up to five years, given two or three times a day; the dose for older children is 0.3 gm. (5 grains) given at the same intervals. Medication should be used only during the first day or two of the cold. Overuse of salicylates may result in salicylate poisoning. Sulfonamides and antibiotics should not be used routinely for the treatment of colds, but are indicated for complications or prolonged infections. Nasal decongestants, antihistaminics, and expectorants are not particularly helpful in young children, but may be ordered. Potent antitussives should be avoided because, if the cough reflex is greatly decreased, the infant may aspirate secretions from the nasopharynx. Nasal drainage must be carried out, since infants cannot blow their noses.

Responsibilities of the Nurse. REST. Rest is important in the acute stage of this disease. The nurse can help the parents understand that the infant must be spared from many of the ordinary day-to-day noises in the home and from the excitement of family visitors or the activities of siblings.

FLUID INTAKE. Water, glucose water, or other clear fluids should be offered frequently in order to maintain hydration and to liquefy secretions, since the infant cannot take large amounts at a time. (Milk tends to make secretions more viscid.) He has great difficulty in sucking and breathing at the same time and should be allowed to rest frequently. The child old enough to drink from a cup needs increased amounts of fluid; small amounts may be given frequently. Little glasses, pretty cups with pictures on the bottom and gaily colored straws make the taking of fluids more interesting to the small child. For children of nursery school age a little pitcher from which a cup can be refilled encourages a greater fluid intake. With a group of children of this age or older an achievement chart may be kept where all can see it. Such a chart shows graphically the fluid intake of each child, and they compete in the race to get ahead of the others.

HUMIDITY. The humidity of the room should be 80 to 90 per cent in order to liquefy the secretions in the respiratory tract and reduce the cough. Excellent mechanical devices to increase the humidity of the atmosphere are on the market. If none is available, a long, shallow pan of water may be placed on a radiator. But unless the radiator is very hot, evaporation is slow, and the moisture in the air is not sufficiently increased. The temperature of the room should be about 70° F. (21.1° C.).

NASAL DRAINAGE. In order for the infant to be able to suck, the nasal airway should be patent during feedings. This can be accomplished by removal of secretions with a hand syringe, gently holding the opposite nostril closed during the procedure. This is done gently so as not to injure the infant. Milking the nose prior to this may be effective. Occasionally a physician will approve the use of a few drops of saline followed by aspiration to clear the nasal passages. Drainage is facilitated by placing the infant on his abdomen and raising the foot of the crib.

NOSE DROPS. Drops are given only when

obstruction is present, not more frequently than every three hours and only for the first two or three days. The therapeutic effect is to shrink the mucous membrane, to relieve the stuffed feeling so characteristic of colds, and to reduce the excessive nasal discharge. The drops are given 15 to 20 minutes before feedings and at bedtime. The nurse must be certain that the infant's nose is cleared of mucus before feeding and when the infant is put to bed.

Because of the danger of cross-infection, each child should have his own bottle of nose drops and medicine dropper. The dropper is kept in the bottle and serves as a stopper. The dropper has a smooth, bulblike tip or is tipped with tubing so that the infant's nose may not be injured. If one bottle must be used for several children, a separate dropper must be provided for each child and never replaced in the bottle after use. The bottle must at all times be kept out of the infant's reach.

To give the drops, the infant is laid on his back, his head over the side of the mattress or his neck extended over a blanket roll. His head may be turned slightly to the side so that the drops do not go directly to the pharyngeal area to be swallowed. His face is held by the nurse's left hand encircling his chin and cheeks, while the drops are inserted with the right hand. If such restraint is not sufficient and a second nurse is not available to assist in the procedure, it may be necessary to "mummy" him. After the drops have been instilled the infant's head is kept below the level of his shoulders for one or two minutes. The nurse or parent may hold the infant on the lap in any way which is comfortable for him, so long as the head is back below the shoulder level.

Only older children should be permitted to use inhalers, and then only under supervision so that they do not overuse them.

PREVENTION OF EXCORIATION OF THE LIP. Excoriation of the upper lip with subsequent infection is caused by the irritating nasal discharge. This may be prevented by applying cold cream or petrolatum to the area.

MEDICATIONS. These are difficult to give to little children. Pills and tablets should be crushed into a powder and mixed with water or syrup, or both. They should be given from a spoon. In giving oral liquid medications to infants, a unit dose bottle with a disposable nipple may also be used.

POSITION. The child's position should be changed frequently. The infant is propped first on one side and then on the other, with his back supported by a rolled blanket.

CLEANSING THE NASAL PASSAGES. As soon as the child is old enough to understand, he can be taught the therapeutic way of clearing the nasal passages. He should learn to keep his mouth open and blow the secretions from both nostrils at the same time. He should never be told, as many adults do tell children, to "close the mouth and blow hard."

CARE BY NONINFECTED NURSES. Nurses can contract colds from the children who are too young to cooperate in the prevention of spread of infection. A nurse with a cold carries the risk of infecting the infants even though good technique is used.

MEDICAL ASEPTIC TECHNIQUE. Infants having acute nasopharyngitis are usually cared for at home. Isolation technique should be maintained as long as a child is infectious. When he is no longer infectious, there is danger of his contracting a secondary infection from organisms carried by nurses or other children. The technique is the same for any condition which can be spread by discharges from the respiratory tract (see p. 95).

Medical aseptic technique *in the home* is difficult to carry out. If possible, the isolation unit should include a bathroom. Members of the family other than the mother should not enter the room. She should use the same technique the nurse uses, making any necessary adaptations to the home environment. The person providing care in such a situation is responsible for cleaning the sick room and for concurrent and terminal disinfection.

Prevention. All patients having infections of the respiratory tract should be isolated so that contact between them and well children will be avoided. A child in good nutritional state is not so likely to catch cold. In older children tonsillectomy and adenoidectomy may be indicated (see p. 649). Vaccines are of questionable value in preventing the common cold. Children acquire resistance to infections upon exposure to them by building up protective antibodies. For this reason the older the child, the more likely is he to resist infection.

OTITIS MEDIA

Etiology and Incidence. Otitis media is an infection of the middle ear. It is usually secondary to a respiratory infection and for that reason occurs in the colder months of the year. It may also follow measles or scarlet fever.

The organism causing the condition in infancy is generally *Hemophilus influenzae*. Acute bacterial infection is usually due to *Diplococcus pneumoniae*, beta-hemolytic streptococci, or staphylococci. In older children infected adenoid tissue around the opening of the eustachian tube may be responsible for recurring otitis media. Allergy may also be involved in recurrent otitis media.

Otitis media is most common in infancy because the eustachian tube, lying between the pharynx and the middle ear, is shorter, wider, straighter, and may be more collapsible than in the older child. A contributing factor is that the infant lies flat in bed during the greater part of the day, and infected material is carried more readily through the tube as well as to other areas, since the mucous membranes are continuous in the respiratory tract.

Clinical Manifestations, Diagnosis, Course, and Complications. The first stage of otitis media is due to swelling of the mucous membrane and consequent closing of the eustachian tube. Congestion, serous exudation, and infection of the middle ear follow.

The *symptoms* are nasopharyngitis (inflammation of the nasopharynx) with pain, which is augmented as exudation occurs and fluid pressure increases in the middle ear.

The *diagnosis* is made by examination of the eardrum with the otoscope. The drum appears bulging and lacks its normal luster. Later the bony landmarks and cone of light are obliterated. If the tympanic membrane has ruptured, a culture may be taken from the drainage from the middle ear behind the tympanic membrane.

The older child will complain of severe, sharp pain in the ear, but the infant often has no great discomfort and may cry very little. He is likely to rub his ear and move his head back and forth, however, as if something annoyed him.

The *course* of the infection is rapid. There is fever, commonly up to 104° F. (40° C.), with possible convulsions in the infant and chills in the older child. The little child is restless and fretful and suffers from gastrointestinal disturbance and anorexia. Fever and pain continue until the inflammation is reduced by adequate treatment, or the eardrum ruptures spontaneously and the exudate is released.

Complications are rare and may result from insufficient therapy. They include chronic otitis media, mastoiditis, meningitis, brain abscess, lateral sinus thrombophlebitis or thrombosis, and septicemia. A chronic condition with a perforated eardrum may lead to impaired hearing or deafness in the affected ear (see p. 586). If mastoiditis occurs, a mastoidectomy may be done.

Treatment. Nose drops are used to shrink the mucous membrane and provide drainage from the blocked eustachian tube. Measures for relief of pain include the application of dry heat to the ear, the giving of aspirin, and the instillation of warm glycerin or oil into the ear. Since the effect of ear drops is variable and since they tend to prevent accurate observation of the tympanic membrane, they are infrequently used. *Myringotomy,* i.e., a clean elliptical incision of

the tympanic membrane, or aspiration of the middle ear may be performed to relieve pressure and prevent the ragged opening made by spontaneous rupture. After a myringotomy, puncture, or spontaneous rupture of the drum the physician will probably order irrigations of the ear with hydrogen peroxide. Cultures of the organism will determine the appropriate antibiotic to use.

Responsibilities of the Nurse. Nursing care is based on both the characteristics of young children and the plan of treatment ordered by the physician. In addition to giving the antibiotic prescribed, the general local treatments will probably include the following.

LOCAL HEAT. A hot-water bottle—the water temperature not above 115° F. (46° C.)—encased in a cotton flannel bag may be placed under the ear and the child kept upon the affected side.

CLEANLINESS OF THE EAR CANAL. The nurse should wash the hands before touching the ear in order to prevent a mixed infection resulting from bacteria carried into the canal. If myringotomy is done or spontaneous rupture of the drum occurs, the physician may request that the purulent material from the external auditory canal be removed by sterile cotton cones or pledgets moistened with physiologic saline solution or hydrogen peroxide. (Some physicians prefer, however, that this not be done.) The area is then wiped dry with sterile cotton.

EAR DROPS OR EAR IRRIGATIONS. If ear drops or irrigations are ordered, it may be necessary to "mummy" the infant unless a parent or another nurse is available to hold him. If the child is under three years of age, the auricle is pulled down and back—if over three years, up and back—in order to facilitate the passage of the fluid onto the drum.

CARE OF THE SKIN. If the discharge is profuse, the skin around the ear can be covered with cold cream, petrolatum, or zinc oxide to prevent impetigo or irritation. If the skin itches, the child's hands are restrained to prevent scratching and spread of the infection.

USE OF AN EAR WICK. If an ear wick is used, it should be small, inserted loosely and changed frequently. If cotton is packed into the ear too tightly, free drainage cannot occur, and infected material may be forced into the mastoid area. If the infant is placed on the affected side, drainage will be promoted. The parents should be cautioned not to wet the wick when shampooing the child's head or when bathing him.

OBSERVATION FOR COMPLICATIONS. The nurse should watch for symptoms of complications such as mastoiditis or meningitis or evidence of the less common complications listed above. In some children after the acute infections have been treated, smoldering, low-grade chronic infections of the mastoid bone lead to loss of hearing (see p. 586). Accurate observation is necessary, therefore, to prevent this problem.

Prevention. The most important means of preventing otitis media is by prevention and treatment of the common cold (see p. 395). In older children it may be necessary to remove hypertrophied and infected adenoid tissue (see p. 649).

SEROUS OTITIS MEDIA

Serous otitis media is manifested by an accumulation of uninfected serous or mucoid material in the middle ear. The cause of this type of otitis media is not known, although it is believed that a respiratory allergy may be involved, or the eustachian tube may be blocked. The child has no pain or fever, but may complain of the ear feeling "full." Permanent hearing loss may result.

Treatment includes the use of nasal vasoconstrictors and oral decongestants containing antihistamines. Audiograms should be done periodically to determine the degree of hearing loss.

If deafness becomes a problem, repeated needle aspiration of the middle ear may be necessary, or as a last resort small plastic tubes may be inserted through the tympanic membranes to provide constant palliative drainage and equilization of pressure. This is a difficult problem which requires the services of the pediatrician and the otolaryngologist.

ACUTE BRONCHIOLITIS AND INTERSTITIAL PNEUMONITIS

These two terms are used interchangeably, especially in speaking of the disease in infants and children. It is difficult to think of a pure bronchiolitis without involvement also in interstitial tissue. In bronchiolitis, expulsion of air from the air sacs is blocked; the result is overdistention of the lung, dyspnea, and cyanosis.

Incidence, Epidemiology, and Etiology. The majority of infections occur in the first six months of life and are infrequent in children more than two years of age.

The condition occurs most frequently in winter and early spring. Many cases occur sporadically, but there is an increase in the number of infants who contract acute bronchiolitis when there is an epidemic of upper respiratory tract infections among school children and adults.

Sex and race do not influence susceptibility to bronchiolitis.

No one organism is always responsible for the disease. A virus would appear to be the causative agent. The respiratory syncytial (RS) virus has been implicated in the illness of infants having bronchiolitis, especially in the winter.

Clinical Manifestations, Diagnosis, and Differential Diagnosis. *Symptoms* of bronchiolitis occur several days after an infection of the upper respiratory tract and vary in severity. Respiratory symptoms are more severe than those of toxicity. The infant has a dry, persistent cough with increasing dyspnea. There is widespread inflammation of the bronchial mucous membrane. The mucosa swells, and a thick exudate is produced. Since air can enter the alveoli on inspiration, but is not expelled on expiration, it is trapped in the lungs each time the infant breathes, and the chest becomes overdistended. There is retraction on inspiration, but the chest collapses poorly on expiration.

The temperature is variable, ranging probably between 100 and 101° F. (37.7 to 38.3° C.). There is no relation between fever and the clinical severity of the disease.

Vomiting and diarrhea are not likely to be severe, but since dyspnea interferes with sucking, feeding may be a problem. The infant is alert, but appears irritable and anxious. The respirations are rapid and shallow and have a characteristic expiratory grunt. The accessory muscles of respiration are used, and there is suprasternal and subcostal indrawing with inspiration. As the lungs become more distended, the alveoli can no longer aerate the blood. Cyanosis may be severe, or the infant may be pale. Rales may not be present or may be scattered and fine, owing to small areas of pneumonia. Chest sounds, termed "wheezing," are common. Dehydration may be severe because of the infant's failure to take fluids and because of loss of water through hyperventilation.

Fluoroscopic and roentgenographic examinations show obstructive emphysema of varying degrees with or without scattered parenchymal infiltration. The white blood cell count is normal. No specific organisms are cultured from the nasopharynx.

The disease has many symptoms which make it difficult to differentiate it from a number of other diseases, among them asthma, cystic fibrosis with pulmonary changes, miliary tuberculosis, pertussis, aspiration of irritating substances and bacterial bronchopneumonia.

Prognosis and Complications. The *prognosis* is usually good if the child has received adequate, prompt supportive therapy. The mortality rate is low, but death may occur because of exhaustion and anoxia.

Complications which may follow the acute condition are bacterial bronchopneumonia, otitis media, pulmonary atelectasis with abscess, and cardiac failure.

Treatment. The treatment is aimed primarily at maintaining full oxygenation of the blood. The child requires an atmosphere of high humidity. (Cold vapor is better than hot steam.) This liquefies the secretions and makes it easier to cough up the mucus which fills the air passages. Oxygen therapy should be given to infants with even moderately severe dyspnea before cyanosis appears. Bronchoscopic aspiration may be done if the exudate has accumulated in the tracheobronchial tree. Positioning is important—by putting the infant on his abdomen, drainage can be better accomplished and air more easily expelled. The infant's head and chest should be slightly elevated. Antimicrobial therapy is used only for infants having a bacterial complication and should be given only after cultures have been taken. Large amounts of sedatives or opiates are dangerous, since they tend to depress the cough reflex and respiratory centers. Small amounts of sedatives, however (e.g., phenobarbital), may be given to quiet a child in a Croupette. The fluid intake is increased. Tachypnea may have a dehydrating effect, and the administration of parenteral fluids may become necessary. Water-soluble vitamins are given.

Responsibilities of the Nurse. In planning the nursing care of the acutely ill child his physical and emotional status must be considered. In addition, the emotional reaction of his parents cannot be disregarded.

The parents are anxious and fearful and possibly blame themselves for the child's condition. They feel helpless because of their lack of knowledge of the disease, its treatment and nursing care. They may be fearful because of separation from the infant. They need to have the plan of treatment explained to them and to receive both emotional support and reassurance.

The nurse watches carefully the infant's respiratory status and observes for any increased respiratory distress. The nurse is attentive also to changes in the pulse rate and temperature.

SPECIFIC CARE. A Croupette is extremely useful in the care of these children (see Fig. 14–3). It provides high humidity and oxygen at a temperature comfortable for the child. The Croupette aids the child's breathing through the higher oxygen content, and the humidity liquefies secretions in the bronchioles, making coughing less distressing to the child. Air under pressure may be used to provide increased humidity if oxygen is not necessary.

The canopy of the Croupette is made of clear plastic; therefore, the nurse can observe the infant easily. Distilled water is used to provide humidity when oxygen or air is passed through it. The bottle containing the water must be

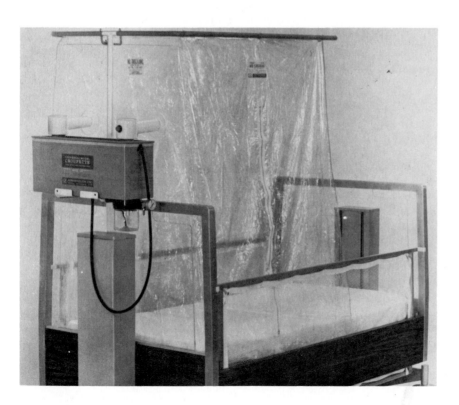

FIGURE 14–3. Croupette cool mist oxygenator tent. Air under pressure instead of oxygen may be used to produce water vapor. (Air Shields, Inc., Moncks Corner, So. Carolina.)

thoroughly cleaned each time it is refilled. The container at the back of the Croupette is for cooling the tent. A blanket may be placed over the sheet to absorb the increased moisture from the humidity in the Croupette. An impervious mattress cover is placed under the sheet to prevent the loss of oxygen, which is heavier than air.

The blankets and the child's clothing must be changed when they become damp so that he may not become chilled. This is done with as little disturbance as possible and is planned to fit into his schedule of feeding and medication.

Complete *charting* of the procedure is important. The date and the time when the child was put into the Croupette and when taken out should be recorded, as well as the amount of oxygen concentration used. It is important to record the infant's response to this therapy as shown by his color, the nature of his respirations, and the degree of his restlessness.

If the child is old enough to understand, the procedure of care in a Croupette is explained to him. A favorite toy may be given to keep with him in the Croupette.

Any secretion in the nostrils is removed. Secretions tend to force the infant to breathe through his mouth. Cotton cones are used for this procedure.

The fluid intake is increased through offering water between feedings. If the infant cannot be taken from the Croupette, the nurse supports his head and back with one hand while holding his bottle with the other. The hole in the nipple should be large enough so that he will not have to suck vigorously to get his feeding, but not so large that there is danger of his aspirating formula coming too rapidly into his mouth.

Water-soluble vitamins, antibiotics, and sedatives are given as ordered by the physician. The nurse should remember that the infant's breathing is labored and medications are given very slowly, while raising the infant's head.

ASPIRATION OF FOREIGN BODIES

Etiology, Pathology, Clinical Manifestations, and X-ray Findings. Small objects which an infant puts into his mouth may be aspirated. Such objects include safety pins, peanuts, beads, parts of broken pacifiers, and parts of toys, such as the button eyes or squeakers of stuffed animals. Carelessness of parents and nurses in leaving small objects within an infant's reach or giving him toys unsuited to his stage of development is most often the cause of such accidents. If an adult is present when aspiration occurs, the child should be placed across the knees, face down in a prone position on an incline, with the head at the lower end, and thumped sharply between his scapulae.

Some objects are radiopaque, others nonopaque. If they can be located by x-ray study, removal is facilitated.

The lesion resulting from aspiration depends upon the object and upon the degree of obstruction of the air passage it causes. Very small objects may cause little difficulty if they do not obstruct the larynx or a bronchus. Yet an obstructive object may produce atelectasis, bronchiectasis, pulmonary abscess, or empyema.

A particle of food may lodge in the bronchus

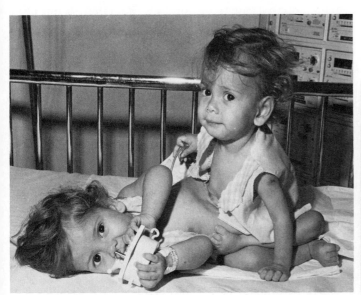
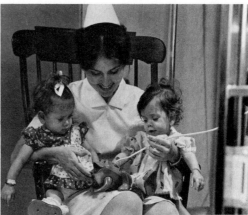

FIGURE 14–4. These Siamese twins, connected at the waist and pelvis when they were born, were separated and cared for by a team headed by Dr. C. Everett Koop, Surgeon-in-Chief at the Children's Hospital of Philadelphia. The team was composed of general surgeons, specialists in urologic and orthopedic surgery, anesthesiologists, and experts in intensive care and pediatric nursing. Although the surgery was overwhelmingly successful, one of the twins choked to death on a piece of bean lodged in her throat after she returned home. (Courtesy of Dr. C. Everett Koop and Children's Hospital of Philadelphia.)

and cause an obstructive inflammatory condition eventually involving the distal respiratory tract. In that case the infant would have a cough, fever, and continued dyspnea.

The *clinical findings* may be given meaning by the parents' description of the infant playing with a small object which later could not be located.

The immediate symptoms are choking, gagging, coughing, and stridor. The signs are laryngeal and tracheal in origin. The child may have dyspnea and hoarseness. If the foreign body is large enough to cause obstruction, cyanosis may occur.

If the foreign body is radiopaque, its location and form can be identified by its shadow on a roentgenogram; the location of a foreign body not radiopaque can be identified by the effects it produces in the trachea or bronchus.

Course. Bronchial obstruction has serious consequences. A foreign body lodged in a bronchus must be removed promptly. If it is allowed to remain more than a few days, it will cause a local purulent infection and a pulmonary abscess. Eventually atelectasis, emphysema, and diminished breath sounds will occur. There will be unequal motion of the sides of the chest on respiration.

Treatment. Laryngoscopy or bronchoscopy, if done in time, will permit removal of the foreign body. If the object has lodged in the larynx or trachea, tracheotomy (see p. 541) may be necessary to keep the airway open until further treatment can be given.

A secondary infection is treated with antimicrobial agents according to the laboratory sensitivity tests done on specimens of the organism involved.

Prognosis. The prognosis is good if there are prompt diagnosis and removal of the object. Nevertheless serious conditions or death may result.

Prophylaxis. Prophylaxis is evident. Keep small objects such as toys with small movable parts, safety pins, small candies, or nuts out of infants' and toddlers' reach. Older children should not give an infant food which he may put into his mouth in such large quantities that he chokes upon it, or objects which may be aspirated if they cannot be eaten. It is not safe for little children to play with the baby unless the mother is there to supervise them. Adults should not set a bad example by putting pins or other objects in their mouths, for small children tend to imitate people about them and will do likewise.

LIPOID PNEUMONIA

Incidence, Etiology, and Clinical Manifestations. Lipoid pneumonia occurs most frequently in weak and debilitated infants. The condition is caused by aspiration of oils or lipoid material. Vegetable oils are less irritating than animal oils. When oily nose drops are used or when the infant is given such substances as cod liver oil while crying, there is danger of aspiration. A child with defective swallowing ability, e.g., a child with a cleft palate, or a child lying flat in bed without his shoulders and head elevated by a pillow or the nurse's arm, is liable to aspirate formula or food while feeding. If this contains lipoid material, lipoid pneumonia may result.

The onset is insidious. There is first an interstitial proliferative inflammation, followed by a chronic proliferative fibrosis. In the last stage there are multiple localized nodules in the lungs.

The *clinical manifestations* are not characteristic of this condition alone. Thus diagnosis is difficult. The infant has a dry and nonproductive cough, his respirations are rapid, and he is dyspneic. Unless there is a superimposed infection, he has no fever or leukocytosis. Bronchopneumonia is a common complication, however.

The roentgenogram shows characteristic features of this condition.

Treatment, Responsibilities of the Nurse, Prognosis, and Prevention. There is no specific remedy for lipoid pneumonia, and a mild form of the disease may persist for several months before the child recovers.

Since there is no specific treatment, *nursing care* is all the more important. The child's position is changed frequently to prevent hypostatic pneumonia. The child is isolated to prevent his contracting a secondary infection from other children or adults.

The *prognosis* depends on the degree of pulmonary damage and on the severity of any secondary infection.

Prevention is negative rather than positive. Intranasal medication with an oil base is not to be used. The child should receive no mineral oil or castor oil.

If the infant is apt to vomit or regurgitate, he is placed on his side or abdomen after being fed to prevent aspiration of fluid.

GASTROINTESTINAL CONDITIONS

FOREIGN BODIES IN THE GASTROINTESTINAL TRACT

Etiology. An infant still in the oral phase of development enjoys putting objects into his mouth. As he sucks upon a small object, he may swallow it. Objects which do not stick in the esophagus, but reach the stomach, will generally pass through the intestinal tract. Some objects, however, do not pass through the pylorus and around the bends of the intestine but become lodged at some point. Sharp objects—needles, bobby pins, hairpins, open safety pins, and the like—may perforate the intestine. Objects within the stomach can usually be removed gastroscopically.

Treatment. There is no specific treatment if gastroscopic removal of the object is not done. A normal diet is continued. Roentgenograms are taken daily. If the object is shown to be moving along in the intestine, perforation is not likely; but if the object is shown to be stationary, operation may be indicated because of the dangers of ulceration and perforation of the bowel. The nurse should watch closely for signs of perforation: nausea, vomiting, blood in the stools, rigidity or tenderness of the abdomen, or evidence of pain. If the physician believes that perforation has occurred, operation is done at once.

Responsibilities of the Nurse. There is no specific nursing care other than close observation of the child for signs of perforation and observation of the stools. The stool is placed in a fine-meshed sieve and water run with force upon it until the fecal matter disintegrates and an object, if present, is easily seen.

BORIC ACID POISONING

Poisoning by boric acid results from either ingestion of the substance or its use as a powder or ointment on the infant's skin. Symptoms of nausea, vomiting, abdominal pain, diarrhea, and a rash with desquamation of the skin occur. Signs of meningeal irritation, convulsions, and coma may follow. The mortality rate in infants is approximately 70 per cent.

Treatment of boric acid poisoning is symptomatic, although exchange transfusion or hemodialysis may be used. Prevention by the avoidance of the use of boric acid in infant care can be accomplished largely through parental education.

VOMITING AND DIARRHEA

Vomiting and diarrhea are clinical manifestations of a variety of disorders of infants and young children. Vomiting and diarrhea are together one of the main causes of morbidity among infants and children in many countries where sanitation and hygiene are poor and children are treated with folk remedies rather than with scientific medicine.

Unsanitary and unhygienic conditions have more serious consequences in infancy than in childhood because of the greater susceptibility to, and lesser ability to combat, infection. Vomiting and diarrhea in the infant cause serious water loss with resulting electrolyte disturbance. Infants are vulnerable to deficits in fluid volume because of their proportionately greater body fluid content and greater extracellular fluid exchange. Fluid imbalances are due to a large surface area, a higher metabolic rate, and functionally immature kidneys. Death is most often due to the effects of dehydration and to acid-base imbalance.

Certain fundamental concepts of fluid and electrolyte equilibrium and acid-base balance must be understood because of their relationship to the problems of vomiting and diarrhea.

Fluid and Electrolytes. Each body cell is bathed in tissue fluid. The water and electrolyte composition of this fluid has a vital influence on the activity of the cell.

WATER. An adequate and continuous supply of water is a requirement for life in all human beings. Dehydration in the infant is more serious than in the adult, however. About 53 per cent of the body weight of the adult male is made up of water. Infants have an even higher proportion of water, in the newborn being 70 to 83 per cent. But in the first six months of life the proportion of water to body weight declines rapidly. Since fat essentially contains no water, there is a greater proportion of water to body weight in the thin person, whether an adult or an infant.

Water within the body is held in compartments separated by semipermeable membranes. These compartments are of three types, according to the kind of fluid they contain.

Cellular or intracellular fluid (water within the cells) represents about 35 to 40 per cent of body weight. Each cell must be supplied with oxygen and the nutrients that it requires; in addition, the water and salt content must be kept within narrow limits.

Extracellular fluid or plasma (water within the blood vessels or intravascular water contained in plasma) represents about 5 per cent of the total body weight of the human being. Plasma, the fluid portion of the blood, contains protein, which normally remains within the walls of the vessels. The water and mineral salts it contains can leave the vessels and enter surrounding tissues. In health the normal fluid volume of the plasma is maintained within relatively narrow limits. If dehydration or hemorrhage occurs, the volume will be reduced and shock will be evident. If overhydration occurs, the heart action may be embarrassed, and fluid will be lost from the vessels to produce edema of the subcutaneous tissues or of the lungs. Plasma contains mineral salts in different concentrations from those of the intracellular water; the predominant components are sodium and chloride.

Extracellular fluid or interstitial fluid is that which is between the vascular spaces and the cells and is similar to plasma except that it contains very little protein. When disease occurs, an increase in interstitial fluid is reflected in edema; a lack of interstitial fluid results in dehydration. Interstitial fluid is relatively greater in volume in infants than in adults. The newborn has approximately 25 per cent of his body weight in interstitial fluid. At two years he will be well on the way to reaching the adult level of 15 per cent of body weight.

The body attempts to keep the composition of each body fluid constant within a narrow range.

Source. The main source of water is through ingestion of fluids and some solid food such as vegetables and meats which contain large amounts of water. A second source is through metabolism. When foodstuffs are broken down into simpler elements, water of oxidation is formed.

Water Losses. Water in the normal healthy person is continually lost through the gastrointestinal tract in stools and saliva; through the skin and lungs, since body heat is removed by the vaporization of water (this volume of water varies greatly, depending on the person's activity, the temperature of the environment and individual make-up); and through the kidneys, whose excretion contains urea and other products of metabolism in combination with water.

In disease these losses may be increased, owing to fever, greater urinary output, diarrhea, and vomiting. If, at the same time, a child ingests insufficient water, he will show signs of dehydration such as thick secretions, dryness of the mouth, loss of skin turgor, sunken eyes, loss of weight, and concentrated urine.

Besides the difference in the proportion of total body water in cellular and extracellular compartments between infants and adults, there is a further difference. The infant takes in and excretes more water than the adult when these amounts are expressed in milliliters per kilogram of body weight. There are two reasons for these differences: (1) the basal heat production per kilogram is twice as high in infants as in adults. Because of this and because he has a greater body surface area in proportion to his size, the infant loses twice as much water per kilogram as does the adult. (2) Because of the infant's greater metabolic rate, there is an increase in the products of metabolism and their elimination. Water must be used to eliminate these in greater urinary excretion.

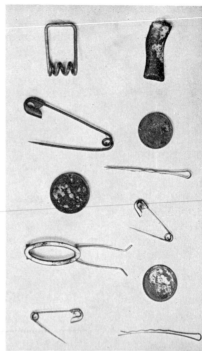

FIGURE 14–5. Some foreign bodies which failed to pass spontaneously and had to be removed by laparotomy, mostly from the stomach and duodenum. (Gross: *The Surgery of Infancy and Childhood*.)

Since the daily turnover of water in the infant is about half of his extracellular fluid volume, any fluid loss or lack of fluid intake depletes his extracellular fluid supply rapidly.

ELECTROLYTES. The movement of fluid in the body is determined in large part by changes in electrolyte balance, especially sodium concentration; however, other forces which are not fully understood are influential. It is easier to understand the scientific basis of fluid balance in the body than the electrolyte balance. The following explanation is given as a review.

Chemical compounds in solution either may remain intact or may dissociate. Examples of those whose molecules remain intact are dextrose, creatinine, and urea. These are nonelectrolytes. Those that dissociate in solution break down into separate particles known as *ions*. Compounds which behave in this manner are known as *electrolytes*. They have gone through the process of ionization and have an important function in maintaining acid-base balance. Each of the dissociated particles, or ions, of an electrolyte carries an electrical charge, either positive or negative.

There are several biologically significant electrolytes. *Cations*, or positively charged ions in body fluid, include sodium (Na^+), potassium (K^+), calcium (Ca^{++}) and magnesium (Mg^{++}). *Anions*, or negatively charged ions in body fluid,

TABLE 14–3. WATER AND ELECTROLYTE IMBALANCES

SUBSTANCE	MAJOR FUNCTIONS	EFFECTS OF TOO LITTLE	EFFECTS OF TOO MUCH	PRIMARY FOOD SOURCES
Water	Medium of body fluids, chemical changes, body temperature; lubricant	Observable symptoms: highly concentrated urine, oliguria, thirst, fever. Others: increase in serum solute and sodium concentration, circulatory failure	Observable symptoms: dilute urine, polyuria, headache, confusion, nausea, vomiting, weakness, muscle twitching and cramps, convulsions, coma. Others: decrease in serum solute and sodium concentration, increase in intracranial pressure	All liquids, fruits, vegetables, eggs, meat
Sodium	Osmotic pressure, muscle and nerve irritability	Observable symptoms: hypotension, nausea, vomiting, diarrhea, headache, muscle weakness, abdominal cramps. Others: decrease in extracellular fluid volume, hemoconcentration, loss of tissue elasticity, microcardia	Observable symptoms: manic excitement, tachycardia, edema. Others: increase in extracellular fluid, congestive heart failure, tendency to potassium deficiency	Salt, meat, fish, fowl, milk, cheese, eggnog, tomato juice, bread, butter, cereals, pickles, cola beverages
Potassium	Intracellular fluid balance, regular heart rhythm, muscle and nerve irritability	Observable symptoms: apathy or apprehension, lethargy, muscle weakness, nausea, tachycardia. Others: ileus or diarrhea, hypopotassemia, metabolic alkalosis	Observable symptoms: muscle weakness, nausea, colic, diarrhea, changes in ECG. Others: hyperpotassemia, cardiac arrest	Meat, fish, fowl, cereals, fruit, juices (grape, apple, cranberry, orange, pear, apricot), bananas, tea, cola beverages
Calcium	Muscle contraction, normal heart rhythm, nerve irritability, blood clotting	Observable symptoms: numbness; tingling of nose, ears, finger tips, or toes; tetany	Few clinical problems	Milk, cottage cheese, ice cream, broccoli, shrimp
Magnesium	Muscle and nerve irritability	Observable symptoms: hypotonic tetany. Others: fibrillary muscle twitching	Few clinical problems	Milk, cereals
Chloride	Osmotic pressure	Occur only after prolonged vomiting; few clinical problems	Few clinical problems	Salt, milk, eggnog
Phosphate	Building of bones and teeth, buffering system, transport of fatty acids, metabolizing of fats and carbohydrates	Hypophosphatemia, poor mineralization of bones, rickets	Observable symptom: tetany. Others: hyperphosphatemia, hypocalcemia	Milk, egg yolk, whole-grain cereals
Bicarbonate	Acid-base balance	Ketosis, augmentation of protoplasmic catabolism, tendency to greater water and electrolyte losses	Hyperglycemia, glycosuria, hepatic failure	Eggs, meat, beef broth, fish, poultry, chicken broth

(From M. A. Berry and C. B. Kerlin: The Drops of Life: Fluid and Electrolytes. *R.N.*, 33:37, September 1970.)

include chloride (Cl^-), bicarbonate (HCO_3^-) and phosphate (HPO_4^{--}).

Each water compartment (see p. 405) has its own electrolyte composition which differs from that of the others. *Milliequivalents* (mEq.) indicate the number of ionic charges or electrovalent bonds in the ionized solution in each compartment. Although the electrolyte composition of the fluid in each of the compartments is known, in treatment of a particular patient measurement is made of electrolytes within the intravascular compartment, because blood samples are more readily obtainable for analysis. This does not give a true measurement of the electrolytes in the cellular space itself.

Sodium. Most of the sodium in the body is extracellular. The average daily intake of sodium equals the output. The average diet meets normal sodium requirements, but if additional amounts are required in therapy, isotonic sodium chloride in 0.85 to 0.9 per cent solutions and whole blood may be given.

Some sodium is excreted through the kidneys and some through the skin in perspiration. It is excreted in large amounts when the temperature surrounding the body is relatively high, and during bodily exercise, fever, or emotional stress. Loss of sodium through the skin does not regulate sodium excretion; it is simply a by-product of temperature regulation of the body. Normally most of the sodium excretion is through the kidneys, which are the chief regulators of body sodium.

Hormones have a definite effect on sodium excretion. The pituitary antidiuretic hormone influences water resorption from the distal tubules. The adrenal cortical hormones, of which aldosterone is the most important, influence reabsorption of potassium and sodium, thus regulating the concentration of these ions in the blood stream.

Water exchange in the infant into and out of the cell is three to four times more rapid than in the adult. Since the sodium exchange is equally rapid, there are special problems in maintenance of a sodium balance in the infant.

Potassium. The main portion of potassium which is exchangeable is intracellular. The serum potassium ranges between 4.1 and 5.6 mEq. per liter. The daily turnover, intake and output of potassium are balanced, however. The average diet meets the potassium requirements of the body.

Potassium balance may be maintained at a low intake. Renal excretion of potassium, however, is accelerated by ACTH, desoxycorticosterone and cortisone, while sodium may be retained.

The activity of all cells is influenced by the potassium concentration in the fluid around them. A high serum concentration of potassium produces a clinical effect on the heart muscle. A low extracellular potassium level may produce complaints of lassitude and weakness, and a loss of tone of both smooth and striated muscle may occur. Circulatory failure may be seen over a period of time.

Potassium should not be given to a patient until his renal function is adequate; otherwise the serum potassium may be raised to high levels. The main contraindications to potassium therapy are adrenal insufficiency and renal failure not relieved by treatment.

Acid-Base Equilibrium. One of the most important considerations in fluid and electrolyte therapy is the acid-base equilibrium or balance. Whether a solution is acid or alkaline depends on the concentration of hydrogen ions (H^+). If the concentration of hydrogen ions is increased, the solution becomes more acid; if the concentration is decreased, it becomes more alkaline. The amount of ionized hydrogen in solution is indicated by the concept of pH. A solution having a pH of 7 is neutral, since at that concentration the number of hydrogen ions is balanced by the number of OH^- ions present. As the hydrogen ion concentration falls, the pH value rises. In other words, an acid solution has a pH value under 7, and an alkaline solution a pH value greater than 7.

The extracellular fluid normally is slightly alkaline, having a pH from 7.35 to 7.45. If the pH rises higher than this, a state of *alkalosis* exists; if the pH drops below, a state of *acidosis* exists. In acidosis the body fluid may still be considered alkaline, although less alkaline than normal. If the pH of body fluid rises above 7.7 or falls below 7.0, the patient's life is in danger.

Normal function of the kidneys and lungs is important in maintenance of the acid-base equilibrium. The kidneys tend to excrete surplus ions and other substances so that acid products of metabolism are lost from the body. The lungs may vary the rate at which carbon dioxide is lost. If the plasma is too alkaline, the respiratory rate will decrease; if the plasma is too acid, the lungs will eliminate carbon dioxide, which is slightly acid, by increasing the depth or rate of respiration.

Another important concept is that of *buffer solutions.* A buffer solution is one which tends to soak up surplus hydrogen ions or to release them as necessary. They are therefore important in regulating the acid-base equilibrium in the body fluid.

There are several buffer systems in the body. Probably the most important one in the extracellular fluid is the carbonic acid $\rightleftharpoons$ sodium bicarbonate system. A disturbance of acid-base equilibrium can be considered to be the result of imbalance in the carbonic acid $\rightleftharpoons$ sodium (or some other base) bicarbonate system. These bicarbonates are found in the extracellular fluid in a ratio of one part of carbonic acid to 20 parts of base bicarbonate. The acid-base equilibrium and the normal pH of the body fluid are changed when this ratio is disturbed.

In a clinical situation a measurement of the blood concentration of bicarbonate will indicate the severity of the acid-base imbalance. The values of the carbon dioxide content or carbon dioxide-combining power are therefore determined. The normal carbon dioxide content of whole venous blood for an infant or child is approximately 18 to 27 mM. per liter. The normal carbon dioxide-combining power of whole venous blood for an infant or child is approximately 40 to 60 volumes per 100 ml. The equivalent values in *serum* from venous blood may be found in Table 4–2 (p. 63). Acidosis is present when these values are below the levels given; alkalosis when the values are above these levels. In certain cases of acid-base disturbance these relations may be reversed.

Purposes of Fluid and Electrolyte Therapy. The physician may order fluid and electrolyte therapy for one or more of the following reasons: to provide for the basic nutrition of the patient, to provide a medium for medication, or to correct an electrolyte imbalance.

Fluid and electrolyte therapy is extremely important in the treatment of vomiting and diarrhea. When a child has either or both of these conditions, a replacement solution is given having an electrolyte content similar to that of the fluid being lost. Many such solutions to meet specific needs are available commercially.

ROUTE OF ADMINISTRATION OF FLUIDS. Size must always be considered when giving fluids to infants and children.

Oral Fluids. The daily intake of oral fluids for an infant if dehydration is present must exceed the normal requirement of 125 ml. per kilogram of body weight. The older child requires an intake of 1500 to 3000 ml. per day if he is to get the amount he needs for replacement purposes. Fluids which contain minerals, such as soup, fruit juices, and milk, should be given as part of the intake. If enough fluid is taken so that the kidneys can produce sufficient urine, they will also be able to correct minor changes in the electrolyte composition of the body fluids. Renal correction of the electrolyte imbalance cannot occur if the urinary output is minimal.

Parenteral Fluids. When oral fluids cannot be given or cannot be given in the quantities required, fluids must be restored parenterally: (1) subcutaneously into the interstitial fluid compartment or (2) into the vascular system by injection into a vein. (For a discussion of parenteral hyperalimentation see page 436.) Commonly used in the past but rare now is clysis, the administration of fluids subcutaneously. Although rare in large medical centers, it may be used in smaller community hospitals. This method of administration has the drawback of possible infection or necrosis of the skin. If fluids are injected into the peritoneal cavity, they are absorbed as they are when given subcutaneously.

Parenteral fluids must be kept sterile throughout the time they are being given. If they are not, either local or general infection may result. They must also be kept nearly neutral chemically when given subcutaneously. Intravenous fluids may or may not be neutral, but are irritating to the veins when they are not. Parenteral fluids must also have nearly the same osmotic activity or isotonicity as the interstitial fluid. (Osmotic activity is a measure of the capacity of a substance to move water across a semipermeable membrane. This, as was shown on page 406, is determined by the concentration of ions and molecules in the solution.)

Isotonic sodium chloride was mentioned on page 407. An isotonic solution of glucose is a substance having a concentration between 5 and 10 per cent. *Distilled water is not an isotonic solution and therefore cannot be given alone subcutaneously or intravenously.* If given accidentally, it may damage the subcutaneous tissue

surrounding the injection site or may hemolyze red blood cells and possibly result in a fatal reaction.

The amount and kind of fluids ordered by the physician to be given parenterally are dependent on their uses and the child's need. These include the amount of fluid and electrolytes the child usually needs per day in health (maintenance therapy), plus the amount he has lost due to his illness (deficit therapy), and the amount he is currently losing or will lose during his illness (concomitant and supplemental therapy). Fluid, electrolytes, calories in the form of glucose solution, plasma, or amino acids prepared for intravenous use may be given.

If insufficient fluids are given, dehydration may continue. If too much fluid is administered by any route, the circulatory system may be overburdened and collapse may occur. In such a situation the child's heart may not pump fluid at the normal rate, and fluid will ooze from the vascular system to produce edema of the subcutaneous tissues or the lungs.

More specifically, fluids containing only water and nonprotein solutes can pass through the blood vessel walls quickly within limits so that pressure is reduced. An infant can tolerate approximately 30 ml. per kilogram in a single injection or up to 150 ml. per kilogram per day in a continuous infusion. When blood or plasma which contains protein is given, smaller amounts are ordered because protein can pass through the blood vessel walls very slowly. The result is that pressure is built up in the vascular space if too much is given too rapidly. The effects of excessive fluid in the body may include convulsions and circulatory failure. For a further discussion of fluid and electrolytes, the student may consult textbooks of anatomy and physiology, chemistry, or specialty books in this field.

DIARRHEA

Metabolic acidosis is associated with a gain of nonvolatile acids or a loss of bicarbonate from the extracellular fluid. For example, in severe diarrheal states with starvation a loss of bicarbonate occurs from the gastrointestinal tract and produces a state of metabolic acidosis.

Incidence. Diarrhea is a symptom of a variety of conditions which together cause *acidosis*, dehydration and malnutrition. Thus it constitutes one of the main causes of morbidity and mortality among infants and children throughout the world.

Contaminated infant foods form a favorable medium for bacterial growth. In countries where the standard of living is low the infant death rate from diarrheal disorders is likely to be high.

Breast feeding safeguards the infant from the main source of infection—contaminated milk. Although these general causes of diarrhea are known, the specific cause in any case is proved only by laboratory studies.

Etiology. In many cases of diarrhea the cause is difficult to determine. The following are generally recognized causes of diarrhea.

Faulty preparation of the infant's formula or other food or the technique of feeding may cause diarrhea. Among such factors are over-feeding, an unbalanced diet (unsuitable combination of protein, fats, and carbohydrates—excessive sugar causes diarrhea), and spoiled food, often because of the lack of refrigeration and unsterile or unclean technique in the preparation of the formula or other foods.

Socioeconomic causes are difficult to determine. The incidence of contaminated milk and other foods as a cause of diarrhea is highest in the lowest socioeconomic group. In the higher socioeconomic groups the cause is more likely to be an infection by direct or indirect contact with someone who has the organism that causes diarrhea in the child. Causative organisms are pathogenic serotypes of *Escherichia coli* and various *viruses,* some of which cause respiratory illness in older children and adults. *Staphylococcus aureus* also causes diarrheal diseases, though sometimes the diarrhea occurs in connection with infections from this organism elsewhere in the body. Other organisms—the Shigella (Shiga, Flexner, Sonne-Duval and others), typhoid, and Salmonella groups of bacteria—may be causative agents. Sometimes diarrhea results from administration of antibiotics; other organisms may overgrow in the intestinal tract because of a change in the normal flora as a result of antibiotic therapy. Such infectious agents include Proteus and Pseudomonas.

Other causes of diarrhea include allergy to certain foods, emotional excitement and fatigue or the unwise use of laxatives in infancy.

Diagnosis, Clinical Manifestations, and Treatment. The *diagnosis* is made from the history and clinical evaluation. The causative factor may be learned from bacteriologic culture from rectal swabs taken at eight- to 12-hour intervals and from bacteriologic cultures of stools. The laboratory studies usually include determining the carbon dioxide- or carbon dioxide-combining power, and the hemoglobin, hematocrit, pH, sodium, chloride, potassium, and nonprotein nitrogen values of the blood.

The *clinical manifestations* of mild diarrhea are different from those of severe diarrhea. Severe diarrhea is of two types, that with a gradual onset and that with an abrupt onset.

MILD DIARRHEA. The clinical manifestations are a low-grade fever, possibly vomiting, irritability and disturbed sleep. The warning that these symptoms are due to diarrhea is a change in the nature and number of stools (two to ten a day), tending to looseness and even fluid consistency. At this stage acidosis and dehydration are not severe, though 10 per cent of the body weight may be lost. Weight loss exceeding this is an indication of severe dehydration.

Treatment is by a reduction in the formula feedings, especially in fat and carbohydrate, in order to put less strain on the gastrointestinal tract. The fluid offered by mouth is increased. Five per cent glucose in saline solution may be given orally every three to four hours. In some cases the physician orders a brief period of starvation (12 to 24 hours) followed by giving glucose in saline solution and, later, half-strength skimmed milk or skimmed lactic acid milk.

SEVERE DIARRHEA. The clinical manifestations of severe diarrhea with a *gradual onset* are elevation of temperature, with vomiting, anorexia, and abdominal cramps. Diarrhea develops, the stools becoming greenish because of unchanged bile content, containing mucus, and possibly tinged with blood. The stools become more frequent—two to twenty a day—and are expelled with force. The infant may be stuporous, may have periods of irritability, and may have convulsions. Because of dehydration, the skin and mucous membranes of the lips become dry and the skin loses its turgor (see Fig. 14–6), the pulse is rapid and weak, the fontanels and eyes are sunken, the output of urine is decreased, and the weight loss may be as great as 25 per cent of the infant's former weight. These signs of dehydration are due chiefly to loss of interstitial fluid.

In *acidosis* the carbon dioxide level may be less than 10 volumes per milliliter. When the amount of urine is decreased and renal function is lost, acidosis is increased, since the kidneys fail to excrete acid-producing metabolites. The depth of respirations increases, while the rate may decrease or increase.

In severe diarrhea with *rapid onset* the temperature ranges from 104 to 106° F. (40 to 41.1° C.). The infant is in extreme prostration; he vomits, and toxic symptoms appear. He is irritable and restless and may have convulsions. Respirations are rapid and hyperpneic. The diarrhea is not as severe as that with gradual onset, but acidosis is present. Collapse is due to loss of intracellular water and diminution of plasma volume. Signs of collapse in the infant are pallor and a flaccid state. The death rate in this kind of diarrhea is high.

The objective of _treatment_ in severe diarrhea with acidosis and dehydration is first to replace the water loss and restore the electrolyte balance. By comparing the child's weight with that before he became ill the approximate amount of water loss is ascertained. Laboratory studies will show electrolyte imbalance and the level of kidney function. Specifically, the objective of this initial therapy is restoration of renal function by means of a hydrating solution (without potassium because of the danger of hyperkalemia as evidenced by changes in the heart sounds), provision of fluid maintenance needs and making up for previous fluid loss by giving a balanced solution. During the initial therapy the infant may be starved for a period of possibly up to 48 hours.

Continuous intravenous therapy is used with the very sick infant because fluid will not be absorbed from subcutaneous spaces. Although whole blood transfusions are not given until the infant has been hydrated because of the greater concentration of blood during dehydration, plasma may be given.

When the infant is hydrated, fluids may be given subcutaneously. Hypertonic solutions should not be given, since they draw fluid into the area of clysis and may precipitate circulatory collapse. Hypotonic or isotonic solutions may be used, and hyaluronidase may be given into the site to promote absorption.

When the number of stools lessens and vomiting ceases, glucose and electrolyte mixtures may be started by mouth. Gradually, if no more diarrhea occurs, the concentration of fluids taken by mouth may be increased and fat and protein may be included until the dietary intake is normal within six to eight days. Diluted skimmed milk, lactic acid milk, or breast milk may be used initially and gradually concentrated as the infant improves.

Specific chemotherapy is given as soon as the organism causing the diarrhea has been determined. If the diarrhea is accompanied by a parenteral infection, this condition must also be treated.

If the child has fever, a tepid sponge bath may be ordered to reduce the temperature and prevent convulsions. No sedatives or cathartics are given, since they may obscure or distort symptoms indicative of the child's condition.

Prevention. The proper method for making, storing, and giving infant formulas should be taught all mothers, and the nurse should help the mother make the necessary adaptations to the equipment in her home. If the mother breastfeeds her infant, such precautions are not necessary. In hot weather the infant is offered water frequently, but the food intake is temporarily reduced. The infant is dressed according to the temperature and not the season of the year.

The child is kept from all contact with adults or children having infection, particularly of the alimentary tract, and an infant sick with diarrhea is isolated to prevent the spread of infection.

Public health measures have a great deal to do with the incidence of diarrhea among infants. Safe sewage disposal, pure water, and control of insects and pests are all part of good sanitation. The parents are taught to make the best use of what they have in protecting the infant from health hazards in the environment which they cannot control. For instance, all water given to the infant should be boiled, his food should be carefully covered to prevent contamination from flies, and a mosquito netting should be placed over him during the seasons when flies and other insects are prevalent.

Responsibilities of the Nurse. NEEDS AS A BASIS FOR CARE. When an acutely ill infant is admitted to the hospital with a diagnosis of diarrhea, he must be isolated immediately until the cause of the diarrhea is established. The nurse must be aware of the needs of the infant, the family, and especially the mother.

The _needs of the infant_ are paramount to all others; they are also more intimately within the nurse-child relationship. The infant must be given the means to satisfy his sucking needs, since feeding by mouth has been discontinued. He may be given a pacifier. If so, he should be bubbled in order to help him expel air which he may have swallowed. He will need to be comforted when his mother is unable to visit him.

He will need comforting also because of his medical isolation and because of restraints necessary during intravenous therapy. An infant just learning to sit up and move about may find restraint very frustrating. Many of the treatments given him will be painful, and he will need the reassurance of his mother's presence. If she is unable to stay with him, one of the nursing personnel should give him the affection and attention he needs.

If nothing is given by mouth, his lips and tongue become very dry, and he will need mouth care. As long as he is dehydrated he will require special skin care to prevent lesions. He will need to have his position changed frequently, and passive exercise should be given, if possible, during periods of restraint.

The _needs of the mother and the family_ cannot be listed in the order of their importance—all are important. The mother needs reassurance if she feels that the child's sickness is in some way her fault. She may feel that she has not been as careful as she should have been in preparing the feeding or in keeping the infant away from other children who had some infection. When she comes to visit the child or telephones to ask about his condition, she should be told of his progress. If his condition becomes worse, the physician should tell her this and take time to answer her questions. The mother may be worried over matters such as shaving the infant's head for intravenous therapy. Such procedures and the need for the treatment should be explained to her.

The nurse must think of the other children in the home and whether any of them may have the same infection as the infant.

ASSISTING WITH VENIPUNCTURE. The nurse will assist with venipuncture to obtain specimens for blood chemistry studies. A sterile syringe must be used because of the risk of reinjection of blood into the vein. Since infants do not have large veins in the antecubital fossa, blood is obtained from the external or internal jugular vein, or the femoral vein (see Figs. 5–14 and 5–15) or, uncommonly, the superior longitudinal sinus. The nurse is responsible for positioning the infant so that blood can be drawn with the least difficulty for the physician and the least discomfort for the child. Firm pressure should be applied for several minutes to the jugular or femoral vein after the needle has been withdrawn. The site should be checked frequently for the next half hour to determine whether any bleeding has occurred.

Mummy restraint is used with infants and young children during treatment and examinations involving the head and neck. The equipment needed is a square sheet or an infant blanket, depending upon the size of the child, and two safety pins. For the method of application see Figure 14–7. Figure 14–8 gives an alternate method. The young child will need to be reassured, for the procedure is more or less frightening, particularly if he knows that it is likely to be followed by an unpleasant or painful experience.

ASSISTING WITH INTRAVENOUS FLUID THERAPY. If the infant has been vomiting, is unconscious, or has anorexia or electrolyte imbalance, or if the physician wants to rest the gastrointestinal tract, intravenous therapy may be necessary. The fluids used for such therapy must be sterile, and have a neutral or nearly neutral chemical reaction and the same isotonicity as the interstitial fluid.

When fluids are given intravenously, the physician must take great care to calculate both the amount and the rate of flow. If the circulation is overloaded by too rapid administration or too much fluid, fatal cardiac embarrassment may occur. With continuous intravenous therapy, up to 150 ml. per kilogram a day can be given. Great difficulty is encountered if the nurse attempts to slow a regular intravenous drip to 4 or 6 drops per minute. Adapting devices should be obtained which produce a "mini" or "micro" drop of $\frac{1}{50}$ to $\frac{1}{60}$ ml. This results in the infant's receiving 50 or 60 mini- or micro-drops per cubic centimeter instead of the 15 drops from the usual intravenous set. Intravenous sets which have a control chamber which prevent the child from receiving too much fluid too rapidly should be used.

The nurse must still, however, keep an accurate record, at least every hour, of the kind

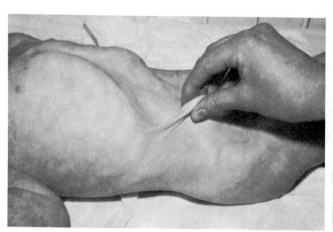
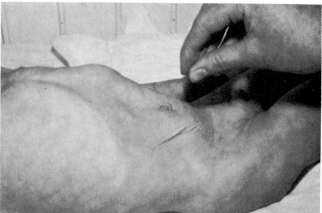

A **B**

FIGURE 14–6. A, Decreased turgor of the skin in parenteral dyspepsia. B, Slow return of lifted abdominal skin. (From Moll, H.: *Atlas of Pediatric Diseases.* Philadelphia, W. B. Saunders Co., 1976.)

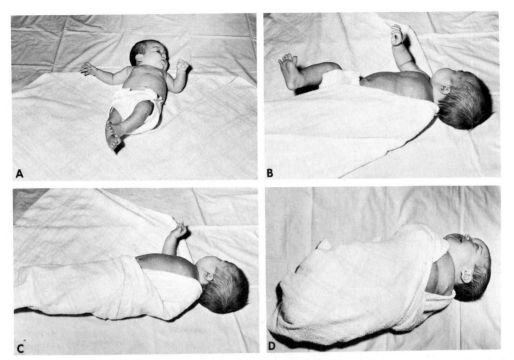

FIGURE 14–7. Mummy restraint. *A*, One corner of a small blanket is folded over. The infant is placed on the blanket with his neck at the edge of the fold. *B*, One side of the blanket is pulled *firmly* over one shoulder. *C*, The remainder of that side of the blanket is tucked under the opposite side of the infant's body. *D*, The procedure is repeated with the other side of the blanket. The blanket should be pinned in place. (Note: When applying a mummy restraint, be certain that the extremities are not forced into an uncomfortable position.)

and amount of fluid given, the amount absorbed, the rate of flow or number of drops per minute and the amount remaining in the bottle. The number of drops must be regulated according to the amount to be given. (There are mechanical devices also available to preset the rate of flow [see Fig. 14–9].) The regulation of drops should be done when the infant is resting quietly. If it

is done when he is crying, the tenseness of his muscles will constrict the blood vessels and cause the fluid to run slowly. Then, when he quiets down, the rate of flow will increase.

The nurse who assists the physician in starting intravenous fluids is responsible for restraining the infant so that the site to be used is immobilized. A mummy restraint can be applied if a scalp vein is to

FIGURE 14–8. An alternate method of applying a mummy restraint so that the infant's chest is exposed. *A*, Pull the blanket firmly over both arms and tuck it under the infant's back. *B*, Wrap the legs in the remainder of blanket on both sides of the body and pin it in place.

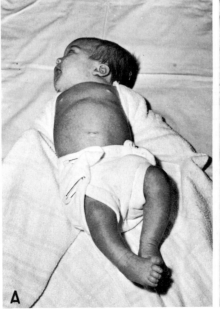
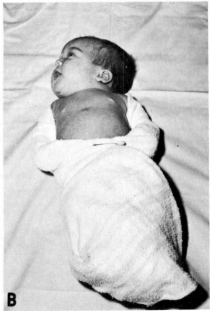

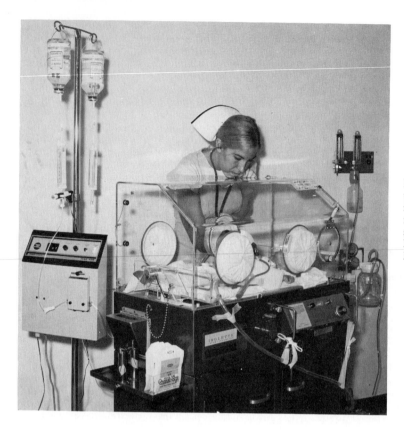

FIGURE 14–9. An infusion pump is particularly helpful in infusing small quantities of fluid. This unit has an electric eye which monitors the drip chamber to ensure a constant flow rate. (Courtesy of D. W. Wilmore, M.D., *Am. J. Nurs.*, 71(12):2335, December, 1971.)

be used; a modified mummy restraint is adequate if another site such as a hand or foot is to be used. Because an infant's veins are very small, it is usual to select one over the temporal region of the skull. If so, the scalp must be shaved over the area. The nurse must hold his head turned to one side as for puncture of the jugular vein. It is best to press the fingers against the bony skull and the prominences of the infant's face rather than putting pressure only on the soft tissue. The head may then be pressed against the pad on the table or bed. Care must be taken to avoid interfering with the infant's breathing while restraining him.

After the physician has inserted the needle it may be supported with folded gauze and taped in place. The infant's head may be immobilized by placing a sandbag on either side; these are held in place by 2-inch strips of adhesive tape. The mummy restraint may be removed and the infant's arms restrained with arm restraints (Fig. 14–10) or clove hitch restraints (see Fig. 11–17).

Other veins in addition to those in the scalp may be used for giving fluids intravenously to infants. Veins in the back of the hands, flexor surfaces of the wrists (see Fig. 15–1), feet, ankles or the antecubital fossa are used. It may be necessary to expose the veins by

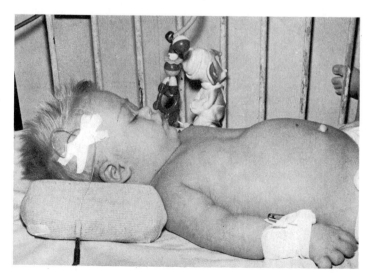

FIGURE 14–10. Venous cannulation. When the need for fluid administration is urgent and superficial veins are inaccessible, a vein must be cannulated with polyethylene tubing. Sandbags placed on both sides of the infant's head, and extremity restraint used to prevent the child's moving and dislodging the tubing. (R. Kaye, J. D. Bridgers and D. M. Picou: Solutions for and Techniques of Parenteral, Oral and Rectal Administration. *Pediat. Clin. N. Amer.*, Vol. 6.)

surgical dissection or a cutdown. A length of sterile plastic tubing is then inserted into the vein and sutured in place. The plastic tubing is connected with the infusion apparatus.

A needle is available that permits the plastic tubing to be threaded through the needle, which is then withdrawn. With this procedure a cutdown is not necessary.

If the flow of fluid during continuous intravenous therapy is stopped for any reason, another vein will probably have to be used when it is started again. Since this involves repeating the entire procedure, the nurse responsible for checking should report any slowing in the flow to the physician, who may be able to establish a free flow again by flushing the needle.

The nurse may be responsible for mixing intravenous fluids and adding medications when ordered. Careful aseptic technique must be used, and precise calculation of dosage of medication must be carried out. Each nurse should know the policy of the institution regarding the giving of intravenous medications. In many hospitals the pharmacy or the physician is responsible for preparing medications for intravenous use.

Sometimes the physician may order oral feedings to be started while the infant is still receiving fluids intravenously. If the needle is in a scalp vein and the physician does not want the infant removed from his crib, it is important that only clear feedings be given. There is serious danger, since the infant's head cannot be raised, that he might aspirate a little of a milk formula, with the possibility of lipoid pneumonia resulting. If the needle is taped securely to the child's scalp, and with the permission of the physician, the infant can and should be held for his feedings.

SUBCUTANEOUS INFUSION OR CLYSIS. When ordering fluids to be given by subcutaneous infusion or clysis, the physician orders the total quantity of an isotonic solution on the basis of the child's size and bodily needs. The rate of flow is not ordered specifically as in intravenous therapy, because the flow is determined by the rate of adsorption from the subcutaneous tissues. In order to facilitate absorption of such fluids, hyaluronidase may be injected into the area.

Various sites may be used for subcutaneous injection. In the infant these are the tissues of the pectoral region, the back, the lower part of the abdomen, or the anterolateral aspects of the thighs. If the pectoral region is used, the child may be immobilized by a mummy restraint which exposes the entire chest (Fig. 14–8). The needles are inserted lateral to and below the nipples. If the subcutaneous tissue of the back is used, the needles are inserted in the upper portion of the back and the fluid is injected from a large syringe. Fluids may be injected into the lower part of the abdomen if the infant is not to have abdominal surgery (such surgery is extremely unlikely in a child with severe diarrhea). The most frequent sites for subcutaneous injection are the anterolateral aspects of the thighs. The infant's arms and legs must be restrained with the clove hitch (Fig. 11–17) or extremity restraint (see Fig. 12–22). Sterile technique must be observed throughout the procedure. Subcutaneous abscesses have sometimes developed after such treatments. The needle point should not be inserted near the femoral or saphenous vessels and should lie between the skin and muscle layers.

Whatever site is used, gentle massage will help to diffuse the fluid into the tissues. If the center of the injected area becomes pale, the position of the needle should be changed.

When an infant is receiving fluids by either the intravenous or subcutaneous route, it is imperative that the nurse recognize his needs for sucking pleasure and for love and attention. A pacifier, unless contraindicated, should be used for the satisfaction of the sucking need. The infant should be bubbled if possible in order to relieve him of swallowed air. This attention, as well as talking to him and playing with him, will relieve his distress so far as is possible during this treatment.

For a discussion of the psychological aspects of the care of the older child receiving intravenous fluids see page 680.

ORAL FLUID THERAPY. If the infant has a mild diarrhea or is recovering from a severe one, fluids may be given orally. The amount of fluid varies with the size and needs of the child. Infants should receive in excess of 125 ml. per kilogram of body weight if their current need and deficit are to be met.

A nurse who is skillful, patient, and kind can usually encourage infants to take adequate amounts of fluid if they are physiologically well enough to do so. The nurse offers at frequent intervals whatever formula or fluid is ordered. An infant who is able to take small amounts frequently probably retains more than the infant who is encouraged to take too much at a time. Forcing fluids is discouraged, because such action too frequently leads to vomiting of all fluid taken.

Before giving the formula the nurse checks the physician's order in case the formula has been changed. After the infant has taken the fluid or formula the nurse charts the following: type of feeding, amount taken, degree of appetite, occurrence of vomiting. Solid foods, such as rice cereal or bananas, are added gradually in the beginning and are increased until a regular diet is given depending on the age of the child.

CHANGE OF POSITION. Change of position and passive exercise are necessary if the infant is restrained for long periods or is too ill to move himself. These measures not only increase his comfort, but also reduce the possibility of intercurrent infection.

SKIN CARE. If vomiting occurs, the skin of the infant's neck and face is cleansed and carefully dried to prevent excoriation. The skin of the buttocks is cleansed after changing the diaper to reduce the danger of irritation and a breakdown of the skin. Oil or a bland ointment may be applied after the cleansing. If the skin does become excoriated, the infant should be placed on his abdomen and his buttocks exposed to the air. The nurse must observe a debilitated infant frequently so as to prevent suffocation when he is lying in this position.

Besides exposing the buttocks to the air, a light treatment may be given. All oil should be removed from the skin before the treatment. A 25-watt bulb is put in a gooseneck lamp clamped to the bed. The lamp should be about 1 foot above the patient, and the buttocks are exposed to the heat for 30 minutes several times a day according to the infant's condition. Care must be taken that the bulb does not touch the bed linen and set fire to it. Many hospitals do not condone the use of the gooseneck lamp because of the danger of burning the infant.

BODY TEMPERATURE CONTROL. The infant's temperature is taken by axilla to prevent undue stimulation of the intestines through irritation of the rectum by a rectal thermometer.

If the infant has a fever, a tepid sponge bath may be necessary. If his temperature is subnormal, additional blankets should be placed over him and tucked in about his body. A hot-water bottle (water temperature 115° F. [46.1° C.]) properly covered may be applied. The hot-water bottle should be examined for leaks before being used. A small infant may be placed in an incubator.

STOOL COLLECTION AND CULTURE. The physician may request that the infant's stools be kept for his inspection. The nurse should wrap the most recently soiled diaper in newspaper or place it in a container for this purpose, discarding the previous specimen. The following characteristics of each stool are charted: color, size, consistency, presence of blood or pus, and odor. If a stool culture is ordered, a culture of the freshly passed stool or from the rectal area is taken, depending on the custom of the hospital. In either case a sterile applicator is used, and the specimen placed in a sterile test tube and sent to the laboratory immediately.

MEASUREMENT OF URINE. The *frequency of voiding* is also recorded. Although the amount cannot be measured exactly, it can be estimated.

One technique for estimating the amount of urine voided is to collect wet diapers in a securely closed plastic bag for each eight hour period. These wet diapers can be weighed and the combined weight of the plastic bag and the number of dry diapers used is subtracted from the total weight. The resulting weight is indicative of the amount of urine voided.

CARE OF THE LIPS. Since the lips are dry, owing to the dehydration, cold cream is applied to the area.

ISOLATION TECHNIQUE. Isolation technique, including gown technique, should be followed if the diarrhea is infectious and is spread by fecal contamination. Strict isolation is necessary to protect other children in the area and personnel. All persons coming in contact with the patient should wear a gown. All equipment used frequently, such as a thermometer or baby oil, is isolated with the infant. Disposable diapers are used. Feces, urine, vomitus, and liquid food waste may be emptied into the sewage in communities with adequate sanitary disposal. In a rural neighborhood or where such facilities are not available contaminated material should be mixed thoroughly with equal volumes of 10 per cent formalin solution or chlorinate of lime, or phenol or cresol in 5 per cent solution, and allowed to stand for at least an hour. Nursing bottles and nipples must be boiled after use. Disposable feeding equipment is discarded. Netting is placed over the infant's bed, and screens are put on doors and windows during the fly season.

Nurses can teach parents the elements of isolation technique, including the correct handwashing technique, so that they can follow the necessary precautions when visiting the infant and avoid carrying infection to the children at home (see p. 95).

If the mother cares for the infant, she must be cautioned to keep her fingernails short so that she will be less likely to carry pathogenic organisms on her hands, and should wash her hands thoroughly after caring for the infant.

PREVENTION OF INFECTION OF THE NURSE. The nurse may become infected through a break in technique when caring for the child or his equipment. Nails are cut short and the hands are washed thoroughly after giving the infant care.

VOMITING

Metabolic alkalosis is associated with the loss of a strong acid from the body. This is most frequently seen in severe persistent vomiting with a loss of hydrochloric acid.

One of the most common symptoms in infancy and early childhood is vomiting. No attention need be paid to the occasional vomiting of the healthy infant, but an infant who vomits frequently requires medical attention. Persistent vomiting may be serious not only because of its etiologic significance but also because it results in dehydration and electrolyte imbalance leading to *alkalosis*. Convulsions and tetany may occur if alkalosis is severe. Alkalosis resulting from severe vomiting is due to a loss of chlorides and potassium. The intracellular fluid has gained sodium ions and lost potassium ions. Potassium ions must be provided in adequate amounts if the normal balance within the cell is to be regained. As soon as renal function and hydration are assured, potassium must be given.

Ultimately, if the infant is not treated and fails to retain any fluid, he may show signs of the ketosis of starvation. Because of the serious consequences of vomiting, every effort should be made to find the cause and to institute immediate treatment.

Vomiting Due to Physical Causes. Faulty feeding technique is the cause of vomiting in healthy, contented infants. Overfeeding leads to gastric distention, which in turn results in regurgitation of the excess formula. *Regurgitation* is a form of vomiting in which the formula comes up in small amounts and drools from the infant's mouth.

The *treatment* for infants who cannot take and retain a large amount of formula is to concentrate the formula so that the stomach will not be overdistended, and yet the infant will ingest the needed calories. If the infant is on a self-demand schedule and takes too much too frequently, reduction of the frequency of feeding tends to reduce vomiting. If he swallows the feeding too rapidly, so that none leaves the stomach before all is taken, overdistention may result. These infants are fed from a nipple with a smaller hole so that the feeding may pass slowly from the stomach into the intestines while they are nursing. If an infant swallows air in large amounts, the stomach will be overdistended, and vomiting will result. The infant should be bubbled frequently to expel air during the feeding. After he has taken all his formula he is placed on his abdomen or right side so that formula may pass from the stomach into the intestines and air may more readily escape; thereby the eructed air will be less likely to force milk before it through the esophagus and out of the mouth. Air forced ahead of the milk into the intestines will cause abdominal distention and pain.

Sometimes infants will vomit because of mucus in the back of the throat. A preventive measure is aspiration of the nasopharynx before offering the feeding.

Improper feeding leading to irritation of the stomach is a common cause of vomiting. Irritation of the stomach may result from a formula which contains too much carbohydrate or fat. Excessive fat slows emptying of the stomach; fermentation takes place, and this leads to irritation. Prevention and treatment are by giving the infant a formula better suited to his nutritional needs.

Foods to which the infant is allergic or which are too highly seasoned, new foods or even lumps in the food, if he is unaccustomed to them, may cause him to vomit.

Vomiting associated with infections or conditions outside the intestinal tract is common. Among these are infections of the respiratory tract, ear, and pharynx. To these should be added acute communicable diseases; e.g., vomiting often accompanies an attack of coughing in pertussis (whooping cough) (see p. 662). When the infectious condition is cured, vomiting ceases. Infections of the gastrointestinal tract which produce diarrhea are likely to be accompanied by vomiting. Such vomiting ceases when the infection is treated successfully.

Conditions other than infections may produce vomiting because of increased intracranial pressure, e.g., hydrocephalus or intracranial hemorrhage. Such vomiting as well as that associated with encephalitis or meningitis is not associated with the feeding time, but is closely related to periods of increased intracranial pressure. The only treatment for this type of vomiting is to reduce the intracranial pressure.

Vomiting may be due to obstruction of the gastrointestinal tract. In the neonatal period vomiting may be due to congenital obstruction (see p. 253) of the intestines or bile ducts. Later, pyloric stenosis (see p. 418), intussusception (see p. 422), volvulus (see p. 253), and strangulated umbilical or inguinal hernia (see pp. 423 and 425) may cause intestinal obstruction and vomiting. Treatment of the intestinal obstruction will cause this type of vomiting to cease.

Vomiting Due to Emotional Causes. Some vomiting is voluntary, as in *rumination*. Rumination is the voluntary bringing up of small amounts of food from the stomach within a short time after feeding. The food is brought back into the mouth by manipulating the tongue or putting the fingers far back into the mouth. The food may be reswallowed, but is more likely to drool from the mouth.

The causes of rumination are not known. It may be that the infant dislikes the food or the person feeding him. Rumination may be due to tension in the environment that prevents the feeding process from being satisfying to the infant. This may indicate disturbed parent-infant relations in which the infant lacks affection and probably attention. Whatever the cause, the habit of rumination may lead to death from starvation.

The treatment suggested at present lies in psychotherapy for the mother and increasing the amount of affection shown the infant. Playing quietly with him for some time after his feeding has often proved helpful. Fortunately it is a habit which he will drop if it can be prevented for a few weeks and the conditions which produced it are changed through a general improvement in his care.

Responsibilities of the Nurse. Vomiting is a symptom, and treatment should be directed toward correction of the cause. In addition to correcting the immediate cause of vomiting, parenteral fluid and electrolyte therapy may be indicated to correct dehydration and alkalosis.

In order to determine the degree of renal function and dehydration, the nurse should chart whenever the infant voids, giving the exact time and estimating the amount of urine voided. Only after the amount and frequency of voiding have been ascertained may potassium be given.

If the vomiting is persistent, drugs of the phenothiazine group may be given in the form of rectal suppositories (see p. 102).

The nurse must make friends with the infant so that he feels secure and is relaxed while feeding. Treatments should never be given at feeding time.

The feeding technique is followed with care. The correct position for feeding resembles the position when feeding at the breast. The infant's head and shoulders are elevated while his body is cradled in the nurse's arms. Affection is shown by gentle pressure on his body. If the infant cannot be moved from the crib, his head and shoulders are raised, if his condition permits, supported by the palm of the hand or forearm. He is fed slowly and bubbled frequently if he is in the nurse's lap. If he is fed in bed, he is bubbled if possible, or allowed frequent intervals of rest. He will probably expel gas before the nipple is again inserted into his mouth. Elevating the head of the bed after feeding mechanically minimizes the tendency to vomit. The infant is handled as little as possible after feeding, since rest inhibits or lessens the probability of expelling the feeding.

It is important to prevent aspiration of vomitus. The infant's head should be turned to the side so that the vomitus may run from his mouth. If the infant is placed on his right side or on his abdomen after feeding, his head is, of course, turned.

Skin care is important. The face is cleansed and dried after the infant has vomited. Particular attention is given to the folds of the neck and the skin behind the ears.

The charting of vomiting must be accurate. The nurse charts the time in relation to feeding, the amount (estimated), odor, type, color, and consistency of the vomitus, whether the infant appeared nauseated before vomiting, and the act of vomiting—whether rumination, regurgitation, vomiting without force, or projectile vomiting.

SALMONELLA INFECTIONS

Incidence, Etiology, Pathology, Clinical Manifestations, and Diagnosis. Salmonellosis is one of the major public health problems in the United States. The highest age-specific attack rates are for infants and young children.

One of the causes of diarrhea mentioned previously (see p. 410) was the salmonella bacteria. These infections are caused by a number of flagellated organisms related because of their antigenic structure. Specific organisms of the group cause typhoid-like infections in human beings. Infection usually occurs after the eating of contaminated food and may last a long time, especially in infants. Recently it was found that the family's pet turtle or Easter chicken may bring the organism causing salmonellosis into the home. For this reason children should be taught to wash their hands thoroughly after handling their pets. The water in the turtle's dish should never be disposed of in the kitchen sink.

The chief pathologic changes include acute enteritis and superficial necrosis of the lymphoid tissue in the intestinal tract.

The *clinical manifestations* are headache, nausea and vomiting, abdominal pain, and diarrhea. Elevation of temperature, drowsiness, and meningismus may occur. Death results from toxemia, extreme dehydration, and circulatory collapse.

Diagnosis is made on the basis of isolation of the organism and demonstration of a significant agglutinating titer of the patient's serum.

Complications and Prognosis. *Complications*

may include osteomyelitis, meningitis, soft tissue abscesses, and bronchitis. The mortality rate depends upon early diagnosis and treatment.

Treatment and Responsibilities of the Nurse. Treatment and nursing care include strict isolation of infected patients, withholding of food by mouth, and adequate administration of parenteral fluids. Chloramphenicol appears to be the drug of choice, although ampicillin may be prescribed. The nursing care is that for a child having diarrhea and vomiting which was discussed previously.

When this diagnosis is made, it should be reported to the local public health department. The public health nurse visits the home to help the mother prevent a recurrence of this infection and to determine whether any other member of the family has symptoms similar to those of the patient.

CONGENITAL HYPERTROPHIC PYLORIC STENOSIS

Incidence and Pathology. This is a common surgical condition of the intestinal tract in infancy. It occurs most frequently in some family strains, in first-born infants, and in males. It is uncommon among black infants.

Pathologically, there is an increase in the size of the circular musculature of the pylorus. The enlargement is usually about the size and shape of an olive. The musculature is greatly thickened, and the resulting tumor-like mass constricts the lumen of the pyloric canal. This impedes emptying of the stomach. The musculature of the stomach then hypertrophies, owing to the effort required to force the formula through the constricted pylorus.

Clinical Manifestations and X-ray and Laboratory Findings. The symptoms appear in infants two to four weeks old, and only then can the congenital condition be diagnosed. The initial *symptom* is vomiting, which occurs both during and after feedings. The vomiting is at first mild, but it becomes progressively more forceful until it is projectile. The vomitus does not contain bile, but may contain mucus and streaks of blood.

Since little of the feeding is retained, the infant is always hungry. He will take formula immediately after vomiting, only to vomit again. There is either failure to gain or loss of weight. Without treatment the infant acquires the typical appearance of the starved child—he looks like a little old man. Because little food passes through the pylorus, the bowel movements decrease in frequency and amount. In some cases, however, a starvation type of diarrhea occurs.

The *signs* of pyloric stenosis are dehydration with poor skin turgor, distention of the epigas-

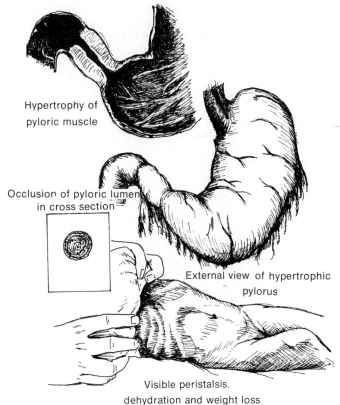

Hypertrophy of pyloric muscle

Occlusion of pyloric lumen in cross section

External view of hypertrophic pylorus

Visible peristalsis, dehydration and weight loss

FIGURE 14–11. Pyloric stenosis. (After Netter.)

trium (in badly malnourished infants the outline of the distended stomach and peristaltic waves passing from left to right may be seen during and after feeding) (Fig. 14–12), and an olive-shaped mass, located by palpation, in the right upper quadrant of the abdomen.

Metabolic alkalosis occurs, owing to loss of hydrochloric acid and potassium depletion. There is an increase in the plasma carbon dioxide content and in pH, and a decrease in serum chloride.

If barium is added to the feeding, an *x-ray* film will show the enlargement of the stomach and the narrowing and elongation of the pylorus, increased peristaltic waves, and an abnormal retention of the barium in the stomach. A film taken several hours after feeding shows that little food has left the stomach.

Laboratory findings show an alkaline, concentrated urine. Hemoconcentration is shown by elevated hematocrit and hemoglobin values.

Diagnosis. The diagnosis is generally made without difficulty; however, pyloric stenosis may be confused with pylorospasm (see p. 421).

Treatment. Few physicians recommend medical treatment for pyloric stenosis. If it is not successful, the infant's condition worsens and the danger from operation increases. If opera-

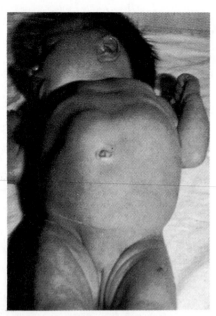

FIGURE 14–12. Typical gastric cramps in pyloric stenosis. Age four weeks; cure by conservative treatment. (From Moll, H.: *Atlas of Pediatric Diseases*. Philadelphia, W. B. Saunders Co., 1976.)

tion is performed early, however, the prognosis is excellent. But if medical treatment is carried out (it is not usually attempted in breast-fed infants), it is an extension of that for pyloric spasm.

Medical treatment is seldom prolonged unless there is definite evidence of improvement in the infant's condition.

MEDICAL TREATMENT. These infants may be given thickened or fine-curd milk feedings, may be lavaged prior to feedings, and may be given antispasmodic drugs (see Pylorospasm, p. 421).

SURGICAL TREATMENT. Surgery consists in performing the Fredet-Ramstedt operation, or pyloromyotomy. This involves a longitudinal splitting of the hypertrophied circular muscle of the pylorus without incising the mucous membrane. When the lumen has been enlarged by this procedure, food can more readily pass through. If the pyloric mucosa is punctured at operation, there is danger of peritonitis due to the leaking of stomach secretions into the peritoneal cavity. If the pyloric muscle is not incised completely, the obstruction will not be relieved.

Preoperative Preparation. The fluid and electrolyte balance must be restored, since a dehydrated infant is a poor surgical risk. If fluid deficiency, electrolyte imbalance, and blood losses are not corrected, shock may occur during operation. After the infant has been hydrated whole blood is given as needed. Vitamins B, C, and K are given parenterally.

Just before operation a catheter is passed through the nose and into the stomach. This may be left in place because removal of stomach secretions and swallowed air ensures a deflated stomach during operation and reduces postoperative vomiting.

Responsibilities of the Nurse. PREOPERATIVE EXAMINATION. The nurse assists the physician in examination of the infant to determine the presence of gastric peristaltic waves visible through the abdominal wall. The equipment needed is a bottle of sterile water, a bib, and a flashlight.

The procedure is simple. The infant is placed on his back with his face toward his left side. The abdomen is exposed. The bib is placed under his face. While the nurse gives the infant water the physician will hold the flashlight over the infant's abdomen from the left side. He stands on the right side of the infant and observes at the level of the abdomen. If peristaltic waves are present, they will be clearly visible.

METHOD OF FEEDING. The infant is fed slowly and bubbled frequently to prevent vomiting. He should also be bubbled before feedings to eliminate gas bubbles in the stomach. After feeding he is handled as little as possible and moved very gently. He should be placed on his right side or abdomen, and the head of the bed raised slightly. An infant seat which elevates the infant's head may be used after feedings. If he vomits after the feeding, he is refed if the physician so orders.

Charting of the feeding is important. His apparent hunger, whether he vomits—including the type and amount—the presence of peristaltic waves, and whether he cries before or after vomiting are all charted.

OTHER PROCEDURES. If drugs are given, the nurse should watch for evidence of overdosage. All symptoms are carefully charted. If the infant has a fever, the physician should be notified at once.

The nurse may be asked to assist the physician with parenteral fluid therapy (see p. 412).

The infant is weighed daily at the same time in the day's schedule. Accuracy is essential, for the weight roughly indicates the degree of dehydration and of malnutrition.

The infant must be protected from infection. Unless all other children with infection are isolated in the pediatric unit, the patient is isolated for his own protection. As is true for all children, nurses and visitors with any infection should not come in contact with him.

The infant's position must be changed frequently to prevent hypostatic pneumonia.

The infant must be kept warm, with blankets and hot-water bottles if necessary.

The charting of output is important and includes the color, frequency, and estimated amount of voiding and the type and number of stools.

POSTOPERATIVE CARE. Fluids may be given intravenously for the first few days after operation to meet the daily fluid requirements.

The infant's position is important. The infant should be kept on his right side or on his abdomen; this position aids digestion of fluids or formula because the pylorus is on the right side of the abdomen, and also prevents the infant from aspirating if he vomits. After the immediate danger of vomiting has passed, a fairly upright sitting position tends to prevent vomiting by making it mechanically difficult. The infant's position should be changed frequently, without disturbing him, if possible.

The nurse should note the indications of shock: rapid, weak pulse, cool skin, pallor, and restlessness. If symptoms of shock appear, the foot of the crib should be elevated and additional warmth provided. It is important to observe the abdomen for distention. Distention might be due to air which the infant has swallowed, but it might also be caused by infection of the peritoneum.

Physicians vary in regard to details of postoperative feeding. Generally, feedings are started four to six hours after operation. The infant is given small amounts, 1/2 or 1 ounce, of 5 per cent glucose and water orally at frequent intervals. This may be increased gradually. A dilute formula of half skimmed milk or Nutramigen and water may be substituted for the glucose solution. The formula may be gradually increased in amount and thickened in consistency until the infant is taking the usual quantity for his size and age. If he vomits, a more gradual increase in volume or a temporary reduction in oral intake should be made.

If the infant was breast-fed, the mother's milk is expressed and given as soon as he can tolerate it. He should be able to feed at the breast three to four days after operation.

The method of feeding is similar to that used preoperatively. A medicine dropper with a soft tip may be used for the initial feedings, but the bottle or breast should be given as soon as possible in order to satisfy the infant's need for sucking. The bottle-fed infant is held in the nurse's lap and cuddled before feeding as soon postoperatively as it is safe to handle him. The breast-fed infant is held as usual, for he derives pleasure from this while satisfying his hunger and his need for sucking.

Prevention of infection of the wound is extremely important if a waterproof collodion dressing has not been used. A pediatric urine collection (PUC) bag may be used to prevent contamination of the incision with urine. If pediatric urine collection bags are not available, the diaper may be placed low over the abdomen so as not to come in contact with the incision. If the penis is large enough, it may be taped to the thigh so that contamination of the incision does not occur when the infant voids.

At the time of discharge the mother is instructed to change his diaper when necessary and to observe for redness around the incisional area. The mother is also instructed not to give the infant a tub bath until the incision is completely healed and to return her infant to his physician's office for follow-up care.

Prognosis. The prognosis is excellent. Complete relief follows successful surgical repair. The mortality rate is low, provided operation is undertaken before the infant has become too dehydrated and malnourished.

PYLOROSPASM

In pylorospasm there is no structural defect of the pylorus. The spasm occurs in hyperactive infants, causing them to vomit frequently and often projectilely as in pyloric stenosis.

The *treatment* of pyloric spasm is by institution of proper feeding technique, lavage before feeding, and administration of antispasmodic drugs such as atropine. Sedation is helpful, and phenobarbital may be used. Some physicians may order the feedings to be thickened or small-curd feedings to be given.

Medical Treatment and Responsibilities of the Nurse. THICKENED FEEDINGS. These are mechanically more difficult to vomit than liquid feedings. Cereal or barley flour can be used to thicken the milk formula. A precooked cereal should be used, since the polysaccharides in it are broken down into simpler sugars. The feedings can be made in any desired degree of thickness. When the infant vomits directly after being fed, he should be refed. Some physicians order small-curd feedings such as those made with lactic acid solution added to whole milk.

PREPARATION AND TYPES OF FORMULAS. *Thickened Feedings.* The formula should be appropriate for the age of the infant. To it are added varying amounts of precooked cereal. The consistency of the thickened formula may be thin or such that it will not drop from a spoon. The physician will order the precise degree of thickening. A very thick formula may be fed from a teaspoon or may be pressed through a nipple with a large hole (or one from which the tip has been cut), with the bowl of a spoon or a tongue blade.

Fine-Curd Milk. Milk containing a very fine curd is usually prepared by adding acid or, less frequently, by fermentation through bacterial action. In fine-curd milk the casein is so altered that a softer and smaller curd is formed in the stomach. Such a curd is easier to digest and can more readily pass through a constricted pylorus. Lactic acid, U.S.P., may be added to a previously boiled cow's milk formula. The amount of acid ordered varies with the fat content; milk having a higher fat concentration requires more acid. Milk containing 3.5 to 4.0 per cent fat requires 6 ml. (1½ fluid drams) to the quart. Both the ingredients and the equipment must be cold to prevent too rapid curd formation. The acid should be diluted with a small amount of sterile water and added to the milk slowly with constant stirring. Commercial preparations of dried lactic acid milk may be purchased instead of preparing it in this way.

LAVAGE. Lavage may be ordered once or twice a day before feeding to cleanse the stomach of formula remaining from previous feedings.

The infant should be placed in a mummy restraint. A pacifier may be used to minimize gagging and to facilitate insertion while the tube is being passed. A basin or pail is put on the chair beside the bed. A sterile catheter (size 10 to 12 French) is used, connected to a funnel by about 2 feet of soft tubing. The catheter is lubricated with sterile water and passed rapidly through the infant's mouth into the stomach to a distance of 9 or 10 inches, i.e., from the tip of the nose to the tip of the sternum. If the catheter should pass into the larynx instead of the stomach, the infant would cough, breathing would become irregular and difficult, and cyanosis would occur. In such event the catheter should be withdrawn *immediately.* The nurse can be certain that the catheter is in the stomach if gastric contents appear in the tube and if the infant breathes normally.

Turn the infant on his left side and siphon off the stomach contents into the basin. Turn the infant on his back and pour an amount of physiologic saline solution or sterile water, a little less than that siphoned off, into the funnel. If the fluid does not flow, owing to air in the tube, "milk" the tube gently. Turn the infant on his left side, invert the funnel over the receptacle, holding it lower than the infant's head, and allow the fluid to drain off. Repeat the procedure until the returning fluid is clear. Usually 500 to 1000 ml. of fluid are used. Upon completion of the procedure, pinch the catheter tightly to prevent fluid from dripping into the pharynx as the catheter is removed.

Lavage is a trying procedure for the infant, and he will need to be held, cuddled, and reassured before he is fed.

DRUGS. Antispasmodic drugs such as atropine or Eumydrin may be ordered to relax the smooth muscle of the pylorus. These drugs are given 15 to 20 minutes before feeding. If atropine is ordered, a freshly prepared solution should be given. Most infants have a relatively high tolerance for this drug, though some may show signs of idiosyncrasy. The initial dose should be small and must be carefully measured to avoid overdosage. The dose is gradually increased until vomiting ceases, when it is gradually decreased. If the drug must be temporarily discontinued, a smaller dose is given when it is again administered. If flushing of the face, dilation of the pupils, or fever occurs, the physician should be notified. He will probably discontinue the medication or reduce the dose.

Phenobarbital may be ordered for its sedative effect upon hyperactive infants. If heavy sedation or excessive drowsiness occurs, the dose should be decreased.

INTUSSUSCEPTION

Incidence and Etiology. Intussusception is an invagination of one portion of intestine into another. Intussusception and incarcerated inguinal hernia are two of the most frequent acquired types of mechanical intestinal obstruction in infancy. More than half of the children having intussusception are under one year of age. Most of the remaining cases occur in the second year, in male infants who were previously healthy.

The *etiology* is questionable. Often no cause is found. Hyperperistalsis may be responsible. Also the intestinal tract of the infant is freely movable, especially the cecum and ileum, making it easier for one portion to invaginate into another. The immediate cause may be diarrhea, constipation, polyps of the intestinal tract which act as a foreign body, or swelling of intestinal lymphatic tissue. Intussusception may at times occur around a Meckel's diverticulum (see p. 761).

Pathology and Clinical Manifestations. Usually the upper part of the intestine invaginates into the lower. Intussusception is classified according to its location. The majority of cases occur at the ileocecal valve.

The mesentery is carried into the lumen of the intestine, and the blood supply is cut off to the invaginated bowel. Edema results. In some cases reduction is spontaneous, but generally necrosis occurs at the site of intussusception. The strangulated portion may perforate, thereby causing peritonitis and death.

The *clinical manifestations* result from the acute intestinal obstruction. The onset in a

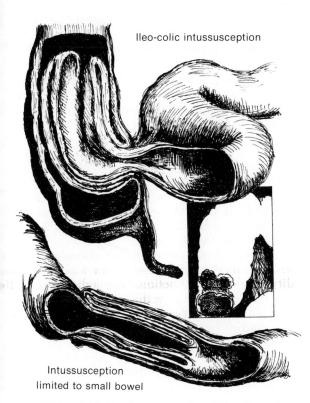

Ileo-colic intussusception

Intussusception limited to small bowel

FIGURE 14–13. Intussusception. (After Netter.)

healthy infant is sudden. The extent and severity of abnormal physical findings depend on the duration of the symptoms. There is paroxysmal pain in the abdomen, evidenced by the infant's kicking his legs and drawing them up upon his abdomen. The infant screams. At first, between pains, he may be comfortable. But the pain becomes progressively more severe. Vomiting occurs, first of the contents of the stomach; then it becomes bile-stained. This may be followed by fecal vomitus, depending on the site of intussusception. There are one or two loose stools followed by a discharge of mixed blood and mucus (currant jelly stools) about 12 hours after the onset. No more fecal matter is passed.

The infant is first restless and then prostrated. His temperature may go up to 106 to 108° F. (41.1 to 42.2° C.). Shock and dehydration occur. A tumor mass may be felt at the site of intussusception; it is usually sausage-shaped. The abdomen is at first soft and then distended or tender. The ring of intestine may be felt on rectal examination if the intussusception is of the ileocecal type. The infant will strain when the intussusception reaches the rectum.

Diagnosis and Treatment. The *diagnosis* is usually easy if there are sudden tenesmus, abdominal pain, vomiting, blood and mucus from the rectum, abdominal tumor, and prostration. After a barium enema a roentgenogram may show the intussusception, which is seen as an inverted cap and an obstruction to further progress of the barium.

MEDICAL TREATMENT. Medical reduction is carried out by a surgeon under fluoroscopic observation after a large barium enema has been given the infant. The intussusception is reduced by hydrostatic pressure. The abdomen is not touched during the process. If the intussusception is reduced, the small intestine will fill with barium and the mass will disappear; if not, operation is performed. This procedure is not without risk. The personnel in the operating room should be alerted to the possibility of a surgical procedure if the medical treatment is not successful.

SURGICAL TREATMENT. The infant is prepared for operation by measures to prevent shock and to correct fluid and electrolyte imbalance. Operation is performed as soon as possible. If gangrene or an irreducible mass is present, the involved segment is resected. Usually all that is necessary is reduction of the intussusception. Surgical intervention is preferred because it is certain to reduce the intussusception and allows inspection to seek for a polyp or other cause of difficulty.

Responsibilities of the Nurse. PREOPERATIVE CARE. Good hydration is necessary preoperatively. The nurse assists in giving parenteral fluid and electrolyte therapy, and whole blood if that is needed to combat shock. Deflation of the stomach by constant gastric suction is necessary. The nurse must observe whether drainage is constant and must measure the amount accurately. Antibiotics must be given in proper dosage so that the blood level of the agents will be adequate at operation.

POSTOPERATIVE CARE. Nursing care after a simple reduction is largely symptomatic. Parenteral fluid therapy may be continued until feedings can be resumed. Usually clear fluid feedings are given soon after peristaltic activity has been heard in the abdomen and distention and vomiting have ceased. It is absolutely necessary to keep the operative area clean and dry.

If bowel resection was done, fluids are given parenterally for several days, and gastrointestinal suction is necessary to prevent distention. Accurate measurement of drainage is important, since whatever fluids and electrolytes are lost must be replaced. The nurse must note symptoms of postoperative shock or peritonitis. Changes in vital signs, color, abdominal distention, or odor from the incision should all be charted and reported.

Since intussusception may occur during the second half of the first year—when the little child not only misses his mother but also is afraid of strangers—the importance of his mother's frequent visits, staying, or rooming-in with the infant (see p. 78) must be stressed. These infants are physically uncomfortable and psychologically hesitant to relate to strangers in the hospital situation. Since intussusception is an emergency, the mother will need an opportunity to verbalize her feelings, her shock on learning of the child's condition, and her self-reproach if she did not immediately take him to a physician at the first signs of pain and the change in his stools.

Prognosis. The prognosis is good if operation is performed at once. The chances of recovery are directly related to the duration of illness before operation. After 24 hours a high mortality rate is expected. Death in untreated cases results from exhaustion in about three to five days after the onset. Spontaneous reduction may occur in some cases. Recurrences are uncommon after operation.

INGUINAL HERNIA

Incidence, Etiology, and Pathology. Inguinal hernias occur much more frequently in boys than in girls. Such hernias may be present at birth or may occur later. They may be unilateral or bilateral.

As the testis descends retroperitoneally from the genital ridge during embryonic life, a sac of peritoneum precedes it into the scrotum, forming a tube. After descent of the testis the tube normally atrophies. If it does not close completely, intestine or peritoneal fluid may descend into it and produce a hernia. The size of the hernia may vary, depending on whether it extends through the external inguinal ring or into the scrotum.

Although a hernial sac is present at birth, the hernia may not appear until the infant is two or three months old. At this time he has a lusty cry, which increases the intra-abdominal pressure sufficiently to open the sac and force peritoneal fluid or intestine into it. As a result a bulge appears in the inguinal region or the scrotum.

In female infants an ovary may descend into a hernial sac as a result of increased intra-abdominal pressure.

Clinical Manifestations. When the hernial sac is empty, there are no symptoms. When abdominal contents are in the sac, incomplete bowel obstruction occurs. The infant expresses his discomfort and pain in fretfulness. Constipation and anorexia may occur.

If a loop of intestine is incarcerated or caught in the sac, all the symptoms of intestinal obstruction appear. There is danger of strangulation of the bowel with cutting off of the blood supply and ultimately gangrene. Incarceration occurs most frequently in the first six weeks of life. The symptom of an incarcerated hernia is the appearance of a firm, irreducible swelling below the external inguinal ring. The infant may vomit, and he becomes highly irritable. Later there may be cessation of bowel movements, abdominal distention, increased vomiting, leukocytosis, and fever.

The physician may be able to reduce the incarcerated hernia within 12 hours after it has occurred. If it cannot be reduced, emergency operation must be done. In severe cases bowel resection may be necessary.

If strangulation occurs before operation, the infant has severe pain and symptoms of complete obstruction. Immediate operation is necessary to relieve the condition.

Diagnosis and Treatment. The *diagnosis* is based on the history of intermittent appearance of a mass in the inguinal region and, on physical examination, the finding of a sac which fills when the infant cries or strains, but which can be reduced easily.

Healthy infants are best *treated* by surgical repair as soon as the condition is diagnosed. Operation involves removing the hernial sac and transfixing the neck at the internal ring. Infants tolerate this operation very well. After operation, in the majority of infants, the danger of strangulation and of edema and gangrene is removed.

If incarceration occurs before operation, an ice bag should be applied over the area to reduce the edema. The foot of the bed is elevated to prevent more abdominal contents from going through the inguinal ring. If manual reduction under sedation is not successful, immediate operation is necessary.

Responsibilities of the Nurse. Preoperatively, as far as possible, the infant should be kept happy and tranquil so that he will not cry. The stools are regulated by diet and possibly medication, since either a constipated or an irritating loose stool will cause the infant to strain. Both crying and straining tend to raise the intra-abdominal pressure and so produce the hernia.

It is often customary to order "nothing by mouth after midnight" for all patients scheduled for operation the next day. With small children, and especially young infants, such an order may result in dehydration. Since fluid metabolism is rapid in infants, those denied normal intake may become very dehydrated, especially if they have been crying, if they have missed previous feedings, or if they are not to be operated on until later in the day.

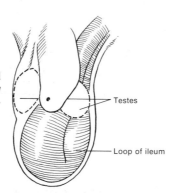

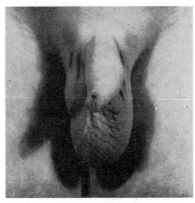

FIGURE 14-14. Child with left inguinal hernia. (Photograph from Gross, R.: *The Surgery of Infancy and Childhood.* Philadelphia, W. B. Saunders Co.)

Testes

Loop of ileum

POSTOPERATIVE CARE. After an inguinal herniorrhaphy the principal nursing problem is prevention of contamination of the wound unless a waterproof collodion dressing has been used. The area should be kept clean and dry.

Feedings are generally resumed a few hours postoperatively unless a bowel resection was done. The infant should be held for feedings and cuddled while being fed. After a simple hernia repair the older child may be as active as he desires to be.

UMBILICAL HERNIA

Etiology, Incidence, and Clinical Manifestations. An umbilical hernia is due to imperfect closure or weakness of the umbilical ring. These hernias occur in all races, but are more common in black children.

The *clinical manifestation* is a swelling at the umbilicus which is covered with skin. This protrudes when the infant cries or strains. It can be easily reduced by gentle pressure over the fibrous ring at the umbilicus. The contents of the hernia are small intestine and omentum (Fig.

14-15). The size varies from less than a centimeter to 5 cm. in diameter.

Prognosis, Treatment, and Responsibilities of the Nurse. Most small umbilical hernias disappear withou treatment, but large ones may require operation. These hernias rarely cause incarceration or strangulation of the bowel.

Physicians differ in their opinions as to the effectiveness of reducing and strapping umbilical hernias. If the physician orders the hernia to be taped, the following procedure may be used.

The area to be taped is painted with tincture of benzoin to protect the skin and to cause the adhesive to adhere to the skin.

The hernia is first reduced by gently pushing the abdominal contents back through the umbilical ring. The sides of the adjacent abdominal wall can be brought together in the midline to make a pleat of skin. A 2-inch strip of adhesive can be applied to the abdomen when the tincture of benzoin is dry, from the far bed line, over the pleat of skin, to the near bed line, covering the umbilical hernia. It should be pulled tightly across the pleat.

Usually operation is not done on an umbilical

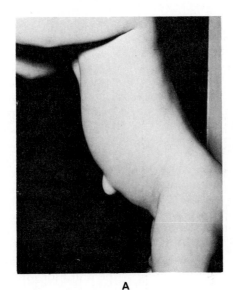

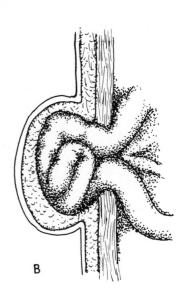

FIGURE 14-15. *A,* Side view of infant with an umbilical hernia. *B,* Diagrammatic representation of an umbilical hernia. (After Netter.)

A

B

hernia unless it becomes strangulated, enlarges, or persists to school age.

Postoperative *nursing care* requires no special technique. The child may be as active as he desires. A normal diet and fluids are given. Pressure dressings, applied at the time of operation, must be kept clean and dry to prevent wound contamination.

GENITOURINARY CONDITIONS

HYDROCELE

A hydrocele is an accumulation of fluid around the testis or along the spermatic cord. It may be a congenital condition or may occur during infancy. In diagnosis a hydrocele causing a swelling of the scrotum must be differentiated from an inguinal hernia. A hydrocele appears as a fluctuant, oval, translucent, tense sac. Fluid may gradually absorb during infancy, but if not, surgical correction is necessary.

PYELONEPHRITIS (PYELITIS)

Incidence and Etiology. Pyelitis is an infection of the renal pelvis. Pyelonephritis is an infection of the renal pelvis and renal parenchyma plus, in most cases, inflammation of the ureters and the bladder. Since infections in infants and children are rarely limited to one part of the urinary tract, the term "pyelonephritis" is probably more applicable than "pyelitis."

The condition is relatively common and is the most common renal disease in childhood. The *incidence* is greatest between two months and two years, the period when diapers are worn. The condition occurs more frequently in girls than in boys.

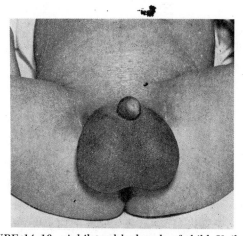

FIGURE 14–16. A bilateral hydrocele of child. Unilateral hydroceles are common and undergo spontaneous regression, rarely requiring intervention. (Davis and Rubin: *DeLee's Obstetrics for Nurses.* 17th ed.)

The female urethra is shorter than the male urethra. Infection entering the urinary tract from the stool in a soiled diaper contaminates the urethra and may be carried to the bladder, causing cystitis. Infection may enter the urinary tract not only through the urethra, but also by way of the blood stream or the lymphatics. Congenital anomalies causing obstruction of urine are predisposing factors because urinary stasis is associated with chronic urinary tract infections.

Organisms most commonly causing acute infection are the colon bacilli. Staphylococci, hemolytic streptococci, and *Streptococcus faecalis* may also cause such an infection. Chronic infections are often caused by multiple types of bacteria. Proteus and Pyocyaneus may also be causative organisms.

Pathology, Clinical Manifestations, and Laboratory Findings. There are inflammatory changes in the renal pelvis and throughout the kidney. In the majority of children there are changes also in the ureters and the bladder. The kidney may be large and swollen. Clumps of bacteria may be present. In chronic pyelonephritis there is loss of function because of scarring of the kidney parenchyma. Eventually the kidney becomes small; kidney tissue is destroyed, and renal function fails.

The *clinical findings* are variable. Symptoms related to the urinary tract may or may not be present. The onset may be gradual or abrupt. Fever may be moderate or as high as 104.5° F. (40.3° C.). Prostration, pallor, and anorexia appear. Vomiting and diarrhea occur; dehydration may result. Urinary urgency and frequency with dysuria are distressing symptoms. The child is irritable, and febrile convulsions may occur.

It is possible that the infant may show none of the symptoms of localizing of the infection to the urinary tract.

Pain and tenderness in the kidney are signs of the condition. If the infection is chronic, it may continue for months or years, causing anemia and failure of growth and development. Eventually renal failure and hypertension result.

Laboratory findings include pyuria, pathologic organisms in the urine, and leukocytosis. Slight or moderate hematuria may occur, and casts may be present.

Diagnosis and Treatment. The *diagnosis* is made on the basis of pus and bacteria in the urine. A catheterized specimen must be obtained. If there is recurring or persistent pyuria, intravenous or retrograde urography should be done. There may be neurologic or structural abnormalities which cause stasis and continued infection. The cystogram is useful for examining the child for ureteral dilatation.

General *treatment* during the febrile period includes rest; analgesic drugs are given if needed. Specific chemotherapy or antibiotic therapy is given to shorten the course of the illness and to avoid progressive renal damage. Sulfonamides are most widely used against urinary tract infections. Methenamine mandelate is effective as a urinary antiseptic only if an acid urine can be maintained. Methionine may be used to acidify the urine sufficiently. Nitrofurantoin (Furadantin) is a bacteriostatic and bactericidal agent against most of the urinary tract pathogens.

During the acute stage the child is encouraged to take more than normal amounts of fluid to dilute the concentration of urine. Transfusions may be indicated for anemia. If there are obstructive lesions, surgical correction may be attempted. Surgical removal is not always possible, however.

Responsibilities of the Nurse. Clean specimens of urine should be obtained, using an infant urine collecting device (for collection of specimens, see p. 96). The genitalia must be thoroughly cleansed before the specimen is collected. Zephiran 1:1000 and, if the physician orders it, hexachlorophene solution may be used for this purpose before the specimen is collected. The area is rinsed with sterile water. If a little girl is old enough to use a bedpan, it should be sterilized before use. If a little boy can control himself during urination, a midstream specimen may be obtained, i.e., he voids a small amount, stops, and then voids into a sterile receptacle for the specimen. Laboratory examination of a clean specimen of urine gives a rough estimate of the number of bacteria present.

For bacterial culture a catheterized specimen is used. The equipment for catheterization is the same as for the procedure in the adult, with the exception of the size of the catheter. For children, size 8 or 10 French is used. Two catheters should be in readiness, since the first to be used may be accidentally contaminated. Various solutions are used for cleansing the genitalia.

The procedure for catheterization of the older child is the same as that for an adult and should be explained to the child. He should be given an opportunity to handle the equipment and should be completely relaxed if catheterization is to be done successfully. The nurse may ask him to breathe deeply through the mouth in order to promote relaxation while the catheter is being inserted into the bladder. For the younger child two nurses are necessary, one to assist him in cooperating and the other to carry out the procedure.

The following points are stressed:

1. The genitalia are cleansed thoroughly with cotton balls dipped in the cleansing solution. *One ball is used for each stroke.* Strokes should be from above downward toward the anus to prevent organisms from the anus from being carried up over the urethral meatus.

2. The tip of the sterile catheter should be lubricated with sterile saline solution before insertion into the urethral meatus.

3. The bladder in the infant lies more anteriorly and higher over the symphysis than in the adult, and the urethra lies under and around the symphysis. The meatus in the young child may be exceedingly difficult to locate because of its small size. Because of these anatomic differences it is essential that the light be good so that the meatus can be seen by inspection without causing the infant unnecessary discomfort by probing with the tip of the catheter. Such probing also contaminates the catheter and necessitates use of the second catheter. The catheter is introduced gently, directed downward, and inserted along the rounded path to the bladder, lying above the symphysis.

During recent years some physicians have utilized the procedure of bladder tap because they believe that this technique presents less chance of introducing infection than does catheterization.

The fluid intake is important. If fluids are ordered in quantity greater than normal, they should be offered between feedings or between meals. The nurse will find it a challenge to discover which fluids the infant likes and his favored way of taking them.

CRYPTORCHIDISM (UNDESCENDED TESTIS)

Pathogenesis, Treatment, and Prognosis. Cryptorchidism is absence of one or both testes from the scrotum. Early in fetal life the testes develop in the abdomen below the kidneys. During the last two months of intrauterine life they descend into the scrotum. If they have not descended by birth, they may descend at any time until puberty. The missing testis or testes may be in the abdominal cavity or inguinal canal.

At puberty, testes normally increase in size and develop increased androgenic and spermatogenic activity. Since an undescended testis is at a higher temperature within the abdomen than in the normal location—the scrotum—the sperm-forming cells degenerate. If both testes are undescended, sterility results.

Normal secondary sex characteristics develop even though both testes are undescended. If the testis is in the inguinal canal, it may be injured more easily than if it were in the scrotum. Emo-

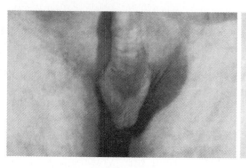 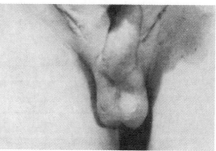

FIGURE 14-17. Undescended testicles. *Left*, Bilateral undescended testes in a ten-year-old boy. The scrotum is underdeveloped. *Right*, Postoperative picture. The testes lie within the scrotum. (From Gross, R.: *The Surgery of Infancy and Childhood.* Philadelphia, W. B. Saunders.)

tional disturbances may occur, especially during the school age, when the young boy finds that he is different from his peers.

Preservation of fertility is the most important factor to be considered in the *treatment.* Either medical or surgical treatment may be used. Some physicians believe that endocrine therapy should be tried during the preschool period. Such therapy is thought to be successful when no hernia is present (hernias are found in more than half the cases). Gonadotropic hormone is used. If excessive amounts of this hormone are given, precocious puberty may result. The defective testes may develop into malignant tumors, even in children who have undergone orchidopexy in the pubertal or postpubertal years.

Many physicians believe that *orchidopexy* should be done in all cases of mechanical interference and prefer to operate on children during infancy because of the problem of preservation of fertility and also because of increased fears during the preschool period. Other surgeons prefer to delay operation until the school age.

When the child returns from the operating room, there will be a traction suture in the lower portion of the scrotum fastened to a rubber band attached to the upper inside aspect of the thigh by a piece of adhesive. This anchors the testis to the scrotum. The infant's leg may be restrained in a straight position without flexing the knee to keep continuous tension on the traction suture. On the physician's order, use of a small ice pack may help prevent swelling and discomfort in the operative area. The nurse should not disturb the tension mechanism in caring for the child and must prevent contamination of the suture line by carefully cleansing fecal material from the perineum. Antibiotics may be given to prevent infection. After about a week, the traction attachment is removed.

If one testis is absent or if a testis must be removed, a silastic prosthesis can be inserted so that the boy will resemble normal boys; thereby no psychologic problem will be induced. This procedure is usually done prior to school age.

The *prognosis* is good if the testis is success-fully placed in the scrotum and if no changes occurred in the testis before treatment.

VIRAL INFECTION

ROSEOLA INFANTUM (EXANTHEM SUBITUM)

Etiology and Incidence. Roseola infantum appears to be caused by a filterable virus, although no one organism has been identified as the causative agent. The mode of spread of this infection is also unknown. This condition occurs equally in both sexes, usually between 6 and 18 months of age, but it may occur in children three years of age or even older. The incidence of this disease is sporadic in a community; no epidemics have been reported.

Clinical Manifestations, Diagnosis, Treatment, and Complications. The onset is acute, with an elevation of temperature up to 103 to 105° F. (39.4 to 40.5° C.). Convulsions may occur. The infant may be irritable, drowsy, and anorexic, but he does not usually appear as ill with such a fever as one might expect. The temperature falls by crisis in two to four days, and a macular or maculopapular rash appears, principally on the trunk and neck and behind the ears, and less often on the face and extremities. Within a few hours the rash begins to fade and within two to three days has usually disappeared. The occipital and postauricular lymph nodes may be enlarged.* *Treatment* is symptomatic, and *complications* such as residual encephalopathy are rare.

Responsibilities of the Nurse. Isolation of the infant is not necessary. By the time the rash appears and the diagnosis is made, the child is probably no longer infectious, if indeed he ever was.

ECHOVIRUS INFECTION

Etiology, Epidemiology, Incidence, Clinical Manifestations, and Diagnosis. Echovirus can be identified by type. At the present time these are numbered from 1 to 33. There is consider-

*This disease may be confused with measles and rubella. In roseola infantum there are no catarrhal symptoms or Koplik spots such as are present in measles, and the temperature is too high for rubella to be present.

able variation between the individual strains of certain types. The echoviruses can be distinguished clearly from other viruses that affect man. Echoviruses have been found in many parts of the world. Infection is more common among children living under poor socioeconomic conditions in warm weather. The virus can be recovered from the oropharynx, urine, feces, and other sources.

Meningitis or exanthems have been associated with various types of echoviruses. When either of these conditions occurs in a community, inapparent infections are also prevalent in the same area. Infection with these viruses disseminates rapidly within families. This indicates a short incubation period and a high degree of communicability. Illnesses due to the echoviruses, with the exception of meningitis and rashes, tend to occur in sporadic rather than epidemic distribution. The manifestations of these infections resemble those seen with other enteroviruses.

Echoviruses may cause clinically inapparent, mild, or rapidly lethal disease in newborn infants. They may be associated with respiratory symptoms, aseptic meningitis, rashes, or diarrhea. In fatal illnesses they are associated with disseminated intravascular coagulation and hepatoadrenal necrosis.

The clinical manifestations in aseptic meningitis caused by these viruses have abrupt onset, with headache and stiffness of the neck or back. The child may also have a sore throat, myalgia of the extremities, and nausea and vomiting. A rash may appear on the face and spread to the trunk or extremities. This illness is usually self-limited and mild in most children.

Some echoviruses produce neuropathy that resembles that of poliomyelitis (see p. 662). Some also produce rashes that may consist of maculopapules, vesicles, urticaria, and petechiae. Rashes are more common in infants and children than in adults. Acute respiratory illnesses have also been produced by echoviruses but are not of significant importance in the cause of respiratory disease.

Diagnosis of these infections can be confirmed in the laboratory by the detection of virus in the blood, feces, urine, oropharyngeal swabbings, cerebrospinal fluid, or other specimens from the patient. Diagnosis can also be confirmed by the demonstration of a related antibody response in the patient's serum.

Treatment, Responsibilities of the Nurse, and Prognosis. Treatment and nursing care are supportive and symptomatic. There is no known way of controlling infection by the echoviruses. Complete recovery is the usual outcome except in newborn infants.

SUDDEN INFANT DEATH SYNDROME (SIDS; CRIB DEATH)

Sudden infant death syndrome has occurred since biblical times, but was not clearly recognized prior to the early 1960's. Since that time it has been established as a specific cause of infant deaths. The Sudden Infant Death Syndrome Act was passed as recently as 1974 (see p. 7). Public funds are now supporting extensive research on this condition.

Incidence, Theories of Etiology, Pathology, and Prevention. Increasing numbers of infants, usually between the ages of one and six months old, are discovered dead in their cribs each year for unexplained reasons. These infants die silently and unexpectedly. The incidence of sudden infant death syndrome may be as high as 2 to 3 deaths per 1000 live births in the urban areas of the United States. More than 8000 to 10,000 such deaths occurred yearly in 1975 and 1976 in this country.

The less the infant weighs at birth, the greater is the possibility of crib death. The more respiratory difficulty the infant had and the lower the Apgar score following birth (see p. 154), the more likely the occurrence of SIDS. This condition occurs in infants who were not completely healthy or who had subtle physical abnormalities before death. There is a possibility that more than one child in a family may die of this cause.

These infants usually appear well developed and nourished at the time of death. Death occurs more often in males than in females, and more frequently during the colder months of the year. More deaths occur between midnight and 9 A.M. than during the rest of the day. Death occurs more frequently among the nonwhite population than among whites, and in infants of lower-income families living in areas where housing and sanitation are poor. It occurs, however, among all socioeconomic groups.

Following the death of an infant, usually in the home, the police arrive to question the parents. An autopsy is performed to determine the cause of death, because it is the only acceptable way to diagnose this condition. At autopsy, only negligible pathologic changes are found. These include a thymus that appears large but is within normal limits; petechiae that may be present in the thymus, lungs, and brain; a larynx that may reveal a moderate amount of subacute inflammation; and small flat adrenals that may be normal for this age. The results of the autopsy should be made available to the parents as soon as possible. The cause of death should be called by its correct name—sudden infant death syndrome—and should appear in that way on the death certificate.

Many theories concerning the cause of this condition have been advanced: accidental aspiration of gastric contents causing laryngospasm, bacteremia, acute spinal injury, or allergy to milk or some other substance. More physicians are beginning to believe, however, that these tragic deaths are almost always due to a sudden and very acute viral infection of the respiratory tract, an unknown inborn error of metabolism, laryngospasm, or failure of cardiac conduction.

Prevention can be aimed only at close medical supervision of infants in the affected age group. Infants with early history of apnea should have apnea monitors available in their homes. If these infants are moved when apnea occurs, respirations may begin again. Living in a home with an apnea monitor may be a horrendous experience, so parents need all the support they can obtain from health professionals.

Responsibilities of the Nurse. If the infant as a newborn is diagnosed as having periods of apnea and is discharged with an apnea monitor, the nurse must teach the parents how to use it. The nurse not only must teach the mechanics of the monitor as they are indicated on the directions for that particular equipment, but must also help parents to think through their course of action should a period of apnea occur.

If an infant dies, the nurse must understand that the grieving father and mother have only recently learned how to care for their new infant. Naturally, when the infant expires unexpectedly they blame themselves. What did they do wrong? The nurse listens, answers their questions honestly and accurately, and helps them to grieve (see p. 109). The nurse must be informed about sudden infant death syndrome and know the local, regional, and governmental resources and organizations as well as parents' groups where help can be obtained.

Death is upsetting to any family (see p. 106), but when an apparently healthy infant is found dead in bed, his parents can be deeply crushed and feel very guilty. They should be assured that *neither suffocation nor obvious infection,* either of which they could blame themselves for, was in any way responsible for the death. One of the most disturbing concerns of these parents is that they will be accused of battering or otherwise neglecting their child (see p. 481). Thus, the parents may become emotional victims of this condition. Some parents do not want to return home if the infant was pronounced dead in the hospital. Some parents withdraw from their friends at the very time they need

people with whom to talk. Nurses must reach out to these parents to listen and to help convince them that the death was not their fault.

Siblings who have regarded the infant as a competitor may quickly have to cope with distorted accusations from those outside the family, with their own possible guilt feelings, and with sudden overprotection from their parents. Questions siblings ask must be answered at the time of questioning. A sibling may ask his parents, "Why did you let my little brother die?" He may be concerned not only about the parents' lack of ability to prevent the infant from dying, but also about whether his parents will be able to prevent the same thing from happening to him. In a situation where the pediatrician who pronounced the infant dead is known to the other children in the family, the siblings may even refuse to return to him for preventive care or for treatment of their own illnesses.

Parents who have lost infants in this way have organized into groups throughout the country in order to support each other during their time of bereavement and to educate the public about the problem of sudden infant deaths. Each parent who has lost an infant in this way needs also the emotional support and compassion of the members of the health team.

The role of the nurse is also directed toward community education: the education of policemen and firemen who are usually the people who respond to the initial call for help when the infant is found. If the child is rushed to the emergency room, the parents must be treated with a caring attitude. Too often the parents are accused of outright neglect or abuse by unthinking personnel. Often the questions of police or hospital personnel leave the parents devastated and without the support they so badly need. Diagnosis of SIDS can only be established as the result of an autopsy and therefore it is important that the parents be helped to understand the need for one. Establishment of the diagnosis is instrumental in helping the parents to deal with their tragedy. Professional counseling may be needed to help parents resolve their feelings concerning the death of their infant.

Nurses should be aware of legislation in their states that deals with victims of sudden infant death syndrome and their families. Nurses can also lend support to new legislation to protect the rights of the parents. They can assist in establishing state and local chapters of the National Sudden Infant Death Syndrome Foundation as another means of humanizing the experience for families of these victims (see References, Audiovisual Media, and Teaching Aids at the end of this chapter).

TEACHING AIDS AND OTHER INFORMATION*

American Academy of Pediatrics

Care of Children in Hospitals.
Infectious Diseases (Red Book).
Parenteral Feeding—A Note of Caution.
The Sudden Infant Death Syndrome.
Vitamin C and the Common Cold.

American Lung Association

Your Child's Lungs Are for Life.

The Children's Hospital Medical Center, Boston, Mass.

Barnett, E.: What to Do About Children's Colds and Sore Throats.

The National Easter Seal Society

Wolinsky, G. F., and Koehler, N.: A Cooperative Program in Materials Development for Very Young Hospitalized Children, 1973.

National Sudden Infant Death Syndrome Foundation

Crib Death, 1974.
Facts About Sudden Infant Death Syndrome.
Home Monitoring.
How Shall We Tell the Children?
Impact on Family and Physician.
La Subita Muerte Infantil.
Nurse's Visit to SIDS Family.
Psychiatric Toll of SIDS.
Psychological Aspects of SIDS.
The Subsequent Child.
Why Did My Child Die?

United States Government

Facts About Sudden Infant Death Syndrome, 1972.
Promoting Community Health, 1975.
Sudden Infant Death Syndrome: Information and Counseling Projects, 1976.

---

*Complete addresses are given in the Appendix.

REFERENCES

Books

Anderson, C. M., and Burke, V. (Eds.): *Paediatric Gastroenterology.* Philadelphia, J. B. Lippincott Company, 1975.

Archuleta, M. J., and Archuleta, A. J.: *Sudden Infant Death Syndrome; An Annotated Bibliography for the Layman.* San Diego, Calif., Current Bibliography Series, 1975.

Camps, F. E., and Carpenter, R. G.: *Sudden and Unexpected Deaths in Infancy-Cot Deaths.* Chicago, Year Book Medical Publishers, 1972.

Collins, R. D.: *Illustrated Manual of Fluid and Electrolyte Disorders.* Philadelphia, J. B. Lippincott Company, 1976.

Dickens, M.: *Fluid and Electrolyte Balance: A Programmed Text.* 3rd ed. Philadelphia, F. A. Davis Company, 1974.

Falconer, M. W., Patterson, H. R., and Gustafson, E. A.: *Current Drug Handbook 1976–1978.* Philadelphia, W. B. Saunders Company, 1976.

Flint, T., Jr., and Cain, H. D.: *Emergency Treatment and Management.* 5th ed. Philadelphia, W. B. Saunders Company, 1975.

Goldberger, E.: *A Primer of Water, Electrolyte and Acid-Base Syndromes.* 5th ed. Philadelphia, Lea & Febiger, 1975.

Gryboski, J. D.: *Gastrointestinal Problems in the Infant.* Philadelphia, W. B. Saunders Company, 1975.

Guyton, A. C.: *Textbook of Medical Physiology.* 5th ed. Philadelphia, W. B. Saunders Company, 1976.

Hardgrove, C. B., and Dawson, R. B.: *Parents and Children in the Hospital: The Family's Role in Pediatrics.* Boston, Little, Brown & Company, 1972.

Harper, H. A.: *Review of Physiological Chemistry.* 15th ed. Los Altos, Calif., Lange Medical Publications, 1975.

Havener, W. H., Saunders, W. H., Keith, C. F., and Prescott, A. W.: *Nursing Care in Eye, Ear, Nose, and Throat Disorders.* 3rd ed. St. Louis, The C. V. Mosby Company, 1974.

Lieberman, E. (Ed.): *Clinical Pediatric Nephrology.* Philadelphia, J. B. Lippincott Company, 1976.

McInnes, M. E.: *Essentials of Communicable Disease.* 2nd ed. St. Louis, The C. V. Mosby Company, 1975.

Plumer, A. L.: *Principles and Practice of Intravenous Therapy.* 2nd ed. Boston, Little, Brown & Company, 1975.

Reece, R. M., and Chamberlain, J. W.: *Manual of Emergency Pediatrics.* Philadelphia, W. B. Saunders Company, 1974.

Reed, G. M. R., and Sheppard, V. F.: *Regulation of Fluid and Electrolyte Balance.* 2nd Ed. Philadelphia, W. B. Saunders Co., 1977.

Rickham, P. P., Soper, R. T., and Stauffer, U. G.: *Synopsis of Pediatric Surgery.* Chicago, Year Book Medical Publishers, 1975.

Shirkey, H. C.: *Pediatric Drug Handbook.* Philadelphia, W. B. Saunders Company, 1977.

Toporek, M.: *Basic Chemistry of Life.* 2nd ed. New York, Appleton-Century-Crofts, 1975.

Williams, H. E., and Phelan, P. D.: *Respiratory Illness in Children.* Philadelphia, J. B. Lippincott Company, 1975.

Winters, R. W.: *The Body Fluids in Pediatrics: Medical, Surgical, and Neonatal Disorders of Acid-Base Status, Hydration, and Oxygenation.* Boston, Little, Brown & Company, 1973.

Periodicals

Barker, W. H.: Perspectives on Acute Enteric Disease Epidemiology and Control. *Bulletin of the Pan American Health Organization,* 9:148, 1975.

Becker, M. H., Drachman, R. H., and Kirscht, J. P.: A New Approach to Explaining Sick-Role Behavior in Low-Income Populations. *Am. J. Public Health,* 64:205, March 1974.

Béhar, M.: The Role of Feeding and Nutrition in the Pathogeny and Prevention of Diarrheic Processes. *Bulletin of the Pan American Health Organization,* 9:1, 1975.

Bergman, A. B.: Psychological Aspects of Sudden Unexpected Death in Infants and Children. *Pediatr. Clin. N. Am.,* 21:115, February 1974.

Bluestone, C. D., and Shurin, P. A.: Middle Ear Disease in Children: Pathogenesis, Diagnosis, and Management. *Pediatr. Clin. N. Am.,* 21:379, May 1974.

Crib Death: Some Promising Leads but No Solution Yet. *Science,* 189:367, August 1, 1975.

del Bueno, D. J.: Electrolyte Imbalance: How to Recognize and Respond to It. Part 1. *RN,* 38:52, February 1975.

Dougall, A. J., Maclean, N., and Wilkinson, A. W.: Histology of the Maldescended Testis at Operation. *Lancet,* 1:771, April 27, 1974.

Drachman, R. H.: Acute Infectious Gastroenteritis. *Pediatr. Clin. N. Am.,* 21:711, August 1974.

Dykes, M. H., and Meier, P.: Ascorbic Acid and The Common Cold. *J.A.M.A.,* 231:1073, March 10, 1975.

Goodman, M. B.: Incidence of Respiratory Infections in Full-Term and Premature Infants During Their First Year. *Nursing Research,* 22:160, March-April 1973.

Guilleminault, C., Peraita, R., Souquet, M., and Dement, W. C.: Apneas During Sleep in Infants: Possible Relationship With Sudden Infant Death Syndrome. *Science,* 190:677, November 14, 1975.

Hamilton, J. R., Gall, D. G., Kerzner, B., Butler, D. G., and Middleton, P. J.: Recent Developments in Viral Gastroenteritis. *Pediatr. Clin. N. Am.,* 22:747, November 1975.

Hogan, G. R.: Hypernatremia—Problems in Management. *Pediatr. Clin. N. Am.,* 23:569, August 1976.

Kee, J. L., and Gregory, A. P.: The ABC's and mEq's of Fluid Balance in Children. *Nursing '74,* 4:28, June 1974.

Khan, A. J., and Pryles, C. V.: Urinary Tract Infection in Children. *Am. J. Nursing,* 73:1340, August 1973.

Kiester, E.: The Black Box That Guards Debbie Whitney's Life. *Today's Health,* 52:52, October 1974.

Kraus, J. F., Franti, C. E., and Borhani, N. O.: Discriminatory Risk Factors in Postneonatal Sudden Unexplained Death. *Am. J. Epidemiol.,* 96:328, November 1972.

Mandell, F., and Wolfe, L. C.: Sudden Infant Death Syndrome and Subsequent Pregnancy. *Pediatrics,* 56:774, November 1975.

Marks, M. I., Marks, S., and Brazeau, M.: Yeast Colonization in Hospitalized and Nonhospitalized Children. *J. Pediatr.,* 87:524, October 1975.

Marx, J. L.: Crib Death: Some Promising Leads But No Solutions Yet. *Nursing Digest,* 4:12, Summer 1976.

McGuckin, M.: Microbiologic Studies: Part 4—What You Should Know About Collecting Stool Culture Specimens. *Nursing '76,* 6:22, March 1976.

Moore, V. B.: I.V. Fluids: Product Survey. *Nursing '73,* 3:32, June 1973.

Naeye, R. L., Messmer, J., Specht, T., and Merritt, T. A.: Sudden Infant Death Syndrome Temperament Before Death. *J. Pediatr.,* 88:511, March 1976.

Nakushian, J. M.: Restoring Parents' Equilibrium After Sudden Infant Death. *Am. J. Nursing,* 76:1600, October 1976.

Ormond, E. A. R., and Caulfield, C.: A Practical Guide to Giving Oral Medications to Young Children. *The American Journal of Maternal-Child Nursing,* 1:320, September-October 1976.

Owen, B., and Portess, M.: Prospective Investigation into Cot Deaths. *Health Visit,* 48:379, October 1975.

Rumack, B. H., and Temple, A. R.: Lomotil Poisoning. *Pediatrics,* 53:495, April 1974.

Snively, W. D., and Roberts, K. T.: The Clinical Picture As An Aid to Understanding Body Fluid Disturbances. *Nursing Forum,* 12:133, 1973.

Soyka, L. F., and others: The Misuse of Antibiotics for Treatment of Upper Respiratory Infections in Children. *Pediatrics,* 55:552, April 1975.

Steinschneider, A.: Nasopharyngitis and Prolonged Sleep Apnea. *Pediatrics,* 56:967, December 1975.

Taylor, J. L.: One Nurse's Baptism of Fire-and Water. *RN,* 39:42, January 1976.

Thong, M. L., and Tay, L. K.: Septicaemia From Prolonged Intravenous Infusions. *Arch. Dis. Child,* 50:886, November 1975.

AUDIOVISUAL MEDIA*

Bandera Productions

To Breathe, To Breathe, To Live
24 minutes, 16mm, sound, color.
Dramatically portrays differences in upper and lower respiratory obstructions—actual scenes of children with epiglottitis, croup, and tracheobronchitis.

Charles Press–Prentice-Hall, Inc.

Crib Death—A Sudden Infant Death Syndrome... A Documentary
Coe, J. I., and Szybist, C.
59 minutes.
Each year 10,000 apparently healthy babies die suddenly and unexpectedly from crib death. Parents who have experienced the loss of a child through SIDS discuss the guilt and self-criticism that exacerbate their normal grief reaction. Recent research findings and suggestions of how to help parents recover from their loss.

Nursing Skills and Techniques Series
Oxygen: Croupette
2–5 minutes, Super-8mm filmloop, color, guide.
Reasons for using a croupette plus procedure and precautions.

Greater Cleveland Hospital Association

Intravenous Therapy Series
Fluid and Electrolyte Balance
28 minutes, videocassette, sound, color, guide.
Presents normal and abnormal mechanisms employed by the human body in maintaining fluid, electrolyte, and acid-base balance.

J. B. Lippincott Company

The Patient and Fluid Balance
64 transparencies with 158 overlays, guide.
Unit 1—The State of Equilibrium: Normal Physiology
Unit 2—Disequilibrium:
Part A: Altered Physiology
Part B: Clinical Application
Unit 3—Fluid Therapy

W. B. Saunders Company

Pediatric Conferences with Sydney Gellis
Adenovirus Vaccines, Parrott, R. H.
Bronchiolitis and Asthma, Gellis, S.
Otitis Media, Klein, J. O.
Sudden Unexpected Death, Gellis, S.
Undescended Testicle, Gellis, S.

Trainex Corporation

Acid-Base Balance—Compensation of Imbalances
35mm filmstrip, audio-tape cassettes, $33\frac{1}{3}$ LP, color.
This program shows how the respiratory system and the kidneys attempt to compensate for excess acids and bases in body fluids. The changes which take place in carbon dioxide and bicarbonate concentrations in body fluids are emphasized.

Acid-Base Balance—Metabolic Acidosis and Alkalosis
35mm filmstrip, audio-tape cassettes, $33\frac{1}{3}$ LP, color.
Metabolic acidosis and alkalosis are defined, and the basic physiology involved in these conditions is presented. The importance of the nurse's knowledge of the underlying con-

ditions that may precipitate metabolic acidosis or alkalosis is stressed. Signs and symptoms of metabolic acid-base imbalances are listed. Nursing care responsibilities toward patients with these imbalances are explained.

Acid-Base Balance—Respiratory Acidosis and Alkalosis
35mm filmstrip, audio-tape cassettes, 33⅓ LP, color.
Respiratory acidosis and alkalosis are defined and the basic physiology involved in these conditions is presented. The importance of the nurse's knowledge of the underlying conditions that may precipitate acidosis or alkalosis is stressed. Signs and symptoms of respiratory acid-base imbalances are listed. Nursing care responsibilities toward patients with these imbalances are explained.

Acid-Base Balance—The Body's Regulation of pH
35mm filmstrip, audio-tape cassettes, 33⅓ LP, color.
A review of the concepts of acid, base, hydrogen ion concentration, and pH. Based on these concepts, the functions of the buffers, respiratory system, and kidneys in the regulation of pH are explained.

Electrolyte Balance
35mm filmstrip, audio-tape cassettes, 33⅓ LP, color.
Defines the ions, and suggests the importance of ionized substances in body fluids. Reviews the milliequivalent measurement of ion concentration, and describes the movement of dissolved substances through membranes by diffusion and active transport. Explains in general terms the function of the kidneys in maintaining normal electrolyte concentrations.

Fluid Balance
35mm filmstrip, audio-tape cassette, 33⅓ LP, color.
Explains how normal fluid volume is maintained through the function of the "thirst mechanism" and the kidneys, with emphasis upon the role of the antidiuretic hormone at the kidney nephron. Describes the distribution of fluid to the cells, tissues and blood plasma. Explains osmosis and osmolarity, and gives examples of the actions of hypertonic, isotonic, and hypotonic fluids.

Functions of Electrolytes
35mm filmstrip, audio-tape cassettes, 33⅓ LP, color.
Includes a brief description of the common electrolytes and their normal laboratory ranges in body fluids. Discusses the functions of sodium, potassium, chloride, calcium, mag-

nesium, and protein in the extracellular fluid. Includes a section on the role of aldosterone in the regulation of sodium and potassium levels, and emphasizes the importance of certain electrolytes within the cells.

Intestinal Disturbances
35mm filmstrip, audio-tape cassettes, 33⅓ LP, color.
Advises parents about the causes of intestinal disturbances and how to treat colic, a "gassy" baby, constipation, and diarrhea.

United States Government

Technical Procedures for Diagnosis and Therapy in Children
Producer: USN
27 minutes, 16mm film, optical sound, color.
Gives step by step procedures for femoral venipuncture, internal jugular puncture, lumbar puncture, subdural tap, gastric lavage, scalp venipuncture, and cutdown.

A Call For Help
Producer: USDHEW
20 minutes, 16mm film, sound, color.
Explores the importance of awareness on the part of those who will respond to the family's initial call for help. Stresses the need for a thoughtful and concerned approach at a time when the family is still in a state of shock and confusion.

After Our Baby Died
Producer: USDHEW
21 minutes, 16mm film, sound, color.
Designed to explore the importance of counseling SIDS parents at the time of loss. It looks at the death through the eyes of the bereaved family.

You Are Not Alone
Producer: USDHEW
25 minutes, 16mm film, sound, color.
Looks at the death of an infant through the eyes of those families and relatives who must cope with a condition that is still unexplained and unpreventable. It follows their progression from confusion and anger to understanding and acceptance.

---

*Complete addresses are given in the Appendix.

Chapter Fifteen

CONDITIONS OF INFANTS REQUIRING LONG-TERM CARE

Infancy covers only a short time. An illness of even a few months may retard an infant in accomplishing his developmental tasks. One of the most important of these tasks is to learn *to trust* people. It is essential that the hospitalized infant keep his trust in his parents' loving protection and learn that others give him physical care and affection. The parents should be encouraged to spend as much time with their child as they can.

The parents reaction to their child's long-term illness depends, naturally, on the seriousness of his condition. If the illness is severe and the prognosis doubtful, the parents are under a prolonged emotional strain. Their reaction may be to overprotect their baby. The infant may respond with a lack of normal attempts to try out new muscular activities by way of self-help and self-amusement. Even an infant is likely to compensate for a lack of control over his environment by a control over adults who will give him what he wants and do for him

what he has not yet learned he can do for himself.

The nurse should understand clearly what activity the physician allows and within that range give the infant opportunity for habilitation. This applies not only to physical activity, but also to psychologic and emotional growth.

The parents should be allowed to verbalize their feelings and thereby relieve to some extent the emotional strain under which they labor. This is not only for their sake, but also because of their influence upon the infant. Unlimited visiting hours in the pediatric unit will give them an opportunity to observe the nurses giving care to their child and to discuss with them the technique of his habilitation, whether it is letting him attempt new physical activities or playing by himself without expecting constant attention.

The mother may become overdependent upon the nurse for emotional support. But as she sees the nurse's care of the infant and his response, she will join the health team and cease to cast her responsibilities upon the other members of the team. When she herself is a member of the team, she loses her sense of frustration at others being able to give the child more and better care than she can, and will understand that they excel in professional service, but that she excels in meeting the child's need for affection and security in the love of one person. Thus with both physical and emotional support from members of the health team, the parents and their child may learn, and in some instances benefit, from the illness.

In order to follow the developmental progress of an infant during hospitalization, assessments of infants requiring long-term care are made at prescribed intervals. On the basis of the developmental assessments a plan for stimulating the infant may be formulated. This plan may be hung by the crib so the parents are aware of its contents and can participate in its execution when possible. Even if the parents are unable to participate in the plan, they know what it contains and the purpose it serves. Such a plan usually includes exercising on a prescribed schedule, planned eye to eye contact, speaking or singing to the infant, and providing him with visual stimuli such as a crib mobile. Such a plan of assessment and stimulation can prevent an infant from lagging developmentally as a result of his hospitalization and the lack of normal contacts that he would have at home.

NUTRITIONAL DISORDERS

The diets of infants and young children may be abnormal in nutriment, i.e., protein, fat, or carbohydrate, or in essential vitamins or minerals. Although several factors may contribute to the production of nutritional disorders, the basic problem is usually a lack of intake, though sometimes there may be poor absorption of one or more components of food after ingestion.

Nutritional disorders are especially harmful during infancy, the period when growth is most rapid and the human organism needs adequate supplies of all essential food elements.

Undernutrition

MALNUTRITION (ATHREPSIA, MARASMUS)

Incidence, Etiology, and Diagnosis. Malnutrition is less prevalent in the United States and Europe than it was a generation ago, but is still a pressing social problem. In underdeveloped countries malnutrition of children is one of the problems in which the World Health Organization is vitally interested.

Malnutrition should be considered secondary to the condition causing it. It is a general term indicating undernutrition. Specific vitamin deficiencies are likely in malnourished infants.

The fundamental cause is that the infant does not receive an adequate diet or is unable to assimilate sufficient nutriment for the metabolic needs of his body, with the result that reserve food elements in the tissues are used. The specific cause may be an inadequate intake or a badly balanced diet; poor feeding habits due to improper training; a physical defect such as cleft lip or cleft palate or other anomalies of the gastrointestinal tract (see Chap. 11), or cardiac abnormalities which prevent the infant's taking an adequate diet; diseases which interfere with the assimilation of food (these are generally chronic diseases such as cystic fibrosis); infections which produce anorexia and decrease the infant's ability to digest his food, and yet at the same time increase his need for food; loss of food through vomiting and diarrhea; or, according to psychologists, emotional problems such as disturbed mother-child relations.

The *diagnosis* of malnutrition may be determined by the obvious symptoms found on physical examination, by failure of growth or by measurement of the blood constituents. Dietary surveys establish the probability of malnutrition in children of any group.

Clinical Manifestations and Laboratory Studies. Failure to gain weight followed by loss of weight is one manifestation of deficiency diseases. Growth of the skeleton and of the brain continues, with the result that the body is long and the head large in proportion to the weight.

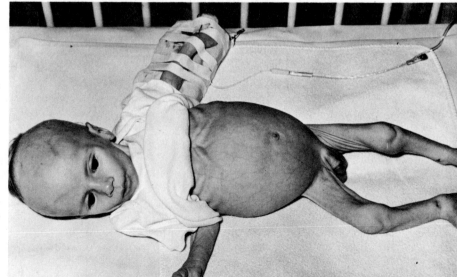

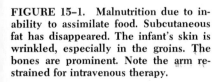

FIGURE 15–1. Malnutrition due to inability to assimilate food. Subcutaneous fat has disappeared. The infant's skin is wrinkled, especially in the groins. The bones are prominent. Note the arm restrained for intravenous therapy.

To maintain metabolism, the body uses its own fat and protein. The subcutaneous fat disappears, but the sucking pads of the cheeks remain, giving the face a factitious roundness. The eyes are sunken. The features have a drawn appearance, and when at last the fat pads have been absorbed, the face takes on an aged look. Tissue turgor is lost, and the skin lies in loose folds on the body. The fat of the abdominal wall and of the buttocks decreases. The skin over the buttocks becomes wrinkled and sags. The skin over the remainder of the body appears loose. The bones are prominent. The infant is no longer active, his muscles are flabby and relaxed, and his cry is weak and shrill.

As his blood volume diminishes and he becomes anemic, his color becomes ashen gray. His temperature is subnormal, the pulse slow, and the basal metabolism tends to be reduced. His digestive capacity decreases, and his appetite is poor. He may have constipation or starvation diarrhea, in which the stools contain mucus and bile. He is subject to infections and has poor resistance. There may be evidence of a specific deficiency disease such as rickets, scurvy, tetany, or iron-deficiency anemia. Nutritional edema may also be present.

The *laboratory findings* show severe hypochromic anemia. The plasma protein level is usually lowered unless hemoconcentration is present. In that case the serum level may be within the normal range.

Complications. Intercurrent infections are frequent; the most common are oral thrush (gastrointestinal tract), pyelonephritis (genitourinary tract), and bronchitis or upper respiratory tract infections (respiratory tract). Skin infections such as furunculosis occur, as well as infected bedsores over the bony prominences, e.g., the occiput, heels, and knees. Nutritional anemia due to a low iron intake may develop. Nutritional edema results when the body, lacking sufficient protein obtained from food, has burnt its own tissues and destroyed the protein in the plasma, so that the level of plasma albumin becomes low. Nutritional edema is seen in infants who have been malnourished for several months. When sufficient protein is given and the infant has recovered so that the body is able to absorb the necessary amount of protein, the edema disappears.

Treatment, Responsibilities of the Nurse, and Prognosis. The basic treatment is to provide sufficient essential nutrients to sustain life and to maintain normal growth and development. In the past intravenous therapy was attempted, but met with only limited success owing to difficulty in prolonged administration, infusate toxicity, or inadequate caloric content. Recently a method of total parenteral nutrition, hyperalimentation, has overcome these difficulties.

Total parenteral alimentation (hyperalimentation) provides an infusate of a mixture of glucose and amino acids (5 per cent fibrin hydrolysate) to which appropriate electrolytes and vitamins are added on the basis of the individual infant's need. This solution is given continuously by means of an infusion pump through a catheter placed in the superior vena cava. This therapy can be given for up to two months while the child is ill. Plasma is also given to provide trace metals and essential fatty acids. Iron can be provided by intramuscular injections of iron dextran or by blood transfusions.

This hypertonic solution must be given at a slow uniform rate into a blood vessel where there is high blood flow for rapid dilution in order to avoid venous inflammation and thrombosis. For this purpose the superior vena cava is cannulated with a silicone rubber catheter from the jugular vein in the neck. The cannula is tunneled subcutaneously from the vein entry point to the scalp. This site of exit facilitates easy cleaning, prevents to a large extent accidental removal, and does not interfere with the total care of the child. An antibiotic ointment and a sterile dressing are applied over a coil of the catheter to prevent infection and to avoid accidental displacement. The catheter does not have to be changed unless it is occluded by blood or by added drugs or is dislodged.

Before the infusion is begun, a Millipore filter is placed in the circuit in order to remove any particles or microorganisms that might have contaminated the solution.

There are potential hazards in the use of this procedure. The large glucose load may overwhelm the infant's insulin production and renal clearance for glucose and produce osmotic diuresis. Because of the relatively large fluid volume used, the child may become overhydrated. The amino acid mixture may produce toxicity or aminoaciduria.

In order to determine the effect of this treatment the following must be done: accurate recording of urine volume, daily weights, daily urinary sugar analyses by the Clinitest method, frequent determinations of serum electrolyte concentrations and blood sugar, hematocrit, and serum osmolarity. Other tests are done to determine the presence of hepatic toxicity.

Constant nursing care for these children is essential. Since the solution used has high nutrient value, it is a good medium for bacterial growth. Septicemia is a great danger; the prevention of infection is of paramount importance from the time the catheter is inserted until it is removed. The intravenous setup must be

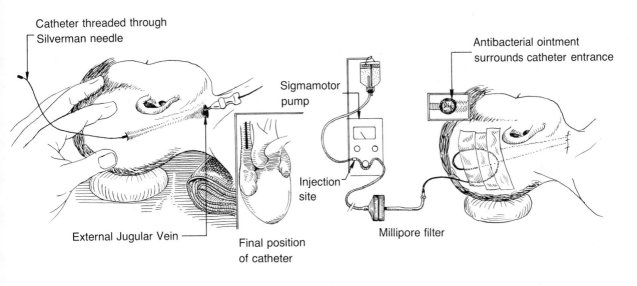

FIGURE 15–2. Technique of delivering hypertonic infusate, showing (*A*) the method of placing the indwelling silicone rubber catheter in the superior vena cava in an infant, and (*B*) the infusate, constant infusion pump and bacterial filter attached to a properly secured "lifeline." (R. M. Filler: Long-term total parenteral nutrition in infants. *New Eng. J. Med.*, 281(11):592 September, 1969.) (Modified from original drawing by S. Rosenthal.)

changed frequently, using sterile technique. The catheter must not be used for the injection of medications or the withdrawal of blood because of the danger of contamination and occlusion.

Infants fed by total parenteral alimentation must be given special care to prevent the emotional consequences of deprivation of experiences and sensations provided by normal feeding methods. Such deprivation results from a lack of stimulation: a lack of the rhythmic sensations of sucking and a lack of the experience and stimulation of feeding itself. In order to prevent such deprivation, the parent or nurse should simulate the actual experience of feeding by offering sucking experiences on a pacifier (unless this is contraindicated) while the infant is held in close contact with the adult's body. Emotional development can be stimulated further by providing eye and verbal contact with the infant. Continuity of care should be provided by having the same person, parent or nurse, care for the child or be with him as much as possible.

The nurse must note any elevation of temperature, because this may indicate infection or an antigenic reaction to the solution.

The quantity of glucose given may cause severe and rapid dehydration by diuresis. For this reason the urine is tested for glucose frequently. If samples reveal a 3+ or 4+ glucose by the Clinitest method, the rate of the infusion or the amount of glucose given may be decreased. Insulin may be added to the solution on the physician's order. The nurse must watch for signs of either hyperglycemia (see p. 781) or hypoglycemia (see p. 279).

The nurse is also responsible for measuring the urinary output, for daily weights of the child, and for assisting with venipuncture for the collection of specimens (see p. 412).

The short-term treatment if hyperalimentation is not used and the long-term treatment of malnutrition are through diet. The initial oral feedings should be low in quantity and in calories, because the digestive capacity is poor. If too much feeding is given too quickly, the infant will probably suffer diarrhea and vomiting. The initial feeding should be diluted breast milk or, if that is not available, skimmed lactic acid milk. The amount of protein and carbohydrate in the formula is slowly increased. It is necessary to increase the fat content more slowly than the carbohydrate, since fat is more difficult to digest. Evaporated or dried milk may be given within a few days, since the curd is smaller than that of fresh milk. Food requirements for such infants may be as high as 75 to 100 calories per pound a day before they gain weight. They must receive increased protein to build body tissue.

Small but frequent blood transfusions may be necessary to correct the anemia and to increase resistance to infection. Medications are aimed at correction of the dietary deficiencies. Intramuscular injections of crude liver extract may be given every two or three days for several weeks, and vitamins A, B, C, and D may be given in usual or increased amounts.

The body temperature must be maintained. If

the infant has a subnormal temperature, he should be placed in an incubator or given extra clothing and covered with blankets or hyperthermia blankets. Hot-water bottles may be placed on both sides of his body for increased warmth. Since he is subject to infection, his feeding equipment should be sterile to avoid danger of contracting thrush. He should be turned frequently to prevent hypostatic pneumonia, pressure areas on the bony prominences, and skin infections. He requires careful skin care. He should be isolated for his own protection, and nursing personnel who care for him should be free from any kind of infection. Since his resistance is low, he should be kept out of drafts.

The feeding ordered by the physician is followed carefully and the order checked before each feeding to see whether it has been changed. The infant is fed slowly and bubbled frequently. During feeding he is handled gently so that he feels secure in his nurse's care, cuddled and surrounded with emotional as well as physical warmth.

Since collapse is possible, the severely ill infant should be watched at all times for the signs of collapse of peripheral circulation, temperature drop, slow pulse, cyanosis or gray-white color of the skin, and coldness of the extremities.

The nurse will assist with administration of parenteral fluids or blood (see p. 412). Accurate, detailed charting is necessary and includes the amount of feeding taken, refused, or vomited, and whether it was taken eagerly or indifferently. It is important for the physician to know the number and kind of stools and whether abdominal distention is present. The infant is weighed at the same time daily to determine the exact gain or loss.

Complications such as concurrent infections or skin conditions are treated as they occur.

The *prognosis* depends on the severity of the condition, its length and on whether infection is present. Severely malnourished infants may go into a state of collapse and die suddenly. This is most likely to happen in infants who have continued to lose weight after institution of treatment and have experienced a sudden drop in temperature accompanied by a slow pulse and evidence of a circulatory crisis. Such infants may have acquired a severe, overwhelming infection against which they have no resistance.

Malnutrition which occurs during the rapid period of brain growth of the fetus or the infant may result in retardation of physical growth and mental development. These children run the risk of brain damage and never catching up or reaching their potential capacity. There may be a lag in their ability to learn. Malnourished children may have anemia and vitamin deficiency diseases also (see p. 441).

Prevention. Prevention of malnutrition is one of the important functions of Child Health Conferences. The amount of the feeding must be adequate. The infant should be fed with good technique so that he may make full use of the feeding ordered by the physician.

Also important in prevention of malnutrition are early treatment of defects, diseases, or infections predisposing to malnutrition, and prevention of emotional disturbances.

If the attack on malnutrition is to be successful, there must also be an understanding of related economic and sociocultural problems, especially the problems of psychosocial deprivation which occur early in life. These problems perpetuate themselves in families; thus generations in a family may be doomed to a marginal existence in society.

KWASHIORKOR (PROTEIN MALNUTRITION)

Kwashiorkor, a widespread syndrome seen among the underprivileged in tropical and subtropical countries, is a form of malnutrition due to a deficiency of protein and other nutrients in spite of an almost adequate caloric intake. Kwashiorkor can be interpreted to mean "red man" because of the hair color, or "deposed child," one whose mother no longer breast-feeds him. It occurs in children from four months to five years of age. Infections cause stress to these children.

In Africa custom dictates that an infant must be weaned the day a new pregnancy is recognized. After her infant has been weaned, the mother feeds him a glutinous root, which is sweet and curbs hunger by swelling the stomach, but has few calories and no protein.

While the infant is growing, sufficient protein must be obtained to maintain a positive nitrogen balance. When adequate amounts of the essential amino acids are not provided, not absorbed, or are abnormally lost, protein malnutrition occurs.

The symptoms of protein malnutrition include a lack of adequate growth, loss of muscle tone, lack of energy, increased susceptibility to infection, and edema. Diarrhea and dermatitis may develop. Dyspigmentation and vitiligo of the skin may occur. The hair is thin and inelastic and may become yellowish, red, or gray because of dyspigmentation. Parasitic infestations, infections such as measles, anorexia, and vomiting are prevalent. The affected children have weak muscles and tend to become irritable and apathetic. Cardiac and liver enlargement may occur.

The serum albumin level is lowered, leading to nutritional edema (see Fig. 15–3). Anemia, vitamin deficiencies, and other blood changes occur.

The treatment of the child having kwashiorkor includes fluid and electrolyte therapy to correct the imbalances. Infections and infestations must be treated with appropriate medications. The long-term treatment is by feeding the child an adequate caloric diet, especially one high in protein of good biologic quality. Unfortunately, if the child survives, the likelihood of retarded growth and irreversible brain damage is great.

MALNUTRITION DUE TO DISTURBED MOTHER-CHILD RELATIONS (FAILURE TO THRIVE)

Etiology, Diagnosis and Clinical Manifestations. The diagnosis of "failure to thrive" is used for infants who have severe malnutrition and faulty physical and emotional development due to a very disturbed mother-child relationship. These infants are usually irritable, apathetic, and anorexic, and may have vomiting and diarrhea. They have distortions of social responses (such as refusing eye contact by holding their arms over their eyes) and are physically underdeveloped. Although these infants are not physically separated from their mothers, their symptoms are similar to the syndrome of anaclitic depression (see p. 359).

These infants present a problem in diagnosis and therapeutic management because a physiopathologic state, i.e., malnutrition due to underfeeding, congenital anomalies, or infections, must be ruled out before the cause can be claimed to be a disturbance in family-infant relations. It is believed that the basic problem of an infant who is normal organically, but who is depressed and fails to thrive is a mother who is immature or neurotic, who cannot claim her infant as her own, who cannot recognize her baby's dependent needs, especially in the area of adequate feeding, and who has self-doubts about her nurturing ability, and a father who is alienated from both the mother and the child. Such a mother fails to provide sensory or tactile, verbal, and play stimulation for the infant.

Treatment and Responsibilities of the Nurse. The *treatment* of these infants is complex, involving pediatrician, nurse, and social worker as a team. An adequate medical history of the family and child should be obtained. In addition, a pediatric and psychiatric evaluation should be obtained. A social service evaluation using an open-ended interview technique is necessary. The physician must provide a setting in which the family can confide stresses that press upon it. He is responsible for the overall diagnosis based on physiologic studies of the child and background investigation of the parents, and for

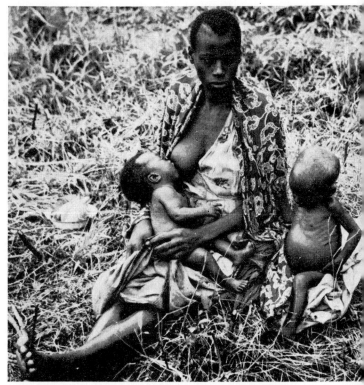

FIGURE 15–3. The baby is nursing and is doing fine, but his deposed elder brother is already a victim of kwashiorkor. (Jane F. McConnell: The Deposed One. *Am. J. Nursing*, Vol. 61.)

management of the family as a whole. The nurse or social worker together with the physician must furnish noncritical, noncompetitive temporary parent-surrogate figures for the parents themselves. They must help the parents to neutralize stress factors that prevent their assumption of parental roles. The mother especially should have help in finding satisfaction in motherhood. The nurse must coordinate infant care, teach proper methods of care to the mother, and pass on to the parents any observations concerning their child. The nurse should also share with the community or public health nurse, if one visits the home, knowledge of ways to help the family. The parents should have ample time to express their feelings to any of the team members. In order for treatment to be successful there must be frank communication between the team and the parents and an accepting attitude on the part of each team member. Such supportive care must be on a long-term basis after the child's hospitalization.

Prognosis and Prevention. The prognosis for infants who have failed to thrive is similar to that for those having extreme malnutrition. Much depends on the severity and length of the condition and on whether infection is present. If the pediatrician-nurse-social worker team could function effectively together in establishing positive parent self-images and appropriate parent-child identification in families in Child Health Conferences, they would promote better mental health and possibly prevent the syndrome of failure to thrive.

Overnutrition

OBESITY

Incidence, Etiology, Clinical Manifestations, and Diagnosis. It has often been said that the "fat" baby is a healthy baby. In many areas in the United States the problem of obesity is more common than that of malnutrition. The prevention of obesity can be called preventive medicine in infancy and childhood because obesity causes such high morbidity and mortality rates later in life.

Just as the cause of undernutrition is due to the infant's not receiving an adequate diet or his inability to assimilate sufficient nutriment for the metabolic needs of his body (p. 435), so the *etiology* of overnutrition is the intake of more calories than are needed to balance energy output. Breastfed infants tend not to overeat because they stop when they are satisfied, while bottlefed infants tend to be more obese because they do not know when to stop sucking since their parents encourage them to finish feedings. The problem of obesity is one reason why infants are doubling their birth weights at an earlier age than they should.

Food intake may be based on the concept of desirable body proportions and size and may differ among families according to social standing and cultural background. Food intake may also vary because of psychological disturbances; hypothalamic, pituitary, or other brain lesions; or hyperinsulinism, which may cause hyperphagia. Metabolic and endocrine disorders such as problems with the thyroid, adrenals, or gonads are rare as causes of obesity. Genetic predisposition to obesity may occur.

Obesity is the result of an increase either in the number or in the size of fat cells, adipocytes. This occurs from the sixth to ninth months of gestation or in infancy. When the infant's weight is reduced, the number of adipocytes remains constant, but the size decreases.

When the parent offers an extra bottle of formula to a crying infant to comfort him or introduces solid food of high caloric density too early, believing that the infant is irritable because of hunger, a habit pattern is formed. If this continues, whenever the child becomes frustrated he expects to receive more food. Such behavior leads to obesity.

The *clinical manifestations* of obesity in the pediatric group occur during infancy, from five to six years of age and during puberty and adolescence. The child is bigger and heavier than his peers, and his bone age is advanced. The facial features may appear small and a double chin may be present. The obese boy of school age may be embarrassed because of adiposity in the mammary regions. The abdomen may appear pendulous and there may be evidence of striae. The penis may appear small because it is imbedded in fatty tissue. The early occurrence of puberty may result in ultimate shortness of stature of the obese individual in comparison with his peers.

The *diagnosis* of obesity is made from the appearance of the child rather than from an arbitrary excess of weight. Infants and children having large skeletal frames and an oversupply of muscular tissue may appear big, but they are not necessarily obese. Obesity is an excessive accumulation of fat that is generalized in subcutaneous and other tissues.

Adipose tissue may be especially noticeable in the upper arms and the thighs. The hand may appear small and the fingers may be tapered. Calipers may be used to measure skinfold thickness or degree of obesity over the right triceps muscle. Orthopedic problems may occur because of excess weight resting on immature bones.

Significant underlying emotional problems are common in obese children. These problems may have contributed to or are the result of the obesity.

Prevention, Treatment, and Responsibilities of the Nurse. Prevention of overnutrition is easier than curing it. Early detection of this condition is dependent on finding those factors in the infant's and later the child's environment or his personality that might predispose him to obesity. Infants whose immediate family members are obese should be given a balanced diet that contains the basic nutritional ingredients but is reduced in calories. Young children should also be helped to find "comforting" measures other than excessive eating. As they grow into the toddler period, children should be encouraged to exercise more than usual.

An ideal weight is important for esthetic reasons as well as for the prevention of diabetes, vascular degenerative disease, orthopedic problems, hypertension, dyspnea, and premature death. An untreated obese infant usually becomes an obese adolescent (see p. 851) and an obese adult.

Vitamin Deficiencies

Although vitamin deficiency diseases are not seen frequently in the United States, they are still being diagnosed in some other countries. It is for this reason they are included in this text.

RICKETS

Etiology and Incidence. Rickets is a deficiency disease of growing children due to a lack of fat-soluble vitamin D (see p. 368).

Since vitamin D increases absorption of calcium and phosphorus from the gastrointestinal tract and decreases renal excretion of phosphate, lack of this vitamin leads to a disturbance of concentration of calcium and phosphorus in the blood and tissue fluids.

Factors predisposing to rickets are (1) heredity. Dark-skinned people living in temperate zones do not receive an adequate amount of vitamin D from the sun's rays. (2) Age. Rickets may occur at any time from three months to three years. (3) Artificial feeding. A breast-fed infant is not likely to suffer rickets, provided his mother is receiving an adequate amount of vitamin D. (4) Prematurity. Prematurity predisposes to rickets because the deposits of calcium and phosphorus at birth are inadequate for the infant's exceptionally rapid growth. (5) Lack of sunshine. Window glass, clouds, fog, and dust or smoke in the air filter out effective ultraviolet rays. (6) Season. The incidence of rickets is greatest in the late winter and early spring.

Pathology and Clinical Manifestations. The manifestations of rickets are most evident in the skeletal system and vary with age and the amount of stress undergone by the affected bone in performing its function in the child's developing body. Deficiency in the structure of the bone is most pronounced in the lack of calcification of the epiphysis. A detectable enlargement occurs here. Besides the bones, the muscles are also affected, lacking normal tone.

The *clinical manifestations* are best described under the various parts of the body affected.

In advanced disease the head appears enlarged and square when viewed from above. The anterior fontanel is late in closing, and the cranial bones are soft and make a cracking sound under pressure. This condition is called *craniotabes* and is primarily apparent in the occipital bones.

The thorax shows the rachitic rosary—beading of the costochondral junctions—and Harrison's groove—a bilateral depression at the sites where the diaphragm is attached to the ribs. When the infant is old enough to sit up, a dorsal kyphosis develops. Scoliosis with deformities of the pelvis occurs frequently. If the pelvis of a female infant is deformed, the constricted inlet and outlet will make childbirth difficult later.

The extremities are likely to be deformed. Bowlegs or knock knees accompanied with flat feet are probably the most obvious deformities. There is epiphyseal enlargement of the wrists and ankles.

Later the infant, on sitting, assumes a crouching, froglike position. Because of the poor bone growth and muscle tone the infant is retarded in motor development and dentition.

The so-called potbelly is caused by relaxed abdominal muscles and may cause the child to be constipated.

The child may have nutritional anemia and a low resistance, especially to respiratory infections.

Diagnosis. Mild and early cases are diagnosed by determining the serum calcium, phosphorus, and alkaline phosphatase levels. Advanced cases are easily diagnosed by the gross clinical manifestations and the history of a lack of vitamin D. Radiographically, changes are evident in the bones.

Treatment and Prevention. *Treatment* is by oral administration of large doses of vitamin D, generally 1500 to 5000 International Units a day for about a month. This usually results in cure of the disease. If deformities are present, corrective appliances are used—splints and braces for bowlegs and knock knees. Osteotomy may be necessary.

Both breast-fed and bottle-fed infants should receive supplemental vitamin D in maintenance amounts of 400 International Units per day. This is of greatest importance during the winter months.

Responsibilities of the Nurse. Before the newborn leaves the hospital his mother should receive an accurate explanation of the need for giving him vitamin D. Such instruction is routine for mothers of infants under the supervision of Child Health Conferences. If the infant already has rickets, the parents should have the treatment explained to her. Only a child with severe late rickets or an accompanying concurrent infection requires hospitalization.

Rachitic children are handled gently and turned frequently. To prevent deformity they are kept from putting their weight on the spinal column or legs during their illness. In lifting the infant undue pressure should never be put on the bones of the chest. The diaper is applied loosely, lest it cause pressure on the long bones of the legs. Proper positioning lessens the danger of deformity. If the infant lies constantly on his back or one side, both his head and chest will be flattened by the pressure of his weight on the soft bones. He should lie on a firm mattress.

Administration of vitamin D presents no problem unless it is in a solution containing oil. Then care must be taken that the infant does not aspirate even a few drops of the substance.

It is important to prevent infection. Frequent changing of his position, required to prevent deformity, will also lessen the danger of lung infection.

Prognosis. Rickets is not a direct cause of death. Minor deformities in general disappear during the preschool period. Severe deformities must be corrected.

INFANTILE NUTRITIONAL TETANY* (TETANY OF VITAMIN D DEFICIENCY)

Incidence and Clinical Manifestations. Infantile nutritional tetany is caused by a deficiency in the intake and absorption of vitamin D. The condition is invariably associated with rickets, but not all rachitic children have tetany. Acquired tetany in a child receiving vitamin D for a rachitic condition is probably due to the rapid deposition of serum calcium in rachitic osteoid tissue and depletion of serum calcium in the blood. It may also result from a decrease in parathyroid activity.

This type of tetany has the same seasonal *incidence* as rickets and occurs in the same age group.

Clinical manifestations are due to increased neuromuscular irritability. There are two stages in tetany—latent and manifest.

In *latent tetany* the child has a low serum calcium level—less than 7 to 7.5 mg. per 100 ml.—but no obvious symptoms other than "jitteriness" or muscular irritability.

There are four main mechanical or electrical means of producing clinical manifestations of tetany which are used in diagnosis.

1. *Chvostek's Sign.* When the skin in front of the auditory meatus, where the facial nerve is close to the surface, is tapped, unilateral contraction of the facial muscles around the nose, eye, and mouth results.

2. *Trousseau's Sign.* If carpal spasm results when the upper arm is constricted for two to three minutes *after the hand has blanched,* the Trousseau sign is positive, showing the presence of tetany.

3. *Erb's Sign.* This test is based on the fact that a patient with tetany has greater muscular irritability than a normal child has. A measured

---

*For other forms of tetany, see page 473.

galvanic current is applied, usually over the peroneal nerve just below the head of the fibula. A positive response consists in dorsiflexion and abduction of the foot.

4. *Peroneal Sign.* This sign is positive when tapping the fibular side of the leg over the peroneal nerve causes abduction and dorsiflexion of the foot.

In *manifest tetany* the serum calcium level is often well under 7 mg. per 100 ml. Muscular twitchings and carpopedal spasm occur spontaneously. In *carpal spasm* the thumb is drawn into the cupped palm. The hands are abducted, the wrists flexed. In *pedal spasm* the foot is extended as in talipes equinus or equinovarus. The toes are flexed, and the sole of the foot is cupped. The arms and legs may be adducted and flexed.

There may be spasm of the larynx—*laryngospasm*—indicated by a high-pitched crowing sound on inspiration, due to spasm of the adductor muscles of the larynx which pull the vocal cords together. If the spasm is severe, respirations may cease and cyanosis may occur. Convulsions—generalized seizures including carpopedal spasm—may occur.

Diagnosis and Treatment. The *diagnosis* is made on the basis of the laboratory data and the clinical manifestations. The laboratory tests show a low calcium level, low, normal, or elevated serum phosphorus level, and increased serum phosphatase.

The objective of *treatment* in hypocalcemic tetany is to raise the serum calcium level above that causing tetany. Calcium may be given in the form of calcium chloride or calcium gluconate. Calcium chloride is given in a 10 per cent solution orally. Calcium gluconate in a 10 per cent solution may be given intravenously if the child cannot take oral medication. Calcium gluconate should not be given intramuscularly or subcutaneously because of the danger of necrosis at the site of injection.

Convulsions may be controlled by oxygen therapy and intravenous administration of calcium gluconate. If these procedures do not give relief, sodium phenobarbital may be administered intramuscularly. Emergency intubation may be necessary if laryngospasm is prolonged and cannot be relieved with sedatives and calcium salt.

After the acute clinical manifestations of tetany have been controlled, calcium therapy should be continued orally; in addition, large amounts of vitamin D should be given daily.

Responsibilities of the Nurse. Nursing care is of utmost importance. The nurse gives the medications as ordered.

The nurse should have padded tongue blades available to prevent the child from biting his tongue during a convulsion, and oxygen ready in case of convulsions and laryngospasm. The nurse must be able to give artificial respiration (see p. 202). Intubation equipment should be in readiness.

Prognosis and Prevention. The *prognosis* is good if treatment is given early. Death may occur from laryngospasm or cardiac failure.

Before the infant is sent home the parents, in conferences with the physician and the nurse, should be told the importance of vitamin D therapy for all growing children.

The *preventive measures* for infantile nutritional tetany are the same as those for rickets.

Scurvy

Incidence and Etiology. Scurvy is due to a lack of the water-soluble vitamin C (ascorbic acid) (see p. 368). The vitamin is unstable and is destroyed by heat, and also by alkaline solutions or by oxidation when in aqueous solutions. Ascorbic acid withstands heat fairly well in an acid solution and in the absence of oxygen. Vitamin C is generally given to infants in the form of orange juice, which should never be boiled.

The newborn has an adequate amount of vitamin C if his mother had a sufficient amount in her diet. Since vitamin C, unlike vitamin D, cannot be synthetized by human beings, the total supply must come from the diet.

Scurvy may occur at any age, but is more frequent in infants from six months to two years of age.

Pathology, Diagnosis, and Clinical Manifestations. Pathologically, there is a defect in the formation and maintenance of intercellular substances in supporting tissues, dentin, bone, cartilage, and vascular endothelium. Clinical manifestations, including a tendency to hemorrhage, can therefore be seen in the teeth and bones. The tendency to hemorrhage may be the specific result of lack of a maintenance amount of cement substance in the walls of the blood vessels or of collagen around the vessels.

The *diagnosis* is usually based on the history, roentgenographic examination, and the symptoms.

X-ray examination shows changes in the distal ends of the long bones. Initially there appears to be atrophy of the bone. In the shaft the bone presents a ground-glass appearance. Subperiosteal hemorrhages of the long bones do not show on the x-ray film *during active scurvy* but are apparent during the healing process.

It is sometimes difficult to distinguish scurvy from arthritis, osteomyelitis, or poliomyelitis because of the tenderness of the limbs and the pain produced on movement. It may also be difficult to distinguish it from dysentery, hemorrhagic nephritis, or blood dyscrasias when the tendency to hemorrhage is the most important clinical manifestation.

The *clinical manifestations* appear slowly after the body has been deprived of an adequate amount of ascorbic acid. The infant becomes fretful, irritable, and apprehensive. He fears to be touched because of the pain when he is moved, as in changing his diaper. He may have anorexia.

Subperiosteal hemorrhage causes great pain, chiefly in the legs. The pain causes a pseudoparalysis. The child assumes a frog position; i.e., the hips and knees are semiflexed with the feet rotated outward.

There may be bluish-purple, swollen, bleeding gums and blood in the vomitus and stools. Hemorrhages may be seen in the soft tissue around the eyes, and petechiae may appear in the skin.

The infant may have the so-called rosary at the costochondral junction. These scorbutic beads are sharper than those of rickets. In rickets they are due to widening of the softened epiphyses; in scurvy they are due to subluxation (partial or complete dislocation) of the sternal plate at the union of the ribs and the sternum.

The infant's temperature may rise to 102° F. (38.9° C.). Anemia develops owing to anorexia and hemorrhage. The infant then becomes very pale. The rate of growth, which is rapid in normal infants, is slowed in those with this condition.

Treatment. The specific treatment for scurvy is large doses of vitamin C. Orange juice, 90 to 120 ml. daily, is given orally, or ascorbic acid, 100 to 200 mg. daily, is given orally or parenterally. After several days of such treatment the normal requirement is all that is needed. An adequate diet is given as a supportive measure. Transfusions may be necessary for severe anemia.

Responsibilities of the Nurse. Nursing care centers about the diet and medications and prevention of pain and infection. During the acute stage the child should be fed in whatever position appears to be most comfortable for him.

The pseudoparalysis of scurvy is the chief problem in nursing. Great gentleness in handling is necessary. Since the infant fears that he will be moved when a nurse approaches him, it is well not to come too close to the bed unless necessary care must be given. In diapering the infant the buttocks may be elevated and the diaper slid under from the side. The buttocks should never be lifted by elevating the legs as is customary with a well child. A bed cradle may be used to prevent painful pressure of the bed clothes upon the child's body.

Nursing care, medication, and treatments should be given at the same time so that the infant may rest without movement between the times when it is necessary to arouse him.

Prevention of infection is of the utmost importance. The infant's position should be changed frequently, and his mouth should be cleansed with water after each feeding.

Prognosis and Prevention. The *prognosis* is excellent if the treatment is adequate. Pain ceases in a few days, and body growth is resumed.

Prevention lies in giving the infant an adequate diet containing an ample supply of vitamin C. An adequate amount of vitamin C is required throughout childhood; older children need 40 mg. of ascorbic acid a day, and adolescents 45 to 60 mg. a day.

RESPIRATORY DISORDERS

CYSTIC FIBROSIS

Incidence and Etiology. Cystic fibrosis is a congenital disease inherited as an autosomal recessive trait. For an infant to have this disease, both parents must be carriers. According to the Mendelian Law, the condition may appear in one fourth of all children of such unions; i.e., each child in the family has a one in four chance of having the disease (see p. 216). A very high concentration of alpha fetoprotein has been found in the blood of children having cystic fibrosis. A higher-than-normal concentration of this same substance has been found in the blood of their parents and some siblings. Current research on blood specimens is attempting to determine a method of identifying carriers of this disease.

Cystic fibrosis is a chronic disease, the most serious lung problem affecting children in this country today. The *incidence* in the general population is from 1:1500 to 1:2000 live births, with equal frequency in either sex. The incidence is greatest among whites and rare in black infants.

Pathology and Clinical Manifestations. There is a widespread change in the mucus-secreting glands of the body, i.e., in the pancreas, lungs, and salivary and sweat glands. The clinical manifesations are therefore respiratory difficulties with problems in the maintenance of an adequate nutritional status.

The pancreatic changes are due to obstruction by inspissated secretion, beginning in the acini and extending to the ducts. Eventually acinar tissue dilates and atrophies and is replaced by connective tissue, resulting in fibrosis of the entire gland. The islands of Langerhans, which produce insulin, usually remain normal. Glucose intolerance may appear with increasing age.

The air passages in the lungs are obstructed by a thick, mucoid secretion, which may produce emphysema or atelectasis and may contain pathogenic organisms causing infection. Later, bronchiolectatic abscesses and areas of bronchopneumonia are found. Eventually pulmonary fibrosis and interstitial pneumonia occur. The acini and ducts of the salivary glands are distended. The saliva contains increased amounts of sodium and chloride. The sweat contains a high concentration of sodium, potassium, and chloride.

The *clinical manifestations* may be present at

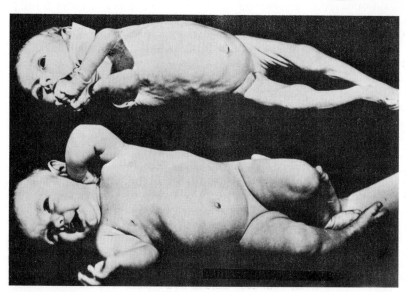

FIGURE 15–4. Cystic fibrosis. This infant before treatment had a protuberant abdomen and emaciated extremities. After treatment her appearance is that of a normal infant. (Courtesy of Pfizer Laboratories.)

birth if the infant has meconium ileus (see p. 254). Most newborns, however, who have cystic fibrosis do not have meconium ileus because the deficiency of the pancreatic enzymes is seldom complete.

If the infant is normal at birth, between the fourth week and the sixth month there may be a failure to gain weight, indicating the onset of the condition. In the early stage the stools are usually loose, but not fatty or frequent. When the infant receives cereals or fish liver oil, the stools become foul-smelling and frothy. Later the stools are light in color and fatty.

There is failure to absorb sufficient food; therefore, the child does not gain weight as he should. At last the fat disappears from the main sites of deposit. There are abdominal distention and emaciation.

During the early part of the first year the child may have persistent severe respiratory infections, usually caused by *Staphylococcus aureus.* The infant may have a spasmodic cough which produces vomiting. He may become dyspneic, may wheeze and become cyanotic. Clubbing of fingers and toes may be seen. Because of persistent obstructive lung disease, the right ventricle of the heart becomes strained and hypertrophied.

Behavior disorders result. The child is irritable and easily fatigued. In spite of these symptoms there may be a good appetite. There is a change in the physical appearance, growth is stunted, the skin appears loose, the buttocks and thighs are atrophied, and the abdomen is protuberant.

Diagnosis. The diagnosis is made on the basis of the history, physical examination, laboratory tests, and roentgenologic studies.

Laboratory examinations show a deficiency of pancreatic enzymes (trypsin, lipase, amylase, and carboxypeptidase). These enzymes are reduced in or absent from the duodenal fluid. Tests for the presence of these enzymes are done on duodenal juices obtained by intubation and aspiration. Usually only a trypsin test is made, because absence of this enzyme is indicative of cystic fibrosis. The test for tryptic activity can be done on a stool specimen.

The sweat is tested for sodium and chloride (and to a lesser extent potassium) content, which is higher than normal in patients with cystic fibrosis. (Note, however, that this abnormality may also occur in siblings and other relatives who have no clinical manifestations of the disease.) In a screening technique the child's hand is placed on agar impregnated with silver nitrate. If the sweat electrolyte level is high, the hand print is seen on the agar.

Diagnosing cystic fibrosis has been simplified by the Cystic Fibrosis Analyzer. A sample of the child's sweat is obtained by iontophoresis. This analyzer features a plastic sweat-generating electrode that eliminates the risk of skin irritation. The generation of sweat takes approximately 30 minutes, while the analysis of its electrolyte content takes one to two minutes. During the pediatric age range a level of more than 60 mEq. per liter of sweat chloride is diagnostic of cystic fibrosis. Values between 50 and 60 mEq. are highly suggestive of the diagnosis. Sweat sodium values are approximately 10 mEq. per liter higher than those for chloride.

Children who have cystic fibrosis have sodium concentrations in their hair and nails about four times greater than those of normal children. Biochemical analysis of infants' fingernails and hair has proved accurate in confirming this diagnosis.

It is possible to test for deficient absorption of fat in the intestines. Microscopic examination of the dilute stool will show excretion of fat in the feces. A low blood cholesterol level may be due in part to poor absorption of fats from the intestines. Since fats are not absorbed, vitamin A given in oily preparations is not absorbed, and some other source of this vitamin must be provided.

Roentgen studies show changes in the intestinal tract and the lungs. A generalized obstructive emphysema, atelectasis, bronchopneumonia, bronchiectasis, and bronchiolectatic abscesses may be apparent. Right ventricular hypertrophy of the heart may be seen in advanced cases.

Treatment. Several members of the health team, including the physician, social worker, dietitian, physiotherapist, respiratory therapist, genetic counselor, and nurse, are involved in the care of the child and his family. Treatment must be planned on a long-term basis, and follow-up care after treatment has been discontinued is extremely important.

Good nutrition is essential. The patient should receive a balanced diet which includes a large amount of protein (4 gm. per kilogram of body weight) and a normal amount of fat. If the child cannot tolerate this, the diet should be limited in order to control the bulk and fat content of the stools. In infancy a protein milk formula to which skimmed powdered milk has been added is good. Banana powder and glucose may also be added to the formula. Other foods which are easily digested and are high in protein or low in fat and starches, such as cottage cheese, lean meats, fruits (especially bananas), and vegetables, may also be given.

THE CHILDREN'S ORTHOPEDIC HOSPITAL AND MEDICAL CENTER
PROCEDURE FOR BRONCHOPULMONARY HYGIENE

UPPER LOBES
APICAL SEGMENTS

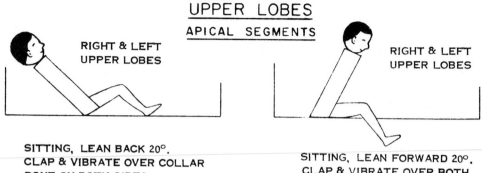

RIGHT & LEFT
UPPER LOBES

SITTING, LEAN BACK 20°.
CLAP & VIBRATE OVER COLLAR
BONE ON BOTH SIDES.

RIGHT & LEFT
UPPER LOBES

SITTING, LEAN FORWARD 20°.
CLAP & VIBRATE OVER BOTH
SHOULDERS.

ANTERIOR SEGMENTS

LEFT UPPER LOBE

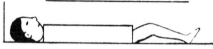

RIGHT UPPER LOBE

LYING ON BACK, PILLOW UNDER KNEES, CLAP & VIBRATE JUST BELOW THE COLLAR BONE
HALFWAY BETWEEN THE NECK AND SHOULDER ON BOTH SIDES.

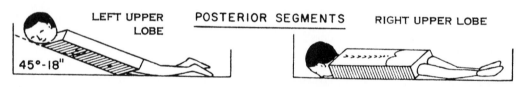

LEFT UPPER
LOBE

POSTERIOR SEGMENTS

RIGHT UPPER LOBE

45°-18"

LYING ON RIGHT SIDE, 3/4 TURN TOWARD
FACE DOWN, (PLACE 3 PILLOWS UNDER
LEFT SHOULDER AND HEAD TO LIFT 12
INCHES OFF BED.) CLAP & VIBRATE OVER
LEFT SHOULDER BLADE.

LYING ON LEFT SIDE, 3/4 TURN (ON TO PILLOW)
FACE DOWN, CLAP & VIBRATE OVER THE
RIGHT SHOULDER BLADE.

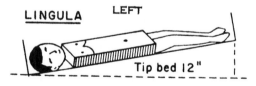

LINGULA   LEFT

Tip bed 12"

LIE ON RIGHT SIDE, ROLL 1/4 TURN BACK ON
TO PILLOWS, CLAP & VIBRATE OVER LEFT
NIPPLE AREA.

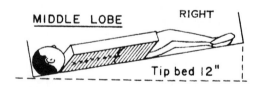

MIDDLE LOBE   RIGHT

Tip bed 12"

LIE ON LEFT SIDE, ROLL 1/4 TURN BACK ON
TO PILLOWS, CLAP & VIBRATE OVER RIGHT
NIPPLE AREA.

ADAPTED FROM DESIGN AND MATERIAL BY ELOISE DRAPER, LPT. FOR PEDIATRIC DEPARTMENT OF THE UNIVERSITY
OF LOUISVILLE MEDICAL SCHOOL.

F36—4   6—65

FIGURE 15–5. Visual aids may be used to teach parents postural drainage procedures to be used at home. Demonstrations of procedures are repeated until parents feel secure in their own proficiency. (Johnson, M. E., and Fassett, B. A.: Bronchopulmonary hygiene in cystic fibrosis, *Am. J. Nurs.*, 69:321, February, 1969.)

LOWER LOBES

SUPERIOR SEGMENTS

LEFT LOWER
LOBE

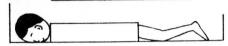

RIGHT LOWER
LOBE

BED LEVEL, LYING FACE DOWN WITH PILLOW UNDER STOMACH, CLAP & VIBRATE JUST BELOW THE SHOULDER BLADES.

BASAL SEGMENTS

ANTERIOR
RIGHT & LEFT LOWER LOBES

POSTERIOR
RIGHT & LEFT LOWER LOBES

Tip bed 18"-20"

Tip bed 18"-20"

LYING ON BACK WITH PILLOW UNDER KNEES
CLAP & VIBRATE OVER LOWER RIBS

LYING FACE DOWN, CLAP & VIBRATE OVER LOWER RIBS

LATERAL

LEFT LOWER
LOBE

RIGHT LOWER
LOBE

Tip bed 18"-20"

Tip bed 18"-20"

LYING ON RIGHT SIDE, CLAP & VIBRATE OVER LOWER RIBS

LYING ON LEFT SIDE, CLAP & VIBRATE OVER LOWER RIBS

PLACE ARMS AND LEGS IN COMFORTABLE POSITIONS.

TREATMENT SCHEDULE

1. CLAP ABOUT A MINUTE IN EACH POSITION.
2. VIBRATE DURING 5 EXHALATIONS; REST ON INHALATIONS.
3. COUGH
4. REPEAT PROCEDURE IF SO ADVISED BY DOCTOR
5. DO 3 TIMES A DAY (UNLESS OTHERWISE ORDERED BY DOCTOR)
    A. MORNING — BEFORE BREAKFAST — DO UPPER, RIGHT MIDDLE & LEFT LINGULA LOBES.
    B. MID—DAY — BEFORE LUNCH OR AFTER SCHOOL — DO RIGHT MIDDLE, LEFT LINGULA, AND LOWER LOBES.
    C. EVENING — BEFORE DINNER OR BEFORE BED DO UPPER AND LOWER LOBES.

ADAPTED FROM DESIGN AND MATERIAL BY ELOISE DRAPER, LPT, FOR PEDIATRIC DEPARTMENT OF UNIVERSITY OF LOUISVILLE MEDICAL SCHOOL.

FIGURE 15–5 *Continued.*

The caloric intake should be high, from 125 to 200 calories per kilogram of body weight per day, since the child cannot utilize food completely (he loses 50 per cent of the caloric value of his food in the stools). Liberal amounts of salt should be given with the food; in summer and hot weather extra amounts should be provided.

The specific medication in cystic fibrosis is pancreatic enzymes, given before each meal to replace the pancreatic enzymes which the child's body cannot produce and which are needed in the digestion of foods. The dose varies with the child's age, his need for the extract, and the kind of product used. In this way the condition of the stools is improved. If the child does not eat, he should not be given the pancreatic enzyme. Vitamins in water-miscible preparations should be given in large amounts.

Prevention of infection, especially respiratory infection, is of the utmost importance. The child should be isolated from other patients and hospital personnel who have respiratory infections. Because of the danger of cross-infection, hospitalization should be as short as possible. This necessitates teaching the mother to care for the child at home.

Antibiotics may be given prophylactically to minimize the danger from a respiratory infection. If, however, the child contracts an infection, appropriate antibiotics should be given in full dosage.

Digitalis and diuretics are given if there is evidence of cardiac failure (see p. 292). Oxygen is used for cyanosis due to bronchial secretions or cardiac failure. Codeine and other medications which suppress the cough reflex or those which dry secretions should not be used. If the child becomes constipated, the diet should be regulated and stool softeners such as Colace may be given.

Treatments aimed at assisting the child to remove thick mucoid secretions from his lungs include postural drainage, clapping, and vibrating.

The specific purpose of postural drainage is to bring the various branches of the bronchial tree into such a position that draining the bronchial branch and the segment of lung it supplies is facilitated. The child is placed in an upside-down position so that the force of gravity will move secretions to the main bronchi and the trachea, from where they can be more easily coughed up. A small child may be placed either on his abdomen on the nurse's lap with his head hanging down or in the same position over pillows in his crib. More effective drainage is obtained if the child's position is changed slightly while clapping and vibrating techniques are used over specific areas of the lungs.

The clapping technique is also called cupping or tapping. The nurse's hand must be in a cupped position, and the wrist is alternately flexed and extended as the child's chest is clapped gently. This percussion dislodges plugs of mucus from the lung. Air can then get behind the mucus and help move it to the trachea.

Vibrating is another technique, done only during exhalation of air from the lungs. The nurse places one hand on top of the other or one hand on either side of the child's rib cage and makes gentle, fine vibratory movements. A thumping-vibrating machine can be obtained and used instead of manual percussion. It can be operated in the home by the parent or by the child himself. After both cupping and vibrating the child is encouraged to cough.

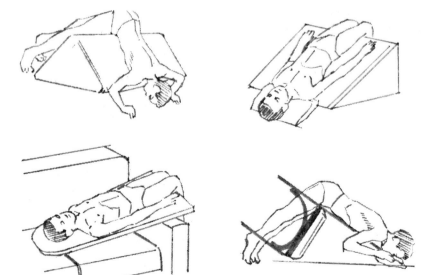

FIGURE 15–6. Improvised equipment for postural drainage. To promote drainage, a triangular cushion, padded wooden frame, ironing board, or padded chair work well. (From Johnson, M. E., and Fassett, B. A.: *Am. J. Nurs.* 69:324, February, 1969.)

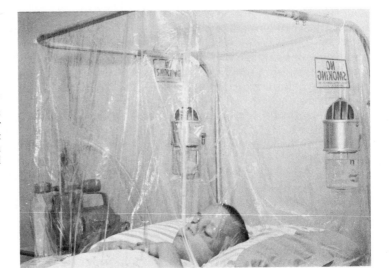

FIGURE 15–7. Home jet-type "mis t tent" nebulization therapy with 2 Mist O₂ Gen nebulizers and a 1/12-horsepower compressor for patients with cystic fibrosis. The fog must be so dense that the patient is not visible when the tent is in operation. (From M. Green and R. J. Haggerty [Eds.]: *Ambulatory Pediatrics*.)

A physical or respiratory therapist can instruct and demonstrate the proper procedure for postural drainage, cupping, and vibrating to nurses and parents caring for children in the hospital or in the home. The therapist may also need to make suggestions for improving facilities in the home for this purpose. The therapist must stress the fact that *gentleness* is necessary in these procedures. Shaking or jarring the child roughly may only result in the child's refusal to have further therapy.

The child may be placed in a humidity chamber in order to dilute the secretions in the lungs and thus make it easier for him to expectorate them.

Aerosol therapy may be given by mask or tent to help remove heavy secretions from the bronchi and to relieve dyspnea. The vapor is given as a fine mist or microparticles at least four times a day. Antibiotic, decongestant, mucolytic, and bronchodilator agents, either alone or in combination, may be added to the aerosol solution. Nebulization under intermittent positive pressure (IPPB) may be used. Since the lungs are inflated by positive pressure during inspiration, the aerosols can be administered to every area where ventilation takes place, with the result that bronchial drainage and pulmonary function are improved. Several kinds of machines may be used for this purpose (Fig. 15–8). It is possible to give this treatment to infants if intubation has been done, but it has proved most successful with children 18 months to two years of age when a mask is used. The treatment is usually given every few hours and continued until the amount of aerosol medication is exhausted. In severe cases aerosol therapy may be given continuously, with pressure maintained on both inspiration and expiration.

Although treatment of children having cystic fibrosis is mainly medical, it may be necessary to perform a tracheostomy or even a pulmonary resection (lobectomy or pneumonectomy) on very ill patients. Intubation may be necessary as noted, but this procedure creates problems owing to the fact that once done it is often extremely difficult to extubate the patient.

Complications. Severe and frequently progressive chronic pulmonary disease is present in the child having cystic fibrosis. Pancreatic insufficiency leads to symptoms of intestinal malabsorption. Rectal prolapse (see p. 454) due to

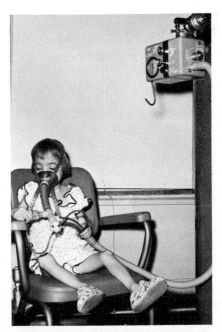

FIGURE 15–8. The Bird machine provides nebulization under intermittent positive pressure. It has proved effective when used on children having cystic fibrosis.

emaciation of the buttocks and weak musculature in the rectal area is a possible complication. It occurs most frequently between six months and three years of age.

Heat prostration may result from a high environmental temperature because the child loses electrolytes in perspiration. Osteoporosis may occur because the child cannot utilize fat-soluble vitamin D and therefore cannot make use of calcium in bone growth as the normal child does. Clinical rickets is not often seen, since rickets is a disease of growing children, and these children do not grow. There is vitamin A deficiency due to the child's inability to absorb fats from which the vitamin is obtained.

Nasal polyps, paranasal sinusitis, intussusception (see p. 422), constipation, and delayed sexual maturation may also be seen. Many males having cystic fibrosis are not fertile. Young women may become pregnant; however, the course of the pregnancy is roughly equivalent to the degree of the pulmonary involvement. The heart is strained by the exertion required to pump blood through the fibrotic lung. Cor pulmonale, in which the right side of the heart becomes enlarged and dilated, is a frequent cause of death.

Responsibilities of the Nurse. The child is usually cared for at home except during periods of complications such as severe respiratory infections. The primary aims of nursing care are to provide care for the child in the hospital and to teach the mother and the child, when he is old enough, the routines of such care at home. The nurse also is in a position to help the family adjust to what may become a new way of life for each member if the child is to receive the care he needs throughout each day.

Conferences with the parents provide for continuation of care the child receives in the hospital. The mother is told of the dietary regimen, and time must be taken to be sure that she understands what the diet consists of and also the best ways of making it acceptable to the child. She will also need to know, and emotionally accept, the physician's plan of treatment, including medical follow-up, hygienic measures, prevention of infection, meeting the child's need for adequate rest and the administration of medication. The nurse not only teaches the mother the necessary procedures but also should explain to her the purpose of each and the expected results. The nurse also explains the necessity for medication which the physician has ordered and the best way to give it to the child.

The child's nutritional state is important. The mother and the nurse must be patient with the child at mealtimes or when giving the infant his bottle. The patient is apt to be irritable, coughs and vomits easily, and often has difficulty in breathing. Small amounts of food are offered slowly but frequently so that he is not tired by his effort to take food. The infant is bubbled frequently so that abdominal distention is not increased. The diet is as varied as possible, with consideration for the child's age and ability to digest various foods. The nurse carefully charts the child's reaction to new foods and the kind of stools which result from additions to the diet.

Preparations of pancreatic enzymes, vitamins, antibiotics, and other medications are given as ordered. Pancreatic enzymes are given with cold foods, since their activity is lessened in hot food, until the child is able to take them in capsule form.

It is imperative that the mother and the nurse accept the personality changes which take place in the child as his illness extends over months. They should give him love and kindness to promote his feeling of security during the discomfort of his illness.

Skin care is required. The buttocks must be carefully cleansed after each stool, and ointment applied to protect the skin from contact with further stools. If the skin becomes irritated, the buttocks should be exposed to the air.

Scrupulous cleanliness of the diaper area will help to reduce the offensive odor from the stools. Soiled diapers should be taken from the unit as soon as they are removed from the infant. An air deodorant is useful, but is never made a substitute for cleanliness.

Because of malnutrition the skin may break down over the bony prominences. The patient is therefore turned frequently, and the entire body kept clean to prevent decubiti. More importantly, changing position lessens the danger of pneumonia. Even if the child is old enough to turn himself, he may be too weak to do so; this is the responsibility of his nurse.

The child is not dressed too warmly, but it is essential that he not become chilled. If he perspires, his clothes should be changed immediately.

The parents or nurse carry out the procedures of postural drainage and manual or mechanical clapping and vibrating as ordered daily, usually before meals to prevent vomiting. The nurse also assists in intermittent positive-pressure and aerosol treatments. The nurse explains to the child, if he is old enough to understand, that he is to take a deep breath under regulated gentle pressure and that a fine mist of medication will reach all areas of his lungs. The child is positioned correctly and helped to sit up straight. This position allows room for movement of the diaphragm and therefore permits deeper respiration. The child is encouraged to breathe slowly and deeply at first and to relax during the treatment. Demonstration by the nurse may help him to understand what is wanted of him.

If the child is afraid of the procedures, he is urged to express his fear. The nurse is then able to give support and encouragement. Eventually most children will cooperate. When medication is used in the mist, the nurse should attend the infant or young child throughout the procedure of intermittent positive pressure. The nurse must use judgment in permitting the older child to use the apparatus alone. The machine is cleaned thoroughly between treatments because of the danger of respiratory cross-infection between children using the apparatus. In some institutions each child has his own apparatus including his own tubing, nebulizer, and mask. Respiratory therapy equipment is cleansed and air dried daily in the home to prevent the growth of bacteria, particularly pseudomonas, on moist equipment or in a standing solution.

Because of the wasted muscles, the site for intramuscular injections presents more problems than in the normal child. Injection sites should be examined carefully for hardened areas, and no further medication given in any area unless it is normally soft and shows no evidence of trauma. Sites are rotated whenever injections are given frequently. Massage may help in absorption of the medication and tends to prevent hardness from developing.

Recording of observations should be complete so that the physician may have a clear picture of the child's condition. The stools are described in detail as to color, odor, consistency, and size. The kind and amount of foods taken, as well as those refused, are charted. Whether the child eats eagerly or indifferently is also noted. Gain or loss of weight is recorded or shown graphically. The color of the skin has diagnostic value. The nurse watches for signs of rectal prolapse and reports all symptoms of this condition. If the child coughs, the physician wants to know the nature and frequency of the cough. Young children cry readily for many reasons, but crying is also a sign of discomfort or pain. The time, kind, and frequency of crying are important both in diagnosis and in judging the effect of treatments and therefore should be recorded in detail. A description of the cry is helpful in appraising not only his physical condition, but also the personality changes which interact with the physical ones.

Severe heat prostration may be prevented if the parent or nurse observes and reports to the physician the first symptoms of this condition.

Prevention of infection, especially respiratory infection, must be a constant aim.

When the mother undertakes the time-consuming and difficult task of caring for her child at home, the nurse can help her to use her affection wisely and set limits to his behavior, even though the prognosis may be poor. The child should be allowed and encouraged to be as active as possible at home as he was in the hospital. Most children can attend school on a part-time or full-time basis. If this is not possible, a tutor may be obtained.

The nurse assists both parents to realize their responsibility in caring for the child and the help they must give him in adjusting to his limitations. The danger lies in overprotection by his parents and therefore deprivation of opportunities for normal development. He should be helped to make the best possible adjustment to his handicap. The affected child should not be permitted to dominate the family. This is unfair to the other family members.

The diagnosis of cystic fibrosis in a child causes emotional and financial problems for a family. Any guilt which the parents may have should be alleviated; otherwise they may have great difficulty in cooperating with the therapy required. The stress in such a family may result in separation or divorce of the parents, especially if more than one child is affected. Therefore it seems that an important role of the nurse is to assess a family for such problems, to provide opportunities for discussion of problem areas, and to assist in coordinating care with other members of the health team, including the physician, social worker, family counselor, religious advisor, and community or public health nurse who may visit in the home. The family should be informed of community facilities available to assist them. They should certainly be informed about the National Cystic Fibrosis Research Foundation and the help it is prepared to give to parents. Since the financial burden may be highly important, organizations and programs which may be helpful should be suggested.

Prognosis. Death may occur in the first year from severe malnutrition or overwhelming respiratory infection. The nurse may be of great support to parents at this time, even though they have known the genetic cause of the disease and the prognosis. Spiritual guidance of such parents may be of great value (see p. 106).

Children having cystic fibrosis who live to young adult life have particular problems in relation to achieving normal maturity. They are very much concerned about their disease and how it will affect their future. Difficulty with their identity crisis is evident during adolescence. They need to be involved in any discussion about their care. They may be disturbed by the need for continued therapy, by their inability to participate in vigorous sports activities, and by their attempts to establish relations with the opposite sex. These problems may become acute because of their image of themselves as smaller in stature and less attractive than others of the same sex. As mentioned previously, the possibility of their having a family and rearing the children to maturity is questionable. Genetic counseling is of great importance for both the parents and the patient having this condition.

Although the life expectancy has been increased with good care, the prognosis is still unpredictable and in severe disease is usually poor.

GASTROINTESTINAL DISORDERS

GLUTEN-INDUCED ENTEROPATHY (CELIAC DISEASE)

Incidence and Etiology. Gluten-induced enteropathy is characterized by chronic intestinal malabsorption resulting in malnutrition and deficiency diseases. The disease may begin during infancy or the toddler period. It occurs in both sexes and has its highest *incidence* in the white race.

Celiac disease in children seems to be related to nontropical sprue in adults and may occur among different members of the same family. The cause is believed to be an inborn error of metabolism with or without an accompanying allergic reaction. The child cannot ingest the gluten or protein portions of wheat or rye flour. Infections and emotional disturbances may lead to exacerbations.

Pathology and Clinical Manifestations. The *pathology* is evident in severe malnutrition and secondary deficiency diseases, of which rickets is the most common, but scurvy or hypoproteinemia may also occur.

Typical *clinical manifestations* appear as early as six months and may last to the fifth year of life. Episodes of diarrhea occur. Anorexia, if it occurs, results in failure of growth. Severe abdominal distention may be caused by collections of gas and by relaxed abdominal musculature. There are fluctuations in weight. Loss of weight is most noticeable in the limbs, buttocks, and groin. The skin over the flattened buttocks may be wrinkled and hang in folds. The face usually remains plump, and the rounded cheeks may be flushed. Tooth eruption is often delayed. The child may show increasing irritability and other changes in behavior.

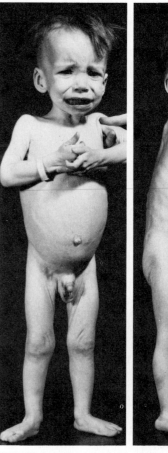
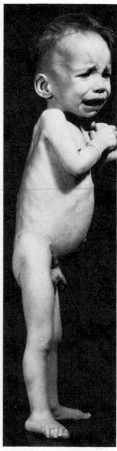

FIGURE 15–9. Characteristic profile of a child with gluten sensitive enteropathy. Note typical facies, "pot" belly, muscle wasting (especially proximal limbs and buttocks). (From Katz, A. J., Falchuk, Z. M., and Shwachman, H.: *Pediatrics.* 57:5, May 5, 1976.)

A *celiac crisis* may be precipitated by a mild respiratory infection. The child has dehydration and acidosis caused by vomiting and large, watery stools. His sleep is restless; sweating is excessive, and his extremities are cold. This condition may result in death if the child is not promptly and adequately treated.

The nature of the stools varies with the diet and the severity of the disease. The typical celiac stools are bulky, heavy and of more than normal frequency (particularly during a crisis), mushy, foul-smelling, pale and frothy. The amount of fat (soaps and fatty acids) in the stool is moderately increased in gluten-induced enteropathy. With improvement in the child's condition the stools become formed and normal in color.

There is a mild hypoproteinemia or protein deficiency. A total serum protein level of less than 5 gm. per 100 ml. indicates that the child is seriously ill. Minerals—calcium and iron—are lost in the stools in amounts depending on the severity of the disease.

Treatment. The treatment consists in controlling the diet. Wheat and rye gluten must be excluded entirely, and the amount of fat must be limited. Approximately 6 to 8 gm. of protein per kilogram of body weight should be given daily. An adequate fluid intake should be assured. If the child is very ill, he is given skimmed or protein milk sweetened with glucose, sucrose or banana powder. Gradually other foods are added, one at a time, at intervals of two or more days. Foods which can be added are eggs, cottage cheese, meat, e.g., chicken and lean beef, fruits, and vegetables.

The diet must meet the child's caloric needs. Monosaccharides and disaccharides may be given, but not polysaccharides (starches). The parents should be given a list of food products which contain the forbidden wheat or rye gluten, such as gravies, meat loaf, puddings and processed meats (cold meat cuts or sausage products), and should be told why these foods are contraindicated for the child.

Treatment during a celiac crisis involves fluid and electrolyte replacement and maintenance therapy. If symptoms of tetany occur, calcium is given until the serum calcium level returns to normal. Liver extract may be given intramuscularly, and large amounts of water-miscible preparations of vitamins A and D should be given to prevent deficiencies. Antibiotics are given if infections develop. Adrenal steroid therapy produces remissions in celiac disease, but a relapse may occur as soon as the medication is discontinued.

Responsibilities of the Nurse. Nursing care involves helping the parents to accept not only the child's physical condition, but also his behavior problems. Typically, the child is irritable and difficult to manage. The nurse must have a sympathetic understanding of their problem. Parents may feel guilty or ambivalent toward the child. They may overprotect him or communicate to him their great concern about his stools.

During hospitalization for diagnosis and treatment the child may need emotional support from the nurses. He is confused and unhappy because of the initial food deprivation. His parents should visit him frequently or, if possible, stay with him. If he becomes hungry in spite of his rye and wheat gluten-free foods, he becomes frustrated and angry and may have temper tantrums or be withdrawn. The understanding nurse will help him to express his feelings in words and will show sympathy if he cries.

Feeding the child is a problem. His appetite is capricious. He should be fed slowly and given small amounts. He should not be forced to eat; when he feels better, he will eat more. New foods should be introduced gradually, one at a time, and may be masked in foods he likes. If he will not take a particular food, this fact is reported to the physician, and the food should be eliminated from the diet and tried again at some future time. Problems with food may occur when the child is at home if he sees the food other children in the family are eating. He may want their food instead of his own.

Recording food intake is important. The nurse should observe and chart the kind and amount of food taken, the child's appetite and his reaction to different foods. With each new addition to the diet she should note the nature of the stools, the child's behavior, and the degree of abdominal distention.

It is imperative to prevent infection. Good hygiene must be maintained, since the child is anemic and malnourished. He perspires freely and must be kept dry. If he is confined to bed and tends to lie in one position, he should be turned frequently.

As the child recovers, every effort should be made to provide him with special treats when he cannot have the food which other children are enjoying.

Children with gluten-induced enteropathy are often withdrawn and do not enter into play with other children. Their play is likely to be passive, since they find active play exhausting. The toddler may retain infantile habits of self-comfort such as sucking his thumb, or he may carry his favorite toy or object wherever he goes to give him a feeling of security. The nurse must be patient and try to provide security for the child in companionship with other children and the unit personnel. As his physical condition improves, his emotional behavior will also change; he will give up infantile habits and seek the companionship of others.

Instructions to the Parents. The parents should learn the underlying concepts of the child's illness and his treatment so that they can give him adequate care after his discharge. In conferences with the mother the nurse stresses (1) the necessity of preventing infection and emotional disturbances from any cause, (2) the importance of strict adherence to the dietary regimen, and (3) the need for follow-up supervision. The dietitian and the nurse can discuss with the parents the foods to buy and various recipes for gluten-free foods. This instruction should be given slowly without frightening the mother, for if she becomes too anxious, she will overprotect the child and restrict his activities beyond the limits set by the physician. Overprotection is harmful to mental health, particularly in the infant or toddler, who has no relations with a teacher or other professional workers to counteract his mother's attentions.

Prognosis. The mortality rate from celiac disease is low, owing to better understanding and more common use of parenteral fluid therapy, dietary management, and control of infection by antibiotics. Recovery takes several months. The course is an intermittent process of exacerbations and remissions. Since celiac disease is a constitutional defect, actual cure does not occur, but clinical manifestations decrease in later life.

PROLAPSE AND PROCIDENTIA OF THE RECTUM AND SIGMOID

Incidence and Etiology. *Prolapse* of the rectum is an abnormal descent of the mucous membrane of the rectum. The membrane may or may not protrude through the anus. *Procidentia* is an abnormal descent of all the layers of the rectum or sigmoid, or both, which likewise may or may not protrude through the anus.

The *incidence* is greatest during infancy, although the condition occurs in children up to three years of age.

Prolapse is precipitated when the intra-abdominal pressure is suddenly increased. Infants and young children who are malnourished, have diarrhea or are constipated are prone to these conditions. Prolapse or procidentia may occur repeatedly with straining at defecation if the sphincter is relaxed and the muscles of the pelvic floor are weak.

Clinical Manifestations. The first manifestation is only protrusion of part of the rectum and sigmoid, which recedes spontaneously. Later, manual replacement may be necessary. The protruding mass is bright red to dark purple, depending on the length of time it has been prolapsed and the degree to which circulation has been cut off. The protrusion may be up to 5 to 6 inches in length. The mass may be a flattened, corrugated tumor or just a fold of mucous membrane protruding from the anus.

Treatment, Responsibilities of the Nurse, and Prognosis. *Treatment* is aimed at the underlying problem, i.e., to correct the child's weight by an adequate diet if he is malnourished, to correct constipation by giving a mild medication (e.g., mineral oil) and instituting proper toilet training, and to correct diarrhea if that is the cause of the difficulty.

During defecation the buttocks should be held together manually or with adhesive tape. If the child is able to indicate when he is about to have a stool, manual pressure is preferable, since it can be adjusted to passage of the stool. The buttocks may be taped together after each bowel movement to prevent repeated prolapse.

For reduction of the protrusion the infant is placed with his head lower than his body. The protrusion may be replaced manually. Toilet paper is put over a gloved finger used to insert the bowel and pressed into the opening of the mass as it is pushed back into the rectum. The finger is then quickly withdrawn, leaving the toilet paper in the rectum. The paper will become soft and be expelled later.

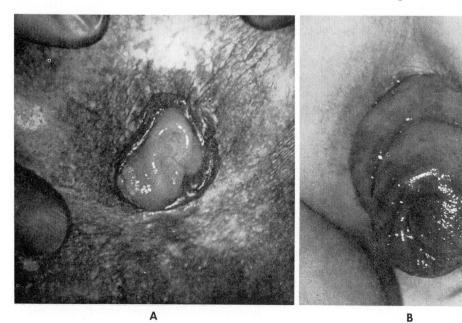

A   **B**

FIGURE 15–10.   Rectal prolapse. *A,* Partial prolapse; only rectal mucosa involved. *B,* Complete prolapse of rectum (procidentia); entire thickness of rectal wall involved. (From P. Hanley and M. O. Hines, in Ochsner and DeBakey: *Christopher's Minor Surgery.* 8th ed.)

Operation may be necessary if other treatment is not successful.

The *prognosis* is usually good with proper treatment.

BILIARY ATRESIA

Etiology, Pathology, Clinical Manifestations, and Prognosis. The cause of biliary atresia is a congenital faulty development of the bile ducts. Bile accumulates in the liver instead of entering the intestinal tract. Bile pigments enter the blood and cause increasing jaundice.

The *pathologic picture* includes jaundice, ascites from portal obstruction, enlarged liver sometimes extending below the umbilicus, absent or deformed gallbladder, and enlarged spleen due to portal obstruction secondary to biliary cirrhosis.

The *clinical manifestation* of jaundice may not be evident until the infant is two to three weeks old. Eventually the skin becomes olive-green. The van den Bergh reaction is direct. The urine is stained with bile, and the stools are white or clay-colored and putty-like because of their high fat content and lack of pigment. Infection seems to cause unusual toxemia. The bleeding and clotting times may be prolonged. The prothrombin level is low. Hemorrhage may occur. Absorption of fat, fat-soluble vitamins A, D, and K, and calcium is poor.

If operation cannot be done to relieve the obstruction, the *prognosis* is hopeless, although some children live for years.

Treatment and Responsibilities of the Nurse. The diet is high in protein and low in fat. Fat-soluble vitamins A and D are given in water-soluble form. Vitamin K is given to prevent hemorrhage. The child is carefully protected from infection. Antibiotics are given when infection occurs.

Surgical reconstructive procedures are done if possible on these children by the age of one to two months. Postoperatively, the child is observed for symptoms of shock. The vital signs are taken as ordered. The child's position is changed frequently and carefully to prevent trauma to the wound. Because healing is impaired, the wound should be inspected for bleeding. The abdomen is observed for distention due to an accumulation of peritoneal fluid or paralytic ileus. Gastric suction may be used until peristaltic movements are heard; therefore, elbow restraints are used to prevent the infant from interfering with the tube. The surgeon may order irrigations of the tube with warm saline solution in order to keep it open. A rectal tube may be needed to further relieve distention.

The child is fed parenterally until he can take feedings by mouth. If surgery has been success-ful, the stools will appear more normal when oral feedings are begun. The appearance of the stools should be described accurately and completely.

The procedure of transplanting a complete liver into a child who has biliary atresia has been done. No conclusive results concerning the long-term success of this procedure are yet known.

CONGENITAL AGANGLIONIC MEGACOLON (HIRSCHSPRUNG'S DISEASE)

Etiology, Incidence, and Pathology. In Hirschsprung's disease there is a congenital absence of parasympathetic ganglion nerve cells from the intramural plexus of a part of the intestinal tract, usually in the distal end of the descending colon.

The condition is more common in males than in females. The symptoms may be present at birth or may appear during infancy.

The involved portion of the intestine has a narrow lumen and lacks peristaltic activity. The portion of the colon above this area is greatly dilated and hypertrophied, and feces and gas accumulate in it. The muscular coat of the dilated colon, at first hypertrophied, may become thin; in infants the mucosa may become ulcerated.

Clinical Manifestations. A newborn infant with Hirschsprung's disease may not pass meconium. Vomiting, abdominal distention, an overflow type of diarrhea or constipation may appear in the first few weeks of life.

The subsequent course shows increasingly obstinate constipation with abdominal distention due to the mass of feces and to gas. Abdominal distention may be so great that respiration is embarrassed. Fecal matter may be expelled in pellet- or ribbon-like form or may be fluid. As the disease progresses spontaneous bowel movements are infrequent. Eventually the abdominal wall becomes thin, and the superficial veins are prominent. The fecal mass may be palpated through the abdominal wall. The more severely affected children may appear malnourished and even stunted in growth. Infants and young children may have periodic attacks of intestinal obstruction due to fecal impaction. As a result there are abdominal pain, vomiting, and fever.

Diagnosis. The diagnosis is based on the clinical manifestations. If diarrhea is one of the symptoms, as is often the case in infancy, it is difficult to differentiate this condition from cystic fibrosis. The determining factors are absence of findings positive for cystic fibrosis in the sweat test and the examination of duodenal secretion for trypsin. Roentgen examination after a barium enema in children over six

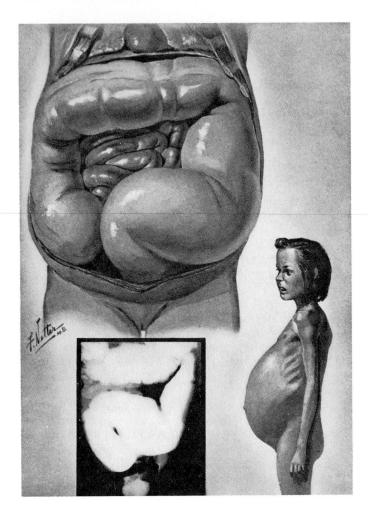

FIGURE 15–11. Megacolon. (Copyright, The Ciba Collection of Medical Illustrations, by Frank H. Netter, M.D.)

months of age shows the narrowed section of the rectosigmoid. After examination the barium must be removed immediately by colonic irrigation.

Rectal examination shows no fecal matter in the colon lower than the obstruction, in spite of pressure in the bowel above.

Treatment. Frequent or daily enemas are given to remove fecal matter as it accumulates. Retention enemas of mineral or olive oil may be used, followed by colonic irrigations. Some of the solution given by enema may be retained; therefore only isotonic solution should be used. If tap water were used and absorbed in large quantities, water intoxication might result.

When the child is in good condition for operation, the narrowed segment of the bowel in the rectosigmoid area is resected. The normal sigmoid section is pulled through and sutured to the anal opening to reconstruct continuity of the bowel lumen.

A more recent operation is the Duhamel procedure. This entails preservation of the rectum and its utilization by means of a long, side-to-side anastomosis (by means of a clamp) between it and the normal ganglion-containing proximal colon. This procedure preserves the sensation of the urge to defecate and normal bowel control.

If the child is not in good condition for operation, a temporary colostomy may be done in preparation for further operation later in infancy or during the toddler period. The colostomy is made in the distal portion of the colon where normal ganglia are found.

Responsibilities of the Nurse. Good general hygiene is important, since these infants are poorly nourished, apathetic, and uncomfortable with distention and nausea. Frequent, small oral feedings are better than three large meals a day. A low-residue diet is given to keep the stools soft so that they can be easily evacuated. Mineral oil or mild laxatives may be ordered for the same purpose.

Because respiration is embarrassed by the abdominal distention, the infant is more comfortable in an upright position. He can be placed in a sitting position and supported with sandbags and pillows. Enemas or colonic irrigations are given as ordered.

The nurse should record the child's appetite and the frequency and nature of the stools.

If the child is to be operated upon, *preoperative care* consists in emptying the bowel by repeated enemas and colonic irrigations with physiologic saline solution. The physician may order chemotherapeutic agents to reduce the bacterial flora.

The procedure for giving an enema is similar to that for the adult, with some alterations necessitated by the anatomy and physiology of the child.

1. A no. 10 to 12 French catheter is used. It should be inserted only 2 to 4 inches into the rectum.

2. The temperature of the solution should be 105° F. (40.5° C.).

3. Physiologic saline solution (never tap water) is used, and is made by dissolving 1 dram of salt in a pint of water.

4. Not more than 300 ml. of solution should be given to an infant unless the physician orders a larger amount.

5. The child is positioned by placing pillows under his head and back. The buttocks are placed upon the pan, which has been covered with a folded diaper to serve as a soft pad under the lower lumbar area. Another diaper is used to restrain the legs in position over the side edges of the bedpan (Fig. 15–12).

6. The enema can should not be more than 18 inches above the level of the child's hips so that the solution will run slowly by gravity and without pressure into the bowel.

7. The results of the enema should be fully and carefully charted.

This is one of the procedures which the parents are taught in order to give the child adequate care when he is discharged from the hospital. (Commercial enemas may be ordered for children. If so, the parents are instructed in their proper use.)

For an oil retention enema a funnel or syringe may be used. From 75 to 150 ml. of oil is usually given at 100° F. (37.7° C.). Pressure over the anus is necessary after a retention enema so that it will not be expelled. A cleansing enema is given 30 to 45 minutes after the oil retention enema.

In *postoperative care* the nurse will probably be asked to assist in the giving of chemotherapeutic agents to reduce the danger of infection.

The infant's temperature after operation is taken by axilla rather than by rectum until healing is complete.

There is careful recording of intake and output of fluids and description of the stools. The perianal area is kept clean and dry at all times, but especially after a corrective surgical proce-

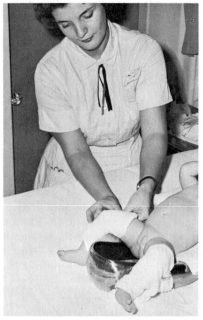

FIGURE 15–12. Positioning the infant for an enema. A pillow is under the infant's head and back. The buttocks are placed upon the bedpan, which has been covered with a folded diaper to protect the infant's back. The legs are restrained in position with a diaper brought under the bedpan and pinned over the legs.

dure. If a colostomy was performed, the infant must be kept clean and dry to prevent excoriation of the surrounding area. The dressing should be changed frequently. If the area around the colostomy becomes irritated, the abdomen is exposed to the air and the skin protected with soothing ointment (see the care of a child having an imperforate anus, p. 248).

Complications. The complications to be feared are ulcers in the mucous membrane of the intestine which will cause diarrhea, perforation, and peritonitis (unusual but possible), and malnutrition.

Course and Prognosis. The child may outgrow the milder forms of megacolon and improve as his body grows. He may have difficulty in controlling flatus. During his early years this creates no serious difficulty, but during school years it may cause him great embarrassment.

Surgical correction has given excellent results.

PSYCHOGENIC MEGACOLON

Psychogenic megacolon may be difficult to distinguish from a true aganglionic megacolon. The cause of this so-called fear-of-the-pot syndrome is a deep antagonism between parents and child. *Treatment* consists of enemas, laxatives, fecal softeners, increased fluids, and proper elimination or toilet training (see p. 496). This condition usually occurs in the preschool period, but is mentioned here since the presenting symptoms may be similar to those of the more serious disease of infancy. The total attitude of the family and child toward bowel training should be understood if treatment is to be successful.

BLOOD DISORDERS

BLOOD FORMATION

Blood cells begin to form in the fetus in the yolk sac about the fourth week of gestation. They form successively in the liver, spleen, thymus, and lymphatic tissues and last in the bone marrow. Although the liver produces the majority of blood cells during the first six months of fetal life, blood formation at term is largely carried on in the bone marrow. During the period of growth nearly all the bone marrow produces blood cells, but after growth has been completed hematopoiesis (blood cell production) is limited to the ends of the long bones, vertebrae, and certain flat bones of the body. If, however, in childhood all the marrow is hematopoietic and more demand is made for blood, other organs (liver, spleen) and lymph nodes produce additional cells. At times these organs may enlarge because of the need for extramedullary hematopoiesis in certain diseases.

Although erythrocytes, granulocytes, and platelets are formed in bone marrow and lymphocytic cells mostly in lymphatic tissue, an examination of peripheral blood may not be adequate for complete understanding of a condition. It is therefore necessary to study by direct or indirect means the states of hematopoietic tissue and the spleen, which is largely an organ of blood destruction.

RED BLOOD CELLS (ERYTHROCYTES). The red blood cells carry hemoglobin, which takes oxygen to the tissues and removes carbon dioxide to be excreted by the lungs. Hemoglobin also acts as a buffer in regulation of the pH of the blood. Production of red cells is stimulated by a reduced oxygen content of the blood as a result of hemorrhage, hemolysis or pulmonary or cardiac disease.

Hemoglobin formation takes place in the reticuloendothelial cells of bone marrow. The red cells are taken from circulation by the reticuloendothelial cells, especially in the spleen. The iron in the hemoglobin is mostly reused; the cell pigment changes into bile pigment and is excreted. When blood is destroyed more rapidly than normal, the liver may not be able to excrete the increased load of bilirubin. Bilirubin accumulates in the plasma, thereby producing clinical jaundice, and may be excreted as urobilinogen in the stools and urine. The spleen and perhaps the liver may enlarge because of increased activity of their reticuloendothelial elements. Rapid formation of new blood cells to replace the old takes place in bone marrow and other tissues.

A mature red cell has no nucleus, but a nucleus is present during the early stage of cell formation. Nucleated red cells are common in fetal blood and may be found in the early days of life, especially in premature infants. Since red cells are constantly being destroyed and created, the presence of some immature cells containing reticulum is to be expected. About 1 to 2 per cent of red blood cells normally are reticulocytes, containing reticulum.

Later in infancy and during childhood the presence of nucleated red cells means that the body is producing them at an abnormally rapid rate in order to meet a demand for them.

The mean number of red blood cells per cubic millimeter of blood is dependent upon the subject's age (see Table 4–1).

The useful life of a normal red blood cell is about 120 days. Factors such as exposure to hemagglutinins or hemolysins (as in erythroblastosis fetalis or transfusion reactions) or anomalies of structure and shape (sickle cell disease or thalassemia) may shorten the life of a cell to as little as a few days.

The Anemias of Infancy and Childhood

Etiology, Clinical Manifestations, and Prognosis. Anemia, a deficit of erythrocytes or hemoglobin, is the most frequent disorder of the blood during childhood. It represents a disturbance in the balance between the production and destruction of these substances.

There are many kinds of anemia, but only the fairly common ones will be considered here. The principal types are due to (1) inadequate production of hemoglobin or red blood cells and (2) excessive loss of blood cells. Causes of underproduction of red blood cells or hemoglobin are (1) lack in the bone marrow of some substance or substances necessary in the formation of cells, (2) depressed functioning of the bone marrow, and (3) specific nutritional deficits in the marrow.

Excessive loss of red blood cells may be due to hemorrhage, e.g., acute hemorrhage in the newborn (see p. 241), chronic ulcerative colitis (see p. 806), or hemolysis of the blood. The most common causes of hemolysis are (1) a congenital anomaly of the erythrocytes or hemoglobin (e.g., thalassemia—p. 461—and sickle cell anemia—p. 463) and (2) acquired anomalies of the erythrocyte or its environment (e.g., toxic hemolytic anemias due to poisons—p. 552—or drugs, and the hemolytic anemias due to burns—p. 556—and immune reactions such as erythroblastosis fetalis—p. 238.

Although the causative factors in anemia are varied, the *clinical manifestations* are similar. In the early stage the child is easily fatigued, weak and listless; later symptoms are pallor, cardiac palpitation, and rapid pulse rate, or tachycardia. Eventually there is mental slowness and physical sluggishness, cardiac enlargement, and inability to carry out the usual activities of childhood.

The *prognosis* varies with the type. When anemia is fatal, it is usually because of weakness of the heart and its inability to maintain the normal circulation of the blood.

Treatment and Responsibilities of the Nurse. The treatment and nursing care depend upon the severity of the condition, its cause, and the age of the child.

Transfusions improve the child's condition his appetite, and his disposition He becomes more active and like other children. Transfusion is lifesaving when anemia has reached the point at which it interferes with cardiac function. The procedure is like that for intravenous therapy (see p. 412). The nurse should note any evidence of discomfort, such as generalized uneasiness, restlessness, crying or chills, which may indicate the onset of a transfusion reaction. There may also be elevation of temperature and changes in the respiratory and pulse rates and in the color of the skin. The child should be observed closely also for changes in the appearance of his urine, the quantity of his urinary output, and for any hemorrhagic phenomena. Whenever the nurse notes such symptoms, she should stop the transfusion and notify the physician immediately.

One problem with transfusions in small children is blocking of the narrow lumen of the needle by the vein wall. To prevent this the blood may be slowly pumped into a small vein by using a syringe. The physician must have assistance to do this procedure. When this technique is used, the blood is given very slowly, with care taken to prevent pumping air bubbles through the needle and also to prevent contamination of the plunger of the syringe.

Medication commonly given includes iron, vitamin C, and liver extract. Iron is given if the cause of the anemia is an insufficient intake of iron or loss of iron supply through hemorrhage. For a discussion of iron therapy see page 460.

Vitamin C is valuable in correction of the anemia caused by scurvy (see p. 443). Liver extract and vitamin B complex may be used in treatment of anemias caused by a megaloblastic bone marrow.

Splenectomy may be performed because of its palliative value or for removal of the pressure of an enlarged spleen upon abdominal viscera.

Preparation of the parents for continued care of the young child having anemia is exceedingly important. In the conference with them, the physician or nurse will take up the whole problem of the general hygiene of the child. Good hygiene includes an adequate diet, rest, sunshine, and fresh air, and will help to build up the child's resistance to infections. The child should be dressed according to the weather and kept from other children and from adults who have colds, sore throats, or other infections.

As the child grows older—out of the age group considered in this chapter—he should be as self-reliant and as independent of help from his parents as his age and physical condition permit. They must further his desire for independence, but keep it within realistic bounds. For instance, when the child is old enough to feed himself, his mother may give him a spoon while she feeds him with another, letting him take turns with her in bringing the food to his mouth. In the hospital the nurse may do the same thing and so accustom him to the procedure before he goes home. Free play activity should be alternated with periods of controlled, quiet play to allow the child to rest. He should never be allowed to exhaust his strength and should be taught gradually as he matures to protect himself against overexertion and emotional strain.

Prolonged hospitalization is to be avoided unless it is necessary because of home conditions detrimental to the child's care or because his condition is such that he cannot be cared for at home. Until recently children who had chronic anemia, such as thalassemia or sickle cell disease, were admitted to the hospital for long periods of blood transfusions. These periods of absence from home and their parents and later from school were detrimental to their normal emotional development. The children often developed a fear of the hospital which made each hospitalization more difficult than the last. They felt insecure as to both their health and the normal pleasures of childhood. Much of this was realistic, but they also developed a chronic anxiety which included fears that were completely illogical and unfounded. In the end their whole lives and indeed those of their parents and siblings revolved around their disease. Hospitalization, if paid for at all, was a great drain on income, often requiring some sacrifice from every member of the family.

Today children are brought to the hospital for diagnostic examination and initial transfusions. They are then admitted to the hospital on a scheduled basis for a one-day stay for further therapy. Children learn quickly about their diseases and feel less threatened by a brief stay in the hospital, during which laboratory studies and transfusions are done, than by prolonged hospitalization. In the pediatric department they are free to talk and play with other children both before the transfusion and afterwards while they are observed for a transfusion reaction. They understand the relation between receiving blood and their feeling of well-being following the transfusion. Children cooperate best when they are familiar with the equipment, the procedure, and the people who carry it out. They should be permitted to handle the equipment initially and to cleanse the area for injection before the transfusion is given.

If a child must be admitted to the hospital for a longer period for examination, laboratory tests, or treatment, the nursing personnel should realize the long-term problem involved and do everything possible to make his stay as pleasant as it can be. Nursing personnel might even keep notes as to his likes and dislikes in food, toys, and bed location. Often such children, on a return admission to the hospital unit, greet the nurses warmly as old friends instead of threats to their security.

The education of the anemic child should be as like that of his peers as his condition permits. If he is not able to attend school, he is taught at home. In many cities and towns the school board sends visiting school teachers to homes or hospitals to teach children who are unable to go to school.

HYPOCHROMIC ANEMIA DUE TO IRON DEFICIENCY

Etiology, Incidence, and Pathology. Iron-deficiency anemia is the most prevalent nutritional disorder among children in this country. It is usually preventable and responds well to therapy.

If hemoglobin is not synthesized, pallor of the erythrocytes results. This hypochromia is accompanied by a decrease in size of the cell—microcytosis. If evidence of anemia is also present, as shown by the red cell count, hemoglobin level and hematocrit value below the normal range for the child's age, a hypochromic anemia can be diagnosed.

The cause is almost always a lack of iron in the diet or the child's inability to use the iron he ingests. The young child can produce hemoglobin only if his diet provides a supply of readily available iron. The minimum daily adult requirement of iron is 15 mg. The infant having iron-deficiency anemia may need 100 mg. of elemental iron each day.

Iron deficiency is most apt to occur at periods of rapid growth. The premature infant (see p. 195) at three to four months of age grows rapidly and is prone to hypochromic anemia. Infants born at term have a greater reserve of iron than has the premature infant, and the results of a diet low in iron, such as one of milk, potatoes, and cereals, are not likely to be severe until the term infant is six months to two years old. At two years the growth rate is slowing down, and children are customarily receiving a varied diet adapted from that prepared for the family.

Behind the poor diet which produces anemia may be social and economic conditions—the low income of the parents or their ignorance of or indifference to dietary needs. They may not know what is an adequate diet or, since the infant will take milk, they do not persist in their efforts at feeding iron-containing foods. This may be because they do not know the technique or lack the time or simply will not take the trouble to accustom the infant to taking into his mouth and swallowing any nourishment which is not in a fluid state.

Only in rare cases is anemia due to abnormal difficulty in swallowing or to prolonged vomiting. Even though an infant ingests an adequate liberal diet suited to his age, there may be insufficient absorption or he may suffer from a chronic disease which diminishes the supply of nourishment, such as celiac disease or a chronic diarrhea. The infant may also have chronic gastrointestinal blood loss due to exposure to a heat labile protein in whole cow's milk.

Clinical Manifestations. The onset of hypochromic anemia is insidious and may occur as a complication of an infection, or the anemia may itself be complicated by an infection. Infants having hypochromic anemia due to iron deficiency are especially susceptible to infections.

Clinical manifestations of severe anemia include poor muscle tone, slow motor development, weakness and waxy pallor. The heart may be enlarged, and a loud, systolic precordial murmur may be heard. The spleen may be palpable. The hemoglobin level is often below 5 gm. The red blood cell count may be below 2,500,000, and stained red cells are pale and microcytic.

Treatment and Responsibilities of the Nurse. *Treatment* is aimed at correction of the underlying cause of the condition. An adequate diet includes vegetables and meat. Vitamin supplements are necessary. Vitamin C (ascorbic acid) appears to enhance the absorption of iron. Iron, especially in inorganic form, should be given. It may be given by mouth in the form of ferrous sulfate, which is absorbed efficiently and is cheap and easily available. It should not be given in too large amounts, since it may produce vomiting. Iron is absorbed somewhat better when given between meals. An adequate response may be obtained when given with food if the child cannot tolerate iron therapy on an empty stomach. Although other iron preparations may be given, many have a smaller iron content, and therefore a larger dose must be given.

Some solutions containing iron should be well diluted and given to older children with a drinking tube or straw to prevent discoloration of the teeth by deposits of iron. The older child should rinse his mouth or brush his teeth after administration of the medication. The solution should be well diluted, and for infants given with a medicine dropper. Iron in pill form or some newer liquid iron preparations may be given without a straw because they have no effect on the teeth. Orange juice may be given with the medication.

Iron may be given parenterally, but this method is seldom used if the child can tolerate oral therapy. Some types of parenteral iron produce irritation at the site of the intramuscular injection and may cause systemic disturbances. The parenterally administered iron preparation of choice is iron dextran. Directions for giving this medication are explicit in the drug package insert and should be followed carefully. Staining of the skin may occur if it is given incorrectly.

Iron overloading or poisoning may occur if too much iron is given or if it is taken by accident. A young child who is attracted to the brightly colored iron tablets may swallow them and cause damage to the intestinal mucosa and a drop in blood pressure.

Blood transfusions are given if the child's condition is serious, especially if the infant has myocardial insufficiency. Repeated small transfusions of concentrated red blood cells are valuable.

Infants suffering from iron deficiency are usually irritable. Feedings must be given slowly. As the anemia improves, the infant's appetite for food other than milk will increase. The infant should receive no more than 1 pint of milk a day. This reduction of milk is likely to result in increased intake of iron-rich foods in the diet. Also, if the infant has gastrointestinal blood loss from intolerance to cow's milk pro-tein, the bleeding is reduced if the amount of milk taken is lowered. Because iron is a constipating medication, the child's diet should contain adequate amounts of roughage and fluids. Semisolid and solid foods can be introduced into the diet in the same manner as for younger children (see p. 369).

The infant must be protected from infection, particularly from nursing personnel who have respiratory infections, and clean technique must be used in his care.

Conferences with the parents are very important, since the prevention of further difficulties lies in the long-term care of the infant. The mother can be helped to manage her daily routine in order to assist her child in establishing a routine pattern of eating. Foods which contain iron are offered. The mother is also encouraged to give the medication until the physician discontinues it. She is told that her child's stools will become dark or black because of iron medication. Parents may become anxious at the color of the stools if they do not know the cause.

Prognosis. Generally the prognosis is good when iron, vitamins and an improved diet are given. Recovery usually takes place in four to six weeks, but treatment is continued for eight to 12 weeks longer. The prognosis is variable if the infant has a concurrent infection.

THALASSEMIA (MEDITERRANEAN ANEMIA, COOLEY'S ANEMIA)

Incidence, Pathology, and Types. Thalassemia is a chronic, congenital hemolytic anemia in which the chief defect seems to be an inability to produce cells capable of normal incorporation of hemoglobin. This condition occurs mainly in children whose parents or ancestors came from countries along the northern shore of the Mediterranean Sea, especially Italy, Sicily, or Greece. Cases occur, however, among blacks, Orientals, Europeans and Jews and their descendants.

The *pathology* is that of chronic microcytic, hypochromic anemia. The specific defect is production of cells of abnormal shape which are deficient in hemoglobin and are destroyed more quickly than normal cells would be. They are not capable of normal incorporation of hemoglobin. The hematopoietic tissue attempts to compensate for this defect by producing more fetal hemoglobin than is normal, but does not produce enough for the effective transportation of oxygen. Large numbers of immature and defective erythrocytes are rapidly destroyed.

There are two types of thalassemia, minor and major. Both are familial conditions.

Thalassemia minor occurs when the gene responsible for the defect is a heterozygous trait (see p. 216). The child with the minor form will show mild anemia, moderate hypochromia, and both anisocytosis and poikilocytosis (a condition in which cells are of unequal size and irregular in shape). Sometimes the spleen is enlarged. These children have no incapacitating symptoms, however, and are able to lead normal lives. Their condition is not likely to be recognized unless blood studies are carried out as part of a family survey.

Thalassemia major is transmitted when both parents have thalassemia minor. On the average, one quarter of their children may be homozygous for the trait of thalassemia major. Such children will have progressive, severe anemia not compatible with long life. This type of anemia responds only temporarily to transfusion therapy. The condition is easily recognized in early infancy because of the onset of a progressive, severe anemia.

Clinical Manifestations. THALASSEMIA MAJOR. Since anemia is not present at birth, the newborn never shows signs of the disease. Severe anemia may develop, however, in the first few months of life. The clinical manifestations are, in general, those of any severe anemia, but certain symptoms peculiar to the condition should be noted.

The infant has a decided pallor, especially of the mucous membranes, and mild jaundice, which later becomes a muddy, bronze color. The enlarged spleen of the young infant increases to an enormous size during childhood. This, with an enlarged liver, causes disabling abdominal distention, which may lead to cardiorespiratory distress and cardiac enlargement with the danger of cardiac failure. Lymphadenopathy occurs, and skeletal changes are noticeable. Not only the physician but also the mother observes the child's retarded physical development, poor posture, abdominal distention, and such skeletal changes as the mongoloid facies—due to the thickened membranous bones of the face and skull, often accompanied with protrusion of the teeth caused by overgrowth of the maxilla—and broad, heavy-appearing hands.

Diagnosis, Treatment, Course, and Prognosis. The *diagnosis* is made on roentgen examination. By the time the infant is one year old there are widening of the medullary spaces, thinning of the cortices and decrease in the size of the bony trabeculae (connective tissue beams which extend from a capsule into the enclosed substances). In older children roentgenograms of the skull show radiating bony trabeculae traversing the widened space, resulting in a hair-on-end appearance.

The laboratory findings show microcytic anemia in both forms of the condition. In thalassemia major there is a severe anemia, a low erythrocyte count and a low hemoglobin level. There is a rapid turnover of erythrocytes, with an elevated reticulocyte count and an increase in nucleated red blood cell precursors. Even in laboratory examination it is sometimes difficult to distinguish thalassemia from anemia of iron deficiency, other hemolytic anemias of infancy, or sickle cell disease. The finding of thalassemia minor in the parents aids in establishing the diagnosis.

There is no *treatment* for thalassemia minor. For thalassemia major frequent transfusions must be given to maintain the hemoglobin level above 40 per cent of normal (6 gm. per 100 ml.). The addition of sedimented cells will increase the efficiency of a transfusion and lessen the danger of cardiac embarrassment due to too much parenteral fluid. These children can live with a relatively low hemoglobin level.

One problem associated with repeated blood transfusions is that of transfusion hemosiderosis (hemochromatosis), or excessive deposition of iron in various tissues. Cardiac failure which may be secondary to myocardial siderosis is a serious problem and may be refractory to the usual treatment for this condition. Experimental attempts are being made to eliminate excessive stored iron through increased excretion via the kidneys by the use of chelating agents.

Aspirin with antihistaminic drugs may be effective as prophylaxis against transfusion reactions. If a severe reaction occurs, cortisone may be of some value. Splenectomy may be helpful, since it lessens the discomfort from the enormous spleen; it may also help to prolong the intervals between transfusions and produces more normal growth.

The parents must be encouraged to accept the child's condition with its poor prognosis, and shown how to give the child as normal a life as possible. As with all children with severe anemias, blood transfusions on a brief inpatient or an outpatient basis are preferable to repeated, prolonged hospitalization.

Thalassemia minor is a benign condition which does not interfere with normal growth and activity. The *prognosis* is therefore good. Since the trait is genetically transmitted, young people with this condition should be made aware of the danger involved if they marry a person with the same trait. Genetic counseling, then, is important for the parents, the patient himself, and potential carriers in the family.

In thalassemia major the earlier the onset and the more severe the symptoms, the more rapidly is the outcome fatal. From early infancy these children must depend upon transfusion therapy. As they grow older the need for transfusions becomes even greater. Growth is stunted, and activity is limited. There is constant danger of cardiac failure. Today more patients survive to adolescence than did in the past. If they do survive, there may be some lessening of the severity of the disease. Death may be due to the severe anemia, to progressive hepatic or cardiac involvement or to intercurrent infection.

SICKLE CELL DISEASE

Incidence, Types, and Pathology. Sickle cell disease is associated with an inherited defect in the synthesis of hemoglobin. It is confined almost exclusively to blacks and is seldom seen in whites. Sickle cell anemia occurs in approximately 1 of every 500 blacks in this country. Large sums of money are currently being used for research on the diagnosis and treatment of this condition, on genetic counseling, and on public education about sickle cell disease.

There are two types of the disease—the severe type and an asymptomatic condition. In the *severe* type there is a persistent hemolytic anemia with periodic episodes of painful crises. This severe condition occurs when the abnormality appears in homozygous form (inherited from both parents) (see p. 215). When the defect is heterozygous (inherited from only one parent), an *asymptomatic* condition is present—the *sickle cell trait* (see below). This is much more frequent among blacks in the United States than is the true disease. If both parents are heterozygous, in each pregnancy there is 1 chance in 4 that the child will have sickle cell disease, 1 chance in four that the child will be hematologically normal, and 2 chances in 4 that the child will have the sickle cell trait.

Pathologically, the hemoglobin in both forms is abnormal (hemoglobin S). Under reduced oxygen tension this hemoglobin is responsible for forming red blood cells into a sickled shape. In sickle cell disease these malformed cells clump together and obstruct capillaries, thereby causing what is known as a crisis in the disease. Capillary obstruction leads to anoxic changes which cause further sickling and thus still further obstruction in the blood vessels. Pain in the area results. Infarcts occur most often in the spleen, but may also occur in bones, kidneys, lungs, gastrointestinal tract, brain, and heart. The spleen may be so badly affected through removing blood cells from the circulation and by these infarcts that it may become fibrotic and may atrophy and finally disappear.

Clinical Manifestations. In children with sickle cell trait there are no clinical symptoms.

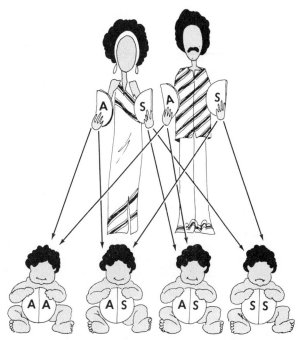

Parents who are carriers of the sickle cell trait do not show symptoms of the disease because hemoglobin A (the normal form of hemoglobin) in their red blood cells protects them from hemoglobin S (the sickling form). But when two carriers become parents, the possibilities are:

☐ One child in four will inherit all normal hemoglobin (AA) and thus be free of the disease.

☐ Two children in four will inherit both hemoglobin A and hemoglobin S (AS) and thus become carriers of the trait like their parents.

☐ One child in four will inherit all sickling hemoglobin (SS) and thus become a victim of sickle cell anemia.

FIGURE 15–13. How sickle cell disease is transmitted from parents to children. (Pearson, H. A.: Progress in Early Diagnosis of Sickle Cell Disease. *Children*, Vol. 18, No. 6, Nov.-Dec., 1971. p. 224.)

In sickle cell disease the onset may be as early as the second or third month of life, when normal fetal hemoglobin is replaced by the abnormal hemoglobin which causes sickling. Approximately half of all children affected by this condition have symptoms by one year of age.

The first clinical manifestation the infant may have is sickle cell *crisis.* This is an acute disturbance in which the infant has severe pain in the abdomen and legs. The abdominal wall may have a boardlike rigidity. The child may also have extreme pallor, fever, vomiting, and severe flank pain, with hematuria, convulsions, stiff neck, coma, or paralysis. Two to three days after the crisis, jaundice may appear. Between crises the manifestations are pallor and anemia. Icterus may be persistent.

Growth of a child with sickle cell disease is not stunted, but he may have long, thin extremities, a short trunk, barrel-shaped chest and protruding abdomen. If he is under nine years of age, the spleen may be palpable. There is cardiac enlargement, and murmurs are common.

Laboratory Findings and Diagnosis. Laboratory examination shows the sickle-shaped cells which are produced under low oxygen tension. This characteristic may be shown on smears of peripheral blood. If it is not seen on a smear, a drop of blood may be placed under a cover slip and sealed off from oxygen by petroleum jelly; if it is kept for one to 24 hours at room temperature, sickled forms of blood cells will appear. Recently a more rapid and equally accurate test tube method has been found that makes screening for this disease easier than it was in the past.

Children having the sickle cell trait can be distinguished from those having the disease. In sickle cell trait the red cell count and hemoglobin level are normal. In sickle cell disease the hemoglobin level ranges from 6 to 9 gm. per 100 ml.; in times of crisis it may fall lower. Each child stabilizes at his own level, and any increase in the level as a result of transfusion therapy is only temporary. The reticulocyte count is elevated to 5 or even 25 per cent, and is usually highest up to a week after a crisis as a result of new cell formation. The leukocyte count is elevated, but the platelets are usually normal in times of crisis.

Roentgenograms of the long bones, skull, feet, and hands show widened medullary spaces and thinning of the cortices.

The *diagnosis* of sickle cell disease is at times difficult to make, since other diseases may appear similar to it. This is especially true during crises when vascular occlusion occurs. Conditions which might be confused with sickle cell disease are thalassemia, syphilis, tuberculosis, osteomyelitis, rheumatic fever, and acute conditions of the abdomen.

Treatment, Responsibilities of the Nurse, Course, and Prognosis. *Treatment* consists of supportive measures such as blood transfusions when necessary, and protection against infection. Treatment during crises includes codeine and aspirin for relief of pain and maintenance of hydration. Antibiotic therapy may be necessary if a bacterial infection such as pneumonia or meningitis is present. Transfusion of erythrocytes may be required. Oxygen is given if the hemoglobin level falls rapidly to as low as 4 gm. per 100 ml. and the child has symptoms of hypoxia. Splenectomy usually has no value in sickle cell disease. In older children autosplenectomy may occur as a result of repeated thromboses.

Urea in invert sugar was advocated in the past for controlling sickle cell crisis. Recent research has shown that giving neither urea nor alkali was superior to giving invert sugar alone in shortening the episodes of crisis. Research on cyanates (sodium or potassium) for the treatment of sickle cell anemia showed significant neurotoxicity and other complications that contradict the use of these substances.

The *nursing care* of a child having sickle cell anemia includes assisting the physician with the treatments mentioned and helping other members of the health team to educate the parents and the child about the disease. The clinical manifestations of the disease such as fatigue, anorexia, pains in the abdomen or extremities, epistaxis, and jaundice can be explained to the parents so that they know when to bring the child to the hospital and when it is necessary only to call the physician for information. The parents need to know that the child should consume huge quantities of liquids, especially in summer, and should also have well balanced meals. They also need to know that the child should be treated immediately when infection occurs. Other children in the family should be tested to find those who may be similarly afflicted.

As with any hereditary condition, genetic counseling is necessary. The parents should also have the opportunity to discuss with members of the health team their feelings about this disease. This is essential to the nurse in helping the parents plan the care of the child.

The *course* depends upon the severity of the sickling tendency, the frequency of crises, and the age of the child. As the child grows older crises occur less frequently. In temperate regions crises occur more commonly in autumn and spring.

The *prognosis* depends on the severity of the disease. The condition may interfere to some extent with the child's growth, nutrition, and activity. The life expectancy of the small child is probably less than the average because of the physiologic handicap, but many of these children grow up to adult life and are able to earn a living. Death is usually the result of severe anemia or intercurrent infection.

ENDOCRINE DISORDERS

CRETINISM (CONGENITAL HYPOTHYROIDISM)

Etiology and Incidence. Cretinism is caused by a congenital insufficiency of the secretion of the thyroid gland due to an embryonic defect in which the gland is absent or rudimentary and unable to produce thyroid hormone. It is one of the most common endocrine diseases of child-

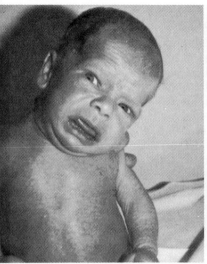 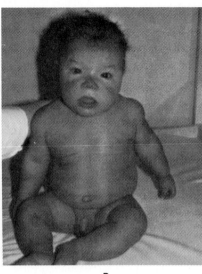 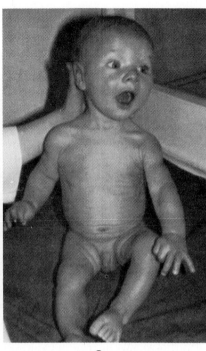

A   B   C

FIGURE 15–14. *A*, Two-month-old infant with hypothyroidism: coarse features, sparse hair, retracted root of nose, large tongue, pale yellow skin, sleepiness, poor drinking, decreased motion, hypothermia, hoarse crying. *B*, Hypothyroidism in a ten-month-old infant. Evident are typical myxedematous aspect, doughy swelling of subcutaneous tissue, shaggy hair, enlarged tongue, apathy, constipation, and hypothermia. *C*, Six weeks after commencing treatment with thyroid extract, the aspect and behavior of the infant shown in (*B*) have changed completely and appear normal. (From Moll, H.: *Atlas of Pediatric Diseases*, Philadelphia, W. B. Saunders Co., 1976.)

hood, occurring in 1 of every 6000 to 7000 births. The condition occurs sporadically in the United States. Cretinism is not to be confused with mongolism, which can be recognized at birth (see p. 308).

Clinical Manifestations and Diagnosis. The infant appears normal at birth, but *clinical manifestations* may appear in the first few weeks or months of life. There is a relationship between breastfeeding of newborns and congenital hypothyroidism. Breast milk provides sufficient thyroid hormone to compensate for the hormone deficiency in some infants and to protect them against neurologic problems and mental retardation. This protection lasts until the infant is weaned.

Early signs of the condition are prolonged physiologic jaundice and feeding difficulties. The infant is pale because of anemia. He is constipated, and an umbilical hernia develops, owing to hypotonic abdominal musculature. There is little perspiration, and the skin is dry and scaly. The child is lethargic, cries little, sleeps most of the time and has little appetite. His temperature is subnormal, his pulse slow. The facial appearance is peculiar, for the eyes are far apart, the bridge of the broad nose is flat, the eyelids are swollen, and the tongue protrudes from the open mouth. The anterior fon-

tanel is widely open because of poor bone development. Dentition is delayed, and the teeth decay rapidly.

The general appearance is abnormal: the arms and legs are short, the relatively large head is supported on a short, thick neck, and the hands are broad and the fingers short. The hair is coarse, brittle, and scanty. The hairline reaches down on the forehead. These infants have an early developmental lag. Bone development is retarded, and physical and motor development is slow. Mental development also is delayed. These children appear lethargic and are late in sitting, standing and walking. They do not learn to talk at the usual time, and sexual maturation is slower than that of the normal child.

They are dull, placid, good-natured babies. Parents who lack knowledge of this condition are often proud of their crying so little and being no trouble. When routine follow-up of newborn infants is neglected, a diagnosis is often not made until much valuable time for early treatment has passed.

Early *diagnosis* may be difficult, for the symptoms appear gradually as the child grows older. Roentgenograms show the retarded bone age in untreated cases; multiple foci of ossification appear in the epiphyses. The basal metabolic rate is decreased. The serum cholesterol level fluctuates, but in general is increased. The normal cholesterol level is 70 to 125 mg. per 100 ml. of serum; in the cretin it is from 250 to 600 mg. The serum phosphatase level is decreased, and the carotene level is many times increased.

A reliable measurement of thyroid function is the protein-bound iodine level of the serum. The values with cretinism are usually under 2 gammas per 100 ml. Another test of thyroid function is the uptake of radioactive iodine by the thyroid gland. In patients with cretinism a normal concentration in the thyroid is not obtained.

Treatment. If treatment is delayed, the infant may become more and more retarded in growth and mental development. The treatment (substitution therapy) is by oral administration of desiccated thyroid. The dose is usually small when the medication is started and is gradually increased to the maximum amount which can be given without producing symptoms of overdosage. This medication must be taken throughout life. The dose may have to be increased at puberty and during the reproductive period.

In addition, the infant should receive a complete diet with adequate amounts of vitamin D. Since thyroid stimulates bone growth, the child will outgrow his supply of vitamin D if additional amounts are not provided.

The anemia is a problem, since it does not respond readily to hematinics. Constipation, another troublesome symptom, is not easily relieved.

Responsibilities of the Nurse. The nurse should observe children being treated with desiccated thyroid for symptoms of overdosage, e.g., rapid pulse, loss in weight, vomiting, cramps, diarrhea, elevation of temperature, and personality changes such as increased excitability and irritability.

Because of the tendency for decay of the teeth, good dental care is provided early to preserve the temporary teeth. As soon as the child is able, he is taught to brush his teeth.

Since one of the main problems in these children is their slowness of mental development, neither the child's parents nor his nurses should attempt to push him beyond his capacity or compare his general development with that of normal children.

Prognosis. The prognosis in untreated cases is likely to be poor. Death may result early from an intercurrent infection, or the child may become a mentally retarded dwarf. If treatment is begun early and continued through life, the child may be normal physically, but probably somewhat mentally retarded (see p. 696). The earlier and more effective the treatment, the better the prognosis. Even with the best therapy,

however, mental development may never be normal.

INBORN ERRORS OF METABOLISM

PHENYLKETONURIA

Incidence, Etiology, and Clinical Manifestations. Phenylketonuria is not a common condition; it occurs in about 1 in every 10,000 births. The condition is equally common in males and females; the majority of affected infants are blue-eyed blonds.

The condition is due to a congenital defect in phenylalanine metabolism. Phenylalanine is an essential amino acid present in all natural protein foods. As the newborn takes in food the phenylalanine accumulates in the blood, and phenylketone bodies are excreted in the urine. The abnormal accumulation of phenylalanine apparently prevents normal brain development.

Phenylketonuria is transmitted by an autosomal recessive gene (see p. 216). The majority of affected infants are offspring of two heterozygous carriers of the gene. With each pregnancy the chance is one in four that the infant will be normal, two in four that he will be a carrier of the defect, and one in four that he will have phenylketonuria. But in some families more than this proportion of children or all the children may be born with this condition.

The *clinical manifestations* begin by about four months of age, when the mother may notice

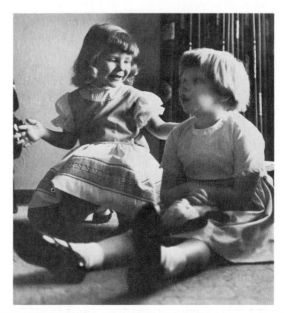

FIGURE 15–15. A comparison of a child having phenylketonuria (*right*) with her sister who has achieved dietary control of the same condition (*left*). (Courtesy of National Association for Retarded Children.)

that the infant has a peculiar odor and is not developing normally. Brain development is arrested, and mental retardation of varying degrees may result; hence the condition is sometimes called *phenylpyruvic oligophrenia.* Neurologic symptoms appear; the child may exhibit schizoid-like, disagreeable personality traits. Eczema or convulsions, or both, occur in about one fourth of these children.

Diagnosis. The diagnosis is made by a simple urine test for phenylketone bodies and by blood tests for phenylalanine. When the plasma phenylalanine level is above approximately 15 mg. per 100 ml., phenylketone bodies usually appear in the urine. The tests are not usually made until the first or second week of life, but are especially necessary on infants born into families with a known history of phenylketonuria or on infants who show signs of mental dullness. The same tests are used for diagnosis and for checking with dietary management. Mandatory laws concerning the testing of infants for phenylketonuria have been enacted in many states.

The *urine test* is made with ferric chloride. One cubic centimeter of urine is placed in a test tube, and 3 drops of a 5 or 10 per cent ferric chloride solution are added. If a green color appears, phenylketone bodies are present. (Phenistix can also be used to test urine.) Normal urine, used in the same combination with ferric chloride, remains yellow.

The *diaper test* is done in many Child Health Conferences (see p. 379), hospitals, and pediatricians' offices for early detection of the condition. A drop of 5 or 10 per cent ferric chloride solution on a recently wet diaper will turn it green if phenylketone bodies are present (a positive result is also obtained with histidinemia). If the urine is normal, it remains yellow. The diaper test should be repeated at intervals, since some children with phenylketonuria do not always give positive results.

For many years the diaper test was the universal method of detecting this disease; however, the screening procedure most prominent at present is the Guthrie test. This test, a simple screening test done on heel blood, can be used to screen newborns for phenylketonuria the day they are discharged from the nursery. Since the blood phenylalanine concentration rises after birth when the infant is given milk feedings, a second test for phenylketonuria should be performed at four to six weeks of age. The earlier the diagnosis can be made, the sooner treatment can be started and the better the prognosis will be. If these tests are not done until after signs of the condition make the physician suspicious, the child will already have suffered damage. Recently physicians have advocated screening programs for pregnant women who may have high phenylalanine levels which could lead to mental retardation in their newborns.

Treatment and Responsibilities of the Nurse. Since the clinical manifestations of phenylketonuria are due to accumulation of unmetabolized phenylalanine, the condition can be controlled by preventing phenylalanine intake from early infancy. Because all natural protein foods contain phenylalanine, Lofenalac (Mead Johnson), a synthetic food providing sufficient protein for growth and repair, yet containing very little phenylalanine, may be substituted. Other foods permitted in the diet include 1 per cent protein fruits and vegetables, tapioca, and cornstarch as cereals, sugar, and butter. Foods which must be omitted include breads, meat, fish, poultry, all types of flour, cheese, milk, nuts, and products made with nuts, eggs and legumes. A table of phenylalanine equivalents is available from Mead Johnson & Company, Evansville, Indiana. Management must be individualized on the basis of response to the therapy, as judged by urine and blood levels of phenylalanine, the level of physical and mental development and the relief of physical symptoms.

The nurse must be aware of the cost of the formula and of the meaning that food has to various cultural groups if she is to understand the reaction of parents to this drastic restriction of diet for their child. Understanding the dietary restriction and the abnormal eating habits may be more difficult than dietary management. Parents have difficulty controlling the diet of an ambulatory child. They are disturbed that usual foods eaten by the child instead of the special diet may result in mental retardation. Parents of such a child need continuous support and guidance from the nurse.

The nutritional status and hemoglobin level are determined frequently, since the infant is on a limited diet. Intelligence tests and other estimates of mental ability are important for infants who have been treated early, to determine the rate of mental growth.

These infants are observed for the onset of dermatologic or neurologic symptoms. Nurses stress in conferences with parents the importance of health checkups of the newborn so that the condition, if it exists, can be treated in the earliest stages. Continued therapy is expensive for the child's family, but they can obtain financial help through federal or state funds or through local health and welfare departments.

Prognosis. The prognosis is at best doubtful, but is far more favorable if a diet with a low phenylalanine content is begun in the early months of infancy. Once brain development has been retarded, the process cannot be reversed; it can only be arrested. If treatment is not given until the child is three years old, he may show improvement in personality and behavior, but not in mental status. Many physicians believe that if the child remains on this diet until he is four to six years old, most of the damage to the brain will be prevented. Termination of the dietary restrictions frequently improves the emotional climate of the family.

GALACTOSEMIA

Incidence, Etiology, Clinical Manifestations, and Diagnosis. Galactosemia represents an inborn error in the metabolism of galactose, a deficiency of galactose-1-phosphate uridyl transferase. It is not a common condition. The defect is transmitted as an autosomal recessive trait (see p. 216). The enzyme that changes galactose to glucose in the liver is missing. Galactose is not found in free form in foods; however, intestinal hydrolysis of lactose from milk products yields glucose and galactose. When the amount of galactose in the blood exceeds the ability of the renal tubules to reabsorb it, galactosuria results. These infants appear normal at birth, but galactosuria occurs one or two weeks later when the infant is taking his milk feeding.

Clinical manifestations at first include feeding difficulties, vomiting, and weight loss. Later, enlargement of the liver and spleen, hepatic failure, mental retardation, and cataracts are evident. Finally lethargy and emaciation increase, and death occurs from infection or hepatic failure.

Diagnosis is made on the basis of finding galactose in the blood and urine of these infants.

Treatment and Responsibilities of the Nurse. This defect must be found early and the infant taken off a diet containing milk before irreversible damage has been done to the brain and the liver. A galactose-free diet of milk substitutes containing casein hydrolysates does not raise the blood galactose level. Milk, milk products, and lactose-containing tablets must be eliminated from the child's diet. Cataracts, if present, require surgical treatment.

AGAMMAGLOBULINEMIA (BRUTON'S DISEASE)

Incidence, Etiology, Clinical Manifestations, and Diagnosis. Congenital agammaglobulinemia is a rare condition in which the child is unable to form gamma globulin (see p. 260). This disorder is transmitted by a sex-linked gene (see p. 217); therefore, it usually affects only boys, although the mother carries the abnormal gene and can transmit it to half of her daughters, who are not affected clinically.

Children having agammaglobulinemia cannot form antibodies against many bacterial antigens or to antigenic substances such as typhoid vaccine and diphtheria toxoid. They therefore have recurrent pyogenic infections, especially with staphylococci, streptococci, pneumococci, and meningococci. Their response to viral infections, however, is normal. Newborn infants acquire gamma globulin from their mothers late in gestation; therefore, infections may not occur until the child is approximately six months of age.

The *diagnosis* is made on the basis of a history of repeated infections, a persistently positive Schick test, or a negative Widal test result after usual immunization procedures have been done, a lack of lymphoid tissue, especially the adenoids, and a lack of gamma globulin in the blood.

Acquired agammaglobulinemia may appear later in life, but this condition is seen in both males and females.

Treatment and Responsibilities of the Nurse. The *treatment* of agammaglobulinemia consists in prevention of infection and immediate treatment of infections when they occur. The patient should receive monthly intramuscular injections of gamma globulin for the remainder of his life. Acute infections may respond to antimicrobial chemotherapy.

Grafts of immunologically competent cells obtained from the bone marrow of a donor have recently shown some success in reversing the course of this disease.

A mother, in an attempt to prevent her child from acquiring infections, may overprotect him. The nurse must help such a mother gain a more positive attitude toward her child's illness.

TAY-SACHS DISEASE (AMAUROTIC FAMILIAL IDIOCY)

Incidence and Etiology. Tay-Sachs disease is one of a group of cerebromacular degenerative disorders. It occurs most frequently among Jewish people originating from eastern Europe. This condition is one that shows autosomal recessive inheritance (see p. 216).

The cause is an absence of the enzyme hexosaminidase component A.

Pathology, Clinical Manifestations, and Diagnosis. The brain becomes atrophic and firm. Stores of lipid are found in the neurons.

The infant is apparently normal at birth. Usually at about six months of age the infant becomes listless, regresses in motor ability, has muscular weakness, and is unable to fix his eyes upon an object. By one year he is flaccid and fat. He has hyperactive reflexes, startles easily at the slightest stimulation, and is *blind*. This degenerative disease continues with muscular degeneration, spasticity, seizures, malnutrition, decerebrate posturing, dementia, and death.

The *diagnosis* can be made prenatally by amniocentesis (see p. 226) and an analysis of the embryonic tissue and fluid obtained. Thus an intrauterine diagnosis can be made and the parents can have a choice concerning the continuation of the pregnancy. Even before the child-bearing period a simple blood test can identify adults who carry the defective gene, but are themselves unaffected by it. Recently research has shown that the enzyme hexosaminidase A, which is absent in Tay-Sachs disease, can be measured in human tears. Adult carriers of the defective genes have low levels of this enzyme.

The diagnosis can also be made after birth when macular cherry-red spots surrounded by a gray-white edematous retina are seen in the fundi of the eyes. Optic atrophy is also noted. Blood and cerebrospinal fluid values usually remain normal.

Treatment, Responsibilities of the Nurse, Prognosis, and Prevention. No treatment is known. The family must be informed of the likely clinical course. They are informed of facilities available in their community for assistance with the child. Genetic counseling about future children is made available to them.

The aim of *nursing care* is to give the child as much comfort as possible. Stimuli are reduced to a minimum, for the child startles easily. Nutrition is maintained by whatever means are possible, including gavage eventually.

The child's emaciated condition necessitates good skin care. He is turned frequently to prevent breakdown of the skin and to lessen the danger of pneumonia. Since the child is blind, the nurse should speak before touching him so as not to startle him.

The gradual deterioration of the child's condition is hard for the parents to bear. They need much understanding and emotional support, particularly since they know that his condition is hereditary. Since it is due to a recessive trait, both parents share the feeling of responsibility for the disease. The rabbi may be a source of comfort and emotional support, but the parents will turn to the physician and the nurse to express their grief at the continued degeneration of the child's condition.

The *prognosis* is hopeless. Death usually occurs before the third or fourth birthday.

The *prevention* of the birth of an infant having Tay-Sachs disease is important. Genetic counseling of the prospective parents or parents of such an infant is essential.

SKIN CONDITIONS

INFANTILE ECZEMA (ATOPIC DERMATITIS)

Incidence. Many different unrelated inflammatory dermatoses may be grouped under the term of "eczema." Here, however, eczema is considered to be an atopic manifestation of a specific allergen, whether ingested or in contact with the skin. Eczema is a common inflammatory skin condition of infants. It is the most frequent evidence of an allergic state seen in infancy. Seborrhea or diaper rash may be frequently associated with infantile eczema.

Eczema is most frequent in the first two years of life. It is uncommon in breastfed infants, but not in infants two or three months old, whether bottlefed or breastfed, who get some additional solid food. Eczema is relatively uncommon after the second year.

An infant, even one well cared for, may receive antigens through contact or by inhalation.

Eczema occurs in both sexes, in any race and at any time of the year. It is most likely, however, to appear in the winter months and to clear up in the summer. It is most frequent in well-nourished, fat infants whose general health is excellent.

Etiology. Several factors may be responsible for the condition. There is a decided familial tendency. Anatomically and chemically, the skin of an infant differs from that of an adult. The infant is likely to show greater response to scratching and to other irritants. His skin has a higher water and sodium chloride content than that of the adult. These attributes are exaggerated in the skin of an infant with eczema. His skin may be abnormally sensitive to irritation from clothes, wool garments, soaps, cold, strong sunlight, or mild skin infections. Some physicians believe that overfeeding, especially of carbohydrates or fat, may have an adverse effect on infants prone to eczema. It is difficult to prove this, although eczema in obese infants has improved when they lost weight as a result of dietary restriction of fat and carbohydrate.

Although there is general agreement that infantile eczema is due largely to allergy, it is difficult to show specific causes for the sensitivity. The most common allergies are due to various foods, e.g., egg white, cow's milk, wheat cereal, and oranges.

Some investigators believe that there is a disturbance in the mother-child relations among infants and children who have eczema. Such children are smothered with love by their parents.

Pathology, Clinical Manifestations, and Diagnosis. *Pathologically,* the capillaries of the skin dilate, thereby producing erythema and edema. Fluid escapes from the capillaries into the tissues. Papules and then vesicles form. These rupture and exude yellow, sticky material, which dries and forms crusts on the skin (see Plate 1, Fig. 5. The infant scratches, and excoriation of the skin results. Mild and severe lesions may exist at the same time on different parts of the body. The skin becomes thickened, and fissures form. Itching is usually intense, and secondary infection results from scratching the lesions. The regional lymph nodes swell in the area. The cervical lymph nodes may swell if there is an infection of the scalp.

The eczema has periods of exacerbation and remission which are discouraging to the mother, who hopes for steady improvement. Eczema most commonly occurs on the cheeks, forehead and scalp, and less frequently behind the ears, on the neck and on the flexor surfaces of the arms and legs. There may be lesions on the trunk, abdomen and back, but these are usually drier and more scaly than elsewhere. The palms of the hands and the soles of the feet are not involved, though the rest of the body may be.

Because of the constant and intense itching the infant may not be able to sleep and may be highly irritable. If the lesions become infected, he may have a low-grade fever. Although most infants with eczema are overweight, malnutrition may be present if an infant has anorexia, dietary restrictions, a chronic infection, or diarrhea.

Eczematous lesions may flare up after prophylactic immunizations. These infants should not be given smallpox vaccination for any reason such as travel because of the possible development of generalized vaccinia (see p. 382). This condition might also occur if the infant were to come in contact with any child who was recently vaccinated. Such contacts should be carefully avoided.

The *diagnosis* is made on the characteristics and distribution of the eruption, the family history, symptoms of severe itching, demonstration of protein sensitivity, and a tendency to improve in summer.

Treatment and Responsibilities of the Nurse. Even the most intensive *treatment* may not produce a cure, but most infants can be helped by therapy.

The parents are instructed as to the course to be expected, the treatment, and the nursing care. They should understand that these infants are prone to infections of the skin and the respiratory tract and that they should be treated at home if at all possible because of the danger of infection in the hospital. Hospitalization may be necessary if the infant already has a secondary infection or if he requires more intensive care and local treatment than the mother can provide. Sometimes there is less external irritation in the hospital environment, and the infant can be kept on a stricter dietary regimen. If the parents are exhausted because of caring for the infant, he may be hospitalized for their sake as well as his own.

If hospitalization is necessary, the infant is isolated for his own protection from infection. These infants are uncomfortable and need mothering. If possible, the parents should visit frequently, and the nurses should give these infants extra attention.

Restraints are important in local treatment, but are applied only when necessary to prevent scratching. These infants scratch their irritated skin instead of crying when they are angry or frustrated. The nurse can help the infant to express his feelings outwardly by encouraging active play or physical movement. Restraints are necessary, of course, when the mother or nurse cannot be with him constantly.

There are many kinds of restraints, and their use depends on the specific type needed. The following are self-explanatory: elbow cuff, abdominal, jacket, face mask, and ankle and wrist restraints.* Any needed combination of restraints may be used, but they must be checked frequently to determine whether they are constricting the circulation. Cotton socks may be put over the hands and feet after the fingernails and toenails have been cut as short as possible to prevent the infant from digging his skin.

Care must be taken to apply the restraints securely but gently. They are removed every few hours to allow free movement. If the infant is extremely uncomfortable because of itching, restraints should be removed from only one extremity at a time so that the nurse or mother can easily prevent him from scratching uncontrollably. If he has a paroxysm of scratching, the improvement of several weeks may be undone, and the skin may be opened to infection.

The infant should be picked up frequently and his position changed as often as possible to prevent respiratory infections, especially pneumonia. He may have supervised periods of play out of his crib to minimize his anger at being restrained and to give him opportunity to learn about his surroundings if he is old enough to walk.

---

*An effective elbow-cuff restraint for an infant may be made with tongue blades inserted into a stitched muslin restraint. This restraint may be secured in place by turning the end of a long-sleeved shirt back over the restraint and pinning it securely (see Fig. 12–2).

To prevent irritation of the skin caused by rubbing against the sheet, heavy plastic sheeting may be placed over the cotton sheet so that the infant can be turned from side to side and lie upon his back without increasing the severity of the lesions. This will also prevent absorption of ointment by the bedclothes. If the parents cannot afford new plastic sheeting, an old pliable plastic table cover can be used. In the hospital large pieces of exposed and washed x-ray film—the sharp edges covered with adhesive tape—may be used beneath the infant's head.

The infant may be bathed in water if it does not irritate his skin. In general it is better not to use soap; a substitute containing hexachlorophene (see p. 163) may be used if it is ordered by the physician. Oil baths may be ordered if both soap and this substitute are irritating to the skin. Oil is applied with a piece of cotton and patted rather than rubbed on. The crusted areas may be soaked with mild antiseptic solution compresses. Saline soaks kept continuously wet for one or two days may be helpful in removing crusts. If large areas are covered with papulovesicles, a soluble starch and sodium bicarbonate bath may be ordered. The water for the bath should have a temperature of 95° F. (35° C.), and the soak should be continued for 15 to 20 minutes. Floating toys may be used to divert the infant's attention. Although the bath is comforting to the irritated skin, the infant may attempt to scratch his body. During the bath only one extremity may be removed from restraint at a time; if both his arms were free, his nurse or mother would be unable to control him.

It is not advisable to take the infant outdoors if the weather is cold or if there is a strong wind. His clothing indoors should be such that he is sufficiently warm, but not overheated. No woolen garments should be used, since he may be sensitive to wool. Diapers are changed promptly to avoid irritation of the buttocks.

The infant is held for his feedings in the same way that healthy infants are held. He needs love for his emotional growth. Holding him will tend to change his position and prevent respiratory difficulties. Allowing him to suck on a nipple or a pacifier provides relaxation and reduces tension during the first year of life.

Local medication applied to the irritated skin is important. Since different kinds of lesions may be present on different areas of the body at the same time, different medications and treatments may be ordered for the various areas. Ointments are not used for weeping areas. On indurated areas the ointment is thoroughly rubbed into the skin. Whatever ointment or lotion the physician has ordered is kept on the skin in a thin layer constantly and applied with long, soothing strokes.

Many kinds of ointments and lotions have been used in the treatment of eczema. It is difficult to apply ointment to the skin of the face so as to be effective, because crusts are usually present. Crusts may be removed by wiping with gauze soaked with liquid petrolatum or by applying saline compresses constantly for one or two days. If an ointment is to be applied to the face, a mask made of gauze or stockinet may be used to keep the medication in close contact with the skin.

To make a face mask, holes are cut in the material to correspond in shape and location to the eyes, nose and mouth. The holes are stitched so that the edges cannot fray. The mask is secured in place on the infant's head by drawstrings. In applying it care must be taken to avoid binding or friction which would irritate the lesions.

If infection has occurred, various lotions or ointments may be used which contain bacitracin, bacitracin with neomycin, or other antibiotics.

If the skin surface is dry, red, and papular, an ointment containing crude coal tar may be ordered. The ointment should be applied as often as necessary to keep the area covered. Before its application, a small area is treated with it to determine the infant's sensitivity to it. All areas treated with tar ointment are constantly bandaged, and uncovered only when new ointment is to be applied. Every day all the ointment is removed with liquid petrolatum, and fresh ointment is applied. A starch bath may be used to remove ointment from large areas of the body covered with papulovesicles.

In teaching parents to use tar ointment the nurse emphasizes that it must be kept in a tightly covered jar to prevent evaporation of volatile ingredients. Stains on linen can be removed by rubbing both sides of the soiled area with lard and washing with soap and water. The parents are also told not to expose the infant to sunlight, since tar ointment contains a photosensitizing fraction that will produce further skin irritation. After the papules and the intense itching have disappeared the tar ointment is often discontinued, and a milder medication such as petrolatum or zinc oxide is used.

Many infants improve under these local applications, but if there is no improvement, further measures must be taken. Treatment involves a search for the specific allergens which cause the condition. Whether these are foods, wool, or inhalants such as dust, they should be removed. Wool should be removed from the child's environment. Neither his clothing nor his blankets should be of wool, and adults caring for him should not wear wool. The area about the crib should be kept free from dust. Carpets and drapes harbor dust and should not be used in his room.

A careful history or an elimination diet can be used to determine allergenic foods. If the infant is on an elimination diet, his mother is given a list of foods he may have rather than a list of foods to be avoided. She should adhere strictly to the diet ordered. Synthetic vitamins may be given to supplement the diet. The diet is increased so as to be as complete as possible. When a new food is added, the mother or nurse should watch for an allergic reaction to it. Such foods and reactions are noted for the physician's consideration.

Skin testing as a means of finding allergenic substances is not very helpful in young infants or in children who have eczematous lesions covering their bodies. It is used with older children.

Many infants with eczema are allergic to cow's milk. Substitutes for this must therefore be provided in their formulas. Some infants can tolerate cow's milk if it has been exposed to a high temperature, thereby altering its protein so that it is less allergenic. For this reason evaporated or dried milk is of great value in the treatment of such children.

Infants sensitive to cow's milk in any form may be given goat's milk, vegetable protein substitutes, formulas made from meat, or products made from hydrolyzed casein. Vegetable protein substitutes, largely made of soybeans, are available commercially in liquid or powdered form. With any substitute formula vitamins C and D, as well as other essentials, must be included in the diet.

Various nonspecific treatments may be ordered. Measures which produce mild dehydration are helpful in the treatment of eczema. If a lowered sodium intake is ordered, water retention may be decreased.

Corticosteroids may be given systemically as well as locally to produce relief in severe cases, and are useful in controlling inflammatory skin reactions. Antibiotic therapy by oral or parenteral administration is essential if infection of the skin or other parts of the body is present. Mild sedation may be necessary if the infant is unable to sleep.

Charting is important and includes the condition of the skin (changes in the appearance and location of the rash and the general appearance of the infected areas), reaction to food (both the articles added to the diet and the formula), treatments given, additional allergic manifestations such as asthma and rhinitis, the amount of discomfort caused by itching of the skin, and alteration in personality characteristics.

The psychologic aspect of nursing is as important as the physical aspect. These infants should receive as much attention and affection as normal infants, if not more. Although their appearance may not encourage the nurse to handle, fondle and play with them, they need loving care to prevent emotional deprivation. A gown or a coverall apron may be worn over the clothing of the nurse or the mother in order to protect it from contact with ointment on the child's skin.

Toys suited to the child's age are provided. The toys must be washable, safe, and soft (if possible) and have a smooth surface. Stuffed toys which contain substances such as wool, feathers, or kapok, to which children may be allergic, should not be used.

The nurse should understand the needs of the parents. Some mothers feel that they have failed to fulfill their maternal role, some are overprotective toward the infants, and others are afraid that their infants have a chronic condition which will result in disfiguring scars and retarded development. The nurse should help each mother to verbalize her feelings about the infant and the care he will need. Helping the mother to overcome her fears about her child while he is in the hospital will ensure better care for him at home.

The nurse must instruct the parents in the methods of local therapy and the diet to be given the infant. The nurse demonstrates the ways of applying restraints and providing exercise and diversion for the child. The nurse helps the parents find ways of giving adequate compensation for the kissing and skin-to-skin contact which other infants enjoy and of providing a happy environment in which the infant can lead as normal a life as is compatible with the necessary restraint of his hands and with local applications of ointments. The child should be permitted to move around his crib, playpen, or room and feel that he is part of the family group. Normal activity and satisfactions are necessary so that he will not feel frustrated by the discomfort of his itching skin. The mother should have an opportunity to care for him in the hospital with the help of the nurses. This will reduce her fears about caring for him after his discharge.

Prognosis. The prognosis is good, but the course is long-drawn out, with remissions and exacerbations. Parents are likely to become discouraged, especially if they have tried their best to care for the child. The nurse must help them to see the situation realistically and without unwarranted anxiety over the child's evident discomfort. Infantile eczema usually clears up spontaneously toward the end of the second year of life. The condition can be controlled earlier if the causative allergens are eliminated. After two years the child may exhibit other allergic manifestations such as asthma and hay fever.

If infection develops during hospitalization of the infant, the prognosis may be poor, but will depend upon the severity of the condition. To prevent this danger these infants should spend as little time as possible in the hospital.

DISORDERS OF THE NERVOUS SYSTEM

Tests used in the diagnosis of conditions of the central nervous system were described in Chapter 12 (see p. 293). The student will find that an understanding of these tests will prove helpful in the discussions of some of the following conditions.

TETANY

Tetany is extreme irritability of the neuromuscular system. It may be caused by any one of a number of conditions. These may be divided into those characterized by a decrease in serum calcium (hypocalcemic tetany) and those in which a state of alkalosis exists (tetany of alkalosis).

Symptoms of *hypocalcemic tetany* occur when the total serum calcium concentration falls below 7 to 7.5 mg. per 100 ml. (normal serum calcium is from 10 to 12 mg.). In tetany of the newborn, i.e., in the first week of life, there is hypocalcemia due to hypofunction of the parathyroid glands. Hypocalcemia also occurs in vitamin D deficiency associated with rickets and is termed infantile nutritional tetany (see p. 442). In celiac disease tetany results because of deficient absorption of vitamin D and calcium (see p. 452).

Tetany of alkalosis occurs when the acid-base balance is shifted to an alkaline level. It is not associated with changes in the serum level of calcium and phosphorus. It occurs with hyperventilation (excessive breathing) and in gastric tetany due to excessive vomiting and the concomitant loss of chloride. It may be observed in pyloric stenosis (see p. 418) or in high intestinal obstruction which causes vomiting.

CONVULSIONS

A convulsion is associated with a paroxysmal burst of electrical activity within the central nervous system which may be detected by the electroencephalogram. The occurrence of a convulsion is suggestive of a cerebral insult.

Incidence and Etiology. A convulsion may be termed a symptom of a disease rather than a disease entity. Convulsive disorders are far more common during infancy and the second year of life than in any other age period.

Convulsions during early childhood are due to a variety of conditions, any of which may affect the nervous system.

In the newborn, birth injury, a congenital defect of the brain, and the effects of anoxia and intracranial hemorrhage are the most frequent causes of convulsions. During later infancy and early childhood acute infections of the central nervous system or other parts of the body, with accompanying elevation of temperature, are the most common causes. Less frequent causes are tetany (see p. 442), pertussis immunization (see p. 380), hypoglycemia (see p. 279), poisoning by a convulsive drug or by lead (see p. 576), asphyxia, fluid and electrolyte imbalance, progressive degenerative diseases, and postnatal intracranial trauma (see p. 475). During later childhood febrile convulsions are infrequent, but convulsions due to idiopathic epilepsy (see p. 692), cerebral damage (see p. 789), brain tumors (see p. 791), and glomerulonephritis (see p. 658) may occur.

Responsibilities of the Nurse. Though children rarely die in convulsions, few other conditions frighten parents to the same extent. The nurse must be understanding of their fear and help them to a realistic attitude toward the child's condition. They should be told that though 7 infants in every 100 have a convulsion, few of them suffer permanent damage. In the remaining cases the condition is indicative of some deep-seated pathologic state.

The nurse places the child who has had a convulsion or in whom a convulsion may occur where continuous observation is possible. The nurse should observe the child frequently so that, if he has a convulsion, care can be given and an accurate report can be made to the physician.

A young child may show changes in behavior indicating the onset of a convulsion, such as irritability, restlessness, or the reverse, listlessness. Such changes are charted with the report of the convulsion. The nurse notes the kinds of movement and whether they are clonic (i.e., twitching, jerking movements) or tonic convulsions (those in which the child becomes stiff and the muscles are in a state of constant contraction), the time the convulsion begins and ends, the areas of the body involved, the amount of perspiration, movements of the eyes and change in size of the pupils, incontinence (this will be influenced not only by the severity of the seizure, but also by the distention of the bladder at the time of the convulsion), the rate of respiration, color, bodily posture, foaming at the mouth due to inability to swallow saliva, vomiting, the apparent degree of consciousness during the seizure, and the infant's behavior after his return to consciousness.

Children whose convulsions are not well conrolled by their medications may need to wear a protective helmet during hospitalization and at home as well. Since the helmet sets them apart because they look different, other children may make cruel remarks about them. This may produce emotional problems caused by isolation from other children.

SEIZURE PRECAUTIONS. The patient must be protected from injury. All hard toys should be removed from the bed, since he might be injured if he fell upon them. A padded tongue depressor should be kept on the bedside stand or taped to the bed to put between the teeth to prevent his biting his tongue. Care should be taken when inserting the tongue depressor to prevent injuring the child's mouth. The sides of the crib are padded if he has had a convulsion recently or is likely to have one. Padding of the crib sides reduces the child's field of vision. The padding is removed as soon as possible so that the child does not feel isolated and is not deprived of sensory stimulation. If the child has repeated convulsions, there should be in readiness an aspirating machine with which to remove accumulated secretions from the nasopharynx, and an emergency oxygen setup in case he has sudden respiratory difficulty.

FEBRILE CONVULSIONS

Incidence and Diagnosis. About 7 per cent of all infants and children have febrile convulsions between six months and two or three years of age. After seven years of age convulsions due to elevation of temperature are usually rare. Males are more affected than females, and there appears to be an increased incidence of febrile convulsions in some families.

Diagnosis of febrile convulsions involves diagnosis of the disease of which fever is a symptom. Most convulsions occurring between six and 12 months of age and in early childhood are initial symptoms of an acute febrile disease. A convulsion in this situation is equivalent to a chill experienced by an adult under the same conditions. Any young child who has a febrile convulsion, however, should be examined to eliminate the possibility of other causative factors.

In order to rule out other factors and to be certain of the cause, a careful history of previous convulsive episodes and illnesses and a com-

plete physical examination, including a neurologic appraisal, should be obtained. Laboratory examination for calcium, inorganic phosphorus and electrolytes in the blood serum and for sugar and urea nitrogen in the whole blood will aid in the diagnosis. If the convulsion is due to fever, the physician will determine whether the infection is intracranial or extracranial and what the specific problem is.

Treatment, Responsibilities of the Nurse, and Prognosis. *Treatment* and *nursing care* are aimed at direct control of the seizures by sedatives such as phenobarbital sodium, the dose depending on the age and size of the patient, and control of the systemic conditions causing the convulsion. Phenobarbital may be continued for a two-year period or longer and then discontinued gradually. Therapy includes antipyretic drugs and measures to reduce the body temperature, such as aspirin and tepid sponge baths; anti-infectious therapy, depending on the organism responsible for the illness; aspiration if the nasopharyngeal secretions are excessive; and oxygen inhalation if the patient is cyanotic.

In addition, the child is offered increased fluids if his condition permits. Medications are given as ordered. He is dressed in as little clothing as possible in a comfortable environment.

The procedure for a tepid sponge bath is as follows.

The water should be tepid.* Long, soothing strokes with a washcloth should follow the course of the large blood vessels of the trunk and extremities. In sponging the extremities the stroke is from the neck to the axilla and down to the palms of the hands, and from the groin to the feet. Gentle friction is used to bring the blood to the surface. Moist cloths should be placed over the superficial blood vessels in the axillae and the groins. A warm water bottle is put to the feet to prevent a feeling of chilliness. This may not be practical with an active infant, but is generally used with an older child. An ice bag is applied to the head for greater comfort.

A sponge bath for an elevation of temperature can be more disturbing to the child than the illness itself. Substitutes for this procedure could be the use of a cold water mattress, or a tepid bath while gradually cooling the water.

If the small child is conscious and refuses to lie down, the nurse may cover herself with a plastic apron and sponge the child in her lap. If he is old enough, he may participate in sponging himself.

---

*Alcohol is added only if it is ordered. Isopropyl alcohol is absorbed by inhalation and may cause coma in a child if the room is not ventilated adequately.

Further nursing care is the same as that for convulsions in general (see p. 473).

The *prognosis* depends upon the cause of the convulsion. A single febrile seizure is not indicative of a later chronic epilepsy, but repeated febrile convulsions increase the probability of subsequent nonfebrile convulsions.

SUBDURAL HEMATOMA

Etiology and Incidence. A subdural hematoma is a collection of blood and fluid within the potential subdural space between the tough dura mater, which lines the inner surface of the skull, and the arachnoid. It may be acute, subacute or chronic. The chronic form is generally seen during infancy. The cause is trauma to the head, either extensive molding at birth or injury after birth. The condition is most frequent in infants who have not received adequate care or have been more often exposed to trauma; it may also be seen in infants who have bleeding tendencies as in purpuric states. If the infant has scurvy, the possibility of subdural hematoma following injury is increased. Meningitis may also cause subdural collections.

Subdural hematomas are not rare. They are more common in males than in females and generally appear between the second and fourth months. The *incidence* decreases thereafter to 14 to 16 months, after which the condition is less common. In about 80 per cent of cases it occurs bilaterally.

Pathology, Clinical Manifestations, and Diagnosis. At the time of the injury the delicate subdural veins are torn, and small hemorrhages occur in the subdural space. Fluid collects, and a sac forms in the subdural space between the dura and the arachnoid layers of the meninges. The sac enlarges with further accumulation of fluid and contains a mixture of old and fresh blood and xanthochromic fluid. The brain beneath the sac becomes compressed, and brain atrophy and clinical signs develop. In the long-standing subdural hematoma the fluid may disappear, leaving a constricting membrane that prevents normal brain growth.

Clinical manifestations are varied. In the *acute* subdural hematoma, usually following trauma, there may be a rapid onset of signs of increased intracranial pressure previously described. In the *chronic* form the manifestations may have an insidious onset. The mother states that the child had anorexia, irritability, restlessness, vomiting, or convulsions. The child who fails to thrive and attain normal developmental milestones may also have a chronic subdural hematoma.

Other signs such as recurrent fever, irritability, changes in reflexes, bulging and tense fontanels, enlarged head, and possibly abnormal eyegrounds may be present when the parents are interviewed. The degree to which these signs are present is important. The sutures may be separated. The infant may have anemia due to loss of blood. The cerebrospinal fluid pressure is increased, and the fluid may contain increased numbers of blood cells and an increased amount of protein. On subdural puncture, a greater than normal amount of fluid can be obtained.

The *diagnosis* is frequently difficult because of the insidious onset of the signs and symptoms and is best made by bilateral subdural taps. In infants this procedure is easily done by inserting the needle in the lateral corner of the fontanel or farther out through the suture line. In older children burr holes must be made through the skull before the needle can be inserted. Computerized axial tomography (CAT scan) is also used in the diagnosis of subdural hematomas.

Treatment and Prognosis. Subdural hematoma is usually treated by a neurosurgeon. The aim of *treatment* is to remove abnormal fluid and the membrane which forms the sac. The three methods of treating a subdural hematoma include repeated subdural taps until dry or the amount of remaining fluid is not clinically significant, subdural shunts such as those used in

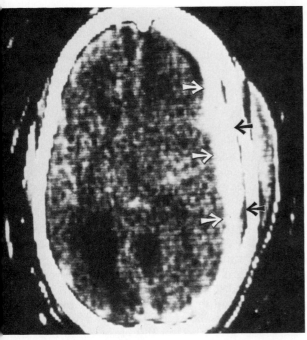

FIGURE 15–16. Subdural hematoma is demonstrated by a CAT scan. There is a large subdural collection of blood (*arrows*) over the surface of the right cerebral hemisphere. (From Gold, A. P., and Carter, S.: *Pediatr. Clin. N. Am.*, 23: 425, August 1976.)

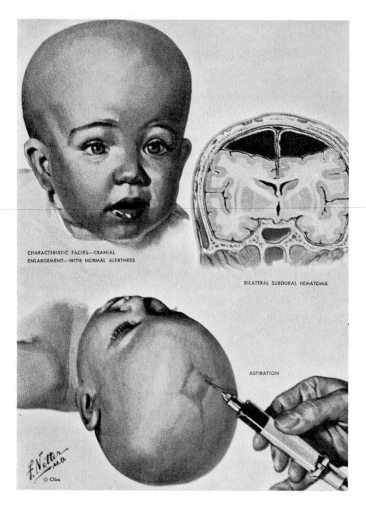

CHARACTERISTIC FACIES—CRANIAL
ENLARGEMENT—WITH NORMAL ALERTNESS

BILATERAL SUBDURAL HEMATOMA

ASPIRATION

FIGURE 15–17. Subdural hematoma. (Copyright, The Ciba Collection of Medical Illustrations, by Frank H. Netter, M.D.)

the treatment of hydrocephalus (see p. 303), and an excision of the membrane by craniotomy. If the hematoma is bilateral, cranotomies are performed at intervals of several days. In some instances aspiration of fluid must be continued or a shunting procedure may be necessary even after craniotomy.

Transfusions are given to correct the anemia. If scurvy is the cause of the condition, vitamin C is administered. Infection is treated with appropriate antibiotics.

The *prognosis* may be determined by the appearance of the brain at craniotomy. If the brain is severely atrophied, the prognosis is poor. After removal there is often a remarkable clinical improvement. The mortality rate varies because of underlying brain damage.

Responsibilities of the Nurse. One of the most important nursing responsibilities is that of early recognition and prompt treatment of the young child suffering from subdural hematoma, so that the brain will be able to grow normally. If the infant does not receive treatment early, the brain will be damaged, and mental retardation will result.

The infant is placed on a sponge rubber mattress and turned frequently to prevent pressure areas on the skin. The physician or nurse who assists in withdrawal of subdural fluid should shave the anterior portion of the child's scalp and cleanse it thoroughly. The nurse should hold the infant securely to avoid injury caused by a sudden movement.

After a subdural tap or a craniotomy the nurse observes the dressing for drainage. If drainage seeps through, the dressing is reinforced to prevent organisms from gaining entrance to the wound, and the physician is notified at once. The nurse differentiates between serous drainage and frank hemorrhage and observes the infant for signs of increased intracranial pressure.

Someone must stay with the infant to prevent his attempting to pull the head dressings off, or else his hands must be restrained with elbow cuffs (see Fig. 12–2) or the clove hitch restraint (see Fig. 11–17). Before applying restraints, every effort should be made to quiet him, since restraints make him more restless and increase intracranial pressure. For more detailed care of the postoperative patient see Chapter 24.

NEUROBLASTOMA

Etiology and Incidence. Neuroblastoma is an embryonal malignant tumor arising from the immature cells of the sympathetic nervous system. The adrenal gland is the most common site of the tumor. Neuroblastomas are probably, next to brain tumors, the most common of all solid tumors in children.

Pathology, Symptoms, Treatment, and Prognosis. *Pathologically,* neuroblastomas are hard, nodular, nonencapsulated tumors which invade adjacent tissues. This condition is often diagnosed late because the symptoms are general. *Symptoms* such as weight loss or lack of gain, abdominal pain, and feeding problems may be due to many causes. Other indications of this condition may be exophthalmos or swelling of the abdomen. The diagnosis is made on the basis of the history, physical examination, and possibly a skeletal survey.

Because of its invasion of other tissues and because it disseminates through blood vascular channels to the liver, skin, and bones, complete surgical removal is difficult and local recurrences are common, as are distant metastases. These tumors may, however spontaneously regress after therapy by surgery, radiation or chemotherapy. Chemotherapeutic drugs include cyclophosphamide (Cytoxan) and vincristine.

In general, children having neuroblastoma have a poorer *prognosis* than those with Wilms' tumor (see p. 311), although they may have spontaneous remissions or spontaneous maturation for unknown reasons.

Responsibilities of the Nurse. The role of the community nurse visiting in the home is largely one of case finding and referral. The nursing care of these children in the hospital is supportive. The nurse, of course, assists with diagnostic tests and gives preoperative and postoperative nursing care. Since the prognosis of many of these children is poor, the nurse may find it helpful to review her role in the support of parents whose young children are facing death (see p. 109).

FAMILIAL DYSAUTONOMIA (RILEY-DAY SYNDROME)

Incidence, Etiology, and Clinical Manifestations. Familial dysautonomia is transmitted to children of both sexes as a simple recessive gene and is most common in Ashkenazi Jews. It is a genetically determined disturbance in autonomic and peripheral sensory functions.

Neuropathologic findings are mostly confined to the peripheral sensory system. The infant's taste buds (fungiform papillae) on the tongue are absent or decreased in number, leading to an absence of the sensation of taste. In addition, the infant may not be able to feel pain. Swallowing movements are poorly coordinated, and as a result, gagging, vomiting, and aspiration of food occurs. Excessive bronchial secretions and repeated aspiration result in pulmonary infection and eventual chronic pulmonary failure.

Autonomic disturbances result in excessive salivation and sweating, decrease or absence of tears, blotching of the skin, urinary incontinence, variable hypertension and hypotension, and faulty temperature regulation.

The problems that arise in association with this condition consist of repeated skin trauma and asymptomatic fractures, due to an absence of pain, and corneal ulcerations, due to a defect in tear formation.

The central nervous system is usually affected and is seen in the infant as possible mental retardation, clumsiness, and lack of emotional stability.

The *etiology* of this condition is not known, but various theories have been advanced. The three tests used to determine the diagnosis are the histamine test, the mecholyl infusion, and examination of the tongue. The diagnosis of familial dysautonomia may be difficult to differentiate from "failure to thrive" (see p. 439) and chronic pulmonary disease.

Treatment, Responsibilities of the Nurse, and Prognosis. Treatment and nursing care of this condition are aimed at controlling recurrent respiratory infections, the use of artificial tears to prevent corneal ulceration, and protection of the child from injuries because of his lack of a pain sensation. Urecholine (bethanecol) has been used to increase tear formation.

As the child grows to adolescence, scoliosis (see p. 870) or kyphosis or both may occur. These conditions cause respiratory difficulties and cardiac strain. A comprehensive understanding of familial dysautonomia is of great value in helping the nurse to support and assist the entire family of a child having this condition.

The *prognosis* in this condition is poor. The majority of patients die before adulthood from chronic pulmonary failure.

Genetic counseling is important in the management of this condition to aid in family planning. There is no method known at present to detect the presence of this disease *in utero* or to test for carriers.

NEUROCUTANEOUS SYNDROMES

Neurocutaneous syndromes include congenital lesions of the central nervous system and the skin. These are often associated with ocular and visceral abnormalities. Three examples of this type of syndrome are discussed: tuberous sclerosis, neurofibromatosis, and Sturge-Weber disease.

TUBEROUS SCLEROSIS

Tuberous sclerosis is an important cause of mental defect and of uncontrollable convulsions. It is inherited as an autosomal dominant trait, but may be caused by a new mutation. Lesions may be seen in the brain, skin, eyes, heart, lungs, kidneys, and bones.

Typical cerebral lesions are tubers or sclerotic patches scattered throughout the cortical gray matter. Small tumor nodules may be present at birth and enlarge gradually, possibly forming masses that may bulge into the lateral ventricles. Sometimes one of these paraventricular tumors undergoes malignant change into an astrocytoma (see p. 791) or a glioblastoma.

More than 90 per cent of these children have convulsions. Myoclonic seizures may occur during infancy; psychomotor seizures or grand mal occur later. More than one half of these children are mentally retarded. Hyperactivity or destructive behavior may be present.

The skin lesion of tuberous sclerosis is *adenoma sebaceum*. These bright red or brownish nodules exist in a butterfly distribution on the nose and cheeks. These appear between two and five years of age. Hypopigmented skin macules of various shapes and sizes are present from birth on the arms, legs, and trunk. These skin lesions on an infant having convulsions suggest the diagnosis of tuberous sclerosis.

Benign tumors are formed in various body organs, especially the kidneys, lungs, heart, liver, and spleen.

The prognosis varies. Children having mild involvement may live a productive life; those with severe mental retardation may require institutionalization. Death may occur as a result of a brain tumor, status epilepticus, a tumor of the heart, or renal failure.

Management of these children includes treatment of the convulsions and assessment of the degree of mental retardation as a basis for future educational efforts. Dextroamphetamine or Ritalin (methylphenidate hydrocloride) may be used to control the hyperactivity of these children. Facial adenomas may be removed if they are cosmetically deforming; however, they may recur. Surgical excision of tumors may be necessary. Genetic counseling is important for parents if the possibility exists that they may have another child with this condition.

NEUROFIBROMATOSIS (VON RECKLINGHAUSEN'S DISEASE)

Neurofibromatosis is inherited as an autosomal dominant trait. The symptoms are hyperpigmented skin lesions (café-au-lait spots) on the trunk and extremities and tumors that develop from elements of the peripheral and central nervous systems. Isolated café-au-lait spots are not uncommon in normal individuals, so the diagnosis of neurofibromatosis can only be made if there are six or more lesions greater than 1.5 cm in diameter. Treatment is not given for the café-au-lait spots and the axillary freckling.

Dermal or subcutaneous neurofibromas are of various sizes and shapes and may even produce hypertrophy of a limb. Surgical removal of these tumors is advised only if there is pain, serious deformity, interference with function, recurrent infection, or malignant degeneration. Local recurrence is common if the lesions are not totally removed. Irradiation of the tumors is not effective.

These children may have a full life expectancy. Mild mental retardation and convulsions may occur. Increased incidence of brain tumors and sarcomas is the principal risk to life.

Genetic counseling is essential. A careful family history and examination of immediate family members is necessary in determining whether neurofibromatosis occurred as a dominant trait or as a mutant. Offspring of a patient having this condition have a 50 per cent chance of inheriting the disorder.

STURGE-WEBER DISEASE

Sturge-Weber disease is not hereditary and occurs sporadically in the population. This is characterized by a congenital capillary hemangioma, which involves the skin of the face and cervical area, mucous membranes, meninges, and choroid on one side. The skin angioma ("nevus flammeus" or "portwine stain") occurs usually in the trigeminal distribution, most commonly in the ophthalmic division. Slow blood flow leads to an anoxic injury in the underlying cerebral cortex. Clinical manifestations of cortical damage are convulsions, mental retardation and hemiparesis on the side opposite that of the lesion. Treatment consists of giving anticonvulsant drugs for seizures, physiotherapy for paretic extremities, and ophthalmoscopic examinations for the early detection of glaucoma. When severe convulsions that cannot be controlled by medications occur, local resection of the cerebral cortical lesion may become necessary. The degree of mental retardation is determined, and plans are made for the child's care on this basis. A cosmetic cream that covers the discoloration of the facial skin may be used.

SKELETAL DEFECTS

CRANIOSYNOSTOSIS

Etiology and Pathology. In the normal newborn infant the bones of the skull are separated. The sutures, which can be located soon after birth, are separated by a layer of fibrous tissue. The bones of the skull grow in this fibrous strip.

In craniosynostosis one or more of the sutures are closed before or shortly after birth. Growth of adjoining bones is stopped, and there is a reduction in the diameter of the skull in this direction. Where open sutures remain, a compensatory growth or enlargement is found. The result is various deformities of the skull, depending on which sutures are closed. Since other defects of the skeleton may be found with craniosynostosis, it is thought the the skeleton is adversely affected early in embryonic life.

Clinical Manifestations. Since most of the brain growth is completed in early childhood, any pressure which interferes with normal expansion may cause brain damage and mental retardation.

In *scaphocephaly* the sagittal suture is closed prematurely. The head develops in a long, narrow shape. Symptoms of intracranial pressure may be evident.

Oxycephaly is a condition in which the coronal suture closes prematurely, either completely or partially. Other sutures may also close and various deformities result. Complications arise since the brain may be severely compressed, with resultant headache, loss of vision, and convulsions. Exophthalmos may occur. Examination is likely to reveal strabismus, nystagmus, and papilledema. Mental retardation is common. Syndactylism may be associated with this deformity.

Roentgenograms reveal the abnormal shape of the skull and absence of one or more sutures.

Diagnosis and Treatment. Craniosynostosis must be differentiated from microcephaly, which results in a small head because the brain fails to grow. Increased intracranial pressure does not occur in microcephaly.

Surgical intervention may prevent mental and visual defects if it is done before compression of the brain occurs. Early repair of the skull also produces a better cosmetic effect. Operation is therefore done as soon as a definite diagnosis is made during infancy. The surgical procedure includes linear craniotomy along the prematurely closed suture with removal of a portion of bone and lining of the edge of the suture with polyethylene film to slow its reunion.

Responsibilities of the Nurse. The nurse has an important role in early finding of these cases. Often the community or public health nurse who visits in the home may be the first person to observe the condition in a supposedly normal infant. Although a diagnosis cannot be made by the nurse, the child can be referred to a physician for evaluation.

The nursing care of a patient after operation is similar to that after a craniotomy for brain tumor (see p. 791). If the nurse has prepared the parents for the fact that their child may have some facial swelling and possible discoloration around the eyes postoperatively, they will be less disturbed by his appearance. The physician may order that the child's head be elevated after surgery to prevent such swelling.

Many parents have the preconception that their child will have brain damage and mental retardation due to craniosynostosis. It is important for the nurse to make certain the parents know that following surgical intervention there should be normal brain development.

Prognosis. The prognosis is excellent if treatment is instituted before permanent brain damage occurs. Because of rapid bone growth resulting in closure of the sutures, revision of the craniotomy may be necessary.

EMOTIONAL DISTURBANCES

Causes of Anxiety in Infancy. Every infant experiences inevitable frustrations because, basically, "he wants what he wants when he wants it." He may desire to suckle when he is supposed to eat solid foods; he may want his parents to carry him around instead of learning to walk.

These frustrations bring him pain, discomfort and anxiety. Gradually he learns that he can rid himself of these uncomfortable states by adopting new methods of behavior, e.g, by learning to eat solid foods and to walk. Infants learn new skills, therefore, because initially they were frustrated and uncomfortable as a result of depending only upon old skills. Learning new skills eventually brings new pleasures and fewer frustrations.

An infant will desire to learn new skills only if he has an optimum period of satisfaction with the old mode of behavior before the period of frustration begins. Infants should be allowed to experience the inevitable frustrations of life slowly and in small doses. Sudden, overwhelming frustrations, such as weaning within a few days, have an adverse effect on the immature personality.

Behavior of the Infant Who Is Anxious. The anxious infant may react in one of three ways: he may resent or fight against the cause of his discomfort; he may turn away or move from it, without fighting; or he may remain immobile and do nothing.

ANXIETY DUE TO FRUSTRATION IN FEEDING. Young infants frustrated in the feeding process will react in the only way they know, by kicking, crying, and constant bodily movement. If the breast-fed infant cannot get adequate amounts of milk because of inverted nipples, he may regurgitate what he has already taken, he may turn away and refuse to suck, or he may fall asleep. Likewise the infant weaned too abruptly may show the same problem behavior.

The infant may react similarly to complementary foods if the food is too hot, if it contains lumps, or if it requires excessive chewing. In such a situation he may vomit repeatedly, may turn his head away from his mother or may become immobile and refuse to participate in the feeding process.

Any of these reactions affects the eating process directly. If the infant blames, as it were, his mother for the discomfort in feeding, he may turn away from her when she approaches him, refuse to eat, cry when she touches him, or when he is a little older, do exactly the opposite of what she requests.

ANXIETY DUE TO FRUSTRATION OF SUCKING. If the desire to suck is frustrated, the infant will suck on non-nutritive objects such as fingers, the blanket, or toys for long periods of time and will continue this activity past the second or third year, when such activity is usually given up.

If the parents permit such sucking on non-nutritive objects, the infant will gain his needed satisfaction. But if the parents disapprove, the infant may reject food or will stop the sucking activity completely and learn to find pleasure in frustration.

ANXIETY DUE TO LACK OF PARENTAL LOVE AND OVERWHELMING FRUSTRATION WHICH THE INFANT CANNOT HANDLE. Degrees of anxiety resulting from frustration in feeding or sucking can be observed in many infants at some time during the first year. The response of infants who have overwhelming anxiety due to a lack of parental love and overwhelming frustration has been discussed earlier (p. 439). Infants who fail to thrive even when they have parents, or those who have no parents to care for them, may ultimately appear to wish death through starvation.

A brief case history may illustrate such a situation.

Timmy, a two-year-old boy, was admitted to the children's unit. He weighed 7 pounds 5 ounces. He had multiple skin infections and suffered from malnutrition and dehydration.

His birthweight was not known. He was the child of an unmarried 15-year-old girl. Shortly after his birth his mother left him with a sister and disappeared. His aunt subsequently married and gave him to a neighbor. During the two years of his life he had eight substitute mothers, neighbors who passed him around at their convenience. Eventually he was given to a woman who really cared for him, but by that time he was so physically retarded and emotionally underdeveloped that her efforts were in vain. He would not suck on a nipple or respond to anyone. She brought him to the hospital, but in spite of gavage feedings, intravenous therapy, antibiotics and the best of nursing care, Timmy died.

The infant equates food with love. Timmy, who received rejection and no love, refused his food and died of starvation.

Symptoms. *Anxiety symptoms* include excessive crying, inability to sleep, restlessness, or rhythmic rocking movements and possibly vomiting. In overwhelming anxiety the infant may experience depression with weeping, screaming when strangers approach, withdrawal, and arrest of physical and emotional development.

Feeding disorders, ranging from refusal of food to air swallowing and repeated vomiting, are common. Eventually marasmus may develop, and the infant may die of starvation.

Antagonistic behavior consists in a lack of enjoyment in the companionship of his parents, in a refusal to enjoy interaction with them, or in doing the opposite of what they request of him.

Treatment and Responsibilities of the Nurse. Prevention of emotional disturbance is much preferred to treatment of the disturbed infant. Many mothers want to be loving and warm to their infants and yet seemingly reject them in some degree because of disapproval by their husbands, relatives, or neighbors of a truly maternal attitude toward the infant. Other mothers want to provide warm loving care for their babies, but are separated from them because of their own illness or that of other members of the family.

Such mothers could be helped to a great degree by education in the emotional needs of infants. Such education, given during the prenatal period, could make them more sure of their own judgment and less sensitive to disapproval by others. Although intellectual understanding is not a cure-all for such problems, the support of an outside authority is reassuring. The physician or nurse can help such women to trust their own maternal feelings as guides in their behavior. Those women discussed earlier who desire to do only things that give them pleasure cannot be good mothers regardless of the guidance they receive. Their immature wish for pleasure causes them to be unaware of the infant's need for love and so they are unable to give love.

In treating an infant for an emotional disturbance, the cause must first be found. The need which is being frustrated must be clearly understood. It is important for both the mother and the physician to treat the child as though he were a little younger than he was when the traumatic experience occurred. For example, if the infant reacts violently to supplementary solid foods, his mother should cease offering them for a while. Then the foods can be introduced gradually *without force* or even undue urging.

Sometimes the feeding difficulty, vomiting, or refusal to eat may become so severe that the infant may need to be removed from his mother for a time. He may be cared for at home by a warm, loving person or may be placed in a hospital. Often such infants may begin to eat well after a brief period of adjustment to the new situation. During the separation the parents should receive guidance so that they may create a more loving environment for the infant when he returns to them.

If the infant is hospitalized, it is the nurse's responsibility to provide the love and tender care he needs. The nurse must hold him closely and show warmth and affection, cuddle him, and be kind and patient in giving him feedings. Often the nurse can demonstrate to the mother how to hold the infant close to her body to feed him and to give him the loving care he needs.

ABUSED- OR BATTERED-CHILD SYNDROME

Incidence, Etiology, Clinical Findings, Diagnosis, and Prognosis. Violence by a husband toward a pregnant wife may be a type of prenatal child abuse, on a conscious or subconscious level, that may lead to handicapping of the child or to his death. Postnatal child abuse is one of the most serious problems confronting the physician and nurse who care for children. The *incidence* is not really known, since many cases go unrecognized, but it appears to be on the increase in our society, especially in large metropolitan areas. It is for this reason that the *Child Abuse Prevention and Treatment Act of 1974* was passed (see p. 7). This Act provides for a National Center on Child Abuse and Neglect and makes funds available for research on methods of identification of causes, prevention, and treatment of these children and for the establishment of regional child abuse centers.

The incidence of child abuse cannot be correlated with educational achievement, social status, or income level of the parents. It is more frequent in situations where family or financial stress exists and where the pent-up frustrations of the parents are focused on the child as a scapegoat.

An abused child (approximately one third of such children are infants or toddlers under three years of age) may have had an earlier diagnosis of failure to thrive (see p. 439). He is one against whom bodily injury and therefore emotional harm also is done by an adult (or less frequently an older child) to such a degree that it comes to the attention of a physician or another member of a helping profession. Child abuse can also occur in institutions such as day-care centers, schools, and child-care agencies.

The *clinical findings* are the result of injuries which may be due to burning, throwing, or knocking the child around or twisting his extremities. They include largely bruises, scratches, burns, hematomas, and fractures of long bones, ribs, or skull. *Neglect*, which is frequently evident in these children, is the chronic failure of adults to protect the child from obvious physical danger or to provide the care he needs. Poor skin hygiene and some degree of malnutrition are usually also evident in battered children.

In *diagnosis* the distinguishing feature of this condition includes variations in stages of healing of several bone lesions as shown on x-ray films. Such lesions were incurred at different times prior to examination and hospitalization.

The principal basis for identifying this problem is the judgment of a professional person, since usually the child is too young to complain and the parents will not admit to abusive practices. The *etiologic factor* is that parents or caretakers have a defect in character structure which allows aggressive impulses to be expressed too freely when they are under tension. In some instances the parent tends to release his rage on one particular child only because he may serve as a symbol of something or someone who once caused the parent unhappiness. A child born out of wedlock is many times the target child. Such parents do not volunteer information about the

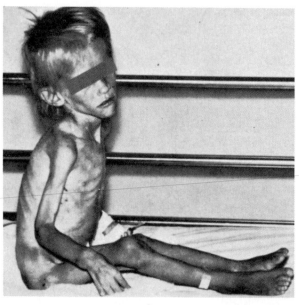

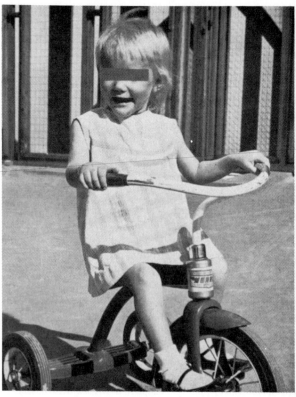

A

B

FIGURE 15-18. *A*, An abused emaciated child who was covered with bruises and abrasions, had fractures of the skull, arm, and hands, and had an intestinal obstruction due to a hematoma in the lumen of the duodenum. *B*, The same child five weeks after admission to the hospital. (From Kempe, C. H.: *Hospital Practice*, 4:56, October 1969.)

child, they contradict themselves when they describe the injury, become irritated when questioned about the child, are angry with him for his injury, and give no indications of feeling guilty about their lack of care of him. They often disappear shortly after the child has been admitted to the hospital, tend not to visit him after admission, and do not involve themselves in his care. These parents are concerned chiefly about themselves, are frequently dependent people who criticize the child, and show no indication of having any perception of how the child might feel. These parents demonstrate role reversal, in which they turn to their infants and small children for nurturing, satisfaction of needs, and protection as they would to their own parents.

There is a so-called "cycle of child abuse." Many parents who abuse their own children were themselves victims of child abuse because they were unable to meet their parents' needs. These individuals, having not received love and security themselves as children, become lonely adults who, when they are of an age to marry, seek a loving parent figure to care for them. Many times the spouse was not abused as a child but is a passive person who permits the abuse of the child or children to occur.

The typical forms of behavior which neglected and battered children show are crying in a hopeless manner or very little crying even when uncomfortable, lack of expectation of assurance or comfort from parents, and apprehension when contacted physically. They seem to seek safety in sizing up a situation, finding out what will happen next, rather than from contact with their parents. Children who are loved and cared for turn to their parents for safety in life; battered children endure life as though they were alone with no real hope of safety in a harmful world.

The *prognosis* is variable. The incidence of death is high among these children, but damaged physical or emotional health or mental retardation is even greater among those who survive.

Treatment, Responsibilities of the Nurse, and Prevention. Nurses in the community, whether in public health, Child Health Conference, or hospital, should provide preventive care for those who are predisposed to physical or emotional illness such as teen-age mothers, unwed mothers, mothers having several pregnancies which were affected by various social or emotional complications, and mothers in an unstable marital situation. The nurse can thus hopefully prevent the mother-infant relationship from becoming critical. Such a nurse can also notice early symptoms of child abuse and refer the child to a protective agency. The nurse's authority is limited, however, and sometimes recommendation to a protective agency is all that can be done.

In any infant with evidence of multiple bone lesions, a subdural tap and x-ray film of the skull must be considered. Fractures of long bones must be reduced and immobilized. The *nursing care* therefore depends on the specific trauma such a child has. These children need good physical care and love.

The nurse must be fully aware of the existence of this syndrome because it is the professional who may first see a child with evidence of trauma. The nurse may also recognize the clues which parents and children give. More specifically, when a child is seen in the emergency room of a hospital or in a Child Health Conference who has severe bruises or other wounds on his body and the nurse suspects that he has been abused, the following should be done. The nurse should chart all observations of his physical condition as on any other patient, but should *not* chart the judgment that he had been beaten. If, however, the adult who accompanied the child made statements about his having been beaten, the nurse may chart these and other statements in quotation marks along with the speaker's identity. The nurse should report all observations to the physician verbally and show him the child's chart. Charting from this time on should include observations of the child's condition and the physician's orders which have been carried out. It is generally the responsibility of the physician or a team of physicians to report violence against children; however, the nurse should be aware of the policy of the agency and the law of the state in which the agency is located.

Prevention of recurrence involves the cooperation of physicians, police department, social service agencies, humane societies, prosecuting attorneys, and nurses. In order to prevent a repeated attack immediately, an abused child may be temporarily placed in a foster home or an institution. This action can provide time for the members of the health team to study the family situation carefully and to help the parents through professional counseling. Thus the family may be preserved, since permanent placement may not be necessary.

The role of the nurse, therefore, consists in casefinding and reporting to the physician any indications of abuse which may be seen, establishing rapport with such families so that insight can be gained into their problems, and caring for the child once he is admitted to the hospital. In working with parents of neglected and abused children a noncritical, nonpunitive approach is necessary in order to prevent them from further acting out their frustrations on their children. This sort of approach may be difficult for the nurse to achieve because of personal feelings of anger or disgust with their behavior.

More specifically, when the abused child is admitted to the hospital, the nurse must help to establish a tone of treatment for the child and his parents rather than one of punishment. A warm and sensitive attitude on the part of the nurse is necessary. The nurse can also help the parents to understand that they are competent in some aspects of childrearing. Parental strengths are acknowledged and praised. It is especially important, therefore, that parents be encouraged to visit and to provide some aspects of the child's care, such as feeding or bathing. In this way the trauma of hospitalization is reduced for both the parents and child. The nurse continues to help the child return to a state of health by giving him physical care and by meeting his developmental needs through sensory stimulation and education, depending on his age. While providing this care, the nurse has many opportunities to demonstrate more positive behavior to the parents when dealing with their child and constructive ways of expressing feelings freely. Such helpful nursing after admission and through hospitalization supports the parents in their coping efforts and may make them more open to other help later.

The nurse must work with other personnel in community services in a coordinated manner. These services include, after prompt reporting, rapid and thorough investigation of each family and maintenance of a central registry, since parents of abused children frequently take them to different physicians or hospitals to avoid identification with previous attacks.

Recently self-help groups called "Parents Anonymous" have been organized across the country. These groups attempt to provide an atmosphere where abusive parents can confess their destructive tendencies and seek a means to stop them without fear of recrimination. Ideally, each such parent should have a normal adult who can assume the role of his or her parent. Since there are few extended families today, a close friend can indeed fulfill a vital role in the life of the family unit. This friend can give support, love, and affection, and can be uncritical and sensitive to the needs of the parent in a way the parent has never known before. These self-help groups need the support and encouragement of the nurse as a professional or as a friend.

In some communities day-care centers have been organized where battering parents and their children can interact and gain support from each other. It must be remembered that most battering parents love their children most of the time. With sufficient support from others they may no longer feel the need to inflict harm.

For those families where more extensive therapy is required, a child abuse team composed of members of the helping professions (physician, psychiatrist, lawyer, nurse, and social worker) should be made available at the community level to deal compassionately with both parents and child. The goal of this team is to provide the child with a secure and safe environment to facilitate his physical and psychosocial growth and development. When possible, the child remains with his family, and close supervision and counseling is provided. If one of the parents or the mother, if no father is present, says in effect or by her actions, "Help me, I'm afraid I'll kill my baby," or if she states that she feels that she cannot cope with the child and does not want him, then society must assume the responsibility for his care. The child may become a ward of the court and be placed in a foster home.

All states have laws that make child abuse a criminal offense, and there are some states in which reporting is mandatory. This legislation, however, leaves much to be desired if children are to be protected from abuse. The law should give full protection to the person reporting the abuse, and it should also provide sufficient protective social services to bear the burden of treating the family and child. If the law is not effective, the nurse should become part of a constructive effort to perfect it.

If the nurse is called to court as a witness, only what was actually observed should be reported. The nurse should remain calm and think out brief, factual answers before responding to questions. Judgmental terms such as "filthy" should not be used. Answers must be specific and consist only of what was actually observed, not what the other children, neighbors, or another nurse has stated. Accurate and detailed nursing notes are important in helping to recall observations and in providing answers to such questioning.

Ultimately most abused children return home with their parents. It is difficult to obtain a conviction in court, since usually the court cannot convict on the basis of evidence of the child alone or on testimony of other young children, nor can a husband and wife be compelled to testify against each other. Unfortunately, indictment without conviction does not prevent further abuse.

Prevention in the long run depends on preventing transmission of the kind of social deprivation which results in the neglect and abuse of children, and contributes through those who survive such treatment to the next generation of parents who will not be able to nurture their children either.

Parental rights are not necessarily sacred. For the benefit of the children sometimes these rights must be terminated.

CLINICAL SITUATIONS

Michael O'Brien, a four-month-old infant, was brought to the Child Health Conference by his mother. He appeared to be well nourished and well developed for his age, although he had had no previous medical supervision. During Mrs. O'Brien's conference with the nurse the mother asked several questions.

1. "Michael has been breastfed since birth, but I have been thinking about weaning him to a cup. When should I do this?"

a. "As soon as you can after he is five months old, because continued sucking may cause his teeth to protrude."

b. "As soon as Michael shows a desire to give up sucking and to drink from a cup."

c. "Before summer comes regardless of his age, because it is difficult to wean an infant in warm weather."

d. "Before he is a year old, because he will have several teeth and will not be able to suck properly."

2. "The doctor said that Michael should eat solid food, but he refuses it after he is breastfed. What should I do?"

a. "Force him to eat, because he will lose weight and develop anemia if he continues to take only milk."

b. "Give him only breast milk as long as he refuses solid food."

c. "Mix the puréed food with some cow's milk and feed it through a large-holed nipple."

d. "Offer small amounts of puréed food before each breast feeding when he is hungry."

3. Michael at four months of age has the following abilities. Select the one that is *not* typical for a child of his age.

a. Enjoys sitting alone.

b. Lifts his head and shoulders at a 90-degree angle when on his abdomen and looks around.

c. Attempts to roll over.

d. Moves his arms rapidly at the sight of a toy.

4. The nurse understands that Michael should be immunized against certain diseases during infancy, including measles (13 to 15 months). These diseases are

a. Measles, pertussis, scarlet fever, chickenpox, diphtheria and possibly tetanus.

b. Pertussis, diphtheria, poliomyelitis, tetanus, measles, and possibly rubella and mumps.

c. Chickenpox, poliomyelitis, measles, diphtheria, typhoid fever and possibly tetanus.

d. Smallpox, tetanus, diphtheria, pertussis, measles and possibly chickenpox.

5. The important point about Michael's *immediate* safety to stress to Mrs. O'Brien at this time would be

a. "Do not give Michael dry toast to chew, because he may aspirate it."

b. "Do not permit Michael to chew paint from the window ledge, because he might absorb too much lead."

c. "When Michael learns to roll over, you must supervise him whenever he is on a surface from which he might fall."

d. "Lock the crib sides securely because he may stand and lean against them and fall out of bed."

Mrs. O'Brien brought Michael back to the Child Health Conference when he was six months old and said that he had been ill for about three days. The physician observed that Michael's anterior fontanel was sunken, his skin turgor was poor, and his skin was warm. Mrs. O'Brien said that he had had about six stools which were watery and foul-smelling each day and that he had vomited all his feedings. He was referred to the local hospital and was admitted promptly with a diagnosis of diarrhea and vomiting.

6. On admission a blood specimen was drawn from his jugular vein. The nurse restrained the infant by using a
   a. Clove-hitch restraint.
   b. Mummy restraint.
   c. Abdominal restraint.
   d. Elbow restraint.

7. Intravenous therapy was started promptly. The most important responsibility of the nurse when caring for such an infant is to
   a. Check frequently the number of drops of solution running into the vein and regulate the flow of solution as ordered.
   b. Remove the needle as soon as the fluid which has been ordered has run into the vein.
   c. Change the bed linen promptly if it becomes moistened from the intravenous solution.
   d. Add a new bottle of solution when the present one is empty, with or without a physician's order.

Mrs. Smith brought her first infant, a five-week-old son, Bruce, to the pediatric clinic because he had been "spitting up" since he was three weeks of age. Bruce had been breastfed for the first four weeks of his life, and then had been put on a formula.

8. The physician made a diagnosis of pyloric stenosis on the basis of the infant's history and clinical manifestations, which included
   a. Projectile vomiting beginning abruptly, normal stools, and malnutrition.
   b. Rumination of feedings, normal stools, and a sausage-like abdominal mass.
   c. Constant abdominal pain with crying, frequent liquid stools, and an olive-shaped abdominal mass.
   d. Gradual increase in vomiting, finally becoming projectile in nature, constipation, and weight loss.

9. The vomitus of an infant having pyloric stenosis is the color of his formula and does not contain bile because
   a. The obstruction is above the opening of the common bile duct.
   b. The liver does not secrete bile, since its functioning is impaired.
   c. The obstruction at the cardiac sphincter prevents the flow of bile to the stomach.
   d. The stenosis of the common bile duct prevents bile from flowing properly.

10. A Fredet-Ramstedt operation was done. Mrs. Smith asks how Bruce will be fed after the operation. In order to answer her question you should know that the feeding regimen after a pyloromyotomy is based on the principle that
    a. Thickened feedings aid mechanically in helping food pass through the pylorus because its weight stretches the hypertrophied muscle.
    b. Clear liquids are tolerated well because they contain no curds which would have difficulty passing through the pylorus.

c. Easily assimilated fluids are given in increasing amounts so that the newly incised muscle can accommodate gradually.
d. Easily digested fluids are given in large amounts in order to combat dehydration.

When Bruce was seven months old, he was readmitted to the hospital with a diagnosis of eczema. He was irritable and restless, and scratched his skin whenever he could. The skin on his face and scalp was secondarily infected. Mrs. Smith said that Bruce had received a wide variety of foods in his diet and that his appetite had been excellent.

11. Eczema is a skin condition caused by
    a. Bacterial invasion primarily by the streptococcal organism.
    b. Excessive secretion of the sebaceous glands.
    c. Inflammation around the sweat glands due to excessive heat.
    d. Allergy to internal or external irritants.

12. When dressing Bruce after his bath, it is important to dress him
    a. In as few cotton clothes as possible according to the temperature of his environment.
    b. In warm woolen clothing, because these infants frequently contract respiratory infections.
    c. In only a diaper, because clothing increases the infant's discomfort.
    d. In cotton clothing, but wrap him in a woolen blanket for warmth.

13. When using restraints, they must be
    a. Kept on constantly to prevent Bruce from scratching.
    b. Removed once a day to allow active motion of his extremities under supervision.
    c. Kept securely in position so that Bruce remains on his back at all times.
    d. Checked frequently to determine whether the restraints are constricting his circulation.

14. Bruce was hospitalized for several weeks. Mrs. Smith was not able to visit him more frequently than twice a month. In order to prevent emotional deprivation during this time, the most important measure the head nurse could take would be to
    a. Place him each day in a playpen near another seven-month-old infant so they could interact with each other.
    b. Place his crib near the entrance to the unit so that he would not become lonely.
    c. Give him many toys to keep him occupied.
    d. Assign the same staff nurse to provide care for him each day.

Mr. and Mrs. Jones had had three children. The first child died at one week of age after an operation for intestinal obstruction due to meconium ileus. The second child is normal. June, their third child, seemed normal at birth and had a good appetite, but she gained weight slowly. At five months bronchopneumonia developed, which responded well to chemotherapy. At eight months she again had bronchopneumonia and continued to have a chronic cough after discharge from the hospital. Upon readmission to the hospital at 11 months because of weight loss, a diagnosis of cystic fibrosis was made.

15. During an evacuation June's rectum prolapsed. After it had been replaced the nurse prevented the recurrence of the prolapse by
    a. Giving a daily colonic irrigation to prevent constipation.

b. Giving a mild laxative each night to prevent constipation.

c. Restraining the child in bed with her head lower than her body.

d. Taping the buttocks together after each defecation.

16. The diet ordered for June during her hospitalization in July and August was

a. Normal protein, high or normal fat, high starch, normal sodium chloride.

b. High protein, normal or low fat, low starch, liberal sodium chloride.

c. Low protein, normal fat, low carbohydrate, low sodium chloride.

d. High protein, high fat, normal carbohydrate, high sodium chloride.

GUIDES FOR FURTHER STUDY

1. During your experience at the Child Health Conference observe several infants under one year of age with their mothers. Note the apparent differences of maternal attitudes toward the infants when their mothers feed them, comfort them or give them physical care. What immediate effects do these various attitudes have on their individual infants?

2. A mother of an apparently normal two-month-old infant at the Child Health Conference has complained to you that in spite of all her efforts to teach him to sit alone, he shows no progress toward accomplishing this ability. What would your response be on the basis of your knowledge of the principles of motor development and your understanding of the interrelatedness of maturation and learning?

3. The women's group of a local church has offered to donate toys for the infants hospitalized at Christmas. List the specific toys you would request for infants of various ages and give the reasons for your choices.

4. Visit a foundling home in or near your community. Observe the infants to determine whether their behavior shows any evidence of maternal deprivation. In terms of your knowledge of the care the infants receive, evaluate your findings and make suggestions in seminar as to how the emotional needs of the infants could be met more adequately.

5. Trace the steps in motor development through which an infant must go before he is finally able to stand alone.

6. During your experience at the Child Health Conference or the pediatric clinic list several questions asked by mothers of infants of various ages. Discuss your answers to these questions in seminar. Evaluate your own progress in being able to establish rapport with these mothers and in being able to answer their questions to their satisfaction.

7. Plan a daily menu for infants of three months, six months and one year. Check each of these diets with the recommended dietary allowances given for infants, on page 367.

8. What are the most recent statistics in your state on infant mortality? What are the most frequent causes of death? After investigating provisions made for the health supervision and care of infants, give suggestions as to how the infant mortality rate in your state could be reduced.

9. Make a study of your state laws and a survey of the organizations and services in your community for the protection and care of the battered child and for counseling his parents. What could you as an individual nurse or as a member of a nursing organization do to improve the effectiveness of these efforts? Discuss your answer in your seminar group.

TEACHING AIDS AND OTHER INFORMATION*

Allergy Foundation of America

Allergy in Children.

American Academy of Pediatrics

Maltreatment of Children: Battered Child Syndrome.
Salt Intake and High Blood Pressure.
Supplemental Feeding Programs for Mothers and Infants.

American Celiac Society

Guide for the Celiac.

The American Humane Association: Children's Division

DeFrancis, V., and Lucht, C.: Child Abuse Legislation in the 1970's, 1974.
De Francis, V.: Children Who Were Helped Through Child Protective Services.
De Francis, V.: Community Cooperation for Better Child Protection.
De Francis, V.: Termination of Parental Rights: Balancing the Equities.
Mulford, R. M.: Emotional Neglect of Children.
Oettinger, K. B., Morton, Rev. A., and Mulford, R. M.: In the Interest of Children: A Century of Progress.
Stoenner, H.: Plain Talk About Child Abuse.

Department of National Health and Welfare: Ottawa, Canada

Report on the Relationship between Income and Nutrition.
Selected Nutrition Teaching Aids.

Dysautonomia Foundation, Inc.

A Nursing Care Plan for the Child Afflicted with Familial Dysautonomia.

Johnson & Johnson

Klaus, M. H., Leger, T., and Trause, M. A. (Eds.): Maternal Attachment and Mothering Disorders: A Round Table, 1974.

Mead Johnson & Company

Cow's Milk Allergy: A Review of Current Scientific and Clinical Findings, 1975.
Galactosemia in Infancy: A Review of the Problem and Its Dietary Management, 1976.

National Cystic Fibrosis Research Foundation

Cystic Fibrosis: Guidelines for Health Personnel.
Cystic Fibrosis: Most Serious Lung Problem of Children.
Educational and Vocational Counseling of the Young Adult with Cystic Fibrosis.
Educational Resource Materials for Pediatric Pulmonary Disease.
Living with Cystic Fibrosis: A Guide for the Young Adult.
Medical Information: Cystic Fibrosis.
Parent's Handbook: "Your Child and Cystic Fibrosis."

---

*Complete addresses are given in the Appendix.

The National Foundation—March of Dimes

Cooley's Anemia & Birth Defects Prevention.
Fast Facts About Sickle Cell Anemia.
Tay-Sachs Disease & Birth Defects Prevention.

Ross Laboratories

Iron Nutrition in Infancy, 1974.
Perinatology—Neonatology—Pediatric Nutrition—Currents, 1976.
The Care of Children with Chronic Illnesses, 1975.

United States Government

Besharov, D. J.: Building a Community Response to Child Abuse and Maltreatment, 1976.
Child Abuse and Neglect: The Diagnostic Process and Treatment Programs, 1975.
Child Abuse and Neglect: The Problem and Its Management: Vol. 1 An Overview of the Problem, Vol. 2 The Roles and Responsibilities of Professionals, Vol. 3 The

Community Team: An Approach to Case Management and Prevention, 1976.
Child Abuse and Neglect Activities, 1975.
Child Neglect: An Annotated Bibliography, 1975.
Comprehensive Emergency Services, 1975.
Listing of National, Regional, and Local Groups Providing Services to Persons Who Have Interest in Sickle Cell Anemia, 1975.
Polansky, N. A., Hally, C., and Polansky, N. F.: Profile of Neglect, A Survey of the State of Knowledge of Child Neglect, 1975.
Russell, F. F. (Ed.): Identification and Management of Selected Developmental Disabilities: A Guide for Nurses, 1975.
Services for Crippled Children, Reprinted 1975.
Sickle Cell Screening and Education Clinics, 1975.
Steele, B. F.: Working with Abusive Parents from a Psychiatric Point of View, 1975.
Studies in Handicapping Conditions: Research to Improve Health Services for Mothers and Children, 1975.
The Extended Family Center, 1974.
WIC Program Survey, 1975, 1975.

REFERENCES

Books

Anderson, C. M., and Burke, V. (Eds.): *Paediatric Gastroenterology.* Philadelphia, J. B. Lippincott Company, 1975.
Archuleta, M. J., and Archuleta, A. J.: *Sickle Cell Anemia: A Selected Bibliography for the Layman.* San Diego, Calif., Current Bibliography Series, 1972.
Boszormenyi-Nagy, I., and Spark, G. M.: *Invisible Loyalties.* New York, Harper & Row, Publishers, Inc., 1973.
Cameron, J. M., and Rae, L. J.: *Atlas of the Battered Child Syndrome.* New York, Longman Inc., 1975.
Creighton, H.: *Law Every Nurse Should Know.* 3rd ed. Philadelphia, W. B. Saunders Company, 1975.
Fischer, J. E. (Ed.): *Total Parenteral Nutrition.* Boston, Little, Brown & Company, 1976.
Fontana, V. J.: *The Maltreated Child: The Maltreatment Syndrome in Children.* 2nd ed. Springfield, Ill., Charles C Thomas, 1974.
Gardner, L. I. (Ed.): *Endocrine and Genetic Diseases of Childhood and Adolescence.* 2nd ed. Philadelphia, W. B. Saunders Company, 1975.
Ghadimi, H. (Ed.): *Total Parenteral Nutrition: Premises and Promises.* New York, John Wiley & Sons, Inc., 1975.
Kelley, V. C. (Ed.): *Metabolic, Endocrine and Genetic Disorders of Children.* New York, Harper & Row, Publishers, Inc., 1974.
Kempe, C. H., and Helfer, R. E. (Eds.): *Helping the Battered Child and His Family.* Philadelphia, J. B. Lippincott Company, 1972.
Luckraft, D. (Ed.): *Black Awareness: Implications for Black Patient Care.* New York, American Journal of Nursing Company, 1975.
McCollum, A. T.: *Coping with Prolonged Health Impairment in Your Child.* Boston, Little, Brown & Company, 1975.
Mitchell, H. S., Rynbergen, H. J., Anderson, L., and Dibble, M. V.: *Nutrition in Health and Disease.* 16th ed. Philadelphia, J. B. Lippincott Company, 1976.
Nathan, D. G., and Oski, F. A. (Eds.): *Hematology of Infancy and Childhood.* Philadelphia, W. B. Saunders Company, 1974.
Oremland, E. K., and Oremland, J. D. (Eds.): *The Effects of Hospitalization on Children.* Springfield, Ill., Charles C Thomas, 1973.

Parrish, J. A.: *Dermatology and Skin Care.* New York, McGraw-Hill Book Company, 1975.
Patterson, P. R., Denning, C. R., Kutscher, A. H. (Eds.): *Psychosocial Aspects of Cystic Fibrosis: A Model for Chronic Lung Disease.* New York, Columbia University Press, 1973.
Rickham, P. P., Soper, R. T., and Stauffer, U. G.: *Synopsis of Pediatric Surgery.* Chicago, Year Book Medical Publishers, 1975.
Scarpelli, E. M., and Auld, P. A. M. (Eds.): *Pulmonary Physiology of the Fetus, Newborn and Child.* Philadelphia, Lea & Febiger, 1975.
Smith, C. H.: *Blood Diseases of Infancy and Childhood.* 3rd ed. St. Louis, The C. V. Mosby Company, 1972.
Till, K.: *Paediatric Neurosurgery.* Philadelphia, J. B. Lippincott Company, 1975.
Wade, J. F.: *Respiratory Nursing Care: Physiology and Technique.* St. Louis, The C. V. Mosby Company, 1973.
Weatherall, D. J., and Clegg, J. B.: *The Thalassaemia Syndromes.* 2nd ed. Philadelphia, J. B. Lippincott Company, 1972.
Weinberg, S., Shapiro, L., and Leider, M.: *Color Atlas of Pediatric Dermatology.* New York, McGraw-Hill Book Company, 1975.
Weldy, N. J.: *Body Fluids and Electrolytes.* 2nd ed. St. Louis, The C. V. Mosby Company, 1976.
Williams, R. A. (Ed.): *Textbook of Black-Related Diseases.* New York, McGraw-Hill Book Company, 1975.
Winick, M. (Ed.): *Childhood Obesity.* New York, McGraw-Hill Book Company, 1975.

Periodicals

Baldwin, J. A., and Oliver, J. E.: Epidemiology and Family Characteristics of Severely Abused Children. *Brit. J. Prev. Soc. Med.,* 29:205, December 1975.
Bassett, L. B.: How to Help Abused Children—And Their Parents. *RN,* 37:44, October 1974.
Besharov, D. J.: Building a Community Response to Child Abuse and Maltreatment. *Children Today,* 4:2, September-October 1975.
Boyle, I. R., et al.: Emotional Adjustment of Adolescents and Young Adults With Cystic Fibrosis. *J. Pediatr.,* 88:318, February 1976.

Burnette, B. A.: Family Adjustment to Cystic Fibrosis. *Am. J. Nursing*, 75:1986, November 1975.

Carter, B. D., Reed, R., and Reh, C. G.: Mental Health Nursing Intervention With Child Abusing and Neglecting Mothers. *J. Psychiatr. Nurs.*, 13:11, September-October 1957.

Carter, Y. A.: Nursing Management in Sickle Cell Disease. *RN*, 38:47, October 1975.

Chamberlain, N.: The Nurse And The Abusive Parent. *Nursing '74*, 4:72, October 1974.

Corey, E. J. B., Miller, C. L., and Widlak, F. W.: Factors Contributing To Child Abuse. *Nursing Research*, 24:293, July-August 1975.

Dharan, M.: The Diagnostic Value of Serum Protein Values. *RN*, 39:73, January 1976.

Ference, R. H.: The Little People: No Small Problem. *RN*, 37:70, September 1974.

Fielding, J., et al.: A Coordinated Sickle Cell Program for Economically Disadvantaged Adolescents. *Am. J. Pub. Health*, 64:427, May 1974.

Ford, R. J., Smistek, B. S., and Glass, J. T.: Photography of Suspected Child Abuse and Maltreatment. *Nursing Digest*, 4:35, Fall 1976.

Friedman, A. L., Juntti, M. J., and Scoblic, M. A.: Nursing Responsibility in Child Abuse. *Nursing Forum*, 15:95, 1976.

Harrison, L. L.: Nursing Intervention with the Failure-to-Thrive Family. *The American Journal of Maternal-Child Nursing*, 1:111, March-April 1976.

Johnson, F. P., and Hatcher, W.: The Patient With Sickle Cell Disease. *Nursing Forum*, 13:259, 1974.

Johnson, J. E., Kirchhoff, K. T., and Endress, M. P.: Altering Children's Distress Behavior During Orthopedic Cast Removal. *Nursing Research*, 24:404, November-December 1975.

Justice, P., and Smith, G. F.: PKU: Phenylketonuria. *Am. J. Nursing*, 75:1303, August 1975.

Kahn, G.: Eczematoid Eruptions in Children. *Pediatr. Clin. N. Am.*, 22:203, February 1975.

Karp, R. J., Haaz, W. S., Starko, K., and Gorman, J. M.: Iron Deficiency in Families of Iron-Deficient Inner-City School Children. *Am. J. Dis. Child*, 128:18, July 1974.

Lloyd-Still, J. D., Hurwitz, I., Wolff, P. H., and Shwachman, H.: Intellectual Development After Severe Malnutrition in Infancy. *Pediatrics*, 54:306, September 1974.

McCormack, M. K., et al.: A Comparison of the Physical and Intellectual Development of Black Children With and Without Sickle-Cell Trait. *Pediatrics*, 56:1021, December 1975.

McCreery, M.: Diet: First-Line Defense Against Celiac Disease. *RN*, 39:50, February 1976.

Marcotte, A. A.: Cystic Fibrosis. *The Canadian Nurse*, 71:33, July 1975.

Neill, K., and Kauffman, C.: Care of the Hospitalized Abused Child and His Family: Nursing Implications. *The American Journal of Maternal-Child Nursing*, 1:117, March-April 1976.

Newberger, E. H., and Hyde, J. N.: Child Abuse: Principles and Implications of Current Pediatric Practice. *Pediatr. Clin. N. Am.*, 22:695, August 1975.

Olson, R. J.: Index of Suspicion: Screening for Child Abusers. *Am. J. Nursing*, 76:108, January 1976.

Osoff, A.: Caring for the Child with Familial Dysautonomia. *Am. J. Nursing*, 75:1158, July 1975.

Roach, L. B.: Color Changes in Dark Skin. *Nursing 77*, 7:48, January 1977.

Rodgers, B., Ferholt, J., and Cooper, C. L.: Screening Tool to Detect Psychosocial Adjustment of Children with Cystic Fibrosis. *Nursing Research*, 23:420, September-October 1974.

Rosman, N. P.: Neurological and Muscular Aspects of Thyroid Dysfunction in Childhood. *Pediatr. Clin. N. Am.*, 23:575, August 1976.

Rutkow, I. M., and Lipton, J. M.: Some Negative Aspects of Sickle Cell Anemia Screening Programs. *Conn. Med.*, 38:257, May 1974.

Schwachman, H.: Gastrointestinal Manifestations of Cystic Fibrosis. *Pediatr. Clin. N. Am.*, 22:787, November 1975.

Smith, S. M., Honigsberger, L., and Smith, C. A.: E. E. G. and Personality Factors in Baby Batterers. *Br. Med. J.*, 2:20, July 7, 1973.

Stainton, M. C.: Non-Accidental Trauma in Children. *The Canadian Nurse*, 71:26, October 1975.

Stokan, R. E.: The Right Formula for the Right Infant: Making Sense of Infant Nutrition. *The American Journal of Maternal-Child Nursing*, 2:101, March-April 1977.

Techlin, J. S.: Evaluation of Bronchial Drainage in Patients With Cystic Fibrosis. *Phys. Ther.*, 55:1081, October 1975.

Tripp, A.: Hyper and Hypocalcemia. *Am. J. Nursing*, 76:1142, July 1976.

Whiting, L.: Defining Emotional Neglect. *Children Today*, 5:2, January-February 1976.

Winick, M., Meyer, K. K., and Harris, R. C.: Malnutrition and Environmental Enrichment by Early Adoption. *Science*, 190:1173, December 19, 1975.

AUDIOVISUAL MEDIA*

American Journal of Nursing Company

Pediatric Nursing Series
21 44 minute classes, black and white.
Class Instructor: Brodie, B.

The Child with Cystic Fibrosis
Participating Instructor: Walter, M.
Clinical manifestations, etiology, diagnosis and treatment are described, with special emphasis on nursing care at home and in the hospital. There are demonstrations of clapping and vibrating techniques and the use of the mist tent.

Psychiatric-Mental Health Nursing
Series Instructor: Mitchell, M.

The Nurse in Child Abuse Prevention
Guest Participants: Shaw, A., and Crawford, M.
30 minutes, videotape, sound, color, guide.

Antecedents and manifestations of the child abuse syndrome are examined and related to the nurse's role in detecting, treating, and preventing this serious disorder of parenthood.

National Cystic Fibrosis Research Foundation

Diagnosis and Management of Cystic Fibrosis
26 minutes, 16mm film, sound, color.
This film emphasizes the variations in clinical manifestations of the disease, offers a guide to diagnostic tests, and explains the rationale of current therapy.

W. B. Saunders Company

Pediatric Conferences with Sydney Gellis
Atopic Dermatitis, Jacobs, A. H.
Cystic Fibrosis and Prolonged Obstructive Jaundice, Gellis, S.

Intensive Transfusion Therapy, Necheles, T.
Problems of Iron Fortified Formulas, Oski, F.
Subdural Hematoma, McLaurin, R. L.
Treatment of Convulsions, Rabe, E. F.
Pediatric Hematology: A Morphologic Approach to Diagnosis
  Naiman, J. L.
  3 35mm filmstrips, 2 audio-tape cassettes, color.
  This program reviews the whole range of hereditary and acquired pediatric blood disorders—from sickle cell anemia to acute myelocytic leukemia to Niemann-Pick disease.

Trainex Corporation

Allergy
  35mm filmstrip, audio-tape cassettes, 33 1/3 LP, color.
  Describes symptoms, causes and possible cures for an allergic child.

Battered Child Syndrome
  35mm filmstrip, audio-tape cassettes, 33 1/3 LP, color.
  Case studies show the results of beatings, mutilation, burns, neglect, kicks, and repeated pulling and twisting of the extremities of children. This program can enhance the viewer's ability to recognize and identify physical and psychological patterns indicative of child abuse.

Clinical Dermatology
  35mm filmstrip, audio-tape cassettes, 33 1/3 LP, color.
  A brief description of the anatomy and physiology of the skin and its accessory organs. Various forms of inflammatory skin eruptions involving the epidermis are illustrated and discussed.

Cystic Fibrosis
  35mm filmstrip, audio-tape cassettes, 33 1/3 LP, color.
  Discusses major features that comprise cystic fibrosis. Individual case studies illustrate variation in clinical manifestations. The significance of roentgenograms, sweat testing, screening meconium for albumin, and testing stool for trypsin and other pancreatic enzymes for the detection and assessment of pathology is explained. Includes discussion of prophylactic and therapeutic management of pulmonary manifestations and gastrointestinal disturbances.

Postural Drainage, Clapping, and Vibration
  35mm filmstrip, audio-tape cassettes, 33 1/3 LP, color.
  In addition to the basic anatomy and physiology of the respiratory system, instructions for breathing retraining, postural drainage positions, proper coughing, clapping and vibration procedures are illustrated. Includes discussion of a pediatric case study.

United States Government

The Battered Child, Part I
  Producer: USNMAC
  27 minutes, 16mm film, optical sound, black and white.
  Discusses patterns of injuries common to the battered child syndrome and interpretation of these patterns. Shows the external symptoms or signs, and cases with no external symptoms but with extensive internal damage, which is obvious at autopsy.

The Battered Child, Part II
  Producer: USNMAC
  26 minutes, 16mm film, optical sound, black and white.
  Discusses patterns of injuries common to the battered child syndrome and the interpretation of these patterns.

---

*Complete addresses are given in the Appendix.

UNIT FOUR

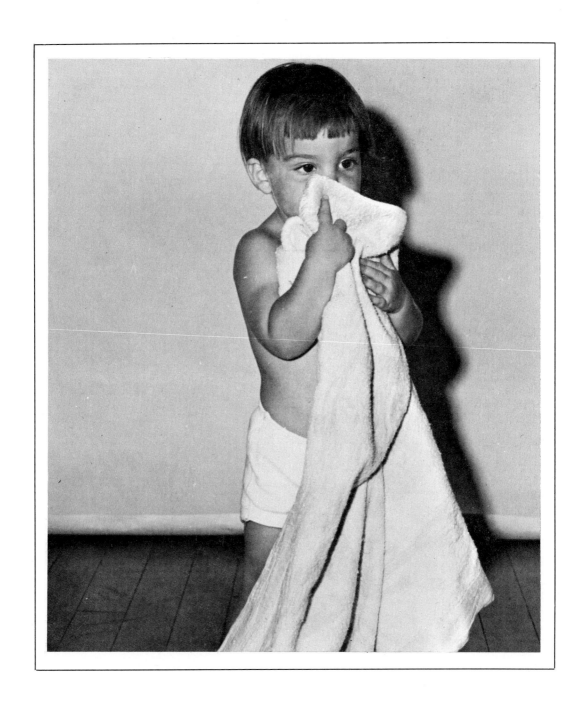

THE TODDLER

DEDICATION

Child! do not throw this book about;
Refrain from the unholy pleasure
Of cutting all the pictures out!
Preserve it as your chiefest treasure.

Hilaire Belloc (1870–1953): *The Bad
Child's Book of Beasts*

Chapter Sixteen

THE NORMAL TODDLER: HIS GROWTH, DEVELOPMENT, AND CARE

The infant by his first birthday has learned to *trust* or *distrust* the adults who care for him. This attitude is modified by experiences throughout childhood and adolescence, but its direct influence on the way he perceives experiences during the toddler stage is evident to all who know him.

As the child moves from passive dependency to active interaction with those about him, society or that small section of it which he knows—his family—guides him in conformity with social norms. The most important demand made upon him during the toddler period is that of toilet training.

During the toddler period parents must learn to accept the changes that occur as the child grows and develops. The child becomes more mobile and begins to assert his independence. Sometimes parents, especially the mother, who enjoyed the total dependency of the infant have difficulty accepting the child's new wish for freedom to explore and to become a person in his own right.

OVERVIEW OF EMOTIONAL DEVELOPMENT

SENSE OF AUTONOMY

As the child passes from infancy into the toddler stage (one to three years) he uses his increasing ability to help himself and to develop his *sense of autonomy*. He makes his desires known to those about him to get what he wants. He shows that he has a mind and a will of his own. If he has learned to trust others, he accepts their gentle, considerate guidance in learning new skills. But when they deny him what he wants, he is angry and hates the very people whom he has learned to love—mother, father, siblings, and nurse. Their response to his anger is important in forming his personality. If they

show him love while refusing him what he wants, he quickly returns to the loving relations which he has learned bring pleasure. He has learned that an angry attitude does not get him what he wants, but that a pleasant response, even when he is denied what he wants, brings him happiness.

Understanding love for the child of his age is shown by giving him all the freedom he can safely use, by giving him all the love and help he needs to keep him safe in an environment which he is unable to control and in which he is dependent upon others for the satisfaction of bodily drives, and by giving him guidance in avoiding hazards in the changing social situations in which he feels himself to be the focal point.

If he has learned by the end of the toddler period to accept and utilize guidance, he has gained a new level of self-control without losing his self-esteem. If he has not learned to be self-helpful, within the limits of his ability and in the way that those about him want, and, equally important, to accept adult direction in situations in which he cannot carry on alone, he is likely to feel insecure in his ability to meet the physical and social problems in his environment. He appears withdrawn and may have a *sense of doubt* about himself and others and a sense of what an adult would feel as shame. He avoids new experiences and thus has fewer opportunities to acquire new skills than has the child with an outgoing personality.

Needs of the Toddler

The basic needs of the toddler are the same as those of the infant. The toddler needs security and love, but he also needs graded independence.

LOVE AND SECURITY

Love enables the toddler to grow up and reach out for more mature goals because he feels secure in his parents' affectionate care of him. Since he feels secure, he can endure the frustrations which come to every child in the process of maturation.

Both boys and girls give their first love to their mothers because mothers give them tender, lov-

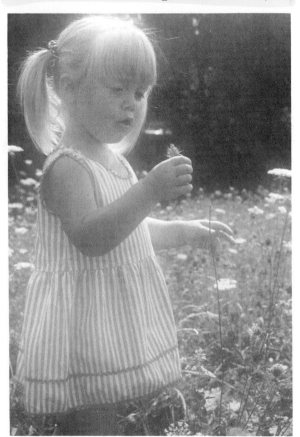

FIGURE 16–1. The young child needs security, but she also needs a degree of independence so she can explore her world. (Courtesy of H. Armstrong Roberts.)

ing care. As the needs of children become more diversified—less for physical care and more for social pleasures—their attachment to a loving father increases. In a family in which the father gives the infant the same care the mother does the infant generally feels as secure with one parent as with the other. But many infants hardly know their fathers until they reach the toddler stage. Then the father plays with them and takes them about with him. These toddlers, however, still turn to their mothers when they want physical care or feel sick.

During the toddler or perhaps even the early preschool period the child may select in addition to his parents an object which has unusual importance and which seems to provide security for him. This *security* or *transitional object,* such as a blanket, diaper, or toy, is affectionately cuddled and loved, but in the process many times becomes dirty and mutilated. The child may become distressed if the object is cleaned or changed in any way.

GRADED INDEPENDENCE

Independence is learned gradually and is given the child only in situations in which he can guard himself from physical and emotional trauma. Independence must be denied him while he is too young to use it successfully, for a painful experience might make him afraid to try out new skills.

FULFILLMENT OF NEEDS

The toddler whose parents give him graded independence which brings pleasurable results develops a sense of self-reliance and adequacy, of *autonomy.* He finds that he is an individual who may make choices under the guidance of his parents. He may decide to play on the floor or on the chair, to eat the food offered him or reject it, to welcome a visitor or cling to his mother's skirt. Sooner or later he learns that there are many things he would like to do, but *can not* or *may not.* He easily learns that he cannot touch all the objects he wants because some are out of his reach. It will take him a little longer to learn that there are some things he *can* do without being hurt, but *may not* do because his parents say "No."

The child wants to do many things he is not physically able to do. Climbing up stairs is an example of his persistence. If he is constantly with a sibling only a few years older than he, he will attempt many activities which he is unable to do successfully.

As his muscular system matures he develops simple muscular skills, but finds that he cannot coordinate these diverse patterns into a purposeful activity such as he sees older children do so easily. Although he has learned to walk, to hold on and let go, to grasp and manipulate objects in various ways, he is often frustrated in his efforts to make his hands and feet do what he wants them to do. The toddler age is a frustrating age.

Regulating the toddler's activities is an important part of his training and is a challenge to the most mature and resourceful adult. The toddler cannot realize the consequences of what he does. Even if there is no danger of being hurt, he may make himself ridiculous so that people laugh at him. This hurts his self-esteem if he cannot also join in the laughter.

A gradually expanding area of growth in a safe environment must be provided for him. Since one reason for adult control is that failure may injure his self-esteem, it is evident that an adult should never use shame or ridicule as a means of punishment or of prevention of forbidden activities. Shaming makes the toddler feel even smaller than he is; if it is used to excess, the child may comply when he is watched, but do as he pleases when he is not observed. This has been the cause of many serious accidents.

A certain amount of defiance is normal and may be more apparent than real. "No, no" does not always mean that he will not do what he is asked to do. It may mean, "Don't look so cross, Mama," or, "I don't know what you mean." "No" is an easy sound to make, and he may use it for personal pleasure rather than for expression of a negative feeling. Even with the two- or three-year-old it may not mean refusal, but rather a bewildered response to injunctions he does not understand. Too often, however, it means that he will not do what the adult asks of him. His defiance is likely to be increased by anger on the part of the adult. This is because the child is likely to become confused, and he follows the adult's lead with expressions of anger. He lacks words to convey his meaning and strikes the adult, has a temper tantrum, cries, or becomes sullen.

Although a certain amount of defiance is part of his growing independence, excessive defiance becomes a habit and, unless wisely corrected, may be a factor in poor adjustment. The repercussion upon himself of the irritation he arouses in others is likely to make him withdraw into himself or become more defiant. If his attitude is not corrected before adolescence, he may find others like himself who are defiant of adult restraint. If he can get along with them, he may become one of the gang whose delinquent acts fill our newspapers and television screens. If he cannot fit into the gang because he will not accept the restraint the gang exercises over its members, he may become a solitary delinquent. He may learn to dislike the real world, in which he is disliked, and turn to day-dreaming. Outwardly he may appear to be a quiet, obedient child in whom defiance is not suspected. He is likely to have poorer mental hygiene than the delinquent has.

Parents or their substitutes should have a deep sense of the value of preserving their own dignity as the child sees it, as well as the child's self-respect.

By building on the sense of trust in others which he developed during his first year of life the child normally gains a sense of autonomy during the toddler stage. He must be respected as an individual and helped to internalize the social norms of his group so that he *wants* to do what is *right* and, conversely, hurts his image of himself if he does what is *wrong*.

This developmental task takes two full years to make even a good beginning on which further guidance can be given as the child grows older.

Three specific areas in which the toddler must be given guidance are (1) elimination control, or control of bodily functions of urination and defecation, (2) learning to talk, and (3) learning social norms.

CONTROL OF BODILY FUNCTIONS

Control of the bodily functions of defecation and urination is important, for it is the most personal phase of the young child's learning, closely related to his sensations. The child would like to continue emptying his bladder and bowels whenever he is conscious of pressure from tension in these organs. Society does not sanction such behavior, and so gradually the toddler must learn to face the frustration of retention, and gain control of defecation and urination with the help of those he loves. Toilet training, or learning elimination control, is at best difficult for the young child, especially if his family places an extreme value on cleanliness. If cleanliness has for his mother a moral aspect (if he dirties himself he is naughty, and if he keeps clean he is good), the child who is not able to keep clean and dry begins to develop feelings of guilt and anxiety because he cannot live up to the expectations of adults who care for him.

The infant, who for the first year received all care, love, and attention, is now asked to assume the responsibility of giving up his comfort and to contribute to the comfort of others. He must learn to excrete urine and feces only at the appropriate time and place, although he cannot understand the necessity for this. He is motivated to try only because he wants to please his mother.

In more technical terms, the infant lives according to the *pleasure principle* (wanting what he wants when he wants it). The toddler must begin to accept the *reality principle* (giving up an immediate pleasure in order to gain another pleasure later). In this instance the toddler must give up the pleasure of excreting where and when he wishes in order to gain his mother's approval. If he does not have a trusting relationship with his mother, he will not be strongly motivated to succeed in toilet training.

Other factors, of course, influence him. If he sees an older sibling using the toilet, he may want to do the same. As he becomes more active his wet clothing is more uncomfortable. If other children point at the puddles he makes and laugh at him, he may laugh too, but he does begin to connect keeping himself dry with part of the life pattern of the older child whom he imitates.

Learning a new skill is difficult before the stage of maturation at which the child is motivated to learn and is physically able without too great an effort. If he is urged to learn before this stage, unfavorable attitudes may develop. To wait beyond the optimum stage when he is ready to learn a new skill is a mistake, because the happiness of using this skill is kept from him. Then, too, skills normal for his age evoke a favorable response from other people, and his self-image, taken from their attitude toward him, is more satisfying.

Toilet Training. The way in which the parents approach the process of toilet training is more important than the actual procedure itself. Their attitude and manner will influence the way the child feels about himself and other people, how he relates to others in the matter of giving and receiving, how he asserts himself with other people, and how he approaches new life situations in the future. The principle of interrelatedness of growth (see p. 28) applies to the matter of toilet training.

Toilet training should be started when the toddler is physiologically and psychologically ready. He is physiologically ready when he can stand alone, i.e., when the tracts of the spinal cord are myelinated down to the anal level. It is useless and too frustrating to the child to attempt toilet training before the neurologic pathways are formed which enable him to control the anal sphincter and the urethra under tension and to excrete when his mother tells him to do so.

The toddler has seen other family members use the toilet, so that he is familiar with the

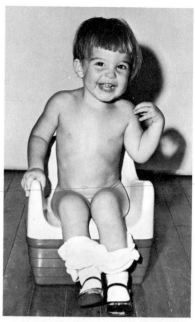

FIGURE 16–2. The toddler should feel secure when placed on the training chair. She should be able to touch the floor with her feet and should be supported adequately by the back and arms of the chair.

process. He will communicate to his mother his own need to excrete by signals that are uniquely his own. Some toddlers grunt or strain, others point to their diapers or tug at them, while those who are more verbal say a special word to communicate their needs.

After the toddler has begun bowel control and when he is physiologically able to retain his urine for a two-hour period, he is usually ready to begin training for urination. Before this time he may have pointed to his puddles on the floor, or tugged at his wet diaper *after* he urinated. Although his mother should commend him for his awareness, she may have to wait a period of time until he can inform her of his need *before* he urinates.

If training is started before the child is physiologically and psychologically ready, it is probable that the child is neither controlling nor expelling excreta at will, but rather that his mother has put him upon the toilet chair at the time when tension caused release of the anal or urethral sphincter, or both. As long as the child's diet and fluid intake are about the same each day this procedure may be successful, but any change in routine is likely to change the time of excretion, and he will soil his diaper or training pants. The mother is then apt to feel that the child has retrogressed and may show her disapproval by a scowling face or severe tone of voice. This leads to a feeling like that of adult shame in the child.

The mother who shows the child what she expects of him when he indicates his readiness for toilet training, who expects success only when he can cooperate, and who approves of him in spite of his failures, will strengthen her relations with him. The toddler will be able to withstand the deprivation of giving up something he wishes to do in order to please his mother, and will not experience feelings of fear, shame, self-doubt, and hostility.

Bowel training is easier to accomplish than bladder training because the number of stools in a day is less than the number of times the child urinates. If the process is begun successfully, but an extraneous factor such as moving to a new house or the birth of a sibling occurs, the mother may expect some regression in behavior and react appropriately.

PROCESS OF TOILET TRAINING. When the toddler communicates his readiness, he should be placed on a comfortable child's toilet seat or training chair on which he feels secure. There should be a rest for his arms and feet. He should not be given food or toys at this time, for these distract his attention from the purpose for which he is put on the chair. The mother or nurse indicates by gestures and tone of voice that he is expected to pass his eliminations in this place and at this time. A specific word indicating the act should be selected, a word easily understood by everyone. This is important, for many a child at nursery school or visiting with friendly adults has not been able to tell the adults that he wants to relieve himself, because he does not understand the words they use and they do not understand what he is saying. The word used by the child or taught to him by his mother often reflects the social class of the parents. Nurses should never show disgust at any word a child may use, though he can be taught a more appropriate one.

Training should not be made a tense issue for either the mother or the child. The mother will find it easier for herself as well as better for the child if she assumes a casual, matter-of-fact attitude. When the child defecates or urinates in the toilet or training chair, he should be praised and cuddled. But when he fails to do so, the mother should never show disappointment or disapproval, for the child of this age has difficulty in releasing the contents of the bowel or bladder at will.

When the child is old enough to go to the toilet by himself, he should have training pants and clothing which he can manage without help so that he can develop increasing independence. A change of panties whenever they are even slightly wet will accustom him to being dry. He feels more grown up and like his siblings when he no longer wears diapers and can be changed while standing. If possible, after he has become accustomed to panties, diapers should not be put on him except at night and at nap time. Children find attractive panties a great incentive to keeping dry. The toddler's pants should be such that he can slip them down or open them with a zipper. A girl's training pants should have elastic at the waist so that they may be easily pushed down below the knees.

Steps which the toddler can climb to reach the adult toilet (with or without the child's toilet seat) are helpful. Boys learn to stand for urination by watching older boys urinate. A step may be necessary for him to urinate into the toilet bowl without wetting the floor.

Enemas, cathartics, or suppositories are not used unless ordered by the physician. The mother can be helped to understand that not all children have a daily bowel movement.

AGE AT WHICH TOILET TRAINING IS ACCOMPLISHED. The average healthy, intelligent child usually accomplishes bowel control by the end of the eighteenth month. Daytime bladder control may be fairly well established by two years of age, and night control by three or four years. Night control is not to be hurried. It is not good to wake the child and take him to the toilet, for he may stay awake for a long time after he has been put to bed again. Withholding fluids in the late afternoon and evening may be tried, but if the child is not physiologically ready, this will not help him to retain urine during the night. Also, he may be thirsty and cry for water during the night.

TRAINING DURING ILLNESS. If the child is not trained when he enters the pediatric unit, he should not be taught to use a bedpan or urinal or toilet chair while he is hospitalized. He would not be motivated to learn, because there would be no one person whom he loves and attempts to please by doing what is asked of him. Then, too, a sick child should not be subjected to the strain of breaking old habits and acquiring new ones.

If the mother on admission of the child says that he is toilet-trained, this is noted in the habit history on the admission chart. The technique used by the mother and the words the child associates with the acts of elimination are recorded. If the child is old enough to understand, he is shown the hospital equipment, such as the bedpan, urinal, and the training chair, if the physician permits him to be out of bed. The nurse should try to keep him on the same schedule as that used at home, but should not be worried if he wets or soils himself and certainly should not show disapproval. The nurse explains to the mother, so that she will not be disturbed by his behavior, that the sick child in a strange environment generally regresses to infantile toilet habits. When he is well again, his mother can help him to resume his former habits of elimination.

MEANING OF TOILET TRAINING TO THE CHILD. The child is now asked to do what his mother wants him to do, whereas when he was a baby, she gave him loving care without asking any other response from him than his loving dependence upon her. Instead of being irresponsible, he is now asked to assume some responsibility for himself.

Fecal Smearing. The child has not yet acquired the adult's distaste for bodily excretions. He likes to manipulate fecal material and smear it upon the floor, wall, or furniture. Such behavior occurs between the ages of 15 and 21 months. The toddler thinks of his feces as coming from him and in this sense regards it as a gift. He does not understand why fecal material is thrown away after he has been urged to expel it into the toilet chair. (This is one advantage of a toilet. He can help pull the handle and see the feces disappear with the swirling water. This is to him a satisfying accomplishment.) The parent or nurse should accept the child's feeling about his excretion and never express strong disapproval of his smearing it upon himself or any object. His desire to smear should be *sublimated,* i.e., be gratified in a socially acceptable way by giving him clay, damp sand, or mud to manipulate. Later he may enjoy smearing in finger painting, using bright, light cheerful colors on large sheets of paper.

Smearing with feces can be reduced if the child is cleaned immediately after a bowel movement. Diapers should be applied securely, so that he cannot put his hands upon the excrement. After he has learned to use the training chair or toilet, smearing is no longer a great problem.

INFLUENCE OF TOILET TRAINING ON THE CHILD'S PERSONALITY. *Ambivalence* toward his mother is common during the training period. He loves her, but now she asks him to give up the comfort of relieving himself when and where he feels the desire to do so. He therefore feels antagonistic toward her. *His ambivalent attitude is composed of love and hate at the same time.* He may strike at her and pull away and a moment later turn to her for comfort. If she maintains an attitude of friendliness and understanding, love will predominate over hostility in him. It is important to minimize his antagonism so that he does not grow out of the training period with feelings of hostility, rebellion and resentment.

SUMMARY. If a mother loves her child, he is normally conditioned to please her and will respond to toilet training without too much difficulty. She will not be discouraged if she has confidence in his intelligence and his desire to do what she asks, and she will give him a reasonable length of time in which to learn.

On the other hand, if the mother shows disgust about the whole process of excretion, the child will feel ashamed of his body. He may feel that he is not lovable. He may even feel that he is a naughty child if he fails in toilet training. Eventually he may acquire the attitude that all physical functions should be brought under rigid control. He may extend this feeling to all his activities and be constantly afraid of doing something which will displease his mother or other adults. In his mind he equates overcleanliness with being good. Unfortunately his desire to keep clean usually inhibits normal active play. Such a child lacks spontaneity and creativity. He is apt to be a child afraid to soil his hands or dirty his clothes when playing. When other children make mud pies, he stands back. Such a child may develop a persistent attitude of anxiously trying to please anyone in authority over him for fear he will lose their approval. Not only must he be perfect himself, but also he

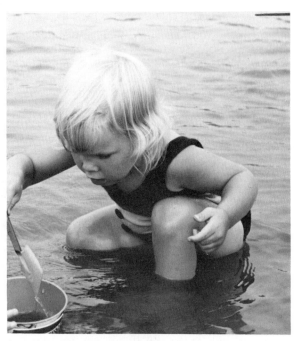

FIGURE 16–3. Toddlers enjoy playing in water and sand. This is a more socially acceptable activity than smearing feces. (H. Armstrong Roberts.)

expects his friends to be likewise. He becomes rigid and inflexible and bound by compulsive rituals which to his mind will minimize the danger of his displeasing someone and thus will lessen his anxiety.

LEARNING LANGUAGE

Learning to talk takes a long time. From the newborn's cry to the first spoken word is the change from a reflex utterance to something which has a meaning for both the child and others. The infant uses motions, particularly movement of the hands, to indicate his wants. Motions are his substitute for speech.

Between the ages of one and three years the child is increasingly able to understand others and to express his feelings and ideas in words. Infants and little children may continue to use gestures, however, such as holding out their arms and smiling when they want to be picked up, even when they are able to say what they want.

Long before a child can use words in sentences he understands the meaning of many words. The mother's facial expression, gestures, and tone of voice help the child to understand the meaning of her words. She may teach him a new word by pointing to an object while she says the word. Or when he is interested in an object, such as a doll, he may say the word as she gives it to him.

Incentives to Speech. In order to speak a child must have satisfying relations with his mother. Unless he feels that she will respond to his words, he is not motivated to speak. He must find it rewarding to talk or he will not be interested in trying. He speaks to express his needs, and to a young child words have magical powers that can make things happen. When he says, "Ma-ma," and points to something, he means, "Please give me that." When he learns the names for objects, he will use the names, e.g., cup, dog. If all his needs are supplied without his asking, he is poorly motivated to speak until he feels the need for words to express attitudes, ideas, and emotions.

Normally a child's first speech is an expression of his wants. This is followed by words or phrases which indicate ideas or what he thinks the function of objects to be. His idea of animals is expressed in terms of what they do; e.g., a dog barks. He early learns the value of speech in pleasant social relations. He takes great pleasure in talking and talks to anyone, his toys, pets, or himself. Even when he can say only a few words, he uses these words to obtain information about himself, other people and things. "Go bye-bye" is not only a request; he is also asking

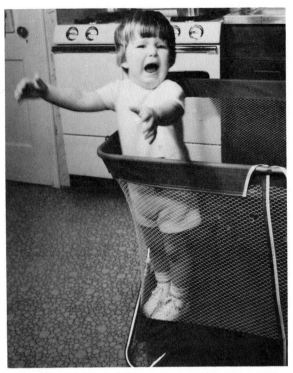

FIGURE 16–4. The toddler cries because he cannot express his needs in words.

whether he is going outdoors. When he says, "Dog," he may be asking where the household pet is.

Methods of Learning. A young child must have a good model or he will not learn to speak correctly. He will imitate poor speech as readily as correct speech, perhaps more easily because it is often more simple and direct and apt to be accompanied with gestures. If an adult uses baby talk in speaking to him, the child has no model for learning the correct words for objects, experiences and attitudes. He needs not only a model talking *to him*, but also the opportunity to use the word immediately in his answer. Talking to toys, to animals and to himself gives him practice in using words, but since he hears only himself, he may be confirmed in his mispronunciation and misuse of words.

There is a plateau stage in learning to talk at which a child makes little progress. The plateau occurs when the child has learned to walk and is so interested in walking that he pays little attention to acquiring new words. Nevertheless he appears to be increasing the number of words he understands.

The child with his limited vocabulary may cry because he is frustrated in his efforts to express his wants or feelings and does not get what he wants. He still hits out when he is angry and cries when he is hurt. He has not yet acquired the ability, physically or psychologically, to control his actions and to use words to express antagonism and unhappiness. Later on, instead of hitting his mother or a playmate, he may express his feeling by saying, "I hate you!" or, "I wish you'd go away," and instead of crying because he may not go out and play he may say, "Why does it rain? I want to play," or simply wail, "I want to go out and play." In either case he is asking for the comfort which crying brought him when he was a baby. Even when he is able to speak, if his emotions are too great for him to control, putting them into words is not a sufficient outlet, and he resorts to the immature outlets of anger and disappointment. Whenever he speaks or cries, the child needs acceptance of himself and his feelings, however unreasonable they appear from the adult's point of view. Crying is a distress signal with him as with an infant.

Examples of this sort of situation are often found in the hospital. When a child thinks that he will be hurt because he will get a needle and is reassured by what we say to him, we see the value of his understanding verbal communication and of his ability to put his fear into words. He needs a simple explanation as a preparation for the procedure and both verbal and physical demonstrations of affection so that he does not feel that these strange adults want to hurt him (technically speaking, that he is being attacked). The nurse in such a situation must not say, "Don't cry." To do so would indicate a lack of understanding of how the child perceives the situation. He is still too young not to be afraid of pain. The nurse or mother should explain the need for the hurt and what is to be done, so far as he can understand the reason or the procedure. If possible, his mother should be there to hold him; if not, one of the nurses whom he knows or at least has made friends with should take her place. The nurse may say to a crying child, "I know you are frightened. It will be over soon."

Vocabulary Building. The child builds a vocabulary in the following ways. The first words he learns are nouns of one syllable, nouns like the sounds he has babbled ("Ma-ma, da-da"). He attempts more difficult words until eventually he can give the names of objects and people in his daily environment. He next learns verbs that mean some form of action which he sees about him and whose meaning he understands (e.g., give, take, run). Adjectives he learns from 18 months on. The first adjectives he learns are usually "good" and "bad," because he hears them frequently. The first adverbs he uses are usually "here" and "where." These are words used by his mother in speaking to him. Last he learns the meaning of pronouns. These are confusing to him because they vary with the person using the word. Johnny is "me" and "I" to himself, but "you" to his mother when she speaks to him, and "he" when she tells his father about him. The same confusion exists with other pronouns.

The size of a child's vocabulary depends on his intelligence, on whether he has had an incentive to learn, and on whether he has been helped to learn new words. At nine months he can say "Ma-ma" and "Da-da," and at one year, two or three more words. From 18 months to three or four years his vocabulary increases rapidly. At two years he can say approximately 300 words, and at three years approximately 900. During school age his general vocabulary increases rapidly as the result of being taught new words and of his pleasure in reading.

Sentence Formation. The child's first attempt at making sentences consists in combining two or more words into a phrase and supplementing these with gestures. Early sentences contain nouns, verbs and, at times, adjectives and adverbs, e.g., "Baby go bye-bye."

Delayed Speech. The normal child will begin to speak by about 15 months of age. If he does not speak by the time he is two years old, the cause for delay should be investigated. Some of the common causes follow.

INTELLIGENCE. Speech is delayed in children of low intelligence. The size of the vocabulary depends to a great extent upon the child's intelligence.

SOCIAL AND CULTURAL ENVIRONMENT. Children of poorer social environments are delayed in speech development because they often have poor models to imitate. Children in an orphanage or a similar institution may have extreme language retardation because adults seldom speak to them individually, and when they do, the subject is likely to be merely what the child is to do or not to do.

ILLNESS. Children who are ill in an institution for a long time have slower speech development than well children because they have fewer contacts with other children and also because their needs are answered before they have to ask for what they want. A child who receives much adult attention at home when he is sick may increase his vocabulary rapidly. It is the hospitalized child who is likely to be retarded.

POOR MODELS. If the child has a poor model to imitate in speaking, his speech will be incorrect or retarded.

NEGATIVISM. The child may decide not to talk because he was forced to talk when he was not mature enough to want to imitate his mother's words. He may have been laughed at for his babyish pronunciation and had his self-image lowered.

DEAFNESS. If the child cannot hear what others say, he cannot imitate them and therefore will not speak unless he has had special training. Even then he will have a smaller vocabulary, poor pronunciation, and a peculiar, flat tone of voice (see p. 586).

SEX. Boys are usually slower than girls in learning to talk. They also have a smaller vocabulary than girls and make more grammatical errors.

Learning two languages at the same time for the child under five years of age is likely to delay his learning to speak and also to cause confusion in both vocabulary and grammatical forms.

CULTURAL DEVELOPMENT

The toddler must learn many other patterns of behavior besides toilet training and language. He learns how to make the simple basic movements in washing and bathing himself and brushing his teeth. He understands what his mother means when she wants him to keep clean, to put his toys away when he has finished playing with them, and to keep his play space neat.

The child is attempting an overall mastery of his world. When he learns to do something by himself, he has a real sense of mastery, independence, and adequacy in meeting his needs. His parents should help him to learn and should approve his success. If parents do not show their approval in ways he can understand, the child experiences a conflict between enjoying what he can do himself (even if this is to get an ashtray and empty it on the floor) and the disapproval of his parents. Since he knows that they will disapprove, he must make a choice between the pleasure of doing what he wants and the pleasure of having his parents' approval. Through such decisions the child eventually learns how to make appropriate judgments, choosing what is considered right in the culture of the group to which he belongs. His basic motivation is love for his parents, a love acquired in infancy and strengthened during early childhood.

Personality Traits of the Toddler

NEGATIVISM

In his desire for independence or autonomy the child wants to do many things he should not do. From infancy through the toddler period he has heard his parents say "No" to his many efforts at self-assertion. Gradually he learns to use the words "No, no" to mean "Don't" and a rather stubborn "I won't." In this way he is substantiating his power as an individual in controlling those who love him. The developmental task of this period is to curb his negative responses and to adjust his conduct to the social norms of those in authority.

Each child goes through this period of negativism during his development toward maturity. Two years is said to be the "No, no" age and has been called "the terrible twos." He wants to act as an individual and appears to want power—to have his own way—more than the pleasure of the forbidden activity. Yet when he is frustrated in achieving what he wants independently of the help of others, or when their reaction toward him leads him to believe that they do not love him, he is likely to turn to the adults against whom his aggression was aimed for comfort in the unpleasant situation he has created for himself.

Sometimes he seems to want to be dependent and independent at the same time. For example, when he is offered ice cream, he may say, "No," and yet eat it quickly in spite of his answer.

A child acts in a negative fashion because he cannot tolerate the frustration of a desire. He cannot accept parental restrictions and at the same time cannot find an acceptable way to gain the results he wants. When he says, "No," he feels as strong as his parents.

Sometimes a child appears to be negativistic when he really is not. He may not object to doing what his parents want, but he does not want to stop what he is doing, e.g., if he is playing happily and is asked to put away his toys and go to bed.

The period of negativism is usually a short one if the child's needs are understood. He needs the support of his parents' love in order to learn how to satisfy his new powers of independence in socially acceptable ways.

Handling Negativistic Behavior. An adult should not use opposition to overcome opposition in a child. Opposition increases the child's desire to show his independence.

An adult should not give the toddler too many commands or interrupt his activities too frequently.

The adult should help the child to participate in what is expected of him by giving physical help, e.g., by putting the toys away when it is bedtime. This allows the toddler to feel that he and the adult are working toward a common goal and not that he is forced to do what the adult wishes. When the mother places food in front of a two-year-old, she may feed him a few spoonfuls, speaking gently to him as she does so. The child may then take the spoon in his hand and feed himself.

The mother must recognize indications of independence in the child. Such recognition increases the child's self-esteem and makes him want to cooperate even more. It helps him to feel self-important. All children learn to know themselves through the attitudes of *significant persons* in their environment (particularly members of their own families) toward them. If the mother has a wholesome concept of the child, he has a wholesome concept of himself. If he accepts himself at this age, he can later accept others.

RITUALISTIC BEHAVIOR

The toddler engages in much ritualistic behavior. He makes rituals of simple tasks because he knows that he can master himself in this way. Ritualistic behavior is most common between the ages of two and four years; it reaches its height at approximately 2½ years. As the child leaves the toddler period he has less and less need of a strict routine because he is more sure of himself and can adapt to changes better than he could when he was younger. Adults should recognize these rituals in such phases as bathing (hanging the washcloth in a certain way), eating (having his bib on always in the same way), and sleeping (always taking his favorite blanket to bed with him). The adult saves time and energy by doing so and also gives the child a feeling of security and mastery of himself.

SLOWNESS IN CARRYING OUT REQUESTS

The toddler is gradually learning the difference between right and wrong. He cannot decide which of two actions to take. He is therefore likely to carry out both actions. For example, when his mother calls him from play to use the training chair, he is likely to finish his play activity first and urinate on the way to the training chair, partly because of his nervousness and haste to do what his mother has asked. When the child learns through experience which action he should take, he will be able to make decisions more wisely and more quickly.

TEMPER TANTRUMS

Temper tantrums occur when the child cannot integrate his internal impulses and the demands of reality. He is frustrated and reacts in the only way he knows—by violent bodily activity and crying. When no substitute solution is available, temper tantrums result. Such situations are most common during the toddler and early preschool

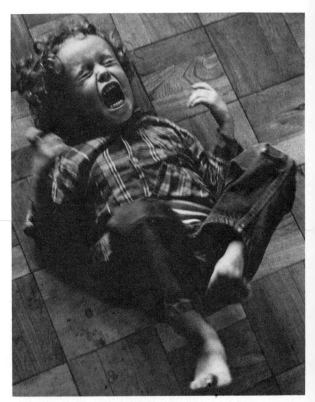

FIGURE 16–5. How well do we understand frustration and rage that lead to temper tantrums when no substitute solution is available to the child. (From *Psychology Today*. 8:101, December 1974.)

periods. If the tantrums are abnormally frequent or continue into school age, the child should be taken to a child guidance center for professional help with his problems or with a deep-seated emotional maladjustment.

In the hospital children may have tantrums because they fear the unknown and are away from those they love. They need help in understanding their environment and care. They also need the security resulting from their mothers' and fathers' frequent visiting.

In a temper tantrum the child is completely oblivious of the reality of the situation. He does not hear or react to what is said to him unless it shocks him so severely that it penetrates his consciousness.

His release of emotion through muscular activity is either aimless or directed against himself. He is likely to bang his head against the floor or otherwise inflict pain upon himself. Only rarely does he attack the adult who provoked the tantrum.

Handling the Child. The child should not be given extra attention, but should be observed and restrained from self-injury or from something in the physical environment which may be a source of injury to himself. Restraint increases the severity of a temper tantrum because it prevents the one outlet which the child knows for his anger. If he hurts another child or an adult or breaks a cherished possession, he may feel guilty when the tantrum is over.

The child's tension will be reduced if he can be removed from the immediate cause of the tantrum and be with one adult who he knows loves him. This adult, usually his mother, should be calm and patient with him, but should not force attention upon him until he indicates that he is ready for the comfort of knowing that he is loved and that his unhappiness can be changed to happiness.

Care After Tantrums. It is advisable to make as few comments as possible upon the child's behavior during a tantrum. He should not be punished in any way. If he will cooperate, it is soothing to wash his face and hands. He may be given a toy to divert his attention from the experience he has undergone. He has been so emotionally upset that he needs to quiet down before he is given food.

Prevention. The mother, knowing the child, may see that a tantrum is imminent. She should try to show him better ways of solving his problem and provide more socially acceptable outlets for his anger and frustration. Also a child often fears his own aggression and the disagreeable state into which it throws him. He should be helped to release his tension in a socially approved way, such as through physical exercise.

The sick child may hammer rubber balls through holes in a board or toss bean bags into a can placed on the floor. In the home a wide range of activities can be used as an outlet for his tension. If he may go outdoors, digging in the garden and helping rake the leaves or shoveling snow are tension-releasing activities. In the house he may use a hammer and pegs or build a block tower which he can then knock down.

If the tantrum is caused by an adult's refusal to grant a request, the adult should be firm and not yield to the child. Only by consistency in adult behavior can a child learn to adjust his own behavior to his expectation of the adult's reaction to what he intends to do. Unfortunately, the child does not and never will live in a world of perfect people, and his own imperfections are less likely to arouse guilt feelings in him if he sees imperfections in those nearest him. One value of a large family is that the children talk over imperfections in their parents—whether real or imaginary—and develop a healthy, realistic love of others even while recognizing their faults. It is a comfort to a two-year-old to know that the four-year-old thinks that mother is sometimes mean. The modern mother knows that she is sometimes mean and that the child knows it, but loves her, just as she loves him with all his naughtiness.

Sometimes when a child feels anger and tensions rising, he isolates himself. This is all right as a temporary measure, but if he always withdraws, he will need help in learning to face problems more directly.

Discipline

Discipline has as its goal *self-control*. It is not merely a way of forcing the child's obedience to adult authority. To be most effective, discipline must be carried out through guidance, helping the child to learn how to live comfortably with others. Discipline, if it is to be constructive, must help the child to direct unacceptable, unrealistic and often futile ways of reaching the goal toward which his impulses are directed into socially approved channels that are effective. This socialization process, begun by the parents, should function without demanding too great sacrifice of the child's individuality and creativity.

As the child learns to control himself in his relations with others, he feels more secure and less anxious. To achieve self-control he needs the help of adults in accepting his feelings and handling them in a constructive way. He needs a positive rather than a forbidding negativistic parent-child relationship.

Discipline is a broad term which includes much of the interaction between the mother or some other adult and the child. A parent uses discipline to establish limits, grant permission, help the child to understand social standards and guide him to direct his impulses into socially acceptable ways of behaving. Much of this is not recognized as discipline by either the parent or the child. It is part of family life or the expression of happy parent-child relations. The way in which a parent approaches the problem of discipline is perhaps the best indication of his feelings toward the child.

Setting of Limits. Limits must be set to the child's behavior if he is to feel secure; otherwise he will constantly suffer the consequences of his mistakes in situations in which he is not old enough to function without guidance. Small children do not know the difference between right and wrong; they must learn the difference from their parents. When limits are imposed, the child will probably be angry momentarily, but he is likely to feel more secure because he knows that his parents can create happier situa-

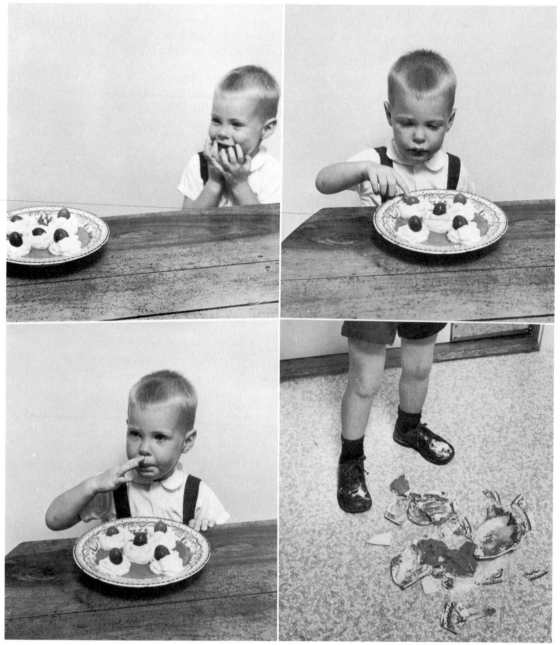

FIGURE 16–6. Mothers sometimes thoughtlessly put such irresistible temptations in the way that they unwittingly lead their children into mischief! (Courtesy of Lew Merrim and *Baby Talk* Magazine.)

tions for him than he can. This is an extension of the sense of trust in adults the infant learned in the first year of life.

It is essential for a child's happiness in relations with other people that he form habits of behavior limited by social approval. Parents who establish habits of behavior which win the toddler friends and give him an acceptable self-image reflected from what others think of him are fulfilling an important part of their function in the training of their child.

The way in which a toddler accepts discipline from his parents or other adults depends upon his love relationship with those adults. Parents who won the trust of their child during his infancy established a relationship in which he was passively cooperative. Passive cooperation lays the foundation for active cooperation.

Constructive Discipline. Parents should be reasonable in their requests and tolerate some delay in the child's response. They should not be overanxious about small details of the child's behavior or say "No" too often. They should never expect from the toddler behavior which is beyond his ability.

The child who has learned the pleasure of cooperating with his parents will carry over the same attitude toward other adults. He will reap the reward of being liked and included in many pleasant situations in which he strengthens his habit of accepting discipline and lays the foundation for self-discipline. Such a child is free to grow, but is given the help he needs with his problems. He is given graded independence, but is not forced to accept more than he can utilize constructively. The adult should do things *with* the child, whenever possible, and not *to* or *for* him, thereby making desirable behavior easy and satisfying to the child.

The child should be shielded from unnecessary fear, but should learn to meet fearful situations courageously. "Courageously" means retaining the ability to think clearly and maintaining full use of all the resources of his body to meet the emergency. This is just what the child loses when he is paralyzed with fear.

If the mother is not *consistent* in her discipline or if the adults about the child do not make consistent demands upon him, he becomes confused and cannot use his developing power of reasoning to determine what will happen if he responds in this way or that. Even if he is motivated to do what the adult says because he loves the adult, he will often disobey because the other parent, whom he also loves, has asked just the opposite of him.

Punishment. Some form of punishment should be given the child who breaks rules which he understands and which are enforced by all adults responsible for his discipline. The child should be allowed to maintain his self-respect when punished, and never be made to feel that his parents do not love him because he has done wrong.

Love should not be used to buy good behavior. Love should call forth love, and the central element in love is furtherance of the welfare, the happiness, of the one loved. Such love is not developed in the child under two years.

Some parents make the mistake of blaming themselves if they feel antagonistic to or angry with (hostile toward) their child. Nurses also may have similar feelings. They never punish a child, because they believe that punishment is an expression of anger. This is a mistake. Punishment is a useful tool in discipline if used with discretion. It often clears the atmosphere for further interaction. The child will not resent it if he feels that he "had it coming to him." He should be punished knowing that the adult still loves him. Punishment should never appear to him as an angry retaliation by the adult. Fear of punishment should be reduced to the minimum which serves to reinforce in the child the habits established during infancy of accepting adult decisions to please the adult. Then the child learns the necessity of obedience as he matures and has decisions to make as to what he will and will not do.

If possible, the child should be shown that punishment is the logical consequence of his wrong decision. When a child burns his hand because he disobeys his mother and touches a hot stove, he sees the result of his disobedience, but he also knows that his mother did not inflict the pain. He remembers not to touch the stove again, for he sees the connection between the pain and his act. The connection is not clear to him when his mother punishes him for disobedience. Only if he has learned to trust his parents' judgment and knows that they do not punish him without good reason does he accept the connection between punishment and what he has done in the same spirit with which he accepted the burnt finger when he touched the stove.

It is even harder for him to learn what is morally right and wrong. Burning his finger had no moral implications (unless his mother had told him not to go near the stove); it was a matter of poor judgment on his part. By being hurt he learned about the physical environment in a painful way. If he has learned that "mother knows best," he believes her when she says that he might get hurt or sick, lose his penny, break his toy or tear his new shirt. But when she forbids behavior which interferes with the rights of other members of the family or of the people he meets when she takes him out with her, the reason for her decision is not clear to him. Nevertheless a child who loves his parents does accept their decisions about what is morally right and wrong as he accepts their decisions on the physical results of behavior. He learns to accept punishment as just when it follows his wrong actions. He learns to fear his own extreme impulses which are followed by unpleasant results in his relations with other people and tries to do right.

If a child feels guilty over something he did which his mother did not find out and for which he was not punished, he may purposely do something naughty in order to be punished and so reduce his feelings of guilt over the first offense. Some children who are ignored and rejected by their parents may actually seek to be punished so as to gain some response from their parents. Although this is not a loving response, it is better than being ignored.

Before condemning what a child does, his

reasoning, motive, and experience must be considered. The child should never be made to feel that the adult condemns *him*. He must be helped to understand that it is what he has done that is condemned and that he is still loved as before. Punishment should relate to the wrong act and follow directly upon the act so that wrong doing and punishment are brought together in the child's mind. Punishment should not be cruel, and corporal punishment should not be used if it can be avoided and never given so as to embarrass the child before others.

Nurses caring for children in the hospital should set limits on their behavior just as mothers do at home. Too often nurses have difficulty in doing this in a hospital setting.

Summary of emotional development

The problems of this period center mostly around the child's need to develop a *sense of autonomy*. He needs to learn to hold on and let go, as in toilet training. He needs help with the conflict between carrying out his new-found abilities and his continuing need for security and parental love. His accomplishments should be praised and his success in self-control noticed.

Parents should remember that the child has many years in which to complete the developmental tasks begun in the toddler period. They should not try to force him too rapidly into more mature behavior. If they do, the child, instead of submitting, may rebel and defeat the parents' attempts to use compulsion. He may become negativistic.

Two kinds of parents fail in guiding a child during this period. The first is the overdemanding parent, the second is the parent whose policy is *laissez-faire*. With such parents the child has no help in his striving for maturity.

The adult must define reality for the child. If adults do not set limits to his behavior, he cannot learn to live satisfactorily in his society.

Mental Development

The *sensorimotor stage* comprising six substages occurs during infancy (birth to one year) and the early toddler period (one to two years) according to Piaget. Four of these substages were discussed in Chapter 13. The last two of the six substages are substage V (12 to 18 months) and substage VI (18 months to two years).

Substage V (12 to 18 months). During this substage the *tertiary circular reaction* is seen. Instead of reproducing events that occur only by accident, the child looks for novel events further away from his environment into a whole new world of experience. If a child enjoys pulling a toy, he will vary his play by pulling larger or smaller toys shorter and longer distances. When he drops or swings objects, he will vary his play in the same way.

The child also learns to imitate behavior of others that he himself has never performed. He can do this only in the presence of the model. When he was younger, he imitated only his own behavior.

The child can now follow complex object displacement, which is an advance in object constancy. He is still limited, however, to following displacements only when he can see them. To understand where an object is when it cannot be seen requires symbolism and thought, neither of which are yet developed in the child.

Substage VI (18 months to two years). The toddler begins to think during this substage. He shows evidence of the beginnings of mental representations of events. He thinks about problems, no longer using only a trial-and-error basis to solve them. Some solutions to problems appear in a quick insightful manner.

The toddler develops *deferred imitation* during this period. The child not only imitates what he sees in the present, but he can now imitate an event that occurred perhaps days before. Thus it can be seen that the event was carried in the child's mind.

Invisible placement implies not only object permanence but also the presence of thought. If the mother, holding a small stick in her closed hand, places it under three different objects, and then shows the child that she no longer has the stick in her hand, the child looks under the last object for it. Thus, according to the child's behavior, he must have known of the existence of the stick even if he could not see it and used thought to infer where it could be found.

Preoperational Stage (2 to 7 years). The preoperational stage is only beginning during the later part of the toddler period from two to three years of age. The child enters a new realm of functioning. He no longer deals with events one at a time and he no longer thinks only in terms of the here and now. The child progresses to the symbolic and perceptual plane. Toddlers are very much influenced by what they see, hear, and experience at a given moment in time. They cannot, however, remember several aspects of a happening at the same time.

Toddlers think mostly about themselves; they are egocentric. To them, what they think is the only way to think; what they want or desire is predominant. They engage in "magical thinking" so that things happen because of their thought or wishes.

The toddler has learned that objects have permanence, existing even when out of sight, thus apart from themselves. This leads the child to progress to the separation of himself from his mother and to begin to develop the concept of "I," which leads him to autonomy.

As the toddler begins to question, he can refer to something another person knows and expect an answer. He can ask his mother, "Where Daddy?" indicating that he can symbolize, that he can remember someone called "Daddy," and that he can verbalize his wish and seek an answer. In other words, what is out of sight is not out of mind to the toddler.

The older toddler begins to ask questions using the words "who," "where," "what," "when," and "why." When the child asks a question beginning with "why," he shows that he is becoming aware of the goals of action. Early questions of this nature do not indicate a real understanding of causality, but with practice in verbal exchange with others, the toddler finally understands how one idea is related to others.

The toddler's memory and attention span are very short. He moves quickly from one activity to another. Since he can stand and walk, he can also move rapidly and randomly through his home, exploring in cabinets and drawers. He can open doors and explore the outside world, leading to his "running away."

OVERVIEW OF PHYSICAL GROWTH AND DEVELOPMENT

Physical growth and motor development are slower between one and three years than during infancy. The toddler period is marked primarily by increasing strength and skill in performance. By the end of the second year the principal types of muscular activities have appeared. Skilled performance in new areas is simply a utilization of old skills in new ways. Old skills become more and more perfected. The result is fewer errors and more speed with smoother, graceful movements. After the basic motor skills have been acquired the repertoire of added skills varies widely, depending upon the child's interest in new activities, his environment, and his ability to learn.

Significance of Delayed Motor Development. Although most children progress through the stages of infantile development at approximately the ages given in Chapter 13, some do not. These are not only late in reaching the stage of independent action characteristic of the toddler period but also are prevented from interacting with other children and from achieving normal social development. The young child whose motor development is retarded cannot join in play with children who can run and climb. He refrains or is excluded from their play and may develop feelings of inferiority which later are the bases for antisocial behavior.

Schedule of Growth and Development. The developmental schedules for toddlers (Table 16–1) are only averages which are in the ranges of ages during which normal children achieve certain levels of development. They are not typical of any one child. There are individual differences. The ages given are *approximate* for the various activities and learnings listed. These developmental schedules provide only a general outline of the growth of a child between one and three years.

DEVELOPMENT OF SEXUALITY IN THE TODDLER

Reinforcement of gender differences and social conditioning increases during the toddler period. Mothers, especially, provide cues to children concerning their gender identity. Mothers encourage active and aggressive play for their sons and less activity for their daughters. The type of clothing and toys purchased and the games encouraged also provide clues to the sex of the child. Parents identify their children by calling them "boys" or "girls." Little girls many times stay closer to their mothers while shopping or while playing outside than boys do. Mothers may arrange their toddler's hair differently depending on the sex of the child, although with our present trend toward unisex hair arrangements, little difference may actually be seen. *Thus the child's self-concept as a girl or a boy is probably completed at about two and one half to three years of age.* Once the core gender identity is imprinted it is usually unalterable. The exact time at which this occurs is not known, but it is generally believed to be when the little boy learns to stand for urination and the little girl learns that she must sit for this purpose.

It is possible that the infant and the toddler can be manipulated into a gender role counter to the genetic sex based on the chromosomes. This may be done for valid medical and psychological reasons such as when the newborn has intersexuality (see p. 314). Gender identity clinics recognize that when a chromosomal male has certain anatomical malformations that result in his being called a female at birth, by the time he is three years old his core gender identity as female is fixed. The child has been psychologically programmed as female. Later, when his anxious parents bring him to the gender identity clinic, it is not possible to reprogram his psy-

Text continued on page 514.

TABLE 16–1. *DEVELOPMENTAL SCHEDULES, 15 MONTHS TO 2½ YEARS*

15 MONTHS

Motor Control (see also Fig. 16–7)

At this age the toddler has reached a plateau of motor development

Walks alone at 14 months, but with a wide-based gait to steady himself. After he has learned to walk it is to him a form of play

Creeps upstairs

Builds a tower of 2 blocks

Throws objects repeatedly and picks them up again. Throwing is evidence of his new ability to release an object in his grasp

Opens boxes

Pokes finger in holes

Holds a cup with fingers grasped about it. He is apt to tip it too quickly and spill the contents

Grasps a spoon and inserts it into a dish. He cannot fill the spoon well. If he brings the spoon to his mouth, it is likely to be turned upside down, and the contents spilled into his lap

Vocalization and Socialization

Uses jargon

Names familiar pictures or objects

Responds to familiar comments

Vocalizes his wants and points to the desired object

Pats pictures in a book and turns pages

Indicates when his diaper is wet

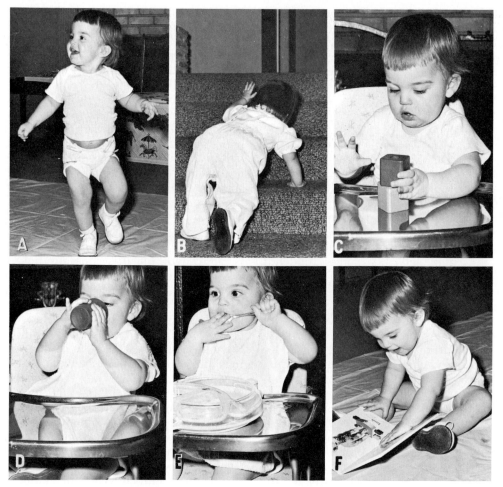

FIGURE 16–7. The 15-month-old (*A*) walks alone, (*B*) creeps upstairs, (*C*) builds a tower of 2 blocks, (*D*) holds a cup with fingers around it, (*E*) grasps spoon, but spills contents, (*F*) pats picture in book.

TABLE 16–1. *DEVELOPMENTAL SCHEDULES, 15 MONTHS TO 2½ YEARS (Continued)*

18 MONTHS

Physical Development
  Anterior fontanel is usually closed (may be closed as early as 12 months)
  Abdomen protrudes
Motor Control (see Fig. 16–8)
  Walks and runs with a somewhat wide stance, but increasingly more like the adult gait. He seldom falls
  Pulls a toy behind him
  Pushes light pieces of furniture around the room
  Can walk sideways and backward (16.7 months)
  Climbs stairs or upon furniture
  Seats himself on a small chair
  Throws ball into a box, puts block in a hole
  Scribbles vigorously. Attempts straight lines. Differentiates between straight and circular strokes
  May build tower of 3 blocks
  Holds cup to lips and drinks well with little spilling. Hands cup to his mother or drops it on the floor
  Can fill his spoon, but has difficulty inserting spoon into his mouth. Is apt to turn the spoon in his mouth. Spills frequently
Vocalization and Socialization
  Knows 10 words
  Uses phrases composed of adjectives and nouns
  Shifts attention rapidly from one thing to another. Moves quickly from place to place. Explores drawers and closets.
    Gets into everything
  Has a new awareness of strangers
  Begins to have temper tantrums if things go wrong
  May resist sleep for some time after he has been put to bed. Calls for his mother
  May control bowel movements
  May smear stool
  Thumb sucking may reach a peak. It usually occurs just before sleep or goes on all night
  Enjoys solitary play or watching others' activities
  Hugs his teddy bear or doll
  Begins to select a favorite toy or object such as a blanket

2 YEARS

Physical Development
  Weight: 26–28 pounds
  Height: approximately 32–33 inches (gain of 3–4 inches in second year)
  Pulse: 90–120 per minute
  Respirations: 20–35 per minute
  Teeth: approximately 16 temporary teeth
  Abdomen protrudes less than at 18 months
Motor Control (see Fig. 16–9)
  More grown up, steady gait
  Can run in more controlled way, has fewer falls and may run away
  Can jump crudely. In initial attempts he usually falls, since his body is propelled forward
  Walks up and down stairs, both feet on one step at a time, and holding onto a railing or the wall
  Builds a tower of 5 or more blocks. Can make cubes into a train
  Can open doors by turning door knob
  Scribbles in more controlled way than at 18 months. Imitates vertical stroke
  Drinks well from a small glass held in one hand
  Can put a spoon in his mouth without turning it
Vocalization and Socialization
  Has a vocabulary of approximately 300 words. Can use pronouns and names familiar objects. Can tell about his ex-
    periences. No longer uses jargon
  Makes short sentences of 3 or 4 words
  Shifts attention less rapidly than child of 18 months
  Behaves as though other children were physical objects. He may hug them or push them out of the way. Would like
    to make friends, but does not know how
  Does not readily ask for help
  Obeys simple commands
  Helps to undress himself. Can pull on simple garments
  Is toilet-trained in daytime. Verbalizes toilet needs
  May still smear with stool
  Thumb-sucking decreased
  Does not know right from wrong
  Number of relatively violent temper tantrums is decreasing
  Is proud of accomplishment of motor skills
  May fear parents' leaving
  Shows increasing signs of sense of individuality
  Enjoys parallel play—no interaction with other children even though their activity is the same. Interaction that does
    occur may consist in snatching toys from one another, kicking or pulling hair
  Manipulates play materials. Dawdles frequently
  Enjoys playing with dolls, placing beads in box and dumping them out, pulling blocks piled in wagon
  Cannot share possessions. Has great sense of "mine," little of "yours"
  Learns to replace toys in their proper place
  Enjoys hearing stories illustrated with pictures
  Begins play which mimics activities of parents
  Takes favorite toy to bed with him, which helps to quiet him. Has many demands before going to bed

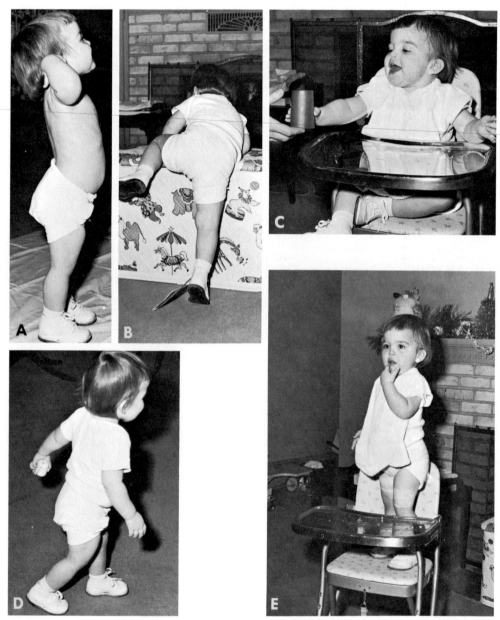

FIGURE 16–8. The 18-month-old (*A*) has a protruding abdomen, (*B*) climbs upon high toy box, (*C*) hands cup to mother, (*D*) moves rapidly from place to place and enjoys pulling toy behind her, (*E*) begins to have temper tantrums. This toddler shows increasing frustration because she wants to get out of her high chair. A temper tantrum occurred shortly after this picture had been taken.

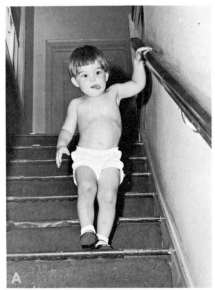
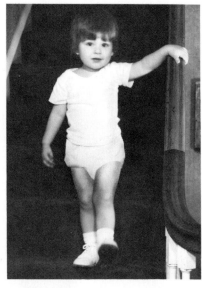
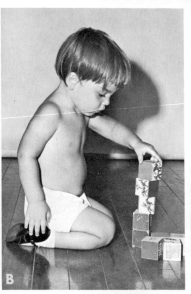
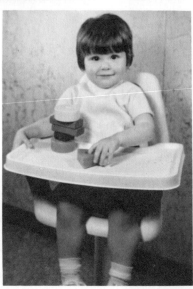
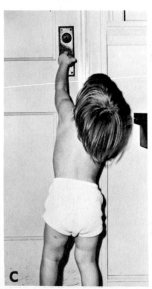
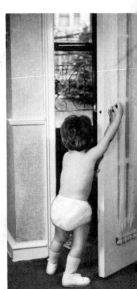
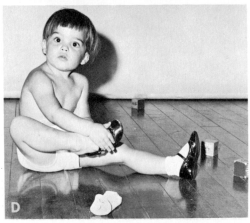
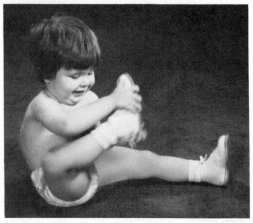

FIGURE 16–9. The 2-year-old. (*A*) walks up and down steps, both feet on one step at a time, and holding onto the rail; (*B*) can build a tower of 5 or more blocks; (*C*) can open a door by turning the door knob; (*D*) helps to undress herself or himself. The stage of development is the same in this girl and boy.

TABLE 16–1. DEVELOPMENTAL SCHEDULES, 15 MONTHS TO 2½ YEARS (Continued)

30 MONTHS (2½ YEARS)

Physical Development
   Has full set of 20 temporary (deciduous) teeth
Motor Control (see Fig. 16–10)
   Walks on tiptoe
   Rides a kiddie car
   Stands on one foot alone
   Can throw a large ball 4 to 5 feet
   Piles 7 or 8 blocks one on top of the other
   Copies horizontal or vertical line
Vocalization and Socialization
   Temper tantrums may continue
During the whole toddler period the child has begun to develop a self-concept from reflected appraisal of significant people—his parents and other adults who care for him. He is beginning to know himself as a separate person, and to have a conscience when he can control some areas of his behavior to conform to social demands

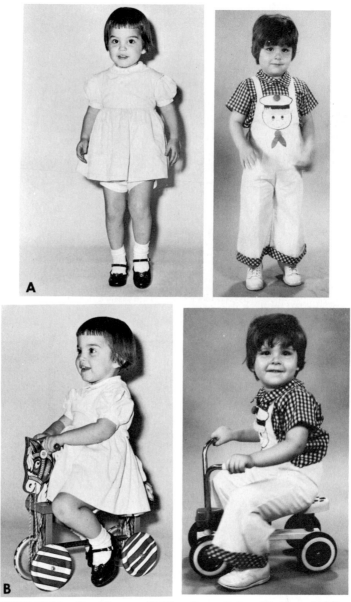

FIGURE 16–10. The 2½-year-old (A) walks on tiptoe, (B) rides a kiddie car.

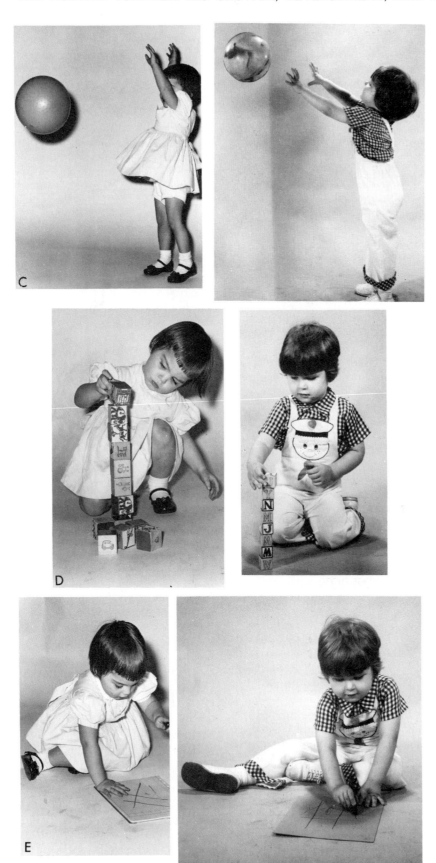

FIGURE 16–10. *Continued.* (*C*) throws a large ball 4 to 5 feet, (*D*) piles 7 or 8 blocks one on top of another, (*E*) copies horizontal or vertical line.

chological gender to that of a male. If the original process is successful, it cannot be reversed.

During the later period of infancy most babies are weaned. This means that the mouth is no longer the major source of satisfaction to the child. Gradually the toddler obtains pleasure from the perineal openings and their functions. The child obtains sensuous pleasure from the feeling of a distended bladder, from masses of feces in the rectum, and from the release of the contents of these organs. As he gains control of these functions through the use of the cerebrum, he gains increased pleasure from his own body.

This so-called *anal phase* coincides with the period of toilet training that has been discussed. This is a time when the small child begins to become self-assertive. While the toddler is learning to control his bodily functions, he develops a primitive sense of power; he can bring upon himself pleasing behavior or approbation from the parent who is training him. The further possible effects of the toilet training process were discussed on p. 498.

Toward the end of the toddler period increased genital stimulation may be observed. The boy discovers his penis and scrotum as part of his normal general bodily exploration. A "No, No" reaction when the infant or toddler first explores the genital area quickly conveys the idea that some parts of the body are bad or dirty while other parts such as the ears or nose are good and clean. Yet every child, no matter how young, needs to learn precisely the opposite, that all parts of the body are good. Parents should have a matter-of-fact acceptance of such body exploration and keep it in proper perspective as they do with all other learning processes. Deliberate genital manipulation for pleasure becomes more common in some children and may assume a sustained form comparable with masturbation during the latter months of the toddler period. Male masturbatory activity is still not as purposeful or goal-directed as it will become later. Ejaculation does not occur until after puberty. This masturbation is an essential precursor and component in the development of the character structure of the adult.

Parents are the first sex educators, not only by what they say, but by the way they treat each other as parents and as male and female persons in the home. By the projection of their own personalities, their feelings about themselves as male or female, the child receives the earliest nonverbal education about sex.

LIFE PERSPECTIVE

The toddler, like the infant, is still totally engrossed in the life of the present. He does not reexperience the past or preexperience the future as a whole; at least he does not in the sense of the development of complex symbolic structures. He has, however, begun to progress to the symbolic and perceptual plane. While the toddler has learned to differentiate between his mother's presence or absence, he believes that he needs her almost constant attention to care for him. The toddler continues developing physically, emotionally, socially, mentally, and sexually. All of these developments contribute to the ultimate emergence of a life perspective.

PLAY

Purposes. The main function of play during infancy is physical development and early association. As the child grows older the importance of play increases. (1) *Physical development* continues through play. Muscles are developed, and exercise is given to all parts of the body. Surplus energy can be worked off during active play. (2) *Social development* occurs when the toddler participates in activity with other children. Although at this age social interaction is limited, he enjoys *parallel play* (playing *beside* another child, but not *with* him). (3) The *therapeutic value* of play is psychological as well as physical, for it sublimates drives so that they are released in an approved way, and helps the child to release emotional tensions. For instance, an angry child may find relief by pounding boards or tossing bean bags. (4) Play is a means of *education*. The toddler who plays with toys of all sorts learns to know colors, shapes, sizes, and textures of play materials. (5) Play develops a beginning understanding of *moral values*. The toddler begins to learn right from wrong. He begins to learn not to hurt other children by rough play.

The toddler has strong feelings about his toys, clutching at them and saying, "Mine, mine." But he slowly learns the importance of sharing, even though it may be difficult for him to do so. He should not be forced to give up his toys until he is older and can understand that play with others involves giving up some pleasures on his part in order to have the greater satisfaction of participation in common projects in which he receives as well as gives pleasure.

Characteristics of Play. Each age group enjoys its own kind of play. Play during childhood follows a pattern of development based on the maturity of the group. Certain play activities are popular at each age no matter what the socioeconomic status, the environment, or the ethnic culture in which the child is brought up.

In general, play with toys is popular until the eighth year. After this children enjoy games which encourage large muscular activity such as running. After this stage, games or sports for which there are strict rules become all-important.

During the toddler period, play is active and is based on the motor and emotional development of the child. Walking in the early toddler period is a delightful game. He has acquired greater skill in the use of his arms. The 15-month-old toddler enjoys throwing objects and picking them up again, putting them into receptacles and taking them out again.

At 18 months the toddler is exceedingly active. Since his attention span is short, he moves freely from place to place and gets into everything. It is difficult to keep him out of drawers. By this age his balance has improved so that he can pull toys behind him or carry a doll or stuffed animal about with him. He enjoys playing alone or watching other children play, but has not learned to play with them in any game requiring group consensus. He notices the activities of his parents and may imitate them.

The two-year-old has less rapid shifts in attention than the younger child. He may dawdle in his play activities. He enjoys manipulating play materials, pounding, patting and feeling mud, sand or clay in his hands. He plays with dolls, strings large beads and puts his blocks into his wagon.

In *parallel play* the toddler plays beside another child in such activities as making mud pies. He wants to be friendly with other children, but does not know how. He may attack another child in his attempt. For this reason adult supervision of toddlers' play is necessary.

The 2½-year-old toddler has developed finer use of his muscles than the two-year-old. He enjoys handling smaller blocks and balls in a sensory way, but he still needs larger blocks and balls for play. He also has enough coordination to ride a kiddie car fairly well.

Play in the early toddler period is mostly free and *spontaneous*. There are no rules and regulations to follow. The child explores as he desires and stops when he pleases. Since he has poor motor coordination, he is apt to be destructive. His toys must be carefully examined to determine whether he might injure himself on broken parts. He does not intentionally break his toys, but his exploration of them—shaking, pushing, rattling—is sometimes more than the toys can stand.

By the end of the second year most children begin to impersonate adults whom they are with and who do what they consider interesting, e.g.,

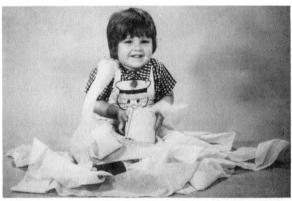

FIGURE 16–11. This toddler has discovered a new kind of play, unrolling toilet tissue.

setting the dinner table. If they play with older children, make-believe use of materials leads to make-believe situations such as playing house. Usually when toddlers play house with preschool children, the toddlers are the children in the family.

Even in the early toddler period *constructive* play is seen, such as making mud pies, making holes in sand, and playing with clay. Toddlers also enjoy crayons and use them in drawing and scribbling on paper. The product usually has no practical use, but its educational value is great. Toddlers enjoy moving their arms in time to music and singing simple songs, but they are unable to coordinate complex movements of their bodies with the music.

Toddlers, because of their short attention span, require a variety of activities and playthings to keep them busy. They spend most of their waking time in play. Since the span of attention of a two-year-old child is so short, they may leave an activity to do something else, but return later to their original play.

Play is informal. The toddler plays when and where he wishes. He needs no special clothes, toys, or play space.

Selection of Play Materials. The toddler's likes and dislikes should be remembered when selecting his toys. He is active and curious. He explores his environment, using his large muscles rather than small ones. He likes to pull and push toys and enjoys pedal-propelled toys, a kiddie car (tip-proof) and low rocking horses. He enjoys toys that open and close. Since he is imaginative, he likes to play with dolls and stuffed animals. His constructive and manipulative activities include playing with sand box toys, water toys, clay, finger paints, blocks, peg boards (large), pounding sets, and thick, large crayons. He enjoys being read to while he looks at the pictures in his book.

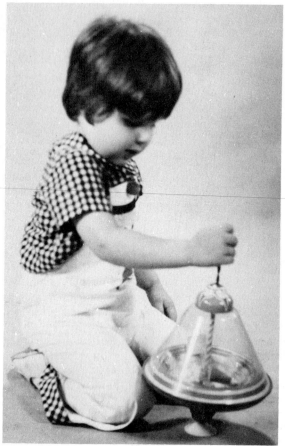

FIGURE 16–12. The 2½-year-old toddler develops further control of the smaller muscles of the body and is proud of this accomplishment.

Safety Factors in Selection of Toys. The toddler needs toys which are safe for him to play with. He should not be given toys that are sharp, have rough edges or small removable parts, nor should he have flammable toys, or beads, marbles, and coins that he can put in his mouth to swallow or aspirate. Toys painted with lead paint are dangerous, since he ingests a little of the paint if he sucks them (see p. 576).

CARE OF THE TODDLER

The parent or nurse should adjust adult procedures to the difference in size between the adult and the child. For instance, *when talking to him, the nurse should squat down so that their eyes are on the same level.* By merely bending over, the adult's image will still be overpowering for the small child. The toddler lacks the adult's resistance to force and loud sounds; he responds best to a light touch and quiet voice.

Procedures should also be adapted to his level

of understanding and endurance of frustration. Although he should be allowed to make decisions on the level of his understanding, he responds best to simple statements or to directions indicating what his mother or nurse wants him to do. Too many choices confuse him, since he does not understand the implications of each choice. He may not ask for what will give him the most pleasure.

The toddler who has learned to trust others knows that the limits they set to his behavior are for his safety and happiness.

Adults often forget that during his daily care the toddler is developing his concept of self, which is formed from the attitudes of others toward him and his behavior. Toddlers are susceptible to the facial expressions of those about them, reading into them their responses to him, to what he does and to his efforts at verbal communication. Because of his ambivalent attitude of love for and aversion to the adults about him, he has difficulty in building his self-image from their behavior toward him. At one time he wants to accept their image of him, at another time to repudiate it. It is during the daily routine contacts with him that loving adults help him build his ego and *conscience,* or super-ego. He internalizes the wishes and demands of others, particularly of those he loves the most. The beginning of a conscience is seen when even to a slight extent he is able to control his behavior in those areas in which he is most mature in order to conform to social norms.

PHYSICAL CARE

The toddler's daily physical care is given as part of a consistent schedule which fits in with that of his mother and the rest of the family. His bath, being part of this care, is given whenever it is most appropriate.

Prevention of tooth decay in the deciduous dentition is important. Proper oral hygiene and an adequate diet are essential for the prevention of decay.

Brushing the teeth should commence as soon as the temporary or deciduous teeth have erupted. By about two years a child should be taught to use a small toothbrush, brushing from the gum line to the edge of the teeth. Tooth-brushing, in addition to cleaning the teeth, also stimulates the gums. He should have a place to keep his toothbrush and be taught how to take care of it. The child of three or four should be taught to brush his teeth after eating and especially before bedtime. Doing it himself stimulates his interest in keeping his teeth clean and helps to establish a routine which is useful as he grows into later childhood. At first he will not be able to use the brush with perfect technique, but he will improve with practice. His parents should supervise his efforts as long as necessary.

Clothing should be light or bright in color, because children like bright colors. Bright colors also have value in accident prevention in that the child is easily seen and is therefore less likely to be injured by vehicles.

Clothing should have large, easily managed buttons and snaps placed where the child can reach them. It should be warm, but not bulky, since the toddler enjoys active play and is irritated when his movements are restricted. All clothing should be easy to put on and remove so that the child can help himself in dressing and undressing.

The infant does not need shoes before he learns to walk; when he walks on warm carpeted floors he may wear no shoes or may wear soft, moccasin type shoes. This aids in the development of the supporting muscles of the feet.

When the toddler begins to walk on hard, cold surfaces, his shoes should be selected with reference to the free development of his feet and posture. Shoes should be wide enough and long enough, have pliable thicker soles, and conform to the shape of the foot, i.e., straight along the inside, with broad toes and relatively narrow heels. The soles should not have even a low heel and should be rough to prevent the child from slipping; they should be 1/2 inch longer and 1/4 inch wider than the foot. The heels should fit snugly.

A little child outgrows his shoes rapidly. It is well to buy inexpensive ones to last until they are too small and are replaced with the next larger size. If expensive shoes are bought, the mother is tempted to have them used until they are worn out. In so doing she is likely to force the child's feet into shoes too small for him. He is then not only uncomfortable, but also in danger of having the shape of his feet distorted by the pressure of tight shoes. Orthopedic shoes are not needed by a child having normal feet.

Toddlers are active, curious, and fond of outdoor play. Although the child of 18 months to two years may be suspicious of strangers, as long as he is with his mother he likes to watch other children play. He enjoys parallel play, but is not yet ready for cooperative play. As he approaches his third birthday he has matured to the stage at which he makes motions of friendliness to other toddlers and some attempt to join in cooperative play. He welcomes a sunshiny day when he may play outdoors, making mud pies, digging in the sand pile, or, on a hot day, splashing in water. In winter he likes to play in the snow for a while, but cannot manipulate it as he can mud and sand.

Toddlers need freedom to play where they can wander without danger of being harmed. An adult should be near, however, for it is impossible to foresee what a child is likely to do. Although he wants to run about freely and does not want anyone to be constantly saying, "No, no," he feels more secure when he knows that an adult is with him.

SLEEP

The amount of sleep the toddler needs depends upon his age, health, emotional tension, activity during the day, and depth of sleep. From one to three years the amount of sleep needed gradually decreases. The child may resist sleep for some time after being put to bed, crying for his mother, or demanding a drink of water or some other form of attention—anything so that he may have company.

At two years the toddler is likely to have a set ritual which he insists on following when he goes to bed. From 1 1/2 to three or four years he likes to take a favorite toy to bed with him. Since this helps him to relax, he should be allowed to have the toy. As he grows older he will voluntarily give up the habit. Other methods to relieve his tension before going to sleep are head-rolling, singing, or talking to himself. He should not be restrained or told to be still, for that only increases his tension and delays his going to sleep. The typical child will outgrow these habits by the time he is three years old or shortly after but may resume them when he is under a strain and anxious, as when he is in the hospital.

Toddlers sleep, on the average, 12 to 14 hours out of the 24, including a daytime nap of one to two hours. Naps may become a source of rebellion in the two-year-old. Few mothers escape the naptime battles, and mothers should not place too much importance on a child's refusal to go to sleep. His outer clothing is removed, he is given a drink of water and taken to the toilet, and then he is placed comfortably in bed. The shades are drawn and the room door closed. He may have one toy in bed with him, but a variety of toys tends to keep him awake, for he handles first one and then another. A cuddly toy is the best kind to take to bed. The parents should be firm in keeping to the daily scheduled time for his nap even if he does not sleep.

Dreams and nightmares or night terrors are common, beginning in a mild form at two to three years of age.

SAFETY MEASURES

Importance of Accident Prevention. Prevention of accidents is an important aspect of the care of children of all ages. Accidents are the principal cause of death among toddlers and account for many permanent handicaps and disfiguring scars. The majority of accidents occur in or near the home. In approximate order of frequency are deaths due to motor vehicles, burns, drowning, falls, poisons and miscellaneous causes.

Careful observation is essential if accidents are to be prevented. Although there has been some advance in the prevention of accidents in early childhood, their incidence has not been reduced as rapidly as has that of serious illnesses which formerly were the main causes of death or permanent disability.

The interests of boys and girls of any age lead them into hazardous situations. When we know the hazards, we are better able to protect the children. Children should be taught what is safe and unsafe for them to do and, until they are old enough to use good judgment, should be under adult supervision.

Nurses as well as physicians can help parents to understand this approach to accident prevention. Then the parents will be able to judge more accurately how much freedom each child can be allowed as he gradually takes over more and more responsibility for his own safety. This applies to the kind of toys given him and to his experimentation in climbing, opening and shutting doors—including slamming the door of the family car—and running ahead of his mother or lingering behind her on the street. If he hurts himself, while sympathizing with him she can point out in terms he can understand the reason why he hurt himself—give him his first lesson in cause and effect of activities which are dangerous for him and cause him pain. In this way his

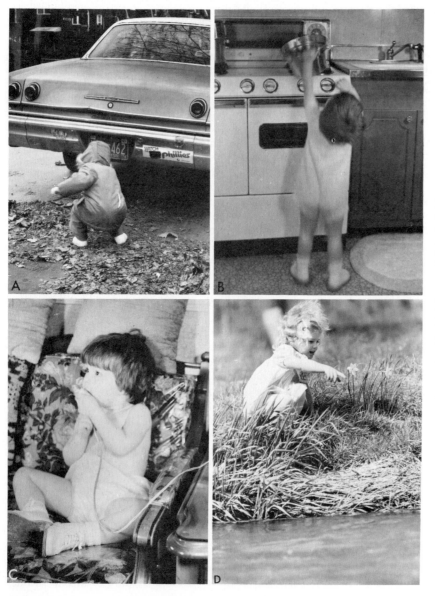

FIGURE 16–13. The toddler's curiosity may lead him into danger. *A,* Automotive safety is doubly important when there is risk to small children. Always check carefully when backing the car from garage or driveway. *B,* Hot, scalding fluids must be kept out of the toddler's reach. Turn handles of pots and pans to back of stove. *C,* Electrical outlets and worn extension cords can be deadly. Plug outlets and keep cords repaired. *D,* A fence around his yard would keep the child from wandering near a pool or fish pond. Teach children to swim early.

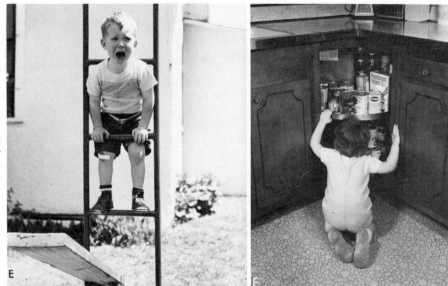

FIGURE 16–13. *Continued. E,* The toddler may climb on high places and possibly fall. *F,* He may eat or swallow anything he finds in his cabinet, which contains cleaning products and insecticides. Medications must be kept out of the child's reach. *H,* The toddler may find a plastic bag and, while playing with it, suffocate. (Photographs courtesy of: *D, E,* H. Armstrong Roberts; *G,* Canada's Health and Welfare, January-February, ...)

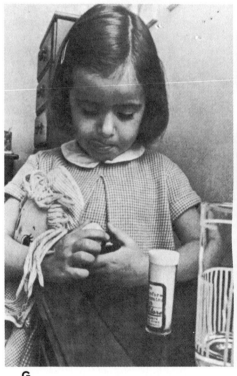

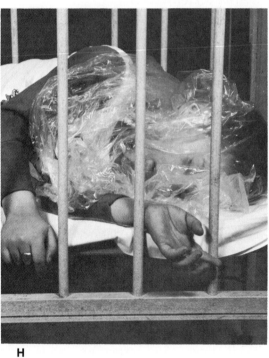

knowledge of what he can safely do will be increased.

Nurses must assume the responsibility of teaching parents and children the importance of accident prevention whenever they meet them, such as in the Child Health Conference, in the home and in the hospital unit or clinic. The most effective way for children to learn is through carefully safeguarded, graded experiences in self-protection. There should be a reciprocal relation between protection of the child and the education appropriate to his stage of maturation.

Specific Hazards of Toddler Years. Toddlers naturally fall frequently. In general they sit down suddenly or fall flat without hurting themselves, but if they fall down steps or from a height, they may injure themselves severely. They also tug at the end of table covers and pull objects such as cups of hot coffee over on themselves because they cannot see the top of the table. The formica-topped table for the family meals is far safer and more convenient to use than the polished wooden dining table covered with a table cloth.

To satisfy a child's curiosity about what is on top of a table and what mother is doing there, he may be lifted up or placed beside her in his high chair. The average child of two years is tall enough to see over the table edge if he stands on tiptoes, holding on to the table, but this is an uncomfortable position and does not give a complete view of what is there. Also he is so unsteady that if he reaches for something, he is likely to sit down suddenly. This is frustrating and may produce a temper tantrum or tears.

The two-year-old's curiosity leads him into danger. When exploring objects, children poke and probe with their fingers, which may be hurt in one way or another. They may be involved in motor vehicle accidents, may be burned or drowned, may fall from a height, may ingest poison, or may be suffocated in a plastic bag or in an empty refrigerator.

Specific Safety Measures: Shared Parent-Nurse Learning. Safety measures are designed to prevent accidents which are likely to occur in the daily life of the child. The nurse can help the mother with her individual problems of accident prevention. Both the mother and the nurse will find it helpful to keep in mind the common sources of accidents among toddlers and the preventive measures which can be taken for their safety.

MOTOR VEHICLE ACCIDENTS. Little children are taught to cross the street holding an adult's hand. Their attention is directed to the custom of crossing at the corner rather than in the middle of the block. If there are traffic lights, they are taught that green means "Go" and red means "Stop." They are too immature to gauge the speed of an oncoming automobile with reference to the time it takes them to cross the street, but they will slowly learn while crossing with adults who do not hurry them while a light is changing.

Toddlers should be supervised to some extent at all times, but especially when playing outdoors on a kiddie car, tricycle, or sled to prevent their darting into the street between parked cars or coasting down a driveway into street traffic. Parents should be careful when backing a car into or out of the garage, for it is difficult to see a small child directly behind the car (see p. 518 Fig. 16–13, A).

The incidence of children injured while riding with their parents is increasing as more family cars are on the road. Children share the adult's danger from collision or overturning of the car. A seat belt should be installed for the toddler so that he is not thrown from the seat if the car stops suddenly or is involved in an accident. When a child stands upon the seat beside the driver, a sudden stop is likely to throw him forward. Modern door catches prevent falls from an open door of a moving car.

BURNS. Matches should be kept away from young children, even though few of them in this age group can strike a safety match. Little children should be watched closely in the kitchen so that they do not touch or fall against a hot stove or investigate the top with its fascinating open flames and pots and pans. Pans with handles extending from side to side or toward the back of the stove are less likely to attract the toddler's attention and are harder for him to reach than pans with handles extending to the front of the stove (see Fig. 16–13, B). Hot radiators are sources of minor burns, particularly if the child falls against one. Recessed radiators protected by built-in screens eliminate this danger. Toddlers are interested in electrical outlets and are likely to poke a pin or other bit of metal into them (see Fig. 16–13, C). Safety plugs may be used to prevent this.

DROWNING. Children like to play in water but if they fall they may be unable to get out of even a shallow pool; if they fall into a swimming pool, they are completely helpless (see Fig. 16–13, D). There is also danger of their drowning in the home. Children should not be left alone in the bathroom after the water for the bath has been drawn. The bathtub may be slippery, and in climbing over the side the child may fall into the water. If he hits his head or falls into very hot water, he might collapse and drown before his mother returns to bathe him. The old-fashioned washtub is seldom used except in rural areas. Serious accidents have occurred when such a tub was filled with hot water and the child's mother went for a pail of cold water. The child investigated the tub in her absence. If he fell in, he was burned even if he was rescued before drowning. Pails of hot water used for mopping floors are also a danger to small children.

FALLS. Children like to climb (see Fig. 16–13, E). Until their muscular coordination and judgment have developed to the stage at which they can climb with safety, special equipment should be provided (e.g., small wooden crates) and all climbing should be under adult supervision.

Children like to look out of windows, but are so short that they often climb on a chair to see what is going on outside. While standing on a chair or a sill they are likely to lose their balance and fall head foremost. Hence all windows should have screens.

Falls on stairs are dangerous. In institutions for children, gates should be placed at the top and bottom of stairways. The ranch type of house or one-floor home has obviated the hazard of falls on stairs. If the house has a basement, the door leading to the stairs should be locked. A child who fell down the basement stairs and was too stunned to cry might lie at the bottom for some time before being discovered.

Falls from open porches were formerly a common source of injury to small children. In buildings today, however, especially in urban housing developments, porches are likely to be omitted or screened and so present no danger.

Falls from shopping carts or strollers while the parent's attention is diverted can cause serious injury. In addition, children can crush their fingers in the adjustable parts of these devices.

Falls from child carrier seats on two-wheeled bicycles are becoming more common as an increasing number of parents want their young children to share the fun of biking. There is also the danger that the child's legs and feet may be caught in the spokes of a turning wheel, causing injury to the child and possibly the adult.

The side gate of a crib should be kept up at all times and fastened securely so that it will not go down if the child leans against its top.

POISONING. The incidence of poisoning in children is greatest between the ages of one and four years. Children are curious about the taste of substances and often ingest poisonous liquids, powders or solids, even indoor plants, which they find in the house. A main source of danger to the child is the household supply of washing powders and detergents, charcoal lighter fluids and similar products, and substances for cleaning sinks, toilets, and the like (see Fig. 16–13, F).

Medicines beneficial in small amounts are often poisonous when taken in larger quantities. If the term "candy" is used when speaking to a child of medicinal pills, or if a medicine has little or no taste or if the unpleasant flavor has been camouflaged with some sweet syrup or sugar coating, the child may finish the bottle. All harmful substances should be kept out of the toddler's reach, and common household poisons and medicines should be kept in locked storage places or on high shelves inaccessible to children. Child resistant containers for medicines are available and should be used (see Fig. 16–13, G). Harmful substances should never be kept in containers intended for food.

Mothers should be taught what to do if a child does take any of these harmful substances. She should telephone the physician or clinic at once or, if she lives close to a hospital, take the child to the emergency ward. If she cannot get medical attention for the child and she lives in a city having a Poison Control Center, she can telephone there for advice. If she knows what substance the child took and the approximate amount, she should give this information clearly and concisely. If the child has taken the contents of a bottle or can whose ingredients are listed, she should give this information. The Center will tell her the emergency treatment and may furnish emergency transportation for the child to the hospital. In most cities the police car is always available. The container from which the poison was taken should be given to the physician who treats the child. If the child vomits spontaneously or after being given an emergency emetic, the vomitus should be examined chemically. This is particularly important if the mother does not know what the child has taken or the ingredients of some commercial product which she knows the child has swallowed.

In some cities the public health nurse is responsible for visiting the home after the child's return from the hospital. The nurse helps the parents to correct the situation which led to the accident and gives them a better understanding of the child's level of growth and development so that further accidents may be prevented.

SUFFOCATION. Plastic bags used to protect items and to cover stored materials may be considered playthings by the young child, who may suffocate as a result of pulling one over his head (see Fig. 16–13, H).

An empty refrigerator is a menace to any child in the vicinity. A refrigerator unit is meant to be airtight to prevent spoilage of food. If a toddler crawls into a refrigerator and the door closes, he may suffocate before he is released. Measures to prevent this accident include completely removing the doors, having the refrigerator destroyed, placing the unit so that the door stands against a wall, or locking the door with a padlock or by other means.

HEALTH SUPERVISION

Visits to the physician or the Child Health Conference, at intervals suggested by the physician, are important during the toddler period. During the second year these visits may be scheduled every two to four months and thereafter twice a year for continued health supervision. During these years, defects may be determined in an early stage. If they yield readily to treatment, they may be prevented from develop-

TABLE 16–2. PRIMARY IMMUNIZATION FOR CHILDREN NOT IMMUNIZED IN INFANCY*

1 THROUGH 5 YEARS OF AGE	
First visit	DTP, TOPV, Tuberculin Test
1 mo later	Measles, Rubella, Mumps
2 mo later	DTP, TOPV
4 mo later	DTP, TOPV
6 to 12 mo later or preschool	DTP, TOPV
Age, 14–16 yr	Td – continue every 10 yr

6 YEARS OF AGE AND OVER	
First visit	Td, TOPV, Tuberculin Test
1 mo later	Measles, Rubella, Mumps
2 mo later	Td, TOPV
6 to 12 mo later	Td, TOPV
Age, 14–16 yr	Td – continue every 10 years

*Physicians may choose to alter the sequence of these schedules if specific infections are prevalent at the time. For example, measles vaccine might be given on the first visit if an epidemic is underway in the community.

From American Academy of Pediatrics: *Report of the Committee on Infectious Diseases.* 17th ed., 1974.

ing into serious handicaps. The physician or nurse also records growth progress and gives advice about safety measures, nutrition, the establishment of desirable habits, and the prevention or correction of objectionable habits in the child. He will give immunizations to continue the program against the communicable diseases discussed in Chapter 13 (see p. 379). If the child was not immunized in infancy, the physician will give immunizations according to the schedule in Table 16–2.

The toddler period is one in which the physician can establish and develop a rapport with the child that will be valuable when the child is sick, particularly if he must be hospitalized.

Dental care and supervision of daily mouth hygiene are important after the child has his full set of temporary teeth, i.e., by about two to 2½ years. Visits to the dentist should be made about every four to six months. The dentist, like the physician, builds up a rapport with the child which is valuable later on when painful dental work must be done. Cleaning the child's teeth, applying a fluoride preparation (see p. 369), and work on superficial cavities in the temporary teeth are seldom painful. The dentist should have a kindly approach to children, explaining procedures to them and allowing them to handle his instruments.

NUTRITION

Nutrition is important in the maintenance of the toddler's health and normal growth and development. Diets for young children should include the essential nutrients in the amounts necessary for maintenance, replacement and increase of tissue and for energy. Children from different cultures may prefer different foods, and allowances should be made for this, but each diet should contain the essential nutrients.

Food is usually offered in three well-spaced meals. The child may also have nutritious snacks between meals if he is very active. He will be ready to eat the well-balanced, varied, yet simple diet offered him at meals if he is not too irritable from intense hunger.

Influence of Growth and Development on Eating Behavior. During his second year of life the child needs less food than during infancy, because he is no longer growing so rapidly. He also has greater interest in the social and physical environment. Many children at this age have anorexia. The mother should remember that the child needs less food per unit of body weight and that this is the primary reason for his anorexia (*physiologic anorexia*). He may have developed food preferences through imitation of his parents or siblings. He may even refuse food for a short time. Food should not be forced upon him. Unless he has some organic disease, serious feeding problems will develop only because adults have tried to impose upon him their ideas of what and how much he must eat. If food is forced upon him when he refuses his meals, he is likely to rebel, and a feeding problem will develop.

Children usually eat well when they are allowed reasonable freedom in both the amount and the kind of food they wish to eat. Strong likes and dislikes are to be respected. The child who dislikes essential food substances is gradually taught to eat them, or they may be included in the diet in some disguised form, e.g., putting mashed carrots in mashed potatoes. The child may take additional milk if it is used in custards.

At times the toddler may be demanding not only in what he wants to eat, but also in the dishes he uses and the way his food is served. His behavior may be bizarre. He enjoys feeding himself even though he may be slow and clumsy. Finger foods are especially helpful in the transition from the use of fingers to the use of a spoon; i.e., dry cereals may be more appealing to a toddler if served without milk and sugar. If the mother is flexible and humors him when the matter is not too essential, this makes him feel important and reinforces good mother-child relations.

Many children are negativistic at this age, especially in eating. A toddler may test his parents to see how far they will let him have his way. Many times a toddler will say "No" to specific foods because of his negativistic trait. This can not be taken seriously, but some limits to his behavior must be set. He feels uncomfortable and often fearful if he is allowed to attempt anything his fancy suggests. A child may refuse his food only to be hungry soon after the meal is over. He may feel sick after eating too much or too rapidly. What an affectionate mother asks her child to do is likely to be what makes him feel good physically and emotionally.

Activity influences a child's appetite. A reasonable amount of running about increases his appetite, but if his curious searching of the environment is continued too long, he becomes overfatigued. A rest period before meals serves to lessen fatigue and his resistance to adult suggestion. Furthermore, mealtime may appear to him as an interruption of his play, and so, even though he is hungry, he may resist being called to the table. His mother determines what is best for him by experimenting with a schedule of meals, snacks, naps, and indoor and outdoor play.

The toddler has such a short attention span that he appears to be even more restless than his biologic need for activity demands. He may wander away from the table before he has finished eating. Forcing him to remain in his place may precipitate a temper tantrum. Often his newly discovered interests may be used to bring him back to the table. If he has gone to get his teddy bear, his mother may say, "Here, let's make a place for Teddy at the table."

The toddler is ritualistic in his eating habits; he may have strong preferences for certain utensils and dishes. He may insist on eating foods in certain sequences. Adults should not impose their own eating habits upon the child, whose ritualistic behavior is a normal part of development at this age. His ritual will tend to coincide with family habits if he is made to feel that he is one of the group and not a baby set apart from the group. There are many reasons why a toddler in his third year may eat with his parents and siblings; he is much less likely to acquire eating whims and fancies if the family has none than if he eats alone.

Handedness becomes evident during this period. The child may be permitted to use either hand in feeding himself. The spoon is placed in front of him so that he can pick it up with the favored hand.

It is well to give a variety of foods so that the child learns to like various tastes. It may be difficult during the toddler period to add new foods because the child is likely to have become discriminating in his tastes and detects and appraises new consistencies and flavors in the foods offered him.

Development of Eating Skills. Children differ in their ability and willingness to feed themselves, but the following represents the typical advances in skill.

12–15 months: Drinks from a cup which he himself holds

15–18 months: Holds his own spoon. The mother can spread newspaper on the floor, and he can wear a coverall bib in case he spills food. Help is not forced upon him, but is offered if he needs it. If dishes are unbreakable rather than china, there is less chance of damage to them and injury to himself if he has an accident.

24 months: Feeds himself fairly well, provided he has had the requisite early experience in helping his mother feed him. The mother should not make the mistake of feeding him in order that he may not spill his food.

Dietary Allowances. Table 16–3 gives the recommended daily dietary allowances for children between one and three years of age.

Specific Suggestions for Feeding. By the time the child is 18 months to two years old he can eat table food and three meals a day. It would be helpful for nurses and mothers to remember the following points.

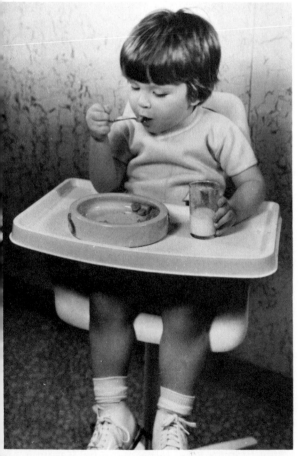

FIGURE 16–14. A 2-year-old child can put a spoon into his mouth without spilling its contents. He can feed himself most foods fairly well, provided he has had earlier experience in doing this.

TABLE 16–3. RECOMMENDED DAILY DIETARY ALLOWANCES FOR CHILDREN 1 TO 3 YEARS OF AGE

	WT.—13 KG. (28 POUNDS) HT.—86 CM. (34 INCHES)
K calories	1,300
Protein	23 g.
Fat-soluble vitamins	
Vitamin A activity	2,000 I.U.
Vitamin D	400 I.U.
Vitamin E activity	7 I.U.
Water-soluble vitamins	
Ascorbic acid	40 mg.
Folacin[a]	100 μg
Niacin[b]	9 mg.
Riboflavin	0.8 mg.
Thiamine	0.7 mg.
Vitamin B$_6$	0.6 mg.
Vitamin B$_{12}$	1.0 μg
Minerals	
Calcium	800 mg.
Phosphorus	800 mg.
Iodine	60 μg
Iron	15 mg.
Magnesium	150 mg.
Zinc	10 mg.

[a]The folacin allowances refer to dietary sources as determined by *Lactobacillus casei* assay. Pure forms of folacin may be effective in doses less than $1/4$ of the RDA.

[b]Although allowances are expressed as niacin, it is recognized that on the average 1 mg. of niacin is derived from each 60 mg. of dietary tryptophan.

From the Food and Nutrition Board, National Academy of Sciences–National Research Council: Recommended Daily Dietary Allowances (1974).

1. Serve food in small portions. The child likes plain food and eats one food at a time.
2. Chop or cut the food into small pieces.
3. The diet for each day should include the following (the particular diet may depend upon the cultural preferences of the family):
   a. Meat or fish, one serving; one egg daily, or cheese
   b. Liver, one or more servings a week
   c. Green and yellow vegetables, two or more servings a day
   d. Citrus fruit, raw or cooked fruit, two or more servings a day (one could be in citrus or tomato juice)
   e. Cereal and bread, enough to meet his caloric needs
   f. Butter or margarine
   g. Milk, 16 ounces to a maximum of 1 quart, part of which may be used in cooking or on cereals
4. Satisfy the child's appetite with nutritious foods and avoid offering him candy, cake, ice cream, and the like. Nutritious snacks may be given between meals.
5. Give vitamins as suggested by the physician.
6. Since the child is growing less rapidly, he may eat less than he did at the end of the first year. Do not force him to eat.

Foods to Avoid. The small child does not miss what he has never had and does not need. Foods to be avoided include chocolate, sugar, large amounts of fat (this is difficult to digest), nuts and seeds (there is danger of inadequate chewing and also of aspiration into the lungs), foods which are highly seasoned, and stimulants such as tea and coffee.

Importance of Good Eating Habits. During the toddler and preschool years eating habits and attitudes toward foods are developed which tend to persist through life. Meals should be served at regular intervals and in a physical and social situation in which the child feels secure. He may have three or four simple meals a day. Some children with small appetites may need a midmorning, midafternoon, or evening snack. Snacks should not be given at a time or in an amount which will interfere with normal appetite at mealtime.

Toward the end of the toddler period most children eat with the family. If his siblings and parents have good or poor eating habits, a toddler will imitate them. Parents who have not already experienced this difficulty with the older children must be told of this problem. They are advised how to handle problems which may arise and be reminded that the basic factor in forming good eating habits is that eating time be made a happy time. Toddlers are too young to learn good table manners. Eating is an enjoyable experience. Mealtime is a family gathering to share this important and pleasurable activity.

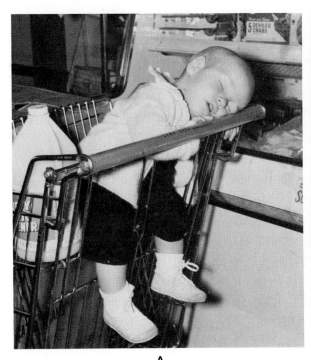
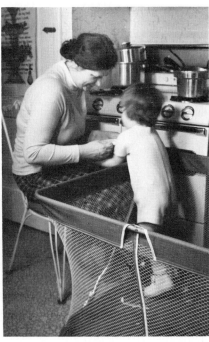

A   **B**

FIGURE 16–15. *A*, Shopping can be tiring, as is illustrated by this toddler as he waits for his mother to complete her grocery shopping at the supermarket. *B*, The young toddler is protected from harm while mother cooks. (*A*, Courtesy of J. Hemenway and *Baby Talk*, October, 1969.)

SEPARATION

Meaning of Separation to the Toddler. The toddler, although his security depends upon both parents, is much closer to his mother than to any other adult or to his siblings. He knows his mother as a very special person. His need for her love is as great as his need for food. His attachment to her is possessive and selfish. She can, he believes, protect him from all harm. His parents, especially his mother, make the toddler's world secure and stable.

By the end of his first year the child realizes that it is his mother who gives him love, protects him from harm and provides pleasurable experiences for him. He believes that he cannot survive without her. Because of this feeling he is fearful when she is out of his sight. The infantile game of peek-a-boo is one way by which the child can master his fear of separation from his mother. Since he can bring her back easily, he finds that he can master his separation anxiety more easily. He discovers later, in the game of hide-and-seek, that his mother will search to find him. In these ways he gradually learns that he can bring his mother back to him through his own activity.

We know from his behavior that a child needs his mother, almost an ever-present companion, until about his third birthday. During the toddler period he gains increasing mastery over his fear of separation, and he learns to share his mother with others.

Reasons for Separation. The young child cannot understand why he is ever separated from his mother. As he matures, however, he becomes increasingly aware that there are others (siblings) whom his mother also loves. He may become resentful of them, and yet his mother expects them to love him and him to love them. At this stage the toddler must be helped to accept his siblings, but he must be shown that he is loved even if he has hostile feelings toward them. He must have all his needs fulfilled, because this means love. Since his mother expects the toddler, who is secure in her love for him, to be like his siblings, he learns one of the first lessons in socialization: to like to be with other people. In this way he gradually matures socially as well as physically. He wins his mother's approval and strengthens her love for him.

As he matures, his mother may work away from home, may continue her studies, and may not be with him constantly. She may become ill or go to a hospital for delivery of another child. The toddler himself may become sick or be injured and be placed in the children's unit of a hospital. His specific response to separation due to hospitalization will be discussed in the next chapter.

TEACHING AIDS AND OTHER INFORMATION*

American Academy of Pediatrics

Car Restraint Devices.
Child Safety Suggestions (Set # 1).
Child Safety Suggestions (Set # 2).
Childhood Diet and Coronary Heart Disease.
Recommendations for Preventive Health Care of Children and Youth.

American Dental Association

Fluoridation Facts.
Parents Want to Help.
The Care of Children's Teeth.
Your Child's First Visit to the Dentist.
Your Child's Teeth.

Child Study Association of America

Auerbach, A. B.: The Why and How of Discipline, 1974.
Family Life and Child Development: A Selective, Annotated Booklist Cumulative Through 1975, 1976.
Reading with Your Child Through Age 5, 1976.

The Children's Hospital Medical Center, Boston, Mass.

Accident Handbook: A New Approach to Children's Safety.
How to Prevent Childhood Poisoning: A New Approach.
What to Do When "There's Nothing to Do."

Consumer Product Information

Safe Toy Tips, 1974.
Young Children and Accidents in the Home, 1974.

Department of National Health and Welfare: Ottawa, Canada

Up the Years from One to Six.
Your Basic List of First Aid Supplies.

The National Association for Mental Health, Inc.

Lo Que Todo Niño Necesita para Criarse Mentalmente Saludable (What Every Child Needs for Good Mental Health).
What Every Child Needs for Good Mental Health.

Public Affairs Committee

Bryant, J. E.: Helping Your Child Speak Correctly.
Freese, A. S.: Protecting Your Family from Accidental Poisoning.
Hymes, J. L.: Enjoy Your Child: Age 1, 2, and 3.

United States Government

Child Development in the Home, 1974.
Cognitive Development in Young Children, 1976.
Dental Health Projects for Children: Demonstrations of Preventive and Remedial Care, 1974.
How Children Grow, Reprinted 1974.
Teach Children Fire Will Burn, 1974.
We Want You to Know About Preventing Childhood Poisoning, 1973.
Young Children and Accidents in the Home, Reprinted 1975.
Your Child from 1 to 3, Reprinted 1973.

---

*Complete addresses are given in the Appendix.

REFERENCES

Books

American Academy of Pediatrics: *Standards for Day Care Centers for Infants and Children Under 3 Years of Age.* Evanston, Ill., American Academy of Pediatrics, 1971.
Boston Children's Medical Center, and Feinbloom, R. I.: *Child Health Encyclopedia: the Complete Guide for Parents.* New York, Delacorte Press, 1975.
Brazelton, T. B.: *Toddlers and Parents: A Declaration of Independence.* New York, Dell Publishing Company, 1974.
Caplan, F., and Caplan, T.: *The Power of Play.* New York, Doubleday Anchor Press, 1974.
Erikson, E. H.: *Childhood and Society.* New York, W. W. Norton and Company, 1964.
Guthrie, H. A.: *Introductory Nutrition.* 3rd ed. St. Louis, The C. V. Mosby Company, 1975.
Helms, D., and Turner, J.: *Exploring Child Behavior.* Philadelphia, W. B. Saunders Company, 1976.
Hurlock, E. B.: *Child Development.* 5th ed. New York, McGraw-Hill Book Company, 1973.
Kenny, T. J., and Clemmens, R. L.: *Behavioral Pediatrics and Child Development.* Baltimore, Williams & Wilkins Company, 1975.
Oliven, J. F.: *Clinical Sexuality.* 3rd ed. Philadelphia, J. B. Lippincott Company, 1974.
Piers, M. W. (Ed.): *Play and Development.* New York, W. W. Norton and Company, Inc., 1972.
Poland, R. G.: *Human Experience: A Psychology of Growth.* St. Louis, The C. V. Mosby Company, 1974.
Rebelsky, F.: *Life: the Continuous Process: Readings in Human Development.* New York, Alfred A. Knopf, 1975.

Recommended Dietary Allowances. 8th ed. rev. Washington, D.C., National Academy of Sciences-National Research Council, 1974.
Roby, P. (Ed.): *Child Care—Who Cares?* New York, Basic Books, Inc., 1973.
Sattler, J. M.: *The Assessment of Children's Intelligence.* Philadelphia, W. B. Saunders Company, 1975.
Saul, L. J.: *Emotional Maturity: The Development and Dynamics of Personality and its Disorders.* 3rd ed. Philadelphia, J. B. Lippincott Company, 1971.
Smith, D. W., and Bierman, E. L. (Eds.): *The Biologic Ages of Man: From Conception Through Old Age.* Philadelphia, W. B. Saunders Company, 1973.
Taichert, L. C.: *Childhood Learning, Behavior and the Family.* New York, Behavioral Publications, 1973.
Toman, W.: *Family Constellation: Its Effects on Personality and Social Behavior.* 3rd ed. New York, Springer Publishing Company, 1976.
Trantham, C. R., and Pederson, J. K.: *Normal Language Development.* Baltimore, Williams & Wilkins Company, 1975.
Watson, R. I., and Lindgren, H. C.: *Psychology of the Child.* 3rd ed. New York, John Wiley & Sons, 1973.
White House Conference on Children 1970: *Profiles of Children.* Washington, D.C., White House Conference on Children 1970, 1971.
Witmer, H. L., and Kotinksy, R.: *Personality in the Making: The Fact-Finding Report of the Mid-century White House Conference on Children and Youth.* New York, Harper and Brothers, 1952.

Periodicals

Alley, R. D., and Heinz, W. C.: Attention, Kids: This Holiday Story Won't Leave You With A Lump in Your Throat. . . *Today's Health*, 51:28, December 1973.

Bruner, J. S.: Child Development: Play Is Serious Business. *Psychology Today*, 8:80, January 1975.

Carlson, S. S., and Asnes, R. S.: Maternal Expectations and Attitudes Toward Toilet Training: A Comparison Between Clinic Mothers and Private Practice Mothers. *J. Pediatr.*, 84:148, January 1974.

Cooperman, G., and Cooperman, E. M.: Two Wheels Unsafe for Two. *The Canadian Nurse*, 71:30, May 1975.

Damerel, P.: How To Choose Shoes That Fit Your Kid's Feet. *Family Health/Today's Health*, 8:36, August 1976.

Gutelius, M. F., Kirsch, A. D., MacDonald, S., Brooks, M. R., McErlean, T., and Newcomb, C.: Promising Results From a Cognitive Stimulation Program in Infancy. A Preliminary Report. *Clin. Pediatr.*, 11:585, October 1972.

Guyer, B., Barid, S. J., Hutcheson, R. H., and Strain, R. S.: Failure to Vaccinate Children Against Measles During the Second Year of Life. *Public Health Rep.*, 91:133, March-April 1976.

Ikeda, J. P.: Expressed Nutrition Information Needs of Low-Income Homemakers. *J. Nutr. Educ.*, 7:104, July-September 1975.

Lipman, A. G.: Child-Resistant Medication Containers to Reduce Pediatric Drug Poisonings. *Conn. Med.*, 36:666, December 1972.

Lystad, M.: From Dr. Mather to Dr. Seuss. *Children Today*, 5:10, May-June 1976.

Malo-Juvera, D.: Seeing Is Believing. *Nursing Outlook*, 21:583, September 1973.

Mayer, J.: Charting A Course To Good Nutrition With Your Children. *Family Health/Today's Health*, 8:30, August 1976.

McBride, A. B.: The Anger-Depression Guilt Go-Round. *Am. J. Nursing*, 73:1045, June 1973.

McCoy, N. L.: Innate Factors in Sex Differences. *Nursing Forum*, 15:277, No. 3. 1976.

Prival, M. J., and Fisher, F.: Adding Fluorides To The Diet. *Nursing Digest*, 3:53, July-August 1975.

Shulman, B. H., and Reddy, G. D.: Purse Poisons. *Pediatrics*, 51:126, January 1973.

Vaillancourt-Wagner, M.: Children's Value To Their Parents. *The Canadian Nurse*, 71:31, August 1975.

Waller, D. A., and Levitt, E. E.: Concerns of Mothers In A Pediatric Clinic. *Pediatrics*, 50:931, December 1972.

Weaver, P.: How Safe Is *Your* Home? *Today's Health*, 52:40, October 1974.

Wolkon, G. H., et al.: Ethnicity and Social Class in the Delivery of Services: Analysis of a Child Guidance Clinic. *Am. J. Pub. Health*, 64:709, July 1974.

AUDIOVISUAL MEDIA*

American Academy of Pediatrics

First Aid Chart
8½ × 11 inch chart.

American Dental Association

Fluoridation: A White Paper
13 minutes, 16mm film, sound, color.
A documentary approach to reporting current information on the safety, effectiveness, and background of community water fluoridation through interviews with six individuals knowledgeable on different aspects of the measure.

It's Up to You
6 minutes, 16mm film, sound, color.
Examples of dental disease are shown in children and adults. The results of dental neglect demonstrate the damaging effects of calculus on teeth and gums. The film explains the formation of plaque and its relation to dental disease, along with the importance of using a disclosing agent. Detailed scenes show flossing and brushing techniques.

The Hands That Help (Las Manos Que Ayudan)
24 minutes, 16mm film, sound, color.
Shows the design and outfitting of the buses into mobile dental clinics, the living conditions of the migrant population in the San Joaquin and Salinas-Santa Clara Valleys, and the dental treatment rendered.

The American Journal of Nursing Company

Growth and Development—Birth Through Adolescence
Series of 23 44 minute classes, black and white.
Class Instructor: Nicolay, R. C.

The Toddler: Origins of Independence
Participating Instructor: Brooker, M.
The needs of the toddler to become more independent with regard to his motor and social skills are shown.

Language Development
Participating Instructor: Crocker, Rev. J.

The processes of the child's acquisition of both speech and language skills are shown and discussed.

Rudiments of Self-Concept
The physical and social influences related to the emergence of a self-concept are presented.

Coping with the Toddler
Some general attitudes and principles are discussed regarding toilet training, enuresis, sibling rivalry, eating, and control of the toddler.

Charles Press—Prentice-Hall, Inc.

Nursing Skills and Techniques Series
2–5 minutes, Super-8mm filmloop, color, guide.

Growth and Development: 15 Months, Part I
Observations for muscle coordination, skills, etc. of a 15-month-old toddler, plus interaction with mother.

Growth and Development: 15 Months, Part II
Further observations of a 15-month-old toddler.

Growth and Development: 18 Months, Part I
Observations of ability, interests, etc. of an 18-month-old toddler.

Growth and Development: 18 Months, Part II
Observations of an 18-month-old toddler.

Growth and Development: 2 Years, Part I
Observations of a two-year-old: activities and negativism.

Growth and Development: 2 Years, Part II
Continued observations of a two-year-old.

Concept Media

Human Development: The First 2½ Years
7 programs of varied length, 35mm filmstrips/tape, sound, color, guide.
Pregnancy, Birth and the Newborn—27 minutes.
Physical Growth and Motor Development—18 minutes.

The Development of Understanding—23 minutes.
Styles of Interaction—22 minutes.
Emotional and Social Development: Part I—17 minutes.
Emotional and Social Development: Part II—17 minutes.
Language Development—21 minutes.

Department of National Health and Welfare: Ottawa, Canada

Insist on Child-Resistant Packaging
Poster.

J. B. Lippincott Company

Growth and Development: A Chronicle of Four Children
Thompson, J. K., and Juenker, D. M.
16mm film and Super-8mm film and/or videotape, sound, color.
Demonstrates the range of normal variation in social, physical, and cognitive development during the first four years of life. The films focus on each child's social and emotional development, identification behavior, motor development, habitual responses, concepts of reality, and body structure and function.

McGraw-Hill Book Company

Language Development
20 minutes, 16mm film or videocassette, color.

Terrible Twos and Trusting Threes
22 minutes, 16mm film, color.

The Child
Kagan, J., and Rabinovitch, M. S.
16mm films or videocassettes.
The Child, Part I: The First Two Months—29 minutes.

The Child, Part II: 2–14 Months—28 minutes.
The Child, Part III: 12–24 Months—29 minutes.

Trainex Corporation

Accidents and Poisoning
35mm filmstrip, audio-tape cassettes, 33 1/3 LP, color.
Defines the most common injury-causing home accidents, and how rooms can be made safer for children.

Growth and Development
35mm filmstrip, audio-tape cassettes, 33 1/3 LP, color.
Provides parents with information on a number of growth patterns including head shape, sleep habits, teething, walking, and talking.

Preventive Dental Care
35mm filmstrip, audio-tape cassettes, 33 1/3 LP, color.
Includes facts about normal and abnormal development of teeth. Explains the medical view of pacifiers and thumbsucking.

Toilet Training
35mm filmstrip, audio-tape cassettes, 33 1/3 LP, color.
Offers constructive do's and don'ts for successful toilet training. Explains how to judge when a child is ready to be trained, and the implications of bed-wetting.

United States Government

For Children—Because We Care
Producer: USNMAC
13 minutes, 16mm film, optical sound, color.
Dr. Benjamin Spock discusses community water fluoridation, its safety, and low cost in reducing dental caries. Photographs of children and adults in fluoridated and nonfluoridated communities show the facts.

*Complete addresses are given in the Appendix.

Chapter Seventeen

CONDITIONS OF TODDLERS REQUIRING IMMEDIATE OR SHORT-TERM CARE

The toddler's major fear is that of being separated from his mother. When he is ill or injured as in an emergency room situation, he protests verbally, "No, no," he cries, and he screams. His nonverbal responses include clinging to his mother, trying to locate her with his eyes, and returning to her if they are separated, even trying to escape in order to find her. With the nurse he may turn away, avoid eye contact, and kick, flail, or bite. The toddler rejects anyone except his mother and father until a trust relationship has been established with him.

HOSPITALIZATION OF THE TODDLER

A great deal of research has been done during the last two or three decades in the area of separation of the toddler from his mother. A summary review is provided here.

In the mind of the toddler his parents are necessary to his very existence. When his parents take him to the hospital and leave him, therefore, he may have a distorted interpretation of the reason for the separation. He may view it as punishment for something he has done or as a complete loss of their love. The child is thus confused about what is expected of him in this strange situation, he is fearful of being hurt physically, and he may become acutely anxious if he thinks that he will not see his parents again. As a result he may revert to infantile behavior, becoming more demanding and self-centered.

The nurse must recognize the child's need to *regress*. The nurse must help him to transfer his trust to those who care for him, at the same time accepting his dependence while he is ill. Illness may cause the toddler, however, to mistrust adults, the negative counterpart of a sense of trust. The nurse should be aware that the child needs help if he is to trust others. The nurse can recognize the ways by which the child learned to trust as an infant and provide loving support as he needs it to achieve again this developmental goal.

Young children between the ages of seven or eight months and three years are most affected by separation from their mothers. This is because the child has reached the point in development at which he knows the difference between himself and others (see p. 352) and has established relationships with those in his environment. Separation at this developmental point may be crucial to his further development. Toddlers who have had a close relationship with their mothers react more to separation than do those who have not had a good relationship with a mothering figure.

The degree to which a young child is disturbed by a period of hospitalization and separa-

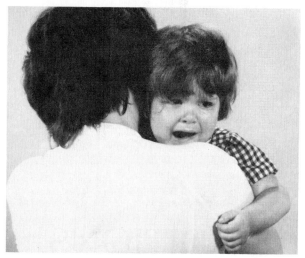

FIGURE 17–1. The toddler is extremely disturbed when mother says that she must leave him.

tion from his mother is dependent on several factors. *Certainly the quality of the child's relationship with his mother and his developmental level before the separation are important. The frequency of previous separations and stresses and the effects these have had on the child are significant. The preparation the child had for the hospitalization and whether his admission was traumatic or not influence his adjustment. The parental response to the separation and the length of his contact with his parents during his hospitalization influence his reaction. During the child's hospital stay the amount of care, support and sensory stimulation he receives from the nursing personnel, influenced in part by his own personality, is important to his coping with this crisis. All these factors also influence his behavior at home with his parents after his discharge from the hospital.*

SPECIFIC RESPONSES OF THE TODDLER

On being hospitalized the toddler experiences basic fears: loss of love, fear of the unknown and fear of punishment. He is too young to be reasoned with; he knows only that his mother or daddy, for whom he calls, does not respond.

More specifically, the stages in the child's apparent adjustment to the hospital when his mother is not present are generally as follows (see also p. 532). The role of the nurse at each stage is included in this discussion.

1. Protest. The child is grief-stricken. He calls for his mother almost constantly. He may reject the nurse when attention is given to him. He may even become hostile to everyone providing care for him. The toddler lives only in the present. He feels that his mother has indeed deserted him. The child feels helpless and may have discomfort from his illness.

The nurse can help the child maintain his emotional tie to his mother and at the same time express his feelings of helplessness and anger. The nurse may feel personally rejected by the child, since efforts at comforting him are not met with immediate success. The nurse may also not approve of his crying. Perhaps the nurse may not have been permitted to cry as a child. Nevertheless the nurse will be most successful during the toddler's period of protest by staying with him while he "protests" and then providing care for him when his tension is reduced.

2. Despair. The child sinks into apparent depression. He is quieter, withdrawn, and apathetic. He mourns deeply for his mother. At this point he may be greatly upset when his mother visits him, because a short visit does not satisfy his need for her. The mother may feel guilty about having left her child with strangers. She can be helped to understand that the release of the child's feelings is important and that he gains comfort from her presence.

The toddler may attempt to comfort himself by sucking his thumb, or other self-comforting measures, or he may hold his favorite blanket securely, curl into a fetal position, and watch anxiously for his mother and for those who may be going to harm him. During this period of despair the toddler may feel that his illness was caused by his own wrong behavior. The nurse can stress the fact that painful treatments are not punishment (see p. 505). In addition, the noises of the hospital unit may frighten him, and so he withdraws.

The child may no longer resist the care of the nurse, but he may regress to his infantile state, soiling himself if he had been partially toilet-trained, ceasing to verbalize if he had begun to talk, and having sleep disturbances and behavioral difficulties.

The nurse can help the toddler most by encouraging his communication of hostility and at the same time showing him by action that he is worthwhile and loved. Instead of withdrawing from him, the nurse can sit quietly with him, waiting for the time when he reaches out for comfort. The nurse can also help by encouraging the mother to bring familiar toys from home and by trying to carry out the daily routine in the hospital as much as possible the way his mother cared for him at home. The child may continue to have hostile outbursts; however, the nurse can set limits to protect him from his own behavior and help him to be as mobile as possible to reduce his aggression. Gradually his feelings of despair will be reduced, and he will have more energy to cope with his illness.

3. Denial. If the child stays in the hospital long enough, he will eventually reach the stage in which he is no longer depressed. He takes greater interest in his surroundings and seems to be happy. At this stage he can no longer tolerate the poignancy of his distress and may repress all feeling for his mother. When she visits him, he barely notices her and does not cry when she leaves.

If the child's stay in the hospital is prolonged, he may eventually settle down to hospital life and apparently require neither his mother nor mothering from nurses. Such maternal deprivation may not result in severe and lasting emotional disturbances; however, some children may be severely emotionally disturbed with no deep attachment for anyone.

The toddler is likely to become a pet of the entire staff. Yet no one has the time or sufficient interest in him to form the loving relation which is needed to stimulate him to learn self-control in order to please his love-object. He is not guided in the development of his habits of self-control and obedience through tutelage and discipline. He is not motivated by love for anyone to do what he does not want to do at the moment.

The nurse can help the child most once he has reached the stage of denial by helping him to trust again in others. It is important that he be helped to establish a relationship with one nurse so that he can reach out to her to express his anger and ultimately face his need for his mother.

If the toddler has not been helped to cope with this period of separation from his mother, on discharge he may not want to go home and clings to the nurse to whom he is accustomed. At home it may be some time before the mother-child tie becomes re-established.

If the toddler receives adequate help from his nurse in expressing his feelings and is encouraged to attain control again in the usual areas of development for a toddler, he may not experience the stages of trauma due to separation from his mother. Certainly every effort the nurse can make will be worthwhile to prevent this threat to his psychosocial development.

THE NURSING HISTORY

If the nurse takes a good nursing history during the initial conference with the parents at admission, several objectives can be reached. The parents can come to understand that the nurse is interested in *their* individual child. Data can be obtained to use in formulating the plan of nursing care. The nurse can ask the mother about her methods of dealing with the child at home so that hospital personnel can follow them as closely as possible. During the conference the nurse can explain hospital policies and routines to the parents. The conference also provides an opportunity for the nurse to come to an understanding with the parents concerning their level of involvement in caring for their child: whether they will or will not be able to visit, or whether the mother or father plans to stay with their child while he is hospitalized.

HOSPITALIZATION OF THE TODDLER WITHOUT THE MOTHER

Some reasons why not all toddlers have their mothers or fathers remain with them in the hospital are as follows: (1) arrangements cannot be made for the care of other children at home; (2) the mother may be the sole means of financial support for the family and cannot afford to remain away from her job; (3) some emotionally disturbed children seem to be more upset when mother is present than when they are left alone; (4) some mothers are too anxious and bewildered and are unable to provide care for their sick children; and (5) some hospitals do not permit or encourage parents to visit. Although some of these reasons are valid, rules that prevent parents from visiting their young children in the hospital should be changed to permit unlimited visiting and rooming-in. Restrictions on visiting by the parents cannot be condoned in the light of recent research in this area.

Tape recorders may be used in some pediatric units. Parents may record messages or bedtime stories to be played to their child when they cannot be present. The familiar voices help to alleviate fear and prevent regressive behavior in the child.

Visiting by the Mother. The toddler separated from his mother has great difficulty in mastering his fear of the loss of her presence. He cannot understand why the separation is necessary. Consequently, he feels that his mother does not want to be with him. He becomes angry, lonely, and frightened. These feelings of anger, fright, or hopeless loneliness are psychologically devastating and, through the psychosomatic interaction, physiologically harmful.

When his mother does visit, he will express strong emotion. This is good, because then his feelings will not be suppressed, to be expressed later. If his mother understands the reasons for the strong reaction, she will not feel that it would be better if she did not come to visit him. His emotional reaction to her presence may occur on first seeing her, during the visit or when she is ready to leave. If, in spite of his anger, he clings to her and cries, she may be so distressed that she may dread visiting again. Yet at the same time she may be gratified by his evident dependency upon her. The nurse must understand and interpret to the mother the meaning of the child's behavior and, when possible, encourage her to stay with her child longer.

Even though the mother is the primary person who takes care of the toddler and is the focus of most of the child's affection, the father is still an important member of the family. Many times in the nuclear family, he is the only one providing emotional support for the mother. He may take turns visiting the hospitalized toddler so the mother can gain relief from the stress of being with the ill child or so she can deal with matters at home.

Unrestricted Visiting. An increasing number of hospitals are permitting unrestricted visiting. Although this arrangement is not as comforting to the child as having his mother with him continually, it is far better than restricted visiting. If unrestricted visiting is permitted, the child is able to vent his feelings of distress and anger frequently instead of suppressing them until he has returned home. Parents, in spite of the tears of their children, are often less anxious than they would be if they could see their children only at restricted intervals.

Hospital personnel often feel that unrestricted visiting hours produce confusion on the unit because of the number of parents present. This does not usually happen if parents are shown how to care for their children and if the unit routine is changed to include their services. In general, unrestricted visiting hours, including encouraging the fathers to visit in the morning before going to work, have improved relations between parents and hospital personnel.

If the mother cannot visit her child frequently, the nurse can exhibit a sympathetic understanding of his loneliness and anxiety. The nurse can share with the child an understanding that he misses his mother and wants to return home. The nurse should not try to help him forget his mother. He can be helped to understand that the close tie with his mother is not broken, even though she is not with him. It is the responsibility of the nurse to make life in the hospital as pleasant as possible for him.

Measures to help the child feel secure in the intervals between visiting hours include permission to have a favorite toy or blanket with him, allowing him to keep a handkerchief, glove or other object belonging to his mother so that he knows she will return, and keeping his shoes with him as a symbol of his returning home. If it is practical, he may speak with his mother over the telephone. Keeping pictures of his family nearby may also help in some situations.

When she must leave, the mother can try to be firm and truthful in telling the child that she must leave and when she will return. She should never sneak out of the unit because she is afraid that he will cry if she tells him the truth. She should not leave while he is sleeping, or he may be fearful of going to sleep again. It is easier for the mother to leave if the nurse anticipates her departure and offers to stay with the child, helping him to wave to her, and reinforcing that she will return. The nurse should stay with him after visiting hours until his initial grief at his mother's departure has passed.

If the mother cannot stay with the child or visit him frequently, he should be assigned to a small group of children whom one nurse regularly attends. The nurse can be relieved by another who is familiar with the children.

PROBLEMS IN THE CARE OF THE TODDLER WHEN THE MOTHER IS NOT PRESENT

Rotation of Personnel. Many different nurses offer the child daily care, with the result that no single one loves and cherishes him. He interests himself in material satisfactions and in superficial relations with any adult who notices him. In a situation in which various nurses must care for a toddler, it is especially important for them all to follow the nursing care plan made for him. By doing so, each nurse will know, among other items of information, his favorite foods and toys, how he prefers to take his medicine, and the best approach to be used in giving him injections. Some semblance of consistency in the care of the child can thus be achieved.

Each nurse caring for the child should recognize the fact that he must adjust to and learn to trust each one as an individual. On the initial meeting each should talk to him from a distance, perhaps walking around the room slowly for a while, before approaching the crib and reaching for him. In this way his level of anxiety may not be increased.

Encouraging Adequate Intake. A sick toddler will often not take the amount of fluids or food he needs to speed his recovery. Some nurses become disturbed when a toddler refuses to eat because this hurts their concepts of themselves as nurturing persons. They must remember that all behavior is caused and that if they can do something about the cause, the behavior can many times be changed. In other words, forcing the child to eat is not the solution to the problem.

A toddler may not eat or drink as much as the nurse believes he should for any of the following reasons: he is not growing as rapidly as he did during infancy and so does not need as much food; he is normally negativistic, in acute conflict between accepting dependency on

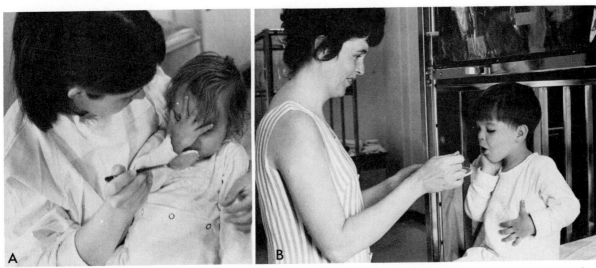

FIGURE 17–2.   A toddler may exert his power by eating or not eating. A, Feeling abandoned by his mother, a hospitalized child may express depression by refusing food. B, A child whom nurses cannot persuade to eat may do so willingly when a member of his family comes in to feed him. (From Snell, B., and McLellan, C. L.: *Am. J. Nursing*, 76:413, March, 1976. Courtesy of Robert Goldstein, Photographer, New Milford, N.J.)

others and being an independent person with a will of his own; he is reacting to the trauma of separation from his mother and of hospitalization; he may not like the kind of food served in the hospital, or he has anorexia caused by his physical illness. If the nurse is aware of these various reasons for his behavior, a possible solution to the problem can be formulated. The nurse can encourage his mother to visit more frequently, especially during mealtimes. The nurse can relax when encouraging the child to eat and can spend more time with him to gain his trust, permitting him the independence of which he is capable and letting him be dependent if he wishes. The mother can be asked for a list of the child's food likes and dislikes and an attempt can be made to serve him the foods he likes. Once the child gains control of himself, his appetite usually improves. The nurse must realize that a happy, healthy child will eat with little help, but an unhappy, ill child will not eat unless assisted by understanding adults.

Elimination Control or Toilet Training.   The child separated from his mother will be hindered in the process of achieving control of both his bodily and his socially acquired actions. He may regress in his ability to maintain sphincter control and wet and soil himself. After his return home he will again feel pride in pleasing his mother by keeping himself clean and dry.

The nurse should know and record on the admission sheet the child's stage of development before his admission to the hospital. The nurse can learn from his mother what methods of training (the equipment, words, and the frequency with which he was placed on the toilet seat or

potty) were used at home so that as far as is possible the same methods can be continued in the hospital. The nurse must not be rigid and demanding, since the child is under an emotional strain due to his feeling of abandonment by his mother. The nurse should sympathetically accept the child's inability to cooperate. He needs to learn about the bedpan and the urinal in his mother's presence. Her approval will motivate him to use the new equipment.

If a young toddler has not started toilet training, the nurse should not feel it necessary to initiate it immediately. If he has a prolonged convalescence, training may be begun when he feels stronger. In order for it to succeed, his mother and one nurse for whom the child feels affection should carry out the training process.

The nurse may have feelings of repugnancy toward soiling by urine and feces on the diaper and the child's clothing (possibly also a soiled bed). An effort must be made by the nurse to understand these feelings and to gain control over them, just as an understanding of the toddler's instinctive pleasure with his own excretory products is necessary.

The nurse should be prepared to forgive "accidents," which are bound to happen. Young children who have achieved control of urination and defecation tend to be upset when an accident occurs. The child needs acceptance. If he knows that the nurse understands and is willing to help, he will more readily cooperate as far as he is able.

Some children use soiling themselves as a means of gaining attention or getting even with the parents who left them in the hospital or as a retaliative measure against the nurses who the child feels lack an understanding of his needs. They may refuse to ask for a bedpan or urinal and then have an "accident" before or even after it is brought to them. If the nurse censures the child because of an "accident," he may repeat the performance to gain attention. The nurse can endeavor to find the reason for his soiling and plan ways to help him cooperate. The child who resorts to such techniques is in a state of emotional turmoil. The nurse, on whom he depends for guidance, can meet his needs, accepting his behavior and yet helping him to gain love and attention in a more appropriate fashion.

HOSPITALIZATION OF THE TODDLER WITH THE MOTHER

It is a truism that the most effective way to prevent trauma to a child from hospitalization is to care for him at home when he is ill. If it is essential that he receive hospital care, every effort should be made to have his mother remain with him.

The child and his mother are first taken to his crib. It is important for the nurse to exhibit an unhurried, friendly, sympathetic attitude. The mother can be provided with a chair and helped to relax. Although the nurse shows an affectionate interest in the child, she must not assume the role of the mother-substitute.

The admission procedure (see Chapter 5) is carefully explained to the mother. The nurse can accept the verbalization of the mother's anxiety and can provide emotional support. The nurse can also explain how the mother can help the child in the hospital milieu.

Since the child gains many of his attitudes from his mother, she should be as calm as possible and in every way provide emotional support for him. By her cooperative attitude toward the nurse she can increase the child's faith in his nurse. The mother can explain to the child the hospital procedures and the use of equipment which is new to him. If he is not to use the potty, but rather the bedpan and the urinal, she can explain this in terms he understands. She can undress him and put on his hospital garments.

If the child's condition permits, the nurse can introduce the mother and her child to other parents and children. The nurse can further orient the mother to the physical facilities of the hospital unit so that the mother can participate conveniently in the child's care. The mother should explain to the child that she will remain with him so that he need not fear abandonment when he sees other children who have been left alone.

A collapsible bed or one of the newer chair-beds can be placed in the room for the mother.

She can then be with her child day and night and provide not only the comfort of being with his mother, but also physical care under the supervision of the nurse.

Many hospitals do not have space for rooming-in facilities. At the very minimum, parents may be permitted to sleep in a chair by the child's bed or, if there is insufficient space, to sleep on a cot in another area of the unit. It is then the responsibility of the nurse to awaken the mother if her child needs her.

Hospital personnel do not always realize the advantages of having the mother stay with the child. They fear that she will be difficult to work with. They are mistaken. The more her maternal feelings are satisfied through providing care for the child (feeding and bathing him), the less anxious she will be. She will help her child to stay on a diet if she understands that one is necessary instead of feeding him candy to compensate for lack of mothering. If his physical condition permits, the mother may continue his toilet training during the hospital stay.

The nurse in a unit where mothers give care to their children can determine how much each mother can be trusted to do for her child and how much guidance she will require. Mothers are generally able to give routine care, but the nurse can instruct them in new skills or in any adaptation of methods which the child's condition makes necessary. A mother should never be urged to attempt procedures she does not feel equal to, for she, like the child, is under a heavy strain which may make her less capable than she is at home. Most mothers will help their children through these difficult experiences if they feel that they themselves have the support of the physicians and nurses. There are times, however, when it would be unwise to permit the mother to be with the child, for if she is unable to control herself the effect upon the child would be disastrous. Whether she stays or not depends upon the situation and upon her reaction and that of the physician and the nurse.

When the mother stays with the toddler, her place at home will have to be filled by the father or older children in the family. Friends and relatives may help keep the home functioning smoothly. If the child is hospitalized for a prolonged period, however, the mother may be encouraged to leave the child's room periodically for meals and to spend some time at home with other members of her family. She needs time for herself in order to gain the strength needed to face her child's illness.

SUMMARY OF THE NURSE'S ROLE IN THE CARE OF THE TODDLER

Although the role of the nurse in the care of the ill child was discussed in general in Chapter

5, significant points in relation to the support of the mother and the toddler are reviewed here.

The experience of hospitalization need not retard the progress of the toddler toward emotional maturity if the nurse helps him integrate the experience of illness and thus increase his ability to adapt to new situations and strengthen the bond between mother and child. The nurse can be a friend who provides emotional support to the patient and his parents. Emotional support will not be accepted if the nurse is not liked, respected and significant to the family members.

Emotional support refers to those aspects of nursing care which help the person's ego to function in an increasingly effective manner. One of the important functions of the ego is to select and carry out a sequence of behavior which will solve a problem faced by the individual so that he will be able to adapt to the situation. In order to provide emotional support to both parent and child, the nurse must be aware of their feelings and ready to respond to them. Recognizing the fact that illness creates stress to which the body reacts in an effort to regain homeostatic balance, the nurse must help to reduce this stress and anxiety by sharing their concerns, showing interest in their problems, and assisting them to adapt to the situation. The nurse must accept the anxiety of the parents and child as appropriate, even though it may cause behavior which seems inappropriate. Any behavior is understood if it is viewed as helping the individual maintain a state of equilibrium.

The manner in which a nurse provides support to the parents has been discussed previously. The way in which she can best provide support to a child is to relieve in a loving, familiar way he can understand any physical pain or emotional distress he may have. It is not enough for the nurse to say that care will be provided for him. The nurse must give the child physical care and assist him to become familiar with his surroundings in the hospital, help him adjust to the routines of the unit and make them flexible if necessary to meet his needs, and prepare him for any discomfort he must face. Through words and actions the nurse must convey to the toddler that he will not be punished for any manifestations of regression or anger he may show, but that he will be accepted as an individual who is loved and respected.

The nurse helps the parents to understand why the toddler behaves as he does when the mother visits or stays with him so that they will continue their close relations with their child. The nurse also discusses with the parents the behavioral changes which may occur when he returns home, such as fear of having his mother out of his sight, demanding behavior, and regression or aggression, as well as suggestions for their behavioral responses should these occur.

PREPARATION FOR HOSPITALIZATION

Preparation for hospitalization is minimal, because children of this age cannot grasp the idea that their mothers will really leave them. Emphasis is placed on how mother and child can be kept together.

The child may be accustomed gradually to being away from his mother for short periods of time by having her leave him in the care of a friend. His mother may also read simple stories about the hospital to him if he is old enough to understand them.

ACUTE CONDITIONS IN THE TODDLER

RETROPHARYNGEAL ABSCESS

Etiology and Incidence. A retropharyngeal abscess is a suppurative lesion involving one or several of the retropharyngeal lymph nodes. It is generally secondary to a nasopharyngeal infection caused by bacteria. It is most common in the first three years of life and is rare after that because of the normal atrophy of these nodes (the nodes are present in the normal newborn). The incidence even in the toddler period has decreased in recent years, owing to better medical supervision of children and more effective therapy.

Clinical Manifestations, Diagnosis, and Differential Diagnosis. Abscess formation is rapid after an acute respiratory infection. The abscess makes it difficult and painful for the child to swallow, and therefore drooling of saliva is prominent. To relieve the pain and facilitate swallowing he tends to keep his mouth open. His head is retracted, and he cries when it is moved. If the lesion is in the upper portion of the pharynx, a bulging of the posterior pharyngeal wall may be visible. Respirations are noisy and are accompanied by a gurgling sound. If the swelling is excessive, obstruction to breathing may occur with stridor and possibly dyspnea. The child's temperature is variable, but tends to be high. Prostration is often severe.

The *diagnosis* is made by inspection with or without a laryngoscope, by palpation or by a lateral roentgenogram.

Differential diagnosis must consider tuberculosis of the cervical vertebrae (cold abscess).

Treatment. If antibiotic therapy is started immediately, regression of the infection often occurs without abscess formation. Local heat in

PEDIATRIC MEDICATION GUIDELINES—12 TO 18 MONTHS

	Developmental Tasks and Behaviors	Nursing Implications
MOTOR	• Advances from standing with support to independent walking.	• Have the child choose a position for taking medication or hold him to provide control and comfort. Forcing the child to take medicine when he is lying down takes away his sense of independence and will frequently result in very resistive behavior.
FEEDING	• Begins independent self-feeding, but is still messy. • Develops voluntary tongue and lip control. • Spits deliberately.	• Home feeding habits should be considered. • Spits out disagreeable tastes effectively. Disguise crushed tablets and contents of capsules in a *small* amount of familiar solid. Be prepared to refeed.
INTERACTIVE	Autonomy versus Shame and Doubt • Indicates needs and wants by pointing. • Speaks 4 to 6 words. Uses individual jargon. • Responds to familiar commands. • Responds to and participates in the routines of daily living. • Exhibits notable independence, resistance, self-assertiveness, and ambivalence. Begins to have temper tantrums.	• Find out what words child uses for drinking, swallowing, and how oral medicines have been given at home. • Let child explore an empty medication cup. He will likely be more cooperative if familiar items are used. • When possible, involve the parents. They are familiar and trusted persons, which is an important factor during an unfamiliar experience. • Tell parents and staff the approach used for medication. Report its effectiveness. • Allow the child as much freedom as possible. • Allow the child to assert himself by choosing a drink to wash down the medicine. • Use games to gain cooperation. • Tell the child what you expect and then follow through. A consistent, firm approach is essential.

EXAMPLE: Eighteen-month-old Simon has been in the hospital 4 days with severe gastroenteritis. He has had nothing orally and has received intravenous (IV) fluids for volume replacement and ampicillin therapy. This morning his IV was discontinued and oral ampicillin started. At shift report the day nurse states he does not take his oral medication well. She reports that she gave the suspension via syringe.

Recognizing that Simon has had experience with a variety of syringes in the last few days, the evening nurse elects to try a different approach. From talking with Simon's mother she knows Simon is used to an assisted self-feeding routine—he has his own fork and spoon and his mother supplements his efforts with another spoon. Also, he enjoys apple juice and can manage a cup fairly well by himself.

Using this "at home" activity and Simon's need to feel familiar with an object to decrease his fear, the nurse allows him to play with a medication cup, drink juice from it, and watch his mother handle and use it. Later she measures the ampicillin into one now-familiar cup and apple juice into another. She allows Simon to hold the juice cup. Simon's sip of ampicillin, given by the nurse, is alternated with a self-fed sip of apple juice. He took the ampicillin without resistance. At night shift report the nurse notes this approach was effective. She encountered no resistive behavior.

FIGURE 17–3.   Guide to administration of oral medications to toddlers. (From Ormond, E.A.R., and Caulfield, C.: *The American Journal of Maternal Child Nursing*, 1:322, September–October 1976.)

PEDIATRIC MEDICATION GUIDELINES—18 TO 30 MONTHS

	Developmental Tasks and Behaviors	Nursing Implications
MOTOR	● Walks, climbs into chair (18 mos.). Advances to running without falling (24 mos.).	● Child is able to run away and kick.
	● Advances to obtaining and throwing small objects.	● Child may throw materials placed within his reach. Never leave medications sitting on the bedside stand.
FEEDING	● Generally feeds self. Advances to proficiency with minimal spilling.	● Allow child opportunity to drink liquids from a medicine cup by himself.
	● Second molars erupted (20-30 mos.). Exhibits increased rotary chewing; manages solid food particles.	● Permits greater flexibility in choosing form of medication.
	● Controls mouth and jaw proficiently.	● Child is effective in spitting out unwanted medications and in clamping mouth tightly closed in resistance.
INTERACTIVE	Autonomy versus Shame and Doubt	
	● Has some sense of time, but no words for time (18 mos.). Then responds to "just a minute" (21 mos.). Advances to understanding, "Play after you drink this." (24 mos.).	● Tell the child getting medicine that any bad taste will only last "a minute."
		● Learn child's level of time awareness from nursing history.
	● Carries out 2 to 3 directions given one at a time.	● Give simplified directions: "Open your mouth, drink, and then swallow."
	● Shows ability to respond to and participate in routines of daily living.	● Include child in establishing medicine-taking routine.
	● Helps put things away; carries breakable objects.	
	● Exhibits independence, resistance, self-assertiveness, and ambivalence.	● Use a firm, consistent approach. Resistive behaviors are at a peak.
	● Throws temper tantrums frequently.	
	● Shows pride in accomplished skills.	● Give immediate, positive tactile and verbal response to cooperative taking of medicine. Ignore resistive behavior.
	● Does not know right from wrong.	
	● Shows conflict between holding on and letting go.	● Give choices when possible: "Do you want to sit in the chair or on my lap to take your medicine?"

EXAMPLE: Barbara, 28 months, has bronchitis and was admitted to the hospital 3 days ago. She has been receiving ampicillin 250 mg by mouth every six hours. Usually a delightful, playful child, she has been labeled a "brat" when it comes time to take her medicine. Nurses have emptied capsules, placed the contents in chocolate syrup, and spoon-fed her with the result of most of the mixture ending up on the nurse. Suspension form has also been tried ineffectively.

Referring to the nursing history for possible help with this child, the nurse discovers that Barbara's favorite food is now candy. Since she has demonstrated proficiency in chewing solid food and candy, the nurse suspects she might take her ampicillin as a chewable tablet. The nurse also feels that involving Barbara in the ritual of medication time might be helpful. At the next medicine time the nurse allows Barbara to pick out two 125 mg tablets herself from a medication cup. Barbara then chews and swallows them. Next she throws the now empty cup into the wastebasket. The nurse gives Barbara a chaser of choice and praises her for her help. Barbara is now a "successful helper" in taking medications.

FIGURE 17-3 *Continued.*

the form of hot compresses to the neck may be used if the child is able to cooperate. When the abscess is ready for incision, this is done by puncture without anesthesia and with the head lower than the chest in order to promote drainage. The opening is then spread apart with a hemostat. Frequent aspiration of the pharynx is performed to remove draining material. The physician must be prepared for respiratory arrest and hemorrhage if these occur. Antibiotic therapy is continued because this condition is usually due to the beta-hemolytic streptococcal bacteria.

Responsibilities of the Nurse. Nursing care includes assisting the physician in his examination of the throat and incising the abscess, and in postoperative care. When the physician examines the throat, the child may be restrained with a mummy restraint (see p. 413). The nurse holds the child's head still with one hand on each side of his head. The child must be securely restrained so that the examination or incision may be done gently and quickly without damage to the wall of the pharynx and with a minimum of pain and fright to the child.

After the incision has been made, a position suitable for drainage from the mouth must be maintained. The foot of the bed is elevated, and the child is placed on his abdomen. A pillow may be placed under his chest and abdomen so that the discharge from the abscess will drain through the mouth rather than down the throat. Restraints may be necessary.

The child is encouraged to take fluids as soon as he can swallow. He must be closely observed for symptoms of respiratory distress and hemorrhage. Frequent swallowing may be an indication of bleeding and should be reported promptly.

Prognosis. The prognosis is good if the abscess is incised as soon as the mass is fluctuant and if proper antibacterial therapy is instituted. An untreated abscess may rupture spontaneously, or death may occur from pneumonia, pulmonary abscess, or anoxia caused by edema of the glottis, pressure upon the larynx, or severe hemorrhage.

Acute Infections of the Larynx

Acute infection of the larynx is more frequent in toddlers than among older children and is more serious because the airway is smaller and therefore more readily obstructed.

Usually other parts of the respiratory tract besides the larynx are involved. Laryngeal obstruction produces clinical manifestations which are the same even though produced by various types of organisms. The clinical manifestations are aphonia, hoarseness, inspiratory dyspnea, stridor, and retraction of various respiratory muscle groups (intercostal, substernal, subcostal, suprasternal) on inspiration.

Diagnosis can be made by laryngoscopic and bacteriologic examinations.

CROUP (ACUTE SPASMODIC LARYNGITIS)

Etiology and Incidence. Croup is a mild inflammation of the larynx. The predominating clinical manifestation is a reactive spasm of the muscles of the larynx which produces a partial respiratory obstruction.

Spasmodic croup is relatively common between the ages of two and four years, but may occur in any child under five. There appears to be a familial and individual predisposition to the condition. The hyperactive and nervous child seems to be affected more often than the quiet one. Susceptible children are likely to have more than one attack, and the attacks invariably occur at night.

Cold air may precipitate an attack in susceptible children, particularly if an upper respiratory tract infection is present. Even moving the child from a warm room where he has spent the day to the cooler bedroom for the night may induce an attack of croup.

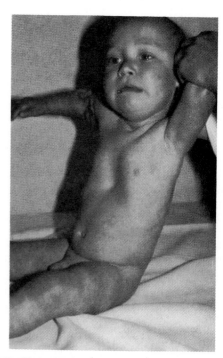

FIGURE 17–4. Eight-month-old infant with pseudocroup: sudden onset of severe dyspnea, gasping hoarse inspirations, deep jugular and sternal retraction, livid skin, and frightened expression. (From Moll, H.: *Atlas of Pediatric Diseases.* Philadelphia, W. B. Saunders Co., 1976.)

Croup has a low order of communicability, and mothers should be told this. Although children seldom, if ever, die of uncomplicated croup, because the child appears to be strangling, croup frightens parents as do few other conditions of like severity.

Clinical Manifestations and Diagnosis. *Clinical manifestations* may appear in a child who has shown no symptoms of an upper respiratory tract infection or other illness. The onset is dramatic, all the more so since it often occurs during sleep.

In a typical attack early in the night the child wakens with dyspnea and coughing. The cough is tight, the sound barking and metallic. Respirations are noisy. The cough wakes the parents, who find the child sitting up in bed, extremely frightened, and struggling for breath. He may grasp at his throat because of his feeling of suffocation. With each inspiration a high-pitched rasp, or a sharp stridor, occurs. The child's face is red, and his lips and nails may be cyanotic. The alae nasi may flare with each inspiration. There may be substernal, suprasternal and supraclavicular retractions. The voice is harsh, the pulse rapid, and the child perspires freely. His temperature is seldom over 101° F. (38.3° C.). After one to three hours the severity of the spasm diminishes, and all clinical manifestations abate. Sometimes more than one attack will occur in a night, or attacks may occur on subsequent nights. The morning after an attack the child may have a loose cough. In a mild attack he may have a croupy cough, but only moderate laryngospasm and dyspnea.

The *diagnosis* is made on the basis of the history, the respiratory difficulty, and lack of other clinical manifestations. The physician must differentiate croup from diphtheritic laryngitis, the laryngospasm of tetany (see p. 442) and acute streptococcal laryngitis.

Treatment. Treatment is directed toward reduction of the spasm of the laryngeal muscles. The child is placed in an atmosphere of high humidity, for this tends to liquefy the secretions in the throat and also reduces the spasm. The physician may order an emetic such as syrup of ipecac to induce vomiting. Vomiting tends to reduce the laryngeal spasm. The dose of the emetic may be repeated once or twice if necessary. A sedative such as phenobarbital may be given after the child has vomited. Chemotherapy may be ordered if the infection is severe, but as a rule is not necessary. Only in rare cases is intubation or tracheotomy needed.

Responsibilities of the Nurse. The nurse carries out the treatment outlined by the physician. The provision of moist air is a primary consideration. The equipment to be used is shown to the child, and the procedure, if he is old enough to understand, is explained to him. The water vapor serves to liquefy secretions, and the warmth, through the use of a croup tent if one is ordered, tends to reduce the spasm of the muscles and to relieve the inflammation of the mucous membrane of the throat. The child is put in a croup tent to concentrate the warm moist air about him. A drug such as benzoin may be added to the water, but actually it is steam vapor that is therapeutic.

The croup tent is made in the following way. The top and sides of the upper half or two thirds of the crib are covered with a blanket (to absorb moisture) and a waterproof plastic covering. Warm moist air is provided by the use of an electric humidifier. The child must be protected from burning himself on the humidifier or from the hot steam. He must have his clothing and bedding changed frequently to keep him dry because the steam condenses and makes them damp. If the child is to be removed from the tent, care is taken that he is not chilled by exposure to air at room temperature. While he is in the tent his condition is observed frequently, and he is kept as content as possible.

Since the end of the bed is not closed, most children are not frightened by a croup tent, but a toddler who is afraid may be helped to imagine that it is his own little house or tent.

The physician may order that the child be given cool moist air, rather than steam, to liquefy the secretions in the larynx. This therapy can be given in the home by the use of a cold steam vaporizer. In the hospital cool mist can be provided through the use of a Croupette, using the pressure of oxygen or, if the child does not need oxygen, compressed air. (For setting up the Croupette, see p. 402.) One reason why cool moist air is ordered rather than hot steam is that cool air may lower the child's body temperature, while the warmth of the steam-heated croup tent may raise it. Some hospitals use devices which mechanically vaporize water and fill the crib, cubicle, or room with mist.

HOME MODIFICATION OF THE HOSPITAL PROCEDURE. The quickest and easiest way to provide warm moist air for the child with an attack of croup is to run hot water in the bathtub or shower, take the child into the bathroom and close the door. This arrangement cannot be continued for long, however, for the steam might damage the paper or plaster on the walls, and the supply of hot water might give out. It does give emergency relief, however, while a hot steam or cool mist tent is being prepared.

The crib may be covered as in the hospital. A plastic table cover may be substituted for the plastic sheeting. If the mother does not have a vaporizer, a kettle of hot water may be used. A gas or electric plate can be used to heat the water. Every precaution must be taken to prevent burning the child. If cool moist air is ordered, a cool mist vaporizer may be used.

If the child does not sleep in a crib, a sheet or blanket may be draped over a baby carriage, or a card table or a large straight-backed chair—tilted—may be placed on an adult's bed, and the child laid under the table or chair. An umbrella may be used instead of the chair, but it does not give a firm support for the tent.

OTHER POINTS IN NURSING CARE. Since syrup of ipecac causes vomiting, the nurse or mother should stay near the child until after he has vomited. He is already anxious because of his respiratory distress, and vomiting increases his anxiety. Soiling his clothing and bed with vomitus may frighten him even if he knows that he will not be blamed for the accident. After he has vomited, a sedative, usually phenobarbital, may be ordered by the physician.

When the child is resting quietly, the nurse can help the parents relieve their anxiety by expressing it in words and can provide sympathetic emotional support. The nurse can explain to the parents the child's condition, why treatments and medications are given, and the progress of his illness. They will then be less frightened if a second attack occurs on the following night.

The nurse is responsible for the administration of any chemotherapeutic agents the physician may order.

So that the physician may have information essential to the diagnosis and treatment of the condition, the nurse must observe and record all signs and symptoms, both objective and subjective, so far as the child is able to communicate. The nurse can also try to teach the mother the importance and meaning of these observations.

The most important symptoms to be observed during the attack are the color of the child, the rate and nature of the respirations, the degree of restlessness, the level of anxiety, the presence of cyanosis, and the degree of prostration.

If the child's respiratory embarrassment increases, intubation or tracheotomy (p. 541) may be necessary. The nurse must promptly report to the physician such a change.

Prognosis and Prevention. The *prognosis* is invariably good, although both parents and child are thoroughly frightened.

There are no specific *preventive measures,* but conditions which increase the probability of an attack of spasmodic croup in children known to be susceptible are to be avoided. If there is evidence of an impending attack, such as coughing or hoarseness, particularly on the night after an attack, general preventive measures which may be taken include keeping the bedroom warm (temperature approximately 70° F. [21.1° C.]), humidifying the air of the room, and giving the child subemetic doses of ipecac, and phenobarbital for sedation.

ACUTE EPIGLOTTITIS

Etiology, Incidence, and Clinical Manifestations. Acute epiglottitis is a severe, rapidly progressive infection of the epiglottis and surrounding areas caused by *Hemophilus influenzae B,* pneumococci, group A streptococci or viruses. It is more prevalent in the temperate zone, more common in winter, and more frequent in areas having high air pollution. It occurs most frequently in young children.

Before the onset of acute epiglottitis the child may have had a slight upper respiratory tract infection. Acute and severe respiratory distress may occur quickly and consists of inspiratory stridor and retractions, cough, muffled voice, dysphagia, drooling, restlessness, and fever of 100 to 105° F. (38 to 40.5° C.). The child may hold his neck in a hyperextended position or sit up with his chin thrust out. Some children may go into a state of shock, having cyanosis or pallor. On examination the epiglottis is edematous and cherry-red in color. An emergency tracheotomy may be necessary to prevent sudden death. If the necessary equipment is not available for a tracheotomy, the child may be kept breathing by inserting a large-bore (12- to 15-gauge) needle through the tracheal wall. Care must be taken that the needle does not penetrate the opposite wall of the trachea.

Treatment and Responsibilities of the Nurse. The treatment and nursing care of a child having acute epiglottitis are similar to the measures taken for a child having croup (see p. 539) and laryngotracheobronchitis (see below).

LARYNGOTRACHEOBRONCHITIS

Incidence and Etiology. Laryngotracheobronchitis is an acute inflammation of the larynx, trachea, and bronchi. The *incidence* is greatest during the first three or four years of life.

Several viral and bacterial agents may cause the infection. The bacteria usually responsible include *Hemophilus influenzae,* hemolytic streptococci, pneumococci, and staphylococci.

Pathology, Clinical Manifestations, and Diagnosis. The *pathology* is manifested in the inflammation and edema of the mucosa and submucosa of the larynx, trachea, and bronchi. A purulent exudate which produces crusts may be present. If these accumulate, they may obstruct the air passages.

Clinical manifestations may follow an acute respiratory infection, or the onset may be sudden and accompanied by prostration, elevation of temperature and severe dyspnea. During the onset respiratory difficulty is usually in the inspiratory phase, since the larynx is involved. Later there may also be expiratory difficulty because of involvement of the bronchi and bronchioles.

The child may become restless, owing to lack of oxygen. Hoarseness or aphonia may be present. The chest shows both substernal and suprasternal retractions. His color may eventually become ashen gray or cyanotic. His temperature may be as high as 104 to 105° F. (40 to 40.5°C.), and febrile convulsions (see p. 474) may occur as the result of the fever. His cough is likely to be persistent. If there is an exudate, the cough is loose, croupy, and noisy, but if the exudate is too thick to move, the child may not cough at all. When obstruction due to exudate is nearly complete, breath sounds may be barely audible, and dyspnea may be severe.

The *diagnosis* is confirmed and the causative organism is found by laboratory examination of a culture of exudate. Sensitivity tests are performed to determine which antibiotic agent is most effective. The material for laboratory examination includes a direct smear and culture to rule out diphtheria. Blood cultures are also obtained. Fluoroscopic and bronchoscopic examinations may be done to rule out the possibility of an aspirated foreign body (see p. 403).

Treatment. The basis of treatment of laryngotracheobronchitis is the provision of (a) sufficient oxygen, given whenever the accessory muscles of respiration are used for breathing, and (b) sufficient humidity to liquefy secretions and so to prevent crusts from forming. Either hot steam (if the child's temperature is not markedly elevated) or cool vapor may be used for this purpose. (c) Drugs to control the infection. Broad-spectrum antibiotics may be given; if the infection is of bacterial origin, they are effective, but if it is caused by a virus, no striking response will be observed.

During the treatment a patent airway must be maintained. When there is severe obstruction, relief can be provided by an emergency tracheotomy. *Tracheotomy*, an incision into the trachea, is made in order to open up a passage for air to enter the trachea proximal to the site of laryngeal obstruction. The incision also aids in the draining of secretions. Indications for a tracheotomy with insertion of a tracheostomy tube are restricted expansion of the lungs (this shows that only a minimal amount of air can enter the lungs), signs of cardiac failure and prostration with severe pallor or cyanosis. The incision is made just below the first tracheal ring (Fig. 17–7).

Drugs such as atropine and opiates are contraindicated because atropine tends to dry up secretions in the respiratory tract, and opiates dull the cough reflex. Digitalization is necessary if clinical signs of cardiac failure (see p. 292) appear.

Parenteral fluid therapy may be required to maintain the proper state of hydration.

Responsibilities of the Nurse. The nurse must observe the child who has laryngotracheobronchitis very carefully for any indication of increasing fatigue or respiratory distress, reporting to the physician immediately the occurrence of increased restlessness, pulse rate, temperature, dyspnea, or retractions. The nurse is responsible for recognizing and reporting indications of increased respiratory distress before cyanosis appears.

While the nurse is observing his physical condition an attempt should be made to make friends with the toddler so that he will accept care more easily in case a tracheotomy becomes necessary. The nurse should help to allay the anxiety of both parents and child caused by the distressing symptoms.

After a tracheotomy, maintenance of this artificial airway is of fundamental importance. It is also the outlet for pulmonary drainage. Accidents arising in maintenance of this airway endanger the child's life. Most of them can be prevented by intelligent nursing care and observation of the child's condition. The nurse must be prepared to care for emergencies as they arise. Sometimes situations can be handled easily. If the physician is needed, the nurse puts in

| mm. | 4 | 5 | 5.5 | 6 | 7 | 8 | 9 |

| size | 00 | 0 | 1 | 2 | 3 | 4 | 5 |

New-born	No. 00-0	3 to 6 years	No. 3
Up to 1 year	No. 1	6 to 12 years	No. 4
1 to 3 years	No. 2	12 to 20 years	No. 5

FIGURE 17–5. Tracheostomy set. *A*, Outer cannula. *B*, Inner cannula. *C*, Obturator. Diagram below shows sizes of tubes (with the diameters in millimeters) usually used for children of various ages.

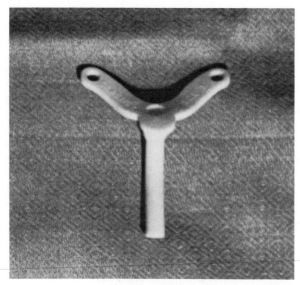

FIGURE 17–6. *A,* The Silastic pediatric tracheostomy tube eliminates the problems of rigid metal tubes. This pliable tube reduces tracheal trauma and tissue irritation. Crusts do not tend to form in these tubes, so it may not require an inner cannula. (From Conner, G. H., Hughes, D., Mills, M. J., Rittmanic, B., and Sigg, L. V.; *Am. J. Nurs.,* 72:68–77, January, 1972.) *B,* The Shiley disposable pediatric tracheostomy tube. (Courtesy of Shiley Laboratories, Inc.)

A

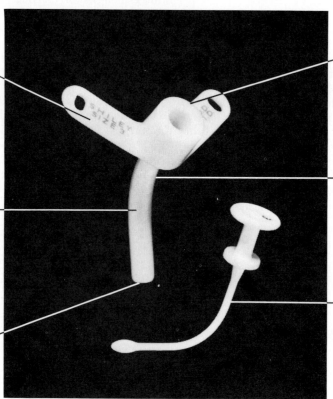

1
Sterile —
Disposable —
Radio-opaque —
5 Sizes (00, 0, 1, 2, 3) to cover the full range of infant and pediatric needs.

2
Maximum airway: special PVC construction allows design which provides maximum internal diameter with minimum external diameter.

3
90-degree end cut to minimize the possibility of blocking against the anterior tracheal wall.

4
Built-in standard 15-mm connector for direct hook-up to ventilation and anesthesia equipment.

5
Soft, flexible, anatomically shaped cannula designed for greater patient comfort during airway maintenance and ventilation.

6
Smoothly tapered obturator to simplify insertion and minimize trauma.

B

a call for him and gives emergency care until he arrives.

Since the situation is frightening, the nurse must use all possible means to reduce anxiety. Self-confidence in the ability to give the child optimum nursing care is essential to inspiring confidence in him and his parents.

After a tracheotomy, the nurse must provide constant care and observe and report indications of respiratory difficulty and the child's reaction to treatment. Observations are made of such danger signals as restlessness, extreme fatigue, dyspnea, cyanosis or pallor, fever, rapid pulse, retractions, and noisy respirations. (Electronic monitoring of the respirations of young tracheostomized children may be utilized.) The nurse must also watch for bleeding or indications of infection around the incision.

Control of the environment is important in prevention of emergency situations. Since in-

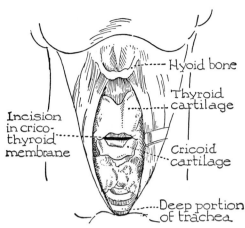

FIGURE 17–7. Diagram showing landmarks and horizontal incision for emergency tracheotomy. (M. G. Lynch, in Ochsner and DeBakey: *Christopher's Minor Surgery.* 8th ed.)

spired air is normally filtered, warmed, and moistened in the upper respiratory tract, the environment must be such that the air the child breathes is to some extent moistened and not too cool before it enters the tracheostomy tube. The room should be warm, the temperature of the air about 80° F. (26.6° C.) (this temperature will also keep the child warm and prevent his being chilled). To moisten the air, a humidifier or croup tent is used. Oxygen may also be necessary. If continuous oxygen is not necessary, an emergency setup should be kept in readiness.

An aspirating machine with good negative pressure is kept at the bedside.

A tray is also kept at the bedside on which is sterile equipment for the routine care of the tracheostomy and for emergency use.

Such equipment includes duplicate tracheostomy tubes* with tapes attached, two curved clamps, scissors, obturator, pipe cleaners or tonsil wire, gauze bandage, gauze dressings, a medicine dropper or syringe and needle, applicators, tongue depressors, an extra catheter (no. 8 to 10 French which has additional holes near the tip to facilitate the process of aspiration of the nasopharynx) and an open-tip catheter, preferably of the whistle tip type (this is used in tracheal aspiration, i.e., clearing the tracheal tube of secretions). In addition, there should be a covered jar of hydrogen peroxide or other solution to cleanse the tracheostomy tube, a covered jar of physiologic saline solution and a covered jar of sterile petrolatum or petrolatum gauze. The jars should be labeled on both sides and on the lids so that the nurse cannot confuse their contents.

A few drops of sterile physiologic saline solution are inserted into the tube to incite a cough

which might dislodge crusts in the lower respiratory passages and to liquefy secretions in the lower respiratory tract and so facilitate aspiration of mucus. The sterile petrolatum may be used to coat the area around the tube. The petrolatum may be applied with a tongue depressor.

Care of the tracheostomy tube and incision involves sterile technique throughout the procedure, including the use of sterile gloves and equipment. The nurse *removes the inner cannula if one is present* and cleans it by soaking it in hydrogen peroxide or other solution and then passing the pipe cleaners or tonsil wire and gauze through the tube. The nurse aspirates the outer cannula and tracheobronchial tree (the depth to which the nurse is permitted to aspirate the tracheobronchial tree depends on the policy adopted by the medical personnel). If the obstruction persists or if the physician has ordered it, a few drops of sterile saline solution may be instilled into the cannula before aspiration. To do this the nurse uses the medicine dropper or syringe.

The aspirating catheter should be pinched so that the lumen is closed while it is inserted into the opening of the outer tube. (A glass Y tube may be used so that the vacuum can be released by fingertip control instead of by pinching the aspirating catheter.) The catheter should be slowly and gently inserted. After withdrawal for rinsing with sterile physiologic saline solution the catheter is rotated 180 degrees between the fingers so that its normal curve will carry it down to another bronchus when aspiration is repeated. The catheter is reinserted and aspiration continued until all drainage has been removed. The inner cannula, thoroughly cleansed, is reinserted and locked in place after the aspiration procedure has been completed.

If the nurse is unable to aspirate the tracheobronchial tree successfully, and if respiratory difficulty or noises on respiration persist, the physician should be notified so that the lower airway can be investigated.

The frequency of aspiration depends upon the need of the child. Immediately after tracheotomy, aspiration is usually performed every 15 minutes, later every 30 minutes or every hour. The need gradually decreases with improvement in the child's condition.

If the nurse is to change the dressing around the tracheostomy tube, the area around the tube is cleansed with hydrogen peroxide. A gauze square cut to the center is slid behind the tube and under the tapes to hold it in position.

The prevention of accidents is important in the nursing care of these children. The toddler is too young to understand the necessity of leaving the tube in place, and so his hands are restrained. Elbow restraints may be used. The older child who is restless and has nothing to occupy his mind may attempt to put bits of food or debris into the tube. The nurse should explain

---

*The plastic Portex tube may be used instead of the tracheostomy set.

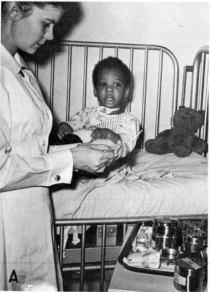

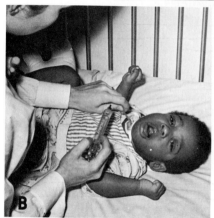

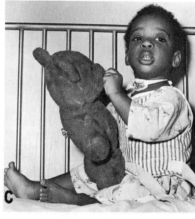

FIGURE 17–8. Tracheostomy care. A, The nurse cleans the inner cannula with a pipe cleaner. Containers are labeled on their tops and sides to prevent accidental interchange of lids. Note the favorite toy of this little boy in the corner of his crib. B, Aspiration is done after sterile saline solution from the syringe has been instilled into the tracheostomy tube. C, The toddler with his tracheostomy tube in place. After his own aspiration he enjoys aspirating his teddy bear. (Gilbert & Ring).

the importance of the tube to such a child. The nurse must be certain that the inner cannula is securely fastened in place so that it will not fall out, and that the tapes are firmly tied so that the child cannot dislodge the tube.

If, by accident, the outer cannula is removed from the trachea, the incision in the trachea must be held open with a hemostat by the nurse while another nurse summons the physician. The physician should insert the extra tracheostomy tube.

If the child stops breathing because of some obstruction of the airway, the inner tube should be withdrawn and the outer tube thoroughly aspirated. The child should be given oxygen through the tracheal tube. If the outer tube has become dislodged, oxygen should be given through the incision. Artificial respiration may be given; the method is that ordinarily given children (see p. 202), with the fundamental difference that the nurse places her mouth to the opening in the neck rather than over the child's mouth. Other methods of artificial respiration may also be used. When the physician arrives, he will attempt to relieve the obstruction by bronchoscopic examination, if need be.

When the child no longer needs the tracheostomy tube, the lumen may be partially obstructed by a cork, or decreasing sizes of tubes may be used to compel the child to breathe through his nose. When he can tolerate a very small tube or complete occlusion of the tube without distress, the tube can be removed, and a sterile dressing can be placed over the incision. In *decannulation,* since the child may not be able to cough up secretions completely, there is danger of their puddling in the lungs with a subsequent rise in temperature and with restlessness. The child should be under close observation for several days. He may be given mild sedation and placed in a mist tent for humidity while he is being decannulated.

There are few conditions in which the nurse's record of observations and the care given are more important than in the nursing of a child with a tracheotomy. Whenever the tube is aspirated, the time should be charted, as well as the amount, consistency, and nature of the return (whether it contains blood, mucus or crusts), and whether the child breathed more easily after the aspiration. The time when the tracheostomy tube is changed should be charted, together with the child's reaction to the procedure.

Psychologic care is extremely important. The child needs his nurse constantly after a tracheotomy because he is in physical danger, and he also needs emotional support. He has a physical basis for his fear of being alone, and his respiration is further embarrassed when he becomes anxious and excited. In his condition he cannot cry or call for his nurse, and is in danger of respiratory obstruction. He must learn to get used to breathing through the tube, which is at first difficult. He needs the love and reassurance of both his mother and his nurse in order to maintain his sense of trust in himself and others. He is afraid, and the nurse increases his fear by aspirating the tube, so that he feels insecure and unhappy. When he becomes accustomed to aspiration of the tube and finds that it makes him more comfortable, he will learn to depend upon his nurse for relief as he does upon his mother for love. He may even play at aspirating his favorite toy (see Fig. 17–8). The importance of the tube can be explained to an older child, but the toddler is too young to comprehend its function until he learns from experience that he feels better after it has been cleared.

Until the toddler becomes accustomed to the tracheotomy tube, he is afraid to swallow. By placing small quantities of fluid or food in his mouth he will learn that swallowing will cause him little or no pain.

Excitement should be avoided, but the child can be amused with toys, or with stories if his hands are restrained and he is unable to play with toys by himself.

OTHER POINTS IN CARE OF THE CHILD. The vital signs are taken as ordered by the physician or more frequently as indicated by the nurse's observations of the child. If the child cannot change his position, the nurse should move him frequently to prevent puddling of secretions. A semi-Fowler's position may be most comfortable for the child. He is helped to get as much rest as possible. It may be necessary to give mouth care if the child is not taking an adequate amount of fluid to keep his mouth moist. It is desirable to give enough fluids—preferably warm—orally to prevent dehydration. His oral intake may be increased by offering small amounts of any fluid he likes at frequent intervals. If the older toddler likes popsicles, these may be given as permitted. If he will not take the required amount, fluids are given parenterally.

As mentioned previously, any treatment for which a needle is used is frightening to a child. The degree of fear he has is in proportion to his age, his past experience with injections, his level of ego strength and cognitive functioning, his anticipation of pain, and his fantasies about any intrusion into his body. The amount of support he receives from his mother or nurse influences the child's response.

Although a young toddler may not have an immediate response to the discomfort of an injection and may not feel it as acutely as an older child, he still feels severe prolonged pain and dislikes being prevented from moving freely because of restraints. When the nurse holds him and comforts him, he is better able to tolerate his discomfort and increase his trust in others.

The hospitalized toddler, who may believe that his parents have deserted him and may feel that his illness is a form of punishment (see p. 505) for being naughty, may view an injection of any needle as a hostile act on the part of the nurse or physician. The preschool child may view an injection as an intrusion into his body also, but at this age he may see it as punishment for masturbation, which his parents may not have permitted (see p. 609).

In order to prevent much of the vigorous response a young child may make to injections, the nurse should explain the equipment and procedure to him on his level of understanding before the injection is given. He may cry at the time, but he can also continue to trust a nurse who has been honest and considerate of his feelings. He can then use whatever ability he has to cope with this experience. *A young child may understand more from the attitude of the nurse who talks to him than he can from the exact meaning of the words used.*

The nurse may give further reason for the treatment and explanation of the procedure to the parents, noting that they can support the child with their presence. If the parents are too anxious (see Infectious Anxiety, p. 617), they may wish to leave the room. In this situation the nurse can encourage the child to express his feelings and provide support for him during and after the procedure.

Drugs and antibiotics are given as ordered by the physician.

The physician may discharge the child before the tracheostomy tube has been removed. In that case the mother must be gradually taught (by demonstration and possibly by film strip) the care of the child before he leaves the hospital.

The father and the child, if he is old enough, should also be familiar with the necessary procedures. The child will probably be referred to a community or public health nurse if he is not under the care of a private physician, and his mother will be instructed to take him for periodic return visits to the outpatient department of the hospital. Not all mothers are sufficiently intelligent and resourceful to undertake the responsibility of such care, but if his mother can be taught to care for him, he is better off at home than in the hospital after he has learned to live with the tube in place and to cooperate in the care it necessitates. The mother is taught not only the procedures she must carry out, but also what observations she should make of his condition, and what she should report to the physician. She can also be told where she can obtain the required equipment such as an aspirator, humidifier, mist tent, and oxygen for emergency use.

The mother must take great care when bathing the child or when he is near a wading pool with other children that he is not momentarily submerged in the water, for liquid will be drawn through the tracheostomy tube directly into his lungs, and he will drown. Caution must also be used in permitting the child to participate in sandbox play because of the danger of aspiration.

Some physicians or nurses introduce mothers of children having a tracheotomy to each other so that they can develop a mutually helpful relationship in solving the daily problems of home care. In addition to these problems, others which may be discussed include how to interpret their child's illness to grandparents, siblings, and friends, how to obtain periodic relief from their daily responsibilities, and how the family budget can be adjusted to meet the additional medical expense.

Prognosis. The prognosis depends upon the age of the child, the severity of the infection, the length of illness before treatment was instituted and the kind of treatment the child receives. Death may occur from the primary infection, from a secondary pneumonia or from respiratory obstruction. Septicemia may cause death, but is an uncommon cause.

Pneumonia

Pneumonias may be classified in several ways on the following bases: anatomic distribution, causative organism, pathologic changes in tissue, and response to antimicrobial therapy. None of these methods of classification is completely satisfactory.

In any type of pneumonia the portions of the lung which are affected are not aerated because the alveoli or air spaces are filled with inflammatory exudate. Because of this fact and also because the child breathes in a shallow manner, often owing to pain on breathing, the oxygen saturation of the blood is invariably reduced.

Since there are many varieties of pneumonia and since some kinds occur principally in one or more age groups, only selected types are discussed in this text. Pneumonia of the newborn and aspiration pneumonia were discussed in Chapter 11, and interstitial pneumonitis or bronchiolitis and lipoid pneumonia in Chapter 14. Pneumonias caused by pneumococci and staphylococci are discussed here, since the nursing care of any other type is essentially the same in the toddler period.

PNEUMOCOCCAL PNEUMONIA

Etiology, Incidence, and Predisposing Factors. Pneumococcal pneumonia is a disease causing more or less consolidation of the affected areas of the lungs. It is caused by the pneumococcus organism, of which there are about 80 types. Certain types are more prevalent among different age groups.

In the past the pneumococcus was the chief cause of pneumonia in infants and young children. Recently the incidence of this type of pneumonia has decreased because of the response of most pneumococcal infections to antibiotic or sulfonamide medications, which are usually given early in the infection. Pneumococcal pneumonia is generally a primary infection. Lobar pneumonia, in which one or more lobes of the lung may be affected, is more common after the period of infancy. The disseminated type, such as bronchiolitis (see p. 401), is seen more often in infancy.

The peak *incidence* is in the late winter and early spring months. In the temperate zone, pneumonia is endemic in the general population. As a result of constant exposure to the infection, most persons have antibodies in their blood against many types of pneumococci.

Predisposing factors are age (the incidence of the disease is highest during the second year of life) and lowered resistance due to malnutrition.

Pathology and Clinical Manifestations. Pneumococci reach the lungs by way of the respiratory passages. The first stage in the attack is termed *engorgement*. During a period of only a few hours the lung becomes dark, bluish-red, and heavy. In the next stage, that of *red hepatization*, the infected lobe becomes solid with red cells and fibrin, and air is displaced. In the third stage, *gray hepatization*, the pleural surface lacks luster and is dull in color. The alveoli are filled with leukocytes and fibrin. In contrast to the two previous stages, the third stage is prolonged. In the final stage, that of *resolution,* a creamy purulent material forms and is evacuated via sputum or resorption.

The typical *clinical manifestations* differ with age and are more variable in children than in adults. The onset is abrupt, although it may be preceded by a mild upper respiratory tract infection. In older children the onset is characteristically preceded by a chill, but in younger children the first symptom may be a convulsion. Symptoms referable to the nervous system are more common in children than in adults.

In the early stages the cough is dry and may cause pain. In the stage of resolution the cough is loose and productive. Fever is a characteristic of the early stage as well as of the course of the disease. The temperature rapidly reaches 103 to 104° F. (39.4 to 40° C.) and may or may not show extreme daily fluctuation. Among untreated older children the temperature drops abruptly, usually on the sixth or seventh day. This marks the crisis of the disease.

The respiratory and pulse rates are characteristic of pneumonia. The rate of respiration may be increased to 40 to 80 per minute in infants and to 30 to 50 per minute in older children. Respirations tend to be increased out of proportion to the increase in the pulse rate. They are shallow in order to reduce the pleural pain. The accessory muscles of respiration may be used, with resulting retractions. In children the alae nasi usually expand and contract with respiration.

The pulse rate is increased. The strength and rate of the pulse beat are indicative of the prognosis of the disease. If the pulse becomes weak and the rate extremely rapid or slow, the prognosis is guarded. Chest pain due to pleural involvement is felt especially on coughing or respiratory movement. The pain may be referred to the abdomen.

Gastrointestinal symptoms are common in the toddler. At the onset of the disease he may vomit or have diarrhea. Anorexia is common during the course of the disease. The older child may complain of a headache. Rigidity of the neck may be present.

Diagnosis, Differential Diagnosis, and Complications. Examination of the chest is paramount in the *diagnosis* of pneumonia. The physician determines the number and extent of the pneumonic areas by the presence of rales, nature of breath sounds and evidence of consolidation. A roentgenogram is taken to corroborate the foci of consolidation found on examination and the presence of any complications such as atelectasis or empyema.

Laboratory tests may show a slight reduction in the red blood cell count and hemoglobin level and an increase in the white blood cell count—commonly from 16,000 to 40,000 per cubic millimeter. The urine has a high specific gravity, is dark amber in color and scanty in amount. There is usually an acetonuria and a mild to moderate albuminuria. The pneumococcus can usually be isolated from the nasopharyngeal and pharyngeal cultures. Bacteria may or may not be seen in the blood cultures.

Lobar pneumonia must be differentiated from atelectasis and pleural effusion and, if there is severe abdominal pain, from gastroenteritis and appendicitis. If nervous symptoms predominate, meningitis may be suspected.

A common *complication* of pneumonia is plastic pleurisy. It exists to some degree in nearly all cases. Abdominal distention or tympanites is a serious complication; if it persists, it may be a reflection of toxic paralytic ileus. Other complications, such as empyema or meningitis, are extremely rare.

Treatment and Responsibilities of the Nurse. The child can be cared for at home if the physical environment is satisfactory and the mother or another adult in the family can nurse him. The physician or nurse has the responsibility of teaching the mother how to nurse the child.

Treatment with sulfonamide or antibiotic therapy, or both, is successful and easily carried out by the mother. When these drugs are given early in the course of the disease, administration of oxygen (difficult and dangerous for the mother to give in the home) is seldom needed. If severe complications arise, the child is hospitalized.

Much of the *nursing care* is symptomatic and geared to the needs of the individual child. He should have adequate rest, both physical and psychological. He should be disturbed as little as possible.

At the first indication of pneumonia the physician orders administration of a sulfonamide or an antibiotic, or both. Penicillin in full dosage seems to be the drug of choice. Drug therapy is important throughout the course of the disease. The antibacterial agent is given for four or five days after the temperature has returned to normal.

An increased fluid intake is necessary to supply the body's increased demand, due to the infection. Fluids are given in sufficient quantities to maintain the normal specific gravity of the urine. This is important for excretion of toxic products and for avoidance of kidney complications when sulfonamides are given. If the child vomits, fluids are administered parenterally (see p. 412). As the child feels better, anorexia becomes less of a nursing problem. He is not encouraged to eat more than he desires, however.

The child tends to lie on the affected side to lessen the pain. His position is changed frequently. Although changing positions causes pain at the time, it ultimately reduces his discomfort and facilitates drainage from the tracheobronchial tree.

For fever, aspirin is given, and cooling sponges (see p. 474) may be ordered. Oxygen is administered for restlessness or severe dyspnea, even though the child is not cyanotic. A Croupette or an oxygen tent may be used. If oxygen is given early, the need for analgesics and sedatives will be reduced. In severe cases aspirin and phenobarbital may be given.

Drug therapy prevents many of the complications which formerly occurred. Abdominal distention is still a serious complication in some affected children. Prophylaxis includes early antibacterial treatment of the infection, oxygen therapy before the appearance of cyanosis, and the avoidance of constipation. If distention occurs, an enema may be given and the rectal tube left in place. Prostigmin is the most effective treatment. It is given for even mild distention and repeated if the distention is not relieved.

An adequate convalescent period is essential even though the child seems well after antibacterial therapy. Before the child is permitted to return to his daily activities he should have gained the weight lost during his illness and not be fatigued by normal exercise. Complete recovery usually takes two weeks.

Prognosis and Prevention. Sulfonamides and antibiotics have dramatically changed the course of pneumococcal pneumonia and reduced the mortality from it. After therapy has begun the temperature usually returns to normal in 24 hours, the child's clinical condition improves, and complications are extremely rare. With early treatment the mortality rate is usually less than 1 per cent in both infants and children.

Prevention consists in isolating the child from contact with patients with pneumonia. This is important in the children's unit of a hospital and in the home if any member of the family has pneumonia.

STAPHYLOCOCCAL PNEUMONIA

Etiology, Incidence, Clinical Manifestations, Pathology, and Diagnosis. The causative organism is *Staphylococcus aureus*. The incidence of this disease has increased in the past ten years, especially in infants and young children.

Staphylococcal infection may be acquired in the newborn nursery (see p. 265), in the hospital unit, in the home, or in the community. It may begin as a skin infection, and the child may then become a carrier of virulent staphylococci in his nasopharynx. Later, either he or another member of his family may suffer from staphylococcal pneumonia.

The onset of the disease is rapid. Multiple lesions occur in the lungs, pulmonary tissue is destroyed, and abscesses are formed. Lesions on the periphery of the lungs may erode into the pleural space and cause tension pneumothorax or empyema. Other *clinical manifestations* are similar to those of pneumococcal pneumonia.

Roentgenograms of the chest often show multiple lesions and confirm the *diagnosis.* Nasopharyngeal and sputum cultures are positive for the organism. Blood cultures are taken and may also prove positive.

Treatment and Responsibilities of the Nurse. Two essential points in the *treatment* of staphylococcal pneumonia are strict isolation and constant nursing care. An antibiotic effective against the strains of staphylococci found in hospitals should be given, such as methicillin or penicillin G among others. The antibiotic patterns of resistance and sensitivity of staphylococci vary in different areas. Sensitivity tests should be done for the particular organism involved, and drugs should be chosen accordingly.

Oxygen therapy and maintenance of the fluid and electrolyte balance are important. The nurse observes the child for any symptom suggesting the development of tension pneumothorax, such as the abrupt onset of pain, dyspnea, or cyanosis.

Prognosis. The prognosis depends on early diagnosis, the use of an appropriate antibiotic, and the lack of complications.

Intestinal Parasites

Children who have intestinal parasites have few if any symptoms. Such symptoms as picking the nose and restlessness in sleep formerly attributed to such infestations are more likely to be due to emotional disturbances.

Several varieties of intestinal parasites infest human beings and frequently infest toddlers. The two most common in the United States are pinworms and roundworms.

ENTEROBIASIS (PINWORM, OR THREADWORM INFECTION)

Etiology. Enterobiasis is a parasitic infection produced by the pinworm, *Enterobius vermicularis,* which invades the cecum and the appendix. The worm is white and threadlike in appearance. The adult male is 2 to 5 mm. in length, the female 8 to 13 mm.

Epidemiology and Pathology.   Enterobiasis is the most common variety of parasitic infestation. It is spread by person-to-person contact. Children are especially susceptible. The condition is frequent where large groups of children are in close contact, as in an institution. The child reinfects himself by contaminating his hands when he scratches the itching skin around the anus where the eggs are lodged, or by handling soiled bedclothes, sleeping garments, or contaminated objects. He then puts his fingers in his mouth, and the eggs repeat the life cycle upon maturing in the intestinal canal. The child may also become infective by breathing airborne ova. Fertile eggs stay infective for about nine days in the average environment.

In short, the route by which reinfestation is accomplished is anus to fingers to mouth or anus to clothing to fingers to mouth.

Pathologically, eggs which are swallowed hatch in the duodenum and migrate directly to the cecum and the appendix. Adult worms develop from eggs in 45 days or less. The worms attach themselves to the mucous membrane of the cecum and the appendix by means of their "lips." Usually at night, gravid worms become detached, migrate down the bowel and crawl out onto the perianal and perineal skin, where they lay thousands of eggs and provoke itching. A few hours after deposition the eggs become infective. Gravid worms entering the vagina may cause vaginitis or a salpingitis and encapsulate in the tubules or migrate to the peritoneal cavity and encapsulate there. The worms cause a severe pruritus, and secondary infection. Scarification may occur from scratching the anal area.

Infestation usually cannot go on without reintroduction of the eggs by mouth.

Clinical Manifestations.   Clinical manifestations are variable. Sometimes there are no symptoms other than itching about the anus at night. There may, however, be symptoms of acute or subacute appendicitis from appendiceal lesions caused by the worms at their sites of attachment. Bacterial infection of the skin may develop from the pruritus ani, which produces weeping, eczematous areas. Vaginitis often occurs, and little girls are frequently irritable, have a poor appetite, lose weight, and suffer insomnia. These difficulties may cause a chronic emotional disturbance. Eosinophilia is present in some affected children.

Diagnosis.   A conclusive diagnosis can be made if, on examination, worms are seen to emerge from the anus. The most practical and effective method of diagnosing the condition is by placing a tongue blade covered with Scotch tape, sticky side out, against the anal or perineal area, where it picks up the eggs. The sticky side of the tape is then placed downward on a slide, which can be microscopically examined at any time by allowing a drop of toluene to filter between the tape and the slide. A tape made especially for this purpose may be used instead of Scotch tape. Anal swabbing is best done in the early morning before arising or just before dressing, bathing or defecation. Eggs are not found readily in the stool.

Treatment.   The aims of treatment are to destroy the ova and worms in the intestine and to prevent reinfection from other persons.

Gentian violet until recently was the drug of choice. This was given for seven to ten days, withdrawn for an equal length of time, and then repeated if necessary. Gentian violet may cause nausea, vomiting (purple), and diarrhea. Two newer medications are now being used more extensively. A harmless and effective drug is piperazine citrate (Antepar), which is available in tablet, wafer, or syrup form. Depending on the child's weight, the dosage is from 250 mg. to 2 gm. once daily before breakfast for seven consecutive days. It produces no side effects when taken as directed. Pyrvinium pamoate (Povan) is an effective single-dose, nontoxic medication. This medication is prepared in tablet or suspension form. The dose is 5 mg. per kilogram of body weight. It will color the stools or vomitus bright red. Since an occasional child may vomit the medication, this possibility should be mentioned to parents. Enemas may also be prescribed.

All infected persons in the household or group must be treated together. After eradication of parasites from the family or group new parasites can be acquired only from outside contacts.

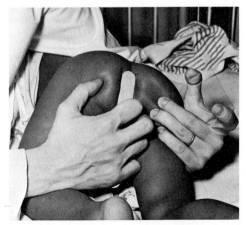

FIGURE 17–9.   Scotch tape test is usually done early in the morning for the purpose of locating the eggs of the pinworm.

Responsibilities of the Nurse. The nurse has an important part in the care of children with enterobiasis. Mothers should be warned of the danger of overdosage of anthelmintic drugs. Some mothers are so anxious to rid the child of parasites that they may give more of the medication than is ordered.

The mother should learn how to give the medication and to carry out any procedures ordered by the physician. If the mother does not know how to give the child an enema, she can be shown the procedure (see p. 457).

The mother needs to know how to prevent reinfestation. The child can wear mitts or socks over his hands so that he cannot pick up the eggs under his fingernails when he scratches about the anus. His nails are cut as short as possible. Hand hygiene should be carried out carefully, especially before meals and in the morning. The child should wear a tight diaper or panties so that he will be unable to reach the infested area. The anus should be cleansed carefully with soap and water after each defecation, and a soothing ointment applied to allay the itching. The toilet seat should be scrubbed daily. Underclothing, bed linen, night clothing, and towels used to dry the child should be boiled to destroy the eggs which are likely to be on the cloth. In the hospital the child should be prevented from contact with others. His bedpan should be cleansed and sterilized after use.

The worms may be removed from the bowel by enema, cathartics, or other drugs prescribed by the physician. This phase of therapy is not often necessary.

The nurse can discuss with the mother the fact that these parasites are not necessarily a sign of uncleanliness so that she need not feel guilty about her child's infection.

Prognosis and Prevention. The *prognosis* is generally good.

Prevention lies in scrupulous personal and group hygiene.

ASCARIASIS (ROUNDWORM INFECTION)

Etiology and Epidemiology. This condition is a parasitic infestation by the giant roundworm, *Ascaris lumbricoides*, found most commonly in the lumen of the small intestine. The mature worm is similar in both shape and size to a white or pink earthworm and is 6 to 15 inches in length. The circumference of the mature female worm is that of a common pencil; it is slightly less in the male.

These parasites are found in warm climates and in the temperate zones up to latitude 40 degrees north or south. The fertile egg is capable of withstanding almost all external conditions except heat. The egg is contained within the feces of an infected person. Where toilets are not used, eggs may be deposited upon the ground, in cracks between stones or on the flooring. The egg embryonates and contains a motile first-stage larva in nine days in a warm environment. A week later the larva moults, and the egg becomes infective, but does not hatch in the soil. It hatches only after having been swallowed by an infected person.

Even if toilet facilities are available, little children may defecate where they are playing rather than take the time to go to the toilet. They spread the eggs where other children are likely to be contaminated. The eggs develop in the top soil, and the children take them into their mouths on toys, contaminated fingers, or food, or by eating dirt. Many children from ages one through ten years have ascariasis where these unsanitary conditions prevail. They are the main source of infestation of older children and adults.

Pathology, Clinical Manifestations, and Diagnosis. In the infective stage the Ascaris is swallowed and enters the duodenum, where it hatches. The larvae penetrate the intestinal wall, mesenteric lymphatics and venules, commonly migrate to the liver and then proceed to the lungs through the right side of the heart.

The larvae invade the air sacs of the lungs by way of the pulmonary capillaries and cause the discharge of minute pools of blood at the sites. This results in an acute cellular infiltration, which blocks passage of the larvae into the respiratory tree. The larvae moult a second time while in the lungs, ascend to the glottis, and are swallowed, becoming established in the small intestine.

The worms may proceed down the intestinal tract and be excreted, or they may migrate into the stomach and be vomited or regurgitated through the nares. Worms may block the appendiceal lumen, perforate the intestinal wall, enter the pleural cavity, block the common bile duct, or migrate to the liver and into its parenchyma.

The *clinical manifestations* are those which would be assumed from the pathology. An atypical pneumonia may occur when many larvae are in the lungs. Migrating larvae may cause an allergy; manifestations include asthma, urticaria, and eosinophilia. Intestinal symptoms may not be present or may include nausea and vomiting, anorexia, and loss of weight. Other symptoms are insomnia, mild fever, nervousness, irritability, and physical and mental lethargy. The most frequent symptom in small children is intestinal colic. Large masses of clumped worms may cause intestinal obstruction, perforation of the intestinal wall, intussusception, or paralytic ileus.

The *diagnosis* is usually made by recovery of eggs in microscopic fecal films. Occasionally the diagnosis is made by examination of the worms which have been passed in the stools, or have been vomited or have emerged from the nares.

Treatment, Prognosis and Prevention. The drug of choice is piperazine citrate (Antepar) (see p. 549), given orally in a dose of 1.0 to 3.5 gm., depending on the size of the child. This dose is given once daily for two consecutive days. It requires none of the auxiliary preparations which other anthelmintics require and has no side effects when given in the recommended dosages.

The *prognosis* is excellent when an appropriate anthelmintic is administered. It is good to fair when secondary complications arise, such as lobar pneumonia or intestinal obstruction or perforation.

Preventive measures are essential where the condition is common. Children and adults must be provided with comfortable, clean toilets and must be taught to use them for every defecation. The infested top soil should be turned under. All infected persons must receive treatment; otherwise preventive measures are not likely to be successful.

Accidents

Although not all varieties of accidents can be discussed here, the care of children who have suffered some of the more common ones can be considered. These include the insertion of foreign objects into the nose or ears, wringer injury, poisoning, burns, and fracture of the femur.

FOREIGN BODIES IN THE NOSE

Incidence and Types. This kind of accident usually occurs in early childhood. The infant does not appear interested in so small an orifice as his nostril, and the older child knows that he should not put anything in it. A toddler puts small objects in his nose, such as beads, pebbles, cherry stones, peas, and watermelon seeds. He is likely to insert any small object if he happens to get hold of it.

Clinical Manifestations and Diagnosis. The child rarely pushes the object far into the nostril because it hurts him to do so. Inexpert attempts to remove it may push it farther in, however. If the mother does not know that the child has put something up his nose, the first symptom which calls her attention to the accident is his complaint of pain when his nose is touched, obvious

obstruction to respiration, and possibly wheezing. If the object is capable of absorbing fluid, it will swell and cause discomfort soon after insertion. If the object is hard and smooth and is not capable of absorbing fluid, it may not produce symptoms for weeks or months. On the other hand, it may irritate the mucous membrane and cause swelling and obstruction. If the object has been lodged in the nostril for some time, a unilateral bloody, purulent discharge may result.

The *diagnosis* is made by examination with a speculum or nasoscope.

Treatment. Sometimes forcible blowing of the nose with the other nostril compressed may dislodge the object. If the foreign body is not easily removed, the physician should spray the nasal cavity with a local anesthetic and attempt removal under direct vision.

FOREIGN BODIES IN THE EAR

Incidence, Types, and Treatment. This kind of accident usually occurs only in early childhood. The child may put any small object, hard or soft, into his ear.

If the object is visible and within easy reach and the child cooperates, it can be gently removed; otherwise it should be removed under general anesthesia.

Ear irrigation should not be done if the foreign material is organic, such as a bean or pea, since it will swell from absorption of water. A postauricular incision may have to be made in some rare cases.

A small mass of tightly packed cerumen, which is technically not a foreign body, may be removed by careful extraction with a curet or hook. If the mass is large, it should be softened with oil or detergent soap solution and removed by irrigation with warm water.

WRINGER INJURY

Incidence, Etiology, and Clinical Manifestations. With the increased popularity of automatic washing machines and the decreased production of the wringer type machine, one would expect a decline in the incidence of household wringer injuries; however, thousands of children sustain injuries of this type each year.

The injury is a result of the child's arm being drawn and crushed between the rollers of wringer type clothes washers. The injury is the result of compression, contusion, heat from the friction of the rollers, and avulsion. The amount of damage is related to the force of the rollers, the amount of the arm that entered the wringer, the length of exposure to pressure, and the forces necessary to remove the arm.

The site of damage to tissues occurs especially

where the rollers stop on the arm: the wrist or the back of the hand, the inside of the elbow, and the axilla. Burning of the skin and subcutaneous tissues and severe bruising of the underlying muscles occur. When a parent or someone else applies traction in an attempt to extricate the extremity, avulsion of the skin and peripheral nerve damage may result. Later, edema and hemorrhage occur in the injured tissues. Fractures are not commonly seen in this type of injury.

Treatment and Responsibilities of the Nurse. When parents bring the child to the hospital, information is collected about the injury. Using aseptic technique, emergency treatment consists of cleansing the injured area with a mild detergent, draining any hematomas that are present, and applying a bulky pressure dressing to the wounds. The extremity must be elevated. Tetanus antitoxin and antibiotics are given. Most of these children are hospitalized for observation for increasing edema or size of the hematomas of the injured part. Circulation in the finger tips is assessed hourly or less frequently, depending on the physician's recommendation.

Dressings are usually changed the day following the injury, after the child has received an analgesic for pain. Areas that have lost full thickness of skin are prepared for grafting; hematomas are drained. If there is increased swelling or paralysis of the injured part, the child remains in the hospital for further observation and treatment.

When the child is discharged, the parents are informed that the extremity must be elevated for two days and that pressured dressings are to remain in place. The nurse can show parents how to elevate the extremity, apply a triangular splint bandage, and rewrap dressings if they become loose at home. If the physician orders medications, the nurse can explain the dosage and the hours they are to be given. The importance of keeping appointments for return visits for changing the dressings is stressed. The extent of activity permitted the child is discussed with the parents at the time of discharge.

POISONING

Poisoning is a morbid condition caused by the ingestion of a toxic substance. A multitude of toxic substances is accessible to the inquisitive or inexperienced child. The immediate treatment of a child who has been poisoned is of the utmost necessity. Although long-term treatment may also be required, poisoning is discussed in this chapter because of the initial emergency nature of the condition.

This discussion is limited to those poisons which children take into their mouths. A child may spit a distasteful poison out, but is also likely to swallow minute particles. He may even swallow repeated mouthfuls. For our purpose we speak of poisons as any substances which, when ingested, even in relatively small amounts, by their chemical action are liable to damage tissues and disturb bodily functions.

Poisons may include (1) those which a child is likely to find in the medicine cabinet, such as aspirin, oral contraceptives, sleeping pills, methadone, or tranquilizers, or in the kitchen cabinet, such as carelessly stored insecticides or potent exterminators for insects, mice and rats; (2) those which have an immediate corrosive effect, such as lye or phenol; and (3) others in which the growth of bacteria produces toxins, as in various foodstuffs.

Food poisoning due to bacterial toxins requires the same kind of nursing care as digestive disturbances (see p. 411) and is spoken of here only in connection with teaching mothers the importance of discarding all spoiled food promptly. Bacterial poisoning from spoiled food is far more common in the low-income groups of large cities than in other social classes or in rural areas because of a lack of adequate refrigeration and a lack of cleanliness in the preparation or storage of food in the home. Custards and salads do not keep well without good refrigeration and are a common source of food poisoning.

For our purpose poisons must also be divided into those which have an effect within a short time, as an overdose of sleeping pills or rat poison, and those which have a slow but cumulative effect, as chronic ingestion of small quantities of paint that contains lead (see p. 576).

The nurse should keep these divisions in mind, since each cannot be discussed separately.

Incidence, Diagnosis, Clinical Manifestations, and Treatment: General Principles. Accidents and poisonings cause the largest number of deaths in the pediatric years in the United States. Children from one to four years are especially prone to ingest a poisonous substance. Poisoning in children is always an accident due to lack of supervision of the child or to carelessness in leaving poisonous substances within his reach. Approximately 800 children under five years of age succumb annually in the United States from the ingestion of poisonous substances commonly found in the medicine chest or kitchen cabinet. Many more have permanent disabilities such as hepatic damage, esophageal stricture or damaged glomeruli. There are a few cases on record of children given poison accidentally by mothers or nurses, but these accidents are so unusual that they need no discussion here.

More than 500 toxic substances are used in the home. These include cleaning agents, detergents, bleaches, insecticides, heavy metals, paint solvents, polishing agents, kerosene, cosmetic preparations, and drugs. The Federal Food and Drug Administration requires that poisonous substances be so labeled. Some commercial preparations have the chemical composition stated on the label, but not always.

Poisoning is more frequent in boys than in girls in the age group under five years, probably because boys are more active and venturesome than girls. The poison which children are likely to take varies with the part of the country and with rural or urban status. There is also a class differential. In tenement areas rat and roach poisons are leading causes of quick poisoning among toddlers. In old sections of many cities poisoning from outmoded lead paint used generations ago on walls and window frames is frequent (see p. 576).

In all cases of ingestion of rapidly acting poisons the *diagnosis* must be made promptly so that the antidote can be administered before the poison is absorbed. For this reason the mother or nurse should endeavor to give the physician a complete history of what has happened. Often, however, she does not know what the child has taken or whether, in fact, he has taken any poison at all. She may think that he has suddenly become sick and take him to the physician for treatment some time after ingestion of the poison. It is essential to know the first indications of poisoning and not make the mistake of believing the child's symptoms to be due to sickness and thereby delay treatment.

Mothers and nurses cannot know the sources, actions and therapy of all known poisons. It is important, however, to know the general principles of management, for in many cases treatment must be instituted before the child can be seen by the physician.

The first step is to identify the poison if this can be done quickly. If it is not known, immediate measures described later should be taken. The mother may see the container from which the child took the poison, or others may give the information. The physician needs this information when he institutes treatment. If the child vomits spontaneously or if the mother has made him vomit by causing him to gag (see below), the vomitus should be saved for the physician's inspection. If the child voids, the urine should also be kept for examination. The physician, nurse, or the mother may be able to identify the poison by its characteristic odor on the child's breath.

If time and facilities are available, laboratory studies should be made. Unfortunately the immediate treatment (induction of emesis or administration of gastric lavage by the physician or nurse) does not always remove all traces of poison from the stomach before a certain amount has been absorbed into the system. It is advisable to give a specific antidote if one is available. Spectroscopic examination of the blood will show the presence or absence of methemoglobin, sulfhemoglobin, and carboxyhemoglobin. The photoelectric colorimeter is used to reveal traces of lead, thymol and many other toxic substances. Later, x-ray studies of the bones can be made to show evidence of lead and bismuth poisoning.

The clinical manifestations and treatment of the different poisons may be found in handbooks on the subject or obtained from the Poison Control Center.

Common clinical *symptoms* of poisoning include (1) gastrointestinal disturbances: (a) abdominal pain, (b) vomiting, (c) anorexia, (d) diarrhea; (2) respiratory and circulatory symptoms: (a) shock, (b) collapse, (c) unexplained cyanosis; (3) central nervous system manifestations: (a) sudden loss of consciousness, (b) convulsions.

These clinical manifestations in a small child are not specific and may indicate acute illness rather than poisoning. The physician must keep in mind the possibility of poisoning; this is essential because he cannot wait for time-consuming laboratory tests to confirm a diagnosis. In most cases of poisoning the effectiveness of the antidote depends upon the time elapsed between ingestion of the poison and administration of the antidote. If the physician does not know the exact nature of the poison or whether the child has actually taken poison, but wishes to rule out that possibility, he may consult the Poison Control Center.

If the poison which the child is believed to have taken is a patent preparation, the ingredients are commonly listed on the container, but if the mother has carelessly put the poison in an old glass jar, its composition may not be known to the mother or physician. The Poison Control Center can usually establish its identity and advise about treatment if there is a clue.

The general principles of *treatment* for ingested poisons may be summed up as follows:

1. Excessive manipulation of the child and overtreatment should be avoided. He should not be treated with large doses of sedatives, stimulants, or antidotes. These may cause more damage than the poison itself.

2. In acute poisoning the mother or nurse should remain calm so that treatment can be instituted and the physician's orders can be carried out.

3. Prompt treatment is necessary, because the amount of poison absorbed depends on the interval between ingestion of the poison and its removal.

At home the immediate procedure is to induce vomiting. If the mother has syrup of ipecac, 15 ml. should be given orally in the home. This may be repeated once within 20 minutes if needed. Vomiting should be induced in all cases except those in which the child is comatose or in which the poison is a petroleum distillate or a corrosive.

After this the child should be taken immediately to a physician in a hospital or clinic. If the mother knows from what container the child got the poison, she should take it with her for the physician's inspection. She should also take any stomach contents which the child has vomited.

If it is not possible to induce vomiting using syrup of ipecac or if there is reason to believe that not all the poison has been vomited, lavage is advisable. Few mothers have the equipment or know how to lavage the child. This is therefore done by the physician or nurse and is often a life-saving measure.

The antidote, if one exists, is then given. The label on the container may state the antidote; if not, the Poison Control Center should be called for information. The antidote is given even if the child's stomach has been emptied by lavage, for some absorption of poison has taken place.

Activated charcoal is an antidote for many poisons. It will absorb large amounts of certain drugs such as morphine and atropine, strychnine, mercuric, and arsenic compounds. It also works on malathion and pentobarbital by mechanical and electrochemical absorption. Tannic acid (strong tea) precipitates alkaloid and metallic poisons. Magnesium oxide suspensions may be used in mineral acid poisoning. Potassium permanganate in a 1:5000 solution oxidizes various organic poisons. After emesis has occurred, the activated charcoal is given in a glass of water, approximately 6 to 8 ounces, using 5 to 10 gm. of charcoal per gram of ingested poison. Burned toast is not an effective substitute for activated charcoal. The use of the so-called universal antidote composed of pulverized charcoal (made from burned toast), magnesium oxide (milk of magnesia), and tannic acid (strong tea) is no longer advised because of its ineffectiveness.

Symptomatic and supportive treatment for shock or metabolic disturbance is given if necessary. The physician may order oxygen therapy and parenteral administration of fluids and electrolytes. Exchange transfusions may be given in certain kinds of poisoning.

SALICYLATE POISONING. Aspirin is used so commonly in homes that parents do not realize its potential danger to children. When aspirin, especially the type prepared in flavored form, is left where children can reach it, excessive ingestion may occur. Several recommendations have been made for the purpose of reducing the number of accidental poisonings involving aspirin: that aspirin tablets be sold commercially in small quantities so that the child can not take a large amount at one time, that they be sold in containers having lids difficult to open, such as those that can be opened only by pushing down and twisting the lid, and that they not be flavored or shaped to look like candy so that they would be less appealing for the young child. Poisoning may also occur from therapeutic overdosage. Aspirin is therefore the most common drug that poisons toddlers. Poisoning may also occur from excessive use of salicylic acid powder or ointment on open, weeping skin lesions.

The clinical manifestations include hyperventilation resulting in respiratory alkalosis which leads to confusion and coma. A metabolic acidosis is also found, due to renal compensation leading to loss of base from the body. Ketosis also follows early symptoms of toxicity. Since salicylates inhibit the formation of prothrombin by the liver, purpuric manifestations may occur. The child may have anorexia, vomiting, sweating, and hyperpyrexia which lead to dehydration.

Immediate treatment includes giving syrup of ipecac and lavage. Fluids containing electrolytes and carbohydrates should be administered intravenously in order to speed excretion of salicylates in the urine. Vitamin K should be given intramuscularly. Peritoneal dialysis, dialysis using an artificial kidney or an exchange transfusion may be used in therapy. It is not possible to discuss these procedures in depth in a textbook of this type. Details may be found in books primarily concerned with emergency or intensive care nursing.

PETROLEUM DISTILLATE (KEROSENE) POISONING. Poisoning from petroleum distillates occurs because toddlers ingest kerosene, benzine, gasoline, naphtha, or some other substance left carelessly around the home. These substances are absorbed quickly from the gastrointestinal tract. Immediate treatment is to have the child swallow quickly 1.5 ml. per kilogram of mineral oil, which reduces absorption, and then begin gastric lavage. Lavage is better than removing gastric contents by an emetic because of the danger of aspiration. The head should be lower than the hips as the gastric contents are removed. Care must be taken that aspiration of the substance does not occur. For this reason some physicians believe that lavage should not be done.

Further treatment consists of stimulants, the use of an antibiotic given prophylactically intramuscularly, oxygen, and transfusion for methemoglobinemia. Pneumonia and kidney complications may occur later.

POISONING FROM CORROSIVE CHEMICALS. A corrosive chemical such as lye destroys the tissues with which the chemical comes in contact. Lye is one of the most common causes of poisoning in children. Sources of lye are washing powders, paint removers, and drainpipe cleaners.

The manifestations of corrosive esophagitis may be seen in the tissue of the alimentary tract from the lips to the stomach. The symptoms are pain, inability to swallow, and prostration. The mucous membranes of the area are white immediately after the accident, but later become brown, ulcerated, and edematous. The edema may be sufficient to obstruct respiration, and tracheotomy may be necessary. The pulse is feeble and rapid, and the child may collapse.

If the child survives, acute symptoms subside, and for a time he may appear well. But esophageal obstruction invariably appears within four to eight weeks as a result of contraction of scar tissue. In severe obstruction the child may be unable to swallow either food or fluids.

The immediate treatment is neutralization of the chemical with dilute vinegar or lemon juice. Pain may be relieved with sedatives. Olive oil or milk taken by mouth may also relieve the pain by its demulcent action. Emetics or lavage should not be utilized for fear of traumatic perforation through the necrotic mucosa. Cortisone may be administered to decrease fibrosis or stricture formation.

If the child cannot swallow, food and fluids must be given parenterally. To prevent stricture of the esophagus, the physician may pass a rubber eyeless catheter of appropriate size and filled with small shot. The first treatment is given about four days after the accident. Dilatation by bougie is continued for at least a year, thus making this a condition requiring long-term care. The size of the catheter is gradually increased. The child may be fed by gastrostomy if obstruction has been complete until the lumen is adequately dilated.

Responsibilities of the Nurse. The nurse should prevent the anxious parents from overstimulating or handling and caressing the child too much.

When the child is brought to the clinic, the nurse will save all vomitus and urine specimens for laboratory examination. The nurse assists the physician with lavage or carries out the order for the procedure (see p. 421).

The child in a mummy restraint is positioned with his face to one side. A well lubricated, large-bore catheter is passed. Size 28 French may be used; the actual size depends upon the child's age and the stomach contents. An Ewald aspirating bulb is attached. A small amount of the lavage solution (150 to 200 ml.) should be injected into the stomach and aspirated as necessary. The procedure is contined until all traces of the poison are removed. In all, 2 to 4 liters of solution should be used.

For immediate emptying of the stomach, water or weak salt and sodium bicarbonate solution may be used until a suitable solution can be obtained. Later, activated charcoal, tannic acid, magnesium oxide or other solution may be used, depending on the poison the child has taken.

Routine lavage is used with the following exceptions: If the child has taken a corrosive poison, there is danger of perforating the esophagus. In strychnine poisoning the stimulation of passing a lavage tube may induce a fatal convulsion.

Good general supportive therapy increases the effectiveness of removing the poison and giving a specific antidote. Supportive therapy will depend, of course, upon the action of the particular poison ingested.

The nurse must watch for evidence of stimulation or depression of the nervous system. Stimulation results in convulsions, restlessness, and delirium. Depression results in stupor and coma.

There may be symptoms of respiratory depression, pulmonary edema or pneumonia. To relieve pulmonary distress, the patient may be given artificial respiration (see p. 202) or oxygen, or establishment of a patent airway may be necessary.

The nurse must watch for peripheral circulatory collapse or cardiac failure. Intravenous administration of fluids or digitalis may be necessary.

Some poisons cause intense vomiting and diarrhea. Water and electrolyte loss must be replaced by parenteral fluids.

The nurse must observe the frequency of voiding and collect samples of urine as ordered by the physician. The extent of renal damage varies. The most important aspect of therapy in relation to the influence of poison on the kidneys is administration of the correct amounts of electrolytes and fluids.

The child's temperature must be taken at frequent intervals, since the physician should be notified if hypothermia or hyperthermia occurs.

The child who is poisoned is prone to infection. He must be isolated from other children, and no nurse who has even a slight infection should care for him. The nurse will give antibiotic therapy as ordered by the physician.

Both the child and his parents are in need of emotional support from the nurse, particularly if the child is in pain. The mother may feel guilty, blaming herself for the accident. Competent, comprehensive nursing care is essential.

Prevention. Most cases of accidental poisoning in young children are due to the carelessness of the adults responsible for their care. The immediate responsibility lies with the child's parents. It is also the responsibility, however, of all members of the health team who teach parents the hygiene and care of children to stress the danger to those active, curious toddlers of leaving poisonous substances in any receptacle within easy reach.

All dangerous substances should be kept out of the toddler's reach, on a high shelf or, better still, in a locked cupboard. All drugs, household chemicals and poisons should be kept in the containers in which they were sold, for these are plainly marked, and no adult is likely to leave them carelessly in easy reach of the child. If poisonous substances are stored in containers used for food, there is danger that someone will leave them where the child can sample the contents.* Children should also be protected from poisoning by spoiled food, thus preventing bacterial poisoning.

BURNS

Immediate care is required by all children who are burned. Although long-term care and rehabilitation are necessary for severely burned children, burns are discussed in this chapter because of the intensive care needed immediately after the injury.

Incidence and Classification. A burn is any destruction of tissue caused by heat primarily. Heat may be either dry as from a hot radiator or stove, from lighted matches, or from the insertion of a live electric wire into the mouth, or wet as from a cup of hot coffee or soup spilled on the child or from the hot tap being turned on while the child is in the bathtub. Other causes of burns are chemical agents, overexposure to ultraviolet or roentgen rays, and radioactive substances. Burns are some of the most frequent accidental injuries of infants and children and are usually preventable. Younger children are apt to be burned at home; older ones may be burned at home or school or during play away from home.

Classification of burns is made according to the degree (depth of tissue destroyed) and percentage of body surface involved. A *first-degree* or *superficial burn* involves only the epidermis. There is redness of the skin, with pain and swelling. Regeneration occurs in superficial burns. A *second-degree* or *partial-thickness* burn destroys superficial skin layers and damages deep tissues. The area is red and blistered and extremely painful. Some scarring may result, but the skin is regenerated from the remaining living epithelial cells. A *third-degree* or *total-thickness* burn produces destruction of the epidermis and some of the dermis. The burned area may appear charred. Nerve endings, sweat glands and hair follicles are destroyed.

Any child having a burn of 5 to 12 per cent or more of his body surface should be admitted to the hospital for treatment. Figure 17–10 shows the rule of nines for the infant and older child or adult.

Problems Associated with Burns; Treatment and Responsibilities of the Nurse. The purposes of treatment of a child having burns are to save his life, to protect him from infection, and to preserve or restore his appearance and functioning as near to normal as possible.

Fluid and electrolyte imbalance presents a serious problem. Shortly after a burn has occurred there is a decrease in the circulatory plasma volume. There is an outpouring of fluid into the burned area during the first 48 hours in addition to a loss of fluid from the surface of the burned and denuded areas. If one fifth to one fourth of the total body skin surface is burned, sufficient fluid may leave the intravascular compartment (see p. 405) so that blood volume is reduced, and the child may have hypovolemic shock. The rest of the body is dehydrated. There is increased concentration of the red blood cells. Erythrocytes are destroyed by hemolysis and bleeding into the burned area. Large amounts of sodium enter the edema fluid of the burned area, where there is consequent replacement of intracellular potassium with sodium. The patient may be in negative sodium balance. At the same time the renal blood flow is lessened just when it is needed to clear potassium and nitrogenous components of the dead cells in the burned area. Acidosis often develops.

---

*This same precaution applies to inflammable materials.

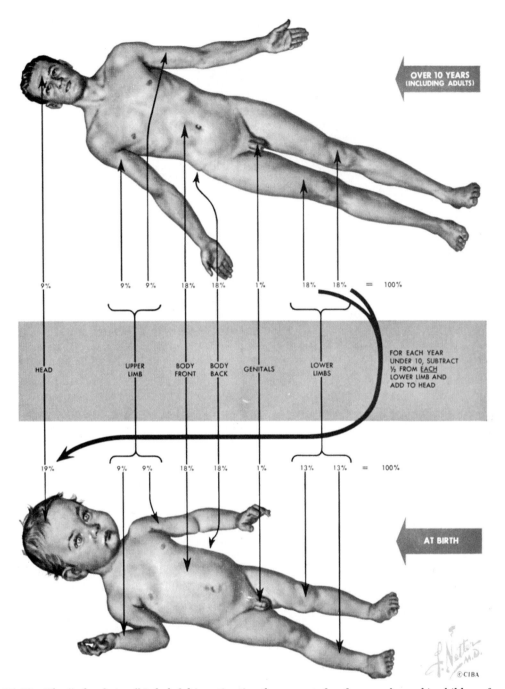

OVER 10 YEARS (INCLUDING ADULTS)

HEAD	UPPER LIMB	BODY FRONT	BODY BACK	GENITALS	LOWER LIMBS	
9%	9% 9%	18%	18%	1%	18% 18%	= 100%

FOR EACH YEAR UNDER 10, SUBTRACT ½ FROM EACH LOWER LIMB AND ADD TO HEAD

HEAD	UPPER LIMB	BODY FRONT	BODY BACK	GENITALS	LOWER LIMBS	
19%	9% 9%	18%	18%	1%	13% 13%	= 100%

AT BIRTH

FIGURE 17–10. The "rule of nines" is helpful in estimating the amount of surface area burned in children of various ages. (Illustrations by Frank H. Netter, M.D., from John W. Chamberlain, M.D., Kenneth Welch, M.D., Thomas S. Morse, M.D. Ciba Clinical Symposia.)

Infection is a problem and may delay reabsorption of edema fluid in the burned area.

Immediate treatment of a first-degree burn consists of cleaning the area and applying a thin layer of an anesthetic ointment and giving analgesics. A bandage may then be applied securely but not too firmly in order to prevent causing pain.

Another method of treatment which can be used immediately after the injury consists in the application of ice water packs or the immersion of the part in ice water. This treatment, which may produce a varying degree of hypothermia, may be used for burns covering an area of up to 20 per cent of body surface. It may be continued until it can be stopped without the return of pain. With the use of this treatment, pain is controlled, and edema, fluid loss, and the rate of infection are decreased.

When a child who has been burned more

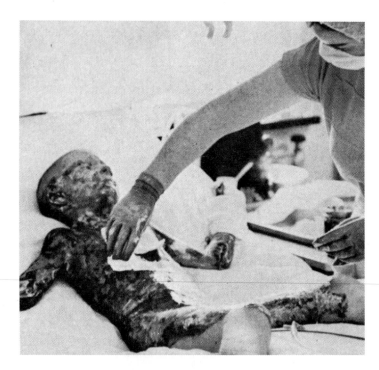

FIGURE 17–11. Sulfamylon acetate is now being used widely in burn treatment. A youngster with burns covering 50 per cent of body surface has the cream applied. (Sister Mary Claudia: *Am. J. Nurs.* 69(4):755–757, April, 1969.)

severely is to be admitted to the hospital, he should be put in a private room which has running water. Sterile technique must be carried out in his care, so that supplies of sterile sheets, towels, cloths, adult isolation gowns, and gloves (sterile disposable gloves may be used) should be obtained. Commercially available disposable burn packs may also be used. Depending on the policy of the hospital, sterile face masks, caps, and shoe covers may be required. Equipment which must be present in the child's room includes an intravenous setup or cutdown tray, intravenous solutions, blood plasma, a catheterization tray with appropriate size Foley catheters, a sterile container to receive the urine, an emergency tracheotomy tray and a tracheostomy tube of appropriate size, a bed cradle if the open technique of therapy is to be used, an aspirating machine with catheters, and a child's size oxygen mask attached to a wall oxygen outlet or tank.

The child may be placed in a laminar-flow, bacteria-controlled unit to help eliminate bacteria from his environment. This is essentially a reverse isolation unit, in which there is a barrier so that the infection-prone child is free from contact with exogenous microorganisms.

In second- and third-degree burns the first problem is to combat shock. The child should be placed on a sterile sheet and the burned area covered with sterile towels. The foot of the bed should be elevated in the case of shock. Morphine, codeine, or another pain-relieving drug is given. Plasma and other fluids are administered intravenously as needed to replace electrolytes

(see p. 406). The child should be kept warm by raising the temperature of the room to 78 to 80° F. (25.5 to 26.6° C.) or by the use of a bed cradle if the open technique or therapy is to be used. Excessive heat, however, may cause dilatation of peripheral blood vessels and aggravate the circulatory disturbance. The hematocrit and hemoglobin levels should be determined as a guide to fluid therapy. Blood chemistry values should be determined frequently.

Typing and crossmatching of blood should be done to prepare for transfusion. A urinalysis is also done. If there is to be débridement, adequate anesthesia is essential. Oxygen should be given to combat anoxia. A tracheotomy (see p. 541) may be done as an emergency procedure if respiratory difficulty occurs. Tetanus antitoxin is given if the patient has not had tetanus toxoid. A booster dose of tetanus toxoid may be given if the child had previous immunization. Gas gangrene antitoxin may also be given. Antibiotics should be given to control infection. A retention catheter is inserted into the bladder so that an accurate output record is possible.

During the first few days after admission to the hospital the child may have increased thirst due to dehydration. Initially, oral administration of fluids will probably be restricted. Although the child will receive fluids intravenously, he may be permitted small sips of water. If fluids are given too rapidly in large amounts, nausea and vomiting will probably result. Ingestion of fluids and nourishment may become a problem later when a bland high protein and high caloric

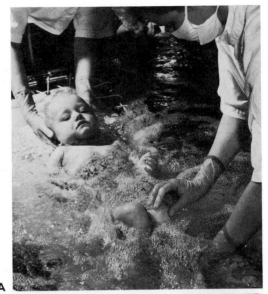

FIGURE 17–12. Treatment of the burn victim. *A*, The whirlpool bath makes the tissues supple, softens the necrotic areas, and allows exercise. *B*, After the bath the nurse (gowned, gloved, and masked) performs superficial debridement of necrotic areas. She then redresses the wounds aseptically. *C*, A cradle prevents the bed clothes from rubbing against the tissues. A plastic tent (or heat cradle) will keep a child at a comfortable temperature. (Courtesy of Saint Justine's Hospital, Montreal.)

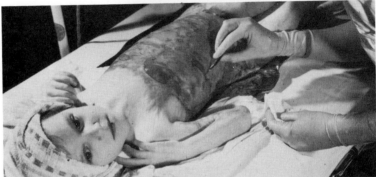

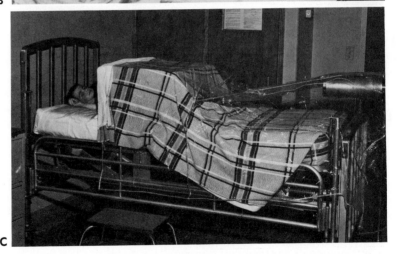

diet with vitamins, especially vitamin C, and iron for tissue repair is necessary. Since many of these children have decreased appetites due to discomfort and inactivity as well as to their general metabolic and physiologic disturbances, gavage may become necessary. Water to which electrolytes have been added may be offered to the child, but this solution may not be well taken because of its unpleasant taste. The services of a nutritionist may be essential in providing an adequate diet for the child with extensive burns.

There is a difference of opinion among physicians about local treatment, and the nurse naturally follows the orders of the individual physician. In the *open technique* of treatment there is no dressing. The burned area is open to the air, so that an eschar forms. The advantages of open

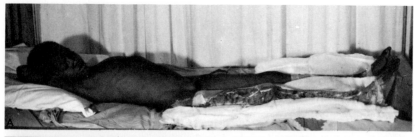

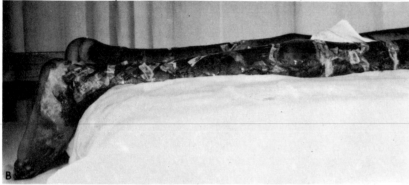

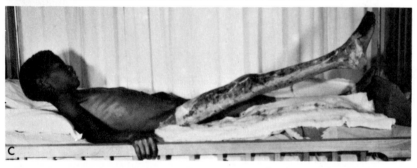

FIGURE 17-13. Third degree burn. *A*, positioning of lower extremities showing symmetric abduction of hips and use of footboard. *B*, When the patient is treated prone, a short mattress placed on top of a regular mattress allows the feet to fall into dorsiflexion. *C*, Active exercise of lower extremity. Hip, knee, and ankle motion were retained throughout the course of treatment. (From Artz, C.P., and Montcrief, J. A.: *The Treatment of Burns.* Philadelphia, W. B. Saunders Co., 1969.)

treatment are that the child has less fever and may be ambulatory if the burned area is not extensive, and there is less odor. The open method of treatment is preferred usually for burns of the hands, face, joints, and genitalia. The danger in using the open technique is that of infection. One method currently used to prevent infection includes reverse isolation of the child in a whole-body isolator bed type of plastic tent with portholes through which care may be given. The real problem in the use of such a device is that of providing emotional support for the child.

Reverse isolation technique can be carried out without using a special isolator through the maintenance of as sterile an environment for the child as possible, including the use of sterile gowns and gloves. All equipment used in patient care should be sterile. Frequent handwashing by personnel and prevention of personnel having infections from caring for the child are essential.

The *closed* or *pressure bandage method* is another method of treatment. In this method the burned area is debrided and gross contami-

nation is removed. A dressing is applied under strict aseptic technique. Pressure is then produced by tightly bandaging the entire dressing. This helps to control plasma loss into the tissues. These bandages should be removed in two or three weeks for grafting , or earlier if the temperature is elevated or there is a foul odor from the dressings indicating infection. Some surgeons apply a light plaster of Paris cast instead of the pressure dressing. The closed bandage method is not used by some physicians because of the danger of infection with Pseudomonas. Research is currently being done on a vaccine to combat Pseudomonas infections in severely burned patients.

Currently various solutions or ointments are used in the treatment of burns, e.g., 0.5 per cent silver nitrate solution, Sulfamylon, silver sulfadiazine, and gentamicin cream. The most frequently used of these is a solution of silver nitrate or Sulfamylon applied locally. Topical creams or burn dressings containing silver sulfadiazine are also being used.

After the burn wound is debrided, a 0.5 per

cent solution of silver nitrate is applied using bulky dressings, which are kept continuously wet with the solution. They are changed one to three times a day, with possible débridement at each dressing change. The advantages of this method are that it decreases bacteria on the burn wound and results in earlier or less necessary skin grafting and a better cosmetic effect. An important disadvantage is that it does not penetrate deeper tissues; the eschar must be removed before the drug can penetrate to the desired level. This method of treatment restricts movement because of the size of the dressing. Another important disadvantage is that the solution dilutes the serum electrolytes with a resultant imbalance. The effects of this dilution can be prevented by providing electrolytes by mouth or vein. There is danger also in the formation of methemoglobin (methemoglobinemia) as a result of a chemical reaction involving silver nitrate and the formation of nitrites.

Having the dressings changed so frequently is emotionally disturbing and painful for the child. It may also be difficult for the nurse to assist with this procedure when the child is so uncomfortable. If the nurse will keep in mind the advantages of this method of therapy, however, optimum support can be given to the child when he is in pain. Because topical silver nitrate stains bedding, clothing and everything else with which it comes in contact, care must be taken in its use.

The advantage of using topical Sulfamylon 10 per cent (mafenide acetate) cream (burn butter) is that it is effective against a wide range of gram-negative and gram-positive organisms. Sulfamylon is applied to the skin approximately twice a day in a layer of cream about one eighth to one quarter of an inch thick. No dressings are needed. Since the open method of treatment is used, there is easy visibility and accessibility to the burn. It penetrates the eschar, so that potent drug levels can be maintained. There may be burning pain in the injured area after application, and skin sensitivity may develop to the drug. The cream is washed off, using sterile technique, once or twice a day. Since this is a painful procedure because of its adherence to the burn wound, the child must be prepared emotionally for it and given supportive care after the treatment is completed. Metabolic acidosis with hyperventilation may occur with the use of this drug. Eschars forming beneath the cream are slow to separate and expose the underlying viable tissue to permit grafting. The survival rate has been improved with this therapy, but because of the problems mentioned above, it is losing favor with some physicians as a form of treatment.

A newer drug, silver sulfadiazine (Silvadene) 1 per cent cream is now being used. This is used to cover the wound in the same manner as Sulfamylon. Either the open or closed methods of treatment may be used. This drug is effective in the control of Pseudomonas aeruginosa infections, as well as infections with other organisms, is painless on application, loosens eschar so débridement is less painful, causes no electrolyte or acid-base disturbances, and does not stain.

Gentamicin cream is used specifically to fight Pseudomonas. This topical agent is easy to apply and has few known side effects. Difficulty has arisen because some strains of Pseudomonas have become resistant to this agent. Still, gentamicin may be used where other topical agents have failed to prevent the growth of strains of this organism.

Subeschar antibiotics are used to control or stop bacterial invasion of healthy tissue adjacent to the burn. Cultures are done on a burn wound biopsy to determine the appropriate antibiotics to use. These are diluted in either isotonic or half-strength saline solution and injected into the area by a needle clysis. This technique controls burn wound sepsis by delivering to the viable-nonviable tissue interface a specific effective antibiotic. This method of treatment is used in addition to topical therapy to treat those infections that escape the control of the topical agents mentioned here.

These very effective chemical agents for topical use have in the recent past been complemented by "biologic" dressings. These include pig skin "xenographs," which can be obtained in lyophilized form; fresh or frozen cadaver skin "allographs"; and fresh amniotic tissue. These all have antibacterial activity superior to the chemical agents when used in appropriate situations. These may be applied to granulating but still infected wounds and to deep second-degree scald burns. They reduce exudative losses and have some beneficial proteolytic action on necrotic detritus. Research is being done on a new skin substitute, a combination of carbohydrates known as mucopolysaccharides and protein collagen, a strong fibrous substance found in skin, bones, and tendons.

In a civilian disaster the best method of treating burns is to expose the area to the air, elevate and immobilize a burned limb, and give the patient prophylactic antibacterial drugs.

With severe burns, anemia may appear by the fifth day or earlier. Transfusions and iron therapy may be given.

The later treatment of burns includes skin grafting and other types of plastic surgery. Skin grafting is successful only if a clean, uninfected, granulating base can be obtained. Eschar formed from open treatment must be softened with sterile wet saline dressings to prepare the wound for a graft. All infection must be cleared before grafting. Necrotic tissue can be soaked off in a tub or by applying wet dressings.

Skin grafts may be of two types: the *homograft*, using skin from another person, and the *autograft*, using skin from the patient. Skin from a donor is used only to cover extensive burns until the patient is in sufficiently good physical condition to have a graft of his own skin.

There are three types of autografts. For a *pedicle graft* a piece of skin is freed from its attachment on three sides, but left in position on one side. The free end is sutured over the burned area. Later, when the sutured portion is attached, the pedicle is freed at its base. *Patch grafts* are small skin grafts. *Split skin grafts* may also be used. Other types of reconstructive plastic surgery may be done after the area has healed and the child's condition has improved.

The plan of *nursing care* depends on the location and extent of the burned area, on the needs of the child and on the kind of treatment ordered. The nurse should observe and record indications of shock (subnormal temperature, low blood pressure, rapid pulse rate, rapid shallow respirations, and extreme pallor) and evidence of toxicity. Toxicity commonly appears in one or two days and is accompanied by high fever, prostration, vomiting, cyanosis, rapid pulse rate, and decreased urinary output with edema. Unless toxicity is combated, coma and death may result. The child should also be observed for abdominal discomfort or bleeding of the gastrointestinal tract indicating a stress or *Curling's ulcer*, which may occur in burned patients.

The child should be protected from infection and injury to delicate epithelium which grows to replace dead tissue. Sterile gown and mask technique should be used. Thorough handwashing is essential, and sterile gloves may be used. All linen used for the child should be sterilized. Pain is relieved by medication ordered by the physician.

If the open technique is used, a cradle covered with a sterile sheet may be placed over the child's body to maintain his body temperature without the need for bed coverings which might stick to the burn sites. If the burned areas on the child's body stick to the sterile cover sheet, spreading the linen with a thin layer of sterile lubricant jelly, with the physician's permission, reduces the sticking and the pain when the child is moved. The room must be kept consist-

ently warm, and the humidity level must be high in the child's room.

A Circ-O-lectric bed or a Stryker or Bradford frame (see p. 298) may be used for children having extensive burns to prevent contamination of the burned areas, to facilitate collection of urine specimens if no catheter has been inserted into the bladder, and to keep the body in good alignment.

A retention catheter may be inserted into the bladder so that an accurate intake and output record can be kept. The urinary output should be 25 to 50 ml. per hour. The nurse should report to the physician if it falls below this minimum, since urinary output is an indication of kidney function as well as a valuable guide to the regulation of parenteral fluid therapy.

Physical therapy should be included in the initial management of the burned child. After the child has stabilized from the initial insult of the burn, the physical therapist can assist with the positioning of the parts of the body. Splints may be used for the extremities, and active and passive exercises may be given.

Body alignment is important to prevent deformity through contractures. If the anterior surface of the neck is burned, a roll placed under the shoulders will prevent contracture. A footboard may be used to prevent foot drop when the child is on his back. When he is on his abdomen, a pillow should be placed beneath each leg to prevent pressure on his toes. The child should be turned every two to four hours, and skin care should be given to prevent pressure areas. The skin around the burned areas should be massaged gently with a soothing lotion approved by the physician. The child should be kept dry to prevent discomfort and contamination of the burned areas. Contracting scars or contractures must not be allowed to form during the healing stage because these are usually the primary reasons for readmission to the hospital for care.

Unless his arms and hands are burned, the child is given toys and equipment for independent play. The nurse can make a sling out of a sheet under the Bradford frame and pin it to the crib sides to support the child's arms and toys.

As a result of fearful and anxious feelings, the child may regress to deal with his stress. The toddler may withdraw, giving up his newly learned autonomy and becoming completely dependent on others. He may also become hostile, uncooperative, and aggressive.

Power struggles over food and eating are common problems among burned children. The child can control whether he will open his mouth or not and whether he will swallow the food or spit it out. Children can also use bowel and bladder control to vent their anger. Thus the child can retaliate against a nurse he perceives to be "against him," even though the nurse is understanding and patient, by urinating or defecating at inappropriate times and places. To be more specific, anger can be shown when the child defecates while the nurse is holding and rocking him. Depending on the extent of immobility, the child can also kick, hit, bite, pick at his wounds or dressings, and scream, thus showing his angry feelings.

If the nurse understands that these types of behavior are due to the child's anger at his situation, responses can be ones of compassion and not guilt. The nurse could consider placing the recovering burn patient nearer to other children so that by watching them, time will pass more quickly for him. Perhaps the parents could visit more frequently to comfort him. An assessment can be made of the things the child can do for himself; thus the nurse can help the child to regain whatever degree of autonomy he had before his injury. Gradually, some of the anger can be vented and dealt with, and new patterns of coping can be developed.

Providing care for a severely burned child may not be easy for his nurses because of his appearance, his possible odor, and his sometimes distressing reaction to care. Nurses must work through their feelings, however, so that they can deal effectively with the child as a person.

Rehabilitation, Response of Parent and Child, Prognosis, and Prevention. The goal of *rehabilitation* in the treatment of a burned child is to help him develop and live to his maximum capacity within the limits of his disabilities. This includes helping the child and his parents to accept disfiguring scars and any handicaps he may have. Loss of function or residual deformities

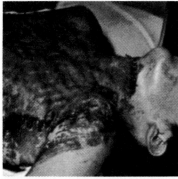

FIGURE 17–14. Hyperextending neck to prevent contracture is accomplished by placing the patient whose neck and chest are burned on a half-mattress. (From Sheehy: *RN*, 37:22, August, 1974.)

may seriously impair the child's self-esteem and body image. Prolonged hospitalization may lead to a dependency reaction that may extend beyond his period of hospitalization. Occupational and physical therapy may be used in the rehabilitation of a child after a burn. He may also be referred to the Social Service Department for an evaluation of his family situation and for aid in providing support to the parents and their child.

The *response of the parent and the child* to his trauma varies. The child may be fearful and anxious because of the fright caused by the accident, his lack of preparation for hospitalization, his extreme pain and his separation from his parents for a long time. The child may also feel guilty if he was hurt while engaged in some activity which was forbidden by his parents or against which they had warned him. This is why a burn may be called the "I told you so" syndrome. Such a child needs much mothering as well as help in becoming involved with his own treatment.

Parents may feel guilty because of lack of supervision of the child—supervision which would have prevented his injury. They may show excessive sympathy for or overprotection of him. These parents should be encouraged to help with the care of the child while he is hospitalized.

The burned child's most difficult and prolonged adjustment is to his scars and possible disfigurement. Young children may believe that when they go home they will look as they did prior to the injury. Parents may believe that plastic surgery will remove all evidences of scars.

Both the child and his parents need reassurance and understanding. The nurse should discover their fears and give them comfort. If the child must return for plastic surgery, he should have encouragement to face another painful period of hospitalization. He should be encouraged to express his aggression in play if he cannot express it verbally. He should be encouraged to cry if he wishes when painful procedures are done to him. If a nurse whom he knows and trusts is with him at such times to support him, he will be better able to withstand the pain. Such expression of his emotions will facilitate his adjustment to his illness and improve his relations with his parents after his recovery.

As the child grows to adolescence, adjustment to his disfigurement becomes most difficult, because children of this age are extremely sensitive about their physical development, attractiveness, and total body image. Parents can provide clothes that cover as much of the scars as possible, such as long-sleeved shirts and blouses to cover the arms and pants outfits to cover scars on the legs. A wig can be provided for the child with scalp involvement and hair loss.

In summary, the rehabilitation of the child involves the cooperative efforts of parents, physician, nurse, physical therapist, mental health professional, and if needed, the reconstructive surgeon. No one can expect treatment and rehabilitation to succeed if the emotional needs of burned children and their families are denied. Knowing the emotional causes of the child's behavior helps in assessing and handling the problems he very naturally exhibits.

In general, the *prognosis* depends on the extent and depth of the burn. Death during the acute phase of the burn results from shock, alterations of blood volume and changes in the electrolyte composition of the blood. Death after the acute phase is the result of toxemia, local or intercurrent infection, or debilitation.

The *prevention* of such painful, often fatal, accidents to children is a broad program of education of adults and children in prevention of fire hazards. Not only should parents be helped to realize the various ways by which children can be burned, but they should also be helped to understand the importance of teaching their children how to put out their burning clothing should they become ignited and how to escape immediately if a fire occurs in their home. The parents and their children should have frequent fire drills so that they become familiar with the various escape routes.

Fractures

The young growing child's bone is resilient; therefore incomplete and *greenstick fractures* are common. A greenstick fracture is one in which one side of the bone is broken, the other side being bent. This type of fracture is common in children because their bones are soft and not fully mineralized. Hence closed (*simple*) fractures of the arms or legs do not always result in pain, obvious deformity, or local swelling. If the child refuses to use a limb after trauma, diagnostic x-ray examination is indicated. Most closed fractures are treated by closed manipulation, traction or casting.

A severe injury, however, will result in a complete break. Open (*compound*) fractures require surgical treatment. These usually heal rapidly, and residual joint disability is rare. Because the child enjoys being active, he usually does not need additional physiotherapy. If de-

formity occurs, this usually disappears during the process of growth.

If the child is immobilized for a long period of time in a body or hip spica, hypercalcemia, a rare complication which may cause renal injury, may occur.

FRACTURE OF THE FEMUR

Incidence, Etiology, Types, and Diagnosis. Many injuries occurring among toddlers are the result of accidental falls. The toddler is learning to climb. He goes up and down stairs and climbs on and off chairs and benches for the sheer joy of it. Although a fracture of the femur is not the only injury he may receive, it is one of the most common serious fractures caused by his many falls. The nurse should stress this danger in her conferences with the mother.

The stairs should have handrails so that the child may hold on to the rail as he goes up or down one step at a time (see Fig. 16–9). Ideally, there should be gates at the top and the bottom of the stairs. Generally there is a door to the basement steps which can be kept shut.

Fracture of the femur, sometimes accompanied by other serious injuries, also results when the child is struck by a passing car as he chases into the street after a ball or by a car being backed out of a driveway or garage. If the driver is the child's parent, that fact adds to the emotional impact of the accident upon the parents. Climbing over the side of the crib or springing on the bed mattress frequently results in severe falls and skeletal injury.

The *diagnosis* is made by his history of inability to bear weight, pain on movement and local tenderness. X-ray examination confirms the findings and the position of the broken fragments.

Treatment and Responsibilities of the Nurse. The child's clothes should be removed gently, first from the uninjured side of the body and then from the injured side. The injured limb should be moved as little as possible. It is sometimes necessary to cut off the clothing.

The physician may order cold applications or ice caps for the first 24 to 36 hours to prevent swelling and edema. Ice caps are placed alongside the leg in the area of the fracture, but not on top of the fracture itself. Aspirin or a salicylate is effective for relief of pain.

The method of fixation of the legs may be by cast if the fracture is undisplaced, but is usually by traction, developed by a system of weights and pulleys and applied to both legs by means of skin traction. Traction is applied to reduce the fracture, to maintain the bones in the corrected position and to immobilize both legs. The traction apparatus commonly used for children up to

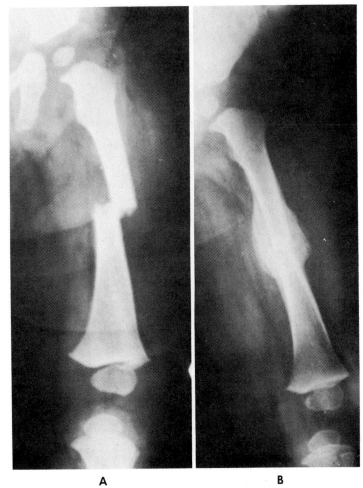

FIGURE 17-15. Fractured femur. Most fractured femurs in childhood are of the spiral type shown. Note comparison of original x-ray films. *A*, Six-month postfracture film. *B*, Callus formation. (From Hilt, N. E., and Schmitt, E. W.: *Pediatric Orthopedic Nursing.* St. Louis, The C. V. Mosby Company, 1975.)

A   B

approximately two years of age having a fractured femur is *Bryant traction,* and the method is by vertical suspension.

The fundamental principle of the Bryant traction system is a bilateral *Buck's extension* applied to the legs. The procedure is as follows:

1. Shave the legs if any hair is present, and paint the skin with tincture of benzoin so that the adhesive will grasp the skin more firmly. Benzoin also serves as a disinfectant for the skin and allays itching and excoriation beneath the tape.

2. A strip of moleskin is cut for each leg, long enough to extend above the knee on each side and under the foot. In the center of each strip, at the level of the sole of the foot, place a thin flat board 3 inches long and an inch broader than the widest distance between the malleoli. There should be a hole in the center of the block through which the traction rope is to be passed. In order to hold the piece of board in place, a second piece of moleskin must be placed on the side facing the child's foot. This piece of moleskin must be as wide as the other and long enough to reach from above the malleoli on one side under the foot to above the malleoli on the other side. This is done to protect the malleoli from pressure from the adhesive. Metal attachments may be used instead of the pieces of wood.

3. Two overhead bars placed longitudinally, or one longitudinal bar with a crossbar, are fastened securely over the crib. One or two pulleys are attached to the bar, in position to apply traction at the desired angle.

4. The moleskin is applied and held in place by gauze, bias-cut stockinet, or Ace bandages. A rope is threaded over the pulleys. Sufficient weights are applied *to elevate the child's hips slightly from the bed.* The legs should be at right angles to the body and the buttocks elevated and clear of the bed. A jacket restraint can be used to keep the child flat in bed and unable to turn from side to side. The child may lie upon the mattress of the bed or be placed upon a Bradford frame within the bed. The nurse should never remove the weights once they have been applied, for the traction should be kept constant. In moving the bed the weights should not be supported, but neither should they be permitted to swing against the bed. After traction has been applied to the child's legs it should be checked carefully in order to prevent constriction of circulation or injury to the feet.

CARE OF THE CHILD IN TRACTION. The nurse should observe the traction ropes to see

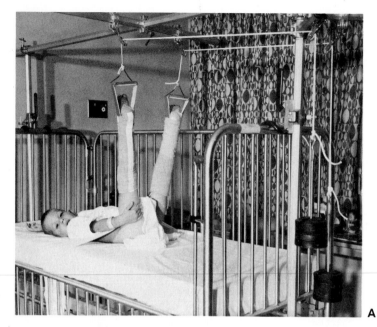

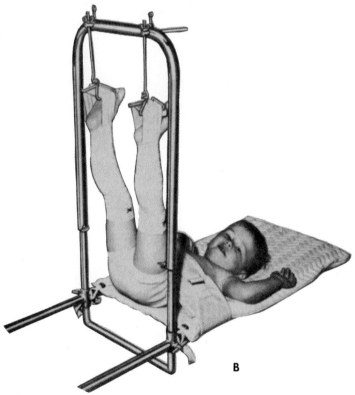

FIGURE 17–16. *A,* Bryant traction is used for the young child who has a fractured femur. Sufficient weights are used to elevate the child's pelvis from the bed. *B,* The Stryker portable Child's Traction Frame is safe for children of all ages. Its portability permits its use in the home. (*A,* H. Armstrong Roberts. *B,* Courtesy of Stryker Corporation, Kalamazoo, Michigan.)

whether the child's body is in correct alignment. The nurse should feel his toes frequently to note any sign of impairment of circulation. The toes should be pink and warm. The nurse can evaluate capillary filling on the toe nails. The nail bed is blanched by exerting pressure on it. When the pressure is released quickly, the nurse observes the period of time it takes for the nail bed to flush to its normal pink color. Usually this occurs immediately. Any cyanosis, tingling, or loss of sensation is an indication that the bandage is too tight, and the physician should be notified to prevent a vascular problem in the extremity. In order to encourage the child to wiggle his toes from time to time to help maintain circulation, foot-fitting puppets may be used. They can be slipped on the feet and the child can make the puppets move by moving his toes. A game can thus be made of this activity. The nurse should be sure that the weights hang free and that the ropes are in the wheel grooves of the pulleys. Little children in Bryant apparatus are tempted to turn from side to side when they are interested in what is going on about them. This interferes with the even traction exerted by the weights. Movement of the body is an indication that the restraining jacket is not fastened correctly.

Lying constantly supine with the friction which the slight movement of the restraining jacket permits is likely to chafe the child's back. Hence he needs good back care. The nurse should reach under his body and rub his back and buttocks. The bed must be kept dry and free from wrinkles and crumbs or other particles of food.

Lack of exercise often results in the child's becoming constipated. His abdomen may become distended. The physician may order a mild cathartic to relieve the distention. Roughage in the diet and the fluid intake should be increased. Enemas may be needed, but continued use of cathartics is to be avoided.

The child in traction may receive overprotection from his nurse, who may believe that he cannot help himself. A child will adapt more easily than an adult to this sort of situation and will learn to feed himself, for instance, with minimal help. The nurse, however, should give him greater attention and approval in order to sustain his ego during his enforced bed rest.

These children need their mothers with them also for ego strength. Application of the Bryant traction is frightening to toddlers, and later, when they are accustomed to it, the restraint makes time pass slowly. Unless amusement is provided for them and their mothers visit them daily, they will find hospitalization a traumatic experience.

Prognosis. Femoral shaft fractures in young children heal quickly. There is usually solid union within three to four weeks after the injury.

TEACHING AIDS AND OTHER INFORMATION*

American Academy of Pediatrics

Accidents in Children.
Care of Children in Hospitals.
New Hazards of Chemicals and Drugs.
Safety Packaging.

American Heart Association

First-Aid in the Home.
The Care and Safety of Children.

The American Journal of Nursing Company

Tracheostomy — Details of Care.

American Lung Association

Your Child's Lungs Are for Life.

American National Red Cross

First-Aid.

The Children's Hospital Medical Center, Boston, Mass.

Rey, M., and Rey, H. A.: Curious George Goes to the Hospital.

Department of National Health and Welfare: Ottawa, Canada

Poisons — Emergency Treatment.

The National Easter Seal Society

Wolinsky, G. F., and Koehler, N.: A Cooperative Program in Materials Development for Very Young Hospitalized Children, 1973.

ROERIG, A Division of Pfizer Pharmaceuticals

Treating Pinworm Infection.
Treating Roundworm Infection.

United States Government

Altshuler, A.: Books That Help Children with a Hospital Experience, 1974.
Fire Accidents Involving the Ignition of Sleepwear Worn by Children Under the Age of Three, 1974.

---

*Complete addresses are given in the Appendix.

REFERENCES

Books

American Academy of Pediatrics: *Care of Children in Hospitals.* Evanston, Ill., American Academy of Pediatrics, 1971.
Arena, J. M.: *Poisoning: Toxicology-Symptoms-Treatments.* 3rd ed. Springfield, Ill., Charles C Thomas, 1974.
Azarnoff, P., and Flegal, S.: *A Pediatric Play Program: Developing a Therapeutic Play Program for Children in Medical Settings.* Springfield, Ill., Charles C Thomas, 1975.
Barnard, K. E., and Erickson, M. L.: *Teaching Children with Developmental Problems: A Family Care Approach.* St. Louis, The C. V. Mosby Company, 1976.
Dreisbach, R. H.: *Handbook of Poisoning: Diagnosis and Treatment.* 8th ed. Los Altos, California, Lange Medical Publications, 1974.
Flint, T., Jr., and Cain, H. D.: *Emergency Treatment and Management.* 5th ed. Philadelphia, W. B. Saunders Company, 1975.
Gellis, S. S., and Kagan, B. M.: *Current Pediatric Therapy 7.* Philadelphia, W. B. Saunders Company, 1976.

Jacoby, F. G.: *Nursing Care of the Patient With Burns.* 2nd ed. St. Louis, The C. V. Mosby Company, 1976.

Miller, R. H.: *Textbook of Basic Emergency Medicine.* St. Louis, The C. V. Mosby Company, 1975.

Petrillo, M., and Sanger, S.: *Emotional Care of Hospitalized Children: An Environmental Approach.* Philadelphia, J. B. Lippincott Company, 1972.

Plank, E. N.: *Working with Children in Hospitals.* 2nd ed. Chicago, Ill., Year Book Medical Publishers, 1971.

Rang, M.: *Children's Fractures.* Philadelphia, J. B. Lippincott Company, 1974.

Reece, R. M., and Chamberlain, J. W.: *Manual of Emergency Pediatrics.* Philadelphia, W. B. Saunders, 1974.

Sevitt, S.: *Reactions to Injury and Burns and Their Clinical Importance.* Philadelphia, J. B. Lippincott Company, 1974.

Sharrard, W. J. W.: *Paediatric Orthopaedics and Fractures.* Philadelphia, J. B. Lippincott Company, 1971.

Shirkey, H. C. (Ed.): *Pediatric Therapy.* 5th ed. St. Louis, The C. V. Mosby Company, 1975.

Silver, H. K., Kempe, C. H., and Bruyn, H. B.: *Handbook of Pediatrics.* 11th ed. Los Altos, California, Lange Medical Publications, 1975.

Strome, M.: *Differential Diagnosis in Pediatric Otolaryngology.* Boston, Little, Brown & Company, 1975.

Surgical Staff, the Hospital for Sick Children, Toronto, and Salter, R. B. (Ed.): *Care for the Injured Child.* Baltimore, Williams & Wilkins Company, 1975.

Varga, C.: *Handbook of Pediatric Medical Emergencies.* 5th ed. St. Louis, The C. V. Mosby Company, 1972.

Vaughan, V. C., and McKay, R. J. (Eds.): *Nelson Textbook of Pediatrics.* 10th ed. Philadelphia, W. B. Saunders Company, 1975.

Williams, H. E., and Phelan, P. D.: *Respiratory Illness in Children.* Philadelphia, J. B. Lippincott Company, 1975.

Periodicals

Bellack, J. P.: Helping A Child Cope With the Stress of Injury. *Am. J. Nursing,* 74:1491, August 1974.

Bennett, R. M.: Drowning and Near-Drowning: Etiology and Pathophysiology. *Am. J. Nursing,* 76:919, June 1976.

Calleia, P., and Boswick, J. A., Jr.: A Home Care Nursing Program For Patients with Burns. *Am. J. Nursing,* 72:1442, August 1972.

Campbell, L.: Special Behavioral Problems of The Burned Child. *Am. J. Nursing,* 76:220, January 1976.

Caudle, J. T.: Emergency Nursing of Near-Drowning Victims. *Am. J. Nursing,* 76:922, June 1976.

Fagerhaugh, S. Y.: Pain Expression and Control On a Burn Care Unit. *Nursing Outlook,* 22:645, October 1974.

Galligan, A. C.: Books For The Hospitalized Child. *Am. J. Nursing,* 75:2164, December 1975.

Gardner, P.: Antimicrobial Drug Therapy in Pediatric Practice. *Pediatr. Clin. N. Am.,* 21:617, August 1974.

Grant, D.: VIP Treatment Proves This Hospital Really Cares. *The Canadian Nurse,* 72:24, July 1976.

Haggerty, R. J.: Childhood Poisoning: An Overview. *Pediatr. Clin. N. Am.,* 17:473, August 1970.

Kunsman, J.: Nursing the Acutely Burned Child: Nursing Care After Primary Excision. *RN,* 37:25, August 1974.

McCulloch, J. H., et al.: Household Wringer Injuries: A Three-year Review. *J. Trauma,* 13:1, January 1973.

Ninman, C., and Shoemaker, P.: Human Amniotic Membranes for Burns. *Am. J. Nursing,* 75:1468, September 1975.

O'Neill, J. A., Jr.: Continuing Care of the Acutely Burned Child. *RN,* 37:93, September 1974.

Ormond, E. A. R., and Caulfield, C.: A Practical Guide to Giving Oral Medications to Young Children. *The American Journal of Maternal Child Nursing,* 1:320, September-October 1976.

Resnick, R., and Hergenroeder, E.: Children and the Emergency Room. *Nursing Digest,* 4:37, September-October 1976.

Rinear, C. E., and Rinear, E. E.: Emergency! Part 3: On-The-Spot Care For Aspiration, Burns, and Poisoning. *Nursing '75,* 5:40, April 1975.

Rodman, M. J.: Poisonings and Their Treatment. *RN,* 35:57, November 1972.

Roskies, E., et al.: Emergency Hospitalization of Young Children. *Nursing Digest,* 4:32, September-October 1976.

Russell, D., and Nevard, D.: Sounding The Alarm For Better Burns Treatment. *Today's Health,* 54:40, March 1976.

Sheehy, E.: Primary Excision: Innovation in Pediatric Burn Care. *RN,* 37:21, August 1974.

Snell, B., and McLellan, C.: Whetting Hospitalized Preschoolers' Appetites. *Am. J. Nursing,* 76:413, March 1976.

Stephens, K. S.: A Toddler's Separation Anxiety. *Am. J. Nursing,* 73:1553, September 1973.

Stinson, V.: Porcine Skin Dressings For Burns. *Am. J. Nursing,* 74:111, January 1974.

Strauss, A., Fagerhaugh, S. Y., and Glaser, B.: Pain: An Organizational–Work–Interactional Perspective. *Nursing Outlook,* 22:560, September 1974.

Talabere, L., and Graves, P.: A Tool For Assessing Families of Burned Children. *Am. J. Nursing,* 76:225, February 1976.

The Do's and Don'ts of Traction Care. *Nursing '74,* 4:35, November 1974.

Wiley, L.: Staying Ahead of Shock. *Nursing '74,* 4:19, April 1974.

Zahourek, R., and Morrison, K.: Help With Problem Patients: Mental Health Nurses as Consultants to Staff Nurses. *Am. J. Nursing,* 74:2034, November 1974.

AUDIOVISUAL MEDIA*

The American Journal of Nursing Company

Play Therapy and the Hospitalized Child
26 minutes, black and white.
Film describes how to aid children in coping with their hospital experience through play therapy.

Bandera Productions

To Breathe, To Breathe, To Live
24 minutes, 16mm, sound, color.
Dramatically portrays differences in upper and lower respiratory obstructions – actual scenes of children with epiglottitis, croup, and tracheobronchitis.

Children's Hospital, National Medical Center, Washington, D.C.

To Prepare a Child
32 minutes, 16mm, sound, color, guide.
Studies have shown that the occurrence of psychological upset from hospitalization is greater in the unprepared than in the prepared child. Child care staff demonstrate the quality of care children need to be well-prepared for this experience.

Medical Electronic Educational Services, Inc.

Pediatric Nursing Series

Prevention of Accidents to Children
22 minutes, 35mm filmstrip/tape, sound, color, guide.
Teaches how to provide a safe environment for the pediatric patient, paying particular attention to child's level of development.

National Institute for Burn Medicine

Teaching Basic Burn Care
40 slides, 35mm, color, guide.
An instructional kit of guides, script, slides, and proficiency examinations. Educators can train medical specialists to provide high-quality burn care. Covers pathophysiology, care, complications, grafting and rehabilitation.

W. B. Saunders Company

Pediatric Conferences with Sydney Gellis
Croup, Gellis, S.
Epiglottitis in Infants and Children, Chasin, W. D.
Staphylococcal Infections, Melish, M. E.

Trainex Corporation

Accidents and Poisoning
35mm filmstrip, audio-tape cassettes, 33 1/3 LP, color.
Defines the most common injury-causing home accidents, and how rooms can be made safer for children.

Introduction to Tracheostomy Care
35mm filmstrip, audio-tape cassettes, 33 1/3 LP, color.
Reviews the anatomy and physiology of the respiratory tract, then shows the changes that take place in the air passages when a tracheostomy is performed. Methods of administering warmth and humidification are demonstrated. Suctioning a patient through an uncuffed tracheostomy tube is shown using the gloved, sterile technique. Care and cleaning of a tracheostomy tube with an inner cannula are included, and dressing changes are discussed.

Management of the Burned Patient
Filmstrip.

Parents and Their Ill Child
35mm filmstrip, audio-tape cassette, 33 1/3 LP, color.
Parents of children who may require diagnostic or surgical procedures in the hospital are given suggestions which will help prepare their child and themselves for the hospital experience.

Preparing the Child for Procedures
35mm filmstrip, audio-tape cassettes, 33 1/3 LP, color.
This program is designed to help health care personnel minimize emotional trauma that a child could experience as a result of hospitalization. It shows ways in which the child might interpret hospital surroundings, procedures, and techniques employed in helping him to make correct interpretations. Included is a discussion of the value of structured play activities.

Tracheobronchial Suctioning
Filmstrip.

Tracheostomy Care — The Cuffed Tube
35mm filmstrip, audio-tape cassettes, 33 1/3 LP, color.
Outlines the care of the tracheostomy patient on controlled ventilation. Step-by-step instruction on cuff deflation, suctioning, and cuff inflation. Minimal-leak inflation and no-leak inflation are shown. Methods to reduce tracheal irritation are demonstrated.

United States Government

Technical Procedures for Diagnosis and Therapy in Children
Producer: USN
27 minutes, 16mm film, optical sound, color.
Gives step-by-step procedures for femoral venipuncture, internal jugular puncture, lumbar puncture, subdural tap, gastric lavage, scalp venipuncture, and cutdown.

°Complete addresses are given in the Appendix.

Chapter Eighteen

LONG-TERM HOSPITALIZATION

Long-term hospitalization of the toddler presents a more serious problem of maternal deprivation than it does in any other age group.

Prevention of Maternal Deprivation. The personnel of the children's hospital or pediatric unit in a general hospital should be educated to understand the toddler's emotional need for his parents so that they appreciate the importance of frequent visiting. If the expense of transportation or loss of time from work is the reason given by parents for not visiting the child, the social service worker may find ways of assisting them. Every effort should be made to keep young children at home, with care given on an outpatient basis. If this is not possible, children should be hospitalized near their homes and, if possible, sent home on weekends and holidays. Arrangements might be made for other young children in the family to go to nursery school so that the mother may be free to visit the sick child. The child's older siblings should be permitted to visit him.

If the mother is unable or unwilling to visit the sick child frequently, the hospital should compensate for his loss of maternal love by supplementing her visits with the long-term care of one of the hospital personnel.

Those caring for toddlers who must stay in the hospital a long time should be permanent members of the staff—graduate nurses, practical nurses, aides or volunteers, foster mothers, or grandmothers, since *it is the separation from a mothering figure that is most detrimental to the child*. Such nursing care helps a toddler to develop autonomy, to establish a relationship that helps him to continue to hope, to retain trust in himself and others, and to learn to handle anger and frustration. Individual care of toddlers prevents much of the emotional trauma seen in hospitalized children who are cared for by a constantly changing series of attendants.

CONDITIONS OF TODDLERS REQUIRING LONG-TERM CARE

1. The case-assignment system should be used exclusively in long-term care of little children.

2. The same personnel should be assigned to a small group of children throughout their period of hospitalization.

3. Children needing long-term hospitalization may be placed in hospital units resembling a children's home where medical attention is provided. The main part of the care should be given by women skilled in meeting the needs of young children; they should be nonprofessional foster-mothers. Each could act as "Mother" to a small group of children. Physicians and nurses would come in only when necessary. In such small family groups a child could form stable relations and lead an emotionally satisfying life.

4. Children confined to the hospital should have as many of the pleasurable activities and as much mobility available to normal children as possible. For instance, they could play with sand and water and do finger painting. In the typical children's hospital unit such play is dif-

ficult to provide. In the model hospitals planned solely for the care of children having chronic and orthopedic conditions and in convalescent hospitals a variety of play materials is provided for the children. A major task for nurses and parents of toddlers having long-term chronic illness is to promote autonomy and independence by teaching self-help skills when they are able to learn them.

LONG-TERM CONDITIONS

"NURSING-BOTTLE MOUTH" SYNDROME

Incidence, Etiology, Clinical Manifestations, Treatment, Prognosis, and Prevention. "Nursing-bottle mouth" syndrome is a phenomenon of extensive caries and discoloration of the teeth that can be observed in young children from 18 months to 4 years old who have had prolonged bottle feedings. These children usually have a history of taking a bottle of milk or juice or a pacifier coated with a sugar substance to bed at night and often at daily nap time, after the earliest tooth had erupted. Since the child does not swallow often during sleep, bacteria and carbohydrate that produce decay remain in the mouth.

Enzymes that are liberated by bacterial flora in the mouth break down carbohydrates to lactic acid and other decay-causing acids that attack the enamel of teeth. The length of time these acids are in contact with the teeth is important in enamel destruction. When the enamel has been decalcified, proteolytic enzymes, also released by the bacterial flora, attack the organic substrate and the dentin and pulp.

The *clinical manifestation* of this condition is unusual and extensive caries formation: the four upper front teeth decay on both the labial, or lip, side and on the lingual, or palate, side; the other teeth (upper and lower back teeth) decay on the tops and the tongue and cheek sides. The lower front teeth are usually unaffected, because of the position of the tongue and the presence of saliva while sucking.

This decay in the temporary teeth results in refusal to eat. Some children refuse all food that requires chewing and will drink only lukewarm beverages. The long-term effects of nursing-bottle mouth are important. The teeth in which there were caries remain very susceptible to decay after nursing ceases. Because of dehydrated and inflamed gingiva, the child may develop herpetic stomatitis.

Although the affected teeth are "only baby teeth," the temporary teeth determine where the permanent teeth will come in. The permanent teeth may erupt in the wrong position

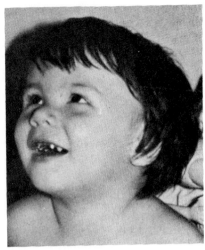

FIGURE 18–1. Bottle-mouth caries. At the age of 2½ years, this child has two teeth missing, four capped, and four filled. (From Rabinowitz, M.: *Children Today*, 3:18, March–April 1974.)

when the roots of the temporary teeth are destroyed. Also, if the temporary teeth must be removed, the child might be completely toothless for the next four or five years. The jaw may become deformed and the permanent teeth may come in crooked, which might result in the need for bracing later.

Without teeth, the young child cannot eat properly. He may develop emotional problems because of the teasing and lack of acceptance by his playmates and later schoolmates. Such children may develop a fear of the dentist that may result in a life-long problem.

Treatment for this condition consists of filling the decayed teeth as early as possible, capping those which can be saved, and removing those which cannot be salvaged. A removable denture may be required to permit the child to masticate and to speak properly. The cost of treatment is great in terms of trauma to the child. The financial cost of treatment may present a tremendous burden for young parents.

Prevention consists in not giving an infant or young child a bottle at night or at naptime. If giving a bottle is absolutely necessary, it should be filled with water.

Responsibilities of the Nurse. Nurses are in a position to teach expectant parents and parents of young children the perils of nursing-bottle mouth syndrome. They can stress that the child's appetite will probably improve if bedtime feedings of carbohydrate substances are eliminated.

Nurses can also teach parents that dental hygiene should be started when the first teeth erupt. The gingival tissue is too tender for brushing before 18 months of age, but the teeth can be cleaned with cotton or gauze moistened with hydrogen peroxide and flavored with a few drops of mouth wash. After 18 months, the child's teeth may be brushed with a small soft or medium toothbrush. The parents should make this an enjoyable experience for the child so that oral hygiene can be viewed positively.

NEPHROTIC SYNDROME (NEPHROSIS)

Types, Etiology, and Incidence. "Nephrotic syndrome" is a term used for a symptom complex having various pathologic findings, clinical manifestations, therapy, and prognosis. All types of nephrosis have in common, however, the clinical manifestations of edema, low blood albumin and high blood cholesterol levels, and severe proteinuria. Although types of nephrosis occur in the neonatal period and in adult life, in this discussion *idiopathic, lipoid, or minimal-lesion* type disease is explored. An example of nephrosis in the toddler and the nursing process can be found in the Appendix.

The *cause* is unknown. It is seldom possible to relate the onset of nephrosis to another condition. Nephrosis may be associated rarely with diabetes mellitus, chronic glomerulonephritis, and syphilis, among other diseases, with dermatitis caused by poison oak or by a bee sting, or with nephrotoxic agents such as penicillamine or trimethadione.

Lipoid nephrosis has been thought by some to be an autoimmune disease, an abnormal immune response of the body. Antikidney antibodies have been found circulating in some children. This disease does respond to the use of adrenocortical steroids and other immunosuppressive agents. Exacerbations of the condition often follow acute infections.

The incidence of new cases under the age of 16 years is approximately 2 per 100,000 population per year in this country. Nephrosis is a disease of childhood, the average age at its onset being 2½ years. It is seldom seen in children under one year of age and for an unknown reason is more common in boys than in girls.

Pathology, Clinical Manifestations, and Laboratory Findings. Pathologically, the kidneys are yellowish and enlarged. The cortices are thickened and the tubules dilated. When a kidney biopsy is done early in the disease, minimal changes are seen in the glomeruli and tubules when an ordinary light microscope is used. When an electron microscope is used, however, a lesion, fusion and swelling of the foot processes of the glomerular epithelium can be seen. These changes are reversible when the proteinuria disappears.

The *clinical manifestations* may be produced by glomerular lesions which permit excessive loss of plasma protein in the urine with resulting reduction in serum albumin. As a result of this reduction in blood proteins, the colloidal osmotic pressure which tends to hold water in the capillaries is reduced. This increases transudation of fluid from the capillaries into the extracellular space, thus producing edema.

At the onset, which is insidious, the child rarely appears ill. Edema is usually the first symptom noted between one and three years of age. The edema, apparent around his eyes and at his ankles, becomes severe and later is generalized. As the fluid accumulates, the child gains weight rapidly. In some cases he may double his normal weight. This state may last from several weeks to months. The common sites of collection of fluid are the peritoneal cavity (*ascites*), the thorax (*hydrothorax*), and the scrotum. In some children the swelling is so great that it seems as if the skin would break. Striae may appear from overstretching of the skin. The edema in the peripheral tissue shifts with postural change. The urinary output varies inversely with the edema.

Pallor may be out of proportion to the degree of anemia.

Anorexia and malnutrition may be severe, but the loss of body tissue is obscured by the edema. Vomiting, diarrhea, and abdominal distention may occur. During periods of edema other clinical manifestations sometimes seen include inguinal and umbilical hernias (see pp. 423 and 425), respiratory distress, rectal prolapse

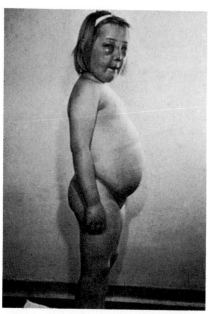

FIGURE 18–2. Ten-year-old girl with lipoid nephrosis. Marked edema, ascites. (From Moll, H.: *Atlas of Pediatric Diseases.* Philadelphia, W. B. Saunders Co., 1976.)

(see p. 454), and decreased motor activity. The blood pressure usually remains normal, but if the child has advanced renal insufficiency, hypertension is seen. The child is generally afebrile. Behavioral concomitants of his condition are irritability and lassitude.

Nephrotic children are susceptible to infection. Interestingly, if the child contracts measles, a remission of the nephrotic condition may result.

A *nephrotic crisis* during the course of the illness may produce such signs and symptoms as fever, abdominal pain, and at times erysipeloid skin eruptions. These subside in a few days, and diuresis may occur.

In the final stage of the disease cardiac failure may occur (see p. 292). The child may have hypertension, azotemia, and hematuria.

The *laboratory findings* on the urine and blood are important in fitting the treatment to the needs of the child. Typical findings include proteinuria (the presence of protein in the urine). There is heavy loss of albumin in the urine, up to 10 gm. or more of protein daily. Diuresis of large amounts of urine results in disappearance of the edema. Persistent hematuria (red blood cells in the urine) may indicate a serious prognosis. Blood changes involve protein and lipids. Sufficient lowering of the serum albumin level takes place to produce a reversal in the normal albumin-globulin ratio. There is an increase in the blood lipids, especially the cholesterol fraction, with levels of 300 to 1800 mg. per 100 ml. A secondary anemia may be present. The erythrocyte sedimentation rate is rapid.

Complications and Treatment. *Complications* are infrequent, since infections are controlled with antibiotics.

The objectives of *treatment* are control of infections, normal adjustment of the disturbed processes, control of edema and promotion of good nutrition and, of equal importance, good mental hygiene.

Control of infection is achieved through prompt antibacterial therapy if an acute infection develops.

The diet should be well balanced, complete, and high in protein to compensate for the constant loss of protein in the urine. It may be advisable to limit salt intake for short periods during the course of the disease. Children do not accept salt-poor diets, however, and their nutrition is likely to suffer if such a diet is all that is given them.

Reduction of the edema is induced through diuresis. Hormonal therapy is widely used in the treatment of nephrosis. Short-term therapy stimulates diuresis, but more prolonged therapy is generally used. Corticotropin is given parenterally, and prednisone is commonly given orally. This therapy is started when the condition is first recognized. Steroid is given daily for about four weeks. Then there is a clinical remission with disappearance of the proteinuria. Diuresis usually occurs in seven to 14 days.

Intermittent hormonal therapy may be given between exacerbations. Smaller doses are ordered than when the child is on intensive therapy during an exacerbation. If the blood pressure is elevated, antihypertensive drugs may be given and hormonal therapy may be withdrawn. Since hormonal therapy masks the signs of infection, the child should be carefully observed for evidence of infection. Antibiotics are not usually given to prevent infection during steroid therapy.

Recently, immunosuppressive agents such as the alkylating agent cyclophosphamide (Cytoxan) and the purine antagonist azathioprine (Immuran) have been used, especially if the child is resistant to or dependent on corticosteroid therapy. These drugs appear to improve the renal lesion and to reduce the frequency of recurrences. When children receive these drugs, they must be observed carefully for the development of leukopenia or bone marrow depression. When Cytoxan is used, alopecia or hemorrhagic cystitis may occur.

Cytoxan and prednisone combined have been used successfully when satisfactory control has not been obtained with corticosteroid therapy alone.

The thiazide diuretics have been used effectively in reducing edema. Chlorothiazide may be given orally. The aldosterone antagonist, spironolactone (Aldactone), may be given with the chlorothiazide to enhance its effectiveness. While these diuretics are being used, the levels of blood electrolytes must be carefully observed. Potassium may be given for potassium depletion if the urinary output is adequate.

Peritoneal drainage may be necessary if a large ascitic collection of fluid is causing respiratory or cardiac distress. If advanced renal failure is evident, fluid intake should vary with the urine volume and the child's capacity to concentrate urine.

Complete bed rest is necessary only during severe edema and when other symptoms are present. The child is allowed out of bed for supervised activity whenever his condition permits, but he must be protected from infectious contacts.

Reduction of anxiety in parents and child is important. The physician gives the parents support and encouragement during the course of the illness. He discusses the nature of the disease with them and the therapy he is using. Whenever possible, children are treated at home and brought to the hospital only for special therapy or expert care.

Responsibilities of the Nurse. Nursing care is the most important element in treatment. The parents are allowed unlimited or frequent visiting and permitted to help in the care of the child. Thereby the harmful effects of maternal deprivation will be avoided, and the parents may express their love for the child in a way which brings relief from their frustrating feeling of helplessness.

The edematous skin must be protected from injury or infection. The child is bathed frequently, with special attention to the moist parts of the body. A boy's genitalia are bathed several times a day and dusted with soothing powder; they may be supported with a soft pad held in place by a T binder. Adhesive should never be used on edematous skin. A pillow can be placed between the knees when the child is lying on his side.

All skin surfaces that are in contact are separated and cotton placed between them, in order to prevent intertrigo (see p. 163).

The child's eyes may be swollen shut. The edematous area about the eyes and lids requires attention. The eyes are irrigated with warm saline solution to prevent a collection of exudate. The child's head is elevated during the day to reduce discomfort from the edema.

In order to prevent respiratory infection the child is kept warm and dry and turned frequently. He should not be exposed to infection through contact with other children in the unit or with personnel who have a cold, sore throat, or other infection.

Nutrition is important, but difficult to maintain, since the child is not hungry during periods of severe edema. The food can be attractively served on colored dishes, with colored straws for the taking of liquids. Small amounts of easily digested foods can be offered, and the child is permitted to help himself to "seconds."

The child is weighed daily and the weight recorded on the child's record. The gain or loss in weight is evidence of the amount of edema present.

An accurate record of intake and output is always valuable. This is difficult, if not impossible, with little children who are only partially toilet-trained and may have regressed during their sickness. If the urine cannot be measured, the amount voided can be estimated by noting the size of the moist area. The color of the urine should also be charted.

If ascites interferes with respiration, the child may be placed in a semi-upright position until paracentesis can be done. Many physicians prefer not to do an abdominal paracentesis on these children because of the danger of infection. When abdominal paracentesis is performed, the nurse explains the procedure to the child in order to gain his cooperation. He should void just before paracentesis so that there will be less danger of puncturing the bladder. The equipment and the exact procedure used vary in different hospitals.

In general, the responsibilities of the nurses are as follows:

Nurse No. 1: Sets up the equipment and prepares the area, collects samples of ascitic fluid for culture, and checks the child's color during the procedure.

Nurse No. 2: Explains the procedure step by step to the child, then places him in a sitting position on the edge of the table and supports his back. The child's hands are clasped in the nurse's. No further restraint is necessary if the child cooperates. The nurse should talk to him, have him close his eyes and turn his head away from the site of the puncture.

Ascitic fluid is not permitted to run too quickly or too copiously from the abdomen, because too rapid reduction of intra-abdominal pressure causes the blood to distend the deep abdominal veins and reduce the normal supply to the heart. This may cause shock.

When the procedure is over, an abdominal binder is applied rather snugly, and the child is put to bed. The nurse must observe and carefully chart the amount of drainage and the child's condition.

During the preschool years the little boy who is prone to fantasy may have real concern about his body image. He may believe that his penis, which is inconspicuous because of the extensive edema, has been cut off. The nurse should remain with the child, help him to verbalize his fears, and reassure him that his body is intact.

When his condition permits, the child is allowed play activities appropriate to his age, interests, and state of health. The Play Lady may visit his bed, or he may be taken to the playroom if there is no danger of contracting an infection from the other children.

Instruction to the Parents on Discharge of the Child. The physician explains the nature of the illness and its therapy to the parents. The nurse may further discuss the child's diet, the administration of medications, prevention of infection, skin care, and the need for continued medical supervision. If the child is to receive corticosteroid therapy at home, the nurse can teach the mother the side effects, such as evidence of masked infection, headache, diplopia, or convulsions, among others, that may occur. The nurse can also teach the mother how to test the urine for protein in order to identify a relapse, so that she can notify the physician.

Discipline is a serious problem in any long-term condition in the toddler. Parents should be consistent in discipline of the child and in setting limits to his freedom. A happy home atmosphere is probably the most important factor in discipline. In a happy situation a child is conditioned to cooperate.

Prognosis. The course is variable and is usually characterized by recurrent edema, which may be of short duration or may last for some time. Since antibacterial therapy has been successfully used to control intercurrent infections, many children survive until nephrosis spontaneously disappears.

If the child does not die from concurrent infection, he has a chance of complete cure, or chronic nephritis or renal failure with a fatal outcome may ensue.

ACRODYNIA (PINK DISEASE, ERYTHREDEMA)

Etiology, Incidence, and Diagnosis. The disease is believed to be caused by poisoning or unusual sensitivity or idiosyncrasy to mercury. The sources of mercury include calomel, mercurial ointment, and diaper rinses. Children must be protected from accidental ingestion of substances containing mercury. Acrodynia is disappearing from most parts of the United States.

The *diagnosis* is based on the distinctive clinical appearance and the course of the disease.

Clinical Manifestations, Laboratory Findings, and Pathology. The *clinical manifestations* form a characteristic pattern. The onset is insidious. The child becomes irritable and at times

apathetic. The palms of the hands and soles of the feet itch and are red and slightly swollen. Later the red skin desquamates. The child experiences perverted sensations, such as burning. The body presents a diffuse erythema and profuse perspiration. The cheeks and nose are pink; the gums are red and swollen. The deciduous teeth, nails, and hair may fall out. The blood pressure is high, the pulse rate elevated. Fever is not usually present unless there is concurrent infection.

The child is hypotonic. He may assume bizarre positions. The knee-chest position is characteristic. Because of photophobia he hides his face.

Anorexia results in malnutrition. Since the child perspires freely, he drinks large quantities of water. He has difficulty sleeping, owing to pain.

The main *laboratory finding* is mercury in the urine.

No characteristic *pathologic changes* have been observed.

Treatment and Responsibilities of the Nurse. Dimercaprol (BAL, British anti-lewisite) is given intramuscularly and is effective against some heavy metal poisons such as mercury. The nurse should watch for undesirable side effects such as lacrimation, nausea and vomiting, salivation, headache, burning sensation, pain in the teeth, sweating, a feeling of tightness in the chest, fever and restlessness. Penicillamine may be given orally for its therapeutic effect in mercury poisoning.

Paraldehyde in olive oil may be given rectally to reduce discomfort. Priscoline may also be given for symptomatic relief. If respiratory infection occurs, it can be treated with antibiotics.

Nursing care must be adapted to the personality changes in the individual toddler. The hyperparesthesia of the skin and muscles results in dislike of and resentment at being handled. The

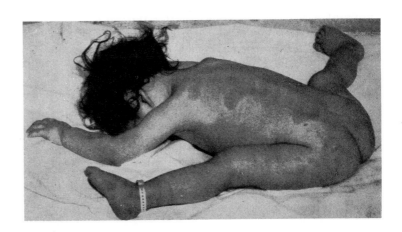

FIGURE 18–3. Extreme hypotonia and photophobia in an infant with acrodynia. This bizarre position may be maintained for hours. (From Vaughan, V. C., III, and McKay, R. J.: *Nelson Textbook of Pediatrics*, 10th ed. Philadelphia, W. B. Saunders Co., 1975.)

nurse attempts to alleviate the child's discomfort and anxiety while he is ill.

To keep the child from injuring himself, the sides of the crib can be covered on the inside with soft padding. The use of a restraining jacket will prevent his falling out of his high chair. Elbow restraints are required to prevent his chewing his fingers or pulling his hair.

Because of his profuse perspiration and to minimize the chances of a secondary pyogenic infection, the child is given frequent tub baths. The clothing is light, preferably of cotton.

Gentle mouth care can be given to prevent infection when the gums are inflamed. Because of photophobia, the child is protected from bright lights.

The diet is high in proteins, minerals, and vitamins. If anorexia is extreme, gavage feedings may be given. He can be offered high vitamin fluids frequently. If the child will not drink fluids in sufficient amounts, parenteral fluid therapy may be necessary.

Every precaution is taken to prevent cross-infection from others who have respiratory infections. The child is weighed routinely to determine weight loss.

Recreation suited to his condition can be provided. During the acute stage these children are seldom eager to play. But the child will enjoy having his nurse read aloud to him or play his favorite pieces on a record player. Recreation helps the child, and also his parents, to adjust to his condition.

Home is the best place for the acrodyniac toddler. The parents can be made familiar with the nature and the course of the disease. They can be taught how to give adequate care.

Complications, Course, Prognosis, and Prevention. *Complications* which may arise are pneumonia, pyuria, diarrhea, and prolapse of the rectum.

The *course* of the disease may extend from several months to a year. Mortality rates are low.

Prevention lies in avoidance of medications containing mercury and in keeping the child safe from the accidental ingestion of mercury preparations.

LEAD POISONING (PLUMBISM)

Etiology, Incidence, and Clinical Manifestations. Lead poisoning is most common between 18 months and three years of age. Lead can enter the body through the gastrointestinal tract, skin, or lungs. The usual route of entrance in children is through the mouth. Little children suck, or chew when teething, painted or lead toys, crib rails, window sills, and furniture. (Paint on repainted wood is apt to come off in

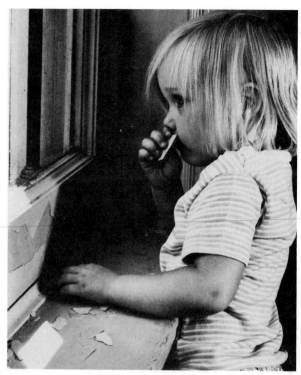

FIGURE 18–4. Prior to 1950, many interior paints contained white lead. In an old building, there may be lead paint on the walls and woodwork. A child can get lead poisoning by eating old paint chips containing lead or by chewing on painted woodwork, railings, windowsills, and similar areas. (Courtesy of National Paint and Coatings Association, Inc.)

flakes.) Toddlers may chew upon painted stair railings, swings, or fences, but are more likely to break off and swallow bits of dried paint from wood surfaces.

Lead may be inhaled with the fumes caused by burning storage batteries, motor fuel (automobile exhaust), or discarded cans containing lead paint, though these are seldom the causes of poisoning in the toddler group.

The *incidence of* lead poisoning appears to be increasing in the tenement areas of large cities, but it is also seen in suburban and rural areas. The walls in old buildings are likely to have layer upon layer of paint. Paints used years ago had a higher percentage of lead than paints used today. Paint for outdoor use today has more lead than that for indoor use, which has less than 1 per cent. In old buildings layers of paint come off in thick flakes which the child may put into his mouth, chew, and swallow. This increase in incidence may be more apparent than real, however, because of federally funded screening programs to locate affected children. Today there are fewer missed cases, because children of the lower-income group receive better health supervision than in the past.

The residual effects of lead toxicity on the nervous system may be permanent and progressive.

The *clinical manifestations* and severity depend upon the degree of cerebral irritation. The onset is insidious except in the rare cases of acute poisoning. Progressive poisoning usually occurs as the result of slow absorption or accumulation of lead in the blood and soft tissues. Lead is transferred slowly from the soft tissues to the bone. Lead is excreted in the urine.

Acute lead poisoning occurs most commonly during the summer and only after accidental ingestion of lead salts or inhalation of lead fumes. The child has nausea, vomiting, abdominal pain, constipation, unusual behavior, convulsions and finally coma. Renal damage is common. Shock may cause death in two or three days. If the child should recover from the acute stage, chronic poisoning may follow.

The clinical manifestations of *chronic lead poisoning* depend on the degree and rate of transport of lead from the intestine or bone (lead is stored in bones) to the blood or soft tissues. In mild cases the child suffers from weakness, loss of weight, irritability, and vomiting. He is pale and suffers from headache, abdominal pain, anorexia, and insomnia.

Encephalitis occurs after a short period of exposure, owing to the extreme vulnerability of the child's central nervous system. Children suffering from lead poisoning are anemic, and have colic, peripheral neuritis, muscular incoordination, joint pains, and a labile pulse rate. Convulsions may occur, followed by stupor and death in coma.

Diagnosis and Treatment. The *diagnosis* is suspected from the history of exposure to lead and the clinical manifestations of poisoning: a lead line at the gums, roentgenographic evidence of increased density at the ends of the long bones, and the presence of radiopaque material in the abdomen indicating the ingestion of foreign substances which may contain lead, basophilic stippling of red blood cells seen on a smear, excessive concentration of lead in the urine, blood or scalp hair, and a mild degree of glycosuria. The metabolism of porphyrin is disturbed in chronic lead poisoning. A laboratory evaluation of free erythrocyte protoporphyrin (FEP) provides an index of the metabolic effect of lead in soft tissues. The normal range for FEP is 20 to 75 μgm/dl. of red cells. Lead causes inhibition of the synthesis of delta-aminolevulinic acid and of the synthesis of protoporphyrin from this acid. The blood and urine contain increased amounts of delta-aminolevulinic acid and porphobilinogen. A proven blood lead concentration of over 50 to 60 μgm/100 ml. is diagnostic of lead

poisoning, requiring further observation and testing of the child and treatment if necessary. Recently, an ultrasensitive portable instrument to detect lead poisoning from a small blood sample has become available. When *lead encephalopathy* is present, the cerebrospinal fluid is under increased pressure and may contain large amounts of protein and a few cells.

The immediate *treatment* of acute lead poisoning is by gastric lavage if poisoning has resulted from the ingestion of lead, followed by catharsis and enemas, and, if necessary, specific measures to counteract shock. The child should be given milk to form insoluble salts in the intestines. To increase the excretion of lead and thereby decrease its concentration in the blood as rapidly as possible, EDTA (ethylenediamine tetra-acetic acid) may be given. This forms a nonionized chelate with lead which is excreted in the urine. EDTA is usually given by intravenous infusion. BAL also causes an increase in the urinary excretion of lead and recently has been used with EDTA in therapy. Penicillamine may be given orally for several days for the purpose of deleading.

Chronic lead poisoning may follow acute poisoning if all traces of lead have not been removed before absorption takes place. For this reason, after emergency care, if there is reason to believe that absorption of lead has taken place, the treatment outlined below is given.

Chronic lead poisoning is commonly the result of taking into the body (with children almost always by ingestion) small amounts of lead over a period of time. A child brought to the hospital for chronic lead poisoning probably has not ingested lead recently. Lead may be in the intestines, but is not likely to be in the stomach. For this reason lavage is not given routinely. The other measures outlined for the treatment of acute lead poisoning may be ordered. One or more courses of drug therapy may be given to increase the excretion of lead from the body. The objective of treatment is to reduce the concentration of lead in the blood and tissues, and to promote its excretion in the urine.

Lead colic is treated with antispasmodics such as atropine, opiates, or calcium salts. Increased intracranial pressure may be treated medically. When *severe encephalopathy* occurs, the child will show rising blood pressure, papilledema, slow pulse, and unconsciousness. Convulsions due to encephalopathy are controlled with phenobarbital given parenterally and paraldehyde administered rectally. Increased intracranial pressure may also be reduced by repeated lumbar punctures, removing a small amount of fluid at a time to prevent brain-stem herniation.

In some children surgical decompression by craniectomy may be necessary. Oxygen may be given for respiratory depression. Parenteral fluids may be administered for fluid and electrolyte imbalance. Urinary retention may be relieved by catheterization.

Treatment to delead the tissues completely takes months, but is essential to prevent recurrence of the symptoms.

Responsibilities of the Nurse. Nursing care is symptomatic. If the child has convulsions, all unnecessary handling should be avoided, since it may stimulate the central nervous system. Nursing care can be planned around periods when medications are to be given. The child who has increased intracranial pressure is observed carefully for respiratory distress. His head is elevated to decrease intracranial pressure.

The child in coma is fed by gavage. He must be turned frequently from side to side, and good skin care is essential. For collection of urine specimens the receptacle must be very clean and free from lead, because the amount of lead found in the urine is exceedingly small.

Prognosis and Prevention. The *prognosis* is generally poor. About half of the affected children have manifestations of encephalitis. The mortality rate is about 25 per cent in these cases. Many of the children who recover have permanent mental or neurologic sequelae, such as mental retardation (see p. 696). Close observation is necessary after treatment for a long time in order to prevent further damage to the central nervous system. The incidence of permanent damage to the central nervous system increases with the duration of exposure to lead.

It is normal for young children of both sexes to mouth and swallow various nonedible substances during the first two years of life, the so-called "teething period."

Children who have *pica* or perverted appetite may continue to ingest lead over long periods. All possible sources of lead should be removed from their environment, and they as well as their siblings should be closely supervised to keep them from obtaining lead from those sources which it is not feasible to remove.

Prevention is doubly important because treatment is not highly successful. Manufacturers in the United States are required to use lead-free paint on all children's toys and furniture. Amateur painters in the home, however, may repaint furniture with paint containing lead. The public is being educated constantly about the danger involved in the ingestion of paint. The community or public health nurse also does this in part while visiting in a home where potential sources of lead poisoning exist.

A simple, inexpensive sodium sulfide spot test has been found to determine the amount of lead in paint. Thus, if areas of paint contain high levels of lead, the paint must be removed or covered in order to prevent children from eating it.

Children living in areas where lead poisoning is prevalent should be screened for lead levels in the blood and urine. If elevated levels are found with or without clinical symptoms, these children should be hospitalized and prophylactically deleaded. A rapid method for screening large numbers of children for lead poisoning requires only a drop of blood obtained from the fingertip.

In many areas the incidence of lead poisoning must be reported to the public health department. The nurse and possibly a sanitarian or housing inspector make a visit to the home to guide the parents and the landlord, if there is one, in removing any source of lead from the environment. In some areas the nurse can teach community residents to do casefinding, education, specimen collection, and follow-up on families in which lead poisoning may be a problem.

The first federal law designed to reduce the lead-poisoning hazard is the Lead-Based Paint Poisoning Prevention Act of 1970. This legislation provides for detection and treatment of lead poisoning, educational programs, and research to find more effective ways to control the lead paint risk.

SYNDROMES OF CEREBRAL DYSFUNCTION

The term "syndrome of cerebral dysfunction" includes the diagnoses of cerebral palsy, mental retardation (see p. 696), epilepsy (see p. 692), autism (see p. 701), hyperkinetic behavior disorders, and visual and auditory perceptual problems (see pp. 589 and 586). The common bond which brings these conditions together is the fact that in all these disorders intellectual impairment is often present as a reflection of poor integration or organization of the neurologic components involved. These neurologic components are neuromotor, state of consciousness, neurosensory, behavioral, and perceptual. Only one of these may be found in a child, or several may be seen in one patient. Usually, since one neurologic component is outstanding for its poor organization, the clinical diagnosis is made on the basis of it.

CEREBRAL PALSY (LITTLE'S DISEASE)

Neuromuscular disability, or cerebral palsy, is the term commonly used for difficulty in controlling the voluntary muscles due to damage to some portion of the brain. There is no common cause, pattern of clinical manifestations, treat-

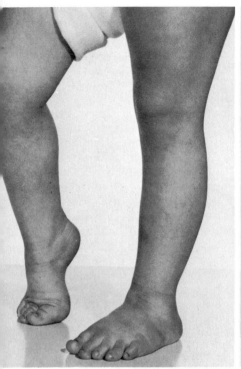
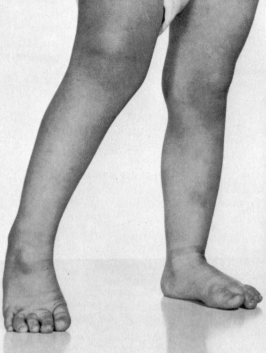
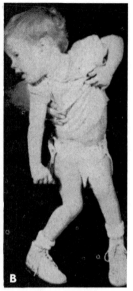

FIGURE 18–5.   Cerebral palsy. A, Spasticity. Right spastic hemiplegia showing equinus deformity. (From Tachdjian, M. O.: *Pediatric Orthopedics.* Philadelphia, W. B. Saunders Co., 1972.) B, Athetosis. (Courtesy of the Association for the Aid of Crippled Children.)

ment, or prognosis for such children. The problem ranges from very mild to severe. The damage is fixed, however, and does not become progressively greater. For this reason it is possible to map out a long-term program of development of those capacities which the child possesses.

Diagnosis and treatment are particularly important during the toddler period if parental attitudes are to be properly formed and the child is to have the foundation of experience necessary for normal emotional development in the years to follow. Although for many years children were treated during infancy for the physical manifestations of the condition, only recently have the intellectual and emotional aspects been studied. Proper handling of the child's intellectual and emotional development is as important as his physical care.

Incidence and Etiology   The *incidence* of the condition is from 100 to 600 cases per 100,000 population. There are almost 300,000 affected children in the United States, making cerebral palsy one of the most common crippling conditions of childhood.

The specific cause is obscure. There are many causes of brain damage which result in this condition; some of these causes are clear, others are not. Damage occurring prenatally, at birth, or during infancy has already been discussed. Ex-

amples of such causes of cerebral palsy are heredity, prenatal infection or anoxia, developmental malformation of the cerebrum, postnatal anoxia (see p. 201), narcosis at birth, erythroblastosis fetalis (see p. 238) with resulting kernicterus, and intracranial hemorrhage (see p. 254). Damage which may occur in infancy or the toddler period includes lead poisoning (see p. 576), head injury with subdural hematoma (see p. 475), brain damage due to febrile illness, encephalitis (see p. 658), meningitis (see p. 660), and hydrocephalus (see p. 301). In many children no single causative factor can be established.

Diagnosis, Types, and Clinical Manifestations.   In some children the *diagnosis* can be made soon after birth. It is based on the following symptoms: asymmetry in motion or contour, difficulty in feeding, i.e., in sucking or swallowing, listlessness or irritability, twitching, stiffening or convulsions, vomiting, excessive or feeble crying, cyanosis or pallor, and failure to follow the normal pattern of motor development (see Chap. 13). In other children the diagnosis is not made until the toddler period, when the question of the child's normal mentality arises.

Two *types* of cerebral palsy account for about 75 per cent of all cases. These types are marked by either spasticity or athetosis. *Spasticity* is characterized by tension in certain muscle groups (Fig. 18–5,A). The stretch reflex is present in the involved muscles. This is the most common type of cerebral palsy. *Athetosis* is characterized by involuntary or excess motion (fine wandering movements) which interferes with normal precision of movement (see Fig. 18–5,B). Various degrees of muscle tension are present.

A third type of cerebral palsy is *ataxia,* characterized by a disturbance of the sense of balance and posture. Children with this condition walk as though they were inebriated. A fourth type, marked by *rigidity,* is characterized by resistance in the extensor and flexor muscles. A fifth type is characterized by *tremor,* in which there are fine muscular movements with a rhythmic pattern. A sixth type is classified as *atonic.*

The *clinical manifestations* vary with the type or types of cerebral palsy present in the individual child. These children as a group are delayed in their developmental milestones such as learning to sit, walk, talk, or feed themselves. During infancy they tend to have high elevations of temperature in response to even mild infections. They tend to be long, thin infants, since their weight gain is usually slow.

Spasticity is the most common evidence of motor disability. The child is unable to control the voluntary muscles, nor can the examiner control them. Certain muscle groups have abnormally strong tonus, which keeps portions of the body, mostly the extremities, in characteristic positions. In severely affected children, deformity of position may occur. The child's voluntary efforts to move such muscles result in jerky motions, making walking, eating and other coordinated movements difficult. The parts of the body commonly affected are the legs, which are in a position of *scissoring* (the child crosses his legs and points his toes), the arms (the fist is clenched, the forearm flexed, the upper arm pressed against the wall of the chest), and the trunk (the head is extended and the back arched).

The spasticity varies from very mild to a severe involvement which produces a helpless child. In very severely affected children, swallowing may be difficult because of involvement of the muscles of the face, jaw, tongue, and pharynx.

In some cases of spasticity, groups of muscles are weakened. Weakness may be present without spasticity, however.

Topographic designations may be identified as follows: *paraplegia,* when only the legs are involved; *hemiplegia,* when half the body is involved; and *quadriplegia,* when all four extremities are involved. Unusual distributions include *monoplegia,* when only one limb is involved, or *triplegia,* when both legs and one arm are involved.

Disturbances other than these physical problems may be due to brain damage, but they may be caused or accentuated by the parents' reaction to the total problem. *Psychologic and emotional problems may be more hampering to the child's development than his motor difficulties.* Speech, sight, and hearing defects or convulsions may complicate the problem and influence the child's interaction with other members of his family and, later, with his social life in the community. There may be varying degrees of mental retardation, but this is not always an accompaniment of cerebral palsy.

The child with cerebral palsy appears to be emotionally unstable, owing primarily to his physical condition, but also to the psychologic treatment he has received. His basic human needs for acceptance, for love from his parents, his peers, and others, for exploration of his environment, for play, for learning as other children do and for the feeling of status which comes through gradually increasing independence are seldom satisfied. He is therefore likely to be chronically emotionally depressed.

If the child has speech problems, he is unable to communicate orally in the normal manner, if at all, with others. If he cannot see well, he is unable to have vicarious experiences through reading or motion pictures—experiences which would enrich the limited use he is able to make of his physical and social environments. If he cannot write, he has further difficulty in establishing satisfactory relations with others. It is in the toddler period that the basis for development of what capacities he has must be laid.

Although the mentality of these children is likely to be affected, many have normal intelligence. With education and special training they may become useful citizens. Even those with intelligence below normal may be trained to earn their living or at least to provide self-care.

Treatment and Responsibilities of the Nurse. The *treatment* of children having cerebral palsy appears to be in a transitional stage. Newer methods of treatment are being proposed. Since there is much discussion and controversy concerning these newer methods of therapy, only the traditional treatment will be explored here.

The aim of *habilitation* is to help the child handicapped since birth to make total use of the abilities he has been able to develop and to help him establish capabilities that the normal child develops automatically. The aim of *rehabilitation* for the child who was once normal, but who because of illness now has a handicap, is to help him relearn or re-establish the abilities he had prior to his illness and to progress in as normal a way as possible. The aim in both habilitation and rehabilitation is to help each person achieve satisfaction in life to the full limit of his capacities.

If children with cerebral palsy are to develop to the fullest extent their capacity to lead normal lives, they should be under the supervision of the cerebral palsy team. This team includes the pediatrician, social worker, surgeon, orthopedist, psychologist or psychiatrist, physiotherapist, speech therapist, teachers, nurses, and the child's parents.

It is difficult to identify all children with cerebral palsy during infancy and the toddler period. Such children may be found at school age, since attendance at school is compulsory. The missed children are usually in the low-income group, particularly in families in isolated rural areas because of their lack of knowledge concerning this condition. Middle-class parents seek help if they see that their child is not normal; also, their children are under the care of a private physician from infancy throughout childhood. Follow-up by community or public health nurses of newborn infants and continued health supervision through clinics and Child Health Conferences have decreased the number of cases in which professional help has been delayed until school age.

Before treatment can be begun, it is necessary to evaluate not only the child's physical condition, but also his intellectual capacity, since treatment will be determined by his needs. It is difficult to evaluate the mental capacity of a child until he is old enough to cooperate on performance tests which use motor abilities. On the best available information realistic short- and long-term programs are planned and re-evaluated as treatment progresses.

No treatment can restore a brain damaged at birth to a normal functioning level. The aim of therapy is *habilitation,* because new habits have to be established rather than lost functions replaced. The goal is to appraise individual assets and potentialities and to capitalize on these in order to create as useful and well adjusted a person as possible. Muscles must be used for new functions, and this training must be made a satisfying, rather than a frustrating, process for the child.

Parents must be helped to accept the child with his assets and liabilities while he is still an infant or as soon as the team is able to evaluate his potentialities. They need help in learning how to care for him and to feel secure in their ability to fulfill the parental role which they have learned to adapt to his needs.

Care includes planning for special problems connected with respiration, feeding, relaxation, play, and education.

Problems of respiration in early life are due to cerebral lesions or to mucus in the infant's throat. Mucus can be removed by aspiration. The infant's position can be changed frequently to reduce his discomfort.

Feeding problems may be caused by difficulty in sucking and swallowing. These are especially hard to manage because these children need more calories than normal children, owing to their increased motion. The child may vomit easily. To help him take his feeding, he can be fed slowly. The nurse must be patient when giving him solid food, since often he cannot control the muscles of the throat. Feeding these children requires skill, acquired only by experience. Helping the child to learn to feed himself is even more difficult. He needs a spoon and a blunt fork (if he is able to control his hand adequately) with special handles so that he can grasp them readily (Fig. 18–6). The plate can be attached to the table so that he does not push it about when he attempts to get food on his spoon or fork.

Problems of relaxation have a special meaning for these children, who are under a constant strain even when attempting to perform the simple acts others carry out unconsciously without giving attention to their movements. Although palsied children tire easily, they find it difficult to relax. They need frequent rest periods in a quiet room with few stimuli of any sort. They should not be excited before rest time

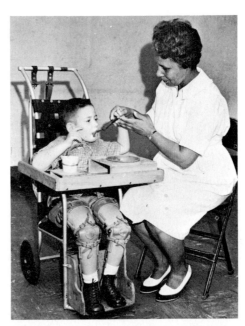

FIGURE 18–6. An ataxic quadriplegic child learns spoon feeding with the help of a recreationist. Adaptations for this child include a bowl holder, a glass holder and straw, and a built-up spoon handle. (United Cerebral Palsy.)

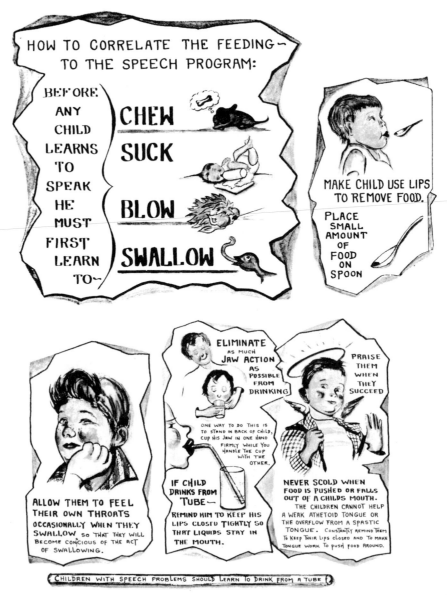

FIGURE 18–7. Feeding the child with cerebral palsy. (Prepared for use at the Walter D. Matheny School for Cerebral Palsied Children, Peapack, N.J.; courtesy of National Society For Crippled Children and Adults.)

or bedtime. The administration of tranquilizers to these children helps to relieve tension and thus promotes relaxation.

These children must be disciplined with understanding. If they feel secure and relaxed, they have far better control over their movements than if they are nervous, angry, or afraid. The adult who can be firm, but not rejecting, in manner and words not only wins their cooperation, but also provides the social environment in which they are physically able to cooperate. The child's success in muscular control reduces his frustration. The palsied child is happier with adults who set limits within which he can function successfully and is thereby less likely to arouse irritation in others. Relaxation is for him a skill which must be learned. After he has learned to relax he can learn purposeful motions which enable him to get the results he desires.

Play problems are many, but can be met successfully. No child leads a normal life if he does not play. But play with these children must be gentle, without excitement, involving only slow changes in stimulation. Mothers and nurses can show creativity and ingenuity in finding toys which will be safe and also have educational value, which foster learning, and encourage self-expression or help in social interaction with other children. When he reaches school age, it is important for him to play in groups so that he

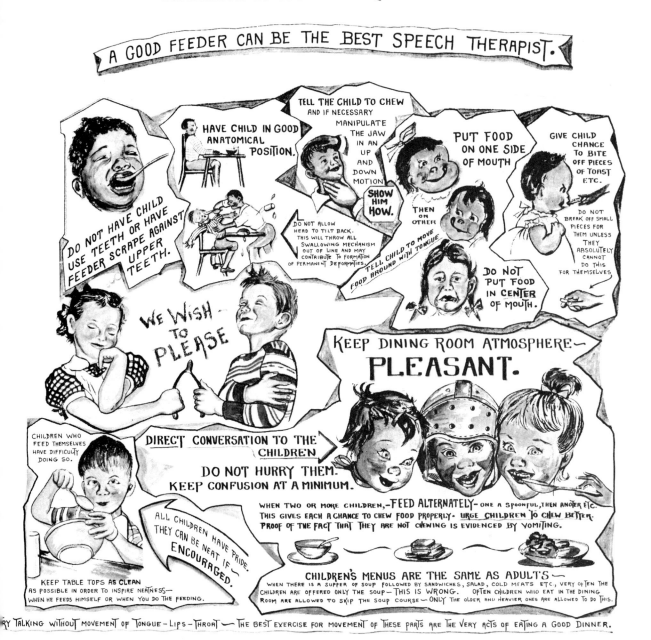

FIGURE 18–7. *Continued.*

will make friends and learn to interact successfully with his peers. He should feel that he is their equal, even if he cannot do all that they do and makes uncouth blunders which interfere with play. Some mothers are afraid to permit their handicapped children to play away from them for fear that they will become lost. Proper identification in the form of a pin, chain, or bracelet locket or a metal "dog tag" is important for any handicapped child away from his parents.

Education includes training in self-care and social relations, as well as formal education. It should begin in nursery school, if not earlier, and can be adjusted to the child's capacity so that he has joy in achieving what is expected of him. When he enters grade school, his work must be adjusted to his mental capacity as well as to his physical limitations. In most cities there are special schools, or special classes in the regular schools, for handicapped children. In these classes or schools, teachers plan the educational programs to meet the needs of small groups of children who have somewhat similar abilities. These schools provide for muscle re-education and physical therapy and often psychologic help for the child who has emotional problems.

The cerebral palsy team may give other forms of therapy either at the school or in conjunction with the school program. Children whose handicap is not too great may attend the regular school classes, or be in special classes for some subjects and in the regular classes for other subjects in which they can be taught with normal children. When education is adapted to individual potential, the child can gain security from being with normal children. Possibly he may excel in some area of study. Working with other children will help to eliminate feelings of inferiority and self-pity. If the child has difficulty in articulation, speech training will be necessary.

One advantage of the special school or classes is that the furniture is designed so that these children can work in comfort.

HOSPITALIZATION. When a child is admitted to the hospital with the diagnosis of cerebral palsy, the nurses who care for him can learn from his mother the methods of care used at home in such areas as feeding techniques, special nutritional needs, relaxation and sleep, and the prevention of constipation and skin breakdown, if pertinent. Such information will not only produce a less traumatic transition from care in the home to care in the hospital for the child, but will also provide the nurse with knowledge that may be utilized in the nursing care of other patients.

Parents may need help in meeting the problems connected with hospitalization of the child. Long-term hospitalization is a financial drain upon the income of the average family. When hospitalization is necessary, the parents, even if they carry hospitalization insurance, may be unable to pay the full hospital and medical bills and still maintain the family level of living which is essential for the other children in the family, as well as for the sick child when he returns home. Such parents are referred to the social worker, who will arrange for financial assistance from a state or community agency.

Parents may not understand why the child must be hospitalized, the treatment he will need or how long he must be away from home. They may be unwilling to leave him in the hospital because they think that he, more than a normal child, will suffer from emotional deprivation. The nurse can do a great deal to help the parents view the child's condition realistically.

Life in the pediatric unit of a general hospital or in a children's hospital should be planned for emotional growth as well as physical improvement of the children. Absence from home may be made a maturing experience, particularly if these children have been overprotected at home.

The physical care of children with cerebral palsy includes the prevention of contractures. This is difficult for the parents to understand. They have tried to make the child as comfortable as possible by allowing him to assume any position and maintain it for as long as he wanted. A qualified physiotherapist can teach parents how to carry out passive stretching exercises depending on the specific needs of the child. Corrective splints may be ordered. Usually these are applied only at night, but leg splints may be used during the day to enable the child to stand.

Appliances can be used in the home and the hospital to help these children lead as normal a life as possible. If the child has difficulty in sitting erect or maintaining his balance, he may need a high-backed chair which has arms and a foot platform. If he still cannot maintain his balance, he may require straps to hold him in the chair securely. Such a chair can be converted to a wheelchair by the addition of wheels and handles on the back. Special equipment is available to enable the child to feed himself. Such equipment includes spoons with large straight or bent handles, plates with rims and suction cups on the bottom to prevent slipping, and covered cups with a hole in the lid through which to insert a drinking tube.

Surgical treatment for orthopedic deformities may be necessary. This may involve the severing of nerves leading to the spastic extremities, lengthening of the tendon of Achilles or other procedures to improve the child's muscular control.

If the child has had a cast applied, the nursing care is that of other patients in casts (see p. 320). If he has not achieved control of bladder and bowel, he may be placed on a Bradford frame (see p. 298). Braces may be used to enable the spastic child to control his motions or to correct his deformity. Medical treatment may include drugs to decrease nervous tension or a tendency to convulsions. Physiotherapy is important to prevent contractures and stimulate control of movement.

Community or public health nurses and hospital nurses are members of the health team caring for children with cerebral palsy. The team serves the children in their homes, in hospitals, schools, and summer camps. Nurses help mothers learn how to give the daily care the child needs and to interpret his needs to other members of the family and to his teachers. As the child grows older, his contacts outside the home increase. Even the toddler is admitted to some nursery schools for handicapped children, and older children go to camp in the sum-

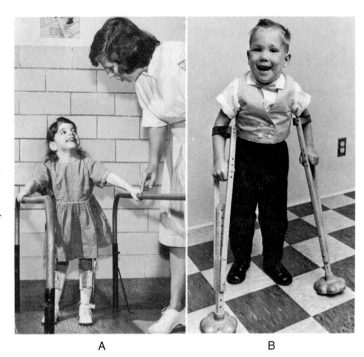

FIGURE 18–8. Learning to walk. *A*, To educate legs to walk properly, parallel bars and perhaps a small flight of steps are brought into play. The physiotherapist helps this child to achieve the goal of the health team. (Courtesy of the National Society for Crippled Children and Adults, Chicago, Illinois.) *B*, "Kenny sticks" with enlarged crutch tips. (Courtesy of Rehabilitation Institute of The Boston Dispensary, and F. H. Krusen: *Handbook of Physical Medicine and Rehabilitation.*)

A

B

mer and join play groups planned particularly for them. Nurses contact professional workers and help them to coordinate these special services with the general plan of treatment made by the cerebral palsy team for the individual child.

In large cities there are organizations which offer guidance to the parents of children with

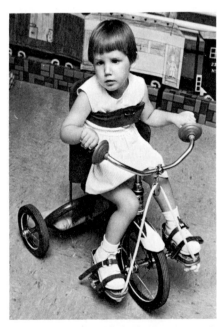

FIGURE 18–9. Tricycle with back, chest strap, foot plates and pulley system to prevent plantar flexion. (Courtesy of the Minneapolis Curative Workshop, and F. H. Krusen: *Handbook of Physical Medicine and Rehabilitation.*)

cerebral palsy. The nurse works closely with the staff of such an organization. Many of these organizations provide group play for children and vocational training for adolescents. Each year more such groups are supporting research on the causes and treatment of cerebral palsy and providing funds for the application of research findings to the habilitation and education of these children.

Prognosis. The prognosis depends upon the severity of the physical condition, the child's mental capacity, and the treatment available. Private, state, and community programs for these children vary in quality and extent of service, and the prognosis in any case must take into consideration the treatment the child will receive. In general, the child with normal intelligence who receives adequate care improves to the extent that he can care for himself and can possibly succeed in a vocation or profession suited to his limitations.

Summary. The role of the nurse includes helping to prevent cerebral palsy, helping to detect it once it has occurred, and helping to provide optimum care for the affected children in cooperation with other members of the cerebral palsy team. The objective in care is that each child develop his potential capacity. In a physically and socially favorable environment many children develop a healthy personality. The foundation is laid during the toddler period. These children must be helped to face reality, to accept themselves objectively, if they are to make a successful adjustment to the problems caused by their handicaps. A child's attitude toward himself and his relations with other people are formed in early childhood, and successful adjustment in adolescence and adulthood is conditioned by his experiences while still a little child. Adults are tempted to make life easy for him rather than helping him face his problems, solve them and go on to the more complex experiences which come with maturation. He needs help with the developmental tasks which come with growing up. Finally he must face the responsibilities of adulthood. If it is possible, he will want to support himself; if he cannot be self-supporting, he must accept support from others. To assume total self-care gives him a feeling of security and of self-respect. He must adjust to his sexual role in life and to the degree of emancipation from his family which is advisable in his condition.

DEAFNESS

Importance of the Problem.   Care of the deaf child is a comprehensive problem which requires teamwork for its solution. There are degress of deafness. Complete bilateral deafness is an extreme handicap. The deaf miss all the pleasure of sound and are without the natural means of communicating with others.

Before the age of one year the nurse may question the infant's ability to hear if he does not awaken from sleep without being touched, if he responds only to comforting when he is held, if he makes few or no babbling sounds or words, or if he does not respond to the sound of speech or to his name when he is spoken to.

A young child who provides irrelevant answers to questions posed to him, who tilts his head or assumes unusual postures when listening, who seems inattentive or has unusual voice mannerisms or speech peculiarities, or who communicates through gestures rather than words may have a hearing loss. Also, the child who is shy and withdrawn with others, who has difficulty in school, or who may have gained the title "problem child" may have some degree of deafness.

Unilateral deafness is different from bilateral deafness and may not be suspected until some accidental occurrence calls the mother's attention to the child's inability to hear in the affected ear. Unilateral deafness, whether partial or complete, is treated with the same care given in bilateral deafness. The child is, of course, not so seriously hampered in his social relations as is the totally deaf child.

Deafness, whether partial or complete, may cause behavior problems and poor adjustment in group relations. Children who are deaf and have no means of communication may become physically aggressive and unmanageable. They may be alert children with normal or above average intelligence and may be remarkably dextrous.

Etiology and Diagnosis.   Deafness may be congenital, owing to anomalies of the ear, or acquired as the result of disease or injury to the auditory nerve or auditory center in the brain. Diseases causing deafness include congenital rubella, congenital syphilis (see p. 262), meningococcal meningitis (see p. 660), encephalitis (see p. 658), and serous chronic otitis media (see p. 401).

Early *diagnosis* is essential. A hearing examination is one of the battery of tests used in institutions participating in the Collaborative Project. With audiologic techniques, the use of the audiometer, it is now possible to diagnose hearing disorders in the newborn; however, these techniques are not used on all children. The new Evoked Response Audiometer can determine a child's ability to perceive and to listen by testing his involuntary reactions to sound and speech at the highest brain level.

Congenital deafness, if complete, is generally recognized in infancy. Unilateral or partial bilateral deafness may not be recognized until the toddler period, when it may be discovered during a routine physical examination (Fig. 18–10). Infants and young children may be tested in a crude manner for their ability to hear. Usually a toy is given to the child. The examiner then stands behind or to the side of the child and produces noise with a buzzer, rattle, or some other noisemaker. A child who hears well will turn toward the sound and forget his play. A deaf child will make no response. In children who are not under health supervision, deafness may not be found until a health examination in nursery or grade school is done. The more refined monaural tests used at this age level include pure tone and speech audiometric tests. These tests are done at all frequencies in a sound-proof room. Detection of impaired hearing by routine audiometric tests should be part of the school health examination and repeated every three years. The school nurse or public health nurse may give these tests. When the child has 70 per cent or less of normal hearing, he cannot hear all that the teacher or his classmates say. He needs special help in order to cover the same amount of material as other children.

Treatment.   Members of the health team necessary for successful treatment of the deaf or partially deaf child are the physician, otologist, audiologist, speech therapist, possibly psychologist or psychiatrist, social worker, nurse, the child's family, and the child himself.

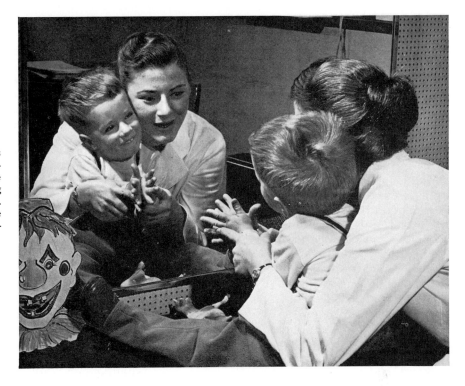

FIGURE 18–10. The child's speech and hearing are evaluated. Gross hearing tests are followed by audiometric testing if hearing loss is suspected. (From M. Stewart: Role of the Nurse in Pediatric Rehabilitation. *Health News*, Vol. 33.)

Early detection of deafness is necessary for proper speech development and for emotional growth. Training is necessary in understanding the facial expression which goes with words of approval or disapproval, of permission or denial, and in lip reading. Lip reading may start as early as 2½ or 3 years of age, the period when a child normally learns to talk in sentences. A specialist in lip reading and in speaking seldom begins this work until the child is of nursery school age. The mother should learn to move her lips correctly when speaking in order to supplement the work of the specialist in lip reading. A hearing aid may be provided for the child at a very early age.

Parents are given instruction in the care of their deaf children, and conferences are held in which they can receive help with particular

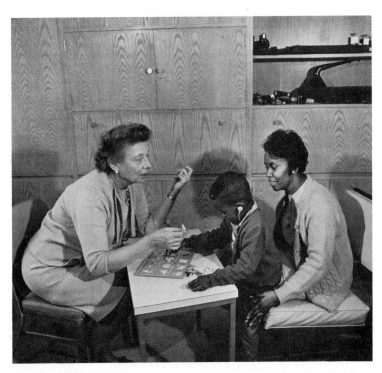

FIGURE 18–11. A child born with defective hearing has been fitted with a hearing aid and is now being taught to identify words with the objects they represent by an audiologist at the Johns Hopkins Speech and Hearing Clinic. (Photograph, Roy Perry, National Institute of Neurological Diseases and Strokes, U. S. Department of Health, Education and Welfare.)

problems. If the parent is deaf (or does not understand the language used), an interpreter can be provided. Many times a parent is reluctant to have a friend interpret because he may not want to share information or have the friend become involved.

If deafness is due to recurrent otitis media (see p. 399) or blockage of the eustachian tube, the services of the otologist should be procured.

If there is a serious hearing loss, special education may be necessary. Nursery schools have been organized for deaf children in many communities, and speech training is often given in connection with them. In some communities instruction in lip reading must be postponed until school age, since there are no facilities for younger children. The sign or finger language may be taught to supplement lip reading. Training to communicate with others lays the foundation for vocational or professional training or for manual labor, skilled or unskilled, in industry. Although the child needs special auditory training, the trend is to combine this with regular school education in order that the child may grow up in a "hearing" world.

Deaf children should be treated as normal children in all respects except their one great handicap; they are normal children who have a hearing loss. Adults who work with them must be patient. Until the child learns to communicate by speech, signs must be used or, if he has learned to write, signs supplemented with written words.

Responsibilities of the Nurse. The nurse helps in discovering deafness or impaired hearing in the infants and children brought to the clinic or Child Health Conference. The school nurse often gives the routine tests for impaired hearing. If a child who has been ill appears to have difficulty in understanding what is said in class, the teacher may send him to the nurse for testing. The school nurse routinely sees children who are known to have impaired hearing so that the physician's program of therapy can be supervised. Nurses work closely with the personnel of special classes and special schools for the deaf. In clinics for deaf children and those who are hard of hearing, nurses have direct contact with both the child and his mother.

Most deaf children do not like others to call attention to their defect or to be made to feel different from their peers. Since there are all degrees of hearing loss, all deaf children cannot be treated the same. In general, however, when caring for a child who does not hear normally, the mother or nurse must take time with him. She should speak to him by facing him in a good light and should speak distinctly without shouting. Shouting does not clarify speech sounds, and exaggerating words or speaking too slowly or rapidly makes it more difficult for the child to understand. Normal well-articulated and well-modulated speech should be used. If the child can read lips, carry on the conversation so that he can see your mouth. Before speaking to the child attract his attention first by touching him lightly. If he does not understand the key word or phrase spoken first, substitute synonyms for clarity. If the child can hear with one "good" ear, favor that side when you talk to him. Facial expressions help to show the meaning of words more than the tone of voice, which the deaf child may not hear. If the older child has difficulty in hearing, jot down key words on a paper for him.

When listening to a deaf child who does not have clear speech, watch his face as he talks and you will be better able to understand what he says. Since a hearing loss affects the language process, the child should be encouraged to take an active interest in language activities such as spelling and reading.

An adolescent who dislikes to be different and is sensitive about his hearing loss may not admit to his handicap. When this situation occurs, repeat your meaning tactfully, but in different words, until he understands.

The mother or nurse should note respiratory infections early in these children so that they can be treated as quickly as possible. The child's ears should be examined at frequent intervals to determine changes in his hearing thresholds.

Prognosis. The prognosis for the improvement or cure of deafness depends on the degree and nature of the pathologic state or structural defect and on whether the child receives optimum treatment. How well a hearing aid and training in lip reading may overcome his physical handicap depends on the availability of such devices and the services of a specialist in teaching deaf children to communicate through speech. If the community does not furnish such help, the child may attend a state school for the deaf or a privately supported institution.

If the prognosis is defined in terms of ability to lead a normal life, then for most deaf children it is excellent. This assumes that deafness is their only handicap. If the child is blind as well as deaf or has low mentality, the prognosis is poorer for social adjustment.

Prevention. The prevention of acquired deafness consists in the prevention of infectious disease which is likely to involve the ear. Respiratory infections are a common example. It is difficult, if not impossible, to prevent all infections, but prompt treatment can be given in all cases of upper respiratory tract infections and otitis media.

Impacted cerumen (wax) impairs hearing and may lead to a lesion of the ear. The wax should be removed by the physician. Sinus infection and infected lymphoid tissue in the nasopharynx should be treated promptly. Drugs which endanger the eighth nerve should not be used indiscriminately.

Relatively few cases of deafness in children are caused by injury. Nevertheless the eardrum can be injured when a child puts something sharp into his ear. Injury to the external ear has little effect on hearing. Injury to the brain can affect the centers of hearing and speech.

BLINDNESS

An infant is usually far-sighted at birth. Although his cornea is almost fully developed, his eyeballs and lenses are not. He has peripheral vision until central vision begins to develop by about six weeks of age. At three months he can follow a moving object with both eyes in all directions. The two eyes should work together. If they do not, the child may have strabismus (see p. 666) or amblyopia (see p. 666).

Etiology and Importance of the Problem. The child may be born blind, possibly as a result of congenital rubella, or may acquire blindness from retrolental fibroplasia (see p. 200), trauma, infection during delivery, ophthalmia neonatorum (see p. 260), or congenital syphilis (see p. 262). Other conditions causing blindness in childhood are numerically of relatively little importance. Accidents caused by exploding soda bottles, fire crackers, or toys may cause injury to the eyes.

Children having visual difficulty may rub their eyes frequently, may squint or frown when trying to see at a distance, or may hold their picture books too close to their eyes when trying to see nearby.

The legal definition of *blindness* is based on a visual acuity of at best 20/200 in the better eye after correction. *Partially* blind children have a visual acuity between 20/70 and 20/200 in the better eye after appropriate correction. Children, like adults, have *myopia* (near-sightedness), *hyperopia* (far-sightedness), or *astigmatism* (variation in the refractive power of the various meridians of the eye resulting in a distorted image).

Children who are blind or have extremely poor vision require special education and training for daily life activities. Their condition may be improved by medical or surgical procedures and the use of glasses. They may need help in acquiring the everyday skills needed in self-care. Instruction must be given through the sense of hearing or touch. If the child has normal mentality, he is able to take the same subjects in school as normal children do, although his progess may be slower than theirs. Without the same education that normal children receive, the blind child does not grow up with the interests, attitudes, and abilities that the sighted possess.

Treatment. The physical condition is treated, if possible, in order to restore or improve sight or to prevent further impairment of vision. If the child wears glasses, they should be made of shatter-resistant lenses set in sturdy well-fitting frames.

Research is currently being done on various electronic methods of helping the blind "see," but none has been perfected for the use of children.

The totally blind child of school age should be enrolled in a school for the blind or, in a school for normal children, in a special class for children with visual problems. Special classes have been established in public and private schools for children whose vision is so poor that they cannot profit from the regular school system of instruction. These schools emphasize the use of auditory instruction and the development of reading skills through touch perception by the Braille system (Fig. 18–12). For children who are not totally blind, books are printed with extra large type so that eye fatigue is minimized. Good lighting and correct posture are emphasized.

Children who have some vision may attend regular classes if a teacher skilled in working with blind children gives them help when it is needed. Such contact tends to develop skill in making friends and joining in the activities of the sighted. Being one of the normal group promotes normal social and emotional development.

Parents must be instructed in the needs of their blind children. Blindness at birth or developing early in childhood prevents the child from knowing what others mean by colors he cannot see and objects he cannot handle (e.g., the sun, a river, or a baby robin). The mother can use such words in context so that the child gets some idea of the meaning. Blind children need to handle as much of their environment as is practical and build up concepts which other children acquire by sight. They can handle modeling clay or play-dough and can weave or paint to learn to "feel." They can listen to bells, music boxes, and record players in order to hear sound. If

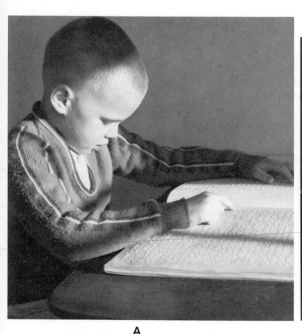

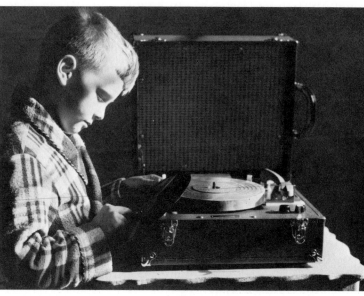

A

B

FIGURE 18–12. The totally blind child needs to develop the senses of touch and hearing, to compensate for his lack of sight. *A*, A blind boy studies his braille. *B*, A blind boy uses a phonograph. (Courtesy of New York State Commission for the Visually Handicapped.)

these children have been protected from hurting themselves while exploring the world about them, meeting their own needs and doing what gives them pleasure, they acquire a skill in self-help which children blinded later in life seldom acquire.

Parents can be helped to understand the special care required by the blind or partially sighted child. The tendency is to overprotect him. They find it hard to give him the freedom he must have to build up skills and experience which are necessary when he reaches adolescence and must prepare himself for adult life. Vocational training is given the blind, and for those who are capable and desire it, a higher education and preparation for the professions which are open to them. Scholarships and maintenance are provided from private or public sources if the student is in need of financial assistance.

Responsibilities of the Nurse. Early detection of impaired vision or of blindness is essential for the treatment and education of the child. Infants who do not reach for their bottle or toys and do not smile when the mother smiles should be examined for blindness. A toddler who walks into the furniture, has no interest in even large pictures and does not respond to the motions of other people should have his eyesight tested by a physician. Undetected cases of blindness are rare, since facilities for health supervision of children in all economic classes have improved, and since physicians and nurses test for vision,

using the Snellen E chart for young children as part of the routine physical examinations given in Child Health Conferences and children's clinics, and the Snellen Chart for children who can read in school.

The blind child needs happiness as all children do and is more dependent than normal children upon the moods of the adults about him. The nurse working with blind children knows that they can interpret moods by the inflection of the voice as other children do by seeing a smile or frown.

In the hospital the nurse interprets the new environment to the blind child until he becomes familiar with the sounds of the unit. The nurse introduces the child to other children near him and helps the sighted children by comments such as, "David cannot see your smile, so try to put a smile in your voice." Before touching a blind child, the nurse should speak to him. Adults must identify themselves to a blind child verbally because he cannot read the name pin or tape they are wearing. Prepare the child carefully for procedures that are planned and let him handle the equipment to be used if possible. The blind child should be encouraged to do all he can for himself. The nurse can provide opportunities for adequate mobility and various kinds of sensory stimulation for the blind child in the hospital.

More specifically, the nurse can help the mother in the following ways. The nurse can discuss with her how to nourish her child's personality by providing love, security, and a sense of belonging in the family. The nurse can also discuss the child's need for body contact and for sensory stimulation. The nurse can help the mother be alert for her child's readiness for new experiences and for his need for freedom of movement and mobility to explore his environment. The nurse can also explain to the mother the reasons why she should talk to her child and encourage his development of other senses. The blind child needs patient parents who can provide time for the establishment of a definite routine of sleeping, eating, and toileting. He needs opportunities to achieve skills, to develop his self-identity, self-reliance and self-respect, and to be free from unnecessary fear or intense feelings of guilt. As the child grows he needs all the experiences of the sighted school child (see Chap. 22) and the adolescent (see Chap. 25).

Community Action. Community action depends upon the attitude of the people in the community toward blindness. Like parents, the community may tend to overprotect children. Part of the nurse's responsibility for blind chil-

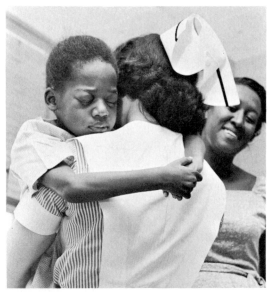

FIGURE 18–14. A blind child feels secure in her nurse's arms. (Dallas Services for Blind Children.)

dren is to channel the community's sympathy for them into helpful activities.

In some communities play groups for children of preschool age have been organized in which blind children can enjoy play with others like themselves. The playground and the equipment are suited to their needs, and adequate supervision is provided. Such play helps these children to make social adjustments, which serve as a basis for contacts with the sighted and which can be developed into a normal ability to participate in group activities.

Prognosis. The outcome of treatment varies with every child, and no general statements can be made. Great strides are being made in the prevention of blindness from gonorrhea and syphilis, and with improved care of premature infants there are very few cases of blindness due to retrolental fibroplasia.

The prognosis for the blind child in the future will be improved because of research being done on new aids for the blind such as a sonar-type electronic device worn on the head that can help the child identify people and objects in the world around him by means of echoes.

The prognosis for mental health is good. The child who is born blind can usually make a happier adjustment to his handicap than a child who becomes blind later because of an infection or injury to his eyes. Parent-child relations are more important than any measure which the community can take to help the blind child. But it is the community which provides education and gives the blind person a position in industry or uses his professional services. Children with

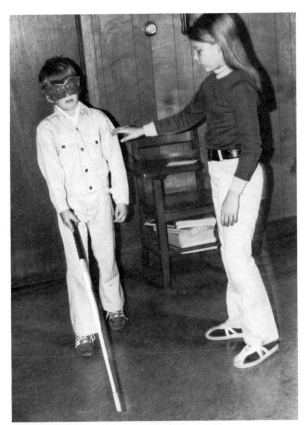

FIGURE 18–13. Difficulties imposed by blindness can be simulated through the use of blindfolds. Such role-playing activities can help children become more sensitive to the feelings of those with a special need. (From Cleary, M. E.: *Children Today*, 5:6, July-August, 1976.)

impaired vision may become self-supporting adults fulfilling all the roles of a normal adult. The totally blind find it more difficult to function in society. Their success depends to a great extent upon their early training.

HELPING THE PARENTS OF THE CHRONICALLY HANDICAPPED CHILD

Parents of chronically physically or mentally handicapped children should be taught that these children need an environment in which they can develop their capacities to the limit, and that the most important element in this environment is the sense of security which loving parents give their children.

Parents may need both financial help and expert counsel in fulfilling their exacting role. It is not easy to be a "perfect parent" to a handicapped child. The children also must be helped to grow up normally. Severe personality handicaps interfere with their social adjustment more than their physical condition limits successful social interaction. A child acquires emotional problems as a result of deprivation of emotional satisfactions and lack of opportunity to use, and so to develop his capacities.

It takes months or years for parents to recover from the shock and frustration of having a child who is not normal. They also fear the additional responsibilities involved in care, and perhaps most of all they fear society's attitude toward them and the child. Anxiety and hostility conflict with their normal love for him.

Such a child disturbs not only parent-child relations, but also all other relations between the members of the family. Parents may manage their feelings in various ways with various reactions on the part of the child. They may deny the existence of his handicap or overprotect him to cover up their negative feelings toward him. Since contact with him causes them anxiety, they may openly reject him and thus not give him the love and security he needs, nor the status of a loved child in the home or that part of

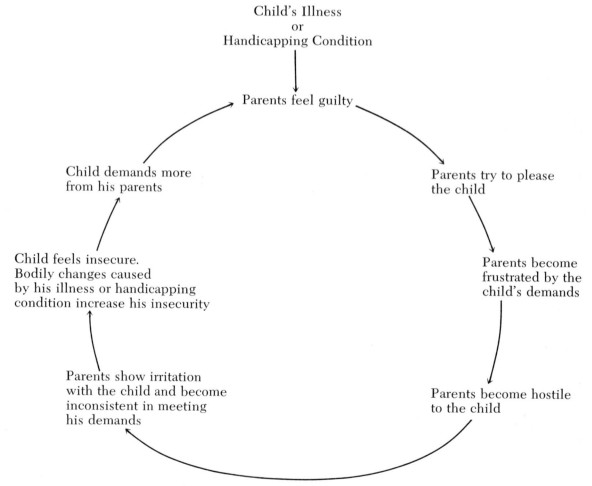

FIGURE 18–15. Possible Parent-Child Interaction. This cyclical interaction may be changed with guidance by members of the health team.

the community outside his home where he is learning to adjust to strangers.

Parents may ignore his cues for readiness to learn because they cannot regard him as a person or because they overprotect him. The child therefore does not develop to his potential level. He may even regress.

Help is given to the parents by the whole team of specialists in the crippled children's program: physician, social worker, psychologist or psychiatrist, nurse, and others, depending on the child's problem. The nurse must understand normal parent-child relations, the normal developmental process and the needs of the child. The nurse must know how to support parents in accepting problems caused by the child's handicaps, and learn to know the parents well enough to give help when they are ready to accept it. To teach a mother techniques of care before she is ready to learn produces frustration and failure.

The nurse can be a great help to parents when they are discouraged by believing in their capacity to care for the child and to give him love and a sense of security. The nurse must communicate to them, not necessarily in words, but by manner, that their feelings are understood and that support and assistance can be provided.

The nurse must help parents see that their responsibility is to help the child to grow up and to develop his capacity, however little it may be, for self-help in daily living. Other professional workers have the function of educating the child and giving him many of the pleasures which normal children enjoy, e.g., going to camp in summer. But it is the parents who give the child experience in daily life within a family. In order to help the parents in their task, the nurse must know the evaluation which the total team makes of the child's potential ability. Without such knowledge the nurse cannot communicate realistic goals toward which the parents and the child can work.

The child's response to the help given him is the final test of its success. If the handicapped child feels that his parents are anxious and frustrated, he will feel unloved and may withdraw into a world of fantasy, never developing to his potential level. Some of these children feel only pity for themselves, some try to hurt others as they have been hurt, and others seek punishment for their own negative feelings.

Children who feel loved and wanted are motivated to overcome the limitations of their handicaps or to compensate through success in activities within their ability. These children are likely to succeed beyond what could be expected of them. The handicapped child does not need pity or sympathy. He needs understanding and a knowledge that others accept his differences and accord him status as an equal.

As the handicapped child becomes able to be away from his parents for longer periods of time, he should be provided with a method of identification such as a Medic-Alert emblem (Medic-Alert Foundation, Turlock, California 95380).

In order for the parents to fulfill their role in the life of their handicapped child they need adequate time for themselves. Relatives and friends may provide care for the child so that the parents can relax away from him periodically. Parents are many times helped through their participation in groups of parents who have children like their own. Mutual problems can be discussed and solutions found.

The role of the parents, and the mother especially, is fundamental to the emergence of all sorts of communication by the child and to the formation of his body image and self-image, although these may be reinforced or negated by pleasurable or painful experiences with other human beings. In spite of a good beginning, since many in our society view disabled persons with disdain or pity, the attitudes of those in his environment may cause a heavy emotional burden to the child and prove to be a hindrance in the process of his development.

The nurse must be aware of personal feelings of repugnance or fear of the handicapped child. The nurse should not be ashamed, for many people have the same feelings toward these children. The first step in changing these feelings to a more positive attitude is to know that they exist.

Probably the most difficult problem faced by some parents of a severely chronically handicapped child is the child's future. Parents can care for, protect, and teach the child when he is young, but as the parents grow older and other children leave home, the severely handicapped child may remain the responsibility of an aging husband and wife. Parents wonder where their child will live out the end of his life when they are not there to give him care. No one can answer this question for them, but they can be assisted in discussing their feelings and in making some plans for the child's future.

Finally, parents of handicapped children need continued counseling about the nature of the child's handicap and his potential for development. They need practical guidance in caring for the child, in obtaining prepared baby-sitters for short-term assistance, and a list of good residential-care facilities where handicapped children can be cared for temporarily, should the need arise. Parents also need a central coordinator such as a physician, social worker, nurse, or later a counselor, some one person who is an advocate to whom they can turn in time of need.

ANXIETY IN THE TODDLER

When a toddler appears anxious, the conflict between his instinctual desires and the demands of his environment is becoming too much for him to endure. Indications of anxiety at his age are refusal to go to bed, "jittery" behavior during the day, restless sleep at night, and disturbance of bowel and bladder functioning.

Toilet training is an acute source of anxiety to many children. Children who have achieved bowel and bladder control may have accidents or may play with feces after they have once discontinued this habit. If a child has been too severely trained, he may become afraid of moving his bowels, with the result that he becomes constipated. Constipation may also develop because he is negativistic toward his mother when she has done something he dislikes.

Feeding problems may result from a child's anxiety over toilet training. The child may regress to infantile pleasures in feeding, e.g., sucking.

Stuttering may develop as part of this general pattern of regression. The child adopts the infantile way of breathing; his respiration may become irregular, and he catches his breath. This sort of respiration produces difficulty in speaking clearly, and stuttering may result. This anxiety reaction has its inception in a sudden fright or shock which produces a startle reflex accompanied by catching of the breath.

Some toddlers, instead of regressing, may appear to grow up suddenly. One evidence of this is masturbation rather than the momentary handling of the genitalia seen in infancy. Some toddlers as a result of too severe toilet training become overclean, not wanting to displease mother by soiling themselves in any way.

A toddler who becomes too anxious over the conflicting desires he experiences will not be able to develop satisfying love relations with an adult, nor a sense of autonomy, which is of vital importance. He will, instead, be overcome by shame and by doubt of his own ability. He can be helped to develop a real love for his mother. She should encourage him to take part in activities which he regards as dirty—playing with mud, sand, plasticine, and finger paints. She should laughingly praise him for getting dirty when it results from play. If he gets dirty as a means of evincing hostility toward his mother, she should accept this hostility as normal in children of his age, in the same way that she accepts his immature love responses.

Adequate *treatment* of anxiety should be instituted early in life so that the prevailing mood during childhood may be happy and emotional development normal. Untreated, the anxiety of a child is cumulative. It becomes a habitual reaction which may persist into adult life.

CRIPPLED (HANDICAPPED) CHILDREN'S SERVICES IN THE UNITED STATES

There are more than 5,500,000 handicapped children in the United States known to official agencies. Many others are receiving care elsewhere, and still others are receiving no care. The objective of the Children's Bureau is to help each state improve services for locating children having a handicap and for providing them with care. Every state and territory has an official program for their help, generally within the health department. Programs have also developed around medical centers, where personnel needed to help the children are taught by specialists and where research is a principal part of the program. Regional clinics are developed in connection with these centers.

A well run program combines (1) locating handicapped children, (2) treatment (correction if possible), (3) management to promote adaptation to their handicaps and to limit the influence of disabilities upon their lives, and (4) prevention of circumstances in which crippling is likely to occur, e.g., safe delivery of the newborn, immunization for poliomyelitis, and prevention of accidents. There is also a secondary aim of attempting to prevent the difficulties in physical, mental, social, and economic areas of living caused by the condition of the child—difficulties which may involve the entire family and even the community.

Programs for handicapped children are broad, covering almost any condition which is a serious handicap in normal living. Each state decides which children are to be eligible for assistance under the handicapped children's program. Programs often include the following: multiple handicaps, hearing defects, rheumatic fever, heart disease (congenital or rheumatic), certain eye defects, and epilepsy. The reasons for the extension of coverage are that there are now fewer children having orthopedic problems and conditions requiring plastic surgery, and new forms of management have been found for children for whom treatment was formerly unknown. Genetic counseling may also be provided.

The first phase in these programs is locating

handicapped children. Certainly the community or public health nurse is assuming more of a responsible role in the case finding and referral of children for care. Necessary treatment follows, either in the agency sponsoring the program or through referral to another agency which can meet the child's needs. The crippled children's team works with the child and the parents, and the community is organized to give many forms of assistance. The public not only gives financial aid for handicapped children, but also supports, through its vote, the crippled children's program in the state, county, and city. The children are provided for in the public school system, and in some localities special teachers may be sent to the home if the child is confined to bed.

This type of service may produce heavier case loads, for more emphasis is placed upon coordination of effort with attempts toward more comprehensive patient care. This newer approach brings together all the resources of the community in prevention, treatment and education. Under this program the child lives as normal a life as is possible and is helped to form positive attitudes toward himself and his problem.

CLINICAL SITUATIONS

When Joanne was 15 months old, Mrs. Wood brought her to the Child Health Conference and complained that her appetite was poor compared with what it had been during infancy. Joanne appeared healthy and was an extremely active child.

1. In discussing Joanne's apparent anorexia with her mother, the nurse would base comments on the fact that
   a. Since Joanne is not growing as rapidly as she did during infancy, she should not be expected to eat as much.
   b. Probably Joanne's anorexia is due to the fact that Mrs. Wood had stopped giving her vitamins when she was a year old.
   c. Perhaps Joanne should have a complete physical examination by the physician.
   d. Perhaps Mrs. Wood should be more firm in urging her to eat.

2. Joanne must have her basic emotional needs met if she is to develop a healthy personality. During the toddler period she should have
   a. Unlimited opportunity to do whatever she wants and as much independence as she desires.
   b. Recognition as a little child and protection from harm through rigid obedience to parental rules.
   c. Realistic limits set on her behavior by her parents and increasing independence as she is ready for it.
   d. Recognition as a miniature adult who is able to set limits on her own behavior.

3. Joanne's social development is best described by stating that she prefers to play

a. Alone, but will share her toys and makes friends quickly with strangers.
b. Alone, but refuses to share her toys and is shy with strangers.
c. With other children, usually shares her toys and makes friends quickly with strangers.
d. With other children, refuses to share her toys and is shy with strangers.

4. The accident rate is high during the toddler period because
   a. Parents tend to neglect children at this age.
   b. Their natural curiosity and activity lead them into danger.
   c. They do not comprehend their parents' warnings of danger.
   d. They are negativistic about everything and refuse to listen to their parents.

One day while Joanne was climbing up the basement steps she fell from the top landing to the basement floor. On her admission to the hospital the physician made a diagnosis of a fractured right femur and multiple bruises.

5. Joanne was placed in Bryant traction. In order to maintain traction, the nurse's most important responsibility was to make certain that
   a. Joanne's hips were resting on the bed and her legs were suspended at right angles to the bed.
   b. Joanne's hips were slightly elevated from the bed and her legs were suspended at right angles to the bed.
   c. Joanne's hips were elevated above the level of her body on a pillow and her legs were suspended in a position of comfort almost parallel to the bed.
   d. Joanne's hips and legs were flat on the bed with the pull of traction coming from the foot of the bed.

6. In order to prevent Joanne from turning to watch activity on the unit, the nurse would
   a. Apply an abdominal restraint and have other children come to her bed to play with her.
   b. Apply clove hitch restraints to her arms and move her bed so that she could watch television.
   c. Apply a restraint jacket and move her bed so that she could watch other children.
   d. Apply no restraints, but move her bed near the center of the unit so that she could watch the activities of the unit personnel.

Mrs. McIntyre called her pediatrician and explained that Betty Jane, age 2½ years, had had a slight cold for two days, but that within the last few hours she seemed to have increasingly difficult respirations and was extremely restless. After examining the child the physician recommended immediate admission to the hospital. She was admitted with a diagnosis of laryngotracheobronchitis.

7. Betty Jane was placed in a Croupette. Cool moist air is effective treatment of this condition because it
   a. Causes dilatation of blood vessels in the bronchi, thus relieving the congestion.
   b. Increases the cough reflex, thus making it easier to expectorate mucus.
   c. Coagulates the mucus, thus relieving the dyspnea.
   d. Relieves the dryness of secretions, making them easier to cough up.

8. Betty Jane became emotionally disturbed when her mother said that she was going home. You as the nurse would suggest that the mother
   a. Omit visiting for a few days until Betty Jane adjusted to the hospital routine.

b. Visit only when Betty Jane was sleeping so that she would not disturb the child

c. Visit as often and as frequently as she could within the hospital visiting policy.

d. Discipline the child because her crying is harmful to her.

Since Betty Jane's respiratory distress became more severe and she showed signs of increasing prostration, an emergency tracheotomy was performed.

9. Immediately after the operation the nurse aspirated Betty Jane's tracheostomy tube

a. As often as secretion appeared at the opening of the tube.

b. Approximately every 15 minutes.

c. Whenever Betty Jane appeared to have difficulty in breathing.

d. Whenever Betty Jane requested that it be done.

10. Betty Jane was afraid to try to swallow after the tracheotomy had been done. The nurse

a. Offered small amounts of her favorite fruit juice or other liquid at frequent intervals and gave approval when she drank it.

b. Explained to her that she would get a "needle" if she did not take some juice by mouth.

c. Told her that her father would give her a dime for every cup of fluid she drank.

d. Told her she would read a story to her each time she took a cup of juice.

11. When the nurse aspirated Betty Jane's tracheotomy, she cleaned the inner cannula

a. By running hot tap water through it and aspirating secretions from it with a catheter.

b. By soaking it in an antibiotic solution and cleaning the outside with a detergent.

c. By soaking it in hydrogen peroxide and passing tonsil wire and gauze through it.

d. By running cold tap water through it and wiping it off with petrolatum.

12. The nurse on one occasion found that Betty Jane had torn off the elbow restraints and had succeeded in pulling out the tracheostomy tube. She was cyanotic, and repirations had apparently ceased. The nurse

a. Went immediately to the telephone to call the physician, held open the incision with a hemostat and gave mouth-to-mouth resuscitation.

b. Inserted another tracheostomy tube into the trachea, aspirated the trachea, asked another nurse to call a physician, and gave oxygen through a nasal catheter.

c. Inserted another tracheostomy tube immediately, asked another nurse to call the physician, gave oxygen through a nasal catheter, and provided artificial respiration.

d. Asked another nurse to call the physician, held open the incision with a hemostat, aspirated the trachea, provided oxygen through the incision, and gave artificial respiration.

13. When Betty Jane was well enough to play in bed, the nurse would assume, on the basis of her understanding of growth and development, that Betty Jane would enjoy

a. Playing with her favorite toy.

b. Constructing a tower of 20 blocks.

c. Listening to popular songs on the radio.

d. Stringing small beads.

Roosevelt Jones, a two-year-old child, was admitted to the pediatric unit with a diagnosis of chronic lead poisoning. His mother stated that he had eaten paint periodically from his crib and from the window sills over a period of several weeks.

14. Roosevelt should be observed carefully by the nurse for

a. Hemorrhage from the rectum.

b. Convulsions.

c. Edema of the extremities.

d. Respiratory difficulty.

15. Roosevelt responded well to treatment. One day when the nurse was bathing him, he said, "My mommy does it *this* way." His comment indicates that

a. He does not like the way the nurse gives a sponge bath.

b. Routines or rituals learned at home are important to him.

c. His mother gives a bath better than the nurse.

d. He hates his nurse.

16. The nurse found Roosevelt in the bathroom, splashing in the water in the toilet. The nurse should

a. Slap his hands and remove him from the room.

b. Explain that children should not play in such dirty water.

c. Give him a basin of clean water in which to splash.

d. Take him back to his unit and lock the bathroom door.

17. During his nap Roosevelt wet his bed. The nurse would

a. Change his clothes and bedding and make no issue of it.

b. Tell him that he will catch cold if he lies in a wet bed.

c. Promise to give him a piece of candy if he has no further accidents.

d. Explain that only babies wet their beds.

18. Roosevelt had frequent temper tantrums during his hospitalization. The best way to deal with them would be to

a. Punish him by putting him back in his crib for the rest of the day.

b. Reason with him and tell him why he should not become angry.

c. Prevent temper tantrums by pampering him.

d. Protect him during his tantrums and attempt to prevent them by helping him meet necessary frustrations.

19. The care which Roosevelt should have after a temper tantrum is

a. Ignore him for the rest of the day because he has been a "bad boy."

b. Wash his face and hands and provide a toy for him.

c. Make fun of him before other children in this group.

d. Make him apologize for his behavior.

20. After a prolonged period of hospitalization Roosevelt became a quiet, withdrawn child who evidenced little interest in his mother when she visited. The nurse should realize that

a. He has accepted his hospitalization well and has matured because of his experience.

b. He has finally been disciplined, and the nurses should expect gratitude from his parents.

c. He had probably become a very disturbed little boy because of his traumatic experience.

d. He was ready to be toilet-trained because he seemed to enjoy playing with his feces.

GUIDES FOR FURTHER STUDY

1. During your experience in the pediatric unit observe the motor development of as many toddlers as you can. Compare the similarities and differences among the children in each age group: 15 months, 18 months, 2 years, and 2½ years.

2. Investigate the resources in your community for the dissemination of information about the treatment of children who have taken poison. If your community has a Poison Control Center, familiarize yourself with its functions. If your community does not have such a facility, discuss with your instructor in seminar your role as a citizen and a nurse in meeting this need.

3. Prepare a plan which you could use to teach a mother the home care of a toddler who has had a tracheotomy. In addition to the content and skills she would need to know, investigate the sources and the approximate cost of the equipment she would need to provide this care.

4. Prepare and give a 20-minute talk on "Accident Prevention" to a small group of mothers of toddlers in your community. Provide pamphlets and a bibliography for them on this subject. Allow time for discussion at the end of your presentation. Make a list of questions which these mothers asked and submit them with your answers to your instructor.

5. What measures are taken to prevent the spread of staphylococcal infections in your hospital?

6. Investigate the programs and services (public and private) offered for handicapped children in your state and community. Discuss in seminar the adequacy of these programs in relation to the need for them.

7. List the functions of the health team members who coordinate their efforts in the care and habilitation of a child with cerebral palsy. If possible, interview the parents of a child having this diagnosis to determine their feelings about this condition and their reaction to the child's treatment. Identify the nurse's specific responsibilities in providing education for the parents and care for this child throughout his growth period. Discuss your findings and conclusions in seminar.

TEACHING AIDS AND OTHER INFORMATION*

American Academy of Pediatrics

Acute and Chronic Childhood Lead Poisoning.
Day Care for Handicapped Children.
Earthenware Containers: A Potential Source of Acute Lead Poisoning.
Lead Content of Paint Applied to Surfaces Accessible to Young Children.
Pediatric Problems Related to Deteriorated Housing.
The Physician and the Deaf Child.

American Foundation for the Blind, Inc.

Brown, J.: Storytelling and the Blind Child.
Dickman, I. R. (Ed.): Sex Education and Family Life for Visually Handicapped Children and Youth: A Resource Guide, 1974.
Froyd, H. E.: Counseling Families of Severely Visually Handicapped Children.
Knight, J. J.: Building Self-Confidence in the Multiply Handicapped Blind Child.
Kurzhals, I. W.: Personality Adjustment for the Blind Child in the Classroom.
Lairy, G. C., and Harrison-Covello, A.: The Blind Child and His Parents: Congenital Visual Defect and the Repercussion of Family Attitudes on the Early Development of the Child.
Moor, P. M.: Toilet Habits: Suggestions for Training a Blind Child, Revised 1974.
Rodgers, C. T.: Understanding Braille.
Tait, P.: Play and the Intellectual Development of Blind Children.

The National Easter Seal Society

Bloodstein, O.: A Handbook on Stuttering, Revised 1975.
Books and Pamphlets for Parents of Handicapped Children.
Brain Injury and Related Disorders in Children.
Denhoff, E.: The Responsibility of the Physician, Parent, and Child in Learning Disabilities, 1974.
Diamond, M.: Sexuality and the Handicapped, 1974.

Directory of Resident Camps for Persons with Special Health Needs, 1975.
Gardner, W. I.: Behavior Modification: An Approach to Education of Young Children with Learning and Behavior Difficulties, 1975.
Henscheid, H.: View of Life, 1975.
Lehman, J. U.: Advertencias para los Padres de Niños Sordos y Medio-Sordos (Do's and Don't's for Parents of Preschool Deaf and Hard of Hearing Children), 1975.
Lehman, J. U.: Do's and Don'ts for Parents of Pre-School Deaf and Hard of Hearing Children, 1976.
Scherzer, A. L.: Early Diagnosis, Management, and Treatment of Cerebral Palsy, 1974.

National Society for the Prevention of Blindness, Inc.

Prevent Blindness: Signs of Possible Eye Trouble in Children, 1976.

United Cerebral Palsy Association

Cerebral Palsy—What You Should Know About It.
Handling the Young Cerebral Palsied Child At Home.
How-to's on Dressing and Feeding.
Social Security and Cerebral Palsy.

United States Government

A Developmental Approach to Casefinding, with Special Reference to Cerebral Palsy, Mental Retardation, and Related Disorders, 1973.
A Handicapped Child in Your Home, 1973.
Feeding the Child with a Handicap, 1973.
Interpreting for Deaf People, 1973.
Lead Poisoning in Children, 1975.
Mercury in the Environment, 1973.
Parents, Are Your Walls Poisoning Your Children? 1973.
Services for Crippled Children, 1975.

---

*Complete addresses are given in the Appendix.

REFERENCES

Books

Azarnoff, P., and Flegal, S.: *A Pediatric Play Program: Developing a Therapeutic Play Program for Children in Medical Settings.* Springfield, Ill., Charles C Thomas, 1975.

Buscaglia, L.: *The Disabled and Their Parents.* Thorofare, N. J., Charles B. Slack, 1975.

Carter, S., and Gold, A. P.: *Neurology of Infancy and Childhood.* New York, Appleton-Century-Crofts, 1974.

Finnie, N. R., et al.: *Handling the Young Cerebral Palsied Child at Home.* 2nd ed. New York, E. P. Dutton & Company, 1975.

Gauchat, D.: *All God's Children.* New York, Hawthorn Books, Inc., 1976.

Gellis, S. S., and Kagan, B. M.: *Current Pediatric Therapy 7.* Philadelphia, W. B. Saunders Company, 1976.

Guyton, A. C.: *Structure and Function of the Nervous System.* 2nd ed. Philadelphia, W. B. Saunders Company, 1976.

Heisler, V.: *A Handicapped Child in the Family: A Guide for Parents.* New York, Grune & Stratton, 1972.

Hofmann, R. B.: *How to Build Special Furniture and Equipment for Handicapped Children.* Springfield, Ill., Charles C Thomas, 1974.

Hughes, J. G.: *Synopsis of Pediatrics.* 4th ed. St. Louis, The C. V. Mosby Company, 1975.

Konigsmark, B. W., and Gorlin, R. J.: *Genetic and Metabolic Deafness.* Philadelphia, W. B. Saunders Company, 1976.

Levine, E. S.: *Lisa and Her Soundless World.* New York, Human Sciences Press, 1974.

Miller, A. L., Rohman, B. F., and Thompson, F. V.: *Your Child's Hearing and Speech.* Springfield, Ill., Charles C Thomas, 1974.

Robinault, I. P.: *Functional Aids for the Multiply Handicapped.* New York, Harper & Row, 1973.

Silver, H. K., Kempe, C. H., and Bruyn, H. B.: *Handbook of Pediatrics.* 11th ed. Los Altos, California, Lange Medical Publications, 1975.

Swaiman, K. F., and Wright, F. S.: *The Practice of Pediatric Neurology.* St. Louis, The C. V. Mosby Company, 1975.

Travis, G.: *Chronic Illness in Children: Its Impact on Child and Family.* Stanford, Calif., Stanford University Press, 1976.

Vaughan, V. C., III, and McKay, R. J. (Eds.): *Nelson Textbook of Pediatrics.* 10th ed. Philadelphia, W. B. Saunders Company, 1975.

Wallace, H. M., Gold, E. M., and Lis, E. H. (Eds.): *Maternal and Child Health Practices: Problems, Resources, and Methods of Delivery.* Springfield, Ill., Charles C Thomas, 1973.

Periodicals

Avey, M.: Primary Care for Handicapped Children. *Am. J. Nursing,* 73:658, April 1973.

Ballou, B., and Todd, T. W.: Understanding Developmental Disabilities: A "Sensitization" Workshop Program. *Children Today,* 2:28, September-October 1973.

Baloh, R. W.: Laboratory Diagnosis of Increased Lead Absorption. *Arch. Environ. Health,* 28:198, April 1974.

Blount, M., and Kinney, A. B.: Chronic Steroid Therapy. *Am. J. Nursing,* 74:1626, September 1974.

Chaiklin, H., Cook, J. J., Hayes, M. E., and Scanland, V. B.: Recurrence of Lead Poisoning in Children. *Soc. Work,* 19:196, March 1974.

Cleary, M. E.: Helping Children Understand the Child with Special Needs. *Children Today,* 5:6, July-August 1976.

Cohen, S., and Gloeckler, L.: Working With Parents of Handicapped Children: A Statewide Approach. *Children Today,* 5:10, January-Feburary 1976.

Cohen, D. J., Johnson, W. T., and Caparulo, B. K.: Pica and Elevated Blood Lead Level in Autistic and Atypical Children. *Am. J. Dis. Child,* 130:47, January 1976.

De La Burde, B., and Reames, B.: Prevention of Pica, The Major Cause of Lead Poisoning in Children. *Am. J. Pub. Health,* 63:737, August 1973.

Doner, F.: Blindness *Can* Be Prevented. *The Canadian Nurse,* 72:27, January 1976.

Eggland, E. T.: Locus of Control and Children With Cerebral Palsy. *Nursing Research,* 22:329, July-August 1973.

Graham, A., and Graham, F.: Lead Poisoning and The Suburban Child. *Today's Health,* 52:38, March 1974.

Haskin, M. R., et al.: Therapeutic Horseback Riding For the Handicapped. *Arch. Phys. Med. Rehabil.,* 55:473, October 1974.

Herth, K.: Beyond the Curtain of Silence. *Am. J. Nursing,* 74:1060, June 1974.

Hosey, C.: Yes, Our Son Is Still With Us. *Children Today,* 2:14, November-December 1973.

Kahn, H.: Visual Dysfunctions. *Nursing '74* 4:26, October 1974.

Klein, J. W., and Randolph, L. A.: Placing Handicapped Children in Head Start Programs. *Children Today,* 3:7, November-December 1974.

Lamm, S., Cole, B., Glynn, K., and Ullmann, W.: Lead Content of Milks Fed to Infants. *Nursing Digest,* 2:66, September 1974.

Lansdown, R. G., et al.: Blood-lead Levels, Behaviour, and Intelligence: A Population Study. *Lancet,* 1:538, March 30, 1974.

Lesser, S. R., and Easser, B. R.: Psychiatric Management of the Deaf Child. *The Canadian Nurse,* 71:23, October 1975.

Lin-Fu, J. S.: An Overview of Lead Exposure and Toxicity in Children. *Nursing Digest,* 2:59, September 1974.

Lockeretz, W.: Lead Content of Deciduous Teeth of Children in Different Environments. *Arch. Environ. Health,* 30:583, December 1975.

Mandleco, B. H.: Monitoring Children's Reactions When They Are Hospitalized for Percutaneous Renal Biopsy." *The American Journal of Maternal Child Nursing,* 1:288, September-October 1976.

Miller, P. G.: Vision Screening for Migrant Children. *Children Today,* 5:6, March-April 1976.

Moor, P. M.: Foster Family Care for Visually Impaired Children. *Children Today,* 5:11, July-August 1976.

Perron, D. M.: Deprived of Sound. *Am. J. Nursing,* 74:1057, June 1974.

Rosendorf, S.: Pa-La-Tee-Sha—They Are Blooming. *Children Today,* 3:12, March-April 1974.

Sabatino, L.: Deaf: Dos and Don'ts of Deaf-Patient Care. *RN,* 39:64, June 1976.

Simon, R.: Delbert Gets A Brain Pacemaker—And A Dream Is Coming True. *Today's Health,* 53:18, November 1975.

Smith, P. J., Nelson, D. M., and Stewart, R. E.: Lead Poisoning Among Migrant Children in New York State. *Am. J. Pub. Health,* 66:383, April 1976.

Steinhauer, P. D., Mushin, D. N., and Rae-Grant, Q.: Psychological Aspects of Chronic Illness. *Pediatr. Clin. N. Am.,* 21:825, November 1974.

Stokoe, W. C., Jr.: Seeing and Signing Language. *Nursing Digest,* 4:40, Summer 1976.

Volpe, J. J.: Perinatal Hypoxic–Ischemic Brain Injury. *Pediatr. Clin. N. Am.,* 23:383, August 1976.

Watt, R. C.: Urinary Diversion. *Am. J. Nursing,* 74:1806, October 1974.

What If Your Patient Is Also Deaf? *RN,* 39:59, June 1976.

AUDIOVISUAL MEDIA *

The American Journal of Nursing Company

Play Therapy and the Hospitalized Child
  26 minutes, black and white.
  Film describes how to aid children in coping with their hospital experience through play therapy.

Long Island Film Studios

Lead Poisoning—The Hidden Epidemic
  10 minutes, 16mm, sound, color, guide.
  Designed to alert all concerned with child care to the disease; sources of lead, detection, diagnosis, treatment and eradication.

The National Easter Seal Society

Feeding the Cerebral Palsied Child
  8½″ × 11″ poster, black and white.
  Demonstrates child development through self-help activities of eating.

Parents' Magazine Films, Inc.

Even Love Is Not Enough: Children with Handicaps
  A series of four 35mm filmstrips, sound, color.
  Provides insight on caring for and working with children with special needs.

Perkins School for the Blind

The World of Deaf-Blind Children—Growing Up.
  29 minutes, 16mm, sound, color.
  Describes social needs of these children and a program designed to meet them.

Trainex Corporation

The Young Spastic Child
  35mm filmstrip, audio-tape cassette, 33 1/3 LP, color.
  Presents detailed training procedures for developing gross motor skills in the young spastic child. Among the training therapies included in this program are head control; weight bearing on elbows, hands, and knees; rolling over and sitting; standing and walking; and carrying the child.

United States Government

International Education of the Hearing Impaired Child Series
  These three films are shown in sequence.
  Developmental Auditory Response Patterns, Parts 1 and 2
  Producer: USBEH
  44 minutes, 16mm film, optical sound, color.
  Shows responses to auditory stimuli in normal children ages 7 weeks to 7½ months, with assessment and commentary by Dr. Kevin Murphy, Royal Berkshire Hospital, Reading, England.

  Auditory Assessment
  Producer: USBEH
  26 minutes, 16mm film, optical sound, color.
  Exhibits techniques of identification and paedo–audiometry currently seen in Denmark, Sweden, England, and the Netherlands.

  The Developing Audio-Vocal System
  Producer: USBEH
  38 minutes, 16mm film, optical sound, color.
  Demonstrates the application of European methods of auditory training and speech in Sweden, the Netherlands, Belgium, England, and Denmark.

  Parent Education
  Producer: USBEH
  24 minutes, 16mm film, optical sound, color.
  Shows home and clinic instruction in Sweden, Germany, England, and the Netherlands.

  Parent Education at Heidelberg
  Producer: USBEH
  11 minutes, 16mm film, optical sound, color.
  Presents Professor Arman Lowe's home teaching and parent education program at the Paedo-Audiological Guidance Center.

  The Deaf-Blind
  Producer: USBEH
  23 minutes, 16mm film, optical sound, color.
  Observes the techniques of evaluation employed by Dr. Ladislav Fisch, Heston Audiology Clinic, England, and the approaches to instruction at Saint Michielsgestel.

  The Multiple Handicapped
  Producer: USBEH
  23 minutes, 16mm film, optical sound, color.
  Shows mentally retarded, cerebral palsied, dysmelia, deaf-blind, and emotionally disturbed deaf children in Sweden, Germany, the Netherlands, and England.

  Parents' Education Programs
  Producer: USDHEW
  30 minutes, 16mm film, optical sound, color.
  Illustrates formal and informal programs for parents of young hearing impaired children. The overview presents issues in family dynamics and parent-child communication and language development.

---

*Complete addresses are given in the Appendix.

UNIT FIVE

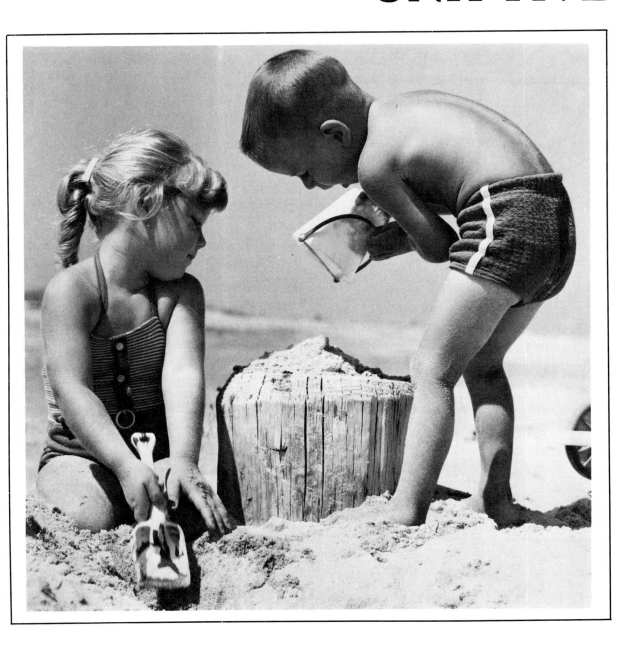

THE
PRESCHOOL
CHILD

THE PRESCHOOL CHILD

Behold the Child among his new-born blisses,
A six years' darling of a pigmy size!
See, where 'mid work of his own hand he lies,
Fretted by sallies of his mother's kisses,
With light upon him from his father's eyes!

William Wordsworth (1770–1850): *Ode on
Intimations of Immortality from
Recollections of Early Childhood* (11. 85–89) Verse VII

Chapter Nineteen

THE NORMAL PRESCHOOL CHILD: HIS GROWTH, DEVELOPMENT, AND CARE

During the last decade one of the most striking societal changes has been the great increase in options available to people in all phases of life. This is particularly true of parenthood; a couple can decide to a large extent if and when they will have one or more natural children or if they will seek to adopt a child.

The arrival of a child or children markedly alters the nature of a couple's marital relations. Children impinge on the time parents have for companionship and for shared leisure with each other. Children also impinge on the sex life of their parents; however, this conflict between the sexual needs of the parents and the selflessness often required of them as parents of young children cannot be avoided. Unless an adequate resolution can be found to this dilemma, parents may become the victims of frustration and guilt.

During the preschool period parents must face the fact that their child is entering increasingly into the activities of the outside world. They then must enter into their own stage of development of learning to separate themselves gradually from their growing child. They must make decisions as to how much free expression and initiative to permit the child, at the same time setting certain limits on his behavior.

OVERVIEW OF EMOTIONAL DEVELOPMENT

The preschool child, having learned to trust others and to know that he is a person in his own right, is ready to find out what he can do. He must learn certain things in order to become the kind of person he wants to be. He watches adults and attempts to imitate their behavior. He longs for the time when he can fully share in their activities.

The preschool child is imaginative and creative. Since he cannot really participate in the adult world, he pretends that he can. The simplest equipment may represent articles used in real life. For instance, a series of wooden boxes or blocks can become a train, or a few small cardboard boxes can furnish a doll's house, the boxes becoming a bed, a chest of drawers, a chair and a table.

The child learns quickly that different materials are suited to specific purposes. He understands language well enough to communicate through speech. This increases his ability to learn from the experiences of others and to understand much that he has not personally experienced. He questions others almost constantly, asking about the world, its people, and their activities. He may become loud and persistent in his questioning and at times annoying. He is searching for explanations of the phenomena in his environment, which to him are problems of causation and function which must be solved in order to do what he wants and get what he wants without adult help.

The preschool child is as vigorous in physical activity as in intellectual explorations. He moves freely and violently. He may attack others on purpose or by accident during play. He enjoys gross motor activity, but may also settle down to tasks which develop the finer muscular skills.

The infant and the toddler are guided in their activity largely by the direction of their parents, but the preschool child shows evidence of having a conscience of his own. The "still, small voice" within him guides him or passes judgment on his deeds. Experts state that children may now begin to feel guilty for their errors or wrongdoing or even for their thoughts. Their unrestricted thoughts and actions frighten them.

The central problem for the preschool child is to learn about the world and other people. He must also learn to assert his own will in such a way that he will not feel too guilty. If he has the knowledge and the ability to solve this problem, he will develop a *sense of initiative* comfortably controlled by conscience. If he fails to solve this problem, he will emerge from this period feeling overwhelmed and with a *sense of guilt*.

Preschool children may feel guilty because of plans they want to carry out, but may not because of parental disapproval, or because of thoughts or fantasies of which conscience disapproves.

If the child is to develop a sense of initiative and a healthy personality, his parents and other adults in his environment must encourage his plans and the use of his imagination. They must

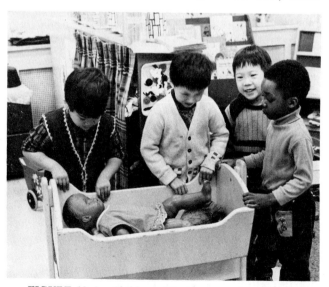

FIGURE 19–1. Children of both sexes enjoy imitating the activities of their parents. Here boys at a day-care center enjoy rocking a doll's cradle. This type of activity combats sex stereotyping. (Courtesy of Gene Maggio, The New York Times.)

limit punishment to those acts which are dangerous, morally wrong, or so socially unacceptable that the result would be unfortunate or harmful to the child or his family.

Preschool children look forward to becoming like their fathers or mothers. They learn adult roles from their parents, who serve as models for behavior. Children enjoy practicing these roles in their play. They begin gradually to learn how to cooperate with their peers and with adults and gain great pleasure from success in their attempts (see p. 629). Parents should encourage the child's efforts to cooperate and let him share in the decisions and responsibilities of family living. If he is denied this opportunity, if his imagination is curbed, and he is frustrated too often in his attempts at growing up, he becomes overanxious and spends too much time and energy in purposeless activity. Such children are apt to develop rigid consciences which exercise strong control over their behavior. At the same time they may feel resentment and bitterness toward the adults who restrict their normal behavior.

The child's sense of initiative must be encouraged throughout childhood and youth. If it is not, the good beginning may end in failure.

THE PRESCHOOL CHILD AND HIS FAMILY

The Family Romance: The Oedipal Period. During infancy and the toddler period children of both sexes tend to love, and to be more dependent upon, the mother, who cares for them most often, than on the father, who is usually not home during the day and may see little of his children except on weekends. Between the ages of three and six, termed the Oedipal period, a change occurs. The little girl becomes more interested in her father. The little boy, however, remains in love with his mother. This change in the love-object influences the children's behavior toward their parents and the role they assume in play. The girl is "Daddy's little girl" and assumes the role of wife and mother in her play. The boy becomes "Mommie's little boy." He gradually becomes more masculine in his play, taking his role from the pattern set by his father.

During this period the little girl may become possessive of her father and may be in competition with her mother for his love. The little boy may likewise become possessive of his mother and may compete with his father for her love. Children feel some aggression toward the parent of the same sex. Usually they keep their feelings hidden, but at times show their attitude in full force, as when they say to the parent of the same sex, "I hate you, go away!" Such feelings make the child feel guilty and anxious, and he may fear retaliation from the parent. The child feels even more conflict within himself, because at the same time that he hates he really loves the parent, though less than the parent of the opposite sex. This conflict of love and hate is also seen in the play of children between three and six years of age. Children love both parents because of the love and attention which parents normally give their children, irrespective of sex.

The parent of the same sex as the child provides a model for the child to imitate as he develops and matures. Parents must give their children much love and understanding during this period of conflict. The child, in order to continue to grow emotionally, must bury his sexual feelings toward the parent of the opposite sex in the unconscious and must identify himself with the parent of the same sex. By the end of this period the boy no longer wants to take his father's place; he simply wants to be like his father. The girl no longer wants to take her mother's place; she wants to grow up to be like mother. The child becomes friends with both parents, not regarding either one as a specific love-object. The *family* then becomes a meaningful love-object. The intensity of response to each member is decreased. The conflict has been resolved.

It is especially important at this stage that the parents be the kind of people that society accepts. If the parents are not acceptable according to society's standards, the child will learn attitudes and feelings which will later be a detriment to his development.

Unfortunately, some children do not make this shift in emotional attachment. The little boy may continue to love only his mother, and the little girl only her father. These children may not then be able to take the next steps in emotional development because of fixation at this preschool level. Such children may in later years need guidance to change this immature relation with their parents.

The Only Child and the Adopted Child. The only child is the object of parental relations in the home; attention is concentrated upon him. The only child of young parents is likely to fare better than one of older parents; he is more likely to have young cousins, and parental attention is less likely to be tinged with anxiety.

The first child is an only child until the second comes along. Young parents are more likely to be expecting a second child. Expectation of another child has somewhat the same influences as his actual presence would have, and the first child is not wholly treated as an only child. This is different from the attitude of older parents

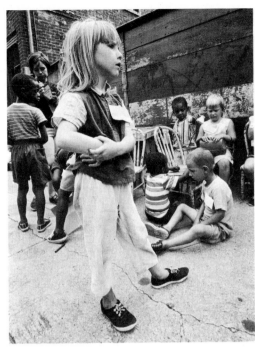

FIGURE 19-2. Without parental guidance the child will learn feelings and attitudes which may later be detrimental to optimum development. (Photograph by Lawrence V. Kanevsky.)

who over a period of years have longed for a child and cannot expect at their age to have other children.

All that has been said about an only child appears to be reinforced through the experience of the death of one or all of the other children.

What has been said of the only child is commonly true of the adopted child. He has in many cases been adopted after the death of a couple's own child or when they find that they are unable to have children. Many child-placing agencies will allow only one child to adoptive parents, since the demand for children to be adopted is greater than the number to be placed. (If twins or siblings are to be placed for adoption, it is customary to give them to parents who desire both children.) Agencies do have many children who are adoptable, but who, because of their being past the age that prospective parents want, because of a physical or emotional disability, or because they are of mixed racial parentage, are not chosen for adoption. Others in institutions are not adoptable because their parents will not give their legal consent to this procedure. The custom of giving adoptive parents only one child works to the detriment of the children, since the life of an only child, lacking contact with brothers and sisters, is not complete unless an effort is made to make it so.

Attendance at nursery school can help to accustom the only child to interacting with his peers.

It is generally considered best to tell the child that he is adopted before this status has any meaning for him. He accepts the parents' attitude that they want him and is satisfied. As he grows older he may feel that he is different from other children and may attribute discipline or punishment to the fact that he is an adopted child whom his parents do not love as they would their own natural child. The increasing number of adoptions during recent years makes the situation more commonplace and less emotionally charged.

Because of the population explosion during the last few decades much has been written about limitation of family size. Small families, whether the children are natural or adopted, can make increasing use of agencies for the purpose of preschool socialization and education in the future.

Effect of the Birth of a Sibling. *Any environmental change may have a traumatic effect on a child.* Even such a change as moving to a new house should be discussed with him. The birth of a sibling is a change of such magnitude that the child should become accustomed before the baby is born to the idea of no longer being an only child. The birth of another child unavoidably deprives the older child of some parental attention, and a child mistakes this for loss of affection. It is difficult for the toddler or child of nursery school age to accept the situation, for his love is still centered almost exclusively on his parents.

The child feels rejected and may become jealous. Infantile expression of jealousy is of two kinds. It may be shown *directly* in open dislike of the baby, or the child may appear to love the baby more than is normal. In so doing he is laying the foundation of a martyr attitude which may persist throughout life. He usually shows his hostility to the new baby openly and directly. He may make derogatory remarks about the baby. If his parents reprove him, he may feel guilty and may rationalize on the childish level. For instance, he may give as an excuse for hitting the baby the fact that the infant has taken his blanket, though the mother has given the blanket to the infant. Later, when the baby is old enough to take his toy, he grabs it back and says, "It's mine." When his mother intervenes, he sulks or hits the baby or her. Such displacement of his anger toward anyone who pets the baby is common.

The child's jealousy may be shown *indirectly* by clumsiness in his contacts with the infant. If his feeling of guilt is great and he is able to express his jealousy openly, he may drop the baby when given him to hold.

The child handles his hostility toward his

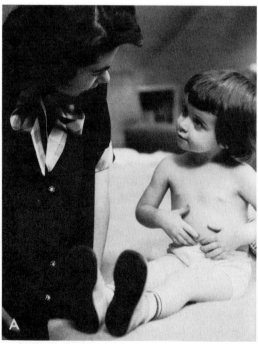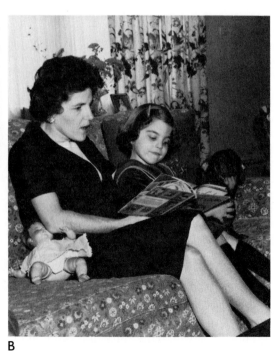

B

FIGURE 19–3. A new infant is coming. *A*, "When I get to be a lady, will I have a baby there too?" (Courtesy of George H. Padginton, Hamburg, New York, and *Baby Talk*, May 1967.) *B*, The child's mother explains to her the coming of the new sister or brother. The use of a book containing pictures of a young infant makes the event seem more real to the child.

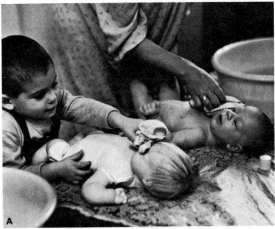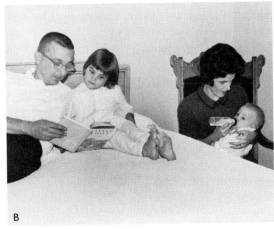

FIGURE 19–4. Ways to prevent possible jealousy of the new infant. A, The preschool child cares for his doll as his mother cares for the new infant. (Photographed by Erika and Bill Stone; courtesy of *Today's Health*, January 1964.) B, The father gives the older child attention while the mother feeds the infant.

mother in different ways. Direct actions against her include physical or verbal attack. On the other hand, he may refuse to have anything to do with her, ignoring her completely because she has brought the new baby home. He may displace his hostility toward her and be hostile to other adults, e.g., his nursery school or Sunday School teacher. He may regress and demand attention similar to that given the baby, refusing to drink from a cup, wanting his milk from a nursing bottle and soiling himself so that his mother must give him the same toilet care she gives "the baby." The mother should accept such temporary regression. If it is too long continued, however, it may be necessary to obtain professional help for the child. The child may repress any outward reaction, without solving his problem. This reaction may interfere with his successful handling of jealousy in later childhood or even throughout life.

Jealousy may begin when the older preschool child learns that the mother is pregnant, possibly during the fourth or fifth month of gestation. It is not wise to tell a young preschool child too early of the pregnancy, since he would have too long a wait before the child's birth. Before the birth of the baby the mother can control the child's jealousy to some extent by giving him as much attention as usual and stressing her pleasure in having him share in loving the coming baby. The baby's coming should be discussed with the child even though he is too young to understand the changes which the arrival of a new infant will make in the family life. Parents can encourage him to talk about his unborn sibling and either to verbalize or express in play his hostility toward the child.

It is a good plan to send the older child to nursery school (see p. 629) in order to develop outside contacts. He may be shown a child's picture book about the arrival of a new baby in the family to help him visualize what his mother means by all the preparations she is making for the coming of the infant.

Jealousy can be handled in a number of ways. A child who shows indications of wanting to hurt the infant is never left alone with him. A more positive measure is to give the child a pet or a doll so that he has something to care for, just as mother is caring for the baby. He may be encouraged to identify with his parents in lovingly protecting the infant.

All sexual questions should be answered frankly, explanation being adjusted to the child's vocabulary and ability to understand sexual processes. The mother may discuss with him the difference between his needs and those of the infant; this may be done in terms of his being more grown up than the baby. For instance, he can clean his teeth, whereas the baby has no teeth; he can walk, holding mother's hand, or run about and play, but the baby must be carried or go in his carriage. The mother can arrange to be alone with the child, or she and his father together with him, while the baby is sleeping in another room. If possible, the child may be with his father when the mother must care for the infant in the evening. Evidence of affection for the infant can be minimized in the presence of the older child.

NEEDS OF THE PRESCHOOL CHILD

The preschool child needs security and independence. He needs the security which comes with the knowledge that he has parents who are with him in the home. He needs their love and understanding. Within this circumscribed world of security and love he needs an opportunity to express his hostility and antagonisms. Because of his growing verbal ability he has increasingly less need to use physical expressions of hostility. As he grows he needs opportunities to assume more responsibility and independence. By expressing his hostility and his growing independence he learns what these feelings are like and how he can deal with them.

The child feels love and security when he has two parents with whom he has daily contact. The parents, besides showing love for him, must teach him and guide him toward maturity: (1) From verbal interaction with them he learns how to express himself so that he can communicate with others on a verbal level. (2) In the home he learns to assume more responsibility and be more independent. (3) He gains from them the knowledge he needs to grow up. Two important aspects of knowledge learned in this age period relate to sex and to religion. *More important than the facts he learns are the attitudes he forms toward this knowledge.*

The preschool child turns his interests to the outside world, to the why's and how's of living.

Guidance. There are few, if any, set rules for the guidance of preschool children, but the following suggestions may be helpful. *Limits to the child's behavior must be set and consistently maintained, thereby giving him a basis for prediction of the reactions of other people to what he does and thus making rational behavior possible.*

Limits set by parents give him a feeling of security which he does not have when he is allowed to decide for himself on matters beyond his ability to decide wisely. Suggestions—not commands—helpful to the child in achieving what he wants at the time, or in forming good relations with other people, are made in positive form. Commands are seldom necessary, but when given in positive rather than negative form are more effective. The child is not spoken to in such a way that he feels guilty or fearful. Rather he is reassured by the sense that his parents are helping him solve problems as they come up in his activities and social relations. A choice of actions may be given him only when he actually may decide which of two or more lines of behavior he may take. A child does not always understand that redirection of his activities is consistent with his own interests. He learns this gradually by experience with the satisfying results which follow parental redirection. He is encouraged to do as much as possible for himself so that he can grow in independence.

Adults should not make the mistake of playing *for* the child. Instead, he is helped to enjoy his own activities. For instance, adults should not make art models for him to copy. He is allowed freely to create his own work. Help is provided whenever necessary, however; this is an important element in his feeling secure in his parents' protecting love. Children live in the present, and suggestion, to be truly helpful, should be provided and reinforced at appropriate times.

DEVELOPMENT OF SEXUALITY IN THE PRESCHOOL CHILD

At the beginning of the preschool period the child has, to a large extent, gained control of his excretory functions and, therefore, is ready to progress from the anal period to the next level of development, the *Oedipal period.* The child's self-concept as a girl or a boy is probably completed also at the beginning of the preschool period.

The Oedipal period was discussed initially as part of the emotional development of the child earlier in this chapter (see p. 604). Although some parents do not recognize the significance of this period, it is the most turbulent period of childhood psychosexual development. Erotic interest in the parent of the opposite sex may range from barely noticeable infatuation to intense erotic impulses and fantasies. At the same time, the child clings to his convictions that there is no physical intimacy between his parents.

As a result of the attachment to the parent of the opposite sex, there is usually some subsurface rivalry. Feelings of guilt may occur, and the child may fear that his rival will punish him for his intense feelings. The normal child may also have *ambivalent feelings* toward the parent of the same sex, because while he loves the parent of the opposite sex, he is also dependent on and loves the parent of the same sex. Thus feelings of love and hate are felt simultaneously toward both parents.

The principal source of sensuous pleasure during this period is the genitalia (i.e., the penis or the vulva). At this time the boy may have fearful fantasies of retaliation by the father in the form of mutilation of his penis, even though in reality no actual hostility has been shown toward him. The girl, in whom the conflict is less intense, may imagine that the mother will retaliate against her.

Under normal circumstances, this competitive sexual conflict is ended by a moderately rapid lysis. The boy perceives that Mother belongs to Father and that when he grows up he will be like Father and find a mate for himself. The girl, going through a similar process, realizes that if she grows up to be like Mother, whom she now wishes to emulate, she will find a husband of her own like Father.

The Oedipus situation had been thought a normal and necessary stage in every child's development. More recent views, however, believe that it is not a universal phenomenon but is subject to and may vary with, social and cultural circumstances.

Sensuous interest becomes centered in the genitalia a little before or after the age of two and a half years. The child has vaguely pleasurable sensations as he discovers and explores this part of his body. The child becomes curious about the presence or lack of a penis in himself and other children. Masturbation of a rather casual nature becomes not too uncommon a behavior for the next few years in children of both sexes.

During the Oedipal period the child progresses from a zone-centered autoeroticism to his first total love object, himself (narcissism). The child becomes fascinated by his reflection in a mirror. The little girl enjoys exhibiting her pretty clothing. Both sexes begin to develop modesty about their own bodies. Narcissism continues to be present to a varying extent, existing along with other object relationships, probably throughout life.

MASTURBATION

Parents find it hard to accept masturbation as an almost universal experience in young children. The infant soon discovers that a pleasant sensation accompanies handling of the genitalia, which has no other significance to him and of course is not accompanied by fantasies (see p. 337). In the preschool child, masturbation may be increased and is commonly accompanied by fantasies. Masturbation is utilized in adolescence to fulfill sexual urges which in our culture generally do not have socially approved release in heterosexual intercourse outside of marriage. It may have a useful part in the ultimate attainment of heterosexual expression of the sex urge.

The child who masturbates excessively for his stage of maturation should not be punished. Rather, he can be helped to work out the problem which is causing him to masturbate more than is normal. The child who has discovered the pleasure derived from masturbation should be given ample opportunity to find other more socially acceptable pleasures outside his body.

Sex education does not solve the problem of masturbation. It does help the child, however, to understand his pleasure in the practice and to understand that the true function of the sexual organs is reproduction.

Although we should not scold the child for masturbating, the habit, if excessive, may keep him from other pleasures which are necessary for optimum growth and development in childhood. Like any pleasure which is practiced in solitude, it interferes with social interaction. If masturbation is excessive, it may become so fixed a habit that it interferes with the normal desire for heterosexual intercourse within marriage.

Poor handling of the problem of masturbation in the preschool child is likely to result in fixation at the autoerotic level, wherein the child seeks pleasure in himself rather than in relations with others.

Parents should be told that masturbation does not produce nervous diseases or weaken the mind or organs of reproduction, but that parental condemnation of the practice in the child may induce lasting psychologic and emotional harm.

Two important aspects of the problem are kept in mind. Masturbation focuses feeling in the genital region. This feeling is necessary for the healthy functioning of men and women. Shame and the threats related to this activity can force children to repress sexual feelings. This might eventuate in impotence in the male and frigidity in the female. Both conditions tend to unhappiness in marriage and to increased susceptibility to mental illness.

The important fact to remember about excessive masturbation in preschool children is that it is a symptom of poor mental hygiene and is not a pathologic process in itself.

There is no one way of helping the child to overcome his tendency to excessive masturbation. He can be assured that he is safe in his parents' affection and should not be afraid or ashamed. Threats or punishment increase his fears. He can be given opportunity for happy relations with playmates and sufficient toys to play with. His parents should be particularly careful to answer all his questions about sex, adapting their answers to his level of understanding.

OBSERVATION OF THE PRIMAL SCENE

Parents vary in their needs for privacy during sexual intercourse, depending on their sociocultural backgrounds and their personal values. Some men and women fear that they will be heard by their children during this act.

The infant or very small child can be fairly well confined to his crib when parents wish to be alone. When a child learns to climb out of his crib, however, he presents a new threat to the privacy of his parents. A child must thus learn that when his parents' bedroom door is closed, they wish to be by themselves.

But, some children are curious and do witness the primal scene. This single event may have no effect on the child if the emotional climate of the family is healthy and there are opportunities for an open exchange between family members.

Because the child may pretend at this age that sex does not exist between his parents, he may become intrigued but frightened by what he observes. He knows that he should not be a witness and is afraid of being apprehended and possibly punished. The child may view the sex act as a struggle between his parents, as if one parent were being physically attacked. The child of this age is neither emotionally nor intellectually prepared for viewing the primal scene.

The actual future effect on the child varies according to his culture, his family circumstances, and his developmental status. In some cultures such events are considered the norm in family life. The individual family climate often contributes more to its potential traumatic significance than the fact of the exposure itself. If aggression or even violence exists within the family, this reinforces the readiness of the young child to interpret sex as a violent interaction. If, on the other hand, love and understanding are the usual modes of interaction among family members, a similar interpretation may be placed on this event. In a rigid, inhibited household in which sexual knowledge and curiosity are stifled, a child's sexual feelings and experience have a greater potential for resulting in anxiety and guilt.

The child's developmental status is also important in determining his reaction to viewing the primal scene. During infancy, observation of parental intercourse may have no effect on a baby. During the preschool years, however, when his sexual interest has increased, the child may be disturbed by the event.

Following such an observation parents should react in a calm, gentle, and understanding way. They should not frighten the child further by scolding or threatening him. Communication patterns must be stimulated within the family and questions must be answered honestly so that healthy family relationships can help to develop in the child a realistic and full concept of sexuality.

Sex Information. The child who learns to trust others and to give as well as receive love has already begun his preparation for a satisfactory marriage and rearing children of his own.

Sex education during the preschool years contributes specific knowledge which the child wants to know and also helps him build desirable attitudes toward this aspect of life. This is especially true when parents love and respect each other and so set a good example for the child to follow. In such a family the child learns that he or she is a boy or a girl and that each sex has its own role to play in life. The attitudes and feelings which children acquire greatly influence their relations with marital partners and with their own children later. It is essential that the child understand that sex is important to his own personality as well as to that of others.

Although the extent and method of sex education must be fitted to the child's needs, certain general principles are applicable to the sex education of all children. Children are likely to ask simple questions about sex by the time they are three to four years of age, although some may not ask until they are six years old. There are individual differences, of course, depending on factors in the child's environment and degree of maturation. *Information on sex should be given in response to the child's interest in the subject, but never as facts which have no connection with the family life.* In general the child is old enough for correct though simplified answers when he is sufficiently mature to ask questions.

Sex information may be given at home, church, or school. The best source of information are sincere and loving parents who feel comfortable in talking about sex. If for some reason this is impossible, the school or church may give the information. Information acquired from acquaintances unfortunately is likely not only to be incorrect but also to give the child a distorted attitude to the whole subject of sexual relations.

Parents should answer the child directly and honestly, basing the amount of information given and the phraseology used on the child's physiologic and developmental level. Information should be given promptly when the question is asked. It is not good to tell more about the subject than is involved in the answer to the question. *The information should be given frankly and unemotionally.* The child will grasp his parents' attitude toward sex more than their answers, and this will free him from worry and preoccupation with sexual problems.

Some questions which preschool children ask concern the birth of a child. They commonly ask, "Where do babies come from?" because curiosity is natural to this age group and because conditions pertaining to sex are obvious in the social life about them. After the child has learned that the infant grows within the mother's abdomen, he may ask, "How does it fit inside there?" or, "Can't he move?" The child sees pregnant women, and mass media treat the subject of sex openly. Household pets deliver their young, and rural children learn early of reproduction in farm animals. When the child asks where babies come from and other questions, he can be helped to clarify his fantasies. If his questions are answered frankly and with a positive attitude of acceptance of his interest in the matter, he will receive the information without shame or anxiety. During the preschool period, emphasis is placed on the physical aspects of sex. The preschool child is too young to understand moral implications, other than the value of doing what his parents ask of him.

In the hospital children many times will ask nurses questions similar to those they ask their parents at home. The same principles just discussed apply in answering such questions; however, if the mother is present, the nurse can discuss the matter with her and have her answer the question. The nurse may answer questions, knowing that the mother understands what is told to her child.

Many of the problems which beset adolescents arise because they dwell on sex and have fantasies about many aspects of sexuality. If answers had been given during the preschool period and enlarged upon as the child grew older, there would be less danger of such turmoil during adolescence.

MENTAL DEVELOPMENT

The *preoperational stage* (two to seven years) began during the toddler period and is completed during the early school years. During this period the child progresses from the sensorimotor stage to the symbolic and conceptual plane. Rather than being guided by sensory and motor events, behavior comes to be guided by mental representations and internalized thoughts. Symbolism enables the child to do more things faster and handle more events in his life than he could before. However, he still does not have what is known as "intelligent" behavior.

Symbolism. With symbolism, a mental event can stand for something in the real world. In symbolic play a piece of wood can represent a car, indicating that the child has an internal representation of what an actual car looks like. Also, the child can repeat an event in play that occurred many hours or days before, showing that there was something in his mind representing the event. This kind of deferred imitation is seen increasingly during the preoperational stage.

Reasoning and Causality. The preschool child cannot do true inductive or deductive reasoning. He tries to reason to explain a causal relationship but fails in his attempt. He has a primitive type of reasoning termed *syncretism* in which he relates several ideas in one confused global mass. Any one idea can be used as a cause for any other element, since they are seen as a global unit. The preschool child may seem to be reasoning, but he is only using a learned association between two events. For example, the child may say, "The sun is shining and the flowers are blooming." In this statement the child really does not understand the causal relationship involved. The child may use another type of reasoning in which his egocentricity is shown. He may say, "This is Thursday because my Mommy takes me to the store on Thursday and I want to go to the store." A faulty conclusion is reached because of the child's wish. *Juxtaposition* is another type of reasoning, in which the child states isolated ideas but makes no effort to determine the cause or links between them. In *transductive reasoning* the child goes from one particular idea to another and reaches a faulty conclusion. For example, a child may say, "It isn't morning because I didn't eat breakfast." Children, however, can reach correct conclusions at times despite their faulty reasoning.

Rules and Moral Development. During the early preoperational stage the child cannot understand rules well. If he plays a game, he makes up the rules and changes them at will because he wants to win. After he does understand the rules, he considers that they are right and cannot be changed. During the later preoperational stage the child learns *moral realism*, in which, for example, he considers that a child who breaks one dish on purpose is not as bad as a child who breaks six dishes accidentally. He believes that breaking one dish is bad, so breaking more must be worse. Not until the end of the *concrete operational period* (7 to 11 years) does the child develop *subjective morality*, by which he begins to think of the intent of the behavior as a way of arriving at moral judgments. Thus the child learns to focus on more than one aspect of a situation. He also learns that other people have motives for what they do and that rules can vary according to the situation.

Concepts of the World. The child in the preoperational stage expresses his ideas about natural events in terms of his three beliefs: (1) *Animism*. He believes that objects such as stars and flowers not only have a life of their own but also have feelings and motives. (2) *Realism*. The child is confused by the physical and psychologic realities of events and believes in the physical reality of psychologic events. For example, when a child dreams he may tell his parents upon awakening, "A horse stepped on me in my crib." (3) *Artificialism*. The young child believes that everything that happens and all objects in his environment are there for the purpose of satisfying human needs. This can be seen in statements such as, "The chair is there because people want to sit down," or "The sun shines because children want to play."

Language Development. The preschool child uses language in a symbolic way. He not only imitates sounds during this stage but he also uses words to represent things. At first, words are utilized in an egocentric way through the use of the *monologue,* in which the child is not trying to communicate with another person. He talks while he plays. The *collective monologue* is like the monologue but occurs when two or more children are playing, as in parallel play. They are spatially close to each other, each talking to himself but not really communicating with each other. At the end of the preoperational period language does become truly socialized and communicative.

Learning Language. The preschool child learns to communicate his feelings and ideas through language in a more precise form than he did as a toddler. He constantly asks questions and learns about the outside world by seeking the meaning of what he experiences through sensory stimulation. He asks how, why, what, when, and where about everything which interests him.

During the preschool period he uses progressively longer and more complex sentences. This is a period of rapid vocabulary growth. Between the ages of two and six years the child learns about 600 words a year, chiefly through the answers given by adults to his questions. He also learns by imitating adults and other children with whom he associates. He may acquire words which his parents do not want him to use, such as ungrammatical terms ("ain't"), slang, or so-called bad words. Usually if adults in his environment ignore unacceptable words and do not give him attention when he uses them, he will cease to use them in his conversation.

An analysis of a child's questions shows his need for information, for relief from anxiety and for attention. Answers to his questions give him increased understanding of his environment and of what is going on about him, as well as a secure feeling that adults can and will help him to learn. Through answers to his questions the child gets not only factual knowledge but also a concept of adult attitudes and feelings about the topics discussed.

The questions of three-year-olds are rather simple when compared with those of four- and five-year-olds, who want to know how things function. These latter questions require more detailed explanations which adults at times may

not be prepared to give. *All adults should remember the guiding principle about answering questions of children and youths: tell the truth to the best of your ability.* If a lie is told, the child will lose his sense of trust in the individual, and his trust in all others may be weakened. *The answer should be in terms of the child's level of understanding.* If an adult does not know the answer, he should tell the child so. Then adult and child are ready to seek the answer together.

SUMMARY OF THE PREOPERATIONAL STAGE

The child in the preoperational stage has limited functioning. Because of his egocentricity he is unable to criticize himself. He believes that he has the best possible views and ideas. Since he cannot appreciate the ideas of others, he cannot make new accommodations. The child shapes his world according to his own needs; he does not shape his behavior according to the demands of reality. As he grows, however, environmental pressures will create a need for him to adapt, and he will be lead to make new accommodations.

Because of *centration or centering,* the preoperational child can only focus on limited aspects of his environment. He cannot view all aspects of situations or objects since he can perceive only the outstanding characteristics of stimuli.

The preschool child also is *unable to trace a process backwards,* that is, he cannot conceptualize that a completed process can be performed in reverse order so that the substances involved are returned to their original state. For example, if the child is shown two round balls of equal size of Silly Putty and he agrees that they are the same size, and then one is flattened, he cannot understand that an equal amount of clay is still in each mass. Because of this inability, his thinking is inflexible and rigid.

The preoperational child can use language and has a memory, and thus he can increasingly understand the meaning of the past, present, and future. He is still, however, not intellectually capable of understanding the basic relationships between and among phenomena.

Religious Development. Close parent-child relations normally extend through the years during which the child is socialized. The greatest influence in a child's life is his parents' attitude about such basic aspects of life as religion, sex, love of country, economic systems, and education. In answering questions parents must be genuine, understanding, objective, and kind, particularly in regard to religion, since faith as well as science is involved.

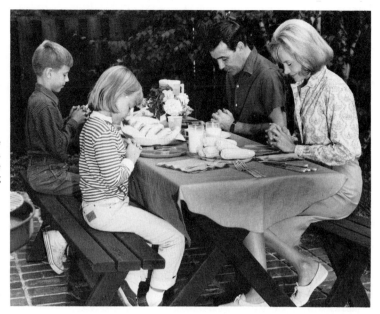

FIGURE 19–5. In a genuinely religious home the spiritual atmosphere pervades all of living. Children learn more by example than from mere verbal explanations. (Courtesy of H. Armstrong Roberts.)

A few general principles pertaining to religious educaton may be given. *A child cannot be kept spiritually neutral.* Whatever his parents may desire, he hears about religion from other children, and he sees churches and pictures of religious objects.

Whatever the parents tell the child about religion has the same force as does information on other subjects. Yet the child observes what his parents do, and if their actions are not in accord with what they teach him, he is quick to notice it.

There are two general methods of religious education: that of indoctrination and that of letting the child follow the religion of his choice. Both methods have many adherents. Neither, taken alone, meets the real issue. The preschool child does not follow any religion because he understands it. Rather, he accepts religion because it is expected of him, because someone he loves influences him to do so, or because it offers some other concomitant pleasures.

Suggestions for religious training in the home include early training in the faith held by the parents. The preschool child is old enough to go to Sunday School. Religion can be made attractive but not forced upon him. He can be taught that God is within our lives, that God loves him. Parents should not give the child the impression that they are condescending to his level when speaking of religion; the discussion can be a shared experience between parents and child. As the child grows up he learns about religions other than that held by his parents.

Religious training in the hospital is difficult, since the child's questions must be answered only by persons of the same faith as his parents.

This avoids confusion of ideas in the child's mind. Furthermore, what the child is told may be a matter of extreme importance to the parents, since the child is not able to think through conflicting statements about religion.

Religious holidays raise many questions in a child's mind. The following explanation of the significance of Christmas may be given unless the policy of the hospital prohibits discussion of the religious concepts involved. The questions most commonly asked are only indirectly of a religious nature.

There is the old question, "Is there *really* a

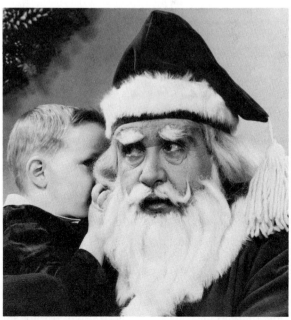

FIGURE 19–6. A young child confides in Santa. (H. Armstrong Roberts.)

Santa Claus?" The answer to be given to a very young child is usually, "Yes." He is too young to understand abstract ideas, and Santa stands for the spirit of Christmas. When the child really begins to question this belief, he is already doubting its truth. He should be allowed to discuss his own ideas on the matter. If he actually doubts whether there is a Santa Claus, he is ready for an explanation of what Santa Claus stands for. He may be told that the spirit of Christmas is that of good will. It is a time to make others happy as Santa Claus made him happy on Christmas Day last year and the year before, as far back as he can remember. The origin of Christmas can be told him, and its religious significance, which he probably already knows if his parents are of the Christian faith. Customs which have developed around the celebration of Christmas in different countries will interest him.

The myth of the Easter Bunny can be explained with similar adaptations.

LIFE PERSPECTIVE

The preschool child has developed some understanding of the meaning of the past, the present, and the future. He can repeat events in play that occurred days before; he knows what he is doing in the present; and he realizes that when the present moment is past there will be more moments coming. But his deep appreciation and understanding of time and what will happen to him in the future are still vague. The ideas of a personal future and ultimate death are not comprehensible to a preschool child; therefore, he cannot yet really form a life perspective.

ANXIETY IN THE PRESCHOOL CHILD

Problems which may cause anxiety and tension in the preschool child may come from within or may arise from his environment. They may be due to lack of satisfaction of a need or to an increase in the number and intensity of the child's fears. His response to the problem is to mobilize defenses to deal with the dangers.

Specific Causes. Several causes of anxiety are common during the preschool period. The child may fear being deserted by his parents, that they no longer love him or that he is being punished for misdeeds or for thoughts which he should not have had. He has a great fear of physical injury.

These specific causes are intensified by the peculiar combination of anxiety-producing circumstances which occur during hospitalization. The main causes of anxiety are separation from his parents and fear of pain.

LOSS OF PARENTAL LOVE. To a preschool child parental love is manifested in his daily life with his parents. Separation from his parents means loss of their love. Hospitalization is for most children only a temporary separation from their parents. Long-term or permanent separation must now be considered.

LOSS OF ONE PARENT. A child may be temporarily separated from his father for business or patriotic reasons. He remains with his mother, who builds up in the child a happy expectation of his father's return. If the father is absent for a long time, good parent-child relations may be difficult to establish.

The child who has lost a parent by death or divorce does not live in a complete home. If the parent has died, there is not the same degree of anxiety which is likely to trouble a child of divorced parents.

Much has been written in recent years concerning the effect of divorce on the children. Actually, if the parents remain together "only for the sake of the children," it may be better for the long-term emotional security of the children that they separate if their differences cannot be resolved. Divorce is generally preceded by a period of unsettled life in which the child may be urged by each parent to love him or her only and to be hostile to the other parent. Generally the court gives the child to the mother, but after the divorce the child may visit his father at times prescribed by the court. The child of divorced parents is confused by the antagonism of each parent toward the other and yet the love of each for him. Of course the child who is loved by only one parent or by neither is deprived of the parental affection which is a child's birthright.

When a boy of preschool age lacks close association with his father, he lacks a male in the home with whom he can identify, against whom he can be aggressive, and from whom he can learn about the role of a man in the home, community, or country. The boy may become a substitute love-object to his mother for her absent husband. He may develop a feminine outlook on life and never learn the typical masculine technique of competition or aggression.

The effect upon the boy of absence of his mother is generally less serious than that due to his father's absence because there is usually a mother-substitute in the home, e.g., a grandmother, aunt, or housekeeper. The boy of preschool age may regress after his mother has left home until he adjusts to her substitute. He may be deeply hurt by his mother's leaving him when he loves her so dearly and may fear loving

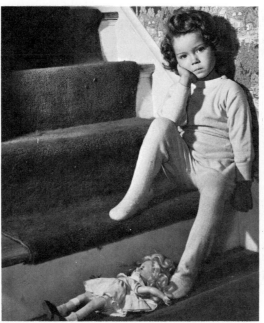 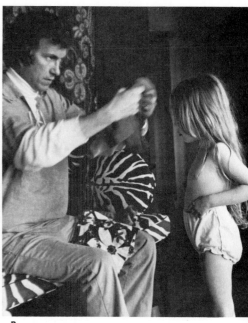

FIGURE 19–7. *A*, A child grieves when her parent has gone away. This overwhelming feeling of loneliness is difficult for her to handle. (H. Armstrong Roberts.) *B*, Men have become more attuned to their nurturing promptings and can therefore assume the responsibility for child care as necessary or desired. (From McBride, A. B.: *Am. J. Nursing*, 75:1653, October 1975.)

A B

a woman who takes her place in the home, lest he be hurt again if she leaves.

The effect upon the girl of absence of the mother is essentially the same as that of absence of the father upon a boy. She will have no one with whom to compete for the father's love, and until a mother-substitute is found she will have no woman with whom she can identify and from whom she can learn the feminine role in life. She may develop a masculine outlook on family and community life.

The effect upon the girl of absence of the father is essentially the same as that of absence of the mother upon the boy. She may become too closely attached to the mother, and also may become afraid of loving a man again and being hurt by his loss. This feeling, if carried over into adolescence, interferes with normal courtship and marriage.

In a situation in which one parent can care for the child, he or she may be assisted by a family member or by the utilization of a homemaker service, or by having the child cared for in a child care center or day nursery or nursery school for part of the day.

Since the upswing in the incidence of communal living in recent years, children have been reared in a new kind of extended family, not one in which different generations live together, but one in which several young adults of the same generation live in the same house. The long-term effects of this living arrangement on the children in the "family" are not yet known.

Homemaker Service. Homemaker services are available in an increasing number of communities in the United States. Homemakers as individuals must be adaptable, reliable, and mature and trained in the field of home management skills and child care.

A homemaker can fulfill an important need in the life of a child who is to continue to live in his own home. Not only can the homemaker care for the child who has lost one parent through death or divorce, but can also provide care for the child who may have two living parents, but whose mother may be ill temporarily or recovering from childbirth, or may be providing care for another seriously ill child. A homemaker could thus help to keep the home together during a period of stress and thus prevent further emotional damage to the child.

Day-Care Centers and Day Nurseries. The Social Security Act of 1935 authorized a program to help each state establish or strengthen public child welfare services for the protection of children. The Public Welfare Amendments of 1962 stated that child welfare services were those public services which supplemented or substituted for parental care and included care of children in foster homes, day-care centers, or other child-care facilities.

Child-care centers and day nurseries are facilities which provide care for children in the absence of their parents. In these centers or day nurseries children whose mothers must be employed outside the home are provided with food, rest, and recreation during the daytime hours. Since many children needing this sort of care come from deprived homes, they may also need intellectual stimulation and cultural enrichment. Thus some sort of program is provided to meet these needs.

Nursery Schools. Nursery schools, on the other hand, are for the primary purpose of educating children on the prekindergarten level. They may be operated for a few hours each day because young children cannot profit from a situation the purpose of which is structured learning for a longer period of time. Nevertheless some nursery schools are extending their periods of service for those who need it (see p. 629).

(see p. 629).

Facilities for care of children are inspected and licensed by state law. Although they must meet certain standards for sanitation facilities, area of space, and equipment for cleanliness, play, and rest, among other requirements, parents should inspect the facility they plan to use in order to determine whether it will be suitable for their particular children. Most parents also like to meet the adults who will be caring for their children and to determine their ability to provide physical care and guidance for them in their absence.

LOSS OF BOTH PARENTS. Separation of a child from both parents has all the effects of the loss of a single parent. The trauma to the child is extreme, and he goes through a period of mourning. Since the child is less verbal than the adult, his feelings must be judged from nonverbal behavior. He may show physical symptoms such as vomiting and diarrhea, or a return to more infantile behavior. For instance, although he is toilet-trained, he may soil himself. He may be uncooperative and naughty.

COUNSELING A CHILD WHO HAS EXPERIENCED PARENTAL LOSS. The experience of losing a loved person during one's lifetime is a universal phenomenon. Following such a loss, grief and bereavement are normal responses. No one can be certain about the age at which a child can begin to master the loss of a parent whether through divorce or death. It is true, however, that future physical and psychologic problems may stem from poorly managed grief at any age.

According to family systems theory, when one part of the system or family is affected by an event, the other parts are also affected in some way. The loss of a parent affects not only the spouse but the children, grandparents, and everyone else in the family in some way.

The young child has fears and fantasies of loss. To the child who has not yet developed a concept of object constancy, even periods of brief separation may cause unbearable anxiety. The child ultimately learns that his parents are permanent and that they have an independent existence apart from himself. Thus, when a parent is permanently lost for whatever reason, the child goes through separation anxiety.

Many variables determine a child's response to parental loss: the sex and age of the child, his level of emotional maturity, the sex of the lost parent, relationships with the departed parent and with the remaining parent, the factors surrounding the loss, the presence of siblings, and his reactions to previous experiences of loss. The ways children view death at various ages are also significant and were discussed on pages 107 to 109. The methods by which other family members cope with loss are also important to the child.

Children do not often express their grief verbally. They displace their feelings on an external situation so that they do not have to deal directly with their internal conflict. Sometimes children appear to accept the death lightly and to go on to other endeavors without the sadness one expects in a more mature response. However, the child does experience grief. This depression may be shown as withdrawal, acting out, or regressive behavior in interactions with others.

Before counseling a child who has experienced parental loss or another surviving family member, the nurse should recognize his or her personal attitudes and feelings regarding grief, loss, and mourning and be able to accept feelings of guilt, anger, and sadness as normal expressions of grief. In order to be effective in this role, the nurse must also have an understanding of the levels of growth and development and a knowledge of loss and mourning. The nurse can assist in a real way by sharing knowledge of community resources that can be of some benefit to the bereaved.

Everyone working with children should know how to help a child who has been separated from one or both parents. No adult should scold or punish a child for his response to parental loss no matter what form it takes. The child is treated with kindness and helped to express his feelings. He is encouraged to talk about the parent (or parents) who has gone away. Preschool children may feel that they have caused the death or departure of the parent of the same sex because they wished him or her to leave and be out of the way. The child must be helped to understand that his wish was not the same thing as a deed of violence against the parent.

Substitute parents should be provided as soon as possible for children who have lost both parents, and should make every effort to win the children's love and confidence. Some children may need psychologic help if the trauma has been too great for them to accept.

If by death or divorce of his parents a child is without a home and there is no other relative to care for him, he will probably be placed by the court in an institution or a foster home, and later, if possible, into an adoptive home.

Institutional Care. The kind of foundling home or orphanage (see p. 5) where many children were crowded together permanently in a situation in which they were not likely to thrive no longer exists in the United States. Today shelters are provided temporarily until foster home care or adoption can be arranged for children having no parents, or homemaker service, day-care center, or day nursery facilities can be arranged for those having one parent. Unfortunately, however, some of the temporary shelters into which children are placed are overcrowded because of the numbers of children needing such care and the length of time necessary to make appropriate plans for placement. Also, some children are kept in institutions because society is unwilling to terminate parental rights even in those instances in which it is obvious that living parents will never take responsibility for the child. Such parents abandon their children, yet because they retain legal control over them the children cannot be adopted and thus cannot gain a measure of happiness from living with adoptive parents who would love them.

Institutions for the temporary care of children are usually organized on the basis of small groups, each group being cared for by "substitute parents." These children are dressed like their peers living in the area, and an attempt is made to provide a homelike atmosphere for them Healthy infants are usually not kept in an institution unless a foster home or an adoptive home cannot be provided.

Foster Home Care. An institution, no matter how well organized, cannot meet the needs of a child as well as good foster parents can. Good foster parents must have a real love for children, must be sensitive to their needs and must have the maturity necessary to let them go from their home when they are to be adopted. Unfortunately, not all foster parents are of this type, and so children may be moved from one foster home to another repeatedly thus preventing them from developing the sense of security they so desperately need. The social worker of a child-placing agency may be the only adult with whom the child establishes a satisfying and continuing relation throughout a childhood spent in institutions or foster homes.

Foster homes must be inspected and licensed in the state in which they are located. They are inspected for cleanliness, sanitation, and adequacy of space among other requirements.

Adoptions. There is a dearth of children available for adoption today, especially the ones most young couples want, the blond, blue-eyed or the dark-haired, brown-eyed, healthy infants may be in short supply. The other children, discussed previously (see p. 360), are indeed the unfortunate victims of circumstances beyond their control.

Nurses who care for infants and children who are to be adopted must remember that, professionally, they are not at liberty to divulge any information either about the biological parents of the child or about the adopting parents, if they are known. If an adoption is handled carefully, an adopted child may have the same love relations with his parents which a child under normal circumstances has with his natural parents.

Children should be adopted through an official adoption agency, rather than independently through a physician or a "friend." These agencies have certain placement practices which deal with the adopting parents and the physical and emotional condition of the child, practices which help to assure a successful adoption.

ANXIETY FROM CAUSES OTHER THAN LOSS OF PARENTAL LOVE. *Conscience anxiety,* in which the child feels that he has done something wrong and expects punishment, is prevalent among children of overparticular or strict parents. The bugbear of the modern child is the person who will punish him if he is naughty.

A common and almost unavoidable kind of *anxiety* is that *arising out of inconsistency* in the do's and don'ts of parents and parental actions. This difficulty is increased when the parents do not lead the kind of life which they teach the child that he must lead. During wartime, for instance, children are taught to sublimate their destructive feelings and direct them to positive ends, and yet they are given toy weapons with which to play soldier. The children are too immature to understand the difference between personal aggression and that prompted by love of country and group morale. This is a great difficulty in the training of little children during a period of national stress.

Infectious anxiety is acquired from an adult, generally the mother. If the mother is relatively free from overt anxiety under severe circumstances, the child also is apt to be free. But if the mother is overanxious even in commonly accepted situations, the child is also likely to be anxious. This sort of anxiety is often seen in hospitalized children. If the mother is anxious about the child, he will be anxious about himself. This is one reason why the nurse should make the mother comfortable and secure about the hospitalizaton of the child.

Real or *objective anxiety* or *fear* is dependent upon the child's ability to understand the nature of the danger which threatens him. Fear of lightning is a needless fear due to the child's not understanding the cause of the lightning. In contrast, a child's fear of needles is gained from experience; he knows that they cause him pain.

Objective fears must be managed with consideration of the preschool child's stage of maturation. Many unreal fears may appear real to little children, and most preschool children have one or another of these fears. This is natural, for they have a limited understanding of the world about them. Adults must help a child to handle his fears if they are not to persist, possibly in a compulsive form, in adult life. A real fear of a situation which is dangerous is logical. The remedy is to show the child what may be done in such a situation and how to avoid dangerous situations. Crossing the street is an example. The child can be taught to cross at the corner with, not against, the traffic light.

Ordinary fears include fear of being injured (or seeing people who have been injured or are crippled), being lost or deserted, and being hurt by animals (particularly those which are large or noisy). Some children fear death, but not as adults do (see p. 107). The child may have had a real experience with any one of these fear-producing situations. Children feel most fearful when they are alone or away from their parents among strangers.

Inner anxiety, in contrast to fear, occurs when a child feels unloved. He may have been punished for masturbation, or deprived of his mother's love because of the arrival of a new sibling. To the child who is anxious many things appear to be dangerous, and vague, unknown dangers appear to be ever present. The adult must understand not only the child's fear of external dangers, but also his inner anxiety, in order to help him.

Night terrors may occur during the preschool period. The child is terrified when he wakens from sleep. Such dreams are usually the result of unresolved emotional conflicts which the child has. If they continue, he should receive therapy for his problems.

The frightened child needs, more than anything else, to be reassured and to gain a feeling of safety. His mother should understand the child's problem, hold him, and let him feel her protection and strength. After he has calmed down, his attention may be directed from the source of his fear. When he appears sufficiently secure, he may want to talk about his fear and even to have contact with the feared object or situation. Perhaps, before contact, he may want to play out the fearful situations as a game. The adult's role in helping a child to overcome fears is to be supportive and understanding.

Common fears can be prevented to a large extent by imagining how new situations seem to a child and talking to him from his point of view. A puppy which is active and playful, not vicious, to a child may appear to be a monster that cannot be controlled. The adult who protects a child from meeting fearful experiences until he is prepared for them and has sufficient self-confidence will prevent many of the common fears of childhood.

Special Problems of the Preschool Child

The common behavioral manifestations of children's feelings are so important that they must be given detailed consideration in order that the inexperienced nurse may learn to give the child comprehensive nursing care. Children may have such behavioral problems as continued thumb-sucking, food likes and dislikes, enuresis, encopresis, selfishness, bad language, hurting others, and destructiveness.

THUMB-SUCKING

The important danger in continued thumb-sucking is not in the habit itself but in the response of parents and other adults to it. Parents tend to feel that if a child sucks his thumb in the preschool period, they themselves have failed in training him. They respond to this feeling of failure by becoming inconsiderate of the child in their handling of the problem. They may alternately punish, love, and ridicule him because he does not overcome the objectionable habit.

Parents need not fear that thumb-sucking will injure the thumb or spoil the shape of the child's jaw unless the habit is continued into older childhood and the child exerts maximum pressure when sucking. In any case the shape of the mouth is likely to return to normal after the thumb-sucking has ceased.

Many children who suck their thumbs probably had too little sucking pleasure during infancy. Thumb-sucking may be a sign that the child feels unloved, that he is in danger or is not good enough. It may be an expression of dissatisfaction with life. When parents or other adults exert pressure upon him to give up the activity, his unhappiness is increased.

In order to help the child, parents and other adults responsible for his care must observe the whole child and try to provide a happier childhood experience for him. Adults should note the occasions when a child sucks his thumb and provide more love and security for him at such times. It is essential to find the basis of the problem. Is the child lonely, too excited or bored? Has he too few toys or does he feel neglected? Although children usually outgrow the habit by the age of five or six years, it is important to find and correct the cause in order to prevent the child from acquiring another habit which serves the same function of giving him pleasure and comfort. The matter may be discussed with a child of five or six years who seems to be trying to overcome the habit. He may be encouraged by assurance that he will probably outgrow the habit.

FOOD LIKES AND DISLIKES

Preschool children may have "food jags" or a liking for certain foods. They may also have dislikes for other foods and vocalize their dismay when the unwanted foods are presented. This sort of situation may lead to bitter family arguments, especially if the parents do not share a similar philosophy of child care. (For a further discussion of this problem, see p. 633).

ENURESIS

Enuresis, an involuntary discharge of urine, or wetting after control should be established (about three years of age), is both a source of embarrassment and a nuisance to the mother of an enuretic child. Mothers should remember that a child can be toilet-trained only when he is physiologically and psychologically ready for control of urine and stool.

Some of the causes of enuresis are lack of training, too early or too severe training or overtraining. If parents would regard this process as only a part of the general training of the child and take it in their stride, there would be fewer problems of enuresis. Children who have achieved control of urine and stool may revert to wetting, especially bed wetting, when they meet problems which they cannot solve, such as those connected with the coming of a new baby.

Adults should not make an issue of toilet training. They should not use bribes or punishment or threaten to stop loving a child because he continues this habit. If enuresis is nocturnal only, giving less fluid in the evening may be tried. But the problem is usually more psychologic than physical. It may be due to a hostile-dependent mother-child relationship. Adults should try to be casual and assure the child that he will outgrow this habit. They should help him to achieve a positive attitude toward enuresis—to want to stay dry—and develop confidence in his ability to control elimination. Wetting will not stop at once, but if the child is more relaxed, dryness will be achieved more easily and with less danger to his personality development.

Nocturnal enuresis, nighttime bedwetting after three or four years of age, may be due to environmental factors, such as a dark hall through which the child must walk to the bathroom, or to his reluctance to get out of a warm bed to go to a cold bathroom.

Enuresis may also be due to a physical cause. For this reason children who do not respond to parental training should be examined by a physician and possibly by a psychiatrist. The child may have an irritable bladder which cannot hold large quantities of urine, or he may have a neurologic defect or a urinary tract infection.

The physician and the parents should analyze the situation in order to determine the child's specific problem. If the problem is not due to a physical cause and if the emotional problem is not too severe, any plan adults use to help the child usually will not succeed if the child is not motivated to gain control. If the child needs to have proof that he can gain control, the parents should arrange to have him spend a night away from home. Because of the social pressure he feels in his new environment, he usually will not wet the bed.

ENCOPRESIS

If there is no physiologic cause and the child continues to have uncontrolled stool passages beyond the time when bowel control is expected, by about three or four years of age, he may be said to have encopresis. This usually is an indication of an emotional disturbance. As with enuresis, encopresis may be due to too rigid toilet training or to a lack of a good mother-child relationship.

On the other hand, if the child has achieved toilet training and he then withholds his bowel movements, a condition may develop which resembles megacolon (see p. 455). His abdomen becomes distended with unpassed feces and gas, and he may have diarrhea due to irritation of the intestinal tract. Although the child should be examined for the possibility of megacolon, he can also be given psychiatric treatment for his unresolved emotional problems.

SELFISHNESS

No child is born with the ability to share with others what is his. He can only slowly learn the joy of giving, or even sharing with others, what he wants to keep for himself. He cannot be forced to share. He must first develop a sense of ownership before he can learn to be generous.

Adults can help him to learn to share with others if they let him have possessions which both they and he recognize as his. He can be allowed to decide whether to give or refuse to give his toy to another child. If a squabble occurs over one child's possession of a toy which another child wants, a substitute toy may be provided so that each has what he wants. Many parents make the mistake of taking a toy from its rightful owner and giving it to a smaller child or to a guest. In order to learn the difficult and often unpleasant lesson of sharing, a child can be helped to enjoy playing with other children. Group play encourages the habit of sharing He will learn first that using things together is fun and then to share and take turns with his toys and those of other children.

BAD LANGUAGE

Children learn improper words just as they learn all the other words in their vocabularies. Parents are horrified when their children call names such as "stinker," "louse" or "stupid." They may be shocked when their children say unapproved words in connection with toilet training. They may be hurt when their children say, "I hate you!" or "I'll shoot you."

Bad language generally has more meaning for the adult than for the child, who, as a rule, has little understanding of what such words mean or their connotations. He may use these words on purpose to annoy adults and enjoy the sensation he creates.

In such a situation adults should relax and not be worried or shocked. The child should not be punished, for punishment emphasizes the importance of the words. The adult may say the same word back to the child in an unemotional way and thus make the word seem of little importance, or give the child a more difficult word such as "Mississippi" to say. The adult may say to the preschool child, "I'm tired of hearing that," or he may request the child not to use the word again because it may hurt others. Since no one method will work in all situations, more than one method may have to be tried.

In a nursery school the teacher may try the methods of nonparticipation with the group, suggestion of other words, distraction, or playing with other words, or sounds. The teacher should not shame or punish the children for using bad language. The less attention is paid to the use of such language, the sooner it will cease.

HURTING OTHERS

Small children hurt others and are themselves hurt when they play together. If the hurting is accidental, the incident should be overlooked. But if a child persistently tries to hurt others, he needs adult help to control his actions or to prevent him from inflicting some serious injury on another child.

The child who repeatedly wants to hurt others by biting, scratching, pulling hair or hitting is a troubled child. He may be jealous or frustrated, and his behavior may result from his mental state. He must not be allowed to hurt other children. He needs to know that someone who loves him deeply will control him and so prevent the unpleasant consequences of his behavior. He needs to feel secure within limits beyond which he is not allowed to go.

The child is not punished by having the same injury inflicted on him which he inflicted on another child. He is not forced to apologize to the child whom he hurt. Under no circumstances is he made to feel rejected by the adult who is in charge of the children. The adult takes positive action in situations in which the child is likely to hurt others. If it is evident that a child intends to thow a stone or hit or bite one of his playmates, the adult restrains him, saying, "Sammy does not want to be hurt." If the harm has already been done, the injured child is soothed and the offender removed to a less emotional environment in which he is helped to control himself. The attention of the other children is directed to some activity which they all enjoy in order that happy play may be resumed. As soon as practical, the offending child can rejoin the play group.

Toys and other objects with which a child can hurt others can be removed if a child who is likely to attack others is participating in group play.

The child who wants to hurt others should be helped to identify with the group, accepting them and being accepted by them. He is given physical outlets in his play through which to work off some of his excess energy and relieve his feeling of frustration. He may be praised for his achievements in group and solitary play and for kindly acts which he does for others.

DESTRUCTIVENESS

All children occasionally break things. Parents must learn to differentiate between accidental and intentional destruction of objects which they may value highly. Much of the child's accidental destructiveness is the result of his boundless energy and endless curiosity. In spite of the damage to property, parents should not too severely limit his outlets for energy and curiosity, for these are valuable qualities which must not be destroyed.

To avoid accidental destruction at home, the parents should remove valuable objects that the child might break or damage. They should provide space for him to play in without danger of his breaking or harming the furnishings of the house.

Toys are apt to be given rough use. Parents should realize that material possessions do not mean as much to a child as to adults. In the course of play children give toys a great deal of wear and tear and may break them by using them in ways for which they were not intended. Adults should set up certain restrictions, however, in the child's use of toys and of objects belonging to adults. He is then able to learn to value his own possessions and those of others. Progress is slow, however. What he values he will learn to use with care. The child who loves his parents is often intensely sorry if he breaks something which he knows they value, even though he also knows that he will not be punished in any way.

An intentionally destructive child is usually an unhappy child unable to control his feelings of jealousy, helplessness, aggression, or anger. He may feel unloved, disliked by his peers, or bored by inadequate playthings. Sometimes such children seem to want to be punished, since it is one way of getting attention. The cause of such destructiveness must be found and appropriate treatment given. The parents should avoid scolding or punishing. They should help him direct his energy into appropriate activities.

INTERRELATIONS OF PHYSICAL, SOCIAL, AND MENTAL DEVELOPMENT

PHYSICAL GROWTH AND DEVELOPMENT

Children grow relatively slowly in the preschool years, but they change from the chubby toddler to the sturdy child. They gain an average of less than 5 pounds a year. The average child of six years of age has doubled his weight at one year of age. During the preschool period the child gains about 2 to 2.5 inches a year. The average height of the six-year-old is 40 inches, or double his birth length. Since the child grows proportionately more than he gains weight during the preschool years, he appears to be tall and thin by the end of his preschool days. With improvement in nutrition for all children the average increase in physical growth may be greater in the future.

Children from three to six years of age gain muscular coordination which enables them to explore the physical environment, just as they acquire the ability to explore intellectually through constant questioning of adults and older children or even their playmates.

The child of six years has learned to walk more as adults do. The lordosis of the smaller child has disappeared. During the preschool years the constantly overactive child may suffer from persistent fatigue and may therefore develop poor posture unless preventive measures are taken.

In general, after the second year the child's motor development consists essentially in increase in strength and ease of performance. No distinctly new types of muscle activities are seen after early childhood. New kinds of performance are based on the use of skills already learned. By the time a child is five years old his skill in the use of muscles and his accuracy and speed allow him to be increasingly independent of others.

The pulse rate is normally 90 to 110, the respiratory rate about 20 when the child is at rest. The blood pressure is approximately 85 mm. of mercury systolic, and 60 mm. diastolic.

SOCIAL AND MENTAL DEVELOPMENT

The child of this age has developed a conscience and has internalized the mores of his group. He has begun to develop for himself such concepts as friendship, acceptance of responsibility, independence (some children show their independence by running away from home), the passage of time, spatial relations, abstract words, and numbers. His attention span has lengthened.

SPECIFIC INTERRELATIONS OF PHYSICAL, SOCIAL, AND MENTAL DEVELOPMENT

Chronologic age is misleading as a basis for child care. The development of the whole child must be considered; this requires individual consideration. Yet chronologic age is useful for any discussion of classified group characteristics. By using the average of each of the characteristics as the norm for the child of any given age, it is possible to tell how far any child deviates from the norm. No child conforms to the average in all areas of development. He may be far above in one area, behind in another and average in all other areas. For this reason a child's behavior at any time is likely to be that of one age group in certain areas and of another age group in other areas.

Although development does not proceed at a uniform rate in all areas, it follows a logical, precise sequence. The rate at which this

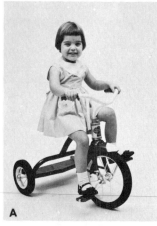

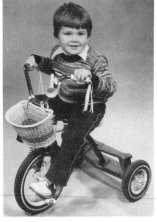

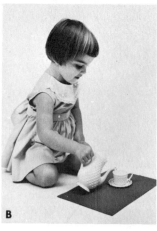

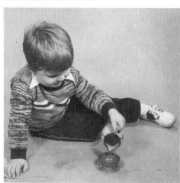

FIGURE 19–8. The 3-year-old (*A*) rides a tricycle, using the pedals, (*B*) pours fluid from a pitcher well, (*C*) begins to use scissors, (*D*) can string large beads.

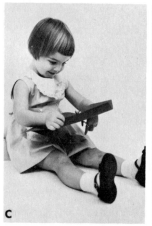

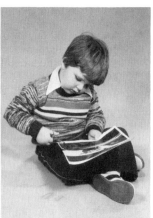

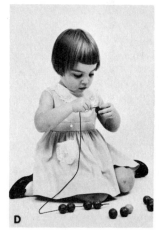

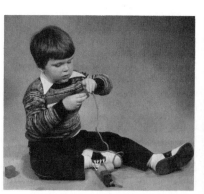

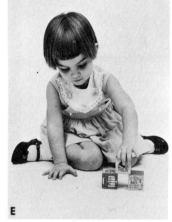
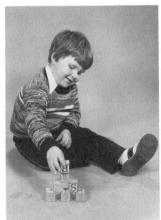

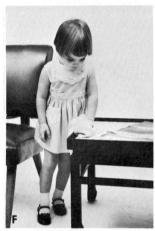
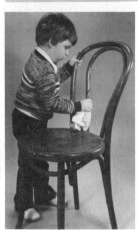

FIGURE 19–8 *Continued.* (*E*) imitates a block bridge, (*F*) can help to dust.

sequence occurs is an individual matter. This is the most important point to remember in applying the concept of growth and development to the care of any particular child.

Three Years.   The three-year-old child is less negativistic and more easily cared for than the toddler. He has fewer temper tantrums, understands words better, and can be given simple reasons and explanations of cause and effect in the phenomena occurring in the world about him. He is interested in new activities; hence this is a period when learning from experience is rapid. Mental activity and verbal expression are increasingly substituted for or reinforce physical activity in the expression of emotions. For instance, a three-year-old is likely to say, "I don't like you," rather than hit someone or throw a stone. Or if he does throw the stone, his emotion is verbalized as he throws.

MOTOR CONTROL. Motor control in the three-year-old is evinced in the following acts:

Rides a tricycle, using the pedals
Walks backward
Walks downstairs alone; walks upstairs, alternating his feet
Can jump from a low step
Can try to dance, but balance may not be adequate

Pours fluid from a pitcher well
Begins to use scissors
Can hit large pegs in a peg board with a hammer
Can string large beads
Builds a tower of 9 or 10 blocks
Tries to draw a picture
Imitates a 3-block bridge
Copies a circle or cross to imitate model
Can undress himself; can unbutton buttons if on front or side of clothing
Helps dress himself
Can go to toilet
Can wash hands
May be able to brush teeth
Can feed himself well
Can help to dry dishes and dust

VOCALIZATION, SOCIALIZATION AND MENTAL ABILITIES. The three-year-old child feels safe in his world because his mother gave him security in the toddler period. His accomplishments are as follows:

Has a vocabulary of about 900 words
Uses language fluently and with confidence
Talks in sentences about things. Does not appear to care whether others listen or not
Repeats a sentence of 6 syllables. Uses longer sentences than the 2-year-old
Uses plurals in speech

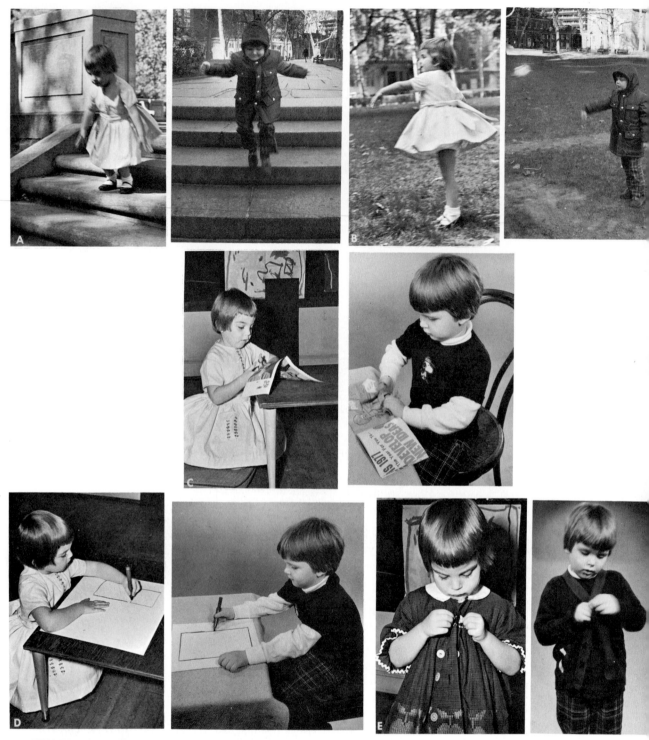

FIGURE 19–9. The 4-year-old *(A)* can jump well, *(B)* throws a ball overhand, *(C)* uses scissors successfully to cut out pictures. *(D)* copies a square, *(E)* can button buttons if on front or side of clothing.

May attempt to sing simple songs
Knows whether he or she is a boy or a girl
Plays simple games with others. Begins to work through the problem of his family relations with other children in play

Begins to understand what it means to take turns
Is toilet-trained at night
Can repeat 3 numbers
Begins to be interested in colors
Knows his family name

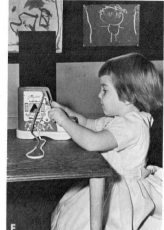 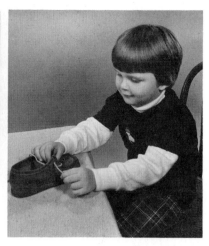

FIGURE 19–9 *Continued.* (F) can lace shoes.

Has little understanding of past, present or future
Can name figures in a picture

The three-year-old may continue to be ritualistic in many of his activities such as arranging toys or going to bed. He is a friendly, laughing child who wants to please others, though he may be jealous of his siblings. He may have fears, usually visual, of the dark or of animals.

Four Years. The four-year-old is not usually as pleasant a member of the group (family, nursery school, or play group) as the three-year-old child. He is more noisy. It is a stormy age. Parents may expect too much of him and clamp down on his manners and the language he uses. *Do's* and *Don'ts* become important. His aggression is turned toward his parents. His emotional tone is likely to change suddenly from gay to unhappy.

MOTOR CONTROL. The four-year-old has the following accomplishments:

Can climb well
Can jump well
Can go up and down stairs without holding the railing, and using his legs alternately like an adult
Throws a ball overhand
Uses scissors successfully to cut out pictures
Copies a square
Can build a 5-block gate when model is given
Can button buttons if on front or side of clothing
Can lace his shoes
Can brush his teeth

VOCALIZATION, SOCIALIZATION AND MENTAL ABILITIES. The four-year-old has the following achievements:

Has a vocabulary of 1500 words or more
Exaggerates, boasts, and tattles on others
Tells family tales outside of home with little restraint
Talks with an imaginary companion, usually of the same age and sex. Projects on this imaginary playmate what is bad in himself. The imaginary playmate is usually forgotten by 6 years of age

May be mildly profane if he associates with older children
Is cooperative in playing imaginative games with several children. Group activities are longer in duration
Can go on errands outside of home
Tends to be selfish and impatient
Takes pride in accomplishments
Aggressive physically as well as verbally
May run away from home
Can name 3 objects he knows in succession
Can count to 3
Can repeat 4 numbers. Is learning number concept
Knows how old he is
Knows which is the longer of 2 lines
Can count 4 coins
Can name one or more colors well
Has poor space perception

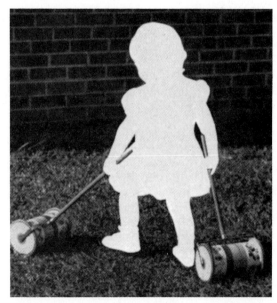

FIGURE 19–10. Imaginary playmates come and go at the whim of a child. "Only" children, who lack real playmates, invent their phantom friends; however, children in large families may create them also. (Courtesy of *Baby Talk*, October, 1970, p. 10).

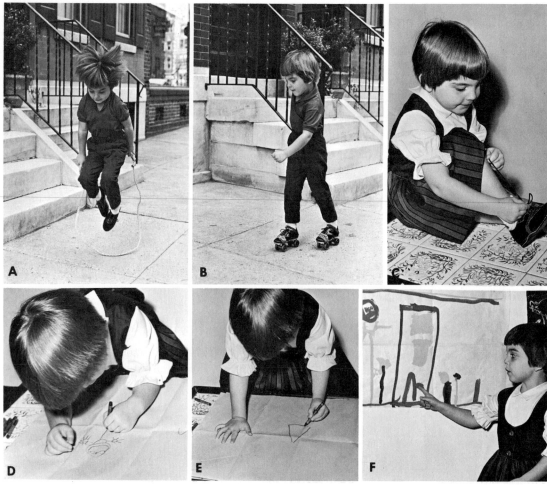

FIGURE 19–11. The 5-year-old (A) can jump rope, (B) can roller skate on 4 wheels, (C) may be able to tie shoelaces, (D) draws a recognizable picture of a man, (E) copies a triangle from model, (F) explains the meaning of her picture to the other children in her kindergarten group.

Five Years. This is usually a comfortable age for the child, and for his parents and kindergarten teacher. He has internalized social norms to the extent that he is likely to want to do what is expected of him. He is less rebellious than at four years. With greater strength, improved muscular coordination and ability to reason, he is less frustrated by obstacles in the environment.

The five-year-old is beginning to take more responsibility for his actions. He still needs reassurance and guidance from adults in adjusting to the needs of his group. Kindergarten is important to him; the experience in group membership in an environment which is planned for learning under professional leadership should supplement home training and experience in the play group. The child of this age has developed a personality which gives an indication of what he will be like when he is older.

The outstanding physical change is that the child is beginning to lose his temporary teeth.

MOTOR CONTROL. This includes the following abilities:

Can run skillfully and play games at the same time
Can hop well
Can jump rope
Jumps from 3 or 4 steps
Skips on alternating feet
Can roller-skate on 4 wheels
Can balance on one foot for about 8 seconds
Puts toys neatly away in a box
Can use a hammer and hit a nail on the head
Can form some letters correctly
Can fold paper diagonally
Prints first name and possibly other words
Draws a fairly recognizable picture of a man
Copies a triangle from model
Can wash himself without wetting his clothes
Dresses himself without assistance
May be able to tie shoelaces

From this age on the child will learn to be more skillful with his hands if he is given assistance and an opportunity to learn. The five-year-old has good poise and excellent motor control.

VOCALIZATION, SOCIALIZATION AND MENTAL ABILITIES. These are as follows:

Has a vocabulary of approximately 2100 words

Repeats a sentence of 10 syllables or more

Talks constantly

Can certainly name 4 colors, usually red, green, yellow and blue. Depending upon his intelligence and his environment, he may learn earlier

Is interested in meaning of relatives—e.g., aunts, uncles, cousins

Asks meaning of words

Asks searching questions

Can determine which of 2 weights is heavier

Can identify penny, nickel, dime

Counts 10 coins

Knows names of days of weeks and a week as a unit of time

Can put together a rectangular card which has been cut diagonally into 2 pieces

No longer runs away from home

The five-year-old is serious about himself and is concerned with his ability. He wants to assume responsibility and glories in his achievements.

SUMMARY

At the close of the preschool period the child's basic personality is formed. He has internalized ideals and standards taught him by his parents and teachers. For this reason his conscience influences his actions more than in a younger child. He is less dependent upon the emotional support and reassuring physical presence of his parents, and is content away from them for longer periods of time. Since he has internalized their attitudes and normally has a strong desire to please them, he is controlled by their wishes, even in their absence, far more than the younger child. His socialization, begun in the home, is reinforced by his teachers. He feels guilty if he acts in an asocial way so as to displease the adults whom he loves.

PLAY

Importance of Play. The progress which the preschool child makes in personality development, ability to deal with reality, and control of his feelings can be seen in his play. Through play the child learns to express his feelings, whether anger or love, less by actions and more by words. Children of this age as they play together are less likely to inflict injury on each other than are toddlers. Through play these children develop concern for their playmates;

they are sympathetic with a child who is knocked down or falls.

By observing children at play the adult gains a view into the child's world.

Beginnings of Cooperative Play. The child gradually shifts from solitary and parallel play to a simple form of *cooperative play.* He begins to exchange ideas with other children and gradually to interact with them in play activities. Among children between the ages of three and five years a loosely organized play group emerges. The activity of the group may be continuous, but the membership changes as children join or leave the group at will. These children enjoy social play, but still feel the need of solitary play at intervals; in solitary play they can do what they want in their own way. This loosely organized play goes on despite the bossiness or aggressiveness of some children in the group.

Toward the latter part of the preschool period a more organized kind of play emerges. The membership of the group changes less frequently. It is still, however, neither complex nor stable in its organization. Within such groups the typical child takes temporary roles of leader or follower.

Characteristics of Play. *Play is the business of children.* Preschool children play actively. They climb, run, hammer, and open doors with a bang and slam them shut. Their developing motor skills require practice so that improvement may be progressive.

These children imitate the social life of adults. Both boys and girls play house, enacting the roles of the different members of the family, or they may imitate firemen, storekeepers, conduc-

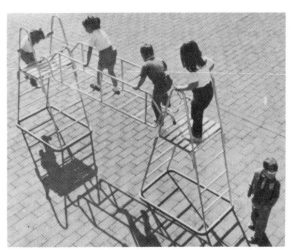

FIGURE 19–12. Preschool children enjoy active play on a gangplank and bridge climber. (Courtesy of Childcraft.)

tors, or their teachers. They change from one role to another as their interest shifts with new experiences.

Preschool play is highly imaginative, but the children are always aware of the difference between the real and their imaginary world. When a child pretends that he is an Indian, he knows that he is not. Yet he plays as if there were no distinction between fact and fancy.

The play of preschool children not only is an imitation of the life about them, but also is repetitive. These characteristics are more notable in some groups than in others. Many play themes stem from a confusion in children's minds about experiences they have had in real life, e.g., the death of a grandparent or the birth of a sibling. The theme may arise from a strong feeling the child has about something in his environment, or from the urge to destroy and demonstrate aggression and power.

A potential problem may arise in the years to come as a result of our present society's emphasis on accuracy in the portrayal of dolls, play furniture, and miniature toy housekeeping and industrial equipment. Children need to be encouraged to express *their own creativity* rather than fitting them within a mold of adult expectation, i.e., forcing them to play only with toys designed for the portrayal of adult life.

THE THREE-YEAR-OLD. Three-year-olds enjoy active games, but they also like to listen to nursery rhymes which they may later dramatize. They are increasingly interested in playing with other children in constantly shifting groups of two or three. Activities shift frequently, but not always with the entrance into the group of a new member or the departure of a child who instituted the activity. These children are beginning to be willing to take turns; this makes cooperative play possible. Such play takes the place of enjoyment in mere physical contact with other children. They enjoy activities with sand and water and playing with toys built for dumping and hauling. Quiet activities which they enjoy are cutting, pasting, and building with blocks.

Three-year-olds like to combine playthings to make a more lifelike situation. For instance, playing with dolls brings into use the doll's bed, tea set, and baby carriage. Imaginative children make substitutes for bought toys; they will use a box for the doll's bed and bits of paper for dishes.

THE FOUR-YEAR-OLD. There is a decided rise in both physical and social activity in the play of four-year-olds. They want to play in groups of two or three and often choose a favorite companion of their own sex. Although they accept the practice of taking turns, they are often bossy in directing others. To be silly in their play, doing things wrongly by intention, is characteristic of this age group.

Four-year-olds have complicated ideas which they are unable to carry out in detail because of lack of skill and of time. They are not able to carry their plan over from day to day as an older child does. They show an increase in the constructive use and manipulation of materials. They are fond of dramatic play and like to dress up. When playing house, the little girl wears her mother's old clothes. Boys as well as girls play house, and each takes the role played by the parent of the same sex. They like not only to play at household activities but also to help mother with cleaning, wiping dishes, dusting, and even ironing and hanging clothes.

Perception of shape in the four-year-old is poor, but he enjoys simple picture puzzles, using the trial and error method of finding the correct place for a piece. He is able to put his toys away but is not likely to do so unless reminded by his mother or teacher. (In nursery school or kindergarten where all the children replace their toys on the shelf, they remind each other and do not need the teacher's direction.)

THE FIVE-YEAR-OLD. At this age children enjoy varied activities. They like to run and jump. Such expressions as "I can and you can't" are common. Now the child plays in groups of five or six, and friendship with his playmates is both stronger and continued over a longer time. He is definitely interested in finishing what he starts, even though it takes several days to complete it. He plays house and likes to dress in adult's clothing to make his game more realistic. He is fond of cutting out pictures and of working with colored paper or on a specific project with his large blocks, e.g., making a store or boat.

In this last year of the preschool period he becomes cooperative, sympathetic, and usually generous with his toys. He is interested in the world outside his immediate environment, likes to go on excursions, and listens to stories of things he has never seen. He maintains interest in stories of greater length than does the three- or four-year-old.

Selection of Play Materials. The choice of play materials for the preschool child should be based on the same general principles of purpose, utility, and safety as the selection of toys for earlier age groups. Play materials especially enjoyed during this period are housekeeping toys and playground apparatus such as sandboxes, jungle gyms, slides, and swings. Toys for active play, such as balls, wagons, tricycles, and other transportation toys, and large blocks for

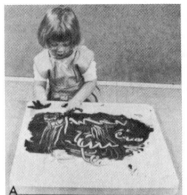
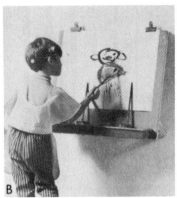

FIGURE 19–13. Preschool children also enjoy painting with finger paints (A) and water colors (B). Note the smocks that protect the children's clothing. Newspapers may be spread on the floor for protection from spills. (Courtesy of Childcraft.)

building steps and bridges are valuable in muscle development and for learning some basic facts and principles of physics. Manipulative materials, e.g., plastic for molding, water colors or finger paints, and musical toys are needed for quiet activities. Children need equipment for cutting and pasting, picture books to color, and illustrated books, both prose and rhyme, which adults or older siblings will read to them.

Role of the Adult in Children's Play. Children need help in learning to find pleasure in being with other children and to share and remember that others have rights which they must recognize. They want to please their mothers or nursery school teachers. If a child fears instead of loving an adult, he may cooperate when the adult is present, but when he or she is not, he knows no limits to his actions.

Some parents encourage their young children

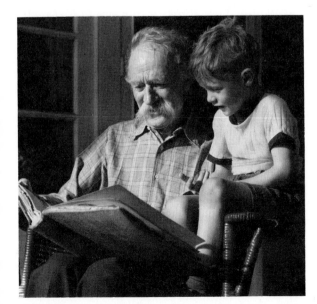

FIGURE 19–14. Grandfather enjoys sharing a story with his grandson. (Courtesy of H. Armstrong Roberts.)

to watch television in order to provide an educational experience for them or to keep them quiet for long periods of time. Studies are being made to determine the relation of this activity to the children's intellectual development and personality characteristics. Questions have been raised about a possible causal relation between viewing violence on television and the degree of childhood aggression, but no final answers have been found to date.

NURSERY SCHOOL

Children from 2½ or three years to five years are accepted in nursery school. There are several reasons why a child is sent to nursery school: when the child needs the educational experience to supplement what he receives at home, when he needs the socializing experience of contact with other children and total care under the guidance of well qualified people, and when the mother must work outside the home to help support the family. Experience is given in a nursery school in investigation, experimentation, exercising the imagination, creative activities, problem solving and socializing. Experience is also given to him in the process of interacting with children of other cultural and socioeconomic groups than his own.

Values. Nursery school promotes growth and development and improves the general health of the child. It increases his capacity for independent action, his self-confidence, and feeling of security in a variety of situations. Since he is in an environment planned to meet his needs and under the supervision of experts in child care, his understanding of himself and of others develops normally, and he is better able to handle his emotions. Nursery school also broadens his appreciation of the avenues of self-expression

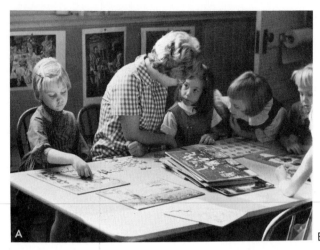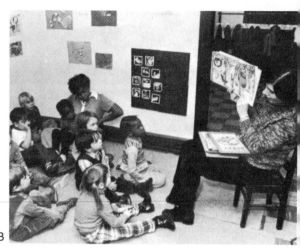

FIGURE 19–15. *A,* At nursery school and kindergarten, younger children are given many opportunities to solve new problems and to interact with their peers. (Courtesy of H. Armstrong Roberts.) *B,* A time for stories is included in play group activities. (From Fenster, S.: *Children Today,* 3:4, September-October, 1974.)

through art, music, and rhythms. As he learns more about the community in which he lives, he is better able to understand the world of which his daily environment is such a small part.

Qualifications. The criteria for the selection of the school include the qualifications of the teachers, the proportion of teachers to children, health policies, physical setup, and educational methods.

Activities. The activities provided at nursery school are first of all those which the child performs daily at home, e.g., eating, toileting, napping, health practices, and play, both indoor and outdoor. The school has equipment for activities appropriate to the child's size and abilities.

Preparation for Nursery School. Even if the child feels secure when separated from his mother for a brief time, she must realize that nursery school may be a very upsetting experience for him. Unless he is adequately prepared, the child may defend himself against the experience by uncooperative behavior or by rejection. Children may adjust in slightly different ways to nursery school, because the school does not present the same situation to all children. Each child has his own past experience and interprets nursery school on the basis of this experience.

Preparation for nursery school generally begins with the mother's own confidence in the school she has selected. If she does not have confidence, it will be almost impossible for her to give the child confidence and make the school a pleasant experience for him. She should take him to the building when the school is not in session so that he may become familiar with the physical surroundings before he is left with strange adults and children. He should

meet his teacher on these visits and learn to trust her (there are, as yet, few male nursery school teachers). He may feel more secure if he brings a toy or something else from home to make concrete the continuity of school life with that at home.

After this preparation, decision is made as to whether the child should attend the school. This depends on whether he will be able to profit from the experience, whether he feels at home there, likes his teacher and feels sure that she will take care of him when his mother is not there, enjoys being with other children, knows the routine and is confident that his mother will return and take him home with her. Children must know these things if they are to feel secure when separated from home and mother for more than a short time. If both the mother and the child feel secure about the school experience, future adjustment will probably be advantageous, and the child will enjoy and profit from the experience.

The mother stays with her child on his first day and should continue to come until he feels secure without her. The time he is in the school without her may be gradually lengthened. She should always tell him when she is leaving and assure him that she will return at the close of the school day. Some children need to have the experience of mother returning after a short period of being without her, to be certain that her return is part of the nursery school routine. The nurse who supervises the health of children in day-care centers, day nurseries (see p. 615) and nursery schools should observe the health of each child in order to make recommendations for care as necessary.

CARE OF THE PRESCHOOL CHILD

PHYSICAL CARE

The preschool child is gaining competency in self-care. A feeling of security in his home environment will help him to become independent in self-care. He learns to feed himself without too much spilling, to dress and undress, to wash his face and hands, to brush his teeth and to toilet himself, but he does not take full responsibility for stopping his play and going to the toilet before urgency makes him unable to control elimination.

Even if it is more convenient for the mother to care for the child than to allow him to be independent, she can encourage him to use his abilities so that he may become steadily more independent and that independence may be the goal he desires. Naturally he is slow and often clumsy in his movements. He needs help in his bath, to tie his shoelaces, and to manipulate buttons or snappers which are almost out of reach. A little child can seldom brush and comb his hair neatly. The mother plans the child's day to give him plenty of time for self-care before breakfast and before going off to nursery school or kindergarten, and for the general cleaning up before dinner. The daily schedule of activities includes time for active play, quiet play, and, for the younger children in this age group, rest periods, if not naps. Time is set aside for mother's meeting his need for cuddling and reassurance that she likes to have him home with her. She holds him on her lap while she reads or sings to him, or as they talk together.

Throughout this carefully planned day his mother protects the child from accidents and from frustrating experiences which retard rather than develop independence.

SLEEP

Certainly by the time the child is of preschool age he should have a room or a portion of a divided room of his own. Privacy in his sleeping area is needed not only for sleep but also for social, sexual, gender identity, fantasy, and individuation development. A private area permits the child to have a place in which to store his own treasured possessions. It also provides him with a place he can go to repair the hurts of everyday events that have produced frustration or disappointment.

The preschool child is normally so interested in whatever he is doing that he does not know when he needs sleep and rest, and resists going to bed.

The sleep of the three-year-old is frequently disturbed at night. He may have frightening dreams due to his real or imaginary daytime fears. He cannot tell the difference between his dream as a private experience and his dream as a shared experience. He may even ask someone whom he had dreamed about whether he remembered what had happened. These children may not stay in their beds, but wander around the house or want to sleep with their parents. Sleeping near the room of a brother or sister who is several years older and has outgrown the fears of the preschool period is often reassuring. Children who sleep poorly at night should have naps during the day; otherwise they are restless.

By the time the child is five years old he usually sleeps quietly and peacefully through the night, but he still may have nightmares. The child who gets adequate rest at night no longer needs a daytime nap. Most children over four years of age reach a stage at which naptime becomes a battle between mother and child. If the child does not sleep, he cannot be forced to do so, but his mother should insist on a rest period in a darkened room. A sleepy-time record played on his toy record player may be helpful, and he may have his favorite cuddly toy in bed with him. Before kindergarten age even the rest period may be eliminated for the average child, although overactive, excitable children may require rest in the afternoon. Most nursery schools and kindergartens have brief rest periods when the children lie on mats upon the floor or on small cots which can be folded or stacked easily and stored away when activity is resumed.

SAFETY MEASURES

Since preschool children have more freedom than the toddler has—playing outdoors alone, frequently away from the safe environment of the back yard—more accidents are likely to occur away from home.

Important causes of accidents in this age group are increased initiative and the desire to imitate the behavior of adults, which lead children into situations hazardous for them.

Their activities often result in falls, and their interest in new things and investigation of what they can do with them often result in serious accidents. They may play with matches, turn on the hot water faucet, lock themselves in unused or abandoned refrigerators or freezers from which the doors have not been removed, or get an electric shock. Their increased freedom, coupled with their immature understanding of danger, results in their playing around motor vehicles, or garden or swimming pools (see p. 518).

Since preschool children cannot be kept in an

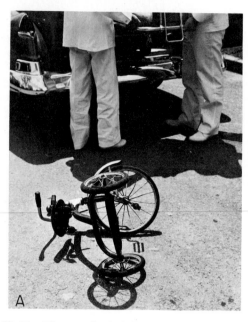
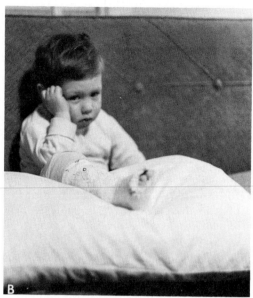

FIGURE 19–16. The preschool child's increased freedom of activity coupled with an immature understanding of danger may result in accidents. A, The child should not have been riding his tricycle in the street. B, Immediate injury may result. (Courtesy of H. Armstrong Roberts.)

accident-free environment, it is important that parents and all adults in charge emphasize safety measures to them. They should explain in terms the child can understand the safety measures adults take and why it is not safe for him to attempt all that his parents can do without injury. As he learns what he can do without danger of injury and how to protect himself, the child should be allowed to take greater responsibility for his own safety. Teachers in nursery school and in kindergarten not only provide a safe environment for the children but also help them to understand the underlying principles of safety measures. The children may play games which teach them the necessary precautions to take in everyday situations such as crossing the street or using safety belts when riding in an automobile or watching where they are going when on a tricycle.

Many children in this age group are accidentally poisoned. The children are less rigidly supervised than they were as toddlers and so are able to investigate all kinds of containers in medicine cabinets, in the kitchen, bathroom or basement. Preschool children are apt to take pills, powders, or liquids because they have seen their parents take them. They may take a substance which looks like food because they think that it will taste good.

The care of the preschool child who has taken poison is similar to that of the toddler (see p. 552). The preschool child, however, is more likely to be able to tell from what container he got the poison and is more cooperative in emergency measures to induce vomiting.

In addition to general sex education, young children should be given information about sex offenders, although this information should not be given at the same time. Preschool children should be taught to protect themselves from child molesters. They should be taught to refuse gifts from strangers, to refuse automobile rides offered by strangers, and to avoid walking alone on lonely streets. Children should learn to know the local policeman to whom they could turn for protection and help should they ever need it in their parents' absence.

HEALTH SUPERVISION

Regular visits to a physician are important, at intervals that he recommends, usually every six months or yearly. The physician or nurse gives the child a complete examination, including, when indicated, tests for visual and auditory perception. The physician or the nurse records the growth, gives advice about nutrition and any problems which occur in the management of the child, and instructs the mother on essential safety factors. Appropriate immunizations against diseases discussed in Chapters 13 and 16 are given.

Tests for visual and auditory perception are important during the toddler and preschool years. For visual testing the simple Snellen eye chart, the "Big E" poster, with letters that diminish in size gradually, tests distance vision. If the child is not old enough to know the alphabet, the eyes are tested with the Snellen Illiterate E Test, which uses only the letter E in different configurations. The preschool child can

THE NORMAL PRESCHOOL CHILD: HIS GROWTH, DEVELOPMENT, AND CARE • 633

tell which way each letter faces. A test for close-up vision is also given to determine how the child discerns letters at reading range.

Eye muscle weakness is checked by observing the child's ability to look in various directions. It is important for the child to be able to focus his eyes and to bring the two images together. Color perception is also measured. The eyes themselves are examined for unexplained irritation, inflammation, or discharge. An ophthalmoscopic examination is essential.

Signs of possible eye trouble in children include rubbing the eyes excessively, covering or shutting one eye, tilting the head or thrusting it forward, difficulty in looking at a picture book or in reading, unusual blinking, inability to see at a distance, or squinting. The child may complain of itching, burning, or scratchy eyes, inability to see, or headaches, dizziness, or nausea. All are indicative of possible eye problems. If the child has strabismus, red-rimmed, encrusted, or swollen eyelids, watery or inflamed eyes, recurring styes, or any of these problems, a thorough eye examination is essential.

The ears are examined with an otoscope to determine the presence of an accumulation of wax and whether there is a perforated eardrum or evidence of middle-ear disease.

Signs of mild hearing loss in children are frequently missed by parents and health personnel. In school or at home the child may be accused of being inattentive or slow in learning. At home the child may turn the television volume up above normal or he may not respond to a caller at a distance. He may also ask the parents frequently to repeat what they have said. If any of these indications of hearing loss are evident, a thorough ear, nose, and throat examination is indicated.

Dental care is important at this age. Caries of the deciduous teeth commonly begin between the ages of three and six and tend to spread rapidly. Since the deciduous teeth act as pathfinders for the growth of permanent teeth, it is essential that the deciduous teeth be kept in good repair until the permanent teeth erupt. If the deciduous teeth are lost, the permanent teeth may drift or be crowded out of position.

Factors in caries formation include a tendency to decay, position of the teeth, the formation of pits or fissures during dental development, the presence of fermentable carbohydrate or acid-producing bacteria which cause decalcification of the teeth, plaque build-up, and the fluoride content of the teeth.

Optimum general health reduces the probability of caries. Dental supervision should be a part of general health supervision, and daily care of

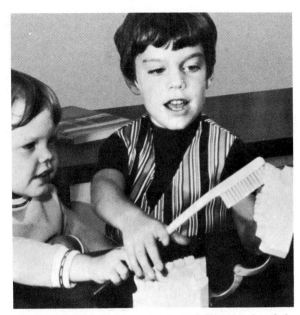

FIGURE 19–17. The preschool child learns to brush his teeth correctly to combat plaque build-up and dental caries. (Courtesy of the American Dental Association.)

the mouth is necessary. The teeth should be brushed after eating, and the child's intake of refined sugar should be limited.

NUTRITION

Because of the preschool child's interest in exploring his environment and because of his relatively slow growth, he is less interested in eating than he was during infancy. Attempts to force him to take food he does not want usually result in more strenuous refusal and in persistent eating problems. His appetite will increase as he nears school age. Measures which have proved helpful in increasing his food intake include serving the meal in a quiet environment with few distractions, providing a rest period before meals, using pretty dishes, providing a comfortable chair and table, and giving small servings.

These children like plain food served attractively in separate dishes. Each child has definite likes and dislikes. New food should be added gradually to increase the variety of his intake. A small amount, e.g., a teaspoonful, should be served and a second helping given if he likes the food. If he refuses the new food, it should be offered again after he has forgotten its taste.

Children of 3½ years use a spoon, and those of four or five years a fork. They often prefer to eat with their fingers, however. Foods which can be picked up in the fingers should be served at every meal.

By the time the child is five or six years old he can eat a simple adult diet. At this age, however,

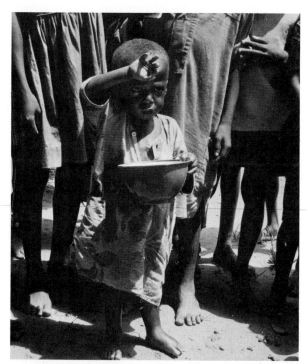

FIGURE 19–18. Millions of children throughout the world exist on an inadequate diet. (Courtesy of UNICEF. Photo by Robison.)

most children dislike creamed or highly flavored food.

Preschool children are influenced by the ex-

ample and expectations of their parents in eating as in other activities. In an atmosphere in which everyone is enjoying the meal, children are likely to eat more than when the father appears critical of the food and the mother is eating sparingly for fear of gaining weight. Children should not be coaxed, bribed, or forced to eat. Distractions should be avoided, and the child should be allowed sufficient time to eat without having attention paid to what he has and has not eaten. He should not be permitted to nibble between meals, although midmorning and afternoon snacks of wholesome food may be given. Children are good imitators and will copy bad eating habits from their parents or siblings just as readily as they follow good habits.

The child identifies with his family. He enjoys eating with them and joining in the conversation. Talk should include the child and not be focused on adult interests alone. It is a good time for parents to answer questions, provided this does not distract the child from eating.

Children of four or five years generally have acceptable manners, but too much emphasis should not be placed on details, and accidents should be accepted without causing the child embarrassment. It is more important that he eat his meal than that he have perfect table manners. The older preschool child wants to help with setting the table and washing the dishes, and should be encouraged to do so. Often help-

TABLE 19–1. RECOMMENDED DAILY DIETARY ALLOWANCES FOR THE PRESCHOOL CHILD 4 TO 6 YEARS

	WT.—20 KG. (44 POUNDS) HT.—110 CM. (44 INCHES)
K calories	1,800
Protein	30 g.
Fat-soluble vitamins	
Vitamin A activity	2,500 I.U.
Vitamin D	400 I.U.
Vitamin E activity	9 I.U.
Water-soluble vitamins	
Ascorbic acid	40 mg.
Folacin[a]	200 μg
Niacin[b]	12 mg.
Riboflavin	1.1 mg.
Thiamine	0.9 mg.
Vitamin B_6	0.9 mg.
Vitamin B_{12}	1.5 μg
Minerals	
Calcium	800 mg.
Phosphorus	800 mg.
Iodine	80 μg
Iron	10 mg.
Magnesium	200 mg.
Zinc	10 mg.

[a]The folacin allowances refer to dietary sources as determined by *Lactobacillus casei* assay. Pure forms of folacin may be effective in doses less than ¼ of the RDA.

[b]Although allowances are expressed as niacin, it is recognized that on the average 1 mg. of niacin is derived from each 60 mg. of dietary tryptophan.

From the Food and Nutrition Board, National Academy of Sciences–National Research Council: Recommended Daily Dietary Allowances (1974).

ing parents at mealtimes results in the child's taking more interest in food and eating more wholesome food, rather than asking for cookies, cakes, potato chips, or pretzels.

If the child refuses to eat sufficient food at mealtimes to keep him healthy, the following factors should be considered: eating too much between meals, an emotional disturbance, over-fatigue, or imitation of adults who have poor appetites. If the child is ill or has dental caries, he may refuse food because it nauseates him or gives him a toothache. Some children use poor eating habits as a means of getting attention or expressing sibling rivalry. These causes are likely to be manifested in other behavior than simply refusal to eat. The cause must be removed to prevent trauma to the child's physical and mental health. He needs reassurance that he is loved.

Table 19–1 lists the food requirements of the preschool child.

EFFECTS OF SEPARATION

The four- or five-year-old child still shows distress when his mother leaves him with strangers, but he has sufficient intellectual maturity to understand her explanation of the separation. He knows enough about the passage of time—the meaning of "soon," "this afternoon," and "tomorrow," or even "the day after tomorrow"—to realize that if he waits, his mother will come back at some fairly definite time.

A child of this age after separation from his mother may cry when he sees her again. This is because seeing her causes his suppressed emotions to be released in tears now that she is there to comfort him. His distress is decreased by crying even if he cries again when she leaves. The child left by his mother in a child care center, nursery school, or hospital is reassured by her visit because it shows that she loves him and will come back to take him home.

TEACHING AIDS AND OTHER INFORMATION*

American Academy of Pediatrics

Identity Development in Adopted Children.
One in Three Pre-Schoolers Aren't Immunized.
Recommendations for Preventive Health Care of Children and Youth.
Selected References on Low Cost Sex Education Publications.
Should Milk Drinking by Children be Discouraged?
Transracial Adoption.
Vision Screening of Pre-School Children.

American Dental Association

What About Fluorides?
What Happened to Mike?
Your Child's First Visit to the Dentist.

The American Humane Association: Children's Division

De Francis, V.: Protecting the Child Victim of Sex Crimes Committed By Adults.

Child Study Association of America

Frank, J.: Television: How to Use It Wisely with Children, Revised 1976.
Olds, S.W.: The Mother Who Works Outside the Home, 1975.
Read Me Another Story.
Reading with Your Child Through Age 5, 1976.
What to Tell Your Child About Sex, Revised 1974.
When Children Ask About Sex, Revised 1974.

Child Welfare League of America, Inc.

Felker, E.H.: Foster Parenting Young Children: Guidelines from a Foster Parent, 1974.
Murphy, L.B.: Growing Up in Garden Court: Children's Hospital, the Menninger Clinic, 1974.
Transracial Adoption Today: Views of Adoptive Parents and Social Workers, 1975.

Consumer Product Information

Backyard Play Equipment, 1975.
Finding the Best Day Care for Your Children, 1974.
One-Parent Families, 1974.
The Thing the Professor Forgot, 1975.
Young Children and Accidents in the Home, 1974.

Department of National Health and Welfare: Ottawa, Canada

Day Care: A Resource for the Contemporary Family.
Family Living and Sex Education: A Canadian Overview.
Family Living and Sex Education: A Guide for Parents and Youth Leaders.
Keep Your Family Safe (safety in the home).
Play for Pre-Schoolers.
Status of Day Care in Canada—1975.
Up the Years from One to Six.

The National Association for Mental Health, Inc.

Family Life and Sex Education.
Glasscote, R.M., and Fishbein, M.E.: Mental Health Programs for Pre-School Children.

National Society for the Prevention of Blindness, Inc.

Signs of Possible Eye Trouble in Children, 1976.
TV and Your Eyes.
Your Child's Eyes Are At Stake . . . Play It Safe, 1975.

Public Affairs Committee

Answers to Questions Parents Ask.
Brenton, M.: Playmates: The Importance of Childhood Friendships.
Hymes, J.L.: Three to Six: Your Child Starts to School.

---

*Complete addresses are given in the Appendix.

Ross, H.: The Shy Child.

Wolfe, A.G.: Differences Can Enrich Our Lives: Helping Children Prepare for Cultural Diversity.

Wolf, A.M.W., and Stein, L.: The One-Parent Family.

United States Government

Cognitive Development in Young Children, 1976.

Daycare: Serving Pre-School Children, 1974.

Day Care: Family Day Care, 1975.

Developing a Statewide Program for Foster Children, 1974.

Fun in the Making, 1973.

Gallagher, U.M.: What's Happening in Adoption? 1975.

Miller, H.M.: Tips on the Care and Adjustment of Vietnamese and Other Asian Children in the United States, 1975.

Older Children Need Love Too, 1973.

One-Parent Families, Reprinted 1975.

Sharing and Caring, 1976.

Super Me, Super You: A Bilingual Activity Book for Young Children, 1975.

Your Child from 1 to 6, Reprinted 1975.

REFERENCES

Books

Bakwin, H., and Bakwin, R.M.: *Behavior Disorders in Children.* 4th ed. Philadelphia, W. B. Saunders Company, 1972.

Baller, W. R.: *Bed Wetting: Origins and Treatment.* New York, Pergamon Press, Inc., 1975.

Baumslag, N.: *Family Care.* Baltimore, Williams & Wilkins Company, 1973.

Berlin, I. N. (Ed.): *Advocacy for Child Mental Health.* New York, Brunner/Mazel Publishers, 1975.

Berman, C.: *We Take This Child: A Candid Look at Modern Adoption.* Garden City, New York, Doubleday & Company, Inc., 1974.

Broman, S. H., Nichols, S. L., and Kennedy, W. A.: *Preschool I.Q.* New York, Halsted Press, 1975.

Chapman, A. H.: *Management of Emotional Problems of Children and Adolescents.* 2nd ed. Philadelphia, J. B. Lippincott Company, 1974.

Comer, J., and Poussaint, A.: *Black Child Care.* New York, Simon & Schuster, 1975.

Creighton, H.: *Law Every Nurse Should Know.* 3rd ed. Philadelphia, W. B. Saunders Company, 1975.

Fein, G. G., and Clarke-Stewart, A.: *Day Care in Context.* New York, John Wiley & Sons, Inc., 1973.

Grunebaum, H., et al.: *Mentally Ill Mothers and Their Children.* Chicago, University of Chicago Press, 1975.

Helms, D., and Turner, J.: *Exploring Child Behavior.* Philadelphia, W. B. Saunders Company, 1976.

Hurlock, E. B.: *Child Development.* 5th ed. New York, McGraw-Hill Book Company, Inc., 1972.

Johnson, E. W.: *Love and Sex in Plain Language:* Revised ed. Philadelphia, J. B. Lippincott Company, 1974.

Kline, D., and Overstreet, H. M. F.: *Foster Care of Children: Nurture and Treatment.* New York, Columbia University Press, 1972.

Knotts, G. R., and McGovern, J. P. (Eds.): *School Health Problems.* Springfield, Ill., Charles C Thomas, 1975.

Langford, L. M., and Rank, H. Y.: *Guidance of the Young Child.* 2nd ed. New York, John Wiley & Sons, Inc., 1975.

National Council of Organizations for Children and Youth: *America's Children 1976.* Washington, D.C., National Council of Organizations for Children and Youth, 1976.

Nilsson, L.: *How Was I Born?: A Story in Pictures.* New York, Delacorte Press, 1975.

Piers, M. W. (Ed.): *Play and Development.* New York, W. W. Norton & Company, Inc., 1972.

Pine, V. R., et al. (Eds.): *Acute Grief and the Funeral.* Springfield, Ill., Charles C Thomas, 1976.

Recommended Dietary Allowances. 8th ed. Rev. Washington, D.C., National Academy of Sciences-National Research Council, 1974.

Robinson, C. H.: *Basic Nutrition and Diet Therapy* 3rd ed. New York, The Macmillan Company, 1975.

Rondell, F., and Murray, A. M.: *New Dimensions in Adoption.* New York, Crown Publishers, Inc., 1974.

Sarason, I. G.: *A Guide for Foster Parents.* New York, Human Sciences Press, 1976.

Starr, B. D., and Goldstein, H. S.: *Human Development and Behavior: Psychology in Nursing.* New York, Springer Publishing Company, 1975.

Wagner, N. N. (Ed.): *Perspectives on Human Sexuality: Psychological, Social and Cultural Research Findings.* New York, Behavioral Publications, 1974.

Wright, G. Z.: *Behavior Management In Dentistry for Children.* Philadelphia, W. B. Saunders Company, 1975.

Zeligs, R.: *Children's Experience with Death.* Springfield, Ill., Charles C Thomas, 1974.

Periodicals

Balter, L.: Psychological Consultation for Preschool Parent Groups: An Educational—Psychological Intervention to Promote Mental Health. *Children Today,* 5:19, January—February 1976.

Baran, A., Sorosky, A., and Pannor, R.: Secret Adoption Records: The Dilemma of Our Adoptees. *Psychology Today,* 9:38, December 1975.

Berkowitz, L., Glickman, J. D., and Friedman, E.: A Mini-community for Young Children. *Children Today,* 3:2, November—December 1974.

Brandwein, R. A., Brown, C. A., and Fox, E. M.: Women and Children Last: Divorced Mothers and Their Families. *Nursing Digest,* 4:39, January—February 1976.

Brennan, E. C.: Meeting the Affective Needs of Young Children. *Children Today,* 3:22, July-August 1974.

Carey, W. B.: Adopting Children: The Medical Aspects. *Children Today,* 3:10, January-February 1974.

Curzon, M. E. J.: Dental Implications of Thumb-Sucking. *Pediatrics,* 54:196, August 1974.

Danoff, J.: Children's Art: The Creative Process. *Children Today,* 4:7, July-August 1975.

Doherty, N., and Hussain, I.: Costs of Providing Dental Services for Children in Public and Private Practices. *Health Serv. Res.,* 10:244, Fall 1975.

Duvall, H. F., Jr.: Beware Refrigerator Entrapment. *Children Today,* 5:24, March-April 1976.

Fenster, S.: Parents and Children Discover Group Play. *Children Today,* 3:2, September-October 1974.

Freyberg, J. T.: Increasing Children's Fantasies: Hold High the Cardboard Sword. *Psychology Today,* 8:62, February 1975.

Galaway, B.: Contracting: A Means of Clarifying Roles in Foster Family Services. *Children Today,* 5:20, July-August 1976.

Galejs, I.: Social Interaction of Preschool Children. *Home Econ. Res. J.,* 2:153, March 1974.

Giarretto, H.: The Treatment of Father Daughter Incest: A Psycho-Social Approach. *Children Today,* 5:2, July-August 1976.

Hammons, C.: The Adoptive Family. *Am. J. Nursing,* 76:251, February 1976.

Harrison, S.: The Most Important 30 Minutes of Your Child's Life. *Today's Health,* 52:42, August 1974.

Heagarty, M., Glass, G., and King, H.: Sex and the Preschool Child. *Am. J. Nursing,* 74:1479, August 1974.

Herron, J.: Southpaws: How Different Are They? *Psychology Today*, 9:50, March 1976.

Inglis, S.: The Nocturnal Frustration of Sleep Disturbance. *The American Journal of Maternal Child Nursing*, 1:280, September-October 1976.

Kadushin, A.: Child Welfare Services—Past and Present. *Children Today*, 5:16, May-June 1976.

Kagan, J.: Future of Child Development Research. *Nursing Digest*, 1:64, December 1973.

Kerr, N.: Neurosis and Primal Therapy. *Nursing Forum*, 15:34, 1976.

Kiester, E.: Should We Unlock The Adoption Files? *Today's Health*, 52:54, August 1974.

Kravik, P. J.: Adopting A Retarded Child: One Family's Experience. *Children Today*, 4:17, September-October 1975.

Lystad, M.: From Dr. Mather to Dr. Seuss: Over 200 Years of American Children's Books. *Children Today*, 5:10, May-June 1976.

McBride, A. B.: Can Family Life Survive? *Am. J. Nursing*, 75:1648, October 1975.

Mark, N.: Some of Television's Finest Minds Offer: The Perfect TV Shows For Your Children. *Today's Health*, 52:47, April 1974.

Nash, A. L.: Reflections on Interstate Adoptions. *Children Today*, 3:7, July-August 1974.

Parness, E.: Effects of Experiences with Loss and Death Among Pre-School Children. *Children Today*, 4:2, November-December 1975.

Phadke, S.: Travelling Child Care for New Delhi's 'Nomad' Workers. *Children Today*, 3:17, January-February 1974.

Safran, C.: What We're Finding Out About Sexual Stereotypes. *Today's Health*, 53:14, October 1975.

Samuels, S. C.: An Investigation into the Self Concepts of Lower- and Middle-Class Black and White Kindergarten Children. *J. Negro Educ.*, 42:467, Fall 1973.

Sgroi, S. M.: Sexual Molestation of Children. *Children Today*, 4:21, May-June 1975.

Sulby, A. B., Diodati, A., and Karsch, B. B.: Family Day Care: The Nutritional Component. *Children Today*, 2:12, May-June 1973.

Zimmerman, B. McK.: The Exceptional Stresses of Adoptive Parenthood. *The American Journal of Maternal Child Nursing*, 2:191, May-June 1977.

AUDIOVISUAL MEDIA*

American Dental Association

Basic Dental Health Education for Parents and Teachers
57 slides, color.
Designed to assist the dentist who is called upon to present a program to an audience of parents or to provide in-service education on dental health to teachers. The basic information and facts concerning dental health and disease and the method of presentation are based on the film *Set the Stage for Dental Health*.

Educacion de la Salud Dental Para Profesores
33 frames, 33⅓ RPM record, color.
This filmstrip, with Spanish titles and sound recording, will assist the dentist who is called upon to present to teachers and parent groups information and facts concerning oral health and disease. Included in the discussion are the process of tooth decay, prevalence of decay among children and the resultant loss of teeth, definitions of dental conditions which contribute to decay and which can be corrected, diet and snacks, and the prevention of oral disease.

Fluoridation: A White Paper
13 minutes, 16mm film, sound, color.
Reports current information on the safety, effectiveness, and background of community water fluoridation through interviews with six individuals knowledgeable on different aspects of the measure.

Learning About Your Oral Health
4 overhead transparencies, 12 prepared spirit masters, detailed content outline.
A dental health education program that can be used from grades K through 12.

The Hands That Help (Las Manos Que Ayudan)
24 minutes, 16mm film, sound, color.
A documentary film describing the design and outfitting of buses into mobile clinics, the living conditions of the migrant population in the San Joaquin and Salinas-Santa Clara Valleys, and the dental treatment rendered.

The American Journal of Nursing Company

Growth and Development—Birth Through Adolescence
Series of 23 44 minute classes, black and white.
Class Instructor: Nicolay, R. C.

Consolidation and Growth
Participating Instructor: Earlywine, J.
Emphasis is placed on the child's acquisition of physical skills, the changes that take place regarding role-playing and goal direction, his learning to distinguish between the real and the unreal, his heightened emotionality and facts pertaining to emotional control.

Preschooler: Psycho-Sexual Development
Participating Instructor: Griffin, M.
Stages of the pre-schooler in his psychosexual development are presented.

Preschooler: Concept Development
The factors influencing concept development are outlined: conditions of sense organs; intelligence; opportunity for learning; types of experience; amount of guidance; sex of the child; and personality.

Concept Media

Human Development: 2½ to 6 Years
8 programs of varied length, 35mm filmstrip/tape, sound, color, guide.
Physical Growth and Motor Development: Part I—19 minutes.
Physical Growth and Development: Part 2—16 minutes.
Language Development—25 minutes.
Intelligence, IQ and Environment—30 minutes.
Cognitive Development—33 minutes.
Sex Differences and Socialization—29 minutes.
The Role of Play in Development—27 minutes.
The World As I Feel It—12 minutes.

Department of National Health and Welfare: Ottawa, Canada

Insist on Child-Restraint Packaging
Poster.

J. B. Lippincott Company

Growth and Development: A Chronicle of Four Children
Thompson, J. K., and Juenker, D. M.
16mm film and Super-8mm film and/or videotape, sound, color.

This series of motion pictures demonstrates the range of normal variation in social, physical, and cognitive development during the first four years of life. The films focus on each child's social and emotional development, identification behavior, motor development, habitual responses, concepts of reality, and body structure and function.

McGraw-Hill Book Company

Frustrating Fours and Fascinating Fives
22 minutes, 16mm film, color.

Jamie: Story of a Sibling
28 minutes, 16mm film, black and white.

The World of Three
28 minutes, 16mm film, black and white.

Trainex Corporation

Accidents and Poisoning
35mm filmstrip, audio-tape cassettes, 33⅓ LP, color.
Defines the most common injury-causing home accidents, and how rooms can be made safer for children.

Preventive Dental Care
35mm filmstrip, audio-tape cassettes, 33⅓ LP, color.
Includes facts about normal and abnormal development of teeth. Explains the medical view of pacifiers and thumbsucking.

Toilet Training
35mm filmstrip, audio-tape cassettes, 33⅓ LP, color.
Offers constructive do's and don'ts for successful toilet training. Explains how to judge when a child is ready to be trained and the implications of bed-wetting.

United States Government

For Children—Because We Care
Producer: USNMAC
13 minutes, 16mm film, optical sound, color.
Dr. Benjamin Spock discusses community water fluoridation, its safety, and low-cost in reducing dental caries. A collection of photographs of children and adults in fluoridated and nonfluoridated communities show the facts.

Parents Are Teachers Too
Producer: USOEO
18 minutes, 16mm film, optical sound, black and white.
Discusses the role of parents as the child's first and continuing teachers, and points out that learning comes easier with a flow of understanding between school and home.

°Complete addresses are given in the Appendix.

Chapter Twenty

THE PRESCHOOL CHILD IN THE EMERGENCY ROOM

The preschool child is more susceptible to injury than the younger child because of his growing curiosity and his increased freedom from close adult supervision. He is more susceptible to acute infections because of his increased contact with other children who may be harboring infection.

The young child who is brought to the emergency room for an acute illness or injury enters a totally new and often frightening situation. How he handles the stress of being in the emergency room depends on his level of development, his past experiences with injury, illness, or hospitalization, his preconceived ideas about physicians and nurses, and his perception of the present situation.

The response of his parents to the child's need for care is important. If the parents are anxious, the child will be anxious also (infectious anxiety). He relies on his parents for security and safety, and if they must relinquish their control of him to hospital personnel who may hurt him, he cannot understand the reason and becomes increasingly upset. The nurse can decrease the anxiety of the parents by showing an understanding of their dilemma. If the parents are kind and compassionate and explain what will happen to him, the child will usually remain relatively calm and cooperative.

The decision as to whether parents should remain with their child during treatment is difficult to determine. Many physicians and nurses believe that a child cooperates better when the parents wait outside the emergency room or clinic while he is given care. They believe that if necessary the child can be threatened into cooperation and restrained more easily if the parents are not present. Actually, most parents, who know their child better than the physicians and nurses do, can help the child to cooperate

CONDITIONS OF THE PRESCHOOL CHILD REQUIRING IMMEDIATE OR SHORT-TERM CARE

through the reassurance of their presence and thus make the experience less traumatic.

If the parents are permitted to remain with the child, they are likely to feel that the nurse has confidence in their ability to be of assistance in his treatment. Their presence also reduces their sense of guilt over what has happened and decreases their feelings of helplessness. If the child sees that the parents trust his physician and nurse, he is likely to cooperate with their requests.

Some parents, however, cannot tolerate seeing their child in pain, and some are too emotionally upset to be of help to the child. In such situations the nurse can ask the parents in the child's presence to remain outside. The physician and the nurse are then responsible for providing the necessary comfort and support to the young patient.

When the child is ill or injured, the physiologic responses to stress include pallor, increased pulse rate, increased rate and depth of respirations, and increased perspiration. These indications of stress may be observed by the nurse.

The preschool child's greatest fear is of bodily harm or mutilation. Because of his increased maturity, when he is under stress he is able to verbalize his fear of harm more than he could when he was a toddler. The preschool child may still cry, protest, scream, groan, whine, or whimper, but he can also use words or sentences to acknowledge the pain or to express his anger or fear. He can try to talk himself out of a situation, such as postponing an event or treatment in an attempt to escape it altogether by saying, "Wait a minute!"

The preschool child may also still show by his actions when he is displeased. He can kick, flail his arms, and try to bite or scratch the physician or nurse. He can also turn his head or body away, hold rigidly still, clench his teeth, or keep his eyes wide open to see everything that is being done or tightly closed to block out the view. He may reach to his parents for emotional support and bodily contact. If his parents have left the area, he may try to escape to find them.

The nurse can lessen the child's anxiety by having a friendly, reassuring attitude. If the nurse is honest and can demonstrate that the persons caring for him are trustworthy, the child will be more likely to cooperate with them.

In the emergency room the nurse can also strengthen the child's ability to cope with his stress by telling him what to expect, by showing him and letting him handle the equipment to be used, and by encouraging his participation in treatment whenever possible. Simple explanations are quite adequate for the preschool child.

Usually the child is asked to remain very still during treatments. A simple explanation of what will be done helps him to cooperate. Giving the child an alternate outlet for his discomfort during treatment is also of value. For instance, if he is given permission to cry or scream, he may be supported in his efforts to cooperate and be quiet. He may be told that he can squeeze the nurse's hand as hard as he can. By doing this his mind is taken off the treatment temporarily. The nurse who offers continued reassurance and helps the child remain still by putting a gentle but firm hand on the affected part may increase the child's ability to cooperate. Appreciation of the child's cooperation can be shown if the nurse says, "The doctor is able to treat you so quickly because you are staying so still."

If the child is unable to cooperate, restraint may become necessary. He should not be made fun of, scolded, or made to feel guilty for his lack of cooperation The child is told the reason for the restraint. If he becomes panic stricken, further reassurance and a brief delay in treatment may help him to regain control.

If a member of the helping team threatens the child to gain his cooperation, the child may remain quiet for the required length of time because of extreme fear, but he may develop fantasies about his treatment that may make therapy more difficult in the future. For instance, the physician while attempting to suture a laceration on the child's hand might say, "If you do not hold still, I am going to cut this hand off!" If the child injures himself again and must be brought for emergency treatment, because of his fear of bodily mutilation he will probably evidence even more panic than he did on his first visit.

Children many times believe that illness or injury is punishment because they did something against their parents' wishes. For instance, parents warn children repeatedly about the dangers involved if they dart out into the street while playing. If a child is struck by a car while he was chasing a ball out into the street, he already feels very guilty about his action. It is not necessary, therefore, for the nurse to reinforce his guilt by saying, "See, this is what happens when you don't do what your Mother and Father tell you." The fact that he has already been injured is punishment enough.

After treatment has been completed young children enjoy handling any clean supplies used during the treatment such as gauze and medicine cups. They may even ask to take these home to "play doctor and nurse" or just to show them to their friends. Such therapeutic play helps children to act out their aggression and fantasies and ultimately to deal with their feelings in a constructive way.

The goal of the nurse in an emergency room situation is to help the child continue his normal development without increasing his fears and fantasies and to make the experience a positive one If the nurse can help him in the ways discussed, he will be better able to deal with his feelings and to meet future stress situations in a realistic manner.

HOSPITALIZATION OF THE PRESCHOOL CHILD

The separation anxiety brought about by hospitalization of the preschool child is likely to be less severe than that in the toddler. Children who have made a satisfactory adjustment to nursery school and have become accustomed to their mothers' being away from home for a time generally make a better adjustment to hospitalization than those who have never left their mothers' side for any length of time. (This is also true for the father if he has had the major responsibility for child care.) Nevertheless preschool children who are ill need the security of mother's presence. The more the mother can be with the child during unrestricted visiting hours or stay night and day with him in his room, the less emotional disturbance will he suffer during and after hospitalization. If she cannot be present, the child may show an excessive desire for affection and even revengeful behavior afterwards.

Preparation for Hospitalization. The preschool child, because of his increased understanding of language, can be better prepared for hospitalization than can the toddler.

Much of the anxiety over details of hospital life can be eliminated if a picture book, pamphlet, or film showing the physical and social environment of the hospital is shown to the child. Such books or films can be obtained from a children's library and are often routinely shown to well children by librarians or nursery school teachers. Some parents and some kindergarten teachers believe it wise not only to discuss a hospital experience with chilren but also to visit the hospital while the child is well. Some pediatric units have parties for well children and their parents, even if the children are not scheduled for admission.

Actual preparation is most likely to be successful when given by the parents. They should assure the child that they will see him as often as they can and take him home again as soon as he is well enough to leave the hospital.

The child can be told why he must go to the hospital. A detailed explanation may be beyond his understanding; *what he is told should be the truth expressed as simply as possible.* Young children may feel that they are ill because they have done something their parents had asked them not to do. This may be literally true, as when a child is burned while playing with matches, when he knew that his parents would not permit it. He needs to be reassured that his pain is not a punishment, but the result of dangerous play. Some parents use this childish concept to threaten the child with illness or injury if he is disobedient. For example, a mother may say "If you do not drink your milk, you will not grow big and strong. You will be sick." When the child is sick, he may believe that he is to blame and that he is being sent to the hospital in punishment, possibly forever. A child should never be threatened in this way, and when hospitalization is necessary, the true reason for it

should be given him. Since preschool children are especially aware of defects, mutilations, and injuries of other children and are fearful of physical injury to themselves, the child can be encouraged to talk of his fears and fantasies and to ask questions about topics which concern him. Truthful explanations will minimize distortions in his thinking and reduce his anxiety.

The child pictures the hospital as very different from any previous experience he has had. He may have heard adults speak of hospitalization, and always with sympathy for the sick. He may have known someone who went to the hospital and did not return. What he sees on entering the hospital when he is ill may not be alarming in itself, but it stands for a life so different from what he knows at home that he is frightened by ideas of what may happen there.

A few days or even a week before a planned hospitalization the mother can tell her child about the pediatric unit and stress the similarity with his daily life rather than the points of difference

Some hospitals have preadmission orientation programs for children who are to be admitted for elective surgery. Some institutions also invite siblings to attend. Such a program may include an invitation to attend a puppet show that may be entitled "Coming to the Hospital," a tour of the areas the child will see during his hospitalization, refreshments, and a discussion of hospital procedures. Coloring books concerning hospitalization may be distributed to the children when the program is over.

Following this the child may ask questions as they occur to him; e.g , when going to bed, he may ask about nighttime in the hospital and be reassured by his mother's explanation. It is not well to talk too much about the hospital far in advance of his admission, so his attention is not centered on the experience to the point that anxiety is built up rather than relieved by what he is told.

The mother can tell the child that he will have a bed in the pediatric unit like his crib at home, but of a different color; that meals will be served him, but that he may eat his meals in bed or perhaps at a table with other children. The use of bedpans and urinals often troubles the child just admitted to the unit. This source of anxiety would be relieved if the mother had explained that they are used when children must stay in bed rather than go to the toilet.

The uniforms of nurses and physicians often frighten a child because uniforms make the people about him look different from the adults he knows at home or sees elsewhere.

If older siblings have been hospitalized, they often reassure a child because he sees that they

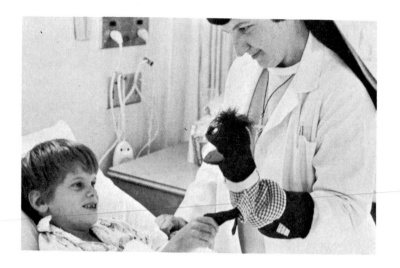

FIGURE 20–1. An anxious and frightened child is calmed through use of a puppet. (Courtesy of Iain Lowrie, Sheepshead Bay, N.Y. © January/February, 1976, The American Journal of Nursing Co. Reproduced from *MCN, The American Journal of Maternal Child Nursing* with permission.)

really did come back home. They may tell him that he will have ice cream there or that a child care worker, recreational therapist, or Play Lady will bring toys to him, or that a nurse made a paper cap like the one she wears for a little girl in the bed next to his. Siblings know the details of hospital life which really interest a child.

The parents can prepare the child for unpleasant experiences. If he is going to have an operation, the parents may play through the experience with him, using puppets, or he may play the patient himself, or a sibling who has undergone surgery may enter into the game. A child is told about going to the operating room and reassured that his parents will be in his room when he is brought back to it. The parents should know something about the anesthetic to be used. If it is to be given through a mask, this may be enacted. A towel may be used for the mask, and the child is told to take deep breaths and then pretend to go to sleep. Depending on his age, the concept of deep breathing may be explained by telling him to pant like a dog running, to breathe as though he were blowing up a balloon or as he does when he runs rapidly. The parents may breathe with him to demonstrate how it is done. He should understand that some discomfort will be involved.

It is not advisable to explain all procedures that might be done. The important thing is that he feels that his parents know what will happen to him. After his admission such procedures as injections are explained to him by his mother or by the nurse immediately before they occur. Then he will be interested in what the nurse is going to do to him and why it is done. He is not interested in the detailed mechanics of the procedure.

The child may enjoy packing his own toothbrush and other articles he will take to the hospital and selecting clean clothes to wear when

he goes home. This provides additional assurance that he will be returning home.

If the child has a toy or blanket which he prizes and which provides a feeling of security when he is afraid or tired, it may be taken with him to his bed in the pediatric area. It will be a

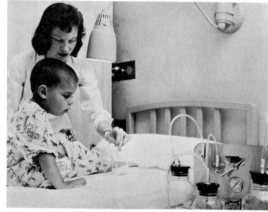

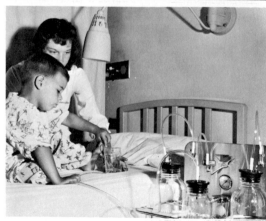

FIGURE 20–2. *A,* The nurse demonstrates the procedure of suctioning to this preschool child. *B,* The child returns the demonstration, thus becoming familiar with the equipment which may be used in his care later. (Margo Smith, University of California School of Nursing.)

link with home and will give him comfort in the strange situation. Nursing personnel should recognize the importance of such a possession and protect it from being lost or damaged by other children

All too often parents are unable to carry out such preparations because of their own anxiety over the child's hospitalization. They may not prepare him at all, or perhaps through ignorance they may give him a misleading impression of what to expect. Such parents might be helped if some member of the health team—the pediatrician, head nurse, supervisor, social worker, or psychologist—were to explain both the life of the children in the particular area where he would be placed and the treatment necessitated by his condition. Nursing students in some pediatric units visit children in their homes, nursery school, or kindergarten to provide such orientation prior to their hospitalization A little time spent in this way might save much anxiety on the part of the parents and the child, and also time of the nursing personnel.

Response of the Child to Hospitalization. The degree of anxiety and fear with which a preschool child responds to acute illness depends on the extent of parental anxiety and on how well he has been prepared by previous experiences for separation. Parents are not able to hide their anxiety completely, and a denial of it confuses the child. The parents should master their anxiety by a full understanding and acceptance of the situation Only then can they build up confidence and courage in the child himself

Children also feel differently toward their parents because, as the child sees it, the protecting role of the parents has weakened. Parents cannot shield a child from the discomfort or pain caused by his sickness, and he does not understand the reason for this. In the hospital he cannot understand why they let physicians and nurses hurt him. He becomes frightened at his parents' impotence and often angry with them for their failure. The parents must understand his feelings and provide support and comfort through meeting his needs, even if they cannot relieve his pain The child needs to feel the warmth of parental empathy, not just to hear it expressed in words.

The preschool child's level of understanding has an important bearing on his response to illness. Because of his lack of exact knowledge of time sequence, he may believe that he will be ill forever. Furthermore, he cannot understand the pain or his feeling of being lost. Because of his physical and emotional state he may have nightmares and lose the ability to evaluate reality that he had when he was well. The very strangeness of his environment arouses fear that new dangers are imminent. These feelings and fears may cause him to become increasingly dependent. He may lose his interest in former activities and center his attention on the part of his body most involved in the pathologic process.

Although preschool children are usually very inquisitive and in many ways intrusive in space, they are fearful of bodily harm during hospitalization. They have only a limited knowledge of body functions and many fantasies about what is happening "inside." For example, when a specimen of blood is drawn, a child may fear that all his blood will be taken and that he will die. In addition, the sight of the laboratory technician "sucking the blood" through a pipet conjures up additional fears. The child may fear the band-aid when it is used because he may believe that it is for more than first aid. The nurse who knows the child can help to minimize these fears by being present for painful procedures.

Intrusive procedures involving the perineal area also may cause considerable distress to the preschool child. For this reason temperatures are taken orally instead of rectally if the child can cooperate during the procedure

Children this age also need opportunities to "play out" hospital experiences which they do not understand. Play equipment should be available, and the children are encouraged to reduce their fears in this way under supervision (see p. 647).

It is important to help the parents handle their own anxiety and then with their aid to assist the child to face reality, understand and accept his illness, and maintain his normal interests in spite of the distraction caused by his condition. The nurse must understand the responsibility in providing emotional support to both the parents and the child. The nurse must realize that an unhappy, anxious child's recovery is retarded by his emotional state, that his progress is not the same as that of a happy child who is neither severely frustrated nor depressed.

In some institutions one person a nurse, social worker, or parent educator, may be responsible for meeting with the parents and their child together or with the parents alone for the purpose of helping them resolve their problems about their child's hospitalization. These meetings are especially important if the child has a long period of hospitalization or a long stay in the intensive care unit.

Parental Role During Hospitalization. If the mother is not permitted to participate in giving care to the child, she may feel guilty and think that she has somehow failed as a mother. She may long to have her child back home with her, thinking of all his lovable traits and forgetting a

PEDIATRIC MEDICATION GUIDELINES—2½ to 3½ YEARS

	Developmental Tasks and Behaviors	Nursing Implications
MOTOR	• Continues to develop proficiency. Basic skills have all been initiated.	• Child may be quite adept in resistive behavior.
FEEDING	• Becoming more proficient in skills. Eating likes and dislikes are definite but changeable. • May be influenced by others' reactions in responding to new food experiences.	• Medication tastes can be disguised with variable effectiveness. • A calm, positive approach is needed to gain a cooperative response from the child; quick tense approach is likely to produce similar behavior in the child.
INTERACTIVE	Initiative versus Guilt • Gives full name. • Is ritualistic. • Has little understanding of past, present, or future. • Shows concrete thinking, egocentricity. • Exhibits early aggressiveness; coercive, manipulative behavior. • Has many fantasies. • May be frightened by his "power."	 • Begin asking for verbal identification of patient before giving medications. • Communicate administration methods. • Use concrete and immediate rewards. • Tolerates frustration poorly. Child's initial response to reason appears positive, but without consistent effect. • Prolonged bargaining is frustrating and frightening to the child because no one is in control of the situation. • Give a choice when possible. Do not give a choice if the child does not have one. • Begin giving simple, honest explanations of why the medication is given (not because the child was bad). • Child's sense of security is dependent upon the nurses' consistent expectations of his behavior.

EXAMPLE: Roger, 3 years old, has otitis media and ampicillin 200 mg is ordered by mouth every 6 hours. He is to get the first dose in the clinic and then treatment is to be continued at home. His mother seems reluctant to agree that he really needs the medication. Finally she says she just cannot face what she knows will be trouble because he is at "that stage" when he won't do anything he is told.

The nurse pours the ampicillin into a cup. Roger is seated on his mother's lap. The nurse says, "Roger, your ears have been hurting. This medicine will help stop the hurting. I have the medicine in a little cup for you to drink. It tastes funny, but I don't think it tastes too bad. You can hold the cup and do it yourself; your mother and I will watch." She hands Roger the cup and watches while he follows through. "Good, it's done in one big swallow. Would you like some apple juice or some water now?" the nurse asks.

When they come back in 10 days, Roger's mother reports changing from juice to gum to ice pops to lemon drops after the medication, but that the medicine all went down.

FIGURE 20–3. Giving oral medications to young children. (From Ormond, E. A. R., and Caulfield, C.: *The American Journal of Maternal Child Nursing*, 1:324–325, September-October 1976.)

PEDIATRIC MEDICATION GUIDELINES—3½ TO 6 YEARS

Developmental Tasks and Behaviors	Nursing Implicatons
MOTOR	
• Develops proficiency of coordination. Can identify the parts of a complete movement or task.	• Child can attempt and master pill taking.
FEEDING	
• Exhibits olfactory, gustatory, and kinesthetic refinement.	• Disguising tastes is generally less effective than it is at younger ages. Child can distinguish medicine tastes and smells.
• Begins to lose temporary teeth (5 yrs.).	• Loose teeth may need to be considered when selecting form of medication.
INTERACTIVE	
Initiative versus Guilt • Makes decisions.	• Child should be active in making decisions which affect him.
• Sense of time allows enjoyment of delayed gratification. • Is able to tolerate frustration. • Seeks companionship. • Shows pride in accomplishments.	• Rewards which are not immediately received and social interaction can be used as effective motivators. Child is able to understand the purpose of medications in simple terms.
• Has ability to follow directions and remember several instructions for a period of minutes to hours.	• Teaching can have long-term benefits.
• Exhibits developing conscience. Needs limits set to help control his frightening sense of "power."	• Prolonged reasoning or arguing may frighten the child; a simple command by a trusted adult may be more effective.
• Exhibits genital interest, general mutilation fears.	• Explain the relationship between cause, illness, and treatment. Use simple terms.
• Illness often seen as punishment.	• Give control when possible—child needs to make choices.
• Shows changeable response to parents.	• Child may be more cooperative in medicine taking for the nurse than for the parent.

EXAMPLE: Orlando, a 4-year-old with repeated pneumonia secondary to cystic fibrosis, has been treated repeatedly with ampicillin. The nurse remembers that previously the suspension form was used with no resistance. But with this admission Orlando has been refusing the familiar suspension.

After watching him swallow whole jelly beans during an afternoon playtime, the evening nurse tries giving him ampicillin capsules at bedtime. She explains the pills are medicine like the pink liquid but that the shells they have stop the medicine from tasting so bad. She points out that they are the same size as the jelly beans he took while playing. Other things she tells him include how he can place the capsules far back in his mouth and swallow water to help "wash" the pills down to his stomach. By bedtime the next day, medication refusal is no longer a nursing problem.

FIGURE 20–3 *Continued.*

few which are undesirable. When he is discharged from the hospital, he may be anything but lovable at home. His behavior is likely to make her feel even less adequate, especially when she remembers how cooperative he was with the nurses. (If he was not cooperative, she may be subconsciously glad.) She should understand that he is not reacting to her, but to the separation experience as a whole. She must not become irritable and too demanding. Rather, she should give him the love and reassurance he needs, and wait until he has recovered from his hospital experience before expecting the pleasing mother-child relations which existed before his hospitalization.

If the mother is permitted to help with the child's care, little of the reaction just described is likely to occur. If maximum contact is kept between them, she will remain realistic about his illness and the kind of child he is. On discharge from the hospital the child will not find it necessary to unload his feelings of anger on his mother, for these will have been kept to a minimum or expressed during hospitalization. Children whose mothers or fathers have stayed with them during hospitalization have a low incidence of disturbances afterwards.

PHYSICAL CARE

Bathing and Dressing. The basic physical care of each child, with the exception of therapeutic procedures, should be similar to what he was accustomed to in his home. It should be based on information obtained from the answers in the questionnaire which was completed at the time of the child's admission.

On the basis of the questionnaire the nurse can learn to what extent the child can bathe himself and brush his own teeth. If he is physically able, he is allowed to care for himself as he did at home. If he expresses his dependency needs by wanting the nurse to carry out these procedures, this is done until he wants to do them himself. The nurse has an excellent opportunity to help him improve his health habits on the basis of what he has learned about such procedures. Children should have their hair shampooed with water and soap or a dry shampoo at least once a week if their condition permits.

As mentioned in Chapter 5, children prefer to select and wear bright colored clothing in the hospital similar to that which they wore at home. It is disturbing to a preschool child to be dressed inappropriately. The nurse should make certain that such clothing fits so that the little boy or girl does not trip over pant legs that are too long or be made uncomfortable by panties that are too tight.

Nutrition. Nutrition may present a challenge to the nurse. While the child is confined to bed it is particularly important that food be made easily available to him and that he be positioned comfortably while eating. If he is permitted to sit up, his back is supported by a backrest or by a pillow placed against the head of the crib. His tray is placed before him on a bed table. (These tables are attractively colored and made with collapsible legs.) The nurse helps him if he finds it difficult to feed himself. Any problems about eating which the nurse cannot solve are referred to the head nurse or to the nutritionist.

The serving of meals for the child who is able to be out of bed follows the pattern used in child-care centers and in nursery schools which provide meals. Regularity is important. A bell may be rung some time before the meal is served. At this warning bell the children stop playing, and preparations for the meal are made. Following the same routine each day makes it habitual, and mealtime is orderly. The meals are preceded by a quiet period of perhaps 15 minutes, during which the children relax, stories are told, and they sing or listen to a record player. A positive attitude toward meals stimulates good eating habits. Children in bed are given bedpans and urinals, and their hands should be washed. Children who are up and about the unit go to the toilet and then wash their hands with soap under running water. Paper towels are used for drying

Children whose condition permits have their meals served at a table. Usually several are seated at one table. Those with special diets or on limited activities may need individual service.

Chairs are of suitable height for the table and such that the child's feet touch the floor. Dishes are attractive and forks and spoons of a size appropriate for the child. All equipment which is not disposable is sterilized. Brightly colored straws encourage a child to take fluids.

Meals should be well prepared, and a wide variety of wholesome food should be served. In some pediatric units children are permitted to select their diets from menus much as is done on adult units. Small servings are preferable, and the nurse should prepare the food so that the child can eat it. Bread and butter may be served in sandwich form so that the child can handle it more easily. His meat and vegetables should be cut up so that he can take a suitable mouthful on his fork or spoon. If the food is served from a cart set up in cafeteria style which can be brought to the table or bed, he may have a choice of foods and, if able, help himself to what he wants. A meal served in this way is likely to be a happier experience than if a tray is set before him and he has no active participation in deciding upon the foods which will give him a balanced meal. For instance, he may choose between string beans and carrots, ice cream and custard, cookies with pink and those with white icing.

The atmosphere should be happy, the children talking pleasantly with one another. It is a good plan to have an adult eat with the children, to give help to those who need it and to provide a more homelike atmosphere.

Some mothers who cannot show their love for their child in other ways bring candy and other snacks for him to keep at the bedside In addition to ruining the child's appetite for more nutritious food, such snacks may not be of a sort to be included in a special diet, if the child has been ordered one. Also, these snacks may attract insects to the area. The nurse should discuss this practice with the parents and seek to help them provide love to their children in more appropriate ways.

REST

Nap time and bedtime may present problems. The child's needs for sleep and his routine at home must be considered in planning his schedule in the hospital. The room is darkened and each child prepared for either sleeping or playing quietly in his crib. A child may like to hold one of his toys. If the nurse demands that all children sleep at nap time, one or two may keep all the others awake by their rebellion against such an unreasonable request.

Children are not put to bed as a form of discipline. This practice makes the process of going to bed for rest appear as a threat to the child.

THERAPEUTIC PLAY

The therapeutic value of play was discussed earlier in this text (see p. 79). There are several reasons for having a recreational therapy program that ultimately benefits the child, his parents, and the total care he receives while in the hospital. The primary purpose is to create a home-like atmosphere which is familiar to the children and to give them an opportunity to express their feelings about being in the hospital. Through play children interact with other children. Anxious parents are reassured when they know that such a program exists. Parents can be helped to appreciate the fact that their child is not limited in his ability to play and to learn, despite possible physical restrictions. They can learn about activities that can be used when their child convalesces at home. Play can also be used as a diagnostic tool to help medical and nursing staff who care for the children.

Children need play activity in the hospital just as they do at home. They need to fill lonely hours and, by expressing their feelings through it, to reduce the trauma caused by hospitalization. While the child is confined to bed it is important for the nurse or child-care worker (Play Lady or recreational therapist) to provide toys selected on the basis of his interests and physical state. When the child is acutely ill and unable to play actively with toys, he may enjoy listening to stories. Telling a story instead of reading it draws children into emotional involvement in it. The story teller can ask questions, insert comments about the individual child and thus make him feel a part of the story itself. If stories about animals or children are told, the child can pretend to be one of the characters and interject his own comments into the narrative. As soon as he is able to be out of bed he can be permitted to play or listen to stories with other children.

The child who is too ill to be permitted out of his crib, as well as the ambulatory patient, enjoys watching the television programs he has become accustomed to watching at home. Such

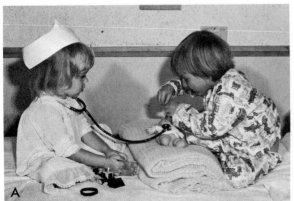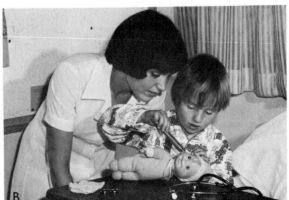

FIGURE 20–4. Therapeutic play by one or more children makes hospitalization easier for the preschool child. *A,* The team approach to learning. *B,* A procedure being carried out by a small patient is supervised. (Reprinted with permission from *The Canadian Nurse,* Volume 71, Number 12, December 1975.)

programs should not be too exciting for the ill child.

Some hospitals have a special nursery school room and an outdoor play area where the children can play together under the guidance of a nursery school teacher. If no other provision has been made, the children may have a place in the unit such as a sun porch away from the acutely ill children and out of the way of physicians making rounds. One of the unit personnel is designated to provide the guidance which such a group needs. In the play area children are free to develop mental, motor, and social skills and to express themselves in a variety of art media, such as finger painting or molding with clay or play dough. In some pediatric units facilities for finger painting may not be available because it is a "messy" type of play activity. Even in the hospital, children enjoy playing with household equipment. They also like equipment peculiar to the hospital which will allow them to work out their feelings about hospitalization (see p. 643).

Children frequently select toys such as doctor or nurse dolls, play syringes, and stethoscopes with which they can imitate the activities they see around them. Old cloth can be used in such play to restrain a doll, to make a doll's sheet, to make bandages, or to improvise a sling for a supposedly broken arm. Much of the equipment which is of value in the play of normal children is also necessary in the hospital play area, particularly simple craft materials, blocks, puzzles, story books, and phonograph records. Children enjoy play telephones because they can pretend that they are calling home.

Children's play areas cannot be kept clean and orderly as judged by adult standards. If the nurses are too concerned about the physical appearance of play areas during playtime, the children feel that the unit personnel do not approve

of their play and are likely to enter only half-heartedly into their make-believe, creative work or games.

Children are taught to take care of toys which they brought from home or had given them by their parents. They may and indeed should let other children play with them if their social growth is to go forward in the hospital as it normally would in their homes, but a place must be provided where their toys can be safely stored. As a child learns to take care of his own toys he also learns to respect those of other children.

Children also need to have holidays celebrated in the hospital much as they would if they were well and at home.

Nurses are responsible for completing all nursing procedures for the children as far as possible prior to the play period. They encourage all children, who are able, to participate in all planned play programs. Nurses themselves may also have an opportunity to participate with the children. In this way they not only learn about children and their play but also have an opportunity to appreciate the contribution of the play supervisor, Play Lady, or recreational therapist to the comprehensive care of their patients.

ACUTE PHARYNGITIS

Incidence, Etiology, Diagnosis, Clinical Manifestations, Complications, and Prognosis. The term "acute pharyngitis" refers to infections primarily involving the throat, however, it may also include acute conditions such as *tonsillitis* and *pharyngotonsillitis*. Involvement of the pharynx is a part of most respiratory tract infections. Acute pharyngitis is uncommon in infancy but increases in incidence, peaking at four to seven years of age. It may occur at any time of life thereafter.

Acute pharyngitis is usually caused by viruses, however, the group A betahemolytic streptococcus may also cause this infection. In addition, group B streptococci or *mycoplasma hominis* may cause some cases.

The *diagnosis* is made on the basis of a throat culture. Conditions that must be ruled out are pharyngitis caused by the pneumococci or *H. influenzae*, diphtheria, infectious mononucleosis, and agranulocytosis.

Although acute pharyngitis is caused usually by either of two groups of organisms, viruses or the group A betahemolytic streptococcus, the clinical manifestations are quite similar.

Viral Pharyngitis. The *clinical manifestations* of viral pharyngitis have a relatively gradual onset and include fever, anorexia, moderate throat pain, and general malaise. Rhinitis,

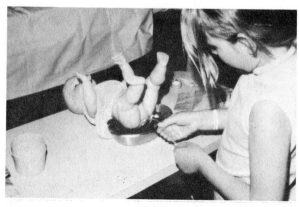

FIGURE 20–5. This preschool child is practicing on her doll a treatment which she must soon undergo herself. (Courtesy of the Medical Center, Laval University, Quebec.)

cough, and hoarseness may also occur. Sore throat may begin after the onset of other symptoms. The cervical lymph nodes may be firm and moderately enlarged. The larynx may also be involved. The white blood cell count is elevated. This condition may last from one to five days. There is a low rate of *complication,* although purulent otitis media may occur.

Streptococcal Pharyngitis. The initial *clinical manifestations* of streptococcal pharyngitis include headache, vomiting, and abdominal pain. An elevation of temperature to 104°F. (40°C.) may be present. The throat may become sore, and pharyngeal erythema and tonsillar enlargement with white or yellow exudate may be seen. Pharyngeal pain causes difficulty in swallowing. The anterior cervical lymph nodes are swollen and may be tender. This condition may continue from one to 14 days.

Complications that may be caused by streptococcal infection include chronic ulcers of the pharynx, peritonsillar abscess, sinusitis, otitis media, and possibly meningitis.

Because acute glomerulonephritis and rheumatic fever may occur after streptococcal pharyngitis, affected children should be examined about 14 to 21 days after recovery to rule out these conditions.

Mesenteric adenitis, which results in abdominal pain with or without vomiting, may occur with either viral or streptococcal pharyngitis and may be diagnosed erroneously as appendicitis.

Treatment and Responsibilities of the Nurse. After a throat culture is obtained, treatment is planned. No specific therapy is given for viral pharyngitis; penicillin is given orally for 10 days for streptococcal infection. Benzathine penicillin G may be given intramuscularly if the child has difficulty swallowing. The disadvantage of giving benzathine penicillin intramuscularly is that there is no way to shorten the length of time the penicillin is in the serum if the child develops allergic manifestations. Erythromycin may be given instead of penicillin.

During the acute illness bedrest is indicated. If the child complains of a sore throat, aspirin and hot or cold compresses to the neck may be ordered. The selection of temperature of the moist compresses depends on which provides the most comfort to the child. If the child is old enough to cooperate, warm saline gargles may offer symptomatic relief for throat pain. For very young children hot steam inhalations may produce the same effect.

Cool bland liquids usually cause less pain on swallowing than hot or solid foods. It is not necessary to encourage the child to eat if his throat is sore.

Isolation precautions are used in the hospital for children having streptococcal pharyngitis, since the condition is spread through contact with nasopharyngeal secretions; however, the child is usually noninfectious within several hours after penicillin therapy is started. It is not possible to prevent the spread of viral pharyngitis. Good hand-washing technique is of utmost importance.

If the child is cared for at home, the parents must be helped to understand the significance of continuing the medication for the entire time it is ordered. Some parents, ignorant of its importance, stop the medication as soon as the child's condition has improved.

If the child has a past history of rheumatic fever, he may be protected against streptococcal disease by giving penicillin or sulfonamide prophylaxis.

CHRONIC TONSILLITIS (CHRONICALLY HYPERTROPHIC AND INFECTED TONSILS)

Chronic tonsillitis may become a problem in the preschool child, but many parents and physicians distort its importance. They may attribute to inflammation of the tonsils many kinds of ills that are not realistic.

Clinical Manifestations. The common clinical manifestations of chronic tonsillitis are recurrent or persistent sore throat and obstruction to swallowing. Dryness of the throat and offensive breath may also be present. An obstruction to breathing is usually due to swollen adenoidal tissue.

Treatment. The surgical procedure of tonsillectomy and adenoidectomy is done if deemed necessary by the physician.

TONSILLECTOMY AND ADENOIDECTOMY

Not all children need to have their tonsils and adenoids removed. These tissues act as a defense against occurrence and spread of respiratory infections. The physician considers the necessity for removal in the individual case, and a conservative approach to this problem is becoming widespread. Antibiotic treatment for respiratory infections has obviated the need for tonsillectomy and adenoidectomy in many children. For an example of tonsillectomy and adenoidectomy and the nursing process in a preschool child, see the Appendix.

Indications. The usual indication is recurrent or persistent sore throat or otitis media. The child may have chronic infection with hypertrophy of the tonsils and adenoids. In considering hypertrophy, it must be remembered that tonsils are normally relatively larger during early childhood than in later years. In some children, however, the tonsils may be small and embedded behind the faucial pillars.

Obstruction to breathing or swallowing is more often due to enlarged adenoids than to tonsils. The adenoid structure, especially on the posterior wall or roof of the nasopharynx, may become hypertrophied and interfere with the passage of air through the nose and obstruct the eustachian tube.

Infection near the tonsils may be an indication for tonsillectomy, such as retrotonsillar and peritonsillar abscesses and suppurative cervical adenitis.

The decision for performing tonsillectomy and adenoidectomy must be based on problems connected with these tissues. Usually the tonsils and adenoids are removed at the same time, though the child's condition may indicate that separate removal is advisable.

If removal of the tonsils and adenoidal tissue is indicated, but operation is contraindicated, as when a child has hemophilia (see p. 682), the physician may recommend radiologic treatment, which results in shrinkage of the tissue.

Age for Operation. Tonsillectomy and adenoidectomy are seldom necessary in infancy or the toddler period, but may be necessary during the preschool period. The operation is postponed as long as possible for two reasons: (1) the condition may correct itself in a year or more as the tissues normally become smaller, and (2) the operation is psychologically more traumatic to a preschool child because of fears prevalent in this age group.

Place for Operation. Tonsillectomy and adenoidectomy may be done on an inpatient basis in the hospital, or the surgery may be done in a day care unit or an ambulatory surgical unit in a hospital, or it may be done in a free-standing ambulatory surgical center outside of a hospital. The term "verticare" has been applied to outpatient surgery for minor operations that require general anesthesia and used to require that the child stay at least overnight in the hospital.

The advantages of these new types of units in the hospital or the free-standing surgical center are that the child does not have to remain away from home for more than a few hours, resulting in less trauma and family disturbance, and that he is less likely to contract infections from seriously ill children in the hospital. This type of surgery has become feasible because of recent improvements in operative techniques, new types of anesthesia, and better control of bleeding.

Preoperative screening tests are usually done the day before admission. The decision to admit a child to a short-term unit is made not only on the basis of the procedure to be done such as tonsillectomy or adenoidectomy, herniorrhaphy and other minor procedures but also on the basis of the child's age, his status in regard to growth and development, and the period of observation required.

When the child is discharged, the parents are informed by the physician or the nurse as to what to expect during his recovery and what to watch for in terms of complications. The parents are told where help can be obtained in case complications occur.

Further advantages of these short-term facilities for low-risk patients include the freeing of inpatient facilities for children having major problems and the lower cost to the patient's family or to the third-party payer.

Time for Operation. Tonsillectomy and adenoidectomy may be done at any time of the year, since immunization against poliomyelitis has become a widespread practice. Colds and sore throats are more prevalent in the winter and spring, but antibacterial agents are given to reduce the danger of secondary bacterial infections.

Tonsillectomy and adenoidectomy are not done until about 14 to 21 days after an acute infection has subsided. If the child has a chronic infection and surgical removal of the tonsils and adenoids is necessary, an antibiotic is given for a few days before and after operation. When an older child has a history of rheumatic fever, penicillin or sulfonamides, or both, is given.

Preoperative Preparation. The child's parents are told of the nature of the operation. The child is prepared for admission to the hospital. He is also told something about the operation he is to have. He should know that it will be in his throat. The nurse in the clinic or physician's office may help the mother if she does not know how to prepare the child in terms he will understand. If the mother has not prepared the child before he comes to the hospital, she is probably incapable of doing so. The nurse must then explain to the child in a general way what will be done in the operating room, particularly with reference to how he will feel when he comes out of anesthesia.

Since these children are of an age when the first teeth are loosened and fall out, the nurse looks for loose teeth and reports them to the physician so that they may be removed before the child is given the anesthetic.

Usually bleeding and clotting times are obtained preoperatively. A barbiturate, together with atropine, is used for preoperative sedation. Food and fluids are withheld for several hours before operation.

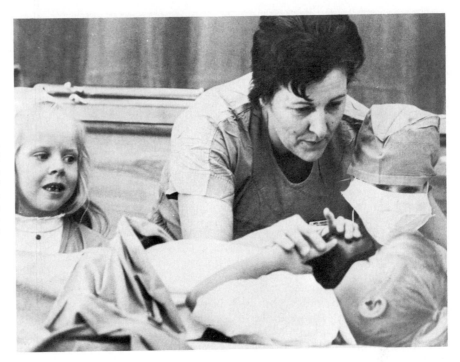

FIGURE 20–6. Preoperative orientation. "Let's pretend" follows children's inspection of equipment. The nurse says, "While Pam is asleep, the doctor will take her tonsils out. Pam will not feel anything." N. Abbott, P. Hansen, and K. Lewis: *Am. J. Nurs.:* 70(11): 2360, November 1970.)

Postoperative Care. On his return from the operating room the child is placed in a prone position with a pillow under his abdomen and chest to facilitate drainage of secretions and to prevent aspiration of vomitus. Since many anesthesiologists believe that positioning of pillows in this way hampers respiratory efforts, the child may be placed partially on his side and partially on his abdomen with the knee of the uppermost leg flexed to hold him in position. He is observed constantly until he is awake and frequently thereafter for several hours. His pulse rate and quality, degree of restlessness, frequency of swallowing and vomiting are noted, since these are symptoms indicative of hemorrhage. Materials necessary for stopping hemorrhage and equipment for suctioning are kept nearby in case of emergency.

Bed rest is indicated for the remainder of the day, and rest periods are necessary for several days after.

Chipped ice may be given when the child wakens. Colored iced popsicles may be more appealing to the child than chipped ice and may encourage his taking more fluids. Synthetic fruit juices are given at first, and later the natural fruit juices. Synthetic juices are less irritating to the throat than most natural juices. Milk, a bland soothing substance, may be given; however, because it coats the mouth and pharynx, the child may try to clear his throat, causing irritation and possible bleeding at the operative site. Soft foods may be started as soon as the nausea following anesthesia is over. All contact with infec-

tion should be avoided. Aspirin may be ordered for discomfort, or acetaminophen (Tylenol) may be ordered if the child is bleeding. An ice collar can be used to relieve discomfort and possibly to reduce hemorrhage unless it makes the child more restless.

Because many parents want to take a major role in their child's care during hospitalization, some surgeons permit them to be present during the anesthetization of the child and to provide care for him after surgery. This parental participation in care does not release the nurse from responsibility for the child's well-being. Indeed, the nurse is responsible for teaching the parents the care to be given postoperatively and for supporting their efforts to provide this care.

Complications. Possible complications are postoperative hemorrhage, lung abscess, septicemia, and pneumonia. Hemorrhage, the most common complication, may be controlled by packing or ligation. If the hemorrhage is severe, anemia, fever, and possibly cardiac dilatation may develop. A transfusion may be indicated.

Reaction of Child to Operation. The value of good preparation (see p. 650) of the parents and child for such surgery is evident when it results in less anxiety for the family, the need for less anesthesia by the child, and later a decreased incidence of hemorrhage. Children who are able to integrate this experience into their personality structure and who have few, if any, emotional ill effects later are those who have been able to transfer positive feelings from the mother to the nurse, to direct their interest away

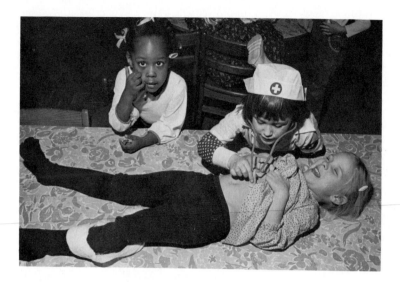

FIGURE 20–7. After hospitalization children may continue their "hospital play" at home. (From West, A. R.: *Children Today*, 5:19, March-April 1976.)

from themselves to other children and to toys and games, and to express themselves freely, either verbally or by crying.

The children most likely to have emotional problems are those who fail to establish positive relations with the nurse, possibly because the mother-child relations are inadequate, who withdraw from the situation or react with panic to it, who are concerned only with their own discomfort and cannot express their feelings about surgery or hospitalization. Parents and nurses may consider these children good during hospitalization, but they are likely to show trauma on their return home.

Discharge of the Child from the Hospital.
Written instructions are given parents about the care of the child after discharge and about symptoms which would indicate that he should be seen at once by a physician. Such symptoms are transient earache, frequent swallowing or the vomiting of blood. The instructions include (1) suggestions for his care, such as keeping him quiet for a few days, fluids and foods to be given, and the necessity of protecting him from infection; (2) information about the giving of medications ordered by the physician; and (3) if the child is not under the care of a private physician, the name and telephone number of the physician to be called in case the parents need advice or emergency care for the child, and the location of the place where the child should be taken for the follow-up examination.

VULVOVAGINITIS

Vulvovaginitis, an inflammatory condition of the vulva and vagina, occurs with some frequency after the toddler period. There are two main types: nongonorrheal vaginitis and gonorrheal vaginitis.

Prepubescent girls tend to acquire vaginal infections more readily than do adolescents or adult females, because the mucosa of the immature vagina is covered with a very thin anestrogenic epithelium, and the vaginal secretions are neutral instead of acidic as in the adult. Since a thick vaginal estrogenized epithelium and an acid medium are protective devices against infections, the child is relatively liable to infection in this area.

NONGONORRHEAL VAGINITIS

Etiology, Clinical Manifestations, Treatment, and Prognosis. Practically any pathogenic organism such as a bacterium, virus, parasite, or fungus can cause nongonorrheal vaginitis.

If the child is not kept clean, if she masturbates, inserts a foreign object into the vagina, has pinworms, or if the area is contaminated with fecal material, vulvovaginitis may result. Organisms from an infected respiratory tract may be transmitted to the genital area by the child's fingers after she has sucked her fingers or picked her nose. If the vaginitis does not respond to therapy, the physician should look for a foreign object causing irritation with subsequent infection.

The *clinical manifestations* are red and swollen genitalia and a vaginal discharge. In some cases a foul odor is present.

Treatment is both systemic and local. The child's general health should be improved and the underlying cause of the infection found. Local application of an estrogenic cream will cure most infections that are nonspecific in 10 days to two weeks. Estrogens may be given by mouth to cornify the epithelium and to produce local tissue resistance. Appropriate antibiotic therapy should be given as needed for specific infections. Monilial vaginitis can be treated with a fungicide such as nystatin. If a foreign body is found, it should be removed and the vagina irrigated. No additional treatment is usually necessary. Pinworm infestation should be treated if present (see p. 548). Douches may be ordered, but are usually unnecessary. Removal of the cause and appropriate treatment assure recovery in most cases.

GONORRHEAL VAGINITIS

Etiology, Clinical Manifestations, and Diagnosis. The *Neisseria gonorrhoeae* causing gonorrhea may gain entrance into the child's vagina during the birth process, from the contaminated hands of the attendants or, later, the hands of the mother. Gonorrhea may also be acquired from unknowing indirect contact with contaminated discharge from an infected child or adult, sexual abuse, or sexual intercourse.

The discharge may vary from a thin, watery type to a thick, yellow, purulent type, depending on the severity of the infection. There is redness and swelling of the vulva and vagina. Although in some cases there is little or no discomfort, there may be dysuria, fever, and excoriation of the skin of the thighs.

Diagnosis is made by laboratory analysis of a sample of the discharge obtained from the vagina or the cervix uteri. Bacterial studies, including culture and a direct smear, should be made.

Complications, Treatment, and Prognosis. *Complications* are much less frequent in children than in adults.

Treatment consists of procaine penicillin given on three successive days. The child should be examined bacteriologically two weeks after completion of therapy because of the possible presence of resistant strains of the organism.

The *prognosis* is good with adequate treatment; without treatment, infection may continue for a long time, possibly until puberty.

VULVOVAGINITIS: RESPONSIBILITIES OF THE NURSE

Case-finding is an important responsibility of the nurse in respect to nongonorrheal or gonorrheal vaginitis. The mother may discuss with the nurse symptoms such as vaginal discharge, irritability, or other indications of an infection mentioned here. A child may complain to the nurse of pain on voiding or defecation. She may also have difficulty in sitting or walking if severe irritation or excoriation of the genitalia and thighs is present.

While bathing a child the nurse examines the genitalia for evidence of a discharge and if any is present reports it to the physician. Individual bedpans and thermometers should be provided. U-shaped toilet seats with paper protectors are used for each child. Showers or spray baths are preferable to tub baths.

The child must be kept extremely clean. The use of a mild soap rather than a detergent is advised. Clean, white, loose-fitting cotton panties should be worn to prevent irritation and binding. Gentle but thorough cleansing of the perineal area is necessary after each urination or defecation.

If the child cannot bathe herself, the nurse or the mother will bathe her. It is important that the perineum be cleansed thoroughly from front to back, rinsed well, and gently and thoroughly dried. An unscented powder may be applied to reduce friction in the area on movement. Both mother and child should be taught to wipe the genitalia *from front to back* after voiding or defecation.

If the vulvovaginitis is due to gonococcus, the child should be isolated until cured. The nurse should be careful in carrying out isolation technique so that no one else becomes infected. The child should not return to kindergarten or nursery school until the infection is completely cured, because of the danger of spreading gonorrhea among the other children.

If the vaginitis has been caused by the insertion of a foreign body, the parents can be counseled that it was probably inserted during normal body exploration just as a foreign body could be inserted into the nose or ear. If there are recurrences, the child may need to be evaluated for a possible emotional problem.

COMMUNICABLE DISEASES

Because of the preschool child's expanding world, his participation in activities with other children in nursery school and play groups, and his exposure to environmental conditions unlike those of his home, he frequently comes in contact with organisms which cause communicable disease. Some of these diseases are preventable, and primary immunizations and booster doses have been given him in infancy (see p. 379), during the toddler period (see p. 522), and during preschool years (see p. 632). Other communicable diseases which are not preventable occur more frequently in this age group than in any other. Serious complications common in past years are less frequent today, however, because of early recognition of the disease and prompt treatment.

COLOR PLATE III

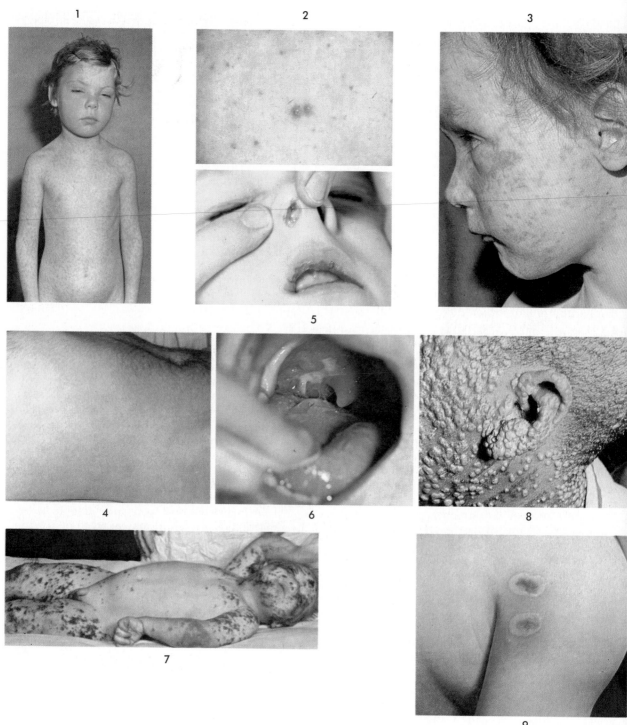

1, **Rubeola.** Small round or oval, red-brown, partially coalescing macules spread over entire body surface. Photophobia (see p. 660). *2*, **Chickenpox.** Note stages of development (macules, papules and vesicles) present at same time (see p. 658). (Courtesy of Dr. P. F. Lucchesi.) *3*, **Rubella** (German measles). See also p. 660. (From Korting, G. W.: *Hautkrankheiten bei Kindern und Jugendlichen.* F. K. Schattauer Verlag, 1969.) *4*, **Scarlet fever** (scarlatina). Diffuse pink-red skin flush with punctate papular lesions (see p. 662). *5*, **Nasal diphtheria** (see p. 658) (Courtesy of Dr. Robert A. Lyon). *6*, **Pharyngotonsillar membrane** of diphtheria (Courtesy of Dr. Robert A. Lyon). *7*, **Fulminating meningococcemia.** Onset 36 hours before admission with vomiting and fever. Death eight hours after admission. (5, 6, and 7 from *Nelson Textbook of Pediatrics*, 10th ed., edited by V. C. Vaughan, III, and R. J. McKay. Philadelphia, W. B. Saunders Co., 1975.) *8*, **Variola vera** (smallpox). Typical umbilicated pustules on erythematous base associated with severe systemic symptoms (see p. 664). *9*, **Smallpox vaccination,** between seven and nine days after the initial vesicle becomes a large necrotic pustule (see p. 382). (*1, 4, 8,* and *9* from *Frieboes/Schonfeld's Color Atlas of Dermatology,* by J. Kimmig and M. Janner. American edition translated and revised by H. Goldschmidt. Stuttgart, Georg Thieme Verlag, 1966.)

654

COLOR PLATE IV

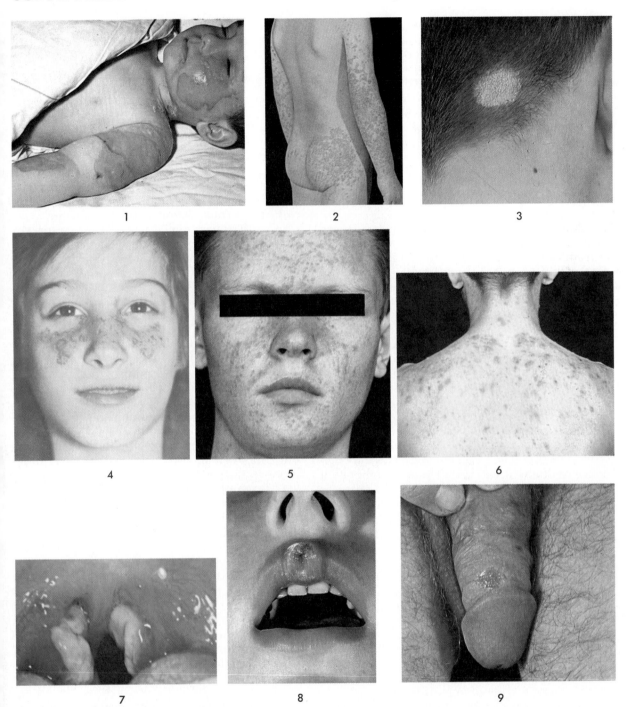

1, **Scald.** Large blisters, erosions, and superficial ulcers caused by hot water (see also p. 556). *2*, **Henoch-Schonlein purpura** (anaphylactoid purpura) See also p. 686. (From G. W. Korting: *Hautkrankheiten bei Kindern und Jugendlichen.* Stuttgart, F. K. Schattauer Verlag, 1969.) *3*, **Tinea capitis.** Sharply marginated round patches with whitish pityriasiform scaling and short broken-off hairs (see p. 754). *4*, Butterfly rash of **systemic lupus erythematosus** (see p. 779). *5*, **Acne vulgaris.** Many papules, with some pustules and comedones in characteristic localization (see p. 849). *6*, **Acne vulgaris.** Infiltrated papules and nodules with some scarring of the upper back. *7*, Pharyngitis, with membrane formation in **infectious mononucleosis** (see p. 868) (Courtesy of Dr. Alex J. Steigman). (*4* and *7* from *Nelson Textbook of Pediatrics*, 10th ed., edited by V. C. Vaughan, III, and R. J. McKay. Philadelphia, W. B. Saunders Co., 1975.) *8*, **Primary syphilis** (chancre). Large indurated lesion on the upper lip. Darkfield positive; STS positive (see p. 887). *9*, **Primary syphilis** (chancre). Smooth, clean exudative infiltrated erosive lesion. Darkfield positive; STS negative. (*1*, *3*, *5*, *6*, *8*, and *9* from *Frieboes/Schonfeld's Color Atlas of Dermatology*, by J. Kimmig and M. Janner. American edition translated and revised by H. Goldschmidt. Stuttgart, Georg Thieme Verlag, 1966.)

The morbidity and mortality rates of communicable diseases have declined dramatically during recent decades but because of the decrease in immunizations of children during the last several years, these rates may rise in the years ahead. Nurses must impress on parents the necessity for full immunization of all children. Continued research and its application in preventive and curative medicine are still necessary.

Definitions. The following definitions are presented as a review of what the student has probably learned in her previous educational experience.

A *communicable disease* is an illness caused by an infectious agent or its toxic products and transmitted from one person to another by direct contact with an infected person, by indirect contact with material containing the causative agent, or by contact with an intermediate host, vector, or inanimate object in the environment. *Sources of infection* may be man, insects, animals, or environmental factors such as dust and contaminated water or food. *Causative agents* include bacteria, yeasts, molds, protozoa, viruses, and rickettsiae.

Communicable diseases may be endemic, epidemic, or pandemic. An *endemic* disease is one that occurs in a proportionately limited number of people in a given area and at a relatively constant rate *Epidemic* disease indicates an incidence of illness which is statistically higher than expected in a given population. A disease is *pandemic* when many cases occur over a large geographic area.

Virulence indicates the ability of the infecting organism to overcome the defenses of the *host*, the body which is involved. The recent habitat of an organism to a large extent influences its virulence. The *incubation period* is the period between exposure to the disease and the appearance of initial symptoms. The *period of communicability* is the time during which an infected person can transmit the disease directly or indirectly to another person.

A *carrier* is a person or animal harboring an infectious agent without manifesting symptoms, although he or it may infect others. A *contact* is a person or animal exposed to an infection through contact with an infected person or animal.

Immunity is the ability of the body to resist the infecting agent. Protection against specific diseases is due to the presence of antibodies which can weaken or destroy the disease-producing agent or neutralize its toxins. *Natural immunity* is present when immunity exists even though the person has not had the disease or been given any form of immunization against it.

Acquired immunity may be either active or passive. *Active immunity* may be acquired by having had the disease or by inoculation with antigens such as dead organisms, weakened organisms, or toxins of organisms. The antigens produce immunity by stimulating the production of antibodies, which protect the body against the infecting agent. Active immunization against common communicable disease has been discussed in relation to health supervision in the various age groups (see p. 381). *Passive immunity* is relatively short-lived and is acquired by transfer of antibodies from mother to child or by inoculation with serum which contains antibodies from immune persons or animals. Passive immunization is used to modify the disease if a person has been exposed or is already infected. Although various types of serums may be used to produce passive immunization, gamma globulin is the most frequent source of human antibodies.

Skin tests may be done to determine immunity against certain diseases. Those most reliable and commonly used are the *Dick test*, which determines susceptibility to scarlet fever, and the *Schick test*, which determines susceptibility to diphtheria.

The *treatment* of communicable disease involves helping the body to resist the invading organisms. Recent research on interferon, a protein produced by the body, shows that interferon-treated cells do not support virus growth well. It would follow, then, that interferon is involved in natural recovery from viral diseases. More study is necessary in this area to determine whether interferon can be used in therapy against some of the viruses causing communicable diseases. *Prevention* is dependent on the establishment of immunity and the prevention of contacts with the causative organism. Because of widespread immunization programs, the spread of many of the childhood diseases has been checked. *Quarantine* means limitation of freedom of movement of persons or animals exposed to a communicable disease for a period of time equal to the longest usual incubation period of the disease.

Children having a communicable disease are hospitalized only if the care they require necessitates hospitalization. They may be admitted to a *general hospital* if proper facilities for *isolation* are available (see p. 95). All personnel caring for such children must be instructed in isolation technique and conscientiously carry it out as a part of medical or nursing care.

Complications. Children who have had encephalitis following a communicable disease such as rubeola, rubella, mumps, pertussis, or meningitis may become mentally retarded (see

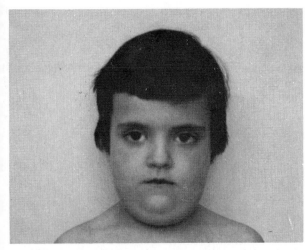

FIGURE 20–8. Mumps. Note the swelling of the glands bilaterally. This child had extreme difficulty in swallowing.

p. 696). Many complications of the common communicable diseases can be prevented if adequate care is given to the child when he initially has his illness.

Classification. Communicable disease entities may be classified into one of four groups: *upper respiratory,* such as pneumonia (see pp. 258, 546), measles, and diphtheria; *gastrointestinal,* such as dysentery and typhoid fever; *dermal* and *membranous,* such as impetigo (see p. 266) and venereal diseases (see p. 887, Chap. 27); and *parenteral,* such as serum hepatitis and malaria. If these diseases are to be controlled, all personnel in medical, nursing, dietary, laundry, housekeeping, and other departments must make combined efforts. Cleanliness is essential in preventing the spread of infection.

Identification of Rashes in Dark Skin. Whether the child is an American Indian, a Negro, a Mexican-American, or simply a deeply suntanned Caucasian, recognition of skin rashes may be difficult. Assessment of changes in skin color requires an alert observer with good color sensitivity.

Adequate lighting is essential. The best illumination is nonglare daylight or a stand light with at least a 60 watt bulb. A newer light that simulates sunlight could also be used. The use of a flashlight or a soft overhead bed light is inadequate for identifying subtle color changes. The part being inspected must be thoroughly but gently cleansed and must have correct light reflection so that rashes may be seen.

The erythema of a rash may not always be accompanied by a noticeable increase in skin temperature. A papular rash may be identified by palpating gently with the fingertips. The nurse may have to rely on the child's complaint of itching or scratching in the case of a macular rash or on observation of the child's having picked, rubbed, or scratched the skin. This behavior may be an indication of skin discomfort. When the skin is not too deeply pigmented, a macular rash may be identified if the skin is gently stretched between the thumb and finger. This technique decreases the normal red tone of the skin and brightens the macules. Since some generalized rashes can also be seen in the mouth, an inspection of the mucosa, the tongue, and the palate may be of value

The Meaning of Isolation to the Child, His Parents, and His Nurse. When a child is isolated, whether for his own protection as when he is burned (see p. 556) or when he has leukemia (see p. 673) or for the protection of others as when he has a communicable disease, he is physically separated from other human beings, both children and adults. In addition, his isolation may psychologically affect the behavior of others toward him. The child may feel forgotten if the nurse does not visit him frequently to care for or to play with him. He may also feel neglected if his parents do not come near him when they visit for fear of carrying infection home to other children in the family.

The child, besides feeling separateness and loneliness, may also be fearful of the gown and possibly the mask and gloves which physicians and nurses wear when they care for him. He may even be disturbed by the strange gowned appearance of his parents when they visit him.

The nurse must explain to both the parents and the child, if he is old enough to understand, the reason for his isolation. If the parents can understand the reason for isolating their child, they are much more likely to be cooperative in following the isolation procedure, much more understanding of the child's need for physical contact and reassurance, and better able to help the child adjust to his hospitalization. If he can understand, the preschool child who is learning to enjoy the presence of other children will appreciate why other children in the unit cannot come near him or exchange their toys with him.

When the child is well enough, the nurse must provide him with opportunities for social interaction and play activities suitable for his age and level of development. Play materials must be of the sort that can be adequately cleaned or disposed of when the child is removed from isolation.

In summary, the nurse must be cognizant of personal feelings toward the isolated child and should be aware of the possible fears lurking in the minds of his parents. The nurse must be perceptive also of the loneliness and fear of the child who is unable to understand this aspect of his care.

Text continued on page 664.

TABLE 20-1. COMMUNICABLE DISEASES

DISEASE	INCUBATION PERIOD	COMMUNICABILITY PERIOD	CAUSATIVE AGENT	METHOD OF SPREAD	CLINICAL MANIFESTATIONS
Chickenpox (varicella) (See Plate 3, Fig. 2)	10–21 days	One day before onset to 6 days after first vesicles appear	Virus	Airborne – droplet infection Direct or indirect contact Dry scabs are not infectious	General malaise, slight fever, anorexia, headache. Successive crops of macules, papules, vesicles, crusts. These may all be present at the same time. Itching of skin. Generalized lymphadenopathy
Diphtheria (See Plate 3, Fig. 5)	2–6 days or longer	Several hours before onset of disease, until organisms disappear from respiratory tract	*Corynebacterium diphtheriae* (bacillus)	Droplets from respiratory tract of infected person or carrier	Local and systemic manifestations. Membrane over tissue in nose or throat at site of bacterial invasion. Hoarse brassy cough with stridor. Toxin from organisms produces malaise and fever. Toxin has affinity for renal, nervous and cardiac tissue
Encephalitis	Dependent on type	Dependent on type Types: 1. Virus encephalitis 2. Postinfectious Occurs with infectious diseases: measles, German measles, mumps, smallpox and following vaccination; pertussis and following immunization 3. Toxic encephalitis Occurs with acute infections or with lead poisoning		1. Virus is maintained in nature by birds and transmitted from bird to bird by mosquitoes and mites. Transmitted to horses and man by bite of infected mosquito 2. Occurs with infectious disease. Cannot be transmitted to others	Encephalitis is an inflammation of the brain. Several types of virus encephalitides, depending on location in which they were found: (St. Louis, Western [U.S.], Eastern [U.S.] and others). Onset is abrupt with vomiting, fever, stiff neck, convulsions, coma Symptoms may appear early or late. Mild symptoms include headache, stiff neck, fever, delirium. More severe manifestations include convulsions, coma, paralysis. Clinical manifestations may be produced by toxin during the course of illness. Child may be very irritable, have muscle twitching or convulsions and abnormal ocular movements
Epidemic influenza	24–72 hours	Not known – possibly during early and febrile stages	Virus types A and B and subtypes; type C	Airborne droplet infection, direct contact	Manifestations in respiratory tract. Sudden onset with chills, fever, muscle pains, cough. If infection is severe and spreads to lower respiratory tract, air hunger may develop
Infectious hepatitis	15–50 days	Few days before to 1 month or more after onset	Virus	Oral contamination by intestinal excretions; contaminated food, milk or water	Manifestations vary from mild to severe, from mild fever, anorexia, generalized malaise, nausea, vomiting, unpleasant taste in mouth, abdominal discomfort and nonexistent or mild jaundice to severe jaundice, coma and death. Early leukopenia is seen. Bile may be detected in urine; bowel movements are clay-colored. Liver function tests are useful for diagnosis

TABLE 20-1. COMMUNICABLE DISEASES (Continued)

TREATMENT AND NURSING CARE	COMPLICATIONS	IMMUNITY
Symptomatic. Prevent child from scratching. Keep fingernails short and clean. Sedation may be necessary. Use soothing lotions to allay itching. If secondary infections occur, antibiotics or chemotherapy may be given	Secondary invasion of pathogenic organisms. Erysipelas, abscesses may occur	*Active immunization:* none *Passive immunization:* none for the normal child. For the ill child human immune serum globulin (ISG) or zoster-immune globulin (ZIG) may be given *Test:* none
Aims of treatment are to inactivate toxins, to kill the organism and to prevent respiratory obstruction. Antitoxin is given against toxin. A broad-spectrum antibiotic may be given against the diphtheria bacilli in addition to antitoxin. Toxoid is given to immunized contacts. Strict bed rest. Prevent exertion. Cleansing throat gargles may be ordered. Liquid or soft diet. Gavage or parenteral administration of fluids may become necessary. Observe for respiratory obstruction. Equipment for suctioning should be available. Oxygen and emergency tracheotomy may be necessary	Vary with severity of disease—bronchopneumonia, circulatory or cardiac failure. Degenerative changes may occur in kidneys	*Active immunization:* one of suitable antigens may be given as part of diphtheria, pertussis, tetanus immunization *Passive immunization:* (1) newborn obtains it transplacentally from immune mother (2) Injection of antitoxin *Test:* Shick test—intracutaneous injection of diphtheria toxin. In susceptible persons, discoloration does and vesiculation may occur at site. If immune, no reaction occurs
No specific treatment can be given. Symptomatic care, adequate nutrition and control of convulsions are essential. Nursing care includes providing a quiet environment, aspiration of nasopharyngeal secretions, gavage or intravenous feedings, oxygen, oral hygiene, good skin care, catheterization and enemas. Sedation and broad-spectrum antibiotics are used to prevent secondary infection. Parents must be helped to understand the prolonged convalescence needed for these children	Incidence of behavioral and neurologic disturbances is higher in young children than in adults. Mental retardation may occur	Immunization is dependent on type of organism involved. Virus encephalitis: some vaccines are available, but not generally used for human patients. Insects such as mosquitoes and mites should be destroyed by insecticides
Symptomatic. Provide bed rest and increased fluid intake. Antibiotics and sulfonamides may prevent secondary infection. Antipyretics, drugs to control cough, and analgesics for pain may be given	In severe cases pulmonary edema and cardiac failure. Secondary invaders may produce bacterial infections of respiratory tract	*Active immunization:* vaccines *Passive immunization:* none *Tests:* none
Symptomatic. Bed rest constitutes basic treatment. Diet should be high protein, high caloric, high carbohydrate and low fat. Food should be served in small, attractive, frequent feedings. Chief reasons for hospitalization are persistent vomiting and toxicity. Fluids may be given parenterally. Enteric precautions are necessary: bedpans should be isolated with the child; disposable gloves may be used when carrying the child's fecal wastes from the room, when giving enemas and taking blood samples. Disposable needles and syringes are advisable in drawing blood samples and in parenteral therapy. Protect from respiratory infections. Observation for indications of increasing severity of disease: unusual somnolence, mental confusion and extreme anorexia. Large doses of adrenal steroids may reverse disease process if irreversible hepatic obstruction has not occurred *Prevention:* thorough washing of hands after bowel movements, adequate cleansing of toilets, decontamination of food and water before use	Liver damage, recurrence of symptoms May be a source of chromosomal damage	*Active immunization:* administration of gamma globulin with subclinical level of disease may produce active immunity. Research is being done to develop a vaccine. *Passive immunization:* pooled gamma globulin after known exposure *Test:* none

Table continued on following page.

TABLE 20–1. COMMUNICABLE DISEASES (Continued)

DISEASE	INCUBATION PERIOD	COMMUNICABILITY PERIOD	CAUSATIVE AGENT	METHOD OF SPREAD	CLINICAL MANIFESTATIONS
Measles (rubeola) (see Plate 3, Fig. 1)	10–12 days	From 4 days before to 5 days after rash appears	Virus	Direct contact and airborne by droplets and contaminated dust	Coryza, conjunctivitis, photophobia are present before rash. Koplik spots in mouth, hacking cough, high fever, rash and enlarged lymph nodes are present. Rash consists of small reddish-brown or pink macules changing to papules; fades on pressure. Rash begins behind ears, on forehead or cheeks, progresses to extremities and lasts about 5 days
Measles— German (rubella) (see Plate 3, Fig. 3)	14–21 days	During prodromal period and for 5 days after appearance of rash	Virus	Direct contact or by contaminated dust particles in air. From secretions of nose and throat of infected persons	Fetus may contract measles *in utero* if mother has the disease. Slight fever, mild coryza. Rash consists of small pink or pale red macules closely grouped to appear as scarlet blush which fades on pressure. Rash fades in 3 days. Swelling of posterior cervical and occipital lymph nodes. No Koplik spots or photophobia as in measles
Meningitis *Aseptic meningitis*	3–5 days or longer	Not really known. Probably 2 to 3 days before to several days after onset	Coxsackie virus Group A viruses (antigenic types 7 & 9) Group B viruses (antigenic types 3 & 5) ECHO virus (types 4, 6, 9 or others)	Direct contact via fecal-oral and pharyngeal-oropharyngeal routes	Onset is fairly acute. Infants are irritable. Older children have headache and hyperesthesia. Fever, nausea and vomiting are common; convulsions rare. Mild, self-limited disease. Nuchal-spinal rigidity occurs. Spinal fluid contains many cells. No organisms are seen on direct smears usually
Bacterial meningitis Meningococcal meningitis (cerebro-spinal fever)	2–10 days	Until meningococci are no longer present in mouth and nasal discharges	Meningococcus or *Neisseria intra-cellularis*	Direct contact or droplet spread from infected person	Sudden onset. Fever, headache, chills, convulsions, irritability, stiff neck and vomiting. Petechial and purpuric areas are seen in skin and mucous membranes in meningococcal septicemia. (See Plate 3, Fig. 5) General muscular rigidity and opisthotonos are seen. Delirium, stupor or coma may occur. Spinal fluid is cloudy and purulent
Hemophilus influenzae *meningitis* (especially from 3 months to 3 years of age)	1–7 days	As long as the pathogen is present in naso-pharynx. No more than 24 hours after beginning effective microbial therapy	Hemophilus influenzae type B	Direct contact or inhalation of infected droplets	Same as meningococcal meningitis
Pneumococcal meningitis	1–7 days	As long as the pathogen is present in naso-pharynx. No more than 24 hours after beginning effective microbial therapy	Diplococcus pneumoniae, especially Types III, V, and XIV	Direct contact or inhalation of infected droplets	Same as meningococcal meningitis

TABLE 20–1. COMMUNICABLE DISEASES (Continued)

TREATMENT AND NURSING CARE	COMPLICATIONS	IMMUNITY
Symptomatic. Keep child in bed until fever and cough subside. Light in room should be dimmed. Keep hands from eyes. Irrigate eyes with physiologic saline solution to relieve itching. Increase humidity in room to relieve cough. Tepid baths and soothing lotion relieve itching of skin. Encourage fluids during fever. Immune serum or gamma globulin may be given to modify illness and reduce complications. Antibacterial therapy given for complications	Vary with severity of disease: otitis media, pneumonia, tracheobronchitis, nephritis Encephalitis may occur	*Active immunization:* (1) live attenuated vaccine; (2) live attenuated vaccine plus separate gamma globulin; (3) killed vaccine (questionable duration of immunity) *Passive immunization:* pooled adult serum, pooled convalescent serum, placental globulin, and gamma globulin of pooled plasma. Newborn obtains immunity transplacentally from mother *Test:* techniques demonstrating rising antibody titers
Symptomatic. Bed rest until fever subsides	Chief danger of disease is damaging effect on fetus if mother contracts infection during first trimester of pregnancy. Newborn may have *congenital rubella syndrome* with permanent defects of cataracts, cardiovascular anomalies, deafness, microcephaly, and mental retardation among others. Virus can be isolated from the blood, urine, throat, cerebrospinal fluid, lens, and other involved organs. Infants may shed virus for 12 to 18 months Severe complications are rare Encephalitis may occur	*Active immunization:* live attenuated rubella virus vaccine *Passive immunization:* gamma globulin *Test:* hemagglutination-inhibition test for detection of rubella antibodies (some states require women to take premarital blood tests to determine their susceptibility to rubella)
No specific treatment. No isolation of patient or quarantine of contacts Aspirin, sponging, and a cool room are helpful Recovery is likely	None usually	*Active immunization:* none *Passive immunization:* none *Test:* none
Crystalline sodium penicillin G is used. Sulfonamides may also be used. Sedatives (paraldehyde) may be needed for restlessness. Intravenous therapy is usually necessary to supply dextrose-electrolyte solutions, plasma, plasma expanders, or blood for dehydration or shock. Symptomatic care includes adequate nutrition (gavage if necessary), frequent turning and good skin care to prevent decubiti, special mouth care to prevent stomatitis, and eye care to prevent drying of conjunctivae. Oxygen administration may be necessary if the child becomes cyanotic. Accurate observation, recording and reporting are necessary if the child has convulsions (see p. 473), drug reactions, urinary retention or constipation. Catheterization or enemas may be required. Cold water mattress may be used to help reduce elevated temperature. Lumbar punctures (see p. 294), are done for diagnosis, intrathecal administration of medication and reduction of intracranial pressure. For severe brain swelling intravenous urea or mannitol may be used. Suction apparatus and stimulants should be kept at the bedside. Observations must be made of return of function to the extremities, or any change in behavior or symptoms or signs indicating the occurrence of otitis media, pneumonia, obstructive hydrocephalus, subdural collections of fluid, paralysis, spasticity or contractures	Otitis media (see p. 399), ophthalmia or pneumonia may occur. Infection may extend to ventricles and cause obstructive hydrocephalus (see p. 301) Subdural collections of fluids may occur. Headache may persist. Intellectual faculties may be impaired (see p. 696). Child may have paralysis, spasticity, contractures	*Active immunization:* none. Research is being done on a vaccine. Three meningococcal polysaccharide vaccines: monovalent A, monovalent C, and bivalent A–C vaccine are licensed for selective use in this country *Passive immunization:* none (mass chemoprophylaxis with sulfadiazine may reduce the meningococcal carrier rate) *Test:* none
Sulfonamides and chloramphenicol or ampicillin. Organism resistance to ampicillin is developing. (same as meningococcal meningitis)	Serious neurologic and mental sequelae. (see above, meningococcal meningitis)	*Active immunization:* none *Passive immunization:* none *Test:* none
Crystallin penicillin G. Relapses may occur. (same as meningococcal meningitis)	Serious neurologic and mental sequelae. (see above, meningococcal meningitis)	*Active immunization:* none *Passive immunization:* none *Test:* none

Table continued on following page.

661

TABLE 20–1. COMMUNICABLE DISEASES (Continued)

DISEASE	INCUBATION PERIOD	COMMUNICABILITY PERIOD	CAUSATIVE AGENT	METHOD OF SPREAD	CLINICAL MANIFESTATIONS
Mumps (infectious parotitis) (see Fig. 20–8)	14–21 days	One to 6 days before first symptoms appear until swelling disappears	Virus	Direct or indirect contact with salivary secretions of infected person	Salivary glands are chiefly affected. Parotid glands, sublingual and submaxillary glands may be involved. Swelling and pain occur in these glands either unilaterally or bilaterally. Child may have difficulty in swallowing, headache, fever and malaise
Pertussis (whooping cough)	5–21 days	Four to 6 weeks from onset	*Bordetella pertussis*	Direct contact or droplet spread from infected person	Coryza, dry cough which is worse at night. Cough occurs in paroxysms of several sharp coughs in one expiration, then a rapid deep inspiration followed by a whoop. Dyspnea and fever may be present. Vomiting may occur after coughing. Lymphocytosis occurs
Poliomyelitis (infantile paralysis)	5–14 days	During period of infection, latter part of incubation period and the first week of acute illness	Virus types 1 (Brunhilde), 2 (Lansing) and 3 (Leon)	Oral contamination by pharyngeal and intestinal excretions	Acute illness. Initial symptoms of upper respiratory tract infection, headache, fever, vomiting. Types of poliomyelitis include abortive, nonparalytic, spinal paralytic and bulbar paralytic forms. Clinical manifestations may vary from mild to very severe after symptomless period following initial symptoms. Later symptoms may include intense headache, nausea, vomiting, muscular soreness, nuchal and spinal rigidity, changes in reflexes, paralysis. Tripod sign is indicative of spinal rigidity. Examination of cerebrospinal fluid shows an increase in protein and in the number of cells, but the fluid is rarely cloudy
Rocky Mountain spotted fever	3–12 days	Not communicable from man to man	*Rickettsia rickettsii*	Spread by wood ticks or dog ticks from animals to man. (If tick is found, it should be removed without crushing it)	Sudden onset of nonspecific symptoms—headache, fever, restlessness, anorexia. One to 5 days after onset, pale, discrete rose-red macules or maculopapules appear
Hemolytic streptococcal infection (streptococcal sore throat and scarlet fever—scarlatina) (see Plate 3, Fig. 4)	2–5 days	Onset to recovery	Beta hemolytic streptococcus, group A strains	Droplet infection or direct and indirect transmission may occur	Initial symptoms of streptococcal sore throat are seen in pharynx. The source of this organism may also be in a burn or wound. Toxin from site of infection is absorbed into blood stream. The typical symptoms of scarlet fever which may result are headache, fever, rapid pulse, rash, thirst, vomiting, lymphadenitis and delirium. Throat is injected, and cellulitis of throat occurs. White tongue coating desquamates, and redstrawberry tongue results. Schultz-Charlton phenomenon is a blanch reaction occurring after intradermal injection of 0.2 ml. of convalescent serum or diluted antitoxin. Other manifestations may include otitis media, mastoiditis and meningitis

TABLE 20–1. COMMUNICABLE DISEASES (Continued)

TREATMENT AND NURSING CARE	COMPLICATIONS	IMMUNITY
Local application of heat or cold to salivary glands to reduce discomfort Liquids or soft foods are given. Foods containing acid may increase the pain. Bed rest until swelling subsides	Complications are less frequent in children than in adults Meningoencephalitis, inflammation of ovaries or testes, or deafness may occur	*Active immunization:* (1) live attenuated vaccine, (2) placentally transferred immunity is possible for newborns *Passive immunization:* Gamma globulin preferably from serum containing high mumps antibody titers *Test:* complement fixation test. Serum amylase determination
Symptomatic. Pertussis immune antiserum may be given. Protect child from secondary infection. Sulfonamides and antibiotics may be given to prevent secondary infections. Provide mental and physical rest to prevent paroxysms of coughing. Provide warm, humid air. Oxygen may be necessary. Avoid chilling. Offer small frequent feedings to maintain nutritional status. Refeed if child vomits. Small amounts of sedatives may be given to quiet the child	Very serious disease during infancy because of complication of bronchopneumonia Otitis media, marasmus, bronchiectasis and atelectasis may occur. Hemorrhage may occur during paroxysms of coughing. Encephalitis	*Active immunization:* vaccine. May be given as part of diphtheria, pertussis, tetanus immunization *Passive immunization:* gamma globulin prepared from hyperimmune human serums *Test:* serum agglutinin titer and by fluorescent antibody technique. Culture of B pertussis from nasopharyngeal mucus
Both parents and child need support and reassurance, for they are fearful of the term "polio." Treatment and nursing care are symptomatic. Avoid overfatigue. Place child on firm mattress with support for feet. Prevent pressure on the toes when child is on abdomen by pulling mattress away from foot of bed and let feet hang over the edge; when child is on back, use a foot board for support of the feet. Change position frequently. Maintain good body alignment. Encourage oral intake of food and fluids appropriate to degree of illness. Physiotherapy may be necessary. Applications of moist heat to alleviate muscular pain. Therapy is required to prevent contracture from muscle shortening and to lessen residual disability. Manipulation of affected extremities within normal range of motion may be done by the nurse with permission of the physician. Antibacterial prophylaxis may be ordered. Catheterization of a distended bladder may be necessary. Since the stools contain the virus, they should be considered infectious. In bulbar poliomyelitis therapy is directed at suctioning of the pharynx and postural drainage to prevent aspiration of secretions, feeding by gavage, parenteral fluids, tracheotomy, use of respirator, oxygen, and prevention of intercurrent infection. Prolonged rehabilitation may be necessary, including braces, splints or surgery.	Emotional disturbances, gastric dilatation, melena, hypertension or transitory paralysis of bladder may occur	*Active immunization* may be acquired from apparent or inapparent infection and from the use of vaccine: trivalent oral polio virus vaccine (TOPV) *Passive:* newborn obtains it transplacentally from mother if immune. Pooled adult gamma globulin *Test:* recovery of poliovirus from feces and throat swabs In epidemic situations children should have limited or no contact with persons outside the family
Early diagnosis and prompt use of chloramphenicol or tetracyclines. Corticosteroid therapy may be given. Supportive therapy, parenteral fluids, oxygen and sedatives may be necessary for seriously ill patients	Central nervous system symptoms, electrolyte disturbances, peripheral circulatory collapse, and pneumonia may occur	*Active immunization:* vaccine *Passive immunization:* none *Test:* serum titer of complement-fixing antibody
Penicillin. Adequate fluid intake, bed rest, drugs to relieve pain, and mouth care are important. Diet should be given as the child wishes; liquid, soft or regular. Warm saline throat irrigations may be given to the older child. Increased humidity for severe infection of upper respiratory tract. Cold or hot applications to painful cervical lymph nodes	Complications are caused by toxins, the streptococcus, or secondary infection. Complications of pneumonia, glomerulonephritis or rheumatic fever may occur	*Active immunization:* none *Passive immunization:* none *Test:* Dick test—intradermal injection of streptococcal toxin. In susceptible persons erythema occurs at site of injection. In immune persons no reaction occurs (Currently, a highly purified vaccine designed to prevent childhood streptococcal infections is being tested, however, its efficacy will not be known for some time)

Table continued on following page.

TABLE 20–1. COMMUNICABLE DISEASES (Continued)

DISEASE	INCUBATION PERIOD	COMMUNICABILITY PERIOD	CAUSATIVE AGENT	METHOD OF SPREAD	CLINICAL MANIFESTATIONS
Smallpox (variola) (see Plate 3, Fig. 8)	12 days	One to 2 days before symptoms until crusts all drop off; usually 3 to 4 weeks	Virus	Direct or indirect contact; possibly air-borne. Crusts are infectious	Abrupt onset with vomiting, headache, high fever and generalized aching. Skin eruption occurs a few days after onset, changing from macules to papules, vesicles, then pustules. Umbilication is characteristic of vesicles. Prostration or convulsions may occur. Individual lesions appear in single crop and progress at same rate. Mucous membranes of mouth and eyes become involved. Degree of scarring depends on severity and extent of eruption
Tetanus (lockjaw)	3–21 days	Not communicable from man to man	*Clostridium tetani* bacillus	Organisms are found in soil and enter body through a wound. Deep puncture wounds are ideal for growth of this anaerobic organism; burns are ideal because of presence of necrotic tissue	Acute or gradual onset. Bacillus produces a powerful toxin having an affinity for nervous system. Clinical manifestations include muscle rigidity and spasm, hyperirritability, convulsions, headache, fever. *Trismus*, or inability to open the mouth, is present. Spasm of facial muscles results in *risus sardonicus*, or the sardonic grin. *Opisthotonos*, a backward arching of the back, develops, due to the dominance of the extensor muscles of the spine. Clonic tetanospasms may be triggered by slight external stimuli. Consciousness is not lost. Urine may be retained, due to spasm of urethral muscles. Cyanosis and asphyxia may occur, due to muscle spasms of larynx and chest. The rate of metabolism is increased because of the intense muscle hyperirritability. Death may result from aspiration pneumonia or exhaustion

Table 20–1 presents in brief form the common communicable diseases found in the pediatric age group and those against which immunization may be given.

ACUTE GLOMERULONEPHRITIS (GLOMERULAR NEPHRITIS)

Incidence, Etiology, and Pathology. Acute glomerulonephritis is the most common form of nephritis in children. Approximately 66 per cent of cases of this disease occur in children under the age of seven years. It is seldom seen under three years of age and is more common in boys than in girls. It does not appear to run in families.

Glomerulonephritis is an antigen-antibody reaction following an infection in some part of the body—usually a group A beta hemolytic streptococcal infection of the upper respiratory tract (see p. 648). Nephritis may follow scarlet fever or a streptococcal infection of the skin such as impetigo or infected eczema. Nephritis may occur from one to three weeks after the onset of the infection.

The kidneys become enlarged and pale. On the cortical and cut surfaces there are small, punctate hemorrhages. The glomeruli appear large and relatively avascular. The glomerular capillaries permit blood protein and cells to pass into the glomerular filtrate. The cells of the tubules appear granular and swollen. Capillary damage occurs. Changes are suggestive of the presence of antigen-antibody complexes on the glomerular capillaries. (Kidney tissue can be obtained by needle biopsy during life and can provide some information about the pathologic process.) There may be generalized edema with cerebral edema.

Clinical Manifestations and Diagnosis. Glomerulonephritis may vary from a mild illness which may go unnoticed to a severe illness having a sudden onset. *Clinical manifestations* in severe cases may include headache, malaise, high fever, hypertension, oliguria or anuria, and possibly cardiac decompensation leading to death.

TABLE 20-1. COMMUNICABLE DISEASES (Continued)

TREATMENT AND NURSING CARE	COMPLICATIONS	IMMUNITY
No treatment except antibiotics and sulfonamides for secondary infections. Eye care, oral hygiene, and diet as tolerated are given. Severe cases may require sedation and parenteral fluid therapy and gavage. Oxygen, blood transfusions and digitalis therapy may be indicated	Laryngitis, bronchopneumonia and encephalitis. Infants having eczema may develop generalized vaccinia if vaccinated	*Active immunization:* vaccination, using multiple pressure method, no longer required (see Plate 3, Fig. 8) *Passive immunization:* vaccinia immune gamma globulin may modify disease *Test:* none
After injury and during illness toxins should be neutralized with antitoxin. Tests for sensitivity to serum must be done before antitoxin is administered. Tetanus immune globulin (human) if available should be used instead of antitoxin (equine). Penicillin is effective against tetanus organisms. Wound should be cleaned thoroughly. Antibiotics should be given to prevent infection of wound. All hospital supplies contaminated with tetanus organism should be adequately sterilized. Good supportive care requires constant attention of the nurse and a physician if possible. Place child in darkened, quiet room. Avoid any stimulation which may cause spasms. A combination of muscle relaxant, sedative and tranquillizing medications will help to control tetanospasms. The child should be relaxed, but not too sedated. Tracheotomy may be necessary if laryngospasm occurs. Parenteral fluid therapy, oxygen, respirator for respiratory failure, suction apparatus, gavage feedings and indwelling catheter may be necessary. After patient recovers, roentgenograms should be taken to detect fractures or avulsion of muscle insertions	Obstruction of larynx, anoxia, atelectasis and pneumonia	*Active immunization:* toxoid is a potent antigen. May be given as part of diphtheria, pertussis, tetanus immunization *Passive immunization:* newborn has placentally transmitted antitoxin, but it is inadequate for protection. Passive immunization results from injection of tetanus immune globulin or antitoxin within a few hours after wound occurs *Test:* none

In the usual case the child is not critically ill, but has hematuria. The urine may appear grossly bloody or may have a smoky color. There may be mild edema around the eyes; only rarely is there generalized edema unless the child has cardiac decompensation. The temperature at first may be elevated to 104° F. (40° C.), but within a week falls to 100° F. (37.8° C.) and continues at this level until the kidneys heal. The child may have a headache, anorexia, vomiting, constipation, or diarrhea. Hypertension may occur. The systolic blood pressure may be elevated to 200 mm. of mercury, the diastolic pressure to 120 mm.

Cerebral symptoms may occur when the blood pressure rises, owing to cerebral ischemia as a result of vasospasm. The child complains of headache, may be drowsy, may have diplopia and convulsions, and may vomit. The pulse is slow. The cerebral symptoms disappear when the blood pressure is reduced.

The urinary output is usually less than normal. The urine contains albumin, red blood cells, some white blood cells and casts, and has a high specific gravity. The blood urea nitrogen value is elevated. Anemia may be present. The corrected erythrocyte sedimentation rate is rapid.

Clinical improvement can be noted between one and two weeks after the onset. The urine becomes normal between six weeks and several months after the onset of the illness.

Approximately three quarters of all children having glomerulonephritis have cardiac involvement. Cardiac failure may cause death, but if the child recovers, there is complete restoration of cardiac function.

The *diagnosis* is based on the history of previous infection, the presence of hematuria, slight edema, and albuminuria. If cardiac failure occurs early in the disease, nephritis may not be the initial diagnosis.

Other diagnoses which must be considered are acute pyelonephritis (see p. 426), scurvy (see p. 443), and blood dyscrasias.

Treatment. The treatment is symptomatic. Bed rest is ordered during the acute stage and until urinary findings are nearly normal. After that, activity does not affect the course of the disease The urine is examined at frequent intervals. The child must be protected from chilling, fatigue, and contact with others having respiratory infections. The diet during the first few days when he may be nauseated consists of clear fluids. As the child recovers, a full liquid, soft, and then a regular diet may be given. If edema is severe, dietary salt may be limited. During the acute phase, protein may be somewhat restricted.

Penicillin should be given during the acute phase because of streptococci found on pharyngeal cultures. It may also be given orally for two to three months following the acute phase in order to lessen the chances of another upper respiratory tract infection. Adrenocortical steroid medication is not usually given.

If the blood pressure is elevated, indicative of vasospasm, cardiac failure or hypertensive encephalopathy may develop. If the systolic blood pressure is above 140 mm. and the diastolic above 95 mm., a combination of reserpine and hydralazine hydrochloride (Apresoline) is given intramuscularly. These hypotensive drugs reduce the blood pressure rapidly. They may be given orally in divided doses after the initial dose. In an acute hypertensive emergency, diazoxide or methyldopa may also be given.

Fluids are restricted if the child has severe hypertension, unless the urinary output is large.

A child having hypertensive encephalopathy with convulsions may need sedation. A lumbar puncture and oxygen therapy may also be ordered. If he has cardiac failure, sedation with opiates, digitalis, and oxygen may be indicated. It is necessary to follow the cardiac status after the symptoms have disappeared.

If the urinary output is decreased, acidosis, edema, and uremia may develop. The need is to increase the urinary output and the excretion of waste products of metabolism Enough water must be taken so that the kidneys can excrete at their maximal capacity. If the child is vomiting, fluids can be given intravenously or subcutaneously to prevent dehydration and acidosis. When nitrogen retention is severe, it may be necessary to eliminate protein from the diet. Solutions containing potassium are not given when oliguria or anuria is present because of the danger of hyperkalemia. If the serum potassium concentration is over 6 mEq. per liter, measures must be taken to reduce it. If other measures fail, peritoneal dialysis is used.

Peritoneal dialysis is useful in correcting acidosis, electrolyte disturbances such as hyperkalemia, and uremia. It is a form of hemodialysis in which the peritoneal lining is used as a dialyzing membrane for filtering waste products from the blood plasma into a dialyzing solution. Strict aseptic technique must be used. Prior to performing peritoneal dialysis, the child's bladder must be emptied. Heparin is added to each liter of dialysis solution. Potassium is added if hyperkalemia is not present or has been corrected by prior dialysis. The dialysis solution should be kept warmed at 98.6 to 100 4° F. (37 to 38° C.). The skin and subcutaneous tissue are anesthetized at the site of insertion of the peritoneal catheter. The trochar and catheter are inserted in the midline just below the umbilicus or just lateral to the rectus muscle at the level of the umbilicus. Care must be taken to determine that the liver and spleen are not enlarged. When the trochar is removed, the catheter is directed into the pelvic cavity. The dialysis fluid is run in slowly, allowed to equilibrate for 20 to 30 minutes and then permitted to drain off. The peritoneal cavity must be drained completely with each cycle. An accurate cumulative record must be kept of the amount of electrolytes and the volume of fluid given and withdrawn. The dialysis fluid should be cultured frequently. Dialysis may be continued for 48 hours. The child's vital signs must be carefully observed for any adverse effect from the procedure. Children tolerate this procedure well. No special equipment is necessary, and an arteriovenous shunt is not required as it is for hemodialysis. A kidney transplant may be done if necessary.

Responsibilities of the Nurse. Bed rest is essential during the acute phase of glomerulonephritis and until the urine is relatively free from blood cells. The nurse prevents chilling of the child by dressing him warmly and, when he is in bed, covering him with light but warm blankets. He should be kept in a well ventilated, warm room away from children with infections.

Vital signs are noted as ordered; the blood pressure is taken frequently because sudden changes may occur. Any rise is reported at once. The nurse observes indications of cerebral manifestations due to hypertension. When these occur, the child is placed in his crib with the gates raised. If he is in a bed, side bars are applied to prevent him from falling. When the blood pressure is elevated, the nurse should have equipment on hand to give the medications which the physician may order.

The skin is kept clean and dry. The diet and fluid intake are as ordered by the physician, and any limitation of salt, fluids, or protein followed exactly. If the fluid intake is restricted, the amount allowed in 24 hours should be divided throughout the day. Small amounts of fluid served attractively are offered at planned intervals. Most of the fluid is given during the day so that the child can sleep as much as possible during the night. The fluid intake and output are measured. The child is weighed at the same time daily to determine progress. The nurse notes the presence of any periorbital edema.

When he is allowed up, he should avoid fatigue. He should have sufficient play activities to keep him quiet and contented.

To prevent disciplinary problems when these children feel better, all the nurses caring for them can establish limits to behavior and be consistent in their care. They allow the child as much independence within limits as he is able to assume If he is sent home for convalescence, the nurse helps the mother plan ways to keep him happy while on prolonged bed rest. The nurse must stress the need for continued medical supervision and continuation of antibiotic therapy if this is ordered.

Prognosis. Glomerulonephritis is usually benign in childhood, and the prognosis is good, but it is unpredictable for the individual child. Second attacks are uncommon, but if healing is not complete, the child may again have symptoms if he has another upper respiratory tract infection or a tonsillectomy. Recurrences of the illness are rare because the child has developed immunity to the specific type of beta-hemolytic streptococcus that caused the original infection. Tonsillectomy and adenoidectomy should not be done for several months after the acute phase, and administration of penicillin should precede and follow the operation to prevent bacterial spread.

The course of glomerulonephritis may last from ten days to a year. Chronic nephritis may develop in a small number of children, or they may die as a result of their illness.

STRABISMUS (SQUINT, CROSS-EYE)

Significance and Etiology. Strabismus is a condition in which the extraocular muscles do not balance; therefore the eyes cannot function in unison. The child seems to be looking in two directions at once. The normal infant many times appears to have a squint at birth, and this may continue until approximately the age of six months, when his eyes become normal. Other infants appear to have strabismus when they have epicanthal folds and a broad nose. This latter condition is termed *spurious squint,* and no treatment is necessary.

The importance of strabismus in the pediatric age group is that (1) one eye is generally not used as much as the other, and therefore poor central vision in that eye results from disuse (*amblyopia ex anopsia*); (2) there is absence of fusion of vision resulting in double images (*diplopia*); and (3) emotional problems occur when the child is taunted by other children about his deformity.

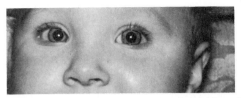

FIGURE 20–9. Pseudoesotropia. Epicanthal folds and a flat nasal bridge frequently give the appearance of esotropia when the infant looks to the side and the entire nasal bulbar conjunctiva is covered. (From Harley, R. D. (Ed.): *Pediatric Ophthalmology.* Philadelphia, W. B. Saunders Co., 1975.)

There are several causes for strabismus, and one or more may be found in any case In some cases it is difficult to ascertain the cause. Strabismus may be congenital or familial, or it may be caused by an acute illness such as encephalitis or diphtheria. It may be due to paralysis of certain muscles or may occur because the muscles do not function together.

Clinical Manifestations and Treatment. The child with strabismus may be able to fuse when he looks in certain directions, but not in others. He may not be able to describe to his mother what he sees. He may tilt his head to bring the images together or close one eye to block out an undesired image. He may appear clumsy and may stumble, or be unable to pick up objects with accuracy.

There are various types of strabismus, each producing slightly different effects on the eyes. In *monocular* strabismus one eye deviates permanently and the other eye is always used. The fixating eye should be patched for months to improve the vision in the other eye. Surgery may be necessary. *Alternating* strabismus is present when either eye may be used for fixation on an object while the other eye deviates. Vision is developed more or less equally in both eyes, but surgery is usually necessary. *Accommodative* strabismus is dependent on the relationship between accommodation and convergence of the eyes. The use of corrective glasses and sometimes occlusion of the eye may be necessary.

When the eyes have a tendency to turn inward, the child is said to have convergent strabismus or *esotropia*. If they tend to turn outward, the condition is called divergent strabismus or *exotropia*. If the eyes are out of vertical alignment, one eye seemingly higher than the other, the condition is known as *hypertropia*.

The first step in *correction* of strabismus is to prevent double vision and to hide the defect by placing a patch over the good or fixating eye. The patch should be kept on all day and cover the eye completely. The patch may be necessary for weeks or months while the child is forced to develop the deviating eye. The patch covering the good eye may prove to be traumatic to the child, since he has difficulty seeing adequately. He may resist wearing it, and parents need help to devise means of having the child keep it on, such as the use of clear glasses with one glass covered. Children as young as 14 months may wear corrective glasses. Orthoptic treatment or muscle exercises may also be effective in developing fusion.

Surgical treatment is carried out on children who do not benefit from exercises or glasses. Operation must be done by the age of three or four years if parallelism of the eyes and binocular vision are to be achieved. Surgery consists in lengthening or shortening extraocular structures.

Strabismus should be corrected before the child goes to school, because other children will laugh at his defect, and he will suffer emotional trauma.

Responsibilities of the Nurse. The nurse can help both the parents and the child to understand the importance of eye exercises and of wearing glasses prescribed by the ophthalmologist. The child who wears glasses must be taught how to protect them when he plays and how to keep them clean. Safety glass should be used in the lenses. A broken lens should be replaced immediately. The child should have his glasses with him when he is hospitalized and keep them in their case, in the bedside table, when he is not wearing them.

A child who is scheduled for operation is hospitalized a few days beforehand. He should be prepared by his parents not only for hospitalization but also before surgery for the postoperative period when his eyes will be covered and his arms restrained. He should also experience having his eyes covered and his arms restrained by his parents or nurse so that he will not be frightened after his return from the operating room. He should know that as soon as possible the eye dressings and restraints will be removed. Some children, when the bandages are removed, may be amazed that they can see, because they may have feared that they would not be a whole person after the operation. The parents should be encouraged to remain with their child postoperatively to provide the sense of security he needs. They or his nurse should read or tell stories to him, play phonograph

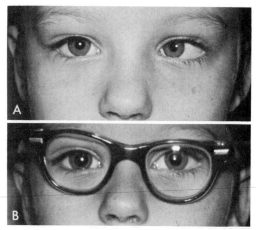

FIGURE 20–10. Accommodative esotropia. *A*, Without glasses there is a left esotropia of 15 degrees (Hirschberg). *B*, Same child wearing single vision lenses, which have aligned the visual axes. (From Harley, R. D. (Ed.): *Pediatric Ophthalmology.* Philadelphia, W. B. Saunders Co., 1975.)

records or turn on the radio, and play simple games with him so that the hours of blindness pass more quickly. The parent or nurse should speak before touching him so that he is not startled.

Therapeutic play is important for these children. The child can act out the role of the helpful or agressive doctor instead of the helpless child. He can bandage his doll's eyes and ultimately his own. When he is able to bandage his own eyes, he has begun to master his anxiety. Observation of a child's play can reveal what part of his treatment the child has accepted and what he is denying psychologically.

A regular diet may be given postoperatively as soon as the child is no longer nauseated. These children enjoy being told about their food while the parents or nurse feeds them. Postoperatively, the nurse can help the parents understand the exercises recommended by the ophthalmologist. The nurse can also notify the nursery school or school nurse so that the same exercises may be continued regularly.

Prognosis. Usually, the earlier treatment is given, the better are the results and personality disorders are prevented. If visual acuity has been affected, permanent reduction of sight may be expected.

TEACHING AIDS AND OTHER INFORMATION[*]

American Academy of Pediatrics

Ampicillin—Resistant Strains of *H. Influenzae*, Type B
Care of Children in Hospitals.
Infectious Diseases (Red Book).
Personal Immunization Record Card.

American Heart Association

Children with Heart Disease: A Guide for Teachers.
Protect Your Child's Heart.

The Children's Hospital Medical Center, Boston, Mass.

Rey, M., and Rey, H. A.: Curious George Goes to the Hospital.

Department of National Health and Welfare: Ottawa, Canada

Immunization—A Guide for International Travellers.

National Kidney Foundation

Acute Glomerulonephritis.
The Artificial Kidney Machine

National Society for the Prevention of Blindness, Inc.

Charlie Brown Detective, 1975.
Crossed Eyes: A Needless Handicap, 1974.

Prevent Blindness: Signs of Possible Eye Trouble in Children, 1976.
Your Eyes for a Lifetime of Sight.

Public Affairs Committee

Graves, J.: Right from the Start: The Importance of Early Immunization.

The Touchstone Center

My Roots Be Coming Back.
Out of My Body.

United Cerebral Palsy Association

Two Kinds of Measles.

United States Government

Altshuler, A.: Books That Help Children with a Hospital Experience, 1974.
Center for Disease Control: Morbidity and Mortality Weekly Report, May 7, 1976.
Kidney Disease and Artificial Kidneys, 1972
Shore, M. F. (Ed.): Red Is the Color of Hurting, 1967.

[*]Complete addresses are given in the Appendix.

REFERENCES

Books

American Academy of Pediatrics: *Care of Children in Hospitals.* Evanston, Ill., American Academy of Pediatrics, 1971.
American Academy of Pediatrics: *Report of the Committee on Infectious Diseases.* 17th ed. Evanston. Ill., American Academy of Pediatrics, 1974.
American Hospital Association: *Infection Control in the Hospital.* 3rd ed. Chicago, American Hospital Association, 1974.
Bell, W. E., and McCormick, W. F.: *Neurologic Infections in Children.* Philadelphia, W. B. Saunders Company, 1975.
Benenson, A. S. (Ed.): *Control of Communicable Diseases in Man.* 12th ed. Washington. D.C., American Public Health Association, 1975.
Briody, B. A.: *Microbiology and Infectious Disease.* New York, McGraw-Hill Book Company, 1974.
Dynski-Klein, M.: *Color Atlas of Pediatrics.* Chicago, Year Book Medical Publishers, Inc., 1975.
Eisen, H. N.: *Immunology.* New York, Harper & Row, 1974.
Falconer, M. W., Patterson, H. R., and Gustafson, E. A.: *Current Drug Handbook 1976–1978.* Philadelphia, W. B. Saunders Company, 1976.
Frobisher, M., et al.: *Fundamentals of Microbiology.* 9th ed. Philadelphia, W. B. Saunders Company. 1974.
Gutch, C. F., and Stoner, M. H.: *Review of Hemodialysis For Nurses and Dialysis Personnel.* 2nd ed. St. Louis, The C. V. Mosby Company. 1975.
Hardgrove, C. B., and Dawson, R. B.: *Parents and Children in The Hospital: The Family's Role in Pediatrics.* Boston, Little, Brown & Company, 1972
Harley, R. D. (Ed.): *Pediatric Ophthalmology.* Philadelphia, W. B. Saunders Company, 1975.
Havener, W. H., et al.: *Nursing Care In Eye, Ear, Nose and Throat Disorders.* 3rd ed. St. Louis, The C. V. Mosby Company, 1974.
Huffman, J. W.: *The Gynecology of Childhood and Adolescence.* Philadelphia, W. B. Saunders Company. 1968.

Hughes, J. G.: *Synopsis of Pediatrics.* 4th ed. St. Louis, The C. V. Mosby Company, 1975.
Kark, S. L.: *Epidemiology and Community Medicine.* New York, Appleton-Century-Crofts, 1974.
Krugman, S , and Ward, R.: *Infectious Diseases of Children and Adults.* 5th ed. St. Louis, The C. V. Mosby Company. 1973.
Lieberman, E. (Ed.): *Clinical Pediatric Nephrology.* Philadelphia, J. B. Lippincott Company, 1975.
McInnes, M. E.: *Essentials of Communicable Disease.* 2nd ed. St. Louis, The C. V. Mosby Company, 1975.
Moffet, H. L.: *Clinical Microbiology.* Philadelphia, J. B. Lippincott Company, 1975.
Moll, H.: *Atlas of Pediatric Diseases.* Philadelphia, W. B. Saunders Company, 1976.
Plank, E. N.: *Working With Children in Hospitals.* 2nd ed. Chicago, Year Book Medical Publishers, Inc , 1971.
Roy, F. H.: *Practical Management of Eye Problems: Glaucoma, Strabismus, Visual Fields.* Philadelphia, Lea & Febiger, 1975.
Royer, P., et al.: *Pediatric Nephrology.* Philadelphia, W. B. Saunders Company, 1974.
Weinberg, S., and Shapiro, L.: *Color Atlas of Pediatric Dermatology.* New York, McGraw-Hill Book Company, 1974.
Youmans, G. P., Paterson, P. Y., and Sommers, H. M. (Eds.): *The Biological and Clinical Basis of Infectious Diseases.* Philadelphia, W. B. Saunders Company, 1975.

Periodicals

Baldwin, D. S., Gluck, M. C., Schacht, R. G., and Gallo, G.: The Long-Term Course of Poststreptococcal Glomerulonephritis. *Ann. Intern. Med.,* 80:342, March 1974.
Baranowski, K., Greene, H. L., and Lamont, J. T.: Viral Hepatitis: How To Reduce Its Threat to the Patient and Others (Including You). *Nursing '76,* 6:30, May 1976.
Brown, M. S.: What You Should Know About Communicable

Diseases and Their Immunizations: A Guide for Nurses in Ambulatory Settings. Part I. *Nursing '75,* 5:70, September 1975.

Brown, M. S.: What You Should Know About Communicable Diseases and Their Immunizations: A Guide for Nurses in Ambulatory Settings. Part II, *Nursing '75,* 5:56, October 1975.

Brown, M. S.: What You Should Know About Communicable Diseases and Their Immunizations: A Guide for Nurses in Ambulatory Settings. Part III. *Nursing '75,* 5:55, November 1975.

Butler, A., Chapman, J., and Stuible, M.: Child's Play is Therapy. *The Canadian Nurse,* 71:35, December 1975.

Carver, D. H., and Seto, D. S. Y.: Hepatitis A and B. *Pediatr. Clin. N. Am.,* 21:669, August 1974.

deBelle, R. C., and Lester, R.: Current Concepts of Acute and Chronic Viral Hepatitis. *Pediatr. Clin. N. Am.,* 22:943, November 1975.

Eden, A. N.: Tonsils—In or Out? *Family Health/Today's Health,* 8:15, April 1976.

Feigin, R. D., and Dodge, P. R.: Bacterial Meningitis: Newer Concepts of Pathophysiology and Neurologic Sequelae. *Pediatr. Clin. N. Am.,* 23:541, August 1976.

Gooden, D.: 'Snorky' Helps to Allay Fears of Children Before Surgery. *Nursing Digest,* 2:80, March 1974.

Grant, D.: VIP Treatment Proves This Hospital Really Cares. *The Canadian Nurse,* 72:24, July 1976.

Green, C. S.: Larry Thought Puppet-Play 'Childish'; But It Helped Him Face His Fears. *Nursing '75,* 5:30, March 1975.

Hedberg, A. G., and Schlong, A.: Eliminating Fainting by School Children During Mass Inoculation Clinics. *Nursing Research,* 22:352, July-August 1973.

Hiles, D. A.: Strabismus. *Am. J. Nursing,* 74:1082, June 1974.

Horoshak, I.: A Special Kind of Kidney Patient. *RN,* 38:55, October 1975.

Hovenden, H. G.: Rocky Mountain Spotted Fever. *Am. J. Nursing,* 76:419, March 1976.

Huffman, J. W.: Indications for Gynecologic Examination in Premenarchal Girls. *Medical Aspects of Human Sexuality,* 7:10, October 1973.

Johnson, B. H.: Before Hospitalization: A Preparation Program for the Child and His Family. *Children Today,* 3:18, November-December 1974.

Judelsohn, R. E., Meyers, J. D., Ellis, R. J., and Thomas, E. K.: Efficacy of Zoster Immune Globulin. *Pediatrics,* 53:476, April 1974.

Katz, H. P., and Clancy, R. R.: Accuracy of a Home Throat Culture Program: A Study of Parent Participation in Health Care. *Pediatrics,* 53:687, May 1974.

Kenny, T. J.: The Hospitalized Child. *Pediatr. Clin. N. Am.,* 22:583, August 1975.

Korsch, B. M., et al.: Kidney Transplantation in Children: Psychosocial Follow-Up Study on Child and Family. *J. Pediatr.,* 83:399, September 1973.

Kunin, C. M., et al.: Detection of Urinary Tract Infections in 3- to 5-Year-Old Girls By Mothers Using a Nitrite Indicator Strip. *Pediatrics,* 57:829, June 1976.

Lee, R. V.: Antimicrobial Therapy. *Am. J. Nursing,* 73:2044, December 1973.

Luciano, K.: The Who, When, Where, What & How of Preparing Children for Surgery. *Nursing '74,* 4:64, November 1974.

Mahler, H. T.: Smallpox: Point of No Return. *Bulletin of the Pan American Health Organization,* 9:48, 1975.

McGuckin, M.: Microbiological Studies: Part 5—Tips for Assisting with Cultures of CSF and Other Body Fluids. *Nursing '76,* 6:17, April 1976.

Melber, S., Leonard, M., and Primack, W.: Hemodialysis at Camp. *Am. J. Nursing,* 76:938, June 1976.

Murray, J. D., et al.: The Continuing Problem of Purulent Meningitis in Infants and Children. *Pediatr. Clin N. Am.,* 21:967, November 1974.

Norberta, Sr.: Caring for Children with the Help of Puppets. *The American Journal of Maternal Child Nursing,* 1:22, January-February 1976.

Nysather, J. O., Katz, A. E., and Lenth, J. L.: The Immune System: Its Development and Functions. *Am. J. Nursing,* 76:1614, October 1976.

O'Grady, R., and Dolan, T.: Whooping Cough in Infancy. *Am. J. Nursing,* 76:114, January 1976.

Ormond, E. A. R., and Caulfield, C.: A Practical Guide to Giving Oral Medications to Young Children. *The American Journal of Maternal Child Nursing,* 1:320 September-October 1976.

Pidgeon, V. A.: Functions and Content of Verbal Contacts Initiated by Disadvantaged and Advantaged Preschool Children with Adults in a Hospital. *The American Journal of Maternal Child Nursing,* 3:247, Winter 1974.

Rachelefsky, G. S., and Herrmann, K. L.: Congenital Rubella Surveillance Following Epidemic Rubella in a Partially Vaccinated Community. *J. Pediatr.,* 84:474, April 1974.

Recommendation of the Public Health Service Advisory Committee on Immunization Practices. Influenza Vaccine. *Morbidity and Mortality.* 24:197, June 13, 1975.

Resnick, R., and Hergenroeder, E.: Children and the Emergency Room. *Nursing Digest,* 4:37, September-October 1976.

Roskies, E., et al.: Emergency Hospitalization of Young Children. *Nursing Digest,* 4:32, September-October 1976.

Sanders, D. Y., and Cramblett, H. G.: Antibody Titers to Polioviruses in Patients Ten Years After Immunization With Sabin Vaccine. *J. Pediatr.,* 84:406, March 1974.

Strangert, K.: Respiratory Illness in Preschool Children With Different Forms of Day Care. *Pediatrics,* 57:191, February 1976.

Visintainer, M. A., and Wolfer, J. A.: Psychological Preparation for Surgical Pediatric Patients: The Effect on Children's and Parents' Stress Responses and Adjustment. *Pediatrics,* 56:187, August 1975.

West, A. R.: Bringing the Hospital to Preschoolers: Teaching Young Children About Hospitals and Health Care. *Children Today,* 5:16, March-April 1976.

Wolfer, J. A., and Visintainer, M. A.: Pediatric Surgical Patients' and Parents' Stress Responses and Adjustment: As a Function of Psychologic Preparation and Stress-Point Nursing Care. *Nursing Research,* 24:244, July-August 1975.

Zweig, I. K.: A New Way to Get Acquainted With the Hospital—Pediatric Open House for Well Children. *The American Journal of Maternal Child Nursing,* 1:217, July-August 1976.

AUDIOVISUAL MEDIA*

The American Journal of Nursing Company

Play Therapy and the Hospitalized Child
26 minutes, black and white.

Describes how to aid children in coping with their hospital experience through play therapy.

---

*Complete addresses are given in the Appendix.

Children's Hospital, National Medical Center, Washington, D.C.

To Prepare a Child
    32 minutes, 16mm, sound, color, guide.
    Studies have shown that the occurrence of psychological upset is greater in the child unprepared for hospitalization than in the prepared child. Demonstrates the quality of care children need to be well-prepared for this experience.

CIBA and Wayne State University

Communicable Disease
    Weinstein, L.
    32 minutes.
    Patients with the following diseases are seen: roseola, rubella, measles, chickenpox, vaccinia, herpes simplex and zoster, mumps, scarlet fever, staphylococcal abscess, pertussis, polio, encephalitis, meningitis, acute tuberculosis, and blastomycosis.

Medical Electronic Educational Services, Inc.

Pediatric Nursing Series
    Prevention of Accidents to Children
    22 minutes, 35mm filmstrip/tape, sound, color, guides.
    Teaches how to provide a safe environment for the pediatric patient, paying particular attention to child's level of development.

National Communicable Disease Center

Stop Rubella
    Producer: National Medical Audiovisual Center
    14 minutes, 16mm, sound, color.
    Urges parents to have their children inoculated against rubella. Traces development of the vaccine

W. B. Saunders Company

Christine Has an Operation
    Wise, D. J.
    30 minutes in English, 30 minutes in Spanish, 35mm filmstrip, tape cassette, color.
    A highly unusual offering, this combination of a tape, filmstrip, coloring book, and instruction guide is designed to help prepare the child between ages four and eight for elective surgery.

Immunology
    Bellanti, J. A.
    35mm slides, black and white.
    These 101 slides graphically portray principles and concepts of immunology, mechanisms of immunologic response, and clinical applications of both principles and mechanisms. The slides help unify many isolated immunologic details into an organized, unified overview.

Pediatric Conferences with Sydney Gellis
    Indications for the Use of Gamma Globulin, Rosen, F. S.
    Infectious Disease, Gellis, S.
    Mumps, Brunell, P. A.
    Pediatric Gynecology, Mitchell, G.
    Rubella Vaccine, Cooper, L. Z.
    Streptococcal Skin Infections, Gellis, S.
    Viral Hepatitis, Krugman, S.

Viral Infections in Childhood
    Sussman, S. J.
    Four 35mm filmstrips, two tape cassettes, color.
    All the essential aspects of differential diagnosis and management of pediatric viral infections are included: skin eruptions, various exudates, swelling, upper respiratory tract inflammations, signs on radiographs, and other visual manifestations. Where appropriate, disease entities have been divided into intrauterine and acquired infections.

Trainex Coporation

Cathy Has an Operation
    35mm filmstrip, audio-tape cassettes, 33 1/3 LP, color.
    Child goes to the hospital for a tonsillectomy. Shows the people Cathy meets and the areas of the hospital. Cathy's doctor and an anesthesiologist visit her preoperatively to familiarize her with the clothing and masks used in the operating room. They explain the kind of sleep used for operations, and describe the recovery room where she will awaken. Then, the filmstrip shows Cathy going through the tonsillectomy procedure.

Immunizations
    35mm filmstrip, audio-tape cassettes, 33 1/3 LP, color.
    Simply and succinctly explains the reasons for immunizations, and the important ones children should receive. Also explains reactions and how to treat them.

Parents and Their Ill Child
    35mm filmstrip, audio-tape cassette, 33 1/3 LP, color.
    Suggestions that will help prepare parents and their child for the hospital experience. Parents are reminded of the frightening misconceptions their child may have, and are shown how they may reduce or eliminate both their child's and their own fears and anxieties.

Peritoneal Dialysis
    Filmstrip.

Preparing the Child for Procedures
    35mm filmstrip, audio-tape cassettes, 33 1/3 LP, color.
    Designed to help health care personnel minimize emotional trauma experienced as a result of hospitalization. Shows ways in which the child might interpret hospital surroundings and procedures, and techniques employed in helping him to make correct interpretations. Included is a discussion of the value of structured play activities.

Principles of Hemodialysis
    35mm filmstrip, audio-tape cassettes, 33 1/3 LP, color.
    Examines the theory and practice of this relatively new therapy. Graphics explain the processes of osmosis, diffusion, and ultrafiltration, by which dialysis accomplishes four vital functions of the normal kidney: removal of metabolic waste products, control of electrolyte levels, maintenance of acid-base balance, and elimination of excess fluid. Different techniques for repetitive access to the bloodstream of the patient in renal failure are seen Shows actual patients undergoing therapy, pointing out the physical and emotional problems, and delineating the intimate, long-term role of the hemodialysis nurse

Principles of Isolation Technique
    35mm filmstrip, audio-tape cassettes, 33 1/3 LP, color.
    Step-by-step demonstrations of techniques basic to effective isolation: preparing the isolation unit, handwashing, putting on and removing protective apparel, discarding disposable items and wastes within the isolation unit, and, doublebagging to remove disposable and nondisposable items from the isolation unit. These principles of isolation technique are applicable to five different types of isolation: respiratory isolation, enteric precautions, strict isolation, protective isolation, and wound and skin precautions.

The Psychological Impact of Isolation
    35mm filmstrip, audio-tape cassettes, 33 1/3 LP, color.
    Emphasizes patient needs, feelings, and behavior at three developmental stages—adult, adolescent, and early childhood. Demonstrates the impact of isolation upon the patient and fosters an attitude of acceptance of each patient's individuality and his unique methods of coping with the isolation situation.

°Complete addresses are given in the Appendix.

Chapter Twenty-One

CONDITIONS OF THE PRESCHOOL CHILD REQUIRING LONG-TERM CARE

MEANING OF LONG-TERM ILLNESS TO THE PRESCHOOL CHILD AND HIS FAMILY

The acutely ill child usually requires a brief period of bed rest, but the chronically ill child requires either a prolonged period in bed or frequent, briefer periods of complete rest. This is trying to the preschool child, for his physical activity and interaction with other children are curtailed. The care of the chronically ill child in the hospital is difficult enough, but in the home it poses a problem which often seems too great for the mother or the father, if he is caring for the child, to handle.

It is usually the mother who is hardest hit when a sick child is cared for at home. She must nurse him, carry on with her household tasks, and also manage the needs of her husband and the other children. Eventually she becomes overtired and irritable; she is no longer able to provide the love and support her family needs.

In some hospitals parents of children having long-term problems such as leukemia meet to discuss difficulties that arise during their children's hospitalization and may continue when the children return home. The medical staff, social worker, or nurses may meet with the parents to discuss their feelings and to help them find answers to their questions. Parents not only get knowledge and support from the professional personnel and from others with similar problems, but sometimes also form friendships that continue outside the meetings and lead to visiting or mutual babysitting arrangements. Some groups have written booklets to be used by new members of the group. These booklets may deal with the initial emotional adjustments to a diagnosis, concerns of fathers and other family members, the care and treatment of the child, the possible return of the child to school, and even the possible reactions of neighbors and friends and some ways to deal with them. Informal meetings may also be held by parents themselves, either inside or outside of the hospital. The rewards of such meetings include increased cooperation from parents, better understanding of the child in the hospital and at home later, and sometimes very valuable suggestions for solving problems.

The nurse can often offer suggestions to ease the mother's burden. The mother must accept the fact that she needs rest and that it is useless for her to attempt the impossible. Perhaps she can rearrange the household duties so that her husband has a greater share of the responsibilities and the other children, family members, or neighbors can give assistance with household duties.

If the child can spend the day on a living

672

room couch instead of in his room on a higher floor, the mother does not constantly have to go up and down stairs.

The mother cannot be with the child at all times, and it is good for him to amuse himself. If he is able to sit up, a bed table over his bed makes a play area on which he can draw, color in his picture book or play with small toys.

It is difficult for the mother, in the midst of housework, to remember when medicine is due. An alarm clock set for the time of the next dose may help. A medicine table near the child's bed with plenty of clean spoons and a pitcher of water saves needless errands to the kitchen or bathroom.

Chronic illness also creates difficulties for the child and his siblings. The sick child often seems to the others to be favored and to get more attention than they do. This heightens the normal sibling rivalry. The children should be helped to understand that the sick child needs extra attention, but is not loved more than they are.

Siblings as well as the sick child may have fears which parents find difficult to understand. Illness frightens children and makes them fear pain. If they are old enough to associate sickness with death, they may develop a real fear of death, not only for the sick child, but also for themselves. Parents should be truthful with the children about the condition of the sick child, within the limits of what children can understand. If restrictions must be placed upon the sick child's activities, the siblings should be told why this is necessary.

Sibling jealousy may sometimes be so strong that the well children may have passing or relatively fixed wishes that something "bad" would happen to the sick child. Such thoughts make the children feel guilty. If the sick child's condition becomes worse, it seems to them as if their wish were responsible for his plight. Then their feelings of guilt may reach disturbing proportions. They need the help of understanding parents who accept such feelings as a natural result of the disturbed emotional relations in a household where the sick child's needs often take precedence over those of his siblings.

As the sick child improves, he may have to make a difficult adjustment. He may look back longingly to the time when his condition secured for him constant attention. He may be demanding and easily upset if he does not get what he wants. His readjustment to healthful living may take weeks. Parents must be patient and understanding and give adequate love, although less attention, while he adjusts to the real tasks of living.

If disability follows a child's illness or if his activity must be curtailed in any way, the family members should understand the reason for this, and teachers and other adults with whom he comes in contact should be told. Then all persons in his environment can exert a consistent influence on the child. He should be encouraged firmly but kindly to derive pleasure from things he can do. Overconcern about the disability must be reduced; the child must be helped to live with his problem. *Emphasis should be placed on the assets he still has rather than on his liabilities, even though these are recognized.*

CHRONIC OR LONG-TERM CONDITIONS

LEUKEMIA

Incidence and Etiology. Cancer is outranked only by accidents as a cause of death in childhood, and leukemia is the principal type of cancer in children. More than 50 per cent of cases of leukemia in children occur before five years of age, the peak of incidence occurring at three to four years of age.

Leukemia is a malignant neoplasm involving all blood-forming organs and causing an overproduction of any one of the types of white blood cells. The normal white blood cell count is 5000 to 10,000 per cubic millimeter; in leukemia it may be more than 50,000 per cubic millimeter.

During childhood acute leukemia is the common form. The disease has no relation to racial,

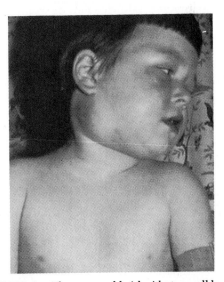

FIGURE 21–1. Three-year-old girl with stem cell leukemia. Classic triad of symptoms: extreme pallor, cutaneous hemorrhage, swelling of lymph nodes. Ecchymosis over nuchal lymphomas, petechiae on flexor surface of left elbow (Rumpel-Leede). (From Moll, H.: *Atlas of Pediatric Diseases.* Philadelphia, W. B. Saunders Co., 1976.)

geographic, or regional factors or to socioeconomic status. The cause is unknown. Research is currently being done on the relation of viruses to the origin of leukemia. The relation of mongolism to leukemia is also being studied. There may be a genetic predisposition to leukemia. It occurs with diseases associated with disorders of immune mechanisms such as agammaglobulinemia and those that produce chromosomal abnormality.

Types, Pathogenesis, and Clinical Manifestations. The type of white blood cell involved offers a basis of classification, but it is sometimes difficult to distinguish which type of leukemia is present in children. The acute undifferentiated or stem-cell type is common, as is acute lymphocytic leukemia. Subacute or chronic forms are rare in childhood; however, the acute form may be changed to a chronic type with the use of suppressive therapeutic agents.

The number of leukemic cells circulating in the blood is not always high, even though there is overproduction of a single cell type. When a high percentage of blast cells is present and the white blood cell count is high, the leukemia is termed "leukemic." When a low percentage of blast cells is present and the white cell count is low, the leukemia is termed "aleukemic." For a diagnosis of aleukemic leukemia a sample of bone marrow, obtained by aspirating marrow fluid, must be examined.

Pathologic changes are related to the increased number of white blood cells and to secondary changes due to disturbed function of the involved organs. Immature white blood cells multiply rapidly, but do not develop into or function as mature cells. The production of normal blood cells is rapidly reduced. The low platelet count is largely responsible for hemorrhagic manifestations. The liver, spleen, and all lymph nodes are enlarged. Renal and osseous changes are seen. Areas of ulceration and secondary infection may be found anywhere in the body.

There are certain common *clinical manifestations* regardless of the type of leukemia. The onset may be rapid or gradual. Widespread petechiae appear. The child is pale and has anorexia, vomiting, weight loss, weakness, and fatigue. The temperature is elevated. Palpitation of the heart and dyspnea are distressing symptoms. Episodic abdominal pain may occur, owing to the enlarged lymph nodes. Anemia becomes severe as the condition progresses. When the platelet count drops, the child bleeds easily and a slight bruise results in large ecchymotic areas; necrotic lesions develop which are apt to become secondarily infected. There are also hemorrhagic areas of the mucous membranes and vital organs.

Clinical manifestations depend on which organ or tissue is invaded by leukemic cells. If the kidney is affected, hematuria results. Necrotic ulcerative lesions may occur around the rectal and perirectal areas, and there is ulceration of the gums. The liver and spleen become enlarged, and lymphadenopathy, especially of deep lymph nodes, develops. The child suffers from leg or joint pain caused by extensive osseous involvement. The pain in the bones is due to the rapidity of osteoblastic and osteoclastic activity along with destruction of the bone by leukemic cells. Increased leukemic foci around the central nervous system may result from the failure of antileukemic agents in effective concentration to cross the blood-brain barrier.

Diagnosis, Complications, and Prognosis. The *diagnosis* is made on the basis of the clinical manifestations. A differential blood smear is done if immature cells are present in the peripheral blood. Anemia is present. Examination of aspirated or surgically removed bone marrow is necessary for a diagnosis of leukemia. The bone marrow shows abnormal leukopoietic tissues and few normal hematopoietic elements. Roentgenograms of the long bones show osseous changes.

Complications arise as a result of lack of normal white blood cells. Intracranial and visceral hemorrhages may occur. Intracranial hemorrhage is the most common immediate cause of death. Death results from the disease itself or from intercurrent infections, or both.

Without treatment the course of acute leukemia is usually that of rapid deterioration, with death occurring in about six months. With treatment acute leukemia may be changed to a chronic form, and the child may survive from two to three years or in some cases even longer. When the child is in the terminal stage of his illness, the question of how long to help him survive by mechanical means is a difficult decision to make.

Impact of a Terminal Illness. Terminal illness makes a heavy emotional impact on the child who is ill as well as on his parents. The effects are also felt by the personnel who provide care for the family. The time the initial diagnosis is made may be the time when grieving begins and actually may be equated with the time of death.

Professional personnel many times ponder the question of whether a child should be told that he has a fatal illness. Whether such information is verbalized, evaded, or denied, many children do sense or "know" the truth. Children of preschool age or older may be aware of the seriousness of their disease and even anticipate their premature deaths. In younger children their fear may be of separation from their parents or of bodily pain.

If parents and children can discuss their mutual concerns on the level of the child's understanding, meaningful communication can be established. The parents can let the child know that they understand and share his problems and that everything possible will be done for his physical and emotional well-being. Through such frank discussion the child feels that others will not lie to him, and that he can verbalize his feelings of fear and anxiety without danger of others deserting him. Older children may be better able to cooperate with therapy if they are told the truth about their disease.

On the other hand, if parents try to protect their children from this knowledge, those children who "know" the truth anyway will in turn attempt to protect their parents from grief. Since the children realize that the parents do not wish to discuss their concerns, they do not establish meaningful communication with them. If such children cannot share their feelings with anyone else, they may become very lonely indeed.

The parents may manifest all types of anticipatory grief reactions. They may become very intellectual about the illness, may deny it or enter into a frenzy of activity, or they may become irritable or depressed. They may worry about exactly how their child will die. The members of the health team should discuss the circumstances surrounding the illness early because parental fantasies may be far worse than the real situation.

The father may appear to wish to flee from his family at a time when they need him desperately. Friends and acquaintances may believe that this behavior shows a lack of interest on his part. In reality, this behavior may be a coping mechanism indicating that he needs increased support so that he in turn can support other members of his family. The father should be helped to express his painful feelings, feelings that make him avoid the ache of a close involvement with the dying child. He should be helped to understand the effect his behavior has on other family members.

In response to the child's illness, siblings may show significant behavioral changes that indicate their problems in coping. They may have evidences of separation anxiety, headaches, abdominal pains, enuresis, depression, learning difficulties in school, or school phobias (see p. 802). They may feel guilty about their actions or feelings prior to the child's illness and may worry lest they too become fatally ill. They may feel that because their parents are preoccupied with the ill child, they are rejecting them. Since the siblings may have anticipatory grief reactions, supportive therapy for them should be included in total family care.

Grandparents, other family members, and friends may be either a source of support or a hindrance during a child's terminal illness, depending on the family relations before the illness was diagnosed. They too may need help in coping with their feelings.

The family members can gain support from each other or from members of the health team. If the family had had a meaningful religious belief before this illness occurred, they may turn to the clergy for support. The referring family physician may be a source of help also, or he may be rejected by the parents because either he was the one who initially made the tentative diagnosis or he was not able to provide total care as could the health team of a large hospital.

The members of the health team can provide significant help in this time of crisis. The physician can interpret the illness and plan the medical care for the child. The social worker can offer practical assistance in solving housing and transportation problems and in planning for the resolution of financial problems. The role of the nurse is of great importance because that is who cares for the child and is with the family for long periods of time. The role of the nurse will be discussed later in this section.

Parents of other leukemic children may also provide significant support because they share common problems with each other. Such parents may meet in the hospital unit when their children are hospitalized or in the clinic setting. Such friendships may continue after their children have died in spite of differences in cultural background, race, socioeconomic status or religious beliefs.

In some hospitals the psychiatrist and other members of the health team meet with the parents, other family members, and the ill child in order to learn more about them as individuals and to help them cope with their problems. Since each family member reacts differently to such stress on the basis of his personality structure, religious beliefs, past experience, his sources of support, and the meaning of the situation to him, the health team members must learn to know each one in order to plan for long-term care. In such meetings family members are able to express their feelings, have their questions answered, and gain an understanding of the depth of concern each health team member has for them.

Nursing personnel are dedicated to helping

their patients recover and return home. When a child is fatally ill, they may feel frustrated and overwhelmed by anxiety and depression concerning the child's death. They may become irritable with each other and with other members of the health team. When death is near, some nurses avoid contact with both the parents and the child because of their own anxieties. Since they know that they are needed, such action leads to intense guilt on their part.

In order to avoid this sequence of events, nurses should talk with each other frequently about their own emotional reactions to their experiences with the children and their parents. In some hospitals the nurses have conferences with the psychiatrist or the child's physician on a regularly planned or an as-needed basis. Such conferences help nurses to cope with their feelings about the situation, thus enabling them to continue to provide their best care for the dying child and his family.

Treatment.   Treatment begins as soon as the diagnosis is made. No cure is known, and treatment is palliative. It is also supportive and specific.

Supportive treatment includes the administration of blood transfusions and antibiotics. Fresh whole blood and blood derivatives such as platelet concentrates and white cells are used for transfusions, whether during a brief or long-term hospital admission, to correct severe anemia, to stop bleeding, and to combat infection. Appropriate antibiotics are given, depending upon the type of infection. Sedatives may also be given whenever needed to make the child comfortable.

CHEMOTHERAPY.   Specific therapy involves the use of chemotherapeutic agents. These drugs can induce or maintain a *remission*, which means that morphologic evidence of leukemia is eradicated from the blood and bone marrow. The child temporarily returns to normal health. Unfortunately, these drugs also produce certain side effects when used.

Corticosteroids have the ability to lyse lymphatic cells. Prednisone or other preparations for parenteral use may be given. The administration of corticosteroids produces Cushing's syndrome, including rounding of the face (moon face), fluid retention, hypertension, and personality changes when heavy doses or prolonged therapy is given. The use of this drug results in rapid relief of signs and symptoms in children who have acute leukemia.

Amethopterin (methotrexate), a folic-acid antagonist, interferes with folic acid metabolism and thus disrupts nucleic acid synthesis in the mitotic process. Cancer cells proliferate rapidly and therefore require exceptionally high nucleic

acid synthesis. Although this drug interferes with the production of DNA and RNA, which are essential for cell reproduction, its use also produces signs of toxicity, including oral and gastrointestinal ulceration and hemorrhage, chills and fever, and hematologic depression. Skin reactions such as a rash or acne, diarrhea, and occasionally alopecia may also be seen.

6-Mercaptopurine (Purinethol) blocks the incorporation of purine into nucleic acids, thus interfering with cell reproduction. The chief manifestations of toxicity of this drug are interference with hematopoiesis and myelotoxicity.

Vincristine (Oncovin) has the ability to destroy both normal and abnormal cells. This drug may produce sensory and neuromuscular toxicity as well as constipation and alopecia. Symptoms of toxicity resemble those of intracranial leukemia.

Cyclophosphamide (Cytoxan) is a potent alkylating agent of the nitrogen mustard group which has the ability to destroy cells. Side effects include nausea, vomiting and anorexia. Depression of bone marrow, myelotoxicity, a sterile hemorrhagic cystitis, and alopecia may also occur.

Daunorubicin (Daunomycin) is a cytotoxic antibiotic which interferes with the biosynthesis of cellular nucleic acids. Its use causes bone marrow damage and complications involving the cardiopulmonary system. Other adverse effects include gastrointestinal disturbance, skin rash and hair loss.

L-*Asparaginase,* an enzyme, has been used experimentally. It is the first clinically useful anticancer drug to be based on a biochemical difference between normal and malignant cells. It kills leukemic cells by preventing them from incorporating L-asparagine, an amino acid essential for protein synthesis. Normal cells make their own. The toxic effects include potentially dangerous blood coagulation and liver-tissue abnormalities. Allergic reactions of the anaphylactic type may occur. Close observation of the child is necessary so that histamine antagonists can be given if a reaction occurs.

Thioguanine and cytosine arabinoside (Cytosar) are newer drugs used for the treatment of leukemia. The predominant toxic effect of both drugs is marrow suppression. Cytosine arabinoside may also produce nausea and vomiting.

Various schedules of drugs are designed for the treatment of children having leukemia. When a remission is rapidly induced with vincristine or a corticosteroid, hyperuricemia and precipitates of uric acid in the kidneys may

TABLE 21-1. DRUGS USEFUL IN THE TREATMENT OF CHILDHOOD LEUKEMIA

GENERIC NAME	PROPRIETARY NAME AND MANUFACTURER	TYPE OF LEUKEMIA*	ROUTE OF ADMINISTRATION	USUAL DOSAGE	PREDOMINANT TOXICITIES
Induction Agents Corticosteroids, e.g., prednisone	Deltasone (Upjohn) Delta-Dome (Dome) Betapar (Parke, Davis) Prednisone (McKesson) Meticorten (Schering)	ALL/AML	Oral	40 mg/M²/day or 2 mg/kg/day	Cushing's syndrome
Vincristine	Oncovin (Lilly)	ALL/AML AML	Intravenous	1.5 mg/M²/week, or 0.075 mg/kg/week (maximum 2 mg per dose)	Peripheral neurotoxicity; alopecia; local necrosis on extravasation
L-Asparaginase	Investigative	ALL/AML ?AML	Intravenous	100–500 IU/kg/day or 500–1000 IU/kg/twice weekly	Anaphylaxis; hypoproteinemia; nausea and vomiting
Daunomycin or adriamycin	Investigative	ALL/AML ?AML	Intravenous		Marrow suppression, alopecia; gastrointestinal irritation
Thioguanine		AML	Intravenous	1.25–2.5 mg/kg/twice daily	Marrow suppression
Cytosine arabinoside	Cytosar (Upjohn)	AML	Intravenous	50–100 mg/kg/twice daily	Marrow suppression; nausea and vomiting
Cyclophosphamide	Cytoxan (Mead Johnson)	AML	Intravenous	50–100 mg/kg twice daily	Marrow suppression; nausea and vomiting
Busulfan	Myleran (Burroughs-Wellcome)	CML	Oral	2.0 mg/day	Marrow suppression
6-Mercaptopurine	Purinethol (Burroughs-Wellcome)		Oral	2.5 mg/kg/day	
Maintenance Agents 6-Mercaptopurine	Purinethol (Burroughs-Wellcome)	ALL/AML AML	Oral	2.5 mg/kg/day	Marrow suppression
Amethopterin	Methotrexate (Lederle)	ALL/AML	a. Oral b. Intravenous c. Intrathecal	a. 1.25–5 mg/day, or 20–30 mg/M² twice weekly b. 50–300 mg/M² weekly to biweekly c. 0.5 mg/kg, or 12 mg/M² (maximum 12 mg) twice weekly until CSF clears	Marrow suppression; nausea and vomiting; gastrointestinal mucosal irritation
Cyclophosphamide	Cytoxan (Mead Johnson)	ALL/AML AML ?CML	a. Oral b. Intravenous	a. 2.5 mg/kg/day or 400 mg/M²/week b. Variable	Marrow suppression; nausea and vomiting
Cytosine arabinoside	Cytosar (Upjohn)	ALL/AML	Intravenous	Variable	Marrow suppression; nausea and vomiting
Thioguanine		AML	Oral	Variable	Marrow suppression
Vincristine	Oncovin (Lilly)	?AML	Intravenous	1.5 mg/M² weekly or biweekly (maximum 2 mg per dose)	Neurotoxicity; alopecia; local necrosis on extravasation

*ALL = acute lymphoblastic leukemia; AML = acute myelogenous leukemia; CML = chronic myelogenous leukemia.
From Vaughan, V. C., III, and McKay, R. J.: *Nelson Textbook of Pediatrics*, 10th ed. Philadelphia, W. B. Saunders Co., 1975.

occur with the lysis of cells. Uric acid can crystallize in the kidneys and cause renal shutdown. In order to avoid this complication, adequate fluid intake and alkalinization of the urine with sodium bicarbonate is essential. Allopurinol, which reduces this material, may also be given. After remission has occurred, vincristine and corticosteroids are discontinued and therapy with doses of 6-mercaptopurine, Cytoxan or methotrexate may be started. Remission is prolonged with the use of these drugs in maintenance amounts. These various drugs may be given in cycles to postpone clinical relapses of leukemia. As the illness progresses, the body becomes gradually resistant to the drugs, and a remission can no longer be obtained.

In *chronic leukemia*, busulfan (Myleran), a nitrogen mustard derivative, may be given. The toxic effect of this drug is marrow suppression.

Approximately one quarter to one half of children having leukemia suffer from leukemic infiltration of the meninges. These children have increased intracranial pressure with vomiting, papilledema, and an enlarged head circumference due to spreading of the sutures. Methotrexate may be injected into the subarachnoid space by lumbar puncture, or roentgen therapy may be used.

BONE MARROW TRANSPLANT. Research has been done recently in large medical centers on a new form of treatment for leukemia, bone marrow transplant. Bone marrow transplant may indeed provide a hope for the eventual cure of this condition. The recipient of a transplant of this type needs a suitable ABO- and HLA-matched donor. This means that the donor is usually a brother or a sister.

Bone marrow transplant is an involved and unpredictable procedure. Each patient responds differently to his new marrow. Prior to the transplant, the patient's marrow cells and all his leukemic cells must be killed by massive chemotherapy and total body irradiation. Cytoxan, with all its side effects of nausea, vomiting, diarrhea, anemia, fluid retention, skin rash, alopecia and uric acid nephropathy, is used. Before treatment a brisk urine flow and an alkaline urine can prevent kidney and bladder problems.

On the day of the marrow infusion the child is given a thorough pHisoHex bath and shampoo on the physician's order. A special antibiotic ointment is applied to every body orifice. The child is wrapped in sterile linen and taken to the x-ray department. Total body irradiation is done. Meanwhile, marrow is removed from the iliac crest of the donor under general anesthesia. After total body irradiation, the child is taken to his isolation room and the marrow infusion is begun. The marrow is given intravenously, and in some unknown manner the cells settle in the marrow cavity of the bone. The child must be observed for an allergic reaction, volume overload, and pulmonary emboli. A rapid flow of alkaline urine is again necessary, because of the amount of cell destruction as a result of total body irradiation. Observation for possible nausea, vomiting, diarrhea, and elevation of temperature following irradiation is necessary. Alopecia may result.

A painful side effect of irradiation is mucositis, a complete denuding of the gastrointestinal tract from mouth to anus. Since the child cannot take fluids or food by mouth, hyperalimentation must be given to fulfill his nutritional needs (see p. 436).

The child must be carefully monitored for infection following a transplant. He is very susceptible to infection because his blood reproductive system and the white blood cells have been destroyed. He is placed in strict sterile reverse isolation and given vigorous antibiotic treatment. The child's body and his environment are kept scrupulously clean. His food, when he is able to eat, is sterilized.

Marrow repopulation may begin within a week. Daily transfusions of red blood cells and platelets may be necessary.

Complications that may occur include rejection of the graft or a leukemic relapse. There may be a graft-versus-host reaction (GVHR), in which lymphocytes from the donor's graft infiltrate the host's body and release a lymphokinin that injures and kills cells by direct contact. Treatment includes hyperalimentation, antibiotics, intravenous methotrexate, and possibly antihuman thymocyte globulin (ATG).

At the present time, if the child survives more than a year after this therapy, he may go on to lead a relatively normal life.

Research on immunotherapeutic modalities for childhood leukemia is also being done.

Responsibilities of the Nurse. The child who has leukemia is usually hospitalized only for diagnosis, for the regulation of therapy, for periods of exacerbation and for terminal care. During the periods of remission he should live at home with his family and lead as normal a life for his age as is possible. Although it may be difficult for them to do, the parents should attempt to provide a happy atmosphere and keep anxiety to a minimum. The child should not be treated too permissively or be overindulged because he is ill.

When the child is admitted or readmitted to the hospital frequent nursing assessments are done, because the condition of a leukemic child may change rapidly in a short period of time. The nursing care of a child having leukemia is based not only on the signs, symptoms, and complications of the disease itself but also on the side effects of the drugs used in treatment.

One of the main areas of concern in the nursing care of a child having abnormal white blood cells, whether due to the illness of leukemia or to its therapy, is protection from the infections of others. Any sign of infection such as increased warmth of tissues, redness, swelling, or drainage is reported immediately. Antibiotics are used to combat bacterial diseases. Resistant organisms may be present in a child who has received prolonged or repeated therapy. Such a child is also protected from exposure to viruses. Should exposure occur inadvertently, gamma globulin may be given if appropriate for the particular virus.

In some pediatric units a child who has leuke-

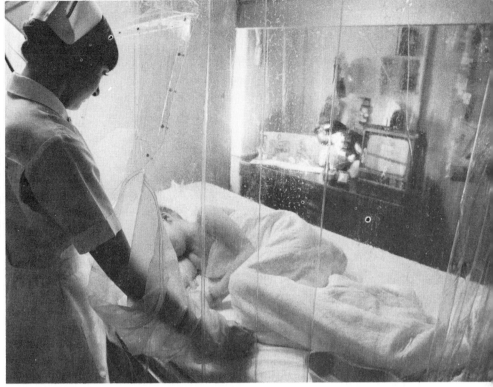

FIGURE 21–2. A plastic "life island" is used to provide a completely sterile environment for children endangered by normal infection. This would include children without normal immunologic function, those suffering burns, and those with very low blood counts because of disease or drug therapy. (Courtesy of Children's Hospital of Philadelphia.)

mia is cared for in a strictly sterile environment. This requires reverse isolation, utilizing a whole-body bed isolator type of plastic tent with portholes through which care may be given (see Fig. 21–2). The child may also be placed in a germ-free laminar air-flow unit (see p. 558). With long-term use such a child is deprived of adequate physical contact and sensory stimulation.

Transfusion therapy using whole blood or blood products is necessary. Before the transfusion the nurse explains the purpose of the treatment, which is to make the child feel better, more like he did before his illness. An explanation about and demonstration of the equipment to be used may be given, depending on the child's level of understanding. The child should be permitted some degree of control during the procedure in order to reduce his feelings of helplessness. Approval is given when the child cooperates. He is encouraged to express his feelings about the procedure freely.

The child's arm is restrained securely on a padded arm board. Other restraints may be used as necessary. The nurse assists the physician in starting the transfusion.

During this treatment the nurse is responsible for positioning the child in as comfortable a manner as possible and providing him with emotional support and diversionary activities. The nurse must be in attendance to regulate the flow of blood in order to prevent circulatory overload and to report any transfusion reaction if it occurs. Indications of a transfusion reaction include a sensation of being chilled, a backache, and general malaise. A young child who cannot describe how he feels may cry and become restless and irritable as an indication of a reaction. Changes in vital signs, color, and urinary output should be recorded. The physician should be notified immediately if any of these symptoms are observed.

Throughout the transfusion the restraints are checked frequently to determine their effectiveness. If they are too loose, the child may work his way out of them; if they are too tight they may restrict his circulation. Vital signs and other essential information are recorded.

The nurse or the parents can provide security and diversion to the child during this prolonged procedure by talking, reading, or playing quietly with him so that the time passes as quickly as possible.

Since the child who has leukemia also has anemia (see p. 458), he tires easily and needs frequent rest periods. He should have well-balanced meals planned from foods he likes. These are served when he is already awake. He is not awakened at meal times, because he needs his rest. Both parents and nurses feel frustrated when a child does not eat, because they see themselves as nurturing persons who are failing in their responsibility. Behavior modification methods may be used when the child is anorexic. If he is praised when he eats, no matter how small an amount, and is not praised when he does not eat, he will probably want to cooperate more fully. The problem of eating should not be made the central focus of the family's concern.

An adequate fluid intake is important. To prevent nausea, small amounts of fluids that he likes should be offered frequently. Commercially prepared or home made high-caloric drinks that he enjoys will increase his caloric as well as his fluid intake. He may prefer soft cool foods to a regular diet. If the child is permitted to select his diet under supervision, he will probably be more interested in eating than if food is merely presented to him.

The intake and output are routinely charted. Because of his anorexia and possibly nausea, vomiting, and diarrhea leading to dehydration and electrolyte imbalance, intravenous therapy may be necessary.

Since the child has a low platelet count, he is observed carefully for hemorrhage, including petechiae and ecchymotic areas in the skin. The nurse handles the child's body *gently*, since the extremities are painful when touched. Oral hygiene is needed and must be done with the utmost care to prevent trauma to the sore and bleeding gums, especially if oral ulcers are present. If the child's mouth is not too sore to have his teeth brushed, the toothbrush is softened under warm running water before use. If his mouth is sore because of his disease or his medications, swabs are used to cleanse the area. His mouth may be rinsed frequently with warm saline solution, plain water, dilute hydrogen peroxide or a mouth-wash as ordered. Because of bleeding or ulceration of the lips, a bland ointment may be applied for comfort. When the child has a sore mouth he may not wish to talk or eat.

Rectal ulcers may occur as a result of damage to the mucosa by chemotherapy or infection. Appropriate antibiotic therapy may be given for any infection, if present. Rectal temperatures should not be taken until the ulcer heals in order to prevent further trauma to the mucosa. The area should be kept clean and dry. A heat lamp may be used to promote healing. The child is positioned so that the pressure on the area is lessened.

Sheepskin may be used beneath pressure points to prevent breakdown of the skin. When injections are ordered, they are given carefully and pressure is applied to the site gently in order to prevent occurrence of hematomas. Intramus-

cular injections or other traumatic procedures may be discontinued if thrombocytopenic bleeding is present.

Accurate charting is important. As mentioned previously, the nurse watches for infection and for bleeding and reports both the site and the amount. It is difficult to get these children to say how they feel, but any complaints are charted, together with the circumstances bearing upon the complaint. The child is observed constantly for indications of central nervous system involvement such as changes in his behavior or physical condition: nausea and vomiting, lethargy or irritability, and headache. These symptoms are reported immediately. Preventive treatment of the central nervous system or administration of irradiation to the cranium and possibly to the spinal axis may become necessary if meningeal complications do occur, as evidenced by the symptoms and signs of increased intracranial pressure. Intrathecal methotrexate, injected into the subarachnoid space, may be given or cytosine arabinoside may be used. The child must be observed for convulsions and any toxic manifestations of the drug used. If this complication is not noted early, ocular palsies and sometimes blindness may occur.

The child is irritable because he is extremely uncomfortable, owing to the organ systems involved in the leukemic process. He should be warned when procedures such as diagnostic tests and intravenous therapy are to be done so that he can mobilize his coping strategies. If the child is permitted to help in some way with the procedures, he will feel less helpless. If he is given approval for his assistance, he will be able to improve his cooperation. He should be encouraged also to express his feelings about such procedures.

Bone marrow aspiration is necessary in the diagnosis and treatment of leukemia. Marrow is obtained from the sternum or iliac crest. The child should be told the purpose and something of the details of the procedure. He will feel the restraint necessary to hold him in position, the cleaning of the area, the injection of a local anesthetic, and the pressure of the needle as it enters the tissue. After bone marrow aspiration the patient should be observed for bleeding from the site.

The nurse observes and records the side effects of any drugs used. When vincristine is used, measures to relieve constipation may be necessary, such as an adequate fluid intake and laxatives. This symptom should be reported early because constipation may be an initial sign of toxicity to the drug. Since this drug may also cause foot drop, a footboard may be utilized. When alopecia occurs as a result of drug therapy, the child is prepared for the possible loss of his hair. Parents many times purchase a wig or a cap for the child to wear when he feels well enough to do so.

If new or research drugs are used, it is important for the nurse to learn their actions and side effects in order to provide good care for the patient and also to teach the parents prior to the child's discharge from the hospital.

During his illness the child may be nauseated, lonely and easily tired. All who care for him can be patient and try to provide a quiet, happy atmosphere in which there are as few frustrations as possible. The mother should be with him as much as possible, both to give him the constant care he needs and to learn how to nurse him during his periods at home. Parents have a natural and positive outlet for their affection when they help in the nursing care of their child while he is in the hospital. Activities are planned that he enjoys. The child should have some control of his environment such as in the selection of toys and in his manner of play. Activities that will frustrate him should be avoided. Some limits on behavior must be set if this long-term therapy is to be as free of distress as possible for the child and his parents.

When the child is cared for at home, he may have diagnostic procedures as well as transfusion therapy given in the outpatient department on an ambulatory basis over a period of months or years. The nurse must gain the trust of both the child and his parents in order to help them through these traumatic experiences. Explanations of new procedures must be made in an understandable manner.

The parents in this situation may contribute to his care by helping to observe, and possibly regulate, the rate of flow of the blood, platelets or white cells being given. The nurse must remember, however, that there is a difference between mothering and nursing and that it is the nurse who is ultimately responsible for the care of the child.

Remissions in children having leukemia are increasing because of the newer forms of treatment being used. During remission the child should be treated as a normal individual of his age. Since the child feels more secure if he is accepted and treated as he was prior to his illness, discipline may become necessary. Parents who are helped to understand the need for discipline will not feel guilty when it is given. Community members who have contact with the child can be informed about the illness

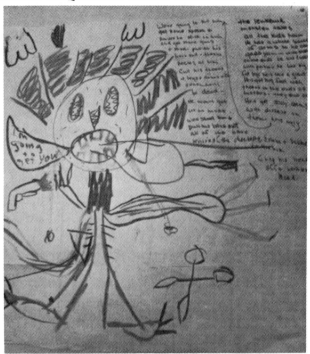

FIGURE 21–3. A child's drawing of the leukemia monster and her accompanying explanation expressed both her fear of the disease and her determination to fight the condition with her doctors and play therapist Estelle Parness, of the UCLA Clinic Play Program. "The leukemia monster," she explains, "takes all the kids' hair ... he can grab you ... He won't get us no more ... All of us have knives. Chop his head off and he'll be dead." (From Azarnoff, P.: *Children Today*, 3:14, July-August 1974.)

by the parents or the nurse in order to reduce apprehension concerning interaction with him.

Terminal nursing care is difficult. Parents may know intellectually that the child will die, but emotionally they continue to hope for a cure. Nurses need to appreciate that parents may be extremely demanding and difficult during their child's illness because of their intense anxiety. The child must be given physical and emotional support, for he is most uncomfortable as long as he is sufficiently conscious of his sensations. His nose and throat should be kept clean, and his lips and mouth moist. Frequent bathing is necessary to keep the skin clean, and his position is changed as often as possible without disturbing him in order to prevent bedsores. Sedatives may be given when necessary.

To minister successfully to the dying child and his parents, the nurse must be able to accept the way in which they express their fear and grief. To do this, personal feelings about death must be faced. When the critically ill child lapses into unconsciousness, the nurse must remain with the parents at his bedside so that they know that everything possible is being done for his comfort. If the nurse leaves them alone with the dying child, they may feel rejection of their grief. If parents cannot be present, the nurse must remain constantly with the dying child to prevent loneliness and the feeling that there is no one to help him when he is suffering and afraid of the change that is coming over him.

The children in the unit sense tension of the nurse and that of the other personnel. They need emotional support, most especially if they know they have the same illness as the dying child. The question as to whether to tell such children that they too will die is one which must be answered on an individual basis. (See page 106 for further discussion of the dying child and his family.)

After the child's death parents may feel a sense of relief as well as grief. They may be relieved that his suffering is over and that they no longer have to worry over how and when the child will die. Since the parents already know this only too well, the nurse should not say, "Your child is better off now that his suffering is over." Some parents may become very angry at members of the health team when death occurs. Such actions should be interpreted as expressions of grief and not as personal attacks.

The siblings may react to the child's death by verbalizing their grief or by crying, by coping with the death through play activities, by evidencing behavior changes, or by intense fears that they will also die of leukemia. Some siblings may feel that they were responsible for the child's death because they may have had hostile feelings toward him in the past. Others may show no reaction immediately, but may have delayed grief reactions later. Since parents may not be able to deal with these reactions at the time they themselves are overwhelmed by grief, professional assistance may be necessary.

Later, parents and other family members who cannot cope with their feelings concerning the child's death may have emotional disturbances of various sorts, such as behavioral changes, depression, conversion reactions, or psychosomatic symptoms. Psychiatric care may become necessary.

It is important to have families return to the hospital at some time after the child's death. At this meeting the autopsy report can be given to them if permission was granted for one to be done. Also, their reactions to the child's death can be discussed and further supportive care for the family members can be planned.

Organizations composed of parents of leukemic children have been formed to help in managing difficult family problems, exchanging information, providing mutual psychologic help, and promoting an effective cancer research program nationally. One such organization is the Candlelighters, 123 C Street S. E., Washington, D.C. 20003.

HEMOPHILIA

Incidence. Hemophilia is not a single disease entity, but a syndrome which represents congenital coagulation disorders. There are defects in any one of several factors in blood plasma needed for thromboplastic activity. It would be well for the student to review the mechanism of normal clot formation before attempting to comprehend the problem in hemophilia.

Blood coagulation (see Fig. 21–4 and Table 21–2) proceeds in three phases. In phase 1, when tissues and blood platelets are injured, materials derived from them react with various accessory factors such as antihemophilic globulin (factor VIII, AHG, AHF) and the Christmas factor (plasma thromboplastin component, PTC, factor IX). These convert an inactive precursor into activated thromboplastin.

In phase 2 the activated thromboplastin reacts with prothrombin and related proteins synthesized in the liver in the presence of calcium ions to form the proteolytic enzyme thrombin. In prothrombin synthesis the liver makes use of several enzymes plus vitamin K.

In phase 3 fibrinogen, which is synthesized in the liver, reacts with the thrombin, thus altering it to a solid form called fibrin. The fibrin precipitates as filaments. These filaments trap blood elements to create a meshlike gelatinous clot.

The clot is destroyed in the following manner. Plasminogen precipitates while the fibrin is precipitating and is incorporated into the clot. Plasma and all other body fluids contain plasminogen. Plasmin results when enzymes called kinases (such as urokinase) work on it. The fibrin of the clot is digested by plasmin into soluble polypeptides, after which the clot resolves.

Hemophilia A is due to deficiency of factor VIII, antihemophilic globulin (AHG); *hemophilia B*, of factor IX (Christmas disease), plasma thromboplastin component (PTC); and *hemophilia C*, of factor XI, plasma thromboplastin antecedent (PTA).

Children may have deficiencies of other factors; however, the two most important types of hemophilia are A and B. Hemophilia A is the true or classic form of the disease. Since the nursing care is approximately the same in all types, the others will not be considered in this text.

Hemophilia A is inherited as a sex-linked recessive trait. Though it appears only in males,

Hemorrhagic Diseases

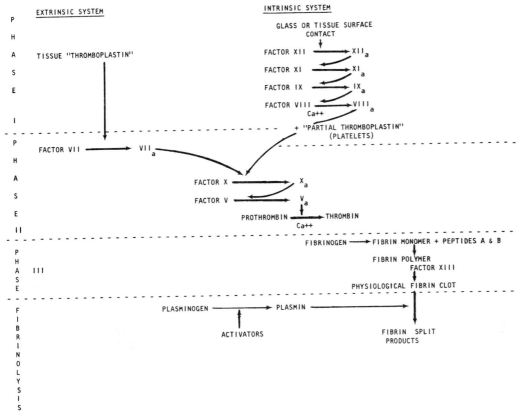

FIGURE 21–4. The coagulation mechanism. (From Vaughan, V. C., III, and McKay, R. J.: *Nelson Textbook of Pediatrics*, 10th ed. Philadelphia, W. B. Saunders Co., 1975.)

it is transmitted by symptom-free females. Male hemophiliacs can transmit a latent form of the disease to female children, however. Spontaneous mutations may have occurred to cause this condition when no other family member has had the disease. It is a congenital defect in the blood-coagulating mechanism leading to severe bleeding.

The disease may be diagnosed in early infancy, when the newborn bleeds from the umbilical cord or after circumcision. This bleeding occurs because factor VIII does not cross the placenta. As children grow older and become more active, the condition is apparent, for even a slight injury produces continued bleeding.

Pathogenesis, Clinical Manifestations, and Treatment. The disease is characterized by a tendency to prolonged bleeding caused by an extremely delayed clotting time. Normal blood clots in three to six minutes; hemophiliac blood may require an hour or more.

The prothrombin time and the bleeding time are normal when a test cut is made because the cut is smooth and small; the incised surfaces are approximated, with the result that adequate

thromboplastin becomes available from damaged cells.

Immediate *treatment* of an open wound consists in cleansing it thoroughly and applying cold and pressure.

In children, hemorrhage frequently occurs into the joints, where repeated hemorrhage may result in permanent crippling. Hemorrhage into the joints is known as *hemarthrosis*, the hallmark of hemophilia. This may occur in joints such as the knees, elbows and ankles, and is extremely painful, since bleeding occurs in a confined space. Therapy consists in the use of sedatives or narcotics, immobilization with splints or traction, and the application of cold to the part. Physicians do not agree on the value of aspiration of blood from the joint. A bivalve plaster cast may be applied for the purpose of immobilization, with physiotherapy after its removal to prevent the development of stiffness and contracture of the joint. A bed cradle may be used to keep the weight of blankets off the affected part. Careful handling is necessary to prevent further bleeding. Anemia, moderate elevation in platelets and leukocytosis may occur if hemorrhages

TABLE 21–2. THE COAGULATION FACTORS

INTERNATIONAL NUMBERS	SYNONYMS	COMMENT
I	Fibrinogen	Number rarely used—congenital deficiency known (afibrinogenemia)
II	Prothrombin	Number rarely used—congenital deficiency known
III	Thromboplastin	No specific factor identified
IV	Calcium	Number rarely used
V	Labile factor proaccelerin	Congenital deficiency known (parahemophilia, Owren's disease)
VI	Activated labile factor, accelerin	No longer differentiated from V
VII	Stable factor, SPCA, proconvertin	Congenital deficiency known
VIII	Antihemophilic factor (AHF) or globulin (AHG)	Hemophilia A (classic hemophilia) results from congenital deficiency
IX	Christmas factor, plasma thromboplastin component (PTC)	Hemophilia B results from congenital deficiency
X	Stuart-Prower factor	Congenital deficiency known
XI	Plasma thromboplastin antecedent, PTA	Congenital deficiency known
XII	Hageman factor	No clinical symptoms associated with congenital deficiency
XIII	Fibrin stabilizing factor	Congenital deficiency known

From Vaughan, V. C., III, and McKay, R. J.: *Nelson Textbook of Pediatrics.* 10th ed. Philadelphia, W. B. Saunders Co., 1975.

have been extensive. Ultimately, after repeated hemorrhages, degenerative changes may occur, leading to fixed joints and muscular atrophy. Orthopedic treatment may become necessary in order to prevent deformity and crippling.

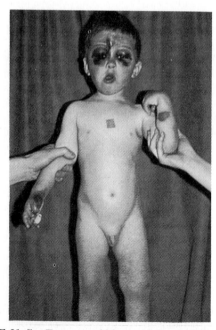

FIGURE 21–5. Two-year-old boy with hemophilia A. First cutaneous hemorrhage at the age of five months. Now, after a fall, extensive subcutaneous hemorrhages of face, lower arms, legs, and hemarthrosis of left knee are evident. (From Moll, H.: *Atlas of Pediatric Diseases.* Philadelphia, W. B. Saunders Co., 1976.)

Hematuria may occur, but is not as serious as intracranial hemorrhage, which may result in death.

When bleeding occurs, replacement therapy to increase the level of factor VIII in the plasma is necessary to stop the hemorrhage. Fresh or fresh frozen plasma or plasma concentrates can be given intravenously. Care must be taken that the circulatory system is not overloaded by giving excessive fluid.

Factor VIII concentrates are available. Cryoprecipitate is one of the most inexpensive of these, since it can be prepared from fresh plasma. Glycine-precipitated factor VIII and factor VIII-rich fibrinogen can be obtained, but these are expensive.

If the child has hemorrhaged in the brain or if he is going to have surgery, factor VIII concentrate therapy should be given. If the child becomes refractory to therapy with factor VIII because of the development of an inhibitor, IgG globulin, massive doses of factor VIII concentrates or exchange transfusions using fresh blood should be administered for hemorrhage.

The choice of an analgesic for use with the hemophiliac is important. It is essential not to use an analgesic that may affect another component of the patient's coagulation mechanism. Aspirin and phenylbutazone inhibit normal platelet function and may prolong bleeding time. Drugs such as acetaminophen or meperidine may be used safely.

Hemophilia is treated largely on an outpatient

basis, with most care given under a home management program. The factor VIII concentrate can be administered intravenously at home by the parent or by the patient himself. The goals of this are the prompt and effective control of bleeding episodes and the increased independence of the patient from hospital care. A patient whose disease is severe and requires frequent transfusions may be placed on a prophylactic infusion program. The goals of the prophylactic infusion program are to maintain adequate levels of the clotting factor and prevent bleeding.

Home care substantially decreases morbidity and hospitalization, thus it decreases the cost. Home treatment in conjunction with counseling and periodic assessment by the professional team including the physician, hematologist, orthopedist, dentist, physical therapist, psychologist, social worker, and nurse represent the optimal management of hemophilia.

Responsibilities of the Nurse. Under a home management program a major responsibility of the pediatric nurse practitioner or the hospital or clinic nurse is to teach the parents and possibly the patient, if he is sufficiently mature, how to administer the factor VIII concentrate at home in an emergency or at regular intervals, depending on the severity of the illness. This instruction may be given when the child is hospitalized or it may be given by the pediatric nurse practitioner or clinic nurse. It includes venipuncture techniques and the manner of monitoring transfusions.

Prior to giving this instruction the physician and the nurse must assess the parents' readiness to assume this responsibility by investigating their knowledge and attitudes about the disease and its treatment and their feelings about follow-up care through periodic clinic visits and telephone consultations.

The nurse teaches the parents and possibly the patient on their level of knowledge and understanding. Teaching sessions and practice periods are necessary until they are secure in their ability to prepare the replacement factor, to carry out aseptic technique, to do a venipuncture, to supervise a slow transfusion, and to recognize complications. Throughout the sessions safety precautions are emphasized in regard to the technique of intravenous therapy. The parents or the patient must keep a record of all bleeding episodes. The nurse on the team may visit the home to provide support and to answer questions that may arise. Continuing support by the members of the team, especially the physician and nurse, is essential for the parents and the child.

The nurse as an educator also teaches the parents and the child methods of preventing injuries that cause bleeding such as in rough and tumble play, or participation in competitive games or contact sports.

During periods of hospitalization due to bleeding, it is necessary for the nurse to understand the attitude of the child and of his family toward the disease and his hospitalization.

Careful handling of the child is necessary. If the child is able to tell the nurse how he would like to be moved, his pain and his feeling of helplessness will be reduced. The nurse must be alert to symptoms of pain or pressure, since bleeding may occur anywhere in the body.

Medication is given orally; however, if injections are necessary, the sites are carefully chosen and rotated. The medication is injected slowly, and pressure is applied for at least five minutes, whether manually or with a pressure dressing. If blood is to be drawn, only superficial veins are used because of the danger of hemorrhage if the femoral or internal jugular veins are used.

If the condition is diagnosed in infancy, the child's toys must be soft and the sides of his crib and playpen padded to protect him from injury. When learning to stand and walk, the child must be protected from falling. He may wear sponge rubber pads on his knees and buttocks and a small football helmet on his head. As he grows older, both he and his parents must understand the danger of trauma in his more active life. His teachers, the school nurse, and his classmates should be informed of his condition and the problems it creates. While adults supervise his activities they must guard against assuming an overprotective attitude and allow the child some activity within the limits of safety.

Normally a boy enjoys physical activity with other children. Since he appears normal, he may conceal his illness in order to gain the acceptance of friends. He may take risks that he knows are dangerous in order to be part of his group. If, instead, he isolates himself, he becomes alienated from his peers, withdraws from other children, and becomes overdependent on adults.

The nurse must provide continued emotional support. During periods of freedom from bleeding his parents may become less conscious of the necessity for medical follow-up. The nurse emphasizes the necessity of medical supervision. He should also receive optimum dental care and supervision early in order to prevent extraction of teeth. If removal of teeth becomes necessary, the child is hospitalized for the procedure.

When a child has a chronic illness such as hemophilia, he may be absent from kindergarten or school many days of the year. When he is not in school, a tutor may be obtained or he may be kept in contact with his class by a school-to-home telephone hookup.

Parents, especially the mother, may feel guilt at having given birth to the child and resentment at having to care for him. The father may resent a son who is not able to compete with other boys on a physical level. If the parents are too anxious, the child will become self-centered and fearful.

The child may use his disease to control his parents, teachers, and other adults and purposely do things dangerous for him. The parents must undertake the difficult task of preparing him for a satisfying role in adult life by helping him to develop his autonomy, initiative and independence.

Because of the long-term nature of his illness, the child and his family may need counseling and financial assistance due to the expense of cryoprecipitate or commercial AHF concentrates. If the child has had repeated episodes of hemarthrosis, he may become so crippled that in order for him to be rehabilitated, surgery or the use of braces, casts, crutches, or a wheelchair may become necessary. The National Hemophilia Foundation can provide assistance in the form of information, the location of parent groups, and clinics as well as other kinds of aid.

Prognosis. The prognosis is uncertain. A cyclic pattern may be noted in which periods of little bleeding and of severe bleeding occur, at times dependent on the amount of stress the child has experienced. Such stress may be caused by interactions with his parents, but it may also be due to situations involving his siblings and peers as well as other adults. Death may follow intracranial hemorrhage or exsanguination from a serious hemorrhage elsewhere in the body.

PURPURA

Spontaneous hemorrhages are characteristic of the condition known as purpura. These may occur in the skin, mucous membranes, or internal organs. Such hemorrhages may develop in any condition in which there is a decreased number of platelets in the blood, defective capillary walls or in which damage is done to normal capillary walls beyond the point at which platelets can stop the bleeding. Petechiae, or minute hemorrhages into the skin, may also occur as an allergic manifestation when a local specific tissue reaction results in capillary stress.

Two specific types of purpura are discussed in this text: idiopathic thrombocytopenic purpura and anaphylactoid purpura.

IDIOPATHIC THROMBOCYTOPENIC PURPURA

Etiology, Incidence, Clinical Manifestations, and Laboratory Findings. Purpura is associated with a deficit in the number of circulating blood platelets. This deficiency is caused by factors outside the platelets themselves.

The disease has its greatest *incidence* in the age group between three and seven years. It is uncommon in black children. The most frequent form of the disease during childhood is the acute, self-limited type.

The onset of the acute type is sudden. It may follow a mild respiratory infection or measles. There are fever and prostration. Characteristic, spontaneous small hemorrhages into the skin, mucous membranes, or other tissues occur. Large ecchymoses may result from trauma. In the severe form of the disease there may be hemorrhages from the vaginal and nasal mucous membranes and from the urinary and gastrointestinal tracts. Cerebral hemorrhages are to be feared.

In the chronic form, infrequent in children, the onset is gradual. The child may have a history of prolonged bleeding following injury and of ready bruising. Periods of good health alternate with periods of excessive bleeding.

The *laboratory findings* confirm the diagnosis made upon the clinical manifestations. The platelet count is always below 100,000 per cubic millimeter of blood (normal is between 200,000 and 500,000). In the chronic form of the disease, iron deficiency may occur from loss of blood. The bleeding time is usually prolonged. The clotting time is normal, but the clot fails to retract in the usual manner. The bone marrow is studied in order to rule out leukemia.

Treatment, Course, and Prognosis. Supportive *therapy* includes transfusions of whole blood to replace blood loss, antibiotic therapy to treat infections, bed rest for moderate or severe bleeding, a well-balanced diet, and vitamin therapy. If severe bleeding occurs, an infusion of platelet-rich plasma or whole blood is necessary. ACTH or cortisone can control severe bleeding, but the effect upon the platelet count cannot be predicted. Splenectomy may be performed if the disease continues for six to 12 months or if hemorrhaging is severe. Splenectomy may induce lasting remissions in children with the chronic form of the disease. The operation modifies symptoms in children who are not cured.

The majority of children who have the acute form of purpura recover in about two months under supportive therapy. Intracranial hemorrhage is uncommon, but is responsible for most deaths from purpura. About 2 per cent of the children with purpura have the chronic form, which is refractory to therapy.

ANAPHYLACTOID PURPURA (SCHÖENLEIN-HENOCH SYNDROME)

Schöenlein-Henoch syndrome is the term used for anaphylactoid purpura because the illness is a polymorphic systemic disease. Skin and visceral lesions are manifestations.

Incidence and Etiology. The disease is not uncommon; it affects all races. It has its highest *incidence* between the ages of three and seven years, the average being about five years.

The cause is unknown. The onset may occur after contact with a specific substance. In such cases allergy seems to be important. It is possible that this is one type of hypersensitivity response to a variety of antigenic stimuli. The onset may follow an upper respiratory tract infection with beta hemolytic streptococci.

Clinical Manifestations and Laboratory Findings. A series of *clinical manifestations* take place, possibly following an infection. Abdominal pain or arthralgia, or both, may occur. After the initial symptom a skin rash appears on the legs and the buttocks, and spreads to the face, arms and trunk. The rash consists at first of urticarial wheals; then a variety of maculopapular erythematous lesions appear. The lesions may finally become petechial or purpuric,

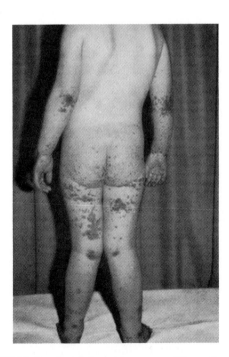

FIGURE 21–6. Anaphylactoid purpura, 30-month-old girl. Distribution of hemorrhagic lesions is typical. Additional finding: knock-knees corresponding to age. (From Moll, H.: *Atlas of Pediatric Diseases.* Philadelphia, W. B. Saunders Co., 1976.)

changing from red to purple, to rust, and then fading. Several kinds of lesions may be present at the same time. Hemorrhage and edema may occur in the gastrointestinal and urinary tracts. There are usually malaise and a low-grade fever.

Other manifestations are acute, colicky abdominal pain, vomiting and melena. In children having renal involvement there may be albuminuria and hematuria. About half of the children with kidney involvement also have hypertension or azotemia. The joints, usually the knees or ankles, may be involved. If so, they are painful and swollen, and motion is limited. These symptoms may be confused with symptoms of rheumatic fever (see p. 767). Cerebral edema and hemorrhage may cause convulsions and coma.

Laboratory findings show no change from the normal in clotting time, platelet count, bleeding time, clot retraction, or in the blood and blood-forming organs. Anemia results if the blood loss is great. The erythrocyte sedimentation rate is elevated.

Treatment, Complications, Course, and Prognosis. There is no specific *treatment.* If a specific allergen (food substance, bacteria, drug, or pollen) is involved, the child should be kept from contact with it. If purpura follows a bacterial infection, antibacterial treatment should be given to eliminate pathogens. During the acute phase bed rest is necessary, and the child should be observed closely for signs of involvement of the kidneys or brain. Corticosteroids may give relief from symptoms and reduce hemorrhage, but they do not shorten the course of the illness. They are usually given on an experimental basis only, since adverse effects may occur. Blood transfusions are given as needed.

Renal *complications* may occur, and renal insufficiency may manifest itself several years after the acute phase of the illness.

The *course* and *prognosis* are extremely variable. The condition may last from about six weeks to one or two years. Death, however, may occur from gastrointestinal and kidney changes, from hypertension or intracranial bleeding.

Responsibilities of the Nurse. When the child has a period of active bleeding he should be observed closely for signs and symptoms of shock and possibly internal or intracranial hemorrhage. If epistaxis occurs, compression and packing measures are used to control the bleeding. If bleeding continues, the nose may be packed with a hemostatic material.

The nurse can emphasize the need for protection of the child from injury since this may precipitate hemorrhaging in various vital organs. If the child returns to kindergarten or school, he should not engage in rough and tumble contact games or physical education.

Both parents and child may become anxious when injury or bleeding occurs. The nurse can support them by explaining the use of transfusions to replace the lost blood.

ALLERGY

Etiology and Predisposing Factors. The term "allergy" denotes an altered tissue reactivity to one or more substances (see immunity, p. 258). When an antigen or a foreign substance enters the body, the individual defends himself by creating an antibody to destroy the foreign material or change it into a harmless substance. Histamine is produced in large amounts by these reactions in allergic persons and is responsible for causing unfavorable allergic effects on body tissues. In nearly all cases the antibody is already present because of the body's responses to previous doses of antigen. Such sensitization may result from inhalation, absorption through the skin, ingestion, or parenteral injection.

The antigen most frequently responsible for the allergic state is a foreign protein, one from a different animal species than man. Carbohydrates, lipids, or chemicals may be protein-linked and may act as antigens in the production of antibodies.

The development of allergic manifestations depends partly on inheritance, in which case the term to be used is *atopy,* partly on the nature of the allergen and partly on the degree and duration of exposure. Although all persons are potentially allergic, susceptibility to allergy varies. Approximately 75 per cent of allergic children have a positive family history of allergy. The child's allergens and his allergic manifestations need not, however, be exactly the same as those of his parents.

The fetus may be passively sensitized *in utero,* but does not exhibit manifestations of the sensitivity until his first exposure to the allergen. Infants and children who have had severe gastrointestinal disturbances may develop sensitivities due to unchanged protein which enters the blood stream because of increased permeability of the intestinal wall. Psychologic factors involved in stress are important in the development of allergy.

Clinical Manifestations, Diagnosis, and Laboratory Findings. *Clinical manifestations* may differ, depending on the age of the child. An infant who has eczema (see p. 469) may suffer allergic rhinitis or asthma as a child. New sensitivities may appear in children, while old ones may continue or be lost.

Children having allergic manifestations should be skin-tested in order to determine the offending substance. Although they react to test allergens as do adults, reactions must be interpreted in the light of clinical findings. The intensity of the reaction does not necessarily indicate the importance of the particular test substance in causation.

The *diagnosis* of an offending allergen may also be made by giving the child an elimination diet. This is effective in determining the causative agent in an infant whose diet includes only a few foods. The mother should understand that certain foods must be eliminated completely from the diet and that the child's reactions to other foods must be accurately observed.

Except in acute asthma, eosinophilia of the peripheral blood is usually present in allergic persons. Eosinophilia of the mucous membranes of the nose may be present in any kind of allergic manifestation.

Treatment, Prognosis, and Prophylaxis. The physician must obtain a detailed history of the child and his family, and the parents must be willing to cooperate in a long-term program of treatment. Three methods of *treatment* may be attempted: the offending allergen may be removed; sensitization to specific known allergens may be decreased; or the response to the offending allergens may be altered.

Probably the most effective way to manage food allergies is to eliminate the particular food from the diet. Care must be taken that the subsequent diet is adequate for a child of his age.

There is no exact method of determining the dosage necessary for desensitization to a known allergen. Desensitization to inhalants is usually done by injection of extracts of the material in gradually increasing doses. The initial dose is usually the smallest amount which, given subcutaneously, will produce a positive intradermal test result. Subsequent doses are given at three- to five-day intervals, and each is larger than the preceding dose. At no time is an amount given which will produce symptoms. Desensitization to foods is accomplished by giving a gradually increasing amount of the substance which causes symptoms.

The third method of treatment is altering the response of the body to the offending allergen. Disturbing emotional factors should be corrected, since the emotional state influences the response of the body. Any endocrine imbalance should be treated. Certain drugs may be beneficial in treatment, including antihistamines, epinephrine and ephedrine. Corticotropin (ACTH) and the cortisones may also be used. Any respiratory infection should be treated, since it may predispose to an allergic state.

Dehydration depresses the allergic response. Allergic manifestations may be reduced by provision for adequate rest and improvement in general health.

An allergy to a substance cannot be cured, but it may be kept sufficiently under control so that no symptoms are produced. Partial or complete removal of the allergen from the environment of sensitive persons can be attempted. It is important that children whose parents are known to have allergies avoid contact with substances which may produce allergy.

If one or both parents is allergic, the newborn is not given cow's milk before he begins breast feeding, since sensitization to cow's milk may occur. Furthermore, during infancy and childhood additions to the diet are in the form of single, simple foods (see p. 367). If a combination of new foods were given at the same time, and an allergic manifestation developed, it would be difficult to know which food was the cause. Children of allergic parents should not be given foods which commonly cause an allergic response, such as cow's milk, eggs, chocolate, wheat, and oranges.

Types of Allergy in Children. The most important clinical manifestations of allergy in children include eczema (see p. 469), asthma, allergic rhinitis (hay fever) and serum sickness. Chronic conditions of the nose, throat and gastrointestinal tract may be due to allergy.

Asthma

Incidence, Etiology and Pathology. Asthma is a pulmonary disorder caused by an allergy. Infantile eczema (see p. 469) is a common forerunner of asthma. The disease is uncommon in infancy; its *incidence* increases in children three years of age and older.

Asthma may be evoked by particular foods, inhalants, or infections, particularly those of the respiratory tract. It may also follow vigorous activity, exposure to cold, or an emotional upheaval. Asthmatic attacks often occur at night after the child has been put to bed, because of his contact with a feather pillow, a wool blanket, a fuzzy, stuffed toy, or even dust in the area.

The smallest bronchioles undergo the greatest change. Initially the bronchiolar musculature goes into spasm, and the mucous membrane becomes pale and edematous. Then thick, tenacious mucus collects, and there is further obstruction of the air passages. During the attack not all the inspired air can be expired, and some collects in the alveoli, thereby causing obstructive emphysema. Wheezing and rales, due to the presence of bronchial secretions, are heard. Atelectasis may develop, caused by obstruction of a bronchus.

The attack may last for a few hours or continue for a few days. The child eventually coughs up the mucus, and the spasm relaxes. If infection is present, further respiratory embarrassment is observed.

Clinical Manifestations, Treatment, and Responsibilities of the Nurse. The onset of asthma frequently follows a traumatic emotional experience. In addition, the parents may have unconscious feelings of rejection of the child. Chronic emotional tension in the child's family and environment may cause him to have repeated attacks. In turn, repeated attacks of severe asthma may become the focus of parental anxiety and set up a continuing struggle be-

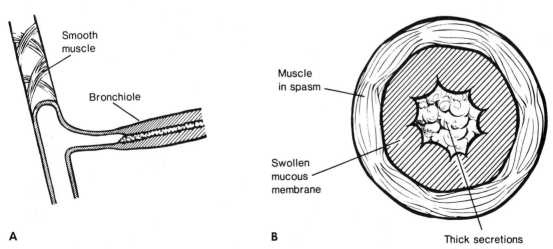

A　　　　　　　　　　　　　　　**B**

FIGURE 21–7.　Bronchiolar obstruction. In an asthma attack, the muscles surrounding the bronchial tubes go into spasm, the walls begin to swell, and abnormally thick mucus accumulates in the air passages. These lead to the trapping of air. A, Longitudinal section of bronchiolar obstruction. B, Enlarged cross-section. (From Fisher, L.: *American Lung Association Bulletin,* 62:3, June 1976.)

tween the parents and the child. In order to reduce the anxiety and tension in the child's environment and thus to help him to lead a more normal life, psychotherapeutic care such as family therapy may be necessary. The physician and the nurse may be instrumental in helping the parents identify the need for such therapy. At times the child may also be helped by residence in an institution where total care is available.

Asthma is characterized by paroxysms of an expiratory type of dyspnea with wheezing and generalized obstructive emphysema. The onset may be gradual with sneezing, nasal congestion, a watery discharge, and a slight cough before the attack. In other cases the onset may be sudden, often at night. The child may sit up in bed to breathe more easily. He perspires profusely and appears anxious. The wheezing occurs largely on expiration. He may cough almost continuously. If a bronchus becomes plugged with mucus, atelectasis occurs in that lobe, and the mediastinum then shifts toward the involved area. The neck veins become distended, and cyanosis is common. During the asthmatic attack the child should never be left alone. The parents become extremely anxious, and their anxiety may further alarm the child, who then becomes increasingly emotionally disturbed. With treatment such an attack may be over quickly. Untreated, it may last several days. In the hospital the nurse should stay with the child during acute episodes of respiratory distress. The nurse's confidence helps to reduce the anxiety of the parents and child. It is essential that the nurse not only assist with therapy, but also observe and report any toxic manifestations of drugs used.

The most effective way to treat asthma is to eliminate the offending allergen, whether food or an environmental allergen. If this cannot be done, desensitization to the allergens involved may be carried out under the care of an allergist. The child should avoid fatigue and chilling and should be kept calm and emotionally at ease.

The most effective drug in the treatment of an acute asthmatic attack is epinephrine given subcutaneously. Epinephrine may also be administered by a pharyngeal spray; it should be sprayed deeply into the larynx as the child inhales.

Other drugs frequently used are ephedrine sulfate or hydrochloride, aminophylline (ethylenediamine), which is a bronchodilator and may be used when epinephrine has lost its effectiveness, and antihistamines. Epinephrine may be given orally at first sign of an attack; however, it may cause vomiting and tachycardia or may stimulate the central nervous system.

Aminophylline is effective in relieving an asthmatic attack; however, it may produce signs of toxicity such as vomiting, irritability, excitement or a convulsion. Anticonvulsant medication such as phenobarbital should be given for such a reaction. The toxic effects of aminophylline may be increased if epinephrine or ephedrine has been given.

A corticosteroid may provide relief quickly when other medications have failed. Prednisone may be given orally. Long-continued use of a corticosteroid may result in suppression of adrenal activity, growth retardation, and dependency on steroids. Potassium iodide is of some value because it liquefies bronchial secretions so that the child can cough them up. Atropine is not used because it tends to dry up secretions.

The asthmatic child should have a generous fluid intake in order to liquefy secretions in the bronchi. Sedation may be needed if he shows indications of becoming exhausted. Sedatives which may be given include phenobarbital, chloral hydrate and paraldehyde. Morphine decreases the cough reflex and makes it difficult for the child to get rid of secretions.

Oxygen may be given to reduce anoxia and cyanosis. Increased humidity in an oxygen tent or in the air of the room may liquefy secretions and enable the child to expectorate. A mist tent is not used, however, because sufficient water does not reach the lower airway. Mist may also have an irritating effect on the respiratory tract of the asthmatic child. If a bronchus becomes plugged and atelectasis results, bronchoscopic aspiration may be necessary to open the airway.

Isopropyl norepinephrine may be used for inhalation therapy. It acts promptly to relieve asthmatic symptoms. A responsible adult gives this therapy, because a child or adolescent may overuse the drug. One or two sprays at half-hourly or hourly intervals should be sufficient to provide relief with the common preparations used.

Antibacterial therapy is given when the child has an infection along with an asthmatic attack. To prevent respiratory infections he may be moved to a warm, dry climate during the winter months. Some physicians recommend giving the child small doses of an antibiotic as prophylaxis against infection during the winter months. Others recommend the use of bacterial vaccines to reduce the incidence of respiratory infections. Some physicians also recommend a tonsillectomy and adenoidectomy when these tissues are the source of repeated respiratory infections or when they cause obstruction.

If the child has *status asthmaticus* (refractory asthma), the attack may continue for several days, both day and night. Death may occur during status asthmaticus. In addition to the administration of the above-mentioned drugs, when a child has status asthmaticus, adequate fluid intake is maintained and acidosis due to the retention of carbon dioxide is corrected. Assisted respiration may become necessary, with the use of positive-pressure breathing, either intermittently or continuously. An endotracheal tube may be used to facilitate aspiration of secretions from the bronchial tree and to do bronchial lavage if necessary. A tracheotomy may also become necessary (see p. 541). Percussion and postural drainage (see p. 446) may help in draining the bronchi. The child who has status asthmaticus needs constant monitoring of his physiologic processes and comprehensive nursing care.

The nurse, besides cooperating in the therapy, also makes accurate observations of the child's behavior when he is with other children or hospital personnel, as well as the interaction between the child and his mother during her visits. A continuous record of observations is of great importance to the physician or psychiatrist in determining the emotional factors involved.

The physician and the nurse are responsible for teaching the mother the long-term care of the asthmatic child. It is important that the child be kept in good health. He should have a balanced diet with vitamins. Since he may eat slowly because of respiratory difficulty, sufficient time should be permitted for meals. Smaller meals at frequent intervals may be less tiring than large meals at longer intervals. The child should have adequate rest. He will probably be more comfortable sitting up than reclining. He is kept as emotionally calm as possible. Simple amusements and quiet play are necessary to keep him happy.

Although the nurse should be patient with the child, limits must be set for his behavior. Inconsistency tends to create emotional conflicts which increase the respiratory difficulty. These children can be permitted to attend a special school for the handicapped and later a regular nursery school or school, provided the teachers and school nurses understand their problem, so that they can live as normal a life as possible.

Prognosis. The prognosis is most favorable if treatment is begun early. Many children cease to have asthmatic attacks at puberty, though others continue having them in adult life. If the asthmatic attacks cease, the child may exhibit some other allergic manifestation.

ALLERGIC RHINITIS (HAY FEVER)

Etiology and Incidence. Hay fever is an allergic manifestation involving the upper respiratory tract. Attacks may be perennial. Allergic rhinitis may be caused by pollen or by exposure to other inhalants. Ragweed and roses cause allergic rhinitis in susceptible persons. The condition is seldom seen in children under three or four years of age.

Clinical Manifestations and Treatment. *Clinical manifestations* include sneezing, which may be paroxysmal, rubbing the nose to relieve itching, and nasal stuffiness. Itching and erythema of the conjunctivae may also occur. The mucous membrane of the nose is pale and swollen. The nasal discharge may at first be clear and profuse, but as secondary infection occurs, it becomes purulent.

Allergic rhinitis is milder than other allergic diseases. The most effective method of *treatment* is elimination of the allergen from the environment if that is at all possible. Air-conditioning and filtering devices may be used. Desensitization may be attempted if the allergen cannot be eliminated.

Antihistamines are frequently used for seasonal hay fever. A side effect of the use of antihistamines is somnolence, which varies in degree, depending on the type of drug used. Epinephrine is seldom used unless asthma is also a problem.

Responsibilities of the Nurse. The nurse who provides routine well child care is in a position to observe a child who may have allergic rhinitis. In addition to the clinical manifestations mentioned, the child may have an allergic salute (a movement of his hand to push his nose up and back), mouth wrinkling, or nose wrinkling, all of which are done to relieve an itching nose. These observations are reported to the physician so that the child can receive therapy. After the diagnosis is made, the nurse can teach the parents environmental control: to make their home allergy-proof and to keep the child away from the offending allergen. The nurse can also teach parents to give medication correctly and ways to prevent infection of the child.

SERUM SICKNESS AND ANAPHYLACTIC REACTIONS

Incidence and Etiology. All persons may potentially get serum sickness if the amount of injected foreign serum is sufficient. It may occur at any age in both sexes.

The most common cause of serum sickness is the prophylactic injection of horse serum, although other serums may also produce clinical manifestations. Injection of the serum incites the production of antibodies, which unite with the rest of the serum to produce the allergic reaction.

The first injection of minute amounts of serum may sensitize a person for years. Total reactions may resemble anaphylactic shock and may occur in persons sensitized to horse serum.

Causes of anaphylactic reactions, less common in children than in adults, include the injection of products containing or derived from penicillin, or insect stings (see p. 757).

Clinical Manifestations, Treatment, Responsibilities of the Nurse, Prognosis, and Prevention. The *clinical manifestations* vary from mild to severe. The onset is usually about two days after the injection of serum, although it may vary from a few hours to a month. The skin eruption, an urticarial wheal, occurs first at the site of the injection, but spreads over the entire body. In more severe cases purpura and exudative eruptions may occur. Angioneurotic edema involving the eyelids, lips, tongue, hands, or feet may occur, and generalized edema may be present. Itching is intense. Generalized lymphadenopathy and enlargement of the spleen may be present. The joints may be swollen and red. Muscular pain, headache, fever, and malaise are frequent. In severe cases neurologic and cerebral complications may be seen. If the person has been sensitized previously, clinical manifestations appear early after serum injection.

When the skin test is done for serum sensitivity or when serum is given, epinephrine should be available to control anaphylactic symptoms and urticarial eruption. Ephedrine may also be used, as may antihistaminic drugs and corticosteroids. Cold compresses, starch baths and antipruritic lotions may be used to relieve itching. Sedatives and salicylates may be ordered to make the child more comfortable.

The reaction to serum is self-limited. It usually lasts from one to three days, but may last a week or longer.

Prevention requires sensitivity tests. It is important that the nurse understand the purpose of this procedure, because serum is frequently used in the prevention of disease.

Before any foreign serum is injected, the child should be tested for sensitivity. An intradermal injection of horse serum, for instance, is made, especially if the child has a history of allergic eczema, asthma, or hay fever. If the child is known to be sensitive, a very weak testing solution should be used at first. If the area becomes red after 20 minutes, the reaction is considered positive. The ophthalmic test may also be used as a guide in determining sensitivity to serum. If the eye becomes red in a few minutes, the reaction is considered positive. An antihistaminic drug may be given prophylactically to prevent serum sickness.

EPILEPSY (CHRONIC OR RECURRENT CONVULSIVE DISORDER)

Convulsions in infancy have already been discussed (see p. 473). Convulsions during the preschool period may indicate that the child has epilepsy.

Epilepsy is characterized by paroxysmal, recurrent attacks of impaired consciousness or of unconsciousness. Tonic or clonic muscular spasms or another type of abnormal behavior occurs. Epilepsy is not a specific disease entity in itself, but rather a general term which includes a variety of recurrent seizure patterns.

People in the community as well as family members sometimes fear those who have epilepsy, or they consider the disease socially disgraceful. Physicians, nurses, social workers, and other team members must educate the public to the real meaning of the disease as a chronic illness. A large amount of information should not be given at once, but slowly so that it does not pose too great a threat.

There are two types of epilepsy–idiopathic and organic.

Idiopathic or Cryptogenic Epilepsy. More than half of the children who have recurrent seizures before puberty have idiopathic epilepsy. The cause of the seizures cannot be found. Heredity may be a factor, but this can seldom be clinically demonstrated. The onset is commonly between four and eight years of age. Treatment to control the seizures is possible in about 85 per cent of these children.

Organic Epilepsy. Organic epilepsy may result from a number of focal or diffuse injuries to the brain which have left residual damage. Such injuries may be caused by direct laceration of brain tissue due to trauma, hemorrhage due to trauma or the hemorrhagic diseases, anoxia (asphyxia neonatorum), infections (e.g., meningitis, encephalitis), or toxic manifestations due to kernicterus or lead poisoning. Degenerative changes may take place in the brain. Congenital problems such as phenylketonuria or hydrocephalus or diseases such as syphilis or toxoplasmosis may result in organic abnormalities in the brain. Organic epilepsy usually shows abnormalities on electroencephalograms.

Clinical Manifestations and Diagnosis. The *clinical manifestations* are used as the basis for the classification of seizures: grand mal, petit mal, psychomotor, focal, and infantile myoclonic seizures.

Grand mal seizures in children are not likely to be preceded by an aura such as is common in adults. Older children may have a headache, may be irritable and lethargic, or may have digestive upsets before seizures. The seizure is a generalized convulsion; a tonic phase and a clonic phase are usually seen. A *tonic spasm* is an involuntary, violent, persistent contraction. In the tonic phase the child falls to the ground, the pupils dilate, and the face is distorted. The

TABLE 21–3. ANTIEPILEPTIC DRUGS

CLASS	DRUG	TRADE NAME	USUAL INDICATION*	COMMENT
Barbiturates	Phenobarbital	Luminal	G	Drug of choice
	Mephobarbital	Mebaral	G	More expensive than phenobarbital
	Metharbital	Gemonil	G	Less effective than phenobarbital
	Primidone	Mysoline	G	Alternate to phenobarbital
Hydantoins	Diphenylhydantoin	Dilantin	G	Drug of choice
	Mephenytoin	Mesantoin	G	Use limited by toxicity
	Ethotoin	Peganone	G	Less effective than diphenylhydantoin
Succinimides	Ethosuximide	Zarontin	P	Drug of choice
	Methsuximide	Celontin	P	Less effective than ethosuximide
	Phensuximide	Milontin	P	Less effective than methsuximide
Oxazolidinediones	Trimethadione	Tridione	P	More toxic than ethosuximide
	Paramethadione	Paradione	P	Alternate to trimethadione
Benzodiazepines	Diazepam	Valium	S	Drug of choice
	Nitrazepam	Mogadon	M	Not available in USA
	Clonazepam	Ro-5-4023	M	Not available in USA
Other	Carbamazepine	Tegretol	G	Not approved by FDA for antiepileptic use
	Phenacemide	Phenurone	G	Use limited by toxicity
	Bromide	-------	G	Use limited by toxicity
	Acetazolamide	Diamox	P	Effectiveness often short-lived
	Quinacrine	Atabrine	P	Occasionally effective
	Dextroamphetamine	Dexedrine	P	Occasionally effective
	Corticotropin	Acthar Gel	M	Drug of choice
	Paraldehyde	-------	S	Largely supplanted by diazepam

* G = grand mal, focal or psychomotor seizures
P = petit mal
M = infantile spasms or minor motor seizures
S = status epilepticus

From Gellis, S. S., and Kagan, B. M. (Eds.): *Current Pediatric Therapy* 7. Philadelphia, W. B. Saunders Co., 1976.

TABLE 21–4. ORAL DOSES OF ANTIEPILEPTIC DRUGS

DRUG	RECOMMENDED ORAL DOSE*	RANGE OF THERAPEUTIC SERUM LEVELS	SERUM HALF-LIFE *Younger Children*	*Older Children*	RECOMMENDED PREPARATIONS
Phenobarbital	100 mg./m²/day (3-6 mg./kg./day) in 3 divided doses	20-40 µg./ml.	60 hours	120 hours	Phenobarbital tablets: 15 mg., 30 mg., 60 mg., 100 mg. Phenobarbital elixir: 20 mg./ 5 ml. (only for young infants when tablets are impractical)
Diphenylhydantoin	200 mg./m²/day (6-12 mg./kg./day) in 3 divided doses	10-20 µg./ml.-	15 hours	30 hours	Diphenylhydantoin tablets: 50 mg. Sodium diphenylhydantoin capsules: 30 mg., 100 mg.
Primidone	500 mg./m²/day (15-30 mg./kg./day) in 3 divided doses	5-15 µg./ml.	4 hours	8 hours	Primidone tablets: 50 mg., 250 mg.
Carbamazepine	400 mg./m²/day (12-24 mg./kg./day) in 3 divided doses†	2-6 µg./ml.	?	?	Carbamazepine tablets: 200 mg.
Ethosuximide	500 mg./m²/day (15-30 mg./kg./day) in 3 divided doses	50-100 µg./ml.	30 hours	60 hours	Ethosuximide capsules: 250 mg.
Trimethadione	1000 mg./m²/day (30-60 mg./kg./day) in 3 divided doses	500-1000 µg./ml. (dimethadione)	150 hours (dimethadione)	300 hours	Trimethadione tablets: 150 mg. Trimethadione capsules: 300 mg.

* When a range of doses (mg/kg/day) is given, the lower dose is for older children and the higher dose is for younger children.
† There is as yet no established dosage of carbamazepine for children, but this schedule has been found effective.
From Gellis, S. S., and Kagan, B. M. (Eds.): *Current Pediatric Therapy* 7. Philadelphia, W. B. Saunders Co., 1976.

neck, abdominal, and chest muscles are held rigidly. The limbs stiffen. As air is forced out of the lungs a brief cry may be heard. The child may bite his tongue and may void or defecate as the result of contracture of the abdominal muscles. Since respiratory movements are arrested, cyanosis occurs. This phase usually lasts up to 40 seconds. The *clonic* phase, which consists in alternate contraction and relaxation of muscles, lasts indefinitely. After this the child goes into a deep sleep. When he wakens, he may complain of headache and may appear confused or stuporous. A child may have seizures at night *(nocturnal epilepsy)* and in the morning find his bed wet or discover that he has bitten his tongue.

A child who has grand mal seizures may become egocentric and negativistic, owing to the attitudes of others toward him and his illness.

Petit mal seizures consist of transient loss of consciousness with possibly rolling of the eyes, lip movements or slight movements of the head, limbs, or trunk. The child does not fall. He usually stares into space. After the age of three years petit mal occurs more frequently in girls than in boys. These attacks last up to 30 seconds. The child may not realize that he had a seizure. He may have as many as a hundred or more in a day or as few as one a month. He is usually confused after an attack.

There is a third type of seizure—*psychomotor seizures*—which cannot be recognized easily because they seem to be purposeful but repetitive inappropriate muscular acts. Usually no tonic or clonic movements are noted. The child may have a slight aura and may sleep after an attack. He is usually not confused.

Focal seizures (jacksonian epilepsy) may be either motor or sensory. The manifestation depends on the location of the focal area in the brain which has the abnormal neuronal discharge. Unilateral jacksonian attacks are usually clonic, indicating that their origin is in the motor cortex. The muscles involved are usually those of the hand, tongue, face, and foot. A focal seizure beginning in one area such as the hand spreads to areas of the body on the same side in a fixed pattern. Consciousness may or may not be disturbed.

Infantile myoclonic seizures or infantile spasms are seen before the age of two years and involve one group of muscles. The child may lower his head and flex his arms innumerable times a day. He may also flex his legs on his abdomen. The electroencephalographic examination shows random high-voltage slow waves and spikes (hypsarrhythmia) suggesting a disorganized state. This type of convulsion usually disappears by the third year, and grand mal seizures appear. The condition is usually accompanied by mental retardation.

Diagnosis is made on the basis of family history and the child's record of convulsive seizures. Different types of epilepsy show a variety of electroencephalographic (EEG) abnormalities. For diagnostic purposes, therefore, whenever a convulsive disorder is present, an electroencephalogram is made. Roentgen studies of the skull are also necessary. Other tests such as pneumoencephalography and examination of the cerebrospinal fluid may be done if indicated (see p. 295).

Treatment and Responsibilities of the Nurse. During an attack the child should be protected from injury. His clothing should be loosened around the neck, and he must be turned to one side so that he does not aspirate secretions. Oxygen should be given if cyanosis occurs and if the convulsion is prolonged.

A prolonged series of grand mal seizures is termed *status epilepticus*. Oxygen is given, and phenobarbital sodium is administered intramuscularly. The environment should be quiet while the child is recovering from a prolonged convulsion. He and his parents need reassurance.

Prolonged therapy has three purposes: control of the convulsions, education of the child's family and others in his environment to accept him, and help so that he may function to full capacity. The treatment includes anticonvulsant drugs, good care of the whole child, diet therapy, and psychotherapy if necessary. The family and the child should have a positive attitude toward his illness. He should lead as normal a life as possible. Anxiety tends to increase the occurrence of seizures. If the child appears anxious, the social worker or child psychiatrist may help the family find the sources of his anxiety. The child should be kept at home rather than institutionalized if his capacities permit home care.

The choice of drugs and the dosage needed to control convulsions depend upon the individual child and the type of seizure. Phenobarbital is often used over a long period for grand mal seizures. If the child has an idiosyncrasy to phenobarbital, a maculopapular skin eruption, drowsiness, and fever may be noted. Mebaral (mephobarbital) is also used in some cases of grand mal seizures. Dilantin (diphenylhydantoin sodium or phenytoin sodium is an effective anticonvulsant, but does not produce excessive drowsiness as barbiturates may. Nonhemorrhagic, painless hypertrophy of the gums may follow administration of Dilantin. No special treatment is required. Drowsiness and ataxia may occur if the child receives too large a dose.

Ethosuximide (Zarontin) is presently the drug

of choice in the therapy of petit mal, since it is less toxic than other compounds. Tridione (trimethadione) is also effective in the treatment of petit mal seizures. This drug may increase the occurrence of grand mal attacks if the child also suffers from such seizures. Phenobarbital or Dilantin may also be ordered. Prolonged or excessive use of Tridione may produce drowsiness, nausea, photophobia or skin eruptions. Aplastic anemia may also occur. Mysoline (primidone) is given for grand mal and psychomotor seizures. Side effects include drowsiness and ataxia.

Corticotropin (ACTH), a corticosteroid, or pyridoxine may be used in the treatment of infantile myoclonic seizures. This therapy, when started early, appears to produce improvement in the clinical status and the electroencephalographic pattern. The nurse's role includes monitoring the blood pressure and administering the medication. The nurse teaches the parents to do these procedures, so that they can provide care for the child at home. If further assistance is needed, the parent can be referred to a community health nurse.

Diet therapy is important. A fasting diet, ketogenic diet, and a reduction of fluid intake tend to prevent seizures. Diet therapy may be used with the older child who cooperates with treatment, but is usually more difficult than with the little child. The diet should be varied and palatable, since a ketogenic diet containing large amounts of fat is not appetizing over a long period.

The nurse must record observations of a convulsion. This is important because the physician is seldom present when the child has a seizure. Although the child must be closely watched, he should not be made to feel that he can never be left alone. The physical aspects of his care are similar to those of the infant during a convulsion (see p. 473). Prevention of injury is a principal concern.

The nurse should keep the child as free from anxiety as possible. Unnecessary stimulation should be avoided. Diversion appropriate to his age and ability should be provided. His play equipment should be such that it will not cause injury during a seizure.

The nurse assists with the diagnostic tests. All procedures should be explained to the child in a way that he will understand. The nurse must see that he swallows his anticonvulsant medications and must watch for side effects of the drugs.

Parent-child relations can be observed for indications of rejection or overprotection of the child. He is watched for traits of egocentricity, emotional instability, and selfishness, and what is noted is reported to the physician. These traits develop as a reaction to adult attitudes toward the child and his illness. The parents and the child must understand the need for continued medical care and supervision to control convulsions.

Since the child is better off at home than in the hospital if the mother can give him the care he needs, it is important that she learn how to care for him. The child should have as normal a life as possible. Safe outdoor activity should be provided. If the convulsions are not too severe and the child is mentally able to profit from the experience, he should go to nursery school and later to school. The attitude of adults and their treatment of him when he has a seizure influence the attitude of other children toward him.

The nurse helps the parents understand the need for giving the medication as ordered and for observing any indications of toxicity or other evidence that the drug or dosage may need to be changed. Other children must be protected from accidental ingestion of the medication by storing it in a safe place. When the child who has a diagnosis of epilepsy goes to school, either the school nurse or his teacher can supervise his medication. If they do not have a supply of the drug in school, the child takes with him only the amount of medication required for one day.

Safety factors must be kept in mind in the case of the epileptic child. In order to prevent head injury if the child has repeated grand mal seizures, it may be necessary for him to wear a protective helmet such as a padded football helmet. This causes him to be different from other children and may create social problems for him in play or school groups. Participation in activities such as swimming, which may be dangerous for him, are permitted only under the supervision of a responsible person.

A Medic Alert identification symbol should be worn by the child having epilepsy. Information on the bracelet or necklace includes the diagnosis and drug therapy being utilized. This is especially important if the child is going to be away from parents and friends who know of his diagnosis.

When the child reaches the adolescent period he may act out his feelings about his illness and test the limits within which he can function. He may "forget" to take his medication and involve himself in activities in which participation was prevented earlier. In this situation the parents can be helped to recognize that his behavior is essentially normal for an adolescent and to assist him in the eventual acceptance of his condition.

The role of parents of an epileptic child is difficult; the child's role is even more difficult. Parents and child need emotional support, reassurance, and praise for their achievements. The seizures can be reduced in frequency so as not to interfere too much with the child's activity. Personality changes can be minimized if parents treat the child as though he were essentially normal. They must prevent him from becoming overdependent on them.

Prognosis. The *prognosis* depends on the mental and physical handicaps the child has and on the adequacy of medical and environmental management. If the child has adequate treatment and was mentally normal at the beginning of his illness, he can be expected to remain essentially normal throughout his life.

As the child grows to adulthood he may find that because of his diagnosis certain of his activities may be limited. Certain states have laws forbidding the epileptic to drive an automobile, to work in certain occupations or to marry. These laws may be changed as the public develops a better understanding of the disease and its therapy.

PSEUDOHYPERTROPHIC MUSCULAR DYSTROPHY (DUCHENNE OR CHILDHOOD FORM)

Pseudohypertrophic muscular dystrophy is a long-term condition of genetic origin that becomes more apparent during the preschool years. This condition was discussed in Chapter 12 (see p. 315).

MENTAL RETARDATION

Incidence and Etiology. Mental retardation is any interference with intelligence that causes a limitation in the way the child is able to adapt to his environment. It is not a disease entity itself, but is a complex of symptoms due to a variety of causes. Between 3 and 4 per cent of all children born in the United States will at some time in their lives be classified as mentally retarded. In this country alone there are approximately 2.4 million mentally retarded children and adolescents under the age of 21 years. More than 100,000 infants born each year will join this group. One of every 10 Americans is directly involved with this problem because a mentally retarded person is in his or her family.

Heredity may be the cause; in some cases mental retardation can be traced through generations and an incidence above average among relatives proved. There are so many other factors, however, that it is difficult to single out heredity. Some of these factors may be classified as follows: (1) *prenatal* causes, including metabolic disorders such as phenylketonuria (see p. 466), hypothyroidism (cretinism) (see p. 464), mongolism (Down's syndrome) (see p. 308), cranial

malformation (see p. 479), maternal infections such as German measles or syphilis, maternal irradiation, anoxia, and isoimmunization (kernicterus) (see p. 240); (2) *neonatal* causes, including intracranial hemorrhage (see p. 254), anoxia (see p. 201), or birth trauma; (3) *postnatal* causes, including intracranial injury or hemorrhage (see p. 475), infections such as meningitis (see p. 660) or encephalitis (see p. 658), poisoning such as with lead (see p. 576), cerebrovascular thrombosis, anoxia, neoplasms (see p. 791), or recurrent convulsions.

Diagnosis. Such factors as epilepsy (see p. 692), cerebral palsy (see p. 578), severe malnutrition (see p. 435), emotional disturbances (see p. 801), blindness (see p. 589), deafness (see p. 586), and speech disorders (see p. 803) may lead to an incorrect diagnosis of mental retardation which may result in the child's being treated as a mental defective and deprived of the opportunity to attain his potential mental development.

A definite diagnosis of mental retardation is made only after a thorough study of the family and the child. Such a study is done by a team composed of members selected from among the following: a pediatrician, a psychologist, a psychiatrist, a social worker, and community or public health and hospital nurses. In order to participate with other team members the nurse should have a good knowledge of community and state resources for such children. The nurse may also help to implement and to interpret the recommendations of the team to the parents. Centers have been established, usually in connection with medical schools of large universities, for research and diagnosis and for the development of plans of care for individual retarded children.

Mental retardation of a severe degree may be recognized as early as birth. It is indicated by failure of the infant to learn to suck at the breast or from a bottle. If a three-month-old infant who has lived in an adequate environment fails to develop normally, mental retardation must be considered. Throughout infancy, before the child learns to talk, rough estimates of his mental ability may be made by testing his motor abilities. Does he sit, stand, and walk within the usual age limits for a physically and mentally normal child? Mentally retarded toddlers may be slow in trying to help themselves, in speaking, in feeding themselves, or in toilet training. Until the child is of preschool age, slowness of development may not be recognized. It becomes a disturbing problem, however, as soon as the child is with normal preschool children living in the same environment. A child who is only mildly mentally retarded may pass through infancy and even the preschool years with no indication of retardation. When he enters school, however, and is expected to understand abstract concepts, his handicap may become apparent.

Causes of delayed development should be sought whenever a child has retarded physical and motor development. The child should have a thorough examination to determine whether there is a physical cause for which therapy can be given.

Intelligence tests and other evaluative devices should be given to provide an estimation of mental capacity. A study of emotional reactions and social adjustments should be made. Personality characteristics of mentally retarded children vary; some children are pleasant and get along well with other children and with adults, but others are restless, irritable, and disobedient. These traits interact with mental capacity in social adjustment. Children of low intelligence are usually clumsy in their movements and slow to respond to stimuli.

Classification and Clinical Manifestations. Mentally retarded children may be classified in three groups. (1) Those children who are *mildly retarded but educable* and have an intelligence quotient between 51 and 75 can reach a mental age of eight to 12 years. (2) Those children who are *moderately retarded but trainable* and have an intelligence quotient between 21 and 50 can reach a mental age of three to seven years. (3) Those children who are *severely retarded and are completely dependent on others for their care* and have an intelligence quotient between 0 and 20 can reach a mental age of zero to two years.

Children who are mildly retarded but educable may learn to function fairly well in the home if they are able to care for themselves, and in the community by learning to perform simple manual services or trades. Children who are moderately retarded but trainable may learn to talk fairly well and understand what is said to them. Their ability to concentrate varies, but is not long upon any one task. They may be able to dress themselves, to acquire socially acceptable elimination control, and to feed themselves without assistance. Some children who are severely retarded may not be able to speak or walk until five years of age, and others may never learn. They require constant care and supervision. Although they may make some progress slowly, they are usually institutionalized.

Management. Management of the mentally retarded child is the responsibility of the home, school, community and state. The initial step is for the physician to inform the parents of the problem. They should not be told, however, until the diagnosis is definitely established. Although parents may have suspected the diagnosis, they face it with great anxiety and, when it is confirmed, may have a feeling of guilt. Parents of a retarded child have a different response to their grief than parents whose child has died. While the parents of a retarded child are grieving over the loss of a desired child, they are required to invest in their handicapped child as a love object and to provide care for him. They need sympathetic understanding of their problems and acceptance of their attitudes in order to free themselves from their feeling of guilt, or at least responsibility for the child's condition, for lack of normal parental love, and the feeling that he is a burden. As soon as possible they are included with other health team members, depending on the child's specific problems and level of functioning, in making realistic plans for the child's care based on their reaction to the handicap, the degree of the child's retardation and the community facilities in the area in which they live.

If the cause of the retardation can be found and is amenable to treatment, every effort should be made to help the child. Thyroid extract is given for cretinism, operation is performed for subdural hematoma, hydrocephalus, or craniosynostosis, and dietary management is provided for phenylketonuria.

Parents can be educated as to a child's potential and should have a realistic concept of his ability. Parents and teachers should not use pressure in an attempt to force a retarded child to learn. Pressure leads only to frustration, which causes further emotional problems. The retarded child needs from parents and teachers the same kind of love, security and help that a normal child needs, but he needs them longer because his dependence extends beyond the usual age.

The plan of management includes environmental arrangements in which the child can utilize his capacities to the best advantage. Although in general the mentally retarded child should be kept in his own environment as long as possible, for some children institutional care is best. For others special training can be given at home. Mentally retarded children as well as those having emotional problems may benefit from foster home care, day care, or the utilization of foster grandparents in long-term care. Some children may profit from attendance at special nursery and grade schools; however, they may also go to a regular school near their homes. Regular schools which have special programs for the retarded and encourage them to socialize with normal children part of the day are excellent for large numbers of retarded children. Some states now have laws regarding the education of the mentally retarded to their fullest potential in public schools. These children

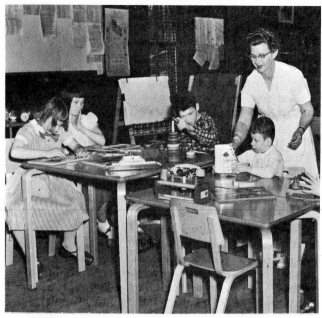

FIGURE 21–8. These retarded children are learning to coordinate their muscular activity through play. (Charles P. Jubenville, Ed. D., Director, Daytime Care Centers.) (*Nursing Outlook*, July 1960.)

should be taught to care for themselves and should learn a vocation if possible. These important decisions must ultimately be made by the parents; however, the health team can give some guidance based on the child's diagnosis.

Before realistic plans can be made the parents of retarded children must accept the diagnosis. If they do not, they may continue to search for a medical reason for the problem and cure of the condition. Once they have accepted the diagnosis and plan for the child's care, they may gain confidence and emotional support by joining a group of parents whose children have the same problem as theirs. They may also become active participants in their local group of the National Association for Retarded Citizens.

Siblings of any handicapped child, but especially those of the mentally retarded, may feel neglected because of the amount of time mother devotes to the retarded child. Some children may regress to the level of the retarded child in order to gain the attention they feel they deserve. When the siblings are older, they may hesitate to bring friends to the home, to date, or to marry because of fear that the condition may be inherited. Adequate explanation should be given to the siblings of a retarded child and free communication established so that misconceptions can be eliminated and anxiety reduced.

Responsibilities of the Nurse. Mentally retarded children have the same basic needs and the same right to respect as all other children do. They have a worth of their own and some capacity for self-realization. The child's self-concept is extremely important in influencing how well he will be able to utilize the abilities he does possess. The nurse can assist each child to reach his maximum potential if he is viewed objectively and as a whole individual.

The major responsibilities of the nurse in the area of mental retardation are prevention, case finding, and management and care.

The nurse may be the first to detect early signs of mental retardation. Often, because of an understanding of normal growth and development, the nurse can observe lack of development of which the parents are unaware. The nurse or the nurse practitioner may utilize the Denver Developmental Screening Test (see p. 31) to evaluate the growing child in the home, well child conference, pediatric medical practice, outpatient department or clinic, or in the hospital. Observations and testing of this kind are reported to the physician, who, with the other team members, can determine the degree of retardation and its possible cause.

The nurse should be a member of the team which plans and carries out recommendations for the care of the child at home and for his education and training. *Operant conditioning, behavior therapy, and behavior modification* utilized in the care of mentally retarded and emotionally disturbed children, are conditioning techniques based on the principle of *reinforcement*. Reinforcement simply means that a reward should be given for a certain response so that the probability of recurrence of that same response will be increased. The reward, such as food, candy, praise, or encouragement, must be given *immediately* and *consistently* after the approved behavior is done. Behavior that is not to be strengthened does not lead to reward. This technique makes it possible to teach complex behavior when it is broken down into small steps which the child can easily achieve. Behavioral changes in the areas of toilet training, feeding, dressing, and the reduction of destructive behavior, among others, are possible with the use of this technique.

Group teaching of behavior modification techniques for several parents and all their adult family members, as well as individual instruction for the parents, is of great value. Group teaching not only makes better use of professional time, but the parents also learn behavioral modification principles and techniques that can be carried out consistently at home. In other words, the nurse teaches the method and the parents carry it out during their daily interaction with their child. Parents can also generalize from their knowledge and experience with more common maladaptive behavior and thus they can deal with less common behavior when it appears.

In helping the mother to provide care the nurse makes it clear that a child, no matter what his chronological age, will proceed in his development and thus needs to be treated according to his mental age. Thus in teaching self-help skills, it is necessary to teach the child at whatever level of mental ability he has at that time. When helping the mother teach the child habit formation, it is essential that the nurse remember the ages at which the average child is ready to perform certain acts successfully, such as elimination control or toilet training, feeding himself, and dressing himself, among others. (See the growth and development charts in Chapters 13, 16 and 19.) Also, any physical handicap must be taken into consideration when teaching a skill. If the child has cerebral palsy (see p. 578), for instance, his progress will be slower than that of a child who has adequate muscular control. The child who is mentally retarded lacks the ability to do abstract reasoning; therefore the purpose of teaching is for habit formation with little expectation of his being able to transfer knowledge from one situation to another. When training for habit formation, it is necessary first of all to help the child to relax, then to proceed through the routine, repeating it sufficiently so that he will eventually be able to do it himself.

When the mother wishes to teach the child elimination control, she first of all keeps a record or schedule of when the child routinely urinates and has his bowel movements. The child is then placed on the toilet approximately every two hours according to his own schedule. Gradually his schedule is modified to fit into the family routine. Each time the mother takes him to the toilet, he is taken to the bathroom. The training chair should not be moved about the house to accommodate his activities. The mother explains simply in words and gestures what he is to do and gives him approval if he succeeds. As when teaching an essentially normal child (see p. 497), if he does not succeed in his attempt, he should not be condemned.

The mother who wants to teach the child to dress himself should provide clothing that is easy to put on and take off and place articles of clothing consistently in an order for his use. As clothing having zippers, buttons, or ties is purchased, the child is guided in practicing these skills.

In helping a mentally retarded child to feed himself, the mother follows the same general principles of teaching as are used for the essentially normal child in addition to the principles of operant conditioning. Special eating equipment may need to be obtained for the child's use.

A new and effective technique for dealing with a variety of deficient eating skills is the *mini-meal* method. In this program regular meals are divided into smaller portions served hourly throughout the day. The nurse or mother can guide the child to proper eating skills. When an appropriate behavior is learned, it is rewarded, and guidance is gradually reduced. Guidance is reinstated if an error occurs. At first, only one utensil is used per meal until all have been utilized correctly. By modifying the child's eating behavior gradually, success may ultimately be attained.

In disciplining the mentally retarded child, the principles utilized for the average child as well as those of operant conditioning are followed. These include consistency in action, the use of simple language to explain what he has done wrong, and the establishment of a routine in his daily living, so that the child learns what is expected of him. If punishment is necessary, it should follow the misdeed immediately so that the two events are connected in the child's mind.

The mentally retarded child needs stimulation from his environment if he is to achieve his potential. He needs as many, if not more, objects to look at, sounds to hear, and items to handle and manipulate as the mentally normal child does.

When such a child is hospitalized, the nurse obtains from the mother an explicit record of the routine she uses for caring for the child at home. Since a mentally retarded child needs to be prepared for each activity and needs repetition in order to learn, the nurse continues with the home routine as much as possible. The nurse's specific functions are provision of physical care as for a normal child and supervision of the child to prevent self-injury. Close restraint is not good for such children. They are given constructive play activity so that their attention is focused on acceptable behavior.

The nurse may help the parents select toys on the basis of the child's mental, not chronologic, age. They may need help to understand that his attention span is short, and that they should give approval for his successes and provide for him simple responsibilities at home.

The age of puberty and adolescence is a time of anxiety and stress for all parents, including those of the retarded child. Meeting the social and emotional needs of the growing child is difficult (see Chap. 25). The nurse will find the teaching aids listed at the end of this chapter of help in guiding parents at this time.

Prognosis, Prevention, and Planning for the Future. Unless the child is severely retarded, the outlook for length of life is about that of normal children. His adjustment to society will depend on the extent of his retardation and on the extent to which he has learned to use his mental resources.

Great strides are being made in the *prevention* of the causes of and the problems due to mental retardation. Research is being done to find means to reduce its incidence such as that related to the *Collaborative Research Project*. During recent years there has been a growing commitment of federal funds to the care of the retarded. Many communities are making strides in providing special services for retarded children. Even greater efforts must be made to increase funds available for research, for the preparation of personnel to care for retarded children, for the organization of more parent groups, and for comprehensive programs to help these children. Nurses are in a unique position to function as advocates for the cause of improving the total care of retarded persons.

EMOTIONAL PROBLEMS

Two emotional disorders that occur most frequently during the preschool period are phobias, or irrational fears, and temper tantrums.

PHOBIAS

Children usually have many fears of dangers in the real world. They learn fear of such things as fire, sharp knives, or a busy street from their parents, who wish to protect them from accidents or harm. But children also fear things which could not possibly cause them harm. They may be afraid of the dark, of the dead, of noises, or of ghosts. Boys are more commonly afraid of injury to their bodies, and girls of the dark and of strange noises. The incidence of these fears is greatest during the preschool period.

When an unreasonable fear produces panic in a child, he is said to have a *phobia*. Not even the reassurance of a loving adult can reduce the emotional feeling about the dreaded object. If the cause of the phobia is close to reality, e.g., fear of a dog which actually is capable of harming a child, the phobia is not too serious. If the cause is not close to reality, the child is emotionally ill. The real problem is not the phobic object, but an insoluble emotional conflict. Most children recover from their phobias, but they may need help to do so.

The most effective way to help a child rid himself of a phobia is to help him slowly cope with the situation or object. The adult should gradually give him an opportunity to be near the feared object and have a chance to inspect or ignore it. The adult should also help him actively to participate in the dreaded situation or with the feared object.

Sometimes reassurance and demonstrations that the object is really harmless or that other children do not fear it will help the child to master his own fear. Under no circumstances is his fear ignored, nor should he be forced to contact the object.

The child is encouraged to be more self-helpful and to spend more time with other children instead of with his parents. He is permitted to express his hostility verbally or to engage in active games in order to work out his feelings.

Children whose activity is seriously limited because of a phobia or whose phobic object is not close to reality should have psychiatric treatment.

TEMPER TANTRUMS

Temper tantrums are normal during the toddler period, but if they continue into the preschool period and become more severe, the child has not learned how to handle the normal frustrations of growing up.

During a severe temper tantrum the child is unconscious of his surroundings and of reality. He uses a great deal of muscular energy, striking out against his surroundings or himself, rarely against the adult responsible for his frustration. The child's reaction is usually out of all proportion to the apparent cause.

In taking his frustration out on himself the child is, in effect, angry with himself. When he becomes exhausted as a result of so much physical activity, he is remorseful because he allowed himself to act like a baby or toddler.

Temper tantrums occur in every child's life. If they are serious or prolonged or recur too frequently, the child is probably not developing as he should. Possibly a child having pathologic temper tantrums has been overindulged and has not learned to control his impulses or to react within normal limits to frustrations. Treatment consists in helping such children to gain more control of their infantile desires and to get pleasure from more mature forms of satisfaction. A nurse can help by causing a child to feel more pleasure in pleasing her than in giving way to every impulse.

Pathologic temper tantrums may occur if the child has been forced too early to be independent and to exert too rigid control over his behavior. He tries hard to behave in a way that will make his parents approve of him. Treatment consists in helping him to lower his own standards of behavior so that he can act in accordance with his age. Under psychiatric care such children learn to control themselves and to function at their age level.

EMOTIONAL ILLNESS

Autism or Childhood Schizophrenia

Incidence of Emotional Illness During the Preschool Period. The number of preschool children having severe mental illness admitted to pediatric units is increasing. More child care units for these patients are being opened in both general and psychiatric hospitals.

The classification of emotional illness in young children is being more clearly differentiated than it was in the past. It is now believed that some children are *autistic* from the early months of life (Kanner). These are the infants who are unresponsive when held, withdrawn from others, and seem to live in a private inaccessible dream world of their own. The young *schizophrenic child*, on the other hand, may have had normal development at first, but then after some months exhibited disordered behavior. He may be confused and anxious but may be responsive to a degree to the care of others. Depending on the degree of retardation, the mentally retarded child (see p. 696) may be difficult to differentiate from those children who have normal intelligence but lack normal emotional development. With better diagnosis, children with mental retardation and those with autism or a schizophrenic illness are being separated and treated in more appropriate ways. The need for nursing personnel in children's psychiatric units remains urgent.

Clinical Manifestations. In general, preschool children who are emotionally disturbed do not have normal personality development for their chronological age. They may have the thinking, behavior, and ways of communicating typical of a younger child. The developmental history of these children is atypical in that the smooth, interrelated pattern of emotional, social, and intellectual development of normal children is not found.

It is the responsibility of the members of the health team to help the parents of these children avoid the feelings of guilt and shame. Many parents recognized that something was wrong with their child early, but because the indications of illness were so vague, the physicians were unable to identify the problem specifically or to provide treatment until the child was past the toddler period.

Withdrawal of these children from contact with people in their environment is generally seen between the third and fifth years, but may be seen as early as the second year. Even though they may have learned to talk, they do not feel the need, nor are they able to communicate in meaningful language.

These children cannot distinguish what is real from what is unreal, and those with severe or very early involvement are unable to differentiate themselves from other persons in the environment. The ability to test what is real develops in the first year of life in a child who receives mature, loving maternal care. In childhood schizophrenics this ability either has not fully developed or has been lost.

Children showing decided withdrawal or *autistic behavior* wander about, hiding in places such as closets where they have little human contact. They enjoy oral activity, mouthing various objects, and must be protected against swallowing harmful substances.

Some markedly autistic children cannot be fitted into organized routines. Such efforts result in increased temper tantrums, masturbation, preoccupation, and anxiety. When they are permitted to remain by themselves, they enjoy solitary play or bodily preoccupations such as sucking or head-banging. Other children cannot tolerate changes in routines and remain inflexible in their behavior.

Management. The severely psychotic child may benefit from residential care and the use of techniques of *operant conditioning*. When he is hospitalized, it is the function of the nurse to provide the love, security, and acceptance that have not been available to him in a healthy, reciprocal relation with his mother, as well as good physical care. Nurses thus become therapeutic agents who act in close cooperation with the child psychiatrist.

Further treatment includes helping the children to identify their own bodies as separate from those of other people, helping them to integrate their concept of self and to develop relations with other human beings, and protecting them from their own destructive impulses. The nurse must try to see the world as the disturbed child sees it, thereby increasing her ability to understand the child and his behavior. As the child improves, routines can be gradually introduced. Those with rigid or stereotyped patterns of behavior should be encouraged to tolerate some flexibility of routines and some innovations in play. The aim of routines is to provide a cycle of rest and activity and to help the child learn to help himself with such functions as bathing, dressing and eating. Young children having lesser degrees of emotional illness are

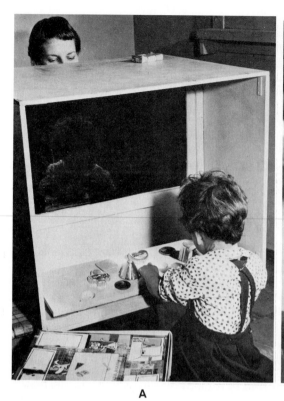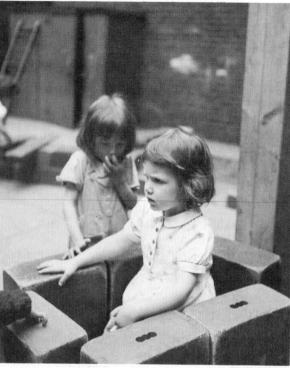

A   **B**

FIGURE 21–9.   A, The observer can note and evaluate the actions of the child at play through the one-way glass screen. Such observations assist physicians in their evaluation of the child's intellectual and emotional status. B, This child, by blocking herself off, may be trying to lessen anxiety brought on by the presence of other children. (A, from Byrd: *Health.* 4th ed. B, from Andronico, M. P., and Guerney, B. G.,: *Children* 16(1): 18, 1969.)

being helped through attendance at centers where they can interact with essentially normal children or with others who also have problems. Many parents of emotionally disturbed children also receive psychotherapy while their children are under treatment.

Prognosis.   The earlier an emotional illness begins, the more guarded is the prognosis because these children present an extremely difficult problem in therapy. They have not developed strength of personality with an ability to relate to others. The psychiatrist must help them to develop their personalities from the earliest foundation. The older the child when his withdrawal occurs, the better is the prognosis.

Most younger children showing profound autistic behavior are considered extremely mentally ill, and only concentrated therapy and care can provide hope for their recovery.

CLINICAL SITUATIONS

Mrs. Rashofer brought her three-year-old son, Barry, to the pediatric clinic. Although her other four children were well, Barry had recently become pale, had been losing weight and seemed to be constantly tired. On physical examination the physician found that the child had widespread petechiae of his skin and ulcerations of his gums. The tentative diagnosis of acute leukemia was made and was later confirmed when a sample of bone marrow was examined.

1. Methotrexate was ordered for Barry. The nurse should know that this drug is
   a. A folic acid antagonist.
   b. An adrenal cortical hormone.
   c. A salicylate.
   d. A purine analogue.

2. When the nurse cares for Barry, it is important to observe him especially for
   a. Vomiting and diarrhea.
   b. Tinnitus.
   c. Cyanosis.
   d. Hemorrhage.

3. The physician has told Barry's parents that although he may have periods of remissions, the eventual prognosis of a child having leukemia is extremely poor. During Barry's illness the nurse would encourage Mrs. Rashofer to assist her in giving him care because
   a. No nurse has time on a busy pediatric unit to provide all the detailed care a child having leukemia requires.
   b. Barry cries whenever his nurse cares for him. He

would probably be happier if his mother gave him care.

c. His mother apparently is not satisfied with the care the child is receiving, since she has several times discussed the possibility of employing private duty nurses for him.

d. His mother needs help in expressing her affection for him and also in learning how to care for him when he is discharged from the hospital.

4. Barry has had a remission of his illness, and the physician has decided to send him home. Just before Barry's discharge from the hospital he and Dickie (three years old also) were playing with blocks in the unit play area. Barry took one of Dickie's blocks, and Dickie began to cry. The nurse would

a. Encourage Barry to return the block to Dickie.

b. Tell Dickie that he cannot play with the blocks unless he can share them.

c. Take the blocks away from both children.

d. Give Dickie another block similar to the one Barry took.

5. In a few weeks Barry was readmitted with his initial symptoms. Mrs. Rashofer assisted the nurse in giving him care as she had on his previous admission. One afternoon the nurse found her crying in the hall outside the pediatric unit. Mrs. Rashofer explained, "I just cannot satisfy Barry any more. Every time I touch him he cries." The nurse would show her understanding in this situation by saying,

a. "I think Barry probably would stop crying if you bought him a new toy. What do you think he would like?"

b. "Perhaps he misses his father. Could he come to care for him awhile this evening.?"

c. "Barry is very uncomfortable now. Perhaps you could help him most by just holding his hand and reading his favorite story to him."

d. "Children sometimes cry when they are feeling better. Why don't you get a cup of coffee? He will be happy to see you later."

6. Barry had lapsed into unconsciousness, and the physician had told the parents the gravity of his condition. Mr. and Mrs. Rashofer sat quietly sobbing beside his crib. To comfort these parents the nurse said,

a. "After Barry dies you'll have to forget him and devote your lives to your other children. They have probably missed you since you have been spending so much time in the hospital."

b. "All of us have done everything possible for Barry. In helping to care for him I have learned to love him too. I believe I can understand to some degree your feelings about your son."

c. "I know you would prefer that I leave you alone with Barry. Please call me if you need me."

d. "I just cannot understand why little children have to suffer. What sin did Barry commit to deserve punishment such as this?"

Martin Schleer, a four-year-old boy, has been admitted to the pediatric unit with a diagnosis of acute glomerulonephritis. Mrs. Schleer said that all three of her children had recently been ill with scarlet fever. Martin's clinical manifestations on admission included slight edema of the face, hematuria and hypertension.

7. When Martin was admitted to the hospital, the head nurse purposely did *not* put him in bed near

a. Barry, who has leukemia.

b. Susan, who is mentally retarded.

c. Wanda, who has a streptococcal tonsillitis.

d. Marsha, who has rheumatic fever.

8. After the nurse had given Martin an intramuscular injection he said, "I hate you. Go away." The nurse should answer,

a. "I hate you, too."

b. "You should not say that. You are a naughty boy."

c. "I am sorry you hate me. I like you."

d. "I won't let your mother come to see you if you say that again."

9. When the nurse took Martin's blood pressure, it was 150 mm. systolic over 110 mm. diastolic. The nurse reported this finding to the head nurse, who said that the physician would probably want to give the child

a. Ammonium chloride.

b. Apresoline and reserpine.

c. Aminophylline and magnesium sulfate.

d. Diamox.

10. One day during visiting hours Martin's mother told him that he had a new baby cousin, Doris. Martin asked his mother where his baby cousin "came from." His mother should

a. Give him a complete description of the normal birth of a baby.

b. Tell him that he must not ask questions like that.

c. Tell him her mother bought Doris at the hospital.

d. Tell him the baby came from inside her mother's body.

11. Martin was in the hospital during the Christmas season. His mother had told him about Santa Claus. Some time during the next few years Martin will question the truth of this myth because Santa could not possibly fit through their chimney. At that time his mother should

a. Insist that there is a person named Santa Claus.

b. Tell him truthfully about the spirit of Christmas.

c. Tell him that Santa will forget him if he persists in asking questions.

d. Feel ashamed that she had told the child a falsehood.

12. Martin was discharged from the hospital. On his first return visit to the outpatient department his mother told the nurse that he had recently become fearful of dogs. In this situation Mrs. Schleer should

a. Force him to touch a dog so that he would get over his fear.

b. Tell him that dogs will not hurt him, that it is a very unusual dog that will bite children.

c. Encourage him to talk about his fear and to play with a small dog in his mother's presence.

d. Ignore the fear because he will outgrow it in a few years anyway.

Mrs. Rinell thought that Susan was slow in developing motor skills in comparison with her two older children, but she did not become too concerned about her until she observed her behavior with other five-year-old children in kindergarten. Although her family physician had said that Susan was a healthy child, she consulted a pediatrician who admitted Susan to the hospital for diagnosis.

13. After a thorough study of the family and the child by the health team members Susan was found to have an intelligence quotient of 65. The nurse should know that she is

a. Within the lower limits of the range of normal intelligence.

b. Mildly retarded, but educable.

c. Moderately retarded, but trainable.

d. Severely retarded and will be completely dependent on others for her care.

14. The nurse should realize that one of her principal objectives in the care of this child is to

a. Help the parents gain a realistic concept of Susan's ability.

b. Encourage her parents in their persistent effort to have Susan learn something new each day.

c. Help her parents to develop a *laissez-faire* attitude toward Susan's training.

d. Encourage her parents to be lenient in their setting of limits on Susan's behavior.

15. Mrs. Rinell, who lives in a community where there is a poliomyelitis epidemic, called the public health nurse and said that Susan was not feeling well. The nurse's advice to her was to

a. Take Susan and her siblings to her grandmother's home in another town so that she would not be exposed to poliomyelitis in her weakened condition.

b. Take Susan to the isolation unit of the local hospital for treatment.

c. Ignore her symptoms since her complaint seemed indicative of an upper respiratory tract infection.

d. Put Susan to bed and call her pediatrician.

GUIDES TO FURTHER STUDY

1. Compare the development of three children during your observation in nursery school according to the following: motor ability, independence in dressing, toileting, and eating, selection of playthings, sociability with adults and children, and ability to rest. Discuss in seminar the similarities and differences in behavior and abilities of these children.

2. During your observation in nursery school observe the behavior of the same three children as in Question 1 as they part from their parents. Note the age of each child and the length of time they had been attending nursery school. Answer the following questions for each child. Did the child hang his outer garments in the coatroom in the parent's presence? Did the parent wait until the child was inspected? Where did the parent actually leave the child? What words did the parent use when parting? Did the child appear unhappy when the parent left the school? What could have been done to make the parting more happy if it was unhappy?

3. Observe the health inspection in nursery school and plan to discuss the following in seminar: the purpose of the daily health inspection, the time it occurred, the procedure of examination, and the way the nurse gained the children's

cooperation. Did the children learn anything from this routine? If the nurse encountered any difficulties in gaining the children's cooperation, discuss each situation as it occurred and make suggestions as to how the problem(s) could have been resolved.

4. As the nurse in The Little Friend's Nursery School it is your responsibility to inform both teachers and children about Rhonda Evans's illness. She has recently been hospitalized with a diagnosis of epilepsy. Discuss what you believe both groups should know about this illness so that positive attitudes can be formed toward this child.

5. Billy Jeffries, three years of age, has been admitted to the hospital for treatment of hemophilia. Describe the role and responsibility of the nurse in relation to both parents and child from the time he is brought to the hospital to the time of his discharge. What guidance should the parents have had by the time of discharge?

6. Preschool children fear bodily injury. During your experience in caring for children collect incidences in which children have shown such fear, expressing it either verbally or nonverbally. How could these manifestations of fear have been prevented? What was your role in reducing these fears?

TEACHING AIDS AND OTHER INFORMATION*

Allergy Foundation of America

Allergy in Children.

American Academy of Pediatrics

Anaphylaxis.
Asthmatic Child and Participation in Sports.
Day Care for Handicapped Children.
Pediatric Aspects of Air Pollution.

The American Cancer Society, Inc.

A Cancer Source Book for Nurses, 1975.

Cancer Incidence; Survival and Mortality for Children Under 15 Years of Age.
Childhood Leukemia: The Family Disease.
Nursing Problems of Children with Cancer, 1974.

The American Humane Association: Children's Division

De Francis, V.: Protecting the Child Victim of Sex Crimes Committed by Adults.
Tormes, Y. M.: Child Victims of Incest.

---

*Complete addresses are given in the Appendix.

Canadian Mental Health Association

Children in Canada: Residential Care, 1971.

Department of National Health and Welfare: Ottawa, Canada

Love, Sex and Birth Control for the Mentally Retarded.

Epilepsy Foundation of America

Because You Are My Friend.
Medical and Social Management of the Epilepsies—An Outline of Diagnosis and Treatment.
School Alert.
You, Your Child, and Epilepsy.

Leukemia Society of America, Inc.

Leukemia—A Guide to Management of the Disease.
Patient Aid Program.

Medic Alert Foundation International

Why Medic Alert?

Muscular Dystrophy Associations of America, Inc.

Around the Clock Aids for the Child with Muscular Dystrophy.
Chart of Differential Diagnostic Characteristics of the Primary Diseases Affecting the Neuromuscular Unit.

The National Association for Mental Health, Inc.

A Child Alone in Need of Help.

National Association for Retarded Citizens

Bijou, S. W.: The Mentally Retarded Child.
Blanton, E.: A Helpful Guide in the Training of a Mentally Retarded Child.
Dybwad, G., and La Crosse, E.: Early Childhood Education Is Essential to Handicapped Children.

Dybwad, G.: The Mentally Handicapped Child Under Five.
Feeding Mentally Retarded Children.
Gardner, J. M., and Watson, L. S.: Behavior Modification of the Mentally Retarded.
Gendel, E. S.: Sex Education of the Mentally Retarded Child in the Home.
Gorelick, M. C.: Toilet Training Your Retarded Child.
How to Provide for Their Future.
Into the Light of Learning.
Mental Retardation & Religion—A Bibliography.
Pattulio, A.: Puberty in the Girl Who is Retarded.

The National Hemophilia Foundation

Control of Pain in Hemophilia, 1975.
New Perspective on Hemophilia.
Psychological Aspects of Hemophilia.
The Hemophilic Child in School, 1975.
The Prophylactic Approach to Hemophilia A.
Your Child and Hemophilia—A Manual for Parents, 1975.

Public Affairs Committee

Bienvenu, M.: Helping the Slow Learner.
Carson, R.: El Asma—Cómo Sobrellevarla (Asthma—How to Live with It).

United States Government

Clinical Programs for Mentally Retarded Children, 1974.
Directory of Inpatient Facilities for the Mentally Retarded, 1975.
Drugs vs. Cancer, 1974.
Kravik, P. J.: Adopting a Retarded Child: One Family's Experience, 1975.
People Live in Houses: Profiles of Community Residences for Retarded Children and Adults, 1975.
The Mentally Retarded Child at Home, Reprinted 1974.

REFERENCES

Books

Ballance, K., and Kendall, D. C.: *Legislation and Services for Exceptional Children in Canada.* Gage, Toronto, Canadian Committee, Council for Exceptional Children, 1970.
Buscaglia, L.: *The Disabled and Their Parents: A Counseling Challenge.* Thorofare, N. J., Charles B. Slack, 1975.
Chinn, P. C., Drew, C. J., and Logan, D. R.: *Mental Retardation: A Life Cycle Approach.* St. Louis, The C. V. Mosby Company, 1975.
Cline, M. J., and Haskell, C. M.: *Cancer Chemotherapy.* 2nd ed. Philadelphia, W. B. Saunders Company, 1975.
Commission on Emotional and Learning Disorders in Children: *One Million Children—The CELDIC Report: A National Study of Canadian Children with Emotional and Learning Disorders.* Toronto, Canada, Commission on Emotional and Learning Disorders in Children, 1970.
Cooper, I. S.: *The Victim Is Always The Same.* New York, Harper & Row, 1973.
Copeland, J.: *For the Love of Ann.* New York, Ballantine Books, 1973.
Downey, J. A., and Low, N. L. (Eds.): *The Child With Disabling Illness: Principles of Rehabilitation.* Philadelphia, W. B. Saunders Company, 1974.
Duthie, R. B., et al.: *The Management of Musculo-Skeletal Problems in the Haemophilias.* Philadelphia, J. B. Lippincott Company, 1973.
Fagin, C. M. (Ed.): *Nursing in Child Psychiatry.* St. Louis, The C. V. Mosby Company, 1972.
Gelfand, D. M., and Hartmann, D. P.: *Child Behavior: Analysis and Therapy.* New York, Pergamon Press Inc., 1975.

Gold, P.: *Please Don't Say Hello.* New York, Human Sciences Press, 1975.
Gordon, B. L.: *Essentials of Immunology.* 2nd ed. Philadelphia, F. A. Davis Company, 1974.
Green, R. (Ed.): *Human Sexuality: A Health Practitioner's Text.* Baltimore, Williams & Wilkins Company, 1975.
Jones, P.: *Living with Hemophilia.* Philadelphia, F. A. Davis Company, 1974.
Jones, P. G., and Campbell, P. E. (Eds.): *Tumours of Infancy and Childhood.* Philadelphia, J. B. Lippincott Company, 1975.
Kempe, C. H., Silver, H. K., and O'Brien, D. (Eds.): *Current Pediatric Diagnosis & Treatment.* 3rd ed. Los Altos, Calif., Lange Medical Publishers, 1974.
Kenny, T. J., and Clemmens, R. L.: *Behavioral Pediatrics and Child Development.* Baltimore, Williams & Wilkins Company, 1975.
Koch, R., and Dobson, J. C. (Eds.): *The Mentally Retarded Child and His Family: A Multidisciplinary Handbook.* Rev. ed. New York, Brunner/Mazel Company, 1976.
Lascari, A. D.: *Leukemia in Childhood.* Springfield, Ill., Charles C Thomas, 1973.
Linman, J. W.: *Hematology: Physiologic, Pathophysiologic, and Clinical Principles.* New York, Macmillan Company, 1975.
McCollum, A. T.: *Coping With Prolonged Health Impairment In Your Child.* Boston, Little, Brown & Company, 1975.
Mitchell, H. S., et al.: *Nutrition in Health and Disease.* 16th ed. Philadelphia, J. B. Lippincott Company, 1976.

Niedermeyer, E.: *Compendium of the Epilepsies*. Springfield, Ill., Charles C Thomas, 1974.

Rapp, D. J.: *Questions and Answers About Allergies and Your Child*. New York, Drake Publishers, 1974.

Roitt, I. M.: *Essential Immunology*. 2nd ed., Philadelphia, J. B. Lippincott Company, 1974.

Ross, A. O.: *Psychological Disorders of Children: A Behavioral Approach to Theory, Research, and Therapy*. New York, McGraw-Hill Book Company, 1974.

Schoenberg, B., et al. (Eds.): *Anticipatory Grief*. New York, Columbia University Press, 1974.

Schoenberg, B., et al. (Eds.): *Bereavement: Its Psychosocial Aspects*. New York, Columbia University Press, 1975.

Sutow, W. W., Vietti, T., and Fernbach, D. J. (Eds.): *Clinical Pediatric Oncology*. St. Louis, The C. V. Mosby Company, 1973.

Travis, G.: *Chronic Illness in Children: Its Impact on Child and Family*. Stanford, Calif., Stanford University Press, 1976.

Vaughan, V. C., III, and McKay R. J. (Eds.): *Nelson Textbook of Pediatrics*, 10th ed., Philadelphia, W. B. Saunders Company, 1975.

Weiss, E. B., and Segal, M. S. (Eds.): *Bronchial Asthma: Mechanisms and Therapeutics*. Boston, Little, Brown & Company, 1976.

Williams, H. E., and Phelan, P. D.: *Respiratory Illness in Children*. Philadelphia, J. B. Lippincott Company, 1975.

Woods, G. E.: *The Handicapped Child*. Philadelphia, J. B. Lippincott Company, 1975.

Periodicals

Aradine, C. R.: Books for Children About Death. *Pediatrics*, 57:372, March 1976.

Armstrong, H., and Patterson, P.: Seizures in Canadian Indian Children: Individual, Family and Community Approaches. *Canadian Psychiat. Assoc. J.*, 20:247, June 1975.

Azarnoff, P.: Mediating the Trauma of Serious Illness and Hospitalization in Childhood. *Children Today*, 3:12, July-August 1974.

Bergner, M., and Hutelmyer, C.: Teaching Kids How to Live With Their Allergies. *Nursing '76*, 6:11, August 1976.

Berman, P. H.: Management of Seizure Disorders with Anticonvulsant Drugs: Current Concepts. *Pediatr. Clin. N. Am.*, 23:443, August 1976.

Bernstein, I. D., and Wright, P. W.: Immunology and Immunotherapy of Childhood Neoplasia. *Pediatr. Clin. N. Am.*, 23:93, February 1976.

Blount, M., and Kinney, A. B.: Chronic Steroid Therapy. *Am. J. Nursing*, 74:1626, September 1974.

Blount, M., and Kinney, A. B.: What to Remember About EEG. *Nursing '74*, 4:36, August 1974.

Bochow, A. J.: Cancer Immunotherapy: What Promise Does It Hold? *Nursing '76*, 6:50, October 1976.

Brandt, E. P.: Dialogue-For-Big-Ears. *Nursing Digest*, 3:19, January-February 1975.

Bruya, M. A., and Bolin, R. H.: Epilepsy: A Controllable Disease. Part I—Classification and Diagnosis of Seizures. *Am. J. Nursing*, 76:388, March 1976.

Bullington, B. P., Sexton, D., and White, P.: Working With Families of Multihandicapped Children in a Residential Institution. *Children Today*, 5:13, September-October 1976.

Closurdo, J. S.: Behavior Modification and the Nursing Process. *Nursing Digest*, 4:27, Fall 1976.

Cohen, D. J., and Caparulo, B.: Childhood Autism. *Children Today*, 4:2, July-August 1975.

Cohen, D. J. Johnson, W. T., and Caparulo, B. K.: Pica and Elevated Blood Lead Level in Autistic and Atypical Children. *Am. J. Dis. Child*, 130:47, January 1976.

Cooper, C. R.: Anticonvulsant Drugs and The Epileptic's Dilemma. *Nursing '76*, 6:44, January 1976.

Dharan, M.: The Immune System: Immunoglobin Abnormalities. *Am. J. Nursing*, 76:1626, October 1976.

Donley, D. L.: Immune System: Nursing the Patient Who Is Immunosuppressed. *Am. J. Nursing*, 76:1619, October 1976.

Evans, A. E., D'Angio, G. J., and Koop, C. E.: Childhood Cancer: Basic Considerations in Diagnosis and Treatment. *Pediatr. Clin. N. Am.*, 23:3, February 1976.

Feldman, G. M.: The Effect of Biofeedback Training on Respiratory Resistance of Asthmatic Children. *Psychosomatic Medicine*, 38:27, January-February 1976.

Fisher, L.: New Frontiers in the Treatment of Asthma in Children. *Am. Lung Assoc. Bulletin*, 62:2, June 1976.

Foley, G. V., and McCarthy, A. M.: The Child with Leukemia: In a Special Hematology Clinic. *Am. J. Nursing*, 76:1115, July 1976.

Foley, G., and McCarthy, A. M.: The Child with Leukemia: The Disease and Its Treatment. *Am. J. Nursing*, 76:1108, July 1976.

Gallagher, U. M.: What's Happening in Adoption? *Children Today*, 4:11, November-December 1975.

Geiger, J. K., Sindberg, R. M., and Barnes, C. M.: Head Hitting in Severely Retarded Children. *Am. J. Nursing*, 74:1822, October 1974.

Greene, P.: Acute Leukemia in Children. *Am. J. Nursing*, 75:1709, October 1975.

Greene, T.: Current Therapy for Acute Leukemia in Childhood. *Nursing Clin. N. Amer.*, 11:3, March 1976.

Gyulay, J. E.: The Forgotten Grievers. *Am. J. Nursing*, 75:1476, September 1975.

Heisel, J. S., et al. The Significance of Life Events as Contributing Factors in the Diseases of Children. III. A Study of Pediatric Patients. *J. Pediatr.*, 83:119, July 1973.

Holaday, B. J.: Achievement Behavior in Chronically Ill Children. *Nursing Research*, 23:25, January-February 1974.

Kikuchi, J.: How the Leukemic Child Chooses His Confidant. *The Canadian Nurse*, 71:22, May 1975.

Knobloch, H., and Pasamanick, B.: Some Etiologic and Prognostic Factors in Early Infantile Autism and Psychosis. *Pediatrics*, 55:182, February 1975.

Leventhal, B. G., and Hersh, S.: Modern Treatment of Childhood Leukemia: The Patient and His Family. *Nursing Digest*, 3:12, July-August 1975.

Liebman, R., Minuchin, S., and Baker, L.: The Use of Structural Family Therapy in the Treatment of Intractable Asthma. *Am. J. Psychiatry*, 131:535, May 1974.

McCalla, J. L.: Immunotherapy: Concepts and Nursing Implications. *Nursing Clin. N. Amer.*, 11:59, March 1976.

Mann, S. A.: Coping With a Child's Fatal Illness: A Parent's Dilemma. *Nursing Clin. N. Am.*, 9:81, March 1974.

Martinson, I.: The Child with Leukemia: Parents Help Each Other. *Am. J. Nursing*, 76:1120, July 1976.

Martinson, I. M.: Why Don't We Let Them Die at Home? *RN*, 39:58, January 1976.

Masagatani, G. N.: Hand-Gesturing Behavior in Psychotic Children. *Nursing Digest*, 2:84, February 1974.

Millspaugh, D., Kremenitzer, M., and Lending, M.: Providing Services for Adolescents Who Live With Seizures. *Children Today*, 5:7, September-October 1976.

Moran, M. J., Niedz, B. J., and Simpson, G. M.: The Resource Family: Helping Emotionally Disturbed Children in Residential Treatment. *Children Today* 4:26, November-December 1975.

Northrup, F. C.: The Dying Child. *Am. J. Nursing*, 74:1066, June 1974.

Nysather, J. O., Katz, A. E., and Lenth, J. L.: The Immune System: Its Development and Functions. *Am. J. Nursing*, 76:1614, October 1976.

O'Regan, G. W.: Foster Family Care for Children With Mental Retardation: Parents of Other Retarded Children Are Ready Resources. *Children Today*, 3:20, January-February 1974.

Orgel, H. A.: Genetic and Developmental Aspects of IgE. *Pediatr. Clin. N. Am.*, 22:17, February 1975.

Pinkel, D.: Treatment of Acute Leukemia. *Pediatr. Clin. N. Am.*, 23:117, February 1976.

Potter, A. E.: Psychiatric Nursing: A Human Experience. *Nursing Forum*, 13:157, 1974.

Price, K. P.: Treating Psychosomatic Disorders with Behavior Therapy. *Nursing Digest*, 3:12, November-December 1975.

Smith, S.: The Family Asthma Program. *Am. Lung Assoc. Bulletin*, 62:6, June 1976.

Spinetta, J. J., and Maloney, L. J.: Death Anxiety in the Outpatient Leukemic Child. *Pediatrics*, 56:1034, December 1975.

Spinetta, J. J., Rigler, D., and Karon, M.: Personal Space as a Measure of a Dying Child's Sense of Isolation. *J. Consult. Clin. Psychol.*, 42:751, 1974.

Steinhauer, P. D., Mushin, D. N., and Rae-Grant, Q.: Psychological Aspects of Chronic Illness. *Pediatr. Clin. N. Am.*, 21:825, November 1974.

Strawczynski, H., Stachewitsch, A., Morgenstern, G., and Shaw, M. E.: Delivery of Care to Hemophilic Children: Home Care Versus Hospitalization. *Pediatrics*, 51:986, June 1973.

Walker, P.: Bone Marrow Transplant: A Second Chance for Life. *Nursing 77*, 7:24, January 1977.

Wiley, L.: The Stigma of Epilepsy. *Nursing '74*, 4:36, January 1974.

AUDIOVISUAL MEDIA*

The American Cancer Society, Inc.

Nursing Management of Children with Cancer
Consultant: Aufhauser, T. R.
22 minutes, color.
Demonstrates the skills, commitment and rewards involved in pediatric cancer nursing. Nursing procedures such as infusions, mouth care, control of infections and fevers, ostomy care, play therapy and emotional support of patients and their families are demonstrated and explained. Alertness in detecting side effects of therapy is emphasized, and methods for managing these are presented.

The American Journal of Nursing Company

Pediatric-Mental Health Nursing
Mental Retardation—The Special 3% (Parts I and II)
Instructor: Cabanski, S., Guests: Carroll, B., and Herzog, T.
Two 30 minute classes, black and white.
Dr. Stanley Cabanski discusses the etiology, care, treatment and future of the six million mentally retarded in our society. Visits are made to four institutions that give care and rehabilitation. Day care schools and residential treatment centers are shown. The nurses discuss the implications for nursing in these conditions and how the nurse can assist families in making use of community resources.

Wednesday's Child (Parts I and II)
Instructor: Mitchell, M. L., Guest: Fischer, L.
Two 30 minute classes, black and white.
Designed to alert the student and general practice nurse to some of the common experiences of childhood that can lead to emotional disturbances. Five case studies are presented.

Psychiatric-Mental Health Nursing
The Crisis of Loss
Series Instructor: Mitchell, M.
Participants: Werner-Beland, Jr., and Mercer, R.
30 minutes, videotape, sound, color, guide.
The commonly encountered nursing problem of loss and mourning is examined within the framework of crisis theory. Examples support the importance of the patient's perception of control and responsibility in coping with loss events.

Charles Press–Prentice-Hall, Inc.

Death and the Family: From the Caring Professions' Point of View
Fredlund, D.
30 minutes.
Discusses children's attitudes toward death. Underscores the need for children to be made aware of death and for them to learn to accept loss in a realistic and healthy manner.

Talking to Children About Death
Williams, G. G.
57 minutes.
Discusses ways to open the channels of communication between parent and child on the sensitive issue of death. Cautions that thwarting children's efforts to understand death can result in serious emotional problems in later life. Offers suggestions on how to help approach the topic of death with children.

Film & Videotape Library, National Institute on Mental Retardation, Canada

Kindergarten
Producer: Communications Resources Division of the National Institute on Mental Retardation
20 minutes, videotape, black and white.
The integration of children with handicaps into regular childhood education programs in Canada, and the effects on the handicapped child, the other children and the teachers, are explored in the videotape. Depicts the experiences of a child with Down's syndrome who attends a normal kindergarten class.

The National Hemophilia Foundation

Almost Miracle Enough
Producer: Texas Central Chapter
28½ minutes, 16mm film, color.
Explores the facts and the misconceptions of hemophilia. Emphasizes research, the critical need for voluntary blood donations and the new-found hope that now exists for all hemophiliacs and their families.

Home Infusion—New Freedom for Hemophiliacs
Producer: Cutter Labs
15 minutes, 16mm film, color.
The film describes a home treatment program, the newest method of managing hemophilia.

If Given a Chance
Producer: Hemophilia of Michigan
15 minutes, 16mm film, color.
Filmed at Hemophilia summer camp at Mill Lake, deals with hemophilia and its treatment.

The Threshold
13½ minutes, 16mm film, color.
This film depicts current modes of treatment, directions of research, and impact on an average family with a young son who has hemophilia.

The Royal College of General Practitioners, Medical Recording Service

Psychiatric Medicine in Family Practice
Uses and Abuses of Children
    31 minutes, (four slides, 2 × 2, 35mm), sound.
    Discusses the role of the child in the family. Explains that a disturbed child is often an indication of a disturbed family.

W. B. Saunders Company

Pediatric Conferences with Sydney Gellis
    Acute Leukemia, Pinkel, D.
    Asthma, Gellis, S.
    Management of the Acute Asthmatic Attack, Berman, B. A.

Trainex Corporation

Allergy
    35mm filmstrip, audio-tape cassettes, 33 1/3 LP, color.
    Describes symptoms, causes and possible cures for an allergic child.

Care of the Patient with Leukemia
    35mm filmstrip, audio-tape cassettes, 33 1/3 LP, color.
    Beginning with blood physiology, progresses through diagnostic tests, care of the child with acute leukemia, central nervous system involvement, bone marrow depression, and care of the patient with chronic leukemia.

More Alike Than Different
    Audio-tape cassettes.
    A candid parent discussion of sexual development in the mentally retarded child. Parents share their feelings, problems, successes and failures, in coping with the physical maturity of their intellectually deprived children. Comments from professionals working in the field of mental retardation and case study dramatizations supplement this discussion.

United States Government

Current Concepts in Epilepsy, Part I, Infants and Children
    Producer: USNMAC
    40 minutes, 16mm film, optical sound, black and white.
    Discusses the definition of epilepsy versus that of seizures. Explains the different etiologies, manifestations, and prognoses. Outlines diagnostic procedures and treatments. (Kinescope)

Diapers Away: Toilet Training the Mentally Retarded at Home
    Producer: USDHEW
    12 minutes, 35mm, sound, color.
    Demonstrates techniques for teaching toilet use to mentally retarded children.

Growing Up at the Table: Teaching Feeding Skills to the Mentally Retarded Child at Home
    Producer: USDHEW
    10 minutes, 35mm, sound, color.
    Demonstrates techniques for teaching self-feeding to non-institutionalized mentally retarded children.

International Education of the Hearing Impaired Child Series
    The Multiple Handicapped
    Producer: USBEH
    23 minutes, 16mm film, optical sound, color.
    Shows mentally retarded, cerebral palsied, dysmelia, deaf-blind, and emotionally disturbed deaf children in Sweden, Germany, the Netherlands, and England.

Teaching the Mentally Retarded—A Positive Approach
    Producer: USNMAC
    22 minutes, 16mm film, optical sound, black and white.
    A documentary following the progress made by four profoundly retarded children during a four month training program. The training emphasis is in areas of self-care—toilet training, dressing, eating, and manners, illustrating that even the profoundly retarded can learn rather complex skills.

---

*Complete addresses are given in the Appendix.

UNIT SIX

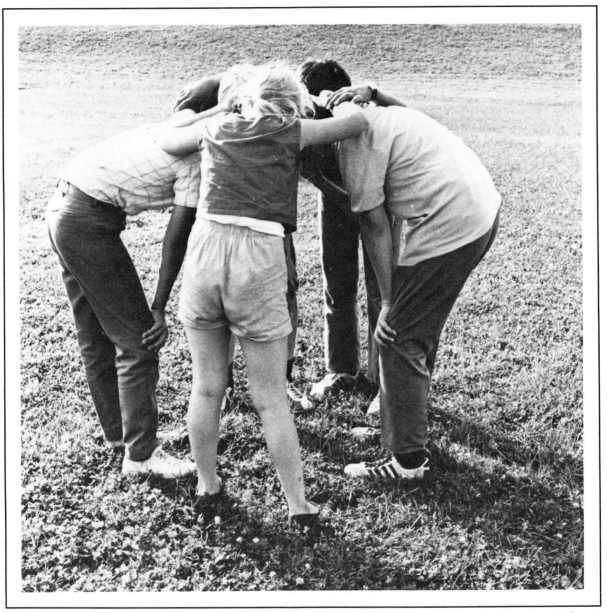

(Courtesy of H. Armstrong Roberts.)

THE SCHOOL CHILD

PARADISE REGAINED

The childhood shows the man,
As morning shows the day. Be famous then
By wisdom; as thy empire must extend,
So let extend thy mind o'er all the world.

Bk. IV, L. 220
John Milton
1608–1674

Chapter Twenty-Two

OVERVIEW OF EMOTIONAL DEVELOPMENT

THE SCHOOL CHILD: HIS GROWTH, DEVELOPMENT, AND CARE

At some time during the school-age period parents must learn to adjust to what appears to be almost total rejection by their child. He may exhibit an overt independence of them and of the standards they have tried to impress upon him. At this time parents may feel hurt, disappointed and angry. Yet, in spite of what appears to be true, the child still needs unobtrusive parental support, given with respect for the child's feelings of independence.

By the time the child reaches his sixth birthday he should have learned to trust others and developed a sense of autonomy. He should also have learned the fundamentals of getting along in his particular environment, through experience in living and through questioning his parents and other adults. He should have developed a sense of initiative, but his activities should be controlled to some degree by his conscience.

These stages which the child passes through before he is six years old are probably the most important for healthy personality development. Children who have not achieved the expected level at each stage are likely to remain handicapped unless help is given them. There are exceptions to this, of course, for experiences in later childhood and in adolescence influence the trend in emotional development.

Sense of Industry. Between the ages of six and 12 years the child develops a *sense of industry* and a desire to engage in tasks in the real world. He is internally motivated to put forth effort on a purposeful activity which will yield a sense of worth. Even before he is six years old a child may show evidence that he enjoys doing socially useful tasks for others, that he wants to do things and to learn to do them well.

These years are usually a calm period, and few overwhelming upheavals are apt to occur. The child continues to learn how to attain the goal of becoming a responsible citizen. He acquires knowledge and skills which will help him to make a worthwhile contribution to society. He learns how to cooperate with others, to play fairly and follow the rules of the game, and to conform to social norms so that his life with others will be a positive experience for him and for those with whom he interacts. With all this, however, the school-age period is characterized by alternate conformity and rebellion against adult authority.

Instead of developing a sense of industry, the child may acquire, or intensify earlier, *feelings of inferiority* and inadequacy. This is more likely to happen if he has not successfully passed through the previous stages of personality development.

The Child and School. The kind of school a child attends is important to his developing a sense of industry, and thus to his future achievements. At school the child has a task, one that

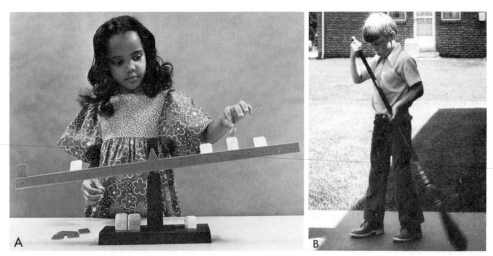

FIGURE 22–1.   The school child wants to learn to do things and to do them well. *A*, Learning how a mathematical balance scale works. (Courtesy of Childcraft.) *B*, Learning household care.

will continue throughout childhood and adolescence. If he is adequately prepared, if his needs as a growing person are regarded and if he is successful, the school experience will have a positive influence on personality development. If he is not successful in school because he is dull, his self-image is that he is stupid. If he is too maladjusted to make friends among his peer group, he feels that nobody likes him. He may stay in school, passively accepting his inferiority, or leave school as soon as the law permits.

Out of school he may find a job in an attempt to feel a sense of accomplishment. To succeed, he needs the sense of industry, which he failed to develop during his school years when it was a main developmental task. If he fails in the job, he may turn to delinquency to gain the status and recognition among his peers which he failed to gain in school and at work. If his delinquency is extreme, he also gains attention from adults which he could not secure by legitimate means.

The importance of adapting the school experience to the needs of the growing child is evident.

School is not the only place where a child may gain a feeling of mastery and acquire a sense of industry. The child may be given useful tasks at home. Parents may delegate to him responsibilities which contribute to the happiness and well-being of all the family. Such tasks and re-

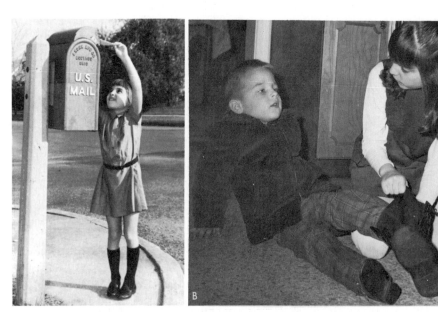

FIGURE 22–2.   The sense of industry is developed as the child learns to assume responsibilities such as (*A*) mailing letters and (*B*) helping with the care of her younger brother.

sponsibilities should not be those which adults do not want to do themselves, but rather are based on a division of labor in which the child's tasks are suited to his abilities. The work should not be so time-consuming that the child has no opportunity to study, to take on status-giving tasks outside the home, and to play with siblings and friends.

Community organizations for children stress both recreation and work, e.g., the 4-H Clubs and the Girl Scouts and Boy Scouts of America.

The school child must grow out of the dependence upon his family which was natural when he was younger, and must find satisfaction in the company of his peer group and adults outside the home. He must develop neuromuscular skills so that he can participate in work and games with others. He must acquire sufficient knowledge to interact with adults outside of school and thereby learn from them about the social life of his society. He must gain some understanding of adult concepts, logic and ways of communicating.

More specifically, during the school years the child develops wholesome attitudes toward himself as a person and learns his or her appropriate masculine or feminine social role. He learns how to get along with his age mates, yet is able to act according to his conscience and his scale of values. He achieves independence in caring for himself. He learns the fundamental skills of reading, writing, and calculating, and the physical skills necessary for ordinary games. *By the time he is 12 years old he should have developed positive attitudes toward his own and other social, racial, economic, and religious groups, and learned the concepts necessary for participation in daily living with adults in his environment.*

THE SCHOOL CHILD, HIS FAMILY AND HIS FRIENDS

Relations with Parents. The child between six and 12 years should have widened his social horizons beyond the confines of his own home. Although he is still dependent upon his parents' love, companionship with his peers and adults outside the home becomes of increasing importance.

The child's relation with the parent of the opposite sex which existed during his preschool years has been resolved. He has come to respect and love that parent, but now identifies with or tries to be like the parent of the same sex. By imitating that parent's role he learns his own social role.

Children gain increasing ideological as well as physical and emotional independence from their parents. They gain new ideas from adults outside the family: teachers, parents of their friends, policemen, television performers, newspaper writers, and authors of textbooks and of fiction. Often these ideas and attitudes conflict with those of their parents. The adults who teach these children must help them to understand this conflict so that they do not become impatient with their parents and lose respect for them.

Health education is a part of modern general education in the public schools. Health measures such as taking a bath every day, accepted by the children, may seem foolish to their parents, who went to school 20 to 30 years ago. Daily baths may be almost impossible in a crowded tenement flat. There is then a conflict between what the child is taught at school and at home, which places a serious strain on parent-child relations.

The school child learns to think of himself as a person in his own right and may resent rigid limits which parents continue to impose on his behavior. Furthermore, he dislikes a show of affection when he is feeling well and in no danger. He often pulls away from the adult's embrace and turns his face from kisses. The parents may be confused and thrown into emotional conflict by the new concepts which children bring home, by their efforts at independence, and by the apparent disinterest in a physical show of parental affection. The parents may be surprised, however, as the well child who refuses to have an adult hovering over him turns to these same adults for affection and protection when he is threatened by illness or injury.

Parents need help in understanding the normal growth and development of their children when such conflicts arise. They may discuss these matters with the child's teacher, alone or during parent-teacher conferences, with their physician, religious advisor or a nurse in the school or one who visits in the home or cares for the child in the hospital.

There are certain guidelines which help parents to counsel and discipline their children in an easier manner. First, parents should invite the confidence of their child as a parent, not as a buddy or school chum. Parents can leave the door open, so to speak, to discussions, but they should never intrude on the privacy of a child, because privacy is the right of every human being. Parents can set a good example for their child to follow in building character traits such as honesty and loyalty. Parents cannot expect their child to obey the rules of society when they themselves do not. Both parents should set consistent limits on their child's behavior, because even though he may be upset at the time, he will ultimately understand that their interest is evidence of their love for him. Parents can also try to see their child as others see him, not as an idealized extension of themselves. Finally, parents should not compare one child with another in the family. Each child is accepted because he is *himself* and different from his siblings or cousins.

Relations with Siblings. Whether the school child is an only child or one of a group of siblings has more and more effect upon his personality. If he is an only child, he tends to cling longer to his concept of being the center of the family. When he goes outside the family to make friends in his peer group, he still expects to be the center of the group and becomes frightened when he learns that he is not. He finds it difficult to learn the give and take of social living with other children. An only child who does not succeed in establishing himself as a group member may find that playing by himself is a lonely existence. He may come to resent being an only child and long desperately for siblings such as his friends have. In addition, since he is the recipient of the undiluted force of his parents' attitudes and feelings he is likely to be limited in his freedom.

Children in a large family find adjusting to children outside the family and sharing with the group easier than does the only child. They learn early that some are given opportunities and restrictions, while others are not. They learn that no one of them, unless it is the youngest child, is singled out as the center of interest, although each in his own way is loved by his parents. Although they may disagree among themselves, each sibling has a deep affection for the other children in the family.

Children in large families have problems, however, which the only child does not have. Sibling jealousy is a problem even in families in which all the members love one another. Although it is more acute in preschool children than among children over six years of age, it still exists. An older child may envy the attention which the younger siblings receive. He may resent the fact that his discarded toys are being broken by a younger child and the fact that, despite his feelings, he is expected to love and often take care of his siblings.

If the school child is a younger sibling, he may envy the older child his freedom and skills. He may strive to be like the older child and be defeated in his attempts. The school child's jealousy of his siblings, younger and older, may actually increase as he strives to keep ahead of the younger child or to catch up with an older one. Scholastic ability is a principal cause of sibling jealousy among school children, particularly in a child who is mentally inferior to his siblings.

School children often prefer to be with their friends rather than their siblings. Relations with a friend are less emotional and freer from parental interference. A child chooses his friends; the sibling relationship is one he is born into and cannot be discontinued when he wishes to be free of it. Ideally, experience with siblings facilitates a child's social adjustment outside the family, but it does not take the place of friendships of his own choice.

Relations with Friends. As the child psychologically moves slowly away from home, his friends become increasingly important to him. He learns to take his place as a member of a group, and his social life begins. In making this adjustment children tend to avoid the company of the opposite sex. Each sex tends to develop its own language and its own activities and behavior. Children of each sex learn to cooperate and to compete with each other in their activities.

Children of school age can be exceedingly cruel to each other. They want to control or feel able to control another person. The state of being "picked on" is common during the school period. Some children are excluded from friendship groups and verbally are made to feel uncomfortable. School children can also be cruel to adults whom they dislike.

Gangs or Groups. Since school children have learned that their parents are not omnipotent, that they make mistakes, and are sometimes afraid, they tend to confide not in them but in their friends. They form close friendships and ultimately join a group of other children of their own sex. Such a group may be merely a friendship group or it may be a secret society or an antisocial gang, depending upon the needs of the children who form it. Among themselves the children discuss the problems they face. They discuss their own theories about life, death, and sexual matters; they share attitudes, values, and beliefs with the peer group. Each child forms his or her own attitudes and values which may later be changed intellectually, but the feelings surrounding them may last through adulthood. Since many school-age children have spent long hours watching television, their own beliefs and those of the group may be influenced by this mass medium.

Much of a boy's hostility and aggression is worked off in his peer group through fighting, either in a supervised, organized game such as

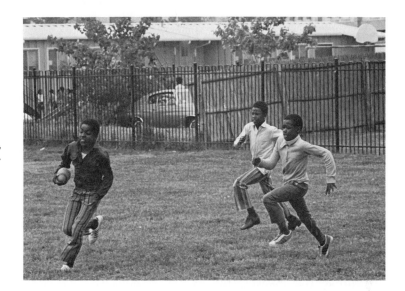

FIGURE 22–3. During school years, friends become increasingly important.

baseball or football or while playing "cops and robbers" or cowboys and Indians. Unfortunately some of these juvenile gangs turn their hostility not against their own age group in play, but against other youths or adults in deadly earnest. When this occurs, the pattern is laid for delinquent behavior.

Girls also form groups and discuss their own problems. They do not, however, as a rule engage in the aggressive and hostile activities common in the boys' gang.

Toward the end of the school period children have learned to compete and to compromise with others and to cooperate so that they can accomplish something in their group which no one child could do without adult help. They have learned how to get along with their own and other groups and to follow the rules of the larger society. They have developed a sense of responsibility about matters which they know are important.

Parents should be understanding and accepting of the activities of their school children and willing to give independence when it is needed. All too often only the mother is interested, and she seldom understands the boy's interests completely. The father often appears disinterested in his children's individual or group activities. This is unfortunate because the boy especially needs his father's loving interest at this time.

DEVELOPMENT OF SEXUALITY IN THE SCHOOL-AGE CHILD

During the beginning of the school-age period the child has emerged from or is in the process of resolving his Oedipal situation. He is moving away from the intense psychosexual upheaval of the genital period and into a somewhat quieter period, termed latency. In the latency period it is especially important for the child to have the parent of the same sex in the home in order for proper identification to occur.

The *latency period* begins at about school age and lasts into early pubescence. The child no longer has the intense erotic fantasizing of the preschool years. He is free to develop new interests and social abilities; thus he makes new companions and with them explores the world beyond his home grounds.

The school-age child becomes much less egocentric and directs his energies beyond himself. During the early latency period children associate with same-sex peers and tend to ignore members of the opposite sex. Girls associate with girls in their play and boys with boys. Girls may fear boys of the same age and tend to draw apart from them. They may think of boys as "dirty" or "messy" persons. Boys, on the other hand, think of and may call girls "sissies." Girls have not traditionally participated in the same kinds of active rough and tumble play as boys. Of course, there have always been exceptions. Today girls may be as vigorous in their play as boys.

Sex Play. Because children engage in more outside activities during the latency period, masturbation plays a less prominent role, though it may continue in some children.

During the later school years sexual behavior is not absent. In the school child the nature of sex play such as genital exploration and masturbation changes. It occurs primarily between peers of the same age and sex. Girls become more hesitant about participation in these activities. After the age of nine years boys tend to surpass girls in their level of sexual activity. Such activity may be caused by social pressure from the group. Parties in which kissing games are played occur and are a rehearsal for activities and feelings to come during the next few years.

Parents and nurses may consider occasional sex play between peers harmless. It is not an indication of precocious eroticism and generally is not a hazard to future attitudes toward sex. When two children separate from their group and are alone together and possibly giggling and then become very quiet, sexual activity may be taking place. If such children are engaging in sex play, they need to be reminded that certain activities are unacceptable under the particular circumstances. The adult should not frighten the children but should explain why the activity is inappropriate at that time and place. The children can be calmly directed toward playing a game or participating in another activity. The best preventive measure for sex play is honesty in answering questions pertaining to aspects of sexuality raised by curious children. Providing children with interesting activities and possibilities for fun will probably reduce the amount of sex play in their group.

Sex play between a brother and a sister is undesirable and potentially harmful. When both children share the same bedroom this practice is not only convenient but may become a regular occurrence, which is repeated for years. The danger lies in the possibility of a psychic fixation on the other sibling throughout life, resulting in a less than good chance of establishing healthy marital relationships. Such children should be given separate rooms for sleeping (see p. 631) especially during the later school years and before pubescence.

Sex Information. Ideally, gradually obtaining the facts of life is a by-product of an affectionate upbringing by two loving parents. The ultimate goal of all education about sexuality is the ability of the individual to merge his biologic impulses with a satisfying family life.

School-age children will continue, as they did during the preschool period, to ask questions concerning reproduction, but the questions will be more specific than they were earlier. While the five-year-old may say, "Daddy put the seed in," as a way of explaining his birth, the seven- or eight-year-old may want an explanation about how Daddy did it. Such questioning is dependent upon the alertness and the ability of the child to articulate and the permissiveness of the parents.

All questions about sex should be answered warmly, directly, and with a comfortable attitude by the parents. The extent of information given should be commensurate with the age and level of emotional maturity of the particular child.

Usually, if a daughter has not asked her mother about the menses by the age of 10 years, the mother should gently introduce the topic. During the time until the child herself menstruates, she should have her questions answered fully and completely. Techniques of self-care during menstruation can be explained and the girl given some choice as to the technique to be used. Although the mother usually informs the daughter about this subject, the father should also let his daughter know that he understands and appreciates the importance of the topic.

Fathers should explore the menstrual cycle with their sons beginning in the prepubertal period if the subject has not been brought up before. The father's attitude about the topic will be shared with his son while he instructs him about this biologic process. Jokes or puns about menses are deprecatory to women and should definitely be avoided.

Knowledge that both parents understand the changes that occur in children of each sex as they mature will help young persons as adults when they communicate sexual feelings and attitudes to a member of the opposite sex. Both parents have a responsibility to respond with warmth and respect to a girl's menstrual cycle as being one of the most positive elements in family organization and human biology. Any misconceptions such as being "dirty" or "sick" during this monthly period should be explored with their children and corrected. Much female deprecation is connected with the menses and is unconsciously agreed to by both men and women. True liberation of women begins in the home with the parents' attitudes toward each other and their children.

Many school curricula guide children toward self-knowledge, self-awareness, and self-fulfillment through studies in history, literature, and biology among other subjects, but they do not usually promote self-knowledge through education for sexuality. If meaningful information concerning sexuality were introduced in the school, it would prevent these children from obtaining erroneous knowledge from their peers, the lay press, or from pornographic material. Sex education during the school years is essentially developing a healthy attitude about sexuality, such as that given in many homes. It is not solely a course that pertains to the physiologic facts of reproduction.

OVERVIEW OF PHYSICAL, SOCIAL, AND MENTAL DEVELOPMENT

PHYSICAL DEVELOPMENT

During the school years the child shows a progressively slower growth in height, but a

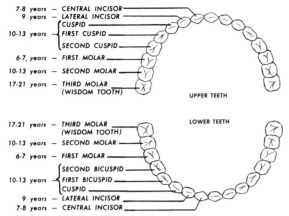

7-8 years — CENTRAL INCISOR
9 years — LATERAL INCISOR
        CUSPID
10-13 years — FIRST CUSPID
        SECOND CUSPID
6-7 years — FIRST MOLAR
10-13 years — SECOND MOLAR
17-21 years — THIRD MOLAR
        (WISDOM TOOTH)   UPPER TEETH

                            LOWER TEETH
17-21 years — THIRD MOLAR
        (WISDOM TOOTH)
10-13 years — SECOND MOLAR
6-7 years — FIRST MOLAR
        SECOND BICUSPID
10-13 years — FIRST BICUSPID
        CUSPID
9 years — LATERAL INCISOR
7-8 years — CENTRAL INCISOR

FIGURE 22–4. Permanent dentition. Eruption of these teeth occurs between six and twenty-one years of age.

rapid gain in weight. He tends to lose the thin, wiry appearance of the earlier years. General growth is slow until the spurt just before puberty. Muscular coordination improves steadily; posture should be good (the earlier lordosis has disappeared). The lymphatic tissue reaches its height of development in the early school period. The frontal sinuses are fairly well developed by six years of age. From this time on all the sinuses are potential foci of infection.

This is the period of eruption and growth of the permanent teeth. The six-year molars are the first to erupt and are the keystone for the permanent dental arch. The receding mandible, characteristic of the younger child, has extended forward to allow room for the permanent teeth.

The temperature, pulse and respiration approach the adult norms. The normal temperature is 98.6 F. (37° C.) The average pulse rate is from 85 to 100 per minute, the blood pressure 95 to 108 systolic and 62 to 67 diastolic. The rate of respiration is 18 to 20 per minute.

The physical changes which indicate pubescence may begin to appear toward the end of the school age.

SOCIAL DEVELOPMENT

In school the child has an opportunity to widen his social contacts while he develops his mental abilities. The school hours of the six-year-old in many places are shorter than those of older school children. This makes the transition from home to school life and the adjustment to new experiences easier for the child.

MENTAL DEVELOPMENT

Concrete Operational Stage (7 to 11 years). According to Piaget, the child is no longer limited in the areas discussed in Chapter 19 concerning the preschool child. During school age the child gives up to a large extent his earlier preoperational egocentricity. He is able to function on a higher level in terms of his mental ability; therefore, he is able to learn in school.

ORDERING OR SERIATION. The school age child is able to arrange things or concrete objects according to their size and relationships to other things. He is thus able to solve an abstract problem when it deals with concrete objects.

CLASSIFICATION. The child is increasingly able to classify objects in a more complex manner than he could during preschool years. While the child in the preoperational stage could classify objects in a single class, the school child can classify objects into classes and subclasses.

THINKING AND REASONING. The school child is no longer limited in his focus on aspects in his environment; he can explore more facets of objects and situations. He can solve problems because he can manipulate symbols. His mental ability permits him to carry on converse and reverse processes. The school child can think problems through; therefore, a new world of logical operations opens before him.

TIME. During the school age period the child thinks not only of the present, but of the past and future. Since the child can recall events that happened in the past, he becomes aware that things exist over a period of time. The child during the preschool period may have indicated his new understanding of time by saying, "Last week I went to the zoo," or "Next year I will go to school," but he really does not have a precise idea about what he meant. To him, "next year" may have meant a few weeks from the present time. When the child is able to understand the concrete operations of seriation, decentration (the ability to focus on many aspects of an experience), and reversibility he is able to understand better the concept of time. During the formal operational stage, or during adolescence, the child will reach full understanding of the concept of time. Then the individual will fully understand the meaning of the concept of "past history" and the real meaning of the concept of "future."

LANGUAGE AND SOCIAL BEHAVIOR. The child's ability to speak and play becomes more socialized and cooperative during the school-age period. Since he is able to perceive how another person feels in a situation, he is able to cooperate with him. Because he has a greater fund of information and the ability to communicate it, the child becomes more social in his relations with others.

LIFE PERSPECTIVE

Since the school child has a greater appreciation of the past, present, and future, he may make plans for his life when he matures. For instance, he may have some idea about what his occupational goal in life will be. Female applicants to schools of nursing many times say, "I have wanted to be a nurse since I was a little girl." This may be quite true for a rare few, but more frequently and at different times they also wanted to be full-time "Mommies" like their mothers, airline stewardesses, teachers, or even engineers or firemen, depending on the individual background. Male applicants may have had similar dreams during childhood about their future vocations but since more vocational choices usually were open to them, the profession of nursing may not have been among their initial choices.

The child, during his elementary school years, may have a rudimentary appreciation of his own nonexistence, but additional years of development are required before he can understand the concept of his own personal mortality. As noted in Chapter 5 (see p. 107) the child's ideas concerning the deaths of other people change during the school years. Further development will be required before he can contemplate his own death.

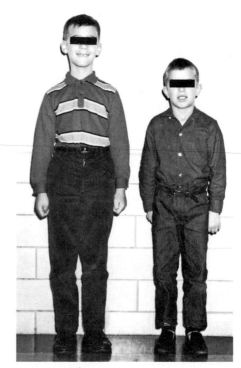

FIGURE 22–5. The older a child becomes, the less it is possible to set norms of physical development, behavior or abilities. These two boys are six years of age, but show an obvious difference in growth.

SPECIFICS OF PHYSICAL, SOCIAL, AND MENTAL DEVELOPMENT

The older a child becomes, the less is it possible to set norms as standards for his behavior or abilities. Such norms illustrate merely the kinds of behavior that often occur at a certain age. The student should recall from Chapter 2 that not all development proceeds on a steady upward curve. It has periods of acceleration, plateaus, and even lags in some areas, while other areas of development proceed normally. Yet all physical growth and mental and emotional development are interrelated in the individual child. Individual differences and the effects of his health status and home, school and community environment become more and more pronounced as the child grows older.

SIX YEARS

The sixth year is a year of transition, of physical and psychologic changes which society has taken as the criterion for readiness to enter school. It is a difficult period for both parents and the child, because he wants to assume increased responsibility and self-direction and yet lacks the basis for making wise decisions. Typically, he is upset and tense, self-centered, and a show-off. He enjoys bossing others, but is easily hurt by the criticism he evokes. He is ready to start anything, but not anxious to finish the task. He may be defiant and rude with adults as a result of his unstable emotional reactions.

Six-year-olds feel tension because they are growing up and are leaving the security of home to go to school. They feel a new wave of separation anxiety, which is felt periodically, even in adolescence. They want the role of the little child again. Parental love and praise are important to them.

Boys and girls play together. Their play is apt to end in chaos. There are disputes and physical battles in which boys and girls take equal parts. The individual child is still more important than the play group as a whole.

The six-year-old may still be troubled by some of the sex questions he asked in the preschool period. He may indulge in sex play. Although he looks forward to marriage, he pays little attention to the sexual aspect and may invite one of his relatives to be his marital partner. He is likely to want his mother to have a baby even if there is already one in the family.

Physical Development and Motor Control. Physical development and motor control are seen in the changing characteristics and abilities of the six-year-old. The loss of the temporary teeth continues, and the first permanent teeth, the six-year molars, erupt. In school, if he did

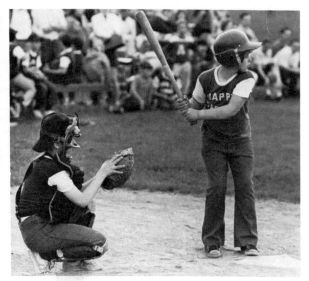

FIGURE 22–6. As the school child grows, his movements become more coordinated and his ability to compete in organized games or sports increases. (Courtesy of H. Armstrong Roberts.)

are common. He appears to be in constant motion. He enjoys physical activity, but his movements may be clumsy because of his fatigue from overactivity—wrestling, playing tag, tumbling, and jumping with other children. His balance is improving; he climbs, skips, hops, and gallops well. Girls jump rope, a single rope, but not double. Both sexes can walk steadily on a chalk mark and learn to skate. Some children can ride a bicycle.

These children can throw and catch a ball. They are aware of their hands as tools, cutting and pasting well. They can hammer, build simple structures, manipulate fasteners on clothing with the aid of sight to guide their hands, and tie shoelaces.

Vocalization, Socialization, and Mental Abilities. The six-year-old has command of practically every form of sentence structure. Speech is fixed, and he is no longer experimenting with its use. He asks questions which show thought and uses language as a tool and less for the pleasure of talking as he did during the preschool age. He may use language aggressively, expressing himself in slang and even swearing. He uses language to share in the experience of others and is interested in learning more about his relatives

not go to nursery school or kindergarten, he is exposed to infection more frequently than he was at home, and ear, nose, and throat problems

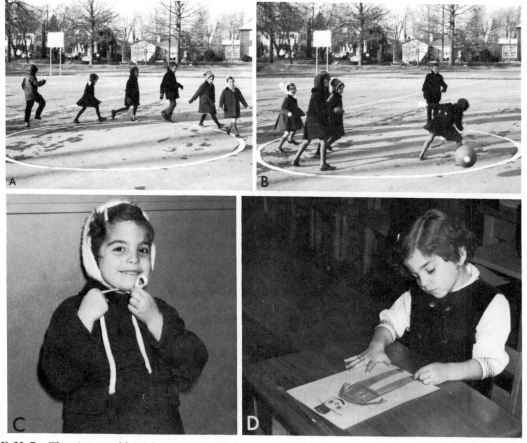

FIGURE 22–7. The six-year-old (A) has improved balance so he can skip and gallop along a chalk mark, (B) can throw and catch a ball well, (C) can tie a bow easily, (D) can draw a man with hitherto absent features.

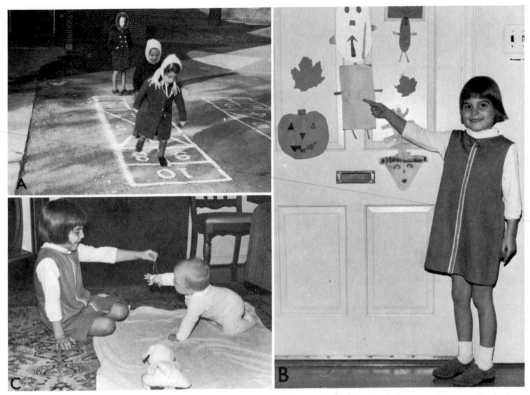

FIGURE 22–8. The seven-year-old (*A*) can play hopscotch, (*B*) knows which month of the year it is, particularly months in which some event such as Halloween occurs, (*C*) is a cooperative member of the family.

and his own and their place in the family tree. He still defines objects in terms of their use: a chair is something to sit on, and a spoon is what he eats with. But he has some concept of abstract words; he knows whether it is morning or afternoon. He knows his right hand from his left, can count to 20 or more, but when printing, he may reverse one or two of the digits or capital letters. Since he can now recognize shapes, he can read, and describe objects seen in pictures. He can draw a man with hitherto absent features such as hands, neck and clothing, and he can distinguish between what he has been taught is attractive and what is ugly when shown a series of faces. He is able to obey three commands given in succession, e.g., "Wipe your hands, put the dishes on the table, and close the door."

Probably his greatest achievement in abstract thought is his beginning interest in the concept of a power greater than himself or his parents—God.

SEVEN YEARS

Seven is an assimilative age, a quieting-down period. The child is less of a problem than he was at six years, more often quiet than boisterous. Many teachers find the second-grade group the easiest to teach in elementary school. The child has less intense relations with others; he does not ask for trouble. But he enjoys teasing, and this often gets him into difficulty with children younger than himself and with adults who take their part. He likes to play alone, although he prefers group play. When playing, he is more passive than the six-year-old.

The seven-year-old sets high standards for his family and feels both a personal inferiority and anger over even their minor failures, as he sees them, in living up to their respective roles. His eithical sense is developing; he is conscious of right and wrong in the conduct of others and in what he himself does. He may tattle on other children from a sense of justice. On the whole he is now a cooperative member of the family and wants the approval of his parents. Parents must respect his inner life, his strains of sadness and his uncalled-for periods of shyness. It is during these periods that he is becoming aware of himself and thus of others.

The seven-year-old is more modest about sexual matters and indulges in less sex play. Many seven-year-olds would like to have a baby brother or sister. The seven-year-old may become involved in an elementary love affair with someone of the opposite sex.

Physical Development and Motor Control. The general level of activity is lower at seven years than at six, but varies widely in individual children. The child has a trait which annoys his elders, but fascinates him and other children—wiggling a loose tooth.

The books he reads need no longer be printed with type larger than average, for his eyes become fully developed between seven and eight years of age. His posture is now more tense and ready for motion than that of the younger child.

Boys and girls enjoy skating and other active sports. There begins to be a diversion, however, between boy and girl sports. Girls jump rope and play hopscotch, games which boys are likely to participate in only in a teasing way. Although seven-year-olds are active, they enjoy games in which they can sit down and rest.

Vocalization, Socialization, and Mental Abilities. The child is becoming oriented in time as well as space. He knows which month it is and the season of the year, particularly months in which some event in which he is intensely interested takes place—Christmas or his birthday. He begins to read the clock, both the hours and the minutes.

His hands are becoming more steady, and he often prefers a pencil with an eraser to a crayon. He can print several sentences, though the letters become smaller toward the end of the line. Reversal of letters is less common, and he is likely to correct such errors. He can repeat five numbers in succession and three numbers backward, count by two's and five's, grasp the basic idea of addition and subtraction, copy a diamond without confusing it with a square, and tell what parts are missing from an incomplete picture of a man. His attention span is lengthening, and he enjoys repeating activities that afford him satisfaction. He is more self-helpful, needing little assistance in dressing, undressing and going to bed. He is increasingly interested in God's place in the world and wants to know where heaven is and what it is like.

EIGHT YEARS

The eight-year-old is at an expansive age and wants to do everything. This is an age of broadening experiences and intellectual exploration. He is more creative and active in his solitary play and work, but he needs other children and

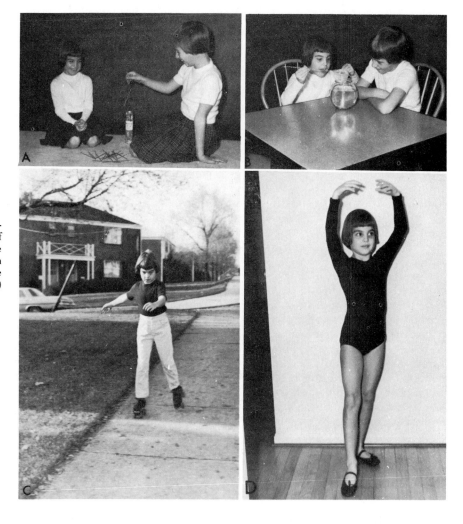

FIGURE 22–9. The eight-year-old (A) enjoys games of skill using small muscles of the hands, (B) evidences interest in science, (C) can move more smoothly when skating, (D) can balance gracefully.

their approval, and he actively seeks their company. He is full of enthusiastic energy and wants to be considered important by adults. He wants to assume responsibility and to spread his influence in the culture of his group by putting on dramatic shows and inventing new ways of doing tasks. He tries to understand adult ideas and standards by listening to what is told him. He learns by experience and from others what is necessary for group living. If his mental ability is average or above average, he becomes very much interested in reading, group activities and school, especially in science as he sees it pictured in space ships and machinery. He likes science fiction. Hero worship begins at this age.

He likes to join clubs if they are not too rigidly organized and takes group fads seriously. Eight-year-olds appear to be sex-conscious, choosing playmates of their own sex. Boys are usually secretive about girl friends, especially if *she* is a new girl in the neighborhood. They show less active interest in sex questions which are beyond their comprehension than does the younger child, but they may ask questions at appropriate times. Parents should suggest to their children that it is better not to discuss the answers to sex questions with siblings or friends.

The eight-year-old behaves best when strangers are present or when he is away from home.

Physical Development and Motor Control. There are subtle changes in the body of an eight-year-old; the arms are growing longer in proportion to the body, and the hands are also proportionately larger. His movements are becoming smoother, more graceful and perfected. His amusements change as he matures. He now likes hiking, playing ball and such games as follow-the-leader. The boy wants to improve his skill in boxing and wrestling, and the girl in jumping rope, hopscotch, and roller skating. Both boys and girls are dramatic in their activities and accompany speech with descriptive gestures.

Vocalization, Socialization, and Mental Abilities. In school the child of eight is writing rather than printing, and enjoys his new skill. In mental tests for his age group are questions such as naming from memory similarities and differences between two objects — e.g., ball and block — and counting backwards from 20. In school and daily life he has new abilities. He is beginning to understand perspective in drawing. He can repeat the days of the week and has some concept of the number of days which must pass before some pleasant event will take place — a holiday, his birthday or, in the hospital, visiting day and that eventful day when he goes home.

Some children enjoy going to Sunday School and are interested in hearing about heaven as "the place you go to when you die."

NINE YEARS

The nine-year-old is neither a child nor a youth. He is only beginning to take part in family group discussions. He is not as restless as the eight-year-old and is more interested in family activities. He is impelled to show others that he is an individual and resists or ignores adult authority when it conflicts with ideas or values of his peer group. Teachers find the children in fourth grade difficult to teach. In broadening his experiences outside the home he grows toward independence. He is better able to accept blame for his acts and assumes responsibility for care of younger siblings and for keeping his room in some sort of order. He is motivated, as well as more likely, to complete the tasks he begins.

He fluctuates between childhood and youth in his actions and thoughts. Hero worship is becoming pronounced. Girls still prefer to play with girls, and boys with boys. They are usually less concerned with the reproductive aspect of sex than when they were eight. This depends, however, on whether their desire for information about the conception and bearing of children was satisfied when they first asked for it. The nine-year-old is in a state of constant urgency, as though he were in a contest with time.

Physical Development and Motor Control. These children have more variation in skills than they had during their first three years of school. Normally, hand-eye coordination is developed, and the child becomes skillful in manual activities. In general, children of this age can use both hands independently.

The child works and plays hard and enjoys displaying his motor skill and strength; he shows great interest in competitive sports such as baseball.

Vocalization, Socialization, and Mental Abilities. New abilities, which show his mental development, include describing common objects in detail, not in terms of use as he did when he was six years old, repeating the months of the year in order, knowing the date, telling time correctly, writing (usually with small, even letters), matching the material which he reads with reality, making correct change from a quarter, arranging five weights according to their heaviness, multiplying and dividing (simple division) and repeating four numbers backward (this is one item in a commonly given mental test).

The child can take care of his bodily needs completely; this is a great step away from early childhood and toward adult self-reliance. He has

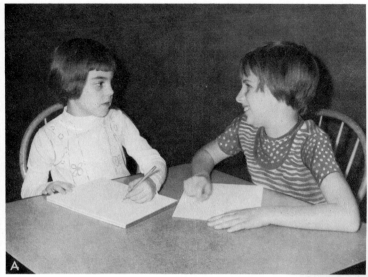

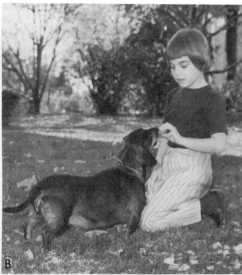

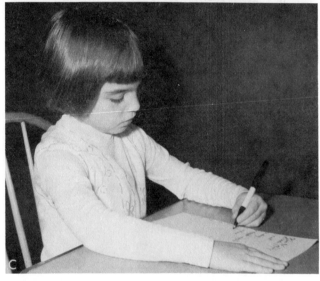

FIGURE 22–10. The nine-year-old (*A*) still prefers to play with others of the same sex; (*B*) provides care for a pet as well as a younger sibling; (*C*) writes with increasing manual dexterity.

developed acceptable table manners and shows them without coaching from his parents. Although he has fewer fears than when he was younger, he has become a worrier. His advance toward adult attitudes is shown in his rejection of the Santa Claus myth, and yet he does not intentionally destroy it for a younger sibling. In contrast to the two preceding years, he may show a lack of interest in God and in religion.

TEN YEARS

The average child of ten years is at the beginning of the preadolescent period. The girl is further advanced than the boy toward puberty. The ten-year-old is even more reasonable than the nine-year-old, for he has acquired greater mastery of himself and his environment. He is courteous and well mannered with adults, and shows more self-direction in his actions. He wants to measure up to a challenge, defined in the social norms of the group. He has broad interests and is beginning to think clearly about social problems and social prejudices. Special talents appear in this age group.

The child adjusts better than before to home routines; he can live by rules and tolerates frustrations. He is entering the age when the need for group activities is at its highest point. To him, attaining a goal for the group is more important than his own ideas or desires. He is capable of great loyalties and intense hero worship; both are qualities making for successful group membership.

The ten-year-old is interested in matters of sex, but is more likely to discuss the subject with his peer group than with his parents. Children of both sexes investigate their sexual organs. Some children are modest, but others present problems of sex play. Outside the classroom the two sexes rarely mix. Although

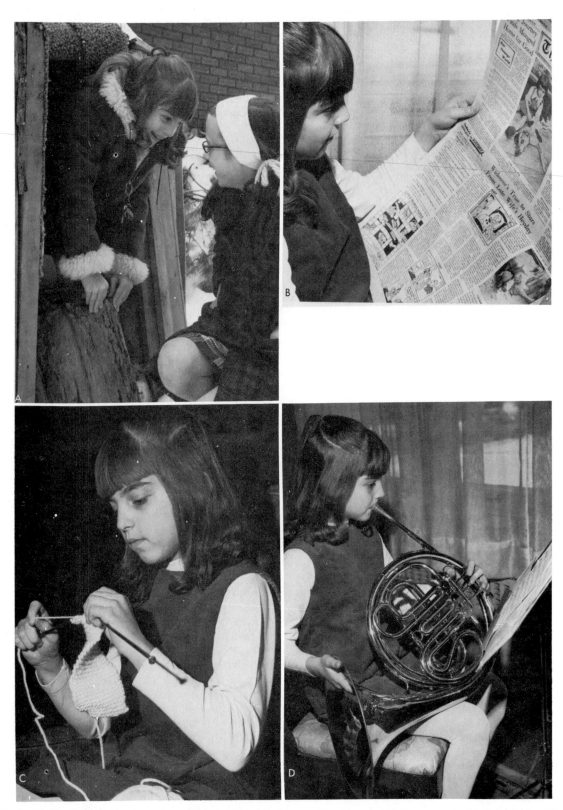

FIGURE 22–11. The ten- to eleven-year-old (*A*) is interested in attaining the goal of the group, in this instance, building a play house in which to talk and share secrets; (*B*) has awakening interest in the world beyond home and community; (*C*) and (*D*) is developing special talents such as knitting and playing a musical instrument.

kissing games may be played in children's entertainments arranged by adults, they are seldom played spontaneously. Children tease each other about friends of the opposite sex.

The ten-year-old wants to be independent. For this reason requests should be made positively and with tact. Negative requests affront his sense of personal worth. The power of suggestion is important at this age and can be used to help the child develop a good character.

Physical Development and Motor Control. As the child's body matures, sex differences are more pronounced. Both boys and girls have perfected most of the basic small motor movements. They desire perfection in their complex abilities. Girls have more poise than boys, partly because of their earlier maturation.

Vocalization, Socialization, and Mental Abilities. The child now thinks of situations in terms of cause and effect. He has some insight into the fundamentals of human relations and wants to accomplish great things in life.

His education is more advanced, and he uses what he knows and the skills he has acquired in his daily life. He can write for a relatively long time and maintains good speed. He likes mystery stories, science fiction, and practical magic. He can use numbers beyond 100 with understanding and can do simple fractions.

TEN TO 12 YEARS (PREADOLESCENCE)

The years between ten and twelve are known as the preadolescent period. It is a time of rapid growth and development, when many problems occur. As he approaches adulthood the child may become overcritical of adults, comparing them with the self-image of the man or woman he or she intends to be. The child wavers be-

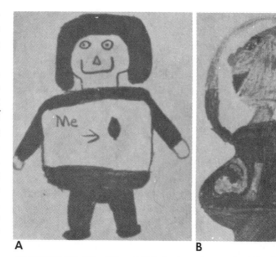

FIGURE 22–12. The child during the early school years visualizes his life before he was born. A, "I was in my mommy before I was born." B, "This is the little egg that's inside my mother's body. This is me inside the egg." (From *Children Today*, March-April 1974.)

tween dependence and independence and is likely to withdraw when he is frustrated instead of voicing his anger. He may rebel against parental standards of bathing and dressing.

Friends in his peer group are extremely important to him; he shares their attitudes and tells them his thoughts rather than confiding in his parents. He enters with enthusiasm into group community projects such as collecting worn clothing for charity or old newspapers for the Boy Scouts.

He is critical of what he does. He wants to become somewhat financially independent of his parents; he is happy to do small jobs after school or during vacations. He seeks an adult

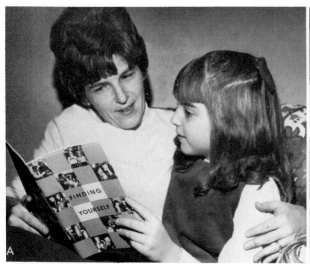
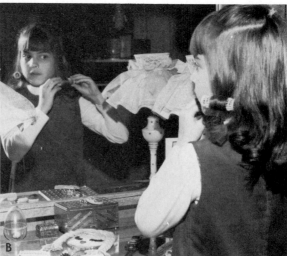

FIGURE 22–13. The twelve-year-old preadolescent (A) is interested in the physical changes she will experience in puberty, (B) is beginning to take pride in caring for her own physical needs.

friend of the same sex with whom to identify and to whom he can express criticism of his parents. The composure and control of the ten-year-old gradually vanish at 11 to 12 years. He becomes annoying, sloppy, exhibitionistic, and negativistic. He tries hard to master reality in preparation for adolescence. He is interested in how things work and is curious about the world in general, but his interest in acquiring academic knowledge may lag.

He needs to gain strength of personality to be able to make healthy solutions to the conflicts of adolescence. The adult who is responsible for the preadolescent at home, in the community, or at school must accept the fact that the child needs to rebel and depreciate others in order to work through his conflict between dependence and independence. He is still dependent, but he does not wish to be made to feel infantile. He rejects his parents because he does not want to feel dependent on them; he meets his dependency needs by relations with other adults. The adult whom the preadolescent selects to fill this role must handle the child through democratic guidance. He must accept the child, yet provide limits to his behavior as the parents did when the child was younger. The preadolescent needs help to channel his feelings and energy in the proper directions—sports and work suitable to his stage of growth and development. He needs help in accepting himself in his new role of preadolescent. Adults in his environment should help him to build up his self-esteem and strengthen his personality in order to prepare him adequately to meet the problems of adolescence.

Physical Development and Motor Control. Children in this age group are filled with energy and are constantly active. Their muscular control is good, and manipulative skill almost equals that of the adult. They appear to be under tension, which is relieved by foot-tapping on the floor or finger-drumming on table tops.

The 12-year molars erupt, the last teeth to erupt during childhood. The preadolescent spurt in growth comes earlier in girls than in boys, but girls lag behind boys in endurance and physical strength.

Vocalization, Socialization and Mental Abilities. Before he is 12 years old the average child is able to define some basic abstract terms such as honesty and justice. His development of vocabulary and his diction depend upon his intelligence, experience, and environmental opportunities. Children in this age group can see the moral of stories. Their interests and intellectual pursuits vary. Intellectual growth is seen in their interest in world affairs, both past and

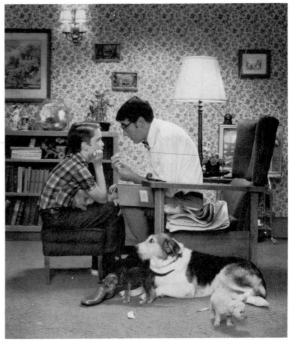

FIGURE 22–14. The older school-age boy also is interested in the physical changes he can anticipate at puberty. (Courtesy of State Farm Life and Accident Insurance Company.)

present, and their attitude toward social problems, especially those which touch their daily lives.

They are eager to learn about health. They want to know why the mouth should be covered when coughing. They are capable of self-care in ordinary situations, but should still be under some supervision of sympathetic adults. They can assume some responsibility for the care of younger children. Their contact with children and adults goes well beyond the limits of home.

The peer group is very close to the 11-year-old. This is a period for sharing secrets. Even a secret language may be devised and used strictly with the close peer group. These children still prefer to play with their own sex group, but accept the opposite sex in their activities. Some boys' groups even accept girls if they wish to join such sports as baseball or football.

SCHOOL

Attendance at school is an important part of the growing child's life. The school is the institution in society specifically designed as the formal instrument for educating its children. Its purpose is to help each child to develop his potential to the fullest. This includes helping each child develop his *sense of industry.*

The basic tools for achieving this objective are

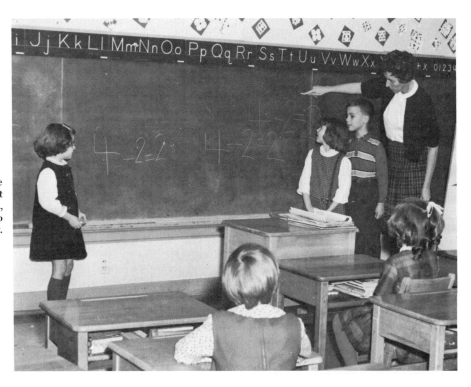

FIGURE 22–15. Attendance at school is an important part of the child's life. In school, children should be helped to develop their sense of industry.

the communication skills and the arithmetic fundamentals. Mastery of these tools then makes it possible for the child to extend his educational horizons to areas such as history, geography, science, social studies, health education, and the creative arts.

From the earliest years the school program provides experience which contributes to the child's social development as a member of a group. It is here that he should be learning to think critically, to make judgments based on reason, to accept criticism, to cooperate with others, and to be both a leader and a follower as the occasion warrants.

The extent to which a child acquires a good self-concept, a sense of personal worth, and a respect for the contribution of others is an important measure of the effectiveness of the school program. Attendance at school is important for all children, irrespective of their socio-economic group and intelligence level. The course of instruction can be such that every child will be able to get a feeling of successful accomplishment in some area.

All children should feel that they can accomplish something both in school and, later, in community life. This does not mean that all children should be passed along with their group in school whether they do well or not. They do not want to be rewarded when they know that they have failed. They need opportunities for success on their individual level of achievement.

Not every child is capable of excelling intellectually in academic courses, but the school can help each child to realize his potential ability and find real satisfaction in his achievement in other areas of living—areas in which the child who does not do well at school may be more successful than those who excel in class work.

Preparation for School. Not all children are emotionally ready for school at the same chronologic age. If the preschool child has attended and adjusted well to nursery school or kindergarten, he probably will have little difficulty with adjustment to school. He will consider school a normal responsibility of childhood.

As soon as school starts there is an enforced separation of the child from his home. The unprepared child, more than those who are prepared, may be uncertain of the expectations of the teacher, a new adult in charge of part of his life. He may be frightened by leaving his parents and by the demands of a group of children different from those he has known before. In general, however, if he has attended kindergarten in the public school of his neighborhood, he will have friends in the first grade and will be accustomed to the school building. If a younger sibling is entering kindergarten, he is protective and tells him all about it. He will go to and from school with siblings or neighborhood friends.

Preparation for school experience is much like preparation for attendance at nursery school (see p. 630). The child should know his full name and address before entering school. He should know certain safety rules, such as how to cross the street safely. He should also know how to care for himself for the most part in matters of dressing and toileting. He should have a physical examination and must meet school requirements for immunization.

The parents can take the child to school before school starts in order to orient him to the physical environment and to meet his teacher. Parents should talk positively about school experience at all times, but particularly to the child entering school. Older siblings will present school as a matter-of-fact experience for all six-year-olds and as something to brag about to younger children. After school has started, if the child appears afraid of the school experience, the mother may stay with him in the classroom for a while until the teacher has established a positive relation with him. Before parents allow a child to go to school alone they must be certain that he knows the way or, if he must take a bus, which bus to ride. Generally the school either is in easy walking distance or sends a bus to collect the children who live too far away to walk to school.

A problem may arise after the child has become familiar with school life in that he pays more attention to the job of gaining friends than to gaining knowledge. This is to be expected, especially if none of his old friends from home, nursery school, or kindergarten are in his class at school.

Parents should not expect too much from children upon their return from school. Children have put in a day of school work and recreation under supervision, both of which are planned to promote growth and development. Nevertheless the child can gradually assume some home responsibilities, planned so that he has time for play with his siblings and friends and also to be by himself. This last is a need often overlooked even by thoughtful parents.

During the orientation period, as well as during all his school life, the child's parents should be willing to listen to his tales about his school experiences. This strengthens his ability to use language and also helps him to become more of a person in his own right. Parents' unflagging interest in school and the child's activities does more than anything else to invest education with its real importance.

If the child refuses to attend school, is chronically unhappy there, or is not learning at the rate he should, his parents may investigate the situation in conjunction with his teacher or other school personnel.

Role of the Teacher. Teachers play a definite role in helping children develop a sense of industry through their assignments, stimulation of group activities and their suggestion that children accept responsibilities for nonacademic duties in the classroom. In addition, teachers can also deepen their students' sense of trust, autonomy, and initiative, or encourage the growth of these traits.

A teacher has a profound influence because, next to the parents, he or she is the most important person in a child's life. This is especially true during the grade-school period when the child needs an older person of his own sex to "worship." This is one reason why it would be beneficial to have more male teachers; the grade-school boy is apt to lack this model. The teacher is the kind of person whom the child can profitably imitate. Unfortunately some parents want the teacher to take too much responsibility for their children; they want relief from their own duty of rearing them. They want the teacher to solve all the child's problems while he is in school. These parents can be helped to understand the proper function of the school and to recognize their own responsibilities as parents.

Parents may seek guidance from teachers or school counselors individually or collectively. Parent-teacher groups are especially valuable for interpreting the function of the school in the child's life, growth, and development at various age levels, and problems such as discipline, sibling rivalry, sex education, and special health problems of children. The leader of such a group may not always give advice, but should let the group solve the mutual problems facing its members.

PLAY AND WORK

Today school age children are becoming increasingly interested in the types of play and work usually associated with those of the opposite sex. For instance, girls are interested in participating in team sports traditionally reserved for boys. Boys are becoming interested in learning to bake and cook. This blurring of interests is healthy, because it teaches members of each sex the value of different types of activities. It may also make it easier later for members of both sexes to adjust to jobs traditionally given to persons of the opposite sex. Sharing at this age may also ultimately lead to a mutual sharing in fulfilling their responsibilities during marriage.

Play is a child's tool for learning, and his play changes with his developmental needs. The child during the school years adds realistic features to his play, yet he becomes at the same time more imaginative. His fantasy and his concept of reality do not now become mixed as they did during the preschool years. He has his day-dreams, but his dreams and fantasies are his secret and are not shared with his parents. Adequate play materials should be provided.

In general, time spent in play and the number of play activities decrease as the child matures. Nevertheless the time spent upon specific activities increases because the attention span becomes longer and the child has a deeper interest in what he is doing. Play during the school years becomes more formal than it was during early childhood, more organized, more competitive and to some degree less physically active. The child begins to have an interest in hobbies or collections of various kinds because in so doing he is actually collecting facts and knowledge about the world in which he lives.

As the child participates in more organized, competitive sports such as football, baseball, or running matches he needs the help of adults in learning the rules. Parents should spend more time with their children. The adult should not be the leader, however. Children respond best when they plan their own play experiences. In this way they learn self-government and self-direction of activities.

Another responsibility of parents during the school years is helping the child learn to work. Children of both sexes should be encouraged to assist with duties in or around the house. Allowing them to help may take more time than doing the work without them, but ultimately the adult's time is saved and the children have developed their sense of industry. If they are not allowed to help when they are young, they may not be interested in helping later in life. The work they are asked to do should definitely contribute to the welfare of the group.

As soon as the child shows interest in earning his spending money—this will be during his later school years—he should be helped to decide the kind of work he would like to do, whether delivering papers, mowing lawns, or baby-sitting. The attitudes toward work which he develops in these early years will be important in shaping the kind of workman he is during adult life.

SIX TO EIGHT YEARS

From six to eight years of age the child is interested chiefly in the immediate environment and the immediate present. He needs, in play, an opportunity to express his feelings and find acceptance. Play must be suited to his interests and concentration span. Since he knows more about family life than any other kind of living, he enjoys playing house. A child also takes the role of a member of various occupational groups with which he comes in contact: nurse, store-keeper, milkman, garage mechanic, or trainman. What a child pretends to be gives the adult insight into his personality.

Six Years. The child six years of age plays with spreading scope and movement. Sex differences in play are defining themselves more clearly. Both sexes, however, enjoy many activities in common. For instance, both girls and boys like to paint and color and to cut out and paste. Boys enjoy drawing airplanes, trains, and boats; girls are more likely to draw people and houses. Boys enjoy digging more than girls do, though it is a favorite activity of both sexes. All children of this age want to learn to ride a bicycle. If they have none of their own, they borrow the bicycles of their older siblings and friends. Both sexes enjoy running games, tag, hide-and-seek, roller skating, and swimming. Girls enjoy jumping rope.

Both boys and girls like to pretend, but there is a sex difference. Boys pretend that they are conductors, astronauts, or soldiers or imitate some other masculine role in which there is plenty of activity. Girls dress up in costumes and play at being mothers or teachers, with younger children or dolls as their children. This is the age when doll play is at its height, and every toy pertaining to the mother role adds to the child's pleasure. Irrespective of sex, these children start collections of miscellaneous items such as bits of pretty paper, pictures, or anything that takes their fancy.

Children six to eight years old like to "read stories from memory," look at comic books, play simple table games, and listen to radio and watch television programs.

Boys and girls may play school and house together, but boys do not do so when playing only with boys. Boys particularly enjoy games characterized by getting under cover and shooting the enemy. They are interested in construction and transportation games.

Suitable toys for girls include dolls, doll clothes, wash baskets, doll strollers or baby carriages, swings, stoves, suit cases, and make-up equipment. Boys like electric trains, airplanes, boats, trucks and automobiles.

Seven Years. Play at seven is approached more cautiously than at six years, and there are fewer new ventures. The child is more obsessive in his play interests. He enjoys funny books and coloring in books with pictures suited to his age. He likes table games, jigsaw puzzles, magic and tricks. He reads simple books fairly well, and enjoys reading. He is content to play by himself when no companions are about and is better able than the six-year-old to plan what he wants to do next. He listens to the radio and watches television programs in which there is plenty of shooting and wild horseback riding. Boys like to invent and then construct playthings and gifts for mother, using cereal boxes, fruit crates, and even packing boxes. Girls enjoy designing dresses for paper dolls.

These children enjoy collecting in quantity, not for quality; they collect stones, bottle caps and almost anything they find which is out of the ordinary.

They demand more realism in their play. They need guns to play cowboys and Indians or "cops and robbers." All seven-year-old "mothers" want dolls the size of a real baby, which can "suck" from a bottle and wet the diaper. These "mothers," who want a realistic family of "children" whose ages range from newborn to four, also love "older" dolls with hair which can be brushed and combed. They like large "sister" dolls, but find them too big for mothering.

Both sexes enjoy active games. Girls like hopscotch, jumping rope, and the quiet game of jackstones. Boys play ball, climb trees, race, and play marbles. Both sexes ride bicycles well, and learn to swim under supervision. If they have the opportunity, many learn to ski. Girls enjoy almost all forms of play which boys engage in, but are not likely to be as proficient as the boys in active sports.

Eight Years. Eight years is an active age, in which there is a wide variety of interests. Unsupervised play among eight-year-olds becomes noisy and may end in a quarrel. They do not enjoy playing alone. With an adult they demand his complete attention; with other children they demand full participation. Their drawings are full of action.

Girls like to mix dough for cookies, make Jello in fancy molds, frost cakes and experiment with simple cooking. Boys enjoy simple chemistry sets and equipment for making telegraph sets and performing magic tricks. They are fond of dramatics, and of fighting and rushing to fires. Girls also enjoy dramatics, though of a less masculine sort, and always want an audience.

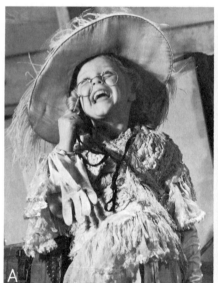
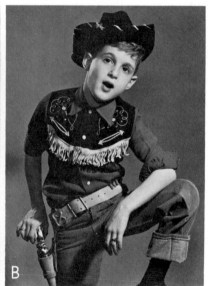
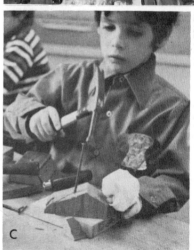

FIGURE 22–16. The eight-year-old (A, B) enjoys dramatic play, (C) enjoys making objects. (Courtesy of H. Armstrong Roberts.)

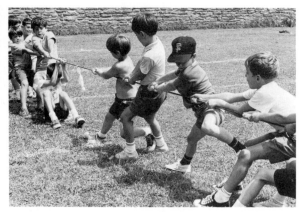

FIGURE 22–17. School-age children enjoy cooperative and competitive sports such as tug-of-war. (Courtesy of H. Armstrong Roberts.)

Boys and girls of this age make collections, but are now conscious of quality, and they classify and organize the items. Boys collect stones and rocks, marbles, cards of baseball stars, or cars. Girls collect paper dolls, valentines, and Christmas cards or similar items.

Eight-year-olds begin to form loosely organized, short-lived clubs. They have secret passwords which must be given before permission is granted to enter the club house, hut, or hangout.

These children enjoy active games. In spite of their fondness for exuberant activity, they respond well to supervision. They enjoy various sports in season. They are interested in table games such as checkers and dominoes. They may invent their own rules for an old game, often to such an extent that it is virtually a new game. Rules may be short-lived, but must be adhered to by all participants while they are in effect. Children of this age do not accept losing a game easily, they argue about decision, and they often walk out of the group if they are beaten.

Most eight-year-olds can read well enough to enjoy childhood classics such as books on travel and geography. Comic books are still prime favorites. These children are at the peak of wanting prizes and objects given with coupons from breakfast cereals plus a small sum of money. They are thrilled to receive mail as adults do. Radio and television are extremely important in their lives. They like stories of adventure and mystery. Science fiction is becoming a favorite.

NINE TO 12 YEARS

The interest of children in this age group expands to distant places, backward into history and forward into the jet age. They like tales which do not point a moral, but give examples of courage, kindness, endurance, and adventure. They feel responsible for performing some ser-

vice as part of their day's activities. They are developing a sense of satisfaction from contributing to group activity, and the beginning of group loyalty which characterizes the gang age of older siblings. They are now able to receive help in understanding the advantage of mature behavior, although they can seldom live up to their ideal of a self-image. They are interested in their future as they say, "What I'm going to be..." Parents should be observant of natural inclinations, although vocational decisions may not be made until the child reaches adolescence or beyond.

Nine Years. The nine-year-old plays and works hard, often to the point of fatigue. He is busy with his chosen activities; he enjoys reading, listening to the radio, and viewing television for prolonged periods. Boys play football or baseball, and girls play with dolls for hours on end.

Both boys and girls enjoy active sports. They are old enough to want to improve their skills, and there is a purpose in their play which they seldom had when younger. Boys often disturb the peace of the home by roughhousing.

Nine-year-olds are great readers, reading their favorite books over and over again. They often read the junior classics, but comic books and books on adventure, war and slapstick domestic humor still fascinate them.

Many children are interested in music and take music lessons in school or from a private teacher. They often apply themselves well to music study and acquire skill through hours of practice. Talents appear at this age, especially in the creative arts. Children have an opportunity to hear music on the radio, television, and record players at home or school. Their choice of the type of music they like depends on their experience on a cultural and socioeconomic level and the influence of their group of peers. They still have favorite programs on the television, but are not as rigid about viewing only these as when they were younger. They all want to go to the motion pictures.

Ten Years. Sex differences in play are pronounced among ten-year-olds. Boys and girls are developing the skills which each sex needs in society. At school the boy works with speed and likes the challenge of mental arithmetic.

The ten-year-old is so conscious of needing the support of his peers that he often esteems the opinions and attitudes of his gang or club more than those of his family. He is interested in social welfare and social justice. He is loyal to his group and does not divulge group secrets. He may indulge in hero worship.

On the radio and television the likes of the ten-year-old are much the same as those of the nine-year-old. Boys spurn romance and love stories. The two sexes are well separated.

Girls enjoy dramatizing life situations, and the subjects they choose are likely to deal with engagements and weddings. They still play with dolls, however, taking the role of mother and "bringing up their children." They are becoming much more interested in their appearance.

Eleven Years. The 11-year-old is full of energy and activity. He experiments with various projects and is intensely interested in the activities of his group. His interest in school may diminish, particularly if he is not a good student. Play is no longer paramount in his life; companionship has become more important than play.

Although these children may seem bungling in motor skill at home, they have acquired new kinds of agility in play. Everything interests them. This is the gang age, and the gang enjoys meeting in its own hut or tree house. The child's interest in reading and motion pictures has increased; the characters he learns about appear to be alive, people he would like to know or perhaps punish in some way.

Twelve Years. The 12-year-old is enthusiastic, so much so that he acts without consideration of consequences. Although he is very much a part of his group, he also likes to be alone. He engages in sports with more team spirit and less wandering of attention to something else in the environment which is of personal interest to him. He has not the same need for praise that he had a year before. His broader interests are seen in his wanting a pen pal from a foreign land.

Twelve-year-olds are becoming interested in earning money, not running errands or little jobs for their parents but in some form of organized project, especially a twosome project, in which they are heavily motivated to succeed. They may be interested in publishing a news bulletin, and many boys have paper routes. Boys and girls still tend to stay apart.

CARE

PHYSICAL CARE

Bathing, Dressing, and Toileting. Children between six and 12 years of age are fairly self-sufficient in bathing, dressing, and toileting, but they need some help with the niceties of manicuring, neatness and even cleanliness. There are, of course, individual differences; some children resent having their ears kept clean, and others do not like to have their hair combed and brushed. Sex differences are apparent: girls are generally more careful of their appearance than boys are.

The six-year-old needs help, through he does not readily accept it. He dawdles and needs management. In undressing he drops his clothes on the floor or flings them aside. The seven-year-old still dawdles, but tends to complete his tasks. The eight-year-old is more efficient in caring for himself. From nine years to the end of the school age children show increased responsibility in selection of clothes, adapted to the occasion and the weather, hanging them up and disposing of soiled garments. They can take care of toileting and bathing, but may still need reminders to brush their teeth or wash their hands thoroughly, and children of both sexes need help with long hair.

SLEEP

The sleep of the school child is rarely quiescent. Fears in the form of night terrors or nightmares prevent his sleeping peacefully because for one reason he has reached the point in his mental development at which he has a concept of death (see p. 107). The bedtime hour should be a quiet time when the parents and the child feel greater interdependency. It is a good time for confidences, questions and answers, and discussions. Routine prayers may be said.

The older child may become self-assertive about the time when he wishes to go to bed. Parents must judge the amount of rest the child needs and see that he is in bed in time for sufficient sleep. The amount needed decreases with age. The six-year-old may need 11 to 12 hours of sleep, while the 12-year-old generally needs only ten hours.

SAFETY MEASURES

Accidents. With the broadening scope of activity among children during the elementary school years, parents cannot hope to be with them constantly in order to prevent accidents. If parents and nursery school and kindergarten teachers have emphasized safety measures, a child should be ready to build on the foundation of past experience and further develop his ability to meet the accident hazards common to school children.

Between the ages of six and 12 years the most common cause of accidental injury and death is *motor accidents.* Children may cross a street against the light or from between parked cars, or be injured while riding in cars.

The second most frequent cause of accidental death is *drowning.* Children should be taught to swim as early as possible. They should also be taught water-survival techniques.

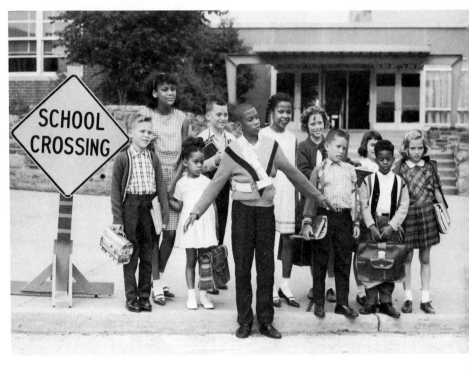

FIGURE 22–18. Motor accidents cause the death of many children each year. This older school-age boy is a member of the safety patrol. He takes his responsibility of protecting other children very seriously. (Courtesy of H. Armstrong Roberts.)

Accidents resulting in injuries to the eyes are not uncommon during the school years. Children should be taught to wear protective devices when doing any activity which is potentially dangerous.

Accidents also occur when children are skating, skateboarding, or riding a bicycle or a minibike. Accidents can occur too when the children are riding the school bus, doing gymnastics, or participating in other sports or games, or playing with other children or with animals.

Sexual Molestation. The purpose of teaching children about sexual molestation is to provide a rational basis for their thinking and action without frightening them. Helping children come to terms with the existence of sexual molestation can help them cope with their ambivalence about sex, which offers on the one hand satisfaction and on the other the risk of injury.

Informing the child about sexual molestation comes under the general heading of warning him about dangers whether they be poisons, pills, or people. Children should be aware of the undesirability of accepting favors from and accompanying strangers. During the school years the child can be introduced to the concept that some older children and adults have problems with their own sexual behavior and that he or she should avoid or leave strange adults who want to befriend them. The child should also be taught to report unusual occurrences with other people to his parents. These matters can then be discussed in an open and supporting manner.

HEALTH

Responsibility for the child's health rests with the parents. Health of the school child is influenced by the health supervision he receives from the family physician and the dentist, by the health instruction given by his parents and teachers, by the environment of his home and school, by the community public health program, and by the direct services he receives in school.

PRESCHOOL HEALTH EXAMINATION

Every child should have a preschool health examination. His height, weight, posture, hearing, and vision are checked carefully. Beginning problems of school children may be due to faulty hearing and vision. Glasses to correct a defect in vision are made of safety glass to reduce the possibility of injury to the eyes. A dental examination and correction of defects are essential. If the child is to gain the optimum benefit from school, he needs to be physically well.

The physician will continue the immunization program against communicable diseases discussed in Chapter 13.

The preschool examination is done in the spring, before the child enters school, so that treatment for any defects or problems can be given before school opens.

Parents should see that the child receives a thorough physical examination every year. If he is not well, he should be taken to a physician.

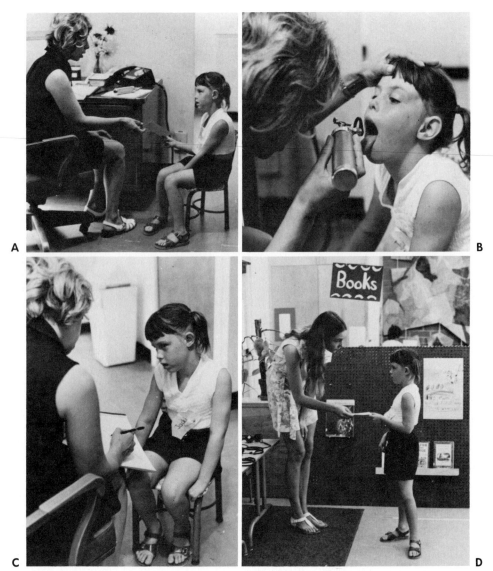

FIGURE 22–19. The child initiates care by (*A*) presenting a card to the school nurse, (*B*) undergoing an examination, (*C*) discussing treatment with the nurse, and (*D*) taking a report to her teacher. (© April 1974, The American Journal of Nursing Company. Reproduced from the *American Journal of Nursing* with permission.)

Dental examinations are made twice a year or as often as the dentist recommends.

SCHOOL HEALTH PROGRAM

The school health program is an important part of the national health program. The main purpose of the school program is to maintain, improve and promote the health of every school child. Adequate supervision of the physical, mental, emotional, and social aspects of school life are included in the program. Routine health appraisals are done on all children, with follow-up on those who need care to see that they receive it. Parent education and parent counseling are also necessary.

The program also includes planning the course content in health education and nutrition, and putting it into effect through instruction and the routine life of the children during school hours. Recreation and physical education should be included. Preventive services are used to control tooth decay, accidents—including those to the eyes—poor nutrition, infectious diseases, unhygienic environment, insufficient care after illness, and drug addiction and emotional disorders.

The School Nurse and the School Nurse Practitioner. The school health program should also include familiarizing school-age children with the concept of a hospital and prepara-

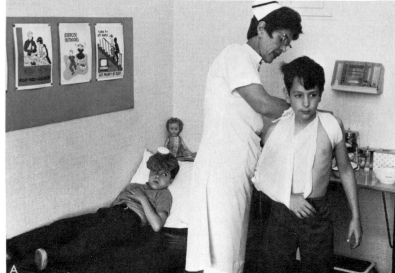

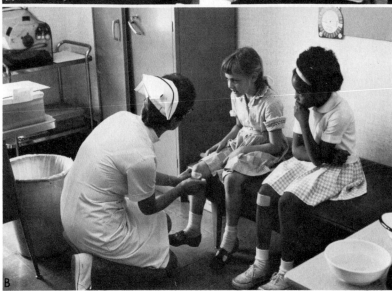

FIGURE 22–20. The school nurse, in addition to her other responsibilities, provides emergency care for the ill or injured child at school: *A*, Adjusting a sling while an ice pack reduces the baseball induced lump on the head of a glum observer. *B*, Bandaging two scraped knees and drying two friends' tears. (Courtesy of M. Ringenberg and *RN*, 32:57–58, September, 1969.)

tion for possible hospitalization in a more thorough manner than was possible at an earlier age. Most children of this age have either been hospitalized themselves or have had a member of their immediate family hospitalized. Even though they have been exposed to hospitals, they still may have specific questions they would like answered. They may also have misconceptions about hospitals that need to be clarified. School nurse practitioners or school nurses are in an excellent position to talk to children and their parents about concepts of hospitalization. Many times the parents cannot talk to their child about going to the hospital. The nurse can educate them in such groups as parent-teacher meetings about the need to talk to their children to prepare them for a specific hospitalization when this becomes necessary.

In certain schools children also learn how it feels to be ill or elderly through an experience called *simulation*. This is an attempt to help children learn how others feel by putting themselves in "the others' shoes." Such learning helps children to bridge the gap between their information and a change in their behavior towards others. As the children discover what it feels like to be old, blind, or chronically ill, they become more interested in staying healthy themselves.

Some schools are also beginning to offer information to the school child on the subject of death. This information may be discussed as part of the school health program or it may be integrated into various areas of the curriculum.

The role of the *school nurse* has changed since the era when a registered nurse was responsible for little more than the application of Band-aids, the screening of children for pediculosis, and the care of children in emergencies. Currently many school systems require the school nurse to have a baccalaureate degree, including general education and specific education in the area of community or public health nursing.

Programs for the specific education of the *school nurse practitioner* have been recently organized. The extended role of the school nurse practitioner in primary care serves to provide improved health care to children in the school setting and to take the basic responsibility for identifying and managing many of the health problems of children. The emphasis is more on preserving wellness within the psychosocial milieu of the child and his family rather than on curing illnesses. These programs should build on previous nursing skills and knowledge.

The role of the school nurse practitioner or school nurse has become complex, being primarily one of offering comprehensive well-child care and assessing factors that may produce problems in learning, as well as of physical disease. The nurse is a member of the school health team, which includes the principal of the school, teachers, school physician, dentist, social worker, psychologist, psychiatrist, guidance counselor, special education staff, and the school custodian and engineer, all of whom are concerned with the physical and mental health of children. It is the nurse's responsibility to develop the kind of relationship with members of the health team that encourages early case finding and referral and also adequate care of children. Local physicians and dentists should understand the school health program and wherein it supplements their services to children. Parents also should be interested in the program and participate, in some situations with their children, on the school health team.

The school nurse or school nurse practitioner many times is coordinator of the activities of the school health team and those of the local board of health, volunteer health agencies, medical clinics, and private physicians in providing the health program of the school. The nurse may also serve on the school's curriculum committee, giving emphasis to health matters in the curriculum. The nurse, in addition, may be the leader of the future nurse's club for those young students interested in nursing as a career.

Since the utilization of the services of the nonprofessional school health aide, the professional nurse is also the leader of the nursing team. The health aide, with the assistance of volunteers, may be responsible for much of the routine office procedures.

The reasons children usually visit the nurse are acute illness, injury or accident, general health evaluation, chronic illness, and behavior problems. The professional nurse is responsible for assessing the health of children as well as for their care during an emergency, such as when a child has a broken bone or an asthmatic attack, and for the care of those children having physical or emotional handicaps, mental retardation, or problems of delinquency.

Much of the nurse's time is taken in conferences with other members of the school health team, parent education and counseling, testing of children, implementation of vision and hearing screening tests, and visits to homes. The nurse visits the homes of children in order to learn more about their diets, living and sleeping accommodations, and interpersonal family relations and conflicts, among other observations. The nurse is attuned to the need for prevention and the need for motivating parents who for some reason do not follow suggestions made by members of the health team. As an observer, health counselor, and consultant the nurse cares for matters relating to the total health of children.

In some situations the school nurse or school nurse practitioner may hold conferences with parents whose children are beginning kindergarten to uncover health problems and to determine the presence of potential learning difficulties. As a health counselor who watches the children's overall well-being as they progress through the school grades, the nurse may also hold conferences with each graduating senior from high school to review his health record with him and to emphasize that his health after graduation is his own responsibility.

The role of the school nurse practitioner or school nurse is changing from one of being child-centered to being family-centered, and the emphasis in school health is truly being placed on strengths rather than weakness and on wellness rather than illness.

HEALTH PROBLEMS DURING SCHOOL AGE

Among the most important health problems of the school child is greater exposure to communicable diseases. Diseases against which he is immunized or which he had in the preschool period present no problem. The parents must be informed of the school regulations about keeping him home from school when he has a fever, cold, rash or other symptoms of communicable disease, to prevent exposing others.

A second health problem is to meet the needs of the handicapped child on entrance to school. His condition poses a special problem for school personnel. They are kept informed of the total habilitation or rehabilitation program being carried out and their specific part in it.

A third problem is presented by the older children, who can be told something about the physical changes they will experience at puberty. Both sexes are informed of this. Although parents talk over these matters with their children in order to maintain good parent-child rela-

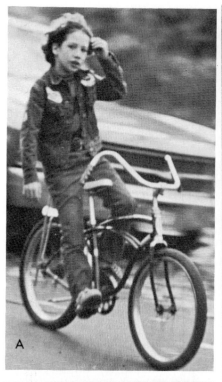

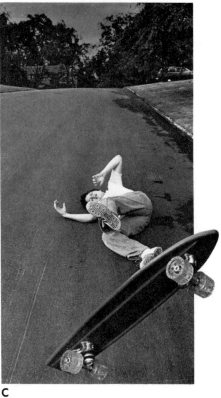

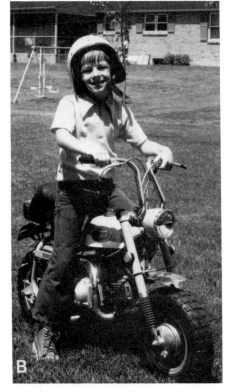

FIGURE 22–21. Accidents occur when children are careless while riding (A) bicycles, (B) motorbikes, or (C) skateboards. (C, Kesselman, J. R.: *Family Health/Today's Health*, 8:34, August 1976.)

tions, the school nurse practitioner, the school nurse, or a teacher may also discuss them individually or in class. The school nurse practitioner or school nurse may also find it necessary to discuss such matters with parents in order to help them educate their own children. Stressing the universality of the experience makes it less personal and more objective. Parents should know what the children are taught in school. Pictorial presentation is supplemented with discussion. The material is selected according to the interest, chronologic age, and level of understanding of the children. It should be factual and presented unemotionally. The child who is unprepared for the physical changes which accompany puberty may be terrified when they occur.

In our speeded-up society, which is overstimulating children of 11 or 12 years to go "steady," many parents are confused about how much restriction to place on their preteen's behavior. Children of this age are not ready emotionally for serious boy-girl involvement and are likely to welcome a firm parental "no" to this sort of behavior.

A fourth problem which has emerged is that of smoking and drug abuse including the increasing use of alcohol. Since the incidence of smoking and drug abuse is increasing even among children who have not yet reached puberty, many physicians and educators believe that programs on these subjects should begin in elementary school.

NUTRITION

During the school age caloric requirements per unit of body weight continue to decrease, but the nutritional requirements remain relatively greater than in a mature person.

Table 22–1 gives the nutritional requirements for children of school age.

School children usually eat well and have fewer food fads than preschool children. Eating problems relate more to the time of eating, e.g., whether it interferes with television programs or group activities, and the manner of eating than to the content and amount of food consumed. Since a child may be hungry after school, nourishment is necessary. Milk and fruit are preferable to candy and cookies.

Because the child wants to be like his peers, the kind of lunch he wants will depend on whether his friends take a lunch box to school or eat in the cafeteria. If the noon meal is not adequate, breakfast and dinner should make up for the deficiency.

School children can be helpful to their mothers at mealtime. They can help plan menus, set the table, shop for food, and wash dishes. Although these activities develop a sense of industry and responsibility, parents should not ask too much of young children, who spend many hours in school and require outdoor play to keep them well.

Eating Habits. Mealtime should be a pleasant, restful period in the day, but many parents do not keep it so because of overemphasis on manners. The child's eating habits will improve as he grows older.

The six-year-old stuffs his mouth, spills food and grabs for it and may be very talkative while eating. He is more interested in eating at the beginning than at the end of the meal. His appetite is good. He may refuse to use a napkin.

The seven-year-old talks less during the meal. He may bolt his food, but he is quieting down. His napkin may not remain in place.

Eight- and nine-year-olds eat more neatly, using napkins as their elders do. They are apt to

TABLE 22–1. *RECOMMENDED DAILY DIETARY ALLOWANCES FOR CHILDREN OF SCHOOL AGE (7 TO 10 YEARS)*

	WT.—30 KG. (66 POUNDS) HT.—135 CM. (54 INCHES)
K calories	2,400
Protein	36 g.
Fat-soluble vitamins	
Vitamin A activity	3,300 I.U.
Vitamin D	400 I.U.
Vitamin E activity	10 I.U.
Water-soluble vitamins	
Ascorbic acid	40 mg.
Folacin[a]	300 μg
Niacin[b]	16 mg.
Riboflavin	1.2 mg.
Thiamine	1.2 mg.
Vitamin B_6	1.2 mg.
Vitamin B_{12}	2.0 μg
Minerals	
Calcium	800 mg.
Phosphorus	800 mg.
Iodine	110 μg
Iron	10 mg.
Magnesium	250 mg.
Zinc	10 mg.

[a]The folacin allowances refer to dietary sources as determined by *Lactobacillus casei* assay. Pure forms of folacin may be effective in doses less than ¼ of the RDA.

[b]Although allowances are expressed as niacin, it is recognized that on the average 1 mg. of niacin is derived from each 60 mg. of dietary tryptophan.

From the Food and Nutrition Board, National Academy of Sciences–National Research Council: Recommended Daily Dietary Allowances (1974).

have better table manners in public than at home.

Ten- to twelve-years-olds eat an adult meal and have table manners similar to those of their parents, whether at home or elsewhere.

Children's eating habits would improve more rapidly if less stress were laid on table manners. A friendly atmosphere and enjoyment of the meal are the best aids to appetite.

EFFECTS OF SEPARATION

If the child has experienced good parent-child relations, he will probably suffer little trauma due to separation from his parents for short periods. The school child has learned to relate to adults and children outside his family and so is not emotionally disturbed when he is left with strange people. He knows the meaning of time gradations and is better able to tolerate separation from his parents. He knows when they will return. Prolonged separation, however, for weeks or months, as during hospitalization, is likely to produce emotional trauma. If his parents do not visit him frequently, particularly if he knows that they are able to come, he feels a sense of rejection which interacts with the physical strain of his illness or injury. The reasons for prolonged separation should be explained to the child in a factual, realistic way by a sympathetic adult, preferably one of his parents. Other evidences of parental love besides visiting should be shown him.

TEACHING AIDS AND OTHER INFORMATION*

American Academy of Pediatrics

Minibike Safety.
Recommendations for Preventive Health Care of Children and Youth.
School Health: A Guide for Physicians.
Smoking and Children: A Pediatric Viewpoint.

American Dental Association

A Visit to the Dentist.
Basic Brushing.
Your Child's Teeth.

American Nurses' Association

Recommendations on Educational Preparation and Definition of the Expanded Role and Functions of the School Nurse Practitioner, 1973.

Child Study Association of America

Brothers and Sisters Are Like That.
Children's Books of the Year 1975, 1976.
Families Are Like That.
Frank, J.: Television: How to Use It Wisely with Children, 1976.
What to Tell Your Child About Sex, Revised 1974.
When Children Ask About Sex, Revised 1974.

Department of National Health and Welfare: Ottawa, Canada

Learning about Family Life.
Playgrounds: A Plea for Utopia, or the Recycled Empty Lot.
Who Knows? (water safety).

Kimberly-Clark Corporation

Very Personally Yours.

National Council on Alcoholism, Inc.

Melquist, E. L.: Pepper, 1974.

National Society for the Prevention of Blindness, Inc.

TV and Your Eyes.

Personal Products Company

Boys: Have You Wondered What Happens When Girls Grow Up?

Estás Creciendo . . . ¡Divierte! (Growing Up and Liking It).
Growing Up and Liking It, 1975.
How Shall I Tell My Daughter?, 1973.

Public Affairs Committee

Archer, J., and Yahraes, D.: What Should Parents Expect from Children?
Barman, A.: Motivation and Your Child, 1975.
Bienvenu, M.: Talking It Over at Home.
Brenton, M.: Playmates: The Importance of Childhood Friendships.
Hill, M.: Drugs—Use, Misuse, Abuse.
Hofstein, S.: Talking to Preteenagers about Sex.
Hymes, J. L.: How to Tell Your Child about Sex.
Lambert, C.: Understand Your Child—From 6 to 12.
Neisser, E. G.: Your Child's Sense of Responsibility.
Ross, H.: The Shy Child.
Wolfe, A. G.: Differences Can Enrich Our Lives: Helping Children Prepare for Cultural Diversity.

United States Government

A Child's World, 1974.
Beautiful Junk, Reprinted 1974.
Body Dimensions and Proportions: White and Negro Children 6-11 Years, U.S., 1974.
Discovering Vegetables, 1975.
Family Background, Early Development and Intelligence of Children 6-11 Years, 1974.
Hazard Analysis of Injuries Relating to Playground Equipment, 1975.
Lettieri, D. J. (Ed.): Predicting Adolescent Drug Abuse: A Review of Issues, Methods and Correlates, 1975.
Research Relating to Children, 1975.
Skeletal Maturity of Children 6-11 Years, U.S., 1974.
Social Development in Young Children, 1976.
Teach Children Fire Will Burn, 1974.
Teaching Children about Safety Belts, 1973.
Your Child from 6 to 12, Reprinted 1974.

---

*Complete addresses are given in the Appendix.

REFERENCES

Books

Boston Children's Medical Center and Feinbloom, R. I.: *Child Health Encyclopedia: The Complete Guide for Parents.* New York, Delacorte Press, 1975.

Bower, E., et al.: *Learning to Play: Playing to Learn.* New York, Human Sciences Press, 1974.

Bryan, D. S.: *School Nursing in Transition.* St. Louis, The C. V. Mosby Company, 1973.

Burt, J. J., and Meeks, L. B.: *Education for Sexuality: Concepts and Programs for Teaching.* 2nd ed. Philadelphia, W. B. Saunders Company, 1975.

Caplan, F., and Caplan, T.: *The Power of Play.* New York, Doubleday Anchor Press, 1974.

Colew, C.: *How to Raise Your Child Without Threats or Violence.* Hicksville, N. Y., Exposition Press, 1974.

Comer, J., and Poussaint, A.: *Black Child Care.* New York, Simon & Schuster, 1975.

Cowen, E. L., et al.: *New Ways in School Mental Health: Early Detection and Prevention of School Maladaptation.* New York, Human Sciences Press, 1975.

Guthrie, H. A.: *Introductory Nutrition.* 3rd ed. St. Louis, The C. V. Mosby Company, 1975.

Helms, D., and Turner, J.: *Exploring Child Behavior.* Philadelphia, W. B. Saunders Company, 1976.

Hernandez, C. A., Haug, M. J., and Wagner, N. N.: *Chicanos: Social and Psychological Perspectives.* 2nd ed. St. Louis, The C. V. Mosby Company, 1976.

Johnson, E. W.: *How to Live Through Junior High School.* Philadelphia, J. B. Lippincott Company, 1975.

Knotts, G. R., and McGovern, J. P. (Eds.): *School Health Problems.* Springfield, Ill., Charles C Thomas, 1975.

Krause, M. V., and Hunscher, M. A.: *Food, Nutrition and Diet Therapy.* 5th ed. Philadelphia, W. B. Saunders Company, 1972.

Lamb, M. W., and Harden, M. L.: *The Meaning of Human Nutrition.* New York, Pergamon Press, 1973.

Lawrence, M. M.: *Young Inner City Families: Development of Ego Strength Under Stress.* New York, Behavioral Publications, Inc., 1975.

Lieberman, F., Caroff, P., and Gottesfeld, M.: *Before Addiction: How to Help Youth.* New York, Behavioral Publications, Inc., 1973.

Nemir, A., and Schaller, W. E.: *The School Health Program.* 4th ed. Philadelphia, W. B. Saunders Company, 1975.

Oliven, J. F.: *Clinical Sexuality: A Manual for the Physician and the Professions.* 3rd. ed. Philadelphia, J. B. Lippincott Company, 1974.

Piers, M. W. (Ed.): *Play and Development.* New York, W. W. Norton and Company, 1972.

Poland, R. G.: *Human Experience: A Psychology of Growth.* St. Louis, The C. V. Mosby Company, 1974.

Race, A. R., Leecraft, J. F., and Crist, T.: *The Sex Scene—Understanding Sexuality.* New York, Harper & Row, 1975.

Rebelsky, F., et al.: *Life: The Continuous Process; Readings in Human Development.* New York, Alfred A. Knopf, 1975.

Recommended Dietary Allowances. 8th ed. rev. Washington, D. C., National Academy of Sciences, National Research Council, 1974.

Sattler, J. M.: *The Assessment of Children's Intelligence.* Philadelphia, W. B. Saunders Company, 1975.

Toman, W.: *Family Constellation: Its Effects on Personality and Social Behavior.* 3rd ed. New York, Springer Publishing Company, 1976.

van der Linden, F. P. G. M., and Duterloo, H. S.: *Atlas on the Development of the Human Dentition.* New York, Harper and Row, 1976.

Vannier, M.: *Teaching Health in Elementary School.* 2nd ed. Philadelphia, Lea and Febiger, 1974.

Willgoose, C. E.: *Health Education in the Elementary School.* 4th ed. Philadelphia, W. B. Saunders Company, 1974.

Periodicals

Anderson, L. S.: When a Child Begins School. *Children Today,* 5:16, July-August 1976.

Auld, M. E., and Ehlke, G. A.: What Camp Nurses Need to Know. *Am. J. Nursing,* 74:662, April 1974.

Backman, H. A., Packard, N. J., and Reiner, A. C.: Camp Nursing: An Opportunity for Independent Practice in a Miniature Community. *The American Journal of Maternal Child Nursing,* 1:88, March-April 1976.

Bewley, B. R., Bland, J. M., and Harris, R.: Factors Associated With the Starting of Cigarette Smoking by Primary School Children. *Br. J. Prev. Soc. Med.,* 28:37, February 1974.

Bland, J. M., Bewley, B. R., and Day, I.: Primary Schoolboys: Image of Self and Smoker. *Brit. J. Prev. Soc. Med.,* 29:262, December 1975.

Boone, S. F.: A New Approach to School Health Records. *J. Sch. Health,* 44:156, March 1974.

Brown, M. S.: Summertime Care for Kids. *Nursing '75,* 5:50, July 1975.

Chinn, P.: Relationship Between Health and School Problems: A Nursing Assessment. *J. Sch. Health,* 43:85, February 1973.

Escalona, S. K.: Children in a Warring World. *Am. J. Orthopsychiatry,* 45:765, October 1975.

Frisch, R. E.: A Method of Prediction of Age of Menarche From Height and Weight at Ages 9 Through 13 Years. *Pediatrics,* 53:384, March 1974.

Green, R., and Fuller, M.: Family Doll Play and Female Identity in Pre-Adolescent Males. *Am. J. Orthopsychiatry,* 43:123, January 1973.

Greene, D., and Lepper, M. R.: Intrinsic Motivation: How To Turn Play into Work. *Psychology Today,* 8:49, September 1974.

Grunberg, E. M.: Standing Orders for the School Nurse. *Nursing '75,* 5:62, February 1975.

Hardin, D.: The School-Age Child and the School Nurse. *Am. J. Nursing,* 74:1476, August 1974.

Hilmar, N. A., and McAtee, P. A.: The School Nurse Practitioner and Her Practice: A Study of Traditional and Expanded Health Care Responsibilities for Nurses in Elementary School, *J. Sch. Health,* 43:431, September 1973.

Hopp, J. W.: Values Clarification and the School Nurse. *Nursing Digest,* 4:60, Fall 1976.

Igoe, J. B.: The School Nurse Practitioner. *Nursing Outlook,* 23:381, June 1975.

Jenny, J., and Frazier, P. J.: Parents' Attitudes About School Dental Services for Children. *J. Sch. Health,* 44:86, February 1974.

Kelson, S. R., Pullella, J. L., and Otterland, A.: The Growing Epidemic. A Survey of Smoking Habits and Attitudes Toward Smoking Among Students in Grades 7 Through 12 in Toledo and Lucas County (Ohio) Public Schools—1964 and 1971. *Am. J. Public Health,* 65:923, September 1975.

Kesselman, J. R.: "The Skateboard Menace." *Family Health/ Today's Health,* 8:34, August 1976.

Koocher, G. P.: Talking With Children About Death. *Am. J. Orthopsychiatry,* 44:404, April 1974.

Koocher, G. P.: 'Why Isn't The Gerbil Moving Anymore?' Discussing Death in the Classroom—And the Home. *Children Today,* 4:18, January-February 1975.

Lewis, C. E., and Lewis, M. A.: The Impact of Television Commercials on Health-Related Beliefs and Behaviors of Children. *Pediatrics,* 53:431, March 1974.

Lewis, C. E.; et al.: An Evaluation of the Impact of School Nurse Practitioners. *J. Sch. Health*, 44:331, June 1974.

Lewis, M. A.: Child-Initiated Care. *Am. J. Nursing*, 74:652, April 1974.

McGrath, P., and Laliberte, E. B.: Level of Basic Venereal Disease Knowledge Among Junior and Senior High School Nurses In Massachusetts: A Survey. *Nursing Research*, 23:31, January-February 1974.

Maxeiner, B. A., O'Rourke, T. W., and Stone, D. B.: Knowledge, Behavior, and Attitudes of Sixth-Grade Students Toward Family Life Education. *J. Sch. Health*, 46:81 February 1976.

Miller, G. P.: Bicycle Safety: A Game of Chance? *Children Today*, 4:12, January-February 1975.

Nader, P. R.: The School Health Service: Making Primary Care Effective. *Pediatr. Clin. N. Am.*, 21:57, February 1974.

Olgas, M.: The Relationship Between Parents' Health Status and Body Image of Their Children. *Nursing Research*, 23:319, July-August 1974.

Pasternack, S. B.: Annual Well-Child Visits. *Am. J. Nursing*, 74:1472, August 1974.

Pelizza, J. J.: A Comparative Study of How Parents From Different Social Classes Perceive School Health Services. *J. Sch. Health*, 43:176, March 1973.

Porter, C. S.: Grade School Children's Perceptions of Their Internal Body Parts. *Nursing Research*, 23:384, September-October 1974.

Quinn, J. M.: Do Animals Have Belly Buttons?: Sex Education at the Elementary School Level. *Children Today*, 5:2, September-October 1976.

Resnick, R., and Hergenroeder, E.: Children and the Emergency Room. *Children Today*, 4:5; September-October 1975.

Rosner, A. C.: Values Clarification and the School Nurse. *J. Sch. Health*, 45:410, September 1975.

Sehnert, K. W.: Understanding the Old or Infirm: Put Yourself in Their Place. *Family Health/Today's Health*, 8:38, April 1976.

Turcotte, C.: How Children See the Nurse. *The Canadian Nurse*, 71:41, April 1975.

AUDIOVISUAL MEDIA*

American Academy of Pediatrics

First Aid Chart
8½ × 11 inch chart.

American Dental Association

Basic Dental Health Education for Parents and Teachers
57 slides, color.
Designed to assist the dentist who is called upon to present a program to an audience of parents or to provide in-service education on dental health to teachers. Parents and teachers will recognize the solutions to problems and realize the importance of preventive dentistry.

Decay in Six-Year Molar Plaque
17¾ × 11¼ inch chart.

Development of the Human Dentition Chart
Schour, I., and Massler, M.
14⅞ × 12 inch chart, color, booklet.
Shows the development of both deciduous and permanent teeth.

Educacion de la Salud Dental Para Profesores
33 frames, 33⅓ RPM record, color.
This filmstrip, with Spanish titles, includes discussion of the process of tooth decay, prevalence of decay among children and the resultant loss of teeth, definitions of dental conditions that contribute to decay and can be corrected, diet and snacks, and the prevention of oral disease.

It's Up to You
6 minutes, 16mm film, sound, color.
Examples of dental disease are shown in children and adults. The results of dental neglect demonstrate the damaging effects of calculus on teeth and gums. Explains the formation of plaque and its relation to dental disease, along with the importance of using a disclosing agent. Detailed scenes show flossing and brushing techniques.

Learning About Your Oral Health
4 overhead transparencies, 12 prepared spirit masters, detailed content outline.
Program can be used from grades K through 12. You can use the entire program or only part of it to suit your particular needs.

Teeth Are for Life
15 minutes, 16mm, sound, color.
Three children help to teach young children about pre-ventive oral care and foster among them favorable attitudes toward dentistry. The function of the incisors, molars, cuspids, and bicuspids are explained and demonstrated. Dental health is discussed, as well as how the dentist helps us maintain healthy teeth.

The American Journal of Nursing Company

Growth and Development—Birth Through Adolescence
Class Instructor: Nicolay, R. C.
Series of 23 44 minute classes, black and white.

Play Activities: Ages 6-13
The importance of the influence of values, culture, seasonal patterns and mass media upon children from 6 to 13 years of age, is emphasized.

Peer Group: Ages 6-13
Participating Instructor: McConner, W. R.
Examples are given of the rise of conforming behavior and the group as a sign of increasing independence from parents; sex cleavages and maturational differences; changes in forms of sibling rivalry.

Sex Roles: Ages 6-13
Participating Instructor: Fitch, F.
The physical and psychological differences of boys and girls in this age group are examined. Effects of certain child rearing tendencies on children of both sexes and principles of sex education are discussed.

Cognitive Functioning: Ages 6-13
A description is given of the child's natural eagerness for learning. Included are symbol differentiation, need for competence and recognition, his learning to deal with abstractions and the increased effectiveness of his overall thought processes.

School and the Child
Participating Instructor: Samuels, I.
The influence on learning ability of the child's initial attitude toward school, relevance of material presented, teacher expectations, influence of cultural differences and cultural inconsistencies are demonstrated and discussed.

American Lung Association

Breathing Easy
27½ minutes, 16mm film, some animation, sound, color, booklet.

A youngster takes a trip into the brain (in reality a U.S. space computer center) and finds out how the human respiratory system works, in health and in the face of such enemies as cigarette smoking and air pollution.

Charles Press–Prentice-Hall, Inc.

The Role of the School in Death Education
Leviton, D.
27 minutes, tape.
Dr. Leviton expresses his views on a need for "formal death education" in the schools. He compares such education to sex education and stresses the value of an academic context. Discussion of the formal classroom situation, teacher and parent education, and the prospect of crisis intervention facilities are included.

McGraw-Hill Book Company

From Sociable Six to Noisy Nine
21 minutes, 16mm film, color.

From Ten to Twelve
26 minutes, 16mm film, color.

Reward and Punishment
14 minutes, 16mm film, color.

Metropolitan Life Insurance Company

The Time of Growing
29 minutes, film.
Depicts the behavior of a group of elementary school children as they interact with their teacher during an ordinary school day. Provides health professionals and parents with an insight into children's mental states. Viewers learn to recognize early signs of emotional difficulties in children and find ways to meet children's particular needs.

National Society for the Prevention of Blindness, Inc.

The Eyes Have It.
8 minutes, film, sound, printed materials.
Introduces children to the principles of eye safety. Stresses such factors as the importance of good lighting and the dangers of being careless with sharp objects.

Personal Products Company

Naturalamente . . . Una Muchacha (Naturally . . . A Girl)
13½ minutes, 16mm, color.
For Students 9 to 14.

Naturally . . . A Girl
13½ minutes, 16 mm, color.
For students 9–14.

Trainex Corporation

Accidents and Poisoning
35mm filmstrip, audio-tape cassettes, 33⅓ LP, color.
Defines the most common injury-causing home accidents, and tells how rooms can be made safer for children.

United States Government

Parents Are Teachers Too
Producer: USOEO
18 minutes, 16mm film, optical sound, black and white.
Discusses the role of parents as the child's first and continuing teachers, and points out that learning comes easier with a flow of understanding between school and home.

---

*Complete addresses are given in the Appendix.

Chapter Twenty-Three

THE SCHOOL CHILD IN THE EMERGENCY ROOM

The healthy school-age child is a very active young person who receives over the years decreasing amounts of supervision from his parents and other adults. In his seemingly endless effort to master new motor skills, he is likely to become injured if he has not learned the principles of safety and their application during his earlier experiences.

The major fear of the child of this age who is brought to the emergency room for injury or illness, in addition to bodily harm, is *a loss of self-control.* He may respond to treatment with verbal protests. He may cry, whimper, whine, groan, or scream. He can use sentences to acknowledge pain, to express fear or anger, and to ask questions to gain information. He may try to postpone treatment in his attempt to gain or maintain self-control and thus to appear brave.

On a nonverbal level the school-age child may evidence his attempt to maintain self-control by sitting or lying very quietly or rigidly still while treatment is being given. He may passively seek support, help, or body contact by changing his facial expression but not by verbally asking for it. When help or comfort is offered, he accepts it gladly. If he becomes very anxious, he may turn or pull away from the physician and nurse and try to escape. If he loses his self-control he may flail, kick, or bang his feet or hands against the table or stretcher on which he is lying.

The care of the school-age child in the emergency room situation is much like that of the preschool child (see p. 639). How the child of this age manages pain and anxiety depends on his level of development and his past experiences with injury, illness, and hospitalization. His perception of what the physicians and nurses are doing or will do to him is also important.

CONDITIONS OF THE SCHOOL CHILD REQUIRING IMMEDIATE OR SHORT-TERM CARE

In an effort to help the child understand what is happening, pictures or simple anatomic chart drawings can be made, and dolls can be used for demonstration purposes. School-age children also appreciate having medical terms or unfamiliar words that are used written down and explained. This shows that the nurse has confidence in their ability to learn and respect for their right to this kind of information. School-age children also enjoy reading about a procedure that is necessary for their care in a simple coloring book with clear step-by-step pictures. The information given should explain the purpose as well as the technique to be used. Many children of eight or nine years know something about the systems of the body and its functions. If they are asked what they think the procedures will be like, their answers provide clues to their fears and conceptual levels.

Although every child responds to stress in his own way, there are certain typical characteristics at each age to guide the nurse in explaining the situation to him. For instance, by the time the child is 11 or 12 years old he can almost reason in an adult manner and can largely control his anxiety under stress. The nurse can talk to a child of this age almost as if he were an adult.

The nurse can encourage the older child to verbalize fears he may have by asking questions such as "How were you hurt, Billy?" This is an invitation to a conversation and shows that the nurse is genuinely interested in him. The child will then talk about his accident. In doing so he will also provide some clues to his understanding of his present situation in the emergency room.

During the procedure or examination the child is given an explanation of when to be still or to lie in a certain position. If the treatment is going to be painful, the nurse can explain to him how much discomfort he will have and about how long it will last. The school-age boy especially needs to be given permission to cry when he is hurt.

After the procedure the child is praised for his cooperation. He may wish to talk about what has happened to him. The child may also play out his feelings by "treating" a doll as he was treated, releasing his positive or negative feelings and possible frustrations at the same time.

The way the child appraises his situation determines his emotional response to it. If he perceives that what is done is for his well-being, he reacts with a feeling of security. If he feels that there is something dangerous in his environment, his response is anxiety or fearfulness. School-age children misunderstand injury and related experiences; thus they may have anxiety. The nurse can help them to attain realistic concepts of bodily injury that help to moderate their fantasies and fortify their reality testing. When the nurse assesses and identifies these harmful misconceptions and fantasies and takes steps to correct them through explanation or other means, the child is helped to adjust to the situation in a more positive manner.

In summary, the nurse who cares for an injured or ill child is responsible for the anticipatory observation of any signs and symptoms of anxieties or fears arising from a loss of body integrity. The nurse can then correct or alleviate these anxieties and fears and help the child to maintain his self-control by comforting him, explaining to him what is happening, and providing any other available means of support.

HOSPITALIZATION OF THE SCHOOL CHILD

Because of medical advances and philosophical changes in thinking, more children are now treated on an outpatient basis in hospitals, and the number of days of hospitalization for each one admitted has been drastically reduced. This is important to the child between six and 12 years because hospitalization causes separation from his family, his school, and his friends.

The school child is usually able to accept his illness and separation from his parents better than does the preschool child. His reaction to hospitalization is related to his previous personality structure and to the nature of the parent-child relation.

Preparation for Hospitalization. Children of school age should have much the same kind of preparation for hospitalization as that given the preschool child (see p. 641). Because of his greater verbal ability the school child usually understands more readily the explanation given him. School children can read booklets about the hospitalization experience. The parents can adapt this material to the needs of the child. He is told the truth about the experience before him. He is assured that his parents will visit him as often as possible, and send cards and telephone so that he knows that they are thinking of him.

Response of the Child to Hospitalization. When a school-age child is admitted to the hospital he is probably outnumbered on the pediatric unit by younger children, and his needs may be overshadowed by theirs. The nurse should therefore understand his needs and respond to them in order to make his hospital experience a positive one, since most school children in spite of the preparation given for this new experience may believe that they caused their own illness, or were to blame for it in some way such as being "bad."

Children between six and eight years of age conform or rebel alternately against adult authority. If the child rebels, he will have guilt feelings and expect to be punished. When the rebellious act results in hospitalization, the therapy he is given may be viewed as punishment. The young school-age child also experiences renewed separation anxiety when he is away from his mother. He may evidence indications of this anxiety by enuresis, night terrors, insomnia, or nail-biting during his hospitalization.

Since the child from eight to ten years of age has a better developed ego, he can respond more appropriately to the limitations and requests of adults responsible for his care. The child has little real knowledge about how his body functions until he is about nine years of age, and even then he may have gross misconceptions mixed with truth. He may believe that he can get diabetes from eating too many desserts, a respiratory infection from not wearing his coat, a nosebleed from exercising too much, or osteomyelitis simply because he fell. He still has little understanding of the specific cause of illness and may feel that he has been singled out from his peer group for punishment.

The child from ten to 12 years of age has already experienced stress in school and is less likely to be disturbed by the problems of hospitalization. He may, however, be disturbed because of the lack of privacy, especially if he is self-conscious about the bodily changes accompanying puberty. He may also be anxious about his absence from school and his loss of friends, and have fear that permanent harm to his body may occur as a result of his illness or injury.

The hospitalized school-age child may be angry or anxious, and have various fears and fantasies. Children in general dislike staying in bed because mobility is important to them. The child's control of the outside world, his inner impulses, and his very self-preservation are achieved to a great degree through his own activity. *Immobilization, then, is probably the most difficult aspect of a child's illness.* When he is restricted in his activity he becomes anxious, and his anxiety leads to a need for greater activity. When he is confined to bed he has little outlet for his deep feelings, and he may become subject to fears and fantasies. He may overexercise when adults are not around or he may be frozen with his fears. If the child must be completely immobilized, he may become depressed and submit with hopeless resignation to his treatment. The child needs help in understanding his illness and must accept some responsibility for his own therapy.

The school-age child many times cannot express his emotion even though he can verbalize well on a variety of topics. He has conflict between being a child and expressing emotion through crying and being a more mature person and telling others how he feels in words. Thus his behavior may vacillate. Depending upon his age, it is difficult for him to express his feelings verbally when he is experiencing so many threats to his well-being at one time. He may

even have difficulty understanding his own fears and threats to his own body.

The fears of mutilation and death are very real for a school-age child. Experiences he has had in real life, read about in fiction, or has seen on television may have increased his fears. Experiences which necessitate "sleep," such as anesthesia with surgery and some diagnostic tests, may evoke fear to a sometimes seemingly unreasonable level unless it is understood from his point of view. When a school-age child says to another child who is leaving the hospital unit to have an appendectomy, "I'll see you in the morgue," he is expressing more than just words in jest.

The child may use several defenses in coping with his anxiety and fear. He may adopt an air of independence and bravado to cover up the fact that he feels helpless and afraid. If an adult whom he trusts, such as his nurse, remains with him, however, his ego is strengthened, and he will be less afraid.

He may want to dress exactly like his friend in the next bed to alleviate his anxiety about being "different," or he may want to engage in dramatic play with other children his age in the hospital unit so that he can approach his problems later with renewed strength. Belief in the use of magic words or actions may also serve to neutralize the child's anxiety about his aggressive feelings and fear of death. He may, for example, cross his fingers and, if possible, his toes before a medical procedure so that no harm will come to him.

In summary, the school child may feel guilty, anxious, angry, and fearful during his hospitalization. Emotions such as these are harmful and may retard his recovery from illness.

The Nurse and the School Child. The school child needs nurses who understand his level of growth and development, his needs, and the experiences he should have for continued personality growth while in the hospital. The nurse is warm, friendly, and fair, yet able to set reasonable limits to his behavior. Each child is seen as an individual who is having unavoidable frustrations due to his illness or injury. The nurse tries to provide satisfactions which make his situation more endurable.

In the hospital as at home friends of his own age are important to the school-age child; therefore he is introduced to other patients his age, and his bed placed near theirs. Since he is old enough to be reasoned with, he is given as many choices as possible in regard to his care. He is not, however, given a choice that the nurse will not accept. For example, the nurse should not ask, "Would you like to go to bed now?" If

Text continued on page 750

NURSING ADMISSION HISTORY 6–11 YEARS

DIAGNOSIS: ______

T ______ P ______ R ______ B.P. ______

HT. ______ WT. ______ ALLERGIES ______

PHYSICAL DESCRIPTION: ______

USE PLATE OR PRINT

M.R. No. ______ DATE ______
PT. NAME ______
PARENT ______
ADDRESS ______
DATE OF BIRTH ______ B.C. No. ______
M.A. No. ______
DIV. ______ CLIN. ______ P.P. DR. ______

Nickname ______ Age ______

Hist. From ______ Lang. ______

1. **FAMILY:** Household composition (i.e., parents, siblings, grandparents) ______

Names and ages of siblings ______

Primary caretaker for child ______

Does mother work ☐ YES ☐ NO If yes, who cares for child ______

How can parents usually be reached ______

Language spoken by parents ______

Any additional problems or changes in the family that might affect this child (i.e., births, deaths, illness, etc.) ______

2. **EATING PATTERNS:**

Example of typical day's meals (including type of food, amounts, and time)

Breakfast @	Lunch @	Supper @	Snacks @

Special likes ______ Dislikes ______

Vitamins ______

Appetite ☐ Good ☐ Fair ☐ Poor Comments ______

Special diet ☐ YES ☐ NO If yes, what ______

Any special religious or cultural preferences ______

Eating problems ______ How handled ______

3. **SLEEPING:**

Bedtime ______ Awakes at ______ Sleeping arrangements ______

Any sleep problems ☐ YES ☐ NO How handled ______

THE CHILDREN'S HOSPITAL MEDICAL CENTER, BOSTON, MASSACHUSETTS 02115

03596

FIGURE 23–1. Nursing admission history, ages 6 to 11 years. (From the Children's Hospital Medical Center, Boston, Mass.)

4. <u>ELIMINATION:</u>

Daily bowel movement ☐ YES ☐ NO If no, how often _____

Any problems with constipation or diarrhea ☐ YES ☐ NO If yes, how handled _____

Has daughter begun to menstruate ☐ YES ☐ NO If yes, any problems _____

_____

5. <u>PERSONAL HYGIENE:</u>

☐ Tub   ☐ Shower   ☐ Other _____

Washes hair - how frequently _____

Needs help with bathing ☐ YES ☐ NO If yes, explain _____

_____

Any dental appliances ☐ YES ☐ NO _____

6. <u>BEHAVIOR AND TEMPERAMENT:</u>

Mother's description of child's usual temperament _____

_____

Special fears _____

What seems to help child when he is distressed _____

_____

How does child usually react to stress (i.e., withdraw, display temper, etc.) _____

_____

Any behavior problems _____

_____

7. <u>INTERPERSONAL COMMUNICATION:</u>

Any problems with communication ☐ YES ☐ NO If yes, explain _____

_____

Uses hearing device ☐ YES ☐ NO Glasses ☐ YES ☐ NO

Is child timid with unfamiliar adults ☐ YES ☐ NO Friendly ☐ YES ☐ NO

How child relates to peers - ☐ Has many friends ☐ Few friends ☐ A loner

Does child have a pet ☐ YES ☐ NO If yes, what _____

Is this the child's first experience away from home ☐ YES ☐ NO

8. <u>ACTIVITY AND RECREATION:</u>

Utilizes - ☐ Wheelchair ☐ Crutches ☐ Braces ☐ Other _____

Favorite recreational activities _____

Does child enjoy T.V. ☐ YES ☐ NO Radio ☐ YES ☐ NO Reading ☐ YES ☐ NO

Favorite T.V. programs _____

Any parental rules regarding T.V. _____

Are there any particular activities that could be done in bed that your child would like_____

_____

Hobbies _____ Clubs _____

FIGURE 23-1 *Continued.*

9. **SCHOOL:**

Grade _____ Name of School _____

Marks ☐ Good ☐ Fair ☐ Poor   Any school problems ☐ YES ☐ NO   If yes, explain _____

_____

10. **PAST AND PRESENT HEALTH CARE:**

Has child been hospitalized before ☐ YES ☐ NO   When _____

Where _____ Why_____

How did he react while in the hospital_____

_____

Any problems after discharge _____

Primary care received from _____

Any other health agencies involved with child or family (i.e., V.N.A., etc.) _____

Has been or is presently involved with any CHMC facility (i.e., clinics, etc.) _____

_____

IMMUNIZATIONS

Has child been properly immunized _____

_____

11. **ADJUSTMENT TO ILLNESS - PARENT AND CHILD:**

What is child's understanding of his illness _____

_____

Have you, or has anyone else, explained any possible procedures, etc., to the child ☐ YES ☐ NO   By whom _____

Explain _____

How has child reacted to his illness (i.e., behavior changes, withdrawn, angry, etc.) _____

_____

Is there anything about his present or past illness which particularly upsets the child (i.e., fears injections, etc.) ☐ YES ☐ NO

_____

Does he take medicines at home ☐ YES ☐ NO   What _____

How _____

Does child administer them himself _____

Any problems _____

What medication has he had today _____

Does the child do any of his care himself (i.e., diabetic – gives injections, tests urine, etc.)

Explain _____

_____

_____

_____

_____

FIGURE 23–1 *Continued.*

PARENT

What is your understanding of your child's illness _____

_____

_____

How are you presently involved in your child's care (i.e., give medicines, do P.T., regulate special diet, etc.)

_____

_____

How would you like to participate in your child's care in the hospital _____

_____

_____

How much time will you be spending with your child in the hospital _____

_____

_____

Are there any aspects of your child's care that you already know you would like to be taught or have reviewed

_____

_____

What changes in your home routine have occurred due to the child's illness _____

_____

_____

12. **QUESTIONS ASKED BY PARENT AND/OR CHILD:**

_____

_____

_____

13. **ADDITIONAL OBSERVATIONS DURING INTERVIEW:**

_____

_____

_____

14. **INITIAL NURSING PROBLEMS FOR CARE PLAN:**

    1. _____

    2. _____

    3. _____

    4. _____

    Comments _____

_____

_____

_____

Date: _____ Nurse Interviewer: _____

FIGURE 23–1 *Continued.*

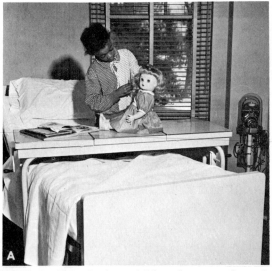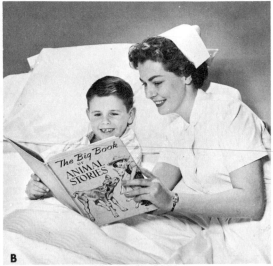

FIGURE 23–2.   The school-age child needs nurses who understand his need for rest and the experiences he should have for continued development while in the hospital. *A*, The nurse may provide toys which the child wants to play with in bed so that she gets the rest she needs. *B*, The nurse may encourage another child to improve his reading skill while he is hospitalized. (Courtesy of H. Armstrong Roberts.)

the child says "No!", then the nurse has the problem of enforcing a hospital rule against the child's decision.

If painful treatments must be done, the understanding nurse will realize how important it is, especially to the boy, to control his tears and "be brave." He is, therefore, moved to an area away from other children so that he can cry without losing "face."

As with the younger child, the school-age child responds best to positive suggestions spoken in a pleasant, encouraging, not bossy, manner. Since the child should have learned to say "Please" and "Thank you," the nurse should reinforce such manners by remembering to say these words.

The nurse should emphasize the positive aspects of the child's behavior, avoiding the use of value judgments such as, "You are a bad boy." Instead, the nurse can specifically say, "You may not hurt Billy." Limits should be set in a nonpunitive way, and love should not be withheld for misbehavior. The child continues his trust in others if he is treated honestly. The nurse who says, "The doctor will not let you go home if you don't eat," or "I will not let your mother come to see you if you do not cooperate with me," is putting little of the knowledge of the growth and development of the child into practice and is certain to fail. If the nurse takes time to listen to the child in a warm, interested manner and talks to him on his level, there will be little trouble gaining his cooperation.

Problems which the nurse must help the child solve are those of his feelings of guilt, fear of

physical harm, anxiety, and anger. The child who is very much affected by his condition will talk less about it than one not so deeply concerned. The nurse must use every bit of ingenuity to break down the emotional barrier set by the child.

If the child cannot verbalize his feelings, the nurse can help him to express himself through drawings or the use of creative materials such as papier-mâché or clay. Many times children can express their thoughts better in a group than they can alone with the nurse. If such a session can be "taped," it can be played back to the group in order to stimulate further conversation. If an older child can write, he may sometimes express his feelings about his hospitalization in a letter to a friend at home. When using any of these methods, the nurse must understand each child and anticipate his individual response to illness. Through perception and appreciation of his subtle cues, the nurse can understand the child's real feelings and his need for comfort and explanation about what is happening to him.

The nurse must help the child understand that illness occurs whether he is "good" or "bad." The nurse should encourage the child to talk of his ideas about the cause of his illness and give him factual information as to the real cause of his condition. The nurse should use various tools to help explain to him the physiologic problem and the necessity for his inactivity. Models or pictures of the heart or other organs of the body, plastic models of the visible man and visible woman, and line drawings of the body may also be used to indicate what is to be done during certain procedures. The nurse must further help the child to overcome his fear by describing what is to be done, by telling him that the treatment will help him to feel better eventually, although it may hurt for a while, by permitting him to handle the equipment used, and by encouraging him to help her with the procedure. Such equipment as syringes and needles, which have hurt him in the past, an oxygen tent, which can cut him off from his friends, and traction, which prevents him from moving, must be completely explained.

Since the child as he grows through school age is curious and eager to learn, the nurse should remember the level of his understanding at various ages and tailor the teaching to his ability to comprehend. Although the six- to 12-year-old child has better ability to cope with stress than a younger child, he still needs the opportunity to discuss his fears and fantasies of illness or injury with a meaningful adult, his parents, or a nurse whom he trusts.

The feeling of anger previously discussed may be shown by the child either verbally or through actions. The child may actually say that he hates the nurse, even though he knows that he has had good care, or he may refuse to comply with requests. The understanding nurse accepts the child's emotion, but sets a limit on his further active expression of it. The nurse might say, "I realize that you are very angry, Joey, but I cannot permit you to throw your books on the floor. Could you tell me how you feel?" If the nurse is calm, the child can verbalize his emotion without acting it out further. Sometimes simply by reflecting the emotion a child shows by saying, "You feel angry, Joey," the nurse can make the child feel understood and perhaps open the door to further communication with him.

When school children have many frustrations during the day and are forced to keep strict self-control, they often release their aggression and tension during the hours when the evening nurse is alone on the unit. This nurse may be faced with pillow fights, arguments, toys thrown on the floor, or paper wads hurled from bed to bed.

The best way to handle this situation is by prevention. The children should have the opportunity during the day to use their aggression in constructive activities. Ambulatory as well as bed patients can have self-directive physical activity under supervision of the Play Lady, recreational therapist, or volunteers.

The nurse can also permit the child to help plan his daily schedule, thereby building up his self-confidence. The nurse should visit him frequently. If the physician permits, another child's bed can be brought close enough for them to play together. The child may also enjoy making his own rules for keeping himself quiet. If he continues to be aggressive, his behavior should be brought to the attention of the physician, who may recommend further psychologic help or treatment.

Children have preconceived notions of what the nurse will be like. If the child perceives qualities of his parents in his nurse, he may react as he does to them. For this reason he may not react to his nurse in terms of how the nurse reacts to him, but rather as he is accustomed to react to his parents. Such behavior gives a clue to his past experience and to his needs for guidance.

The school child normally does not like an adult hovering over him and protecting him; but when he is injured or ill, he wants adult protection and support. A boy especially may think of nurses as a threat to his independence, yet when a painful procedure is to be done, even he will seek the nurse for strength and support.

Hospital and community nurses should learn ways to help convalescent children to be constructively happy. Hospitalized children enjoy continuing the collections they started at home themselves and starting new collections better adapted to items found in the hospital. They may collect empty antibiotic bottles, paper cups or greeting cards. They may enjoy reading, playing table games, listening to the radio, and watching television. The nurse must supervise these activities so that they will not be too exciting for the children.

School children who enjoy assuming responsibility and caring for younger children may help in the hospital unit during convalescence. This will help them gain confidence and recognition and acquire skills. They may cooperate in cleaning up the playroom and the schoolroom in the afternoon. They may help to put away supplies and pass nourishment. Often they can help feed younger children, read to them, or play with them. This enables the older children to identify with adults in the unit and gives them a feeling of self-confidence.

Physical Care of the Child. School children who have become fairly independent in caring for themselves become embarrassed when they are ill because they are physically cared for by the nurse. This is especially true of boys ten years of age or older. The nurse should remember that the school-age child can contribute to his own physical care in the matters of bathing, feeding, and dressing unless he is too ill or handicapped to do so. If he cannot care for himself, the nurse should help the child to accept the situation and cooperate rather than feel that he is forced to submit because it is the custom in the hospital. The child associates such care with being a baby and feels threatened by his loss of power. It is a good plan to speak casually of the care adult patients receive, asking a young boy or girl whether he or she would like to be a nurse or telling a boy of nursing in the military service. The child should be encouraged to regain his independence as soon as he is physically able to do so. Normally he is anxious to do all that he can for himself. This, in part, is the reason why children of school age enjoy wearing regular clothing instead of hospital gowns, because this indicates that they are no longer very ill. The nurse should also recognize the fact that the older school child can and should have an opportunity to participate and cooperate with his parents in the efforts of the health and nursing teams.

School children have learned the terminology of their group, especially in connection with urination, defecation, and the organs of reproduction. The nurse should understand that the child learned his attitudes and expressions at home and from his friends. To make him feel ashamed of the only terms which sound familiar to him would cause a younger child to feel that he was among strangers who did not love him. He might be afraid to tell the nurse when he again needed to go to the toilet. In school he asks to be excused, but that request does not fit the hospital situation. The older child may feel that the nurse rejects him because he comes from a low socioeconomic class. His sense of worth, his self-image, is hurt, and he may withdraw from the situation.

The child from eight to 11 years may have sleep phobias associated with fears of dying, especially when he first realizes the irreversibility of death. These may occur in the hospital when he is physically ill, especially when he is frightened because of impending surgery and possible loss of control of body functions. The nurse should comfort the child and remain with him until he is quiet.

School in the Hospital. Children hospitalized for short-term care may not have the time to become actively involved in school work as do those children requiring long-term hospitalization. Nevertheless the individual child may need the support of a visiting teacher even though he is in the hospital for only a few days. The nurse needs to understand the importance of school to the child and should encourage communication between the child and his teacher, if possible, so that he can return to his class when he is discharged. For a more complete discussion of the education of the hospitalized child see Chapter 24.

ACUTE CONDITIONS

EPISTAXIS (NASAL HEMORRHAGE, NOSEBLEED)

Incidence, Etiology, Clinical Manifestations, Treatment and Responsibilities of the Nurse. Epistaxis is common throughout childhood, especially during the school age, but the incidence decreases after puberty. It is caused by external trauma, foreign bodies, forcible blowing of the nose, or picking the nose. Allergic rhinitis or sinusitis may also lead to nosebleed. The strain of emotional excitement or physical exercise may be enough to start nasal bleeding. A circulatory, renal, or emotional condition which produces an elevation of blood pressure may cause nasal hemorrhage. It may also result from rheumatic fever, a blood dyscrasia, or an infection. As girls reach puberty, epistaxis may occur as vicarious menstruation.

The onset is sudden. Blood may flow from one or both nostrils. Bleeding is usually minimal and stops spontaneously, but it may be fatal if the child has a hemorrhagic disease.

The child is kept in a semi-erect position, with his head tilted forward to prevent blood trickling posteriorly into the pharynx. If the child swallows blood, he may become nauseated and vomit "coffee-ground" material.

His clothing is loosened around the neck. He should not blow his nose. An ice bag over the bridge of the nose is helpful. Gentle but firm compression of the nasal alae against the septum is made. A solution of epinephrine may be applied to the nasal mucous membrane with a cotton applicator (epinephrine is a vasoconstrictor). A tampon made of a piece of salt pork (fatback), which has been shaped to fit the nostril may be used to stop the bleeding. In more severe cases packing the nares may be necessary. If a bleeding site can be found, the physician may cauterize the point of bleeding with silver nitrate. In hemorrhagic disease blood transfusion may be required if much blood is lost.

RESPIRATORY INFECTIONS AND COMMUNICABLE DISEASES

Incidence and Care. If the child has not had the common communicable diseases in the preschool period, he is likely to get them when he goes to school because of close contact with many children. For the same reason the child is prone to respiratory infections. This is especially true if he comes from a small family in which he is overprotected or has been brought up in a rural area where infections are less common. The greatest *incidence* of infections is in the first grade.

Health teaching should begin in the early grades. The child is taught to cover his mouth with his handkerchief when coughing and to turn his face toward the floor. This is particularly necessary at the table, where coughing would spread droplets on food. He should not contaminate his hands and then contaminate toys, books, door knobs, and other objects which others touch.

Children should be dressed according to the temperature and protected from rain and snow with raincoats, hoods and boots. They can be taught to come home to change their clothing if they get wet. (If the mother scolds them for getting wet, they will not come home at once, but will wait, hoping to dry off before she sees them.) Teachers can make provision for children caught in the rain on the way to school.

Every teacher can tell classes to report symptoms of a cold, sore throat, or other illness. The children should be taught to wash their hands when contaminated and always before eating. It is essential, but difficult, to teach them not to offer each other bits of candy, apples, laps of ice cream cones, and sucks of pop from the bottle or common straw, because they think it friendly and generous to share what they have with another child.

Children should be kept away from others who have respiratory infections. The child with an infection is not sent to school. If he comes and the teacher finds that he is sick, the teacher or the school nurse may send him home, provided there is someone there to care for him, or should telephone for his mother to come for him. If there is no adult at home to receive him, the child may be kept in the infirmary. If the school has no infirmary, and his condition permits, he is placed in the rear of the classroom away from other children. If someone comes for the child, he should be told how to care for him. Such instruction includes home isolation technique and how to make paper bags to receive the child's paper handkerchiefs. Immunization techniques should be recommended if necessary. If the child is so sick that he will need considerable nursing care, the mother is helped to schedule her time so that she gets enough rest.

SINUSITIS

The sphenoidal sinus, the maxillary antrums, and the anterior and posterior ethmoid cells are present at birth. The frontal sinuses develop from the anterior ethmoid cells. Although sinusitis may occur at any time, it is most common during childhood in the school-age period.

ACUTE PURULENT SINUSITIS

Clinical Manifestations, Diagnosis, Complications, and Treatment. The sinuses may be involved during acute nasal infections (see p. 395), but there may also be acute inflammations and empyema of one or more sinuses that may be of greater importance clinically.

Clinical manifestations of sinusitis include rhinitis, elevation of temperature, localized pain or tenderness to pressure over the sinuses, a sense of fullness, headache, and perhaps edema over the area of the infected sinus. A purulent discharge may be seen through a nasoscope. When the infant or small child has acute ethmoiditis, periorbital cellulitis with redness of the skin and edema of the soft tissues may be present.

Diagnosis is made by roentgenography (the frontal or maxillary sinus is filled with pus and is opaque), or transillumination of the sinuses.

Complications of sinusitis include otitis media (see p. 399), meningitis (see p. 660), optic neuritis, orbital cellulitis and abscess, cavernous sinus thrombosis, and nephritis (see p. 664).

Treatment of sinusitis consists of shrinking the nasal mucous membranes to increase drainage from the sinus, gentle suction or aspiration of the purulent material, antibiotic therapy on the basis of nasal and nasopharyngeal cultures and smears, and drainage of the affected sinus if there are persistent symptoms.

CHRONIC SINUSITIS

Etiology, Clinical Manifestations, Complications, and Treatment. Chronic sinusitis occurs when there is a local or generalized problem that encourages the persistence of infection, such as nasal deformities, infected hypertrophied adenoids, allergy, or infected teeth. Children who have cystic fibrosis (see p. 444) with a lack of secretory antibodies and children with other immunodeficiency states may also have chronic sinusitis.

Clinical manifestations include low-grade fever, malaise, fatigue, anorexia, and nasal discharge. Complete nasal obstruction may occur because of swelling of the middle turbinates. Frequent sneezing, postnasal drip or constant purulent discharge leading to a chronic cough, pharyngeal irritation, mouth-breathing, headaches, and tenderness on palpation of the sinuses may also occur.

Complications of acute sinusitis may also occur in children having chronic sinusitis. In addition, "sinobronchitis" or a chronic infection of the bronchi may occur. This is especially true in children who have cystic fibrosis.

Treatment is based on the results of a culture of the drainage from the involved sinus. The usual organisms found are pneumococci, staphylococci, streptococci, and *H. influenzae.* Systemic antibiotics and nasal decongestants are of value. The mucous membranes can be shrunken through the use of ephedrine or Neo-Synephrine nose drops, given in such a way that the solution can enter the sinuses. Local heat may be applied to the sinus areas two to three times a day. If necessary, obstructive nasal deformities are corrected and hypertrophied infected adenoid tissue is removed.

Responsibilities of the Nurse in the Care of the Child Having Sinusitis. The goal of therapy is to facilitate the drainage of purulent material from the affected sinus. The instillation of nose drops, the application of local heat, and an increase of humidity in the air are important methods for achieving this purpose.

Nose drops are administered after the nasal passages are gently but thoroughly cleaned. For the procedure of giving nose drops to an infant, see page 399. In order to give nose drops to an older child he can be placed on his side with a folded blanket under his shoulder and with his head in a dependent position. The nasal solution is instilled and the child is instructed to breathe through his mouth in order to prevent the medication from being drawn into the pharynx. This position is maintained for approximately five minutes. If the child then sits up and puts his head down between his knees, drainage of the nasal contents can be expected.

Local heat may be applied to the affected area in the form of warm moist compresses. A humidifier may be used to increase the water vapor in the air in order to liquefy the secretions and to facilitate the process of drainage.

Since these patients have an elevation of temperature, the temperature should be monitored frequently. Cool sponge baths and antipyretics may be given to reduce fever. Increased fluid intake should be encouraged.

If periorbital edema is present, warm moist compresses may be applied. Any drainage from the eyes should be reported, in addition to the extent of tissue swelling and the ability of the child to open his eyes.

The nurse is responsible for assessing the child's response to treatment, including the degree of his temperature, the amount of purulent nasal drainage and its change of consistency to more watery and clear drainage as his condition improves, and the condition of his eyes and the

periorbital tissue around them. The nurse also observes for evidence of complications such as crying, complaining of an earache, tugging at his ear, or holding his hand over his ear, all of which may be indications of otitis media. Indications of neurologic problems must be reported promptly.

If the child is hospitalized, the nurse is responsible for providing the nursing care, but if the child is to be cared for at home, the nurse is responsible for teaching the parents the general care and the prescribed treatments to be given.

RINGWORM (TINEA)

Ringworm is a superficial fungus infection of the skin. Ringworm is classified according to the area of the body affected or the shape of the lesion produced. Since several fungi may cause ringworm, laboratory examination is often necessary before adequate treatment can be carried out. All types of ringworm are contagious.

RINGWORM OF THE SCALP (TINEA CAPITIS)

Incidence and Etiology. This condition, practically limited to children, is common among neglected children. It is a serious problem in schools of disorganized, low-income urban areas.

In the United States the most common causative agent is *Microsporum audouini.* This infection is transmitted by human beings and is highly infectious. *Microsporum canis* is transmitted from an animal. These conditions tend to disappear spontaneously at puberty.

Infection may begin at the base of a single hair, but it spreads in a circular fashion, forming lesions up to 2 inches in diameter. The spores of the fungus invading the hair at the base cause the hair to break off close to the skin, leaving a bald area. The scalp here becomes red, and grayish scales appear. A secondary infection may occur. The child may complain of mild itching.

Diagnosis, Treatment, Responsibilities of the Nurse, and Prognosis. The *diagnosis* is made by examination of the scalp under a beam of ultraviolet light from a Wood's lamp. Microscopic examination of extracted hairs may also be made.

The response to *treatment* with griseofulvin administered orally is good. The lesions can be cured in seven to ten days. Locally, a strong antifungal ointment such as Whitfield's ointment can be used. The nurse can teach parents that the head should be covered with cloth or a stockinet skull cap. This is washed and boiled each day to prevent spread of the infection. The child can be considered cured when a direct microscopic examination and a culture are negative.

The *prognosis* is good.

RINGWORM OF THE SKIN (TINEA CORPORIS; TINEA CRURIS)

There are two types of ringworm of the skin: tinea corporis and tinea cruris.

The lesions of *tinea corporis* are on the neck, face, forearms, and hands. The lesions begin as rounded or slightly irregular, reddish-pink, pea-sized, slightly raised, scaly patches. The centers of the patches clear, and the periphery spreads. The outline takes on the form of a ring. Mild itching is present.

The lesions of *tinea cruris* (jockstrap itch) occur in the groin. Local warmth in the affected area causes inflammation, itching, and infection, with small pustule formation.

Treatment, Responsibilities of the Nurse, and Prognosis. The response to *treatment* with griseofulvin and topical therapy such as an ointment containing hydrocortisone is good. Whitfield's ointment may also be used. The nurse can teach parents that the intertriginous areas are to be kept clean and dry. Frequent bathing with careful removal of the soap is necessary. Aeration of the affected areas can occur if loose-fitting, absorbent, nonbinding clothing is worn.

With treatment, the *prognosis* is excellent.

RINGWORM OF THE FEET (TINEA PEDIS) (ATHLETE'S FOOT)

Etiology and Incidence. Tinea pedis is usually caused by *E. floccosum, T. rubrum,* and *T. interdigitale.* This condition is common among school children during the summer months. The infection comes from other children and adults. It is acquired at swimming pools and other places where people go barefoot. The infection usually appears between the toes. There is no scale formation, but the superficial epithelium is macerated and desquamates. The raw surface is often fissured. Itching is intense, and pain may follow if the child rubs or scratches the area.

Treatment, Responsibilities of the Nurse, and Prevention. Ointment such as Desenex or Whitfield's ointment should be applied. The feet may also be soaked in Burow's solution. The nurse can teach parents that stockings and other foot coverings contaminated by the fungus should be sterilized or discarded. Light, ventilated shoes which reduce sweating are less aggravating to the condition than heavy footwear.

As a preventive measure children should wear shoes when walking where others are going barefoot and contaminating the area. Infected persons should stay away from swimming pools, gymnasium dressing rooms, and all places where they may spread infection.

PEDICULOSIS

Types, Etiology, and Incidence. There are three types of pediculosis in children: (1) pediculosis capitis, or infestation with the head louse, which is exceedingly common among neglected children; (2) pediculosis corporis, or infestation with the body louse; and (3) pediculosis pubis, or infestation with the crab louse. Since pediculosis capitis is the most common type in children, only this will be discussed here.

Pediculus capitis, or head louse, is present on the scalp, and the ova (eggs) or nits are attached to the hair. The ova are grayish, translucent, oval bodies which adhere to the shaft of a hair. They hatch in three or four days. The lice are usually seen on the heads of neglected, unclean children. They are easily transferred from child to child in schoolrooms and in tenement areas. They are more common among children wearing their hair long.

Clinical Manifestations, Treatment, and Responsibilities of the Nurse. There is severe itching of the scalp. Scratching leads to excoriation with serous, purulent, or sanguineous exudation. Crusts form, and the hair is matted.

The posterior cervical lymph nodes become infected from the scalp lesions. Excoriations may be present on the face and neck.

Treatment and *nursing care* are effective. The aims of therapy are to kill the pediculi, devitalize nits, and bring relief to the child. All inflamed areas must be healed. Clothing is dry cleaned or laundered and ironed. Treatment in the evening with a 2 per cent benzyl benzoate–20 per cent benzocaine emulsion or with gamma benzene hexachloride, followed by a shampoo in the morning effects a cure. Treatment may be repeated as often as necessary on the physician's order. Nits may be removed by combing the hair with a fine-tooth metal comb dipped in hot vinegar. If the hair is heavily infested, it may be advisable to cut it. If pustules are present on the neck and face, an antibiotic may be used. Children are cautioned not to exchange hats with other children. The remainder of the family is also examined for infestation. They are referred to the local public health agency so that the home can be evaluated and so that the nurse can encourage the family to go to the clinic for examination. Depending on the situation, this may lead into general health teaching of the total family unit.

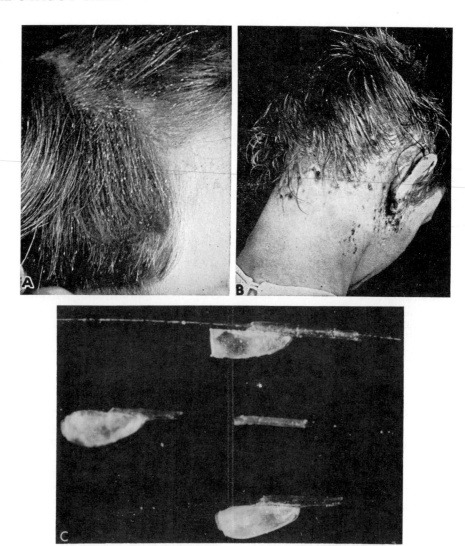

FIGURE 23–3. Pediculosis capitis. *A*, Numerous nits are visible. *B*, Impetiginous lesions frequently develop secondary to scratching, especially in children. (Lewis and Wheeler: *Practical Dermatology.* 3rd ed., Philadelphia, W. B. Saunders Co., 1966.) *C*, Nits on hairs. (Moschella, S. L., Pillsbury, D. M., and Hurley, H. J.: *Dermatology.* Philadelphia, W. B. Saunders Co., 1975.)

SCABIES

Etiology and Clinical Manifestations. Scabies is caused by *Acarus scabiei (Sarcoptes scabiei)*, or itch mite. The female acarus burrows under the skin to deposit her eggs. The itch mite is easily transmissible from person to person. The body is involved where the skin is moist and thin, between the fingers or toes, on the wrists, in the axillae and around the abdomen and genitalia. The path where the mite burrows under the skin, about ½ inch in length, but superficial, may be seen easily. Secondary infections with papules, vesicles or pustules may occur. Itching is intense.

Treatment and Responsibilities of the Nurse. The objectives of care are to kill the parasite and to relieve the itching. *Treatment* consists of a prolonged hot soaking bath followed by two applications of 15 per cent benzyl benzoate emulsion or a 1 per cent gamma benzene hexachloride lotion or cream at intervals of 12 hours. Twelve hours after the last application another hot bath should be taken. Treatment is effective within 48 hours. A broad-spectrum antibiotic can be used to treat secondary bacterial infection. Hydrocortisone cream 0.5 per cent can be applied to counteract the irritative reaction. Treatment includes all infected persons in the household so that all mites are killed simultaneously. All contaminated clothing and bed linen must be dry cleaned or boiled.

For **impetigo contagiosa** (see Plate 2, Fig. 6) and **Furunculosis** see page 266.

CONTACT DERMATITIS (POISON IVY)

Incidence, Etiology and Clinical Manifestations. Contact dermatitis is the most frequent

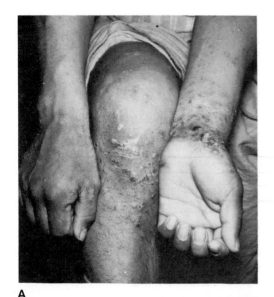

A

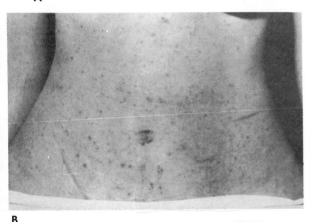

B

FIGURE 23-4. Scabies. *A,* Scabies with bacterial infection. (Moschella, S. L., Pillsbury, D. M., and Hurley, H. J.: *Dermatology.* Philadelphia, W. B. Saunders Co., 1975.) *B,* Excoriations over abdomen and lesions in the umbilicus. (Lewis and Wheeler: *Practical Dermatology.* 3rd ed. Philadelphia, W. B. Saunders Co., 1966.)

type of dermatitis which occurs during the school-age years. Although airborne allergens, chemicals found in clothing and shoes, and toys may cause allergic reactions, vines and weeds, particularly poison ivy *(Rhus toxicodendron),* are the most common offenders. School-age children are not as closely supervised by adults as they were when younger and may roam into areas where weeds are prevalent. Thus they come into repeated contact with potentially poisonous plants.

The skin response depends on the level of the child's sensitivity. The response may vary from reddening of the skin and edema to the formation of blisters with severe itching. The dermatitis occurs on exposed surfaces, but may be carried to covered surfaces by the hands. If no further contact is made with the plant, the dermatitis disappears in about two weeks.

Treatment, Responsibilities of the Nurse, and Prevention. The *treatment* of poison ivy contact dermatitis consists in eliminating further contact with the weed, and the use of corticosteroids locally or systemically to reduce the inflammatory reaction. These drugs are most effective when given before the formation of blisters. Soothing substances such as calamine lotion may be used to relieve the itching.

This type of dermatitis can be prevented best by avoiding contact with the plant. The child should learn to recognize this particular weed by the shape and configuration of its leaves, although they are by no means uniform. If the child does come in contact with the plant, immediate and thorough cleansing of the skin can reduce the possibility of a dermatitis. Hyposensitization to the allergen may be attempted during the spring months.

INSECT ALLERGY

Etiology, Clinical Manifestations, and Diagnosis. Insects can cause allergy in children in three ways: (1) a respiratory allergy may occur as a result of inhaling debri of insects; (2) local cutaneous reactions may occur as a result of insect bites; (3) anaphylactic reactions may occur as a result of the sting of an insect.

The *clinical manifestations* of insect allergy depend on the etiology of each. The child who has an inhalant allergy may develop conjunctivitis, rhinitis (see p. 691), or asthma (see p. 689). One who has been bitten by an insect may develop urticaria or papular, vesicular, and erythematous eruptions. Delayed hypersensitivity reactions may also occur.

The child who has been stung by an insect may have pain and a local papule or wheal with erythema at the site, and he may have edema of

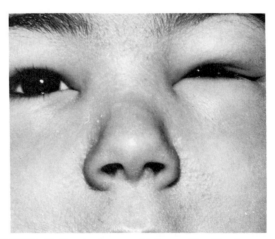

FIGURE 23-5. A six-year-old boy with allergic contact dermatitis, showing erythema, edema, and vesicles 72 hours after contact. (Vaughan, V. C., III, and McKay, R. J. (Eds.): *Nelson Textbook of Pediatrics.* 10th ed. Philadelphia W. B. Saunders Co., 1975.)

the area, but he may also have a life-threatening anaphylactic episode. In an anaphylactic episode the child may have generalized urticaria, upper and lower airway obstruction, and circulatory collapse leading to rapid death without prompt treatment. Serum sickness or the nephrotic syndrome may occur some time after the child has been stung.

Diagnosis can be made on the basis of the history of contact, a bite or a sting, and the appearance of the skin lesions. Skin testing using extreme caution because of severe sensitivity to the insect may be done. This procedure is of value not only to verify IgE-mediated sensitivity but also as a beginning point for therapy to hyposensitize the child.

Treatment, Responsibilities of the Nurse, and Prevention. Avoidance of the insect is the best preventive measure against insect allergy. The use of insect repellents and destroying the insects at their breeding sites are very helpful.

Treatment after contact with an insect may consist of hyposensitization. For the child who has been *bitten* by an insect, treatment consists of topical medicants to relieve local discomfort and itching. An antihistamine may also be given.

If an anaphylactic reaction occurs following a Hymenoptera *sting* (bees, wasps, yellow jackets, and hornets), epinephrine may be given subcutaneously or by aerosol. An antihistamine is also given. Commercially prepared kits containing a tourniquet, syringe filled with epinephrine, and an antihistamine tablet are available. Such a kit should be available to parents of any child who has had a severe or anaphylactic reaction to a stinging insect. Epinephrine in an aerosol unit (Medihaler-Epi) may be used as a substitute for the epinephrine in the kit. After the sting and upon the completion of this emergency first aid procedure, medical assistance should be sought. The application of cold to the area reduces discomfort, decreases the circulation in the part, slows down the absorption, and reduces the development of edema. Stingers left by bees can be removed with tweezers or by scraping the area with a knife.

A course of hyposensitization is administered to a child who has had a severe or anaphylactic reaction to a stinging insect. Since the individual insect cannot usually be identified, a very dilute solution of allergens consisting of bee, hornet, wasp, and yellow jacket extract is generally used.

Methods of protection against stinging insects consist of wearing light-colored clothing and avoiding the use of odors such as those found in hair sprays or oils and perfumes or colognes. Children are also cautioned not to walk barefoot through grass, especially through clover. If in proximity to insects, an aerosol spray can be used as a deterrent.

OSTEOMYELITIS

Incidence, Etiology, and Pathogenesis. The *incidence* of osteomyelitis is highest among children five to 14 years of age and twice as frequent among boys as among girls. Acute osteomyelitis is due to deposition in the bone of bacteria by way of the blood stream from some primary source, usually on the skin, as furunculosis, impetigo, or infected burns.

The causative organism commonly is hemolytic *Staphylococcus aureus*, although other pathogenic bacteria may be involved. Lesions occurring prior to the development of osteomyelitis may include impetigo (see p. 266), furunculosis (see p. 266), burns (see p. 556), and infected chickenpox lesions (see p. 658).

Bacteria enter the blood stream and are carried to the metaphysis of a bone. Infection spreads laterally along the epiphyseal plate, penetrates the cortex and locates *under the periosteum*, causing an abscess. The medulla of the bone may become infected. Dead bone forms a *sequestrum*, which may be extruded or absorbed. The periosteum forms new bone and may completely cover the dead shaft with an *involucrum*.

Clinical Manifestations and Diagnosis. The first *clinical manifestation* is a furuncle or other infection of the skin. One or two weeks later malaise, septicemia, fever, chills, and vomiting may develop abruptly. The child suffers a sharp, localized pain in the affected bone, usually the knee, elbow, hip, or shoulder, but the flat bones of the skull, spine, or pelvis may also be involved. Signs of inflammation—swelling and redness—are present over the bone. The child may become very ill with fever and toxic symptoms.

The *diagnosis* is made on a leukocyte count of 15,000 to 25,000 or more cells. A blood culture is usually positive. If so, the causative organism is located. Roentgenograms may be made after changes in the bone have occurred, i.e., in ten days or more after the onset of symptoms.

Treatment, Prognosis, and Complications. *Treatment* consists in giving antibiotics intravenously or orally, according to the organism found on blood culture. Usually antibiotics effective against several strains of *Staphylococcus aureus* are used until the specific organism is proved. A splint or traction is applied to the affected extremity to immobilize it and lessen the pain. Analgesics are given for pain. If an abscess forms, it is drained, and the purulent material is cultured. If extensive destruction of bone has occurred, the lesion must be removed surgically before healing can occur.

The course and *prognosis* depend on early therapy and its continuance over an adequate time. If the condition is treated early and adequately with antibiotics, the prognosis is excellent. Inadequate treatment may lead to chronic osteomyelitis. Long-term care may be required if the legs are involved. The child may have residual shortening of the involved leg. The mortality rate has decreased greatly since specific antibacterial agents have become available.

If the osteomyelitis is not adequately treated and the infection invades the joint cavity directly or is carried to a joint space by way of the blood stream, *septic arthritis* may occur. Fluid from the joint may be aspirated and cultured to determine the appropriate antibiotic to be used. The symptoms and treatment are similar to those of osteomyelitis. If antibiotic therapy is not successful, surgical drainage of the joint may become necessary. Destruction of the tissues in the joint space may later interfere with the function of the joint itself. Surgical drainage is especially important if the hip joint is involved, because septic arthritis may lead to destruction of the femoral head and eventual dislocation of the hip. Postoperatively, closed infusion and drainage are used until the drainage is sterile. A cast may be applied to prevent dislocation.

Responsibilities of the Nurse. In both osteomyelitis and septic arthritis the nurse's role is one of early detection through assessment of the child's condition. By knowing the etiology and the clinical manifestations of these conditions the nurse can recognize the possibility of these diagnoses and refer the child to a physician for diagnosis and treatment.

If the child is hospitalized, the necessity for bed rest is explained to him. The nurse can assist the physician in obtaining cultures from the blood and the wound for diagnostic purposes. The nurse can also assist with intravenous therapy through which antibiotics are given. Analgesics are given for discomfort or pain. When a splint is used for immobilization, it is applied as ordered. When skin traction or a cast is used for immobilization, it is the nurse's responsibility to check the circulation in the limb for signs of circulatory impairment (see p. 323). When the temperature is elevated or if surgery is done, the vital signs are taken every four hours. If closed infusion and drainage are necessary, the nurse is responsible for monitoring the fluids. An accurate record of intake and output is necessary.

When the child feels better, he needs appropriate recreation and socialization with his peers. The recreation therapist can either provide such activities for him in his crib or bed or he may be taken to the play area in his bed or wheelchair. The child's parents are involved in his care so that they understand the reasons for the treatment given.

SUPRACONDYLAR FRACTURE OF THE HUMERUS

Incidence, Etiology, Pathology and Clinical Manifestations. Supracondylar fractures are common injuries of childhood and are most likely to occur when the child is climbing or engaged in a competitive sport that requires physical skill. Supracondylar fracture of the humerus occurs just above the elbow and is due to direct trauma to the arm.

The distal fragment is displaced posteriorly and presses on the brachial artery, thus interfering with the circulation to the forearm. Swelling and bleeding in the area also hamper the return of venous blood from the forearm. The combination of these two factors can produce serious ischemic paralysis.

Diagnosis, Treatment, Responsibilities of the Nurse, and Complications. The *diagnosis* is made by roentgenogram. It is essential to reduce the fracture promptly and adequately and re-establish the circulation and drainage to and from the forearm. The surgeon may manipulate into place bones with only slight displacement. A splint is applied to hold the elbow in flexed position. The arm may be placed in an overhead suspension apparatus to reduce edema. X-ray films should be taken to check the position of the fragments. The arm is immobilized for three to four weeks. After the fracture has healed, the child can re-establish motion with his own muscles without forceful manipulation.

If swelling was great at the time of injury, traction and suspension are used to reduce the fracture. The color of the skin and the quality of the radial pulse must be checked with both kinds of treatment.

Upon admission to the hospital the child is usually apprehensive, unhappy, and perhaps feeling guilty because the injury occurred while he was doing something he should not have done. Since there was no time for preparation for hospitalization, he needs a nurse who is a friend.

The nurse should check the radial pulse and the color of the skin of the arm frequently—usually every 30 to 60 minutes. Observations are continued for the first 24 to 48 hours after the injury. Because of the possibility of Volkmann's ischemia, if the child complains of persistent pain, or numbness, or if the fingers are

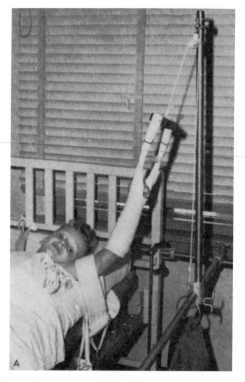
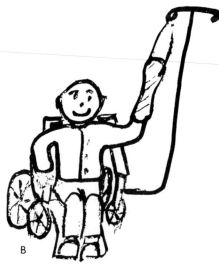

FIGURE 23–6. *A*, Dunlop traction used in treatment of supracondylar fracture of the humerus. *B*, Treatment as seen through the eyes of a child. Drawing this impression of his therapy assisted the child to overcome his anxiety. (*A*, From Wilson, J. C.: *Pediatr. Clin. N. Am.* 14:3, 659, 1967. *B*, Courtesy of Public Relations Dept., Children's Hospital of Philadelphia.)

discolored or cold, or if the radial pulse is weak, the physician should be notified immediately.

Upon admission, the child is placed on a firm mattress. Proper positioning is important and depends on the treatment to be given. Ice bags may be ordered to aid in the control of swelling and to relieve pain. The bags should be well covered and only partially filled with small pieces of ice. They are placed under, not over, the arm, since their weight should not rest on the injured area.

Volkmann's ischemia may result from interference with the peripheral circulation. Peripheral nerve injury and faulty union of the bone may also occur. The prognosis of peripheral nerve injury is good because the nerves are not divided. If faulty union of the bones occurs with deformity, a supracondylar osteotomy is necessary to restore elbow functioning.

To prevent a feeling of dependency, the child should be encouraged to do as much as possible for himself. Various kinds of activity appropriate to his physical limitations can be provided.

Prior to discharge, the nurse demonstrates to the parents and child the treatment ordered: the triangular sling or the collar and cuff neck sling so that the arm is held in alignment properly. If a cast has been applied, the nurse can explain its care (see p. 323).

APPENDICITIS

Incidence, Etiology, Pathology, and Clinical Manifestations. Appendicitis is rare during the first two years of life, but the *incidence* increases throughout the school years and adolescence.

Obstruction, especially with fecal concretions, is the principal factor in the majority of cases. Obstruction may also be caused by infection or allergy. Organisms found in the appendix include streptococci, *Staphylococcus aureus,* and coliform bacilli. Pinworms may be an initial cause of inflammation (see p. 548).

The mucosa is inflamed and ulcerated. The lumen becomes distended, thereby impairing the blood supply. Bacteria may escape through the wall and cause diffuse peritonitis or an abscess confined by adjacent intestine and omentum.

The *clinical manifestations* may be variable. The onset may be abrupt or may follow gastroenteritis. The manifestations may include nausea, vomiting, abdominal pain, constipation or diarrhea, localized tenderness, and absence of peristalsis unless diarrhea is present. Abdominal pain in children may not be localized in the lower right quadrant. The child may not be able to report accurately the site of the pain.

Other manifestations are anorexia, mild leukocytosis (12,000 to 15,000 cells), fever of 99 to

102° F. (37.2 to 38.8° C.), flushed face, increased pulse and respiratory rates, restlessness, irritability, and sleeplessness.

Diagnosis, Treatment, Responsibilities of the Nurse, Complications, and Prognosis. The *diagnosis* of appendicitis in childhood is difficult, since a number of other conditions produce somewhat similar symptoms. If the child has a respiratory infection, abdominal pain may be due to incipient pneumonia. Inflammation of a Meckel's diverticulum (see below), mesenteric adenitis, or gastroenteritis (see p. 409) may also cause symptoms suggestive of appendicitis. Irritation of the peritoneum may occur in rheumatic fever (see p. 767) and resemble appendicitis. Repeated examinations may be necessary before a definite diagnosis is made.

Appendectomy—surgical removal of the appendix—should be done as soon as possible after the diagnosis has been made and the child is in condition for operation. Both the parents and the child may be apprehensive because of their lack of preparation prior to hospitalization and surgery. A brief simple explanation with an opportunity for questioning helps them to cope with their situation.

Preoperative preparation is routine and consists in withholding of food, establishment of hydration by the intravenous route, and reduction of temperature below 102° F. (38.8° C.) (rectally). Administration of antibiotics, to prevent or minimize the danger of peritonitis, and enemas may be ordered, but cathartics are not given. Operation is done immediately after admission or as soon as possible.

After appendectomy intravenous fluids, nothing by mouth, and gastric decompression are continued until peristalsis is heard. The nurse observes and reports indications of the development of an abscess or peritonitis such as irritability, continued postoperative pain, and anorexia. If all is well, diet and activity return to normal quickly and the child usually returns to school in one or two weeks. Strenuous activity is restricted for several weeks.

If the child had peritonitis or a peritoneal or appendiceal abscess, continuous gastric suction, chemotherapy and parenteral fluids may be ordered. The child may be placed in semi-Fowler's position to assist in localizing the infection. He is ambulated as early as possible even if he still has a gastric suction tube in place. Recovery, naturally, will be slower than in the uncomplicated case.

Complications include a localized abscess and diffuse secondary peritonitis. The appendix may perforate because the parents gave the child a cathartic (lay treatment for any abdominal pain in childhood) or because the child, interested in play and not wanting a cathartic, did not tell his mother of his discomfort.

The operation is practically without risk if it is performed before perforation occurs. Even after perforation has occurred the risk is relatively slight, although hospitalization is prolonged.

MECKEL'S DIVERTICULUM

Etiology, Pathology, and Clinical Manifestations. When the intestinal remnant of the omphalomesenteric duct from the terminal ileum to the umbilical cord persists and does not close, a Meckel's diverticulum is formed. It arises from the ileum, but usually does not have a connection with the umbilicus. A Meckel's diverticulum may be ½ to 3 inches in length and may be lined with intestinal mucous membrane. In some cases it may also contain gastric mucosa.

The diverticulum usually is not responsible for symptoms. When its gastric mucosa secretes gastric ferments, complications arise. It may produce ulceration in the ileum or in the diverticulum which may lead to massive hemorrhage, perforation and peritonitis. The diverticulum may cause intestinal adhesions, strangulation or intussusception (see p. 422), and this may result in intestinal obstruction.

When hemorrhage occurs, the stools may be black at first, and then bright red. With hemorrhage there will be pallor and an increased pulse rate. If transfusions are not given immediately, collapse and death may occur.

Finding the diverticulum is the only way of confirming the diagnosis.

Treatment, Responsibilities of the Nurse, and Prognosis. Observation by the nurse is important to determine the child's condition. The vital

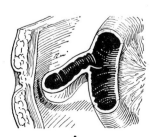 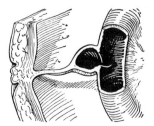 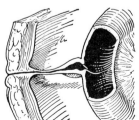

FIGURE 23–7. Meckel's diverticulum of the ileum. *A,* Ordinary blind sac. *B,* Diverticulum continued to umbilicus as a cord. *C,* Diverticulum with fistulous opening at umbilicus. (Arey: *Developmental Anatomy.* 7th ed. rev. W. B. Saunders Co., Philadelphia, 1974.)

A   B   C

signs and blood pressure are taken and the child's skin color is observed. Tests are done by the nurse on each of the child's stools to determine the amount of blood being lost. Transfusions are given for hemorrhage, and surgical excision of the diverticulum is necessary. After surgery the child will require gastric decompression by the use of a nasogastric catheter and intravenous fluids. Nursing care after the removal of a diverticulum is similar to that given after other abdominal surgery.

The *prognosis* is good, and no further problems or recurrence are usually anticipated.

REYE'S SYNDROME (ACUTE ENCEPHALOPATHY AND HEPATOMEGALY WITH FATTY INFILTRATION) (ENCEPHALOHEPATITIS)

Etiology, Incidence, Clinical Manifestations, Diagnosis, and Prognosis. Reye's syndrome is an acute and frequently fatal condition of childhood. This illness follows a mild viral infection from which the child appears to be recovering. The cause is unknown, but it seems to be associated with an infection caused by influenza B, herpes simplex, varicella, echovirus, or other viruses. There is a current theory, but certainly not the only one, that links an interaction between a toxin such as an insecticide or a herbicide and a virus as the causative factor. Other theories include disruptions of mitochondrial function, problems with lipid metabolism, and a genetic metabolic predisposition to the syndrome.

Reye's syndrome is relatively rare, although its incidence seems to be increasing, probably because of improved diagnosis. The age range of affected children is from two months to adolescence, with peaks occurring at six and 11 years. It occurs most often in winter and spring.

The *clinical manifestations* of Reye's syndrome have abrupt onset and consist of protracted vomiting with dehydration. A few hours later there is a change in the state of consciousness, and the child becomes confused, delirious, and stuporous. The child may have a slight tachycardia and a normal temperature and blood pressure. Neurologically, the child may have pupillary changes, a decreasing sensorium, and hyperactive reflexes. The electroencephalogram (EEG) is markedly abnormal. Metabolic derangements, an irregular respiratory pattern with an acute interstitial pneumonia, and cerebral edema with increased intracranial pressure occur.

Four stages of the illness can be defined. In stage I the child is comatose but can be aroused. In stage II the child cannot be aroused but responds to stimuli with avoidance movements.

In stage III the child responds to pain by decerebrate posturing. He still has pupillary reflexes. In stage IV the child is flaccid with no response to painful stimuli. In this stage there are no spontaneous respirations or pupillary light reflexes.

Diagnosis is made on the basis of clinical examination and laboratory studies. Clinical examination reveals an encephalopathy or cerebral swelling without evidence of inflammation and fatty degeneration of the viscera, notably the liver, which is a bright yellow fat-filled organ. There is no clinical jaundice. Laboratory studies include an elevated serum glutamic-oxaloacetic acid transaminase (SGOT), an elevated serum glutamic-pyruvic acid transaminase (SGPT), and an abnormal prothrombin time. The blood ammonia level may be elevated. The blood urea nitrogen (BUN) is elevated and the blood glucose is usually normal, although some children develop hypoglycemia. If a liver biopsy is done, it shows microvesicular fat droplets. These are diagnostic of the syndrome.

This syndrome mimics other disease states such as drug ingestion, meningitis encephalitis, and brain abscess. Toxicity after the ingestion of aspirin causes many similar symptoms.

The *prognosis* is guarded, but Reye's syndrome is not necessarily the fatal disease that some have suggested. The course of the disease is about 7 to 10 days, ending with recovery or death.

Treatment and Responsibilities of the Nurse. The multifaceted nature of Reye's syndrome necessitates utilization of the team approach. The treatment and nursing care consist of providing supportive care and intensive clinical monitoring of all systems on an hourly basis and reducing the increased intracranial pressure.

When the child is admitted to the hospital, treatment consists of the intravenous administration of glucose, glucose with insulin and therapy with electrolytes, neomycin cleansing enemas to reduce ammonia production by the intestinal flora, citrulline drug therapy, peritoneal dialysis to reduce the blood ammonia level, and exchange transfusions. Double volume blood exchange transfusion is the treatment of choice. Corticosteroids or mannitol may be given if there is increased intracranial pressure. Phenobarbital or another anticonvulsant may be given for seizures. The child may need to be intubated and placed on a respiratory-cardiac monitor.

Neurologic checks, including pupillary responses and the vital signs and blood pressure, are taken frequently. The child is also observed for his response to simple verbal commands and to painful stimuli, his corneal and gag reflexes, his ability to move, and the absence or presence of decerebrate posturing.

If the child is irritable, convulsing and disoriented, he is restrained with clove hitch and jacket-type restraints, the siderails of his bed are padded, and seizure precautions are instituted. Fluids are administered intravenously, usually through a cutdown tube. If the child continues to vomit, a nasogastric tube is passed. A Foley catheter is inserted in order to measure the urine output accurately. The child on a respirator requires suctioning, good skin care, and oral hygiene. A skin care program is started early, and the child is turned every hour or two to prevent skin breakdown. If his pupils are fixed and dilated, his eyelids are kept closed with gauze and tape to prevent corneal abrasions. Oxygen, suction equipment, and other emergency equipment should be kept at the bedside.

If the decision is made to transfuse the child, a CVP line, through which the double volume exchange will take place, is inserted and the position of the catheter is checked by x-ray. The child's total blood volume using fresh whole blood is exchanged twice. Calcium gluconate is given intravenously to prevent a deficit of calcium. During the procedure the monitor should be observed closely for evidence of cardiac arrhythmias, and the nurse should observe the child for evidence of a transfusion reaction (see p. 459).

One major problem in helping families to deal with their child's illness is that little is known about this condition. Children who survive the illness do so quickly. It is known and can be shared with parents that children who survive this disease have no apparent after effects. Parents who have had a child who was vomiting, then became comatose, and shortly after taking him to the hospital became critically ill, blame themselves for not seeking care sooner. These families need great support and reassurance that the care they gave was sufficient for the degree of illness observed.

From the patient's point of view he does not remember being taken to the hospital and wakes up in a strange place with no clothes on, tubes in his arms, a catheter in place, and surrounded by strange people. The child needs to establish trust in these people and to obtain a feeling of security. He needs to be reoriented as to time and place. His modesty should be maintained by covering him as much as is possible and using a bedside screen or a curtain. These measures will preserve his dignity. He needs honest explanations about what is happening and why. During recovery the child is helped to show his feelings through play therapy or through verbal expressions of feelings. The nurse can correct any misconceptions he may have about his experiences. When the child feels better, he is helped to interact with his peers and to begin to carry on activities which interest him and are within his ability.

It is the nurse's responsibility to be alert to the possibility of Reye's syndrome when a child who has had a viral infection begins to vomit persistently, becomes prostrate, and appears sicker than usual with this type of infection.

TEACHING AIDS AND OTHER INFORMATION*

Allergy Foundation of America
Insect Sting.

The American Journal of Nursing Company
Care of the Well Child.

American Lung Association
Your Child's Lungs Are for Life.

American Medical Association
Poison Plant Rashes.
Your Friend the Doctor.

Canadian Mental Health Association
Suddenly It Happens—Your Child Is Ill, 1967.

The Children's Hospital Medical Center, Boston, Mass.
Accident Handbook.
Rey, M., and Rey, H. A.: Curious George Goes to the Hospital.

Consumer Product Information
Poison Ivy, Oak, and Sumac, 1971.
Typical Poisonous Plants, 1973.

Department of National Health and Welfare: Ottawa, Canada
Help! (first aid).

Play Schools Association, Inc.
Play in a Hospital.

Ross Laboratories
Common Orthopedic Conditions in Childhood, 1973.

The Touchstone Center
My Roots Be Coming Back.
Out of My Body.

United States Government
Altshuler, A.: Books That Help Children with a Hospital Experience, 1974.
Leaves Mean Poison Ivy, 1972.
Red Is the Color of Hurting, 1967.

---

*Complete addresses are given in the Appendix.

REFERENCES

Books

American Academy of Pediatrics: *Care of Children in Hospitals*. Evanston, Ill., American Academy of Pediatrics, 1971.

Brunner, N. A.: *Orthopedic Nursing: A Programmed Approach*. 2nd ed. St. Louis, The C. V. Mosby Company, 1975.

Fisher, A. A.: *Contact Dermatitis*. 2nd ed. Philadelphia, Lea & Febiger, 1973.

Flint, T., Jr., and Cain, H. D.: *Emergency Treatment and Management*. 5th ed. Philadelphia, W. B. Saunders Company, 1975.

Fregert, S.: *Manual of Contact Dermatitis*. Chicago, Year Book Medical Publishers, 1975.

Gellis, S. S., and Kagan, B. M.: *Current Pediatric Therapy 7*. Philadelphia, W. B. Saunders Company, 1976.

Gross, R. E.: *An Atlas of Children's Surgery*. Philadelphia, W. B. Saunders, Company, 1970.

Hardgrove, C. B., and Dawson, R. B.: *Parents and Children in the Hospital: The Family's Role in Pediatrics*. Boston, Little, Brown & Company, 1972.

Hertzler, J. H., and Mirza, M.: *Handbook of Pediatric Surgery*. Chicago, Year Book Medical Publishers, 1974.

Hilt, N. E., and Schmitt, E. W., Jr.: *Pediatric Orthopedic Nursing*. St. Louis, The C. V. Mosby Company, 1975.

Hughes, J. G.: *Synopsis of Pediatrics*. 4th ed. St. Louis, The C. V. Mosby Company, 1975.

Jones, P. F.: *Emergency Abdominal Surgery in Infancy, Childhood and Adult Life*. Philadelphia, J. B. Lippincott Company, 1974.

Larson, C. B., and Gould, M.: *Orthopedic Nursing*. 8th ed. St. Louis, The C. V. Mosby Company, 1974.

Maddin, S. (Ed.): *Current Dermatologic Management*. 2nd ed. St. Louis, The C. V. Mosby Company, 1975.

Moschella, S. L., Pillsbury, D. M., and Hurley, H. J., Jr.: *Dermatology*. Philadelphia, W. B. Saunders Company, 1975.

Oremland, E. K., and Oremland, J. D. (Eds.): *The Effects of Hospitalization on Children*. Springfield, Ill., Charles C Thomas, 1973.

Petrillo, M., and Sanger, S.: *Emotional Care of Hospitalized Children*. Philadelphia, J. B. Lippincott Company, 1972.

Rang, M.: *Children's Fractures*. Philadelphia, J. B. Lippincott Company, 1974.

Rickham, P. P., Soper, R. T., and Stauffer, U. G.: *Synopsis of Pediatric Surgery*. Chicago, Year Book Medical Publishers, 1975.

Sharrard, W. J. W.: *Paediatric Orthopaedics and Fractures*. Philadelphia, J. B. Lippincott Company, 1971.

Shirkey, H. C.: *Pediatric Drug Handbook*. Philadelphia, W. B. Saunders Company, 1977.

Silver, H. K., Kempe, C. H., and Bruyn, H. B.: *Handbook of Pediatrics*. 11th ed. Los Altos, California, Lange Medical Publications, 1975.

Surgical Staff/The Hospital for Sick Children, Toronto, Canada, and Salter, R. B. (Ed.): *Care for the Injured Child*. Baltimore, Williams & Wilkins, 1975.

Vaughan, V. C., III, and McKay, R. J. (Eds.): *Nelson Textbook of Pediatrics*. 10th ed. Philadelphia, W. B. Saunders Company, 1975.

Periodicals

Anspach, E., et al.: Johnny and the School Nurse Practitioner. *Am. J. Nursing*, 74:1099, June 1974.

Bellack, J. P.: Helping a Child Cope With the Stress of Injury. *Am. J. Nursing*, 74:1491, August 1974.

Brown, S.: Easing the Burden of Traction and Casts. *RN*, 38:36, February 1975.

Corey, L., et al.: A Nationwide Outbreak of Reye's Syndrome: Its Epidemiologic Relationship to Influenza B. *Am. J. Med.*, 61:615, November 1976.

DeVivo, D. C., Keating, J. P., and Haymond, M. W.: Acute Encephalopathy with Fatty Infiltration of the Viscera. *Pediatr. Clin. N. Am.*, 23:527, August 1976.

Flammang, M., and Hahn, J.: The Child with Reye's Syndrome. *Nursing '76*, 6:80C, March 1976.

Hogan, K. M., and Sawyer, J. R.: Fracture Dislocation of the Elbow. *Am. J. Nursing*, 76:1266, August 1976.

Itkin, I.: Bee Sting. *Am. Fam. Physician*, 13:124, May 1976.

Reeves, K. R.: Beware of Reye's Syndrome. *Am. J. Nursing*, 74:1621, September 1974.

Reisman, R. E., and Arbesman, C. E.: Stinging Insect Allergy: Current Concepts and Problems. *Pediatr. Clin. N. Am.*, 22:185, February 1975.

Resnick, R., and Hergenroeder, E.: Children and the Emergency Room. *Nursing Digest*, 4:37, September-October 1976.

Roskies, E., et al.: Emergency Hospitalization of Young Children. *Nursing Digest*, 4:32, September-October 1976.

Rice, A. K.: Common Skin Infections in School Children. *Am. J. Nursing*, 73:1905, November 1973.

Samaha, F. J., et al.: Reye's Syndrome: Clinical Diagnosis and Treatment With Peritoneal Dialysis. *Pediatrics*, 53:336, March 1974.

The Do's and Don'ts of Traction Care. *Nursing '74*, 4:35, November 1974.

U.S. Center for Disease Control: Increased Scabies Incidence—United States. *Morbidity Mortality*, 25:10, January 17, 1976.

Weeks, H. L.: What Every ICU Nurse Should Know About Reye's Syndrome. *The American Journal of Maternal Child Nursing*, 1:231, July-August 1976.

Zweig, I. K.: A New Way to Get Acquainted With The Hospital—Pediatric Open House for Well Children. *The American Journal of Maternal Child Nursing*, 1:217, July-August 1976.

AUDIOVISUAL MEDIA*

The American Journal of Nursing Company

Play Therapy and the Hospitalized Child
26 minutes, black and white.
Film describes how to aid children in coping with their hospital experience through play therapy.

Children's Hospital, National Medical Center, Washington, D.C.

To Prepare a Child
32 minutes, 16mm, sound, color, guide.
Studies have shown that the occurrence of psychological upset after hospitalization is greater in the unprepared than in the prepared child. The child care staff in the film demonstrate the quality of care children need to be well-prepared for this experience.

Health Sciences Communication Center, Case Western Reserve University

Ethan Has an Operation
16mm film, 16 minutes; Super-8 film, 16 minutes, videotape cassette, sound, color.
Filmed during the hospitalization of a seven-year-old boy

for a hernia operation. It is primarily to reduce anxiety in children about to undergo surgery. Coverage includes: the admission process, orientation to the ward, examinations by surgeon and anesthesiologist, meeting other children in the playroom, a blood test, preoperative medication, separation from the mother, the operating room, anesthesia, return to the recovery room, the child's reunion with his parents, and discharge from the hospital.

W. B. Saunders Company

Christine Has an Operation
    Wise, D. J.
    30 minutes English, 30 minutes Spanish, 35mm filmstrip, tape cassette, color.
This combination of a tape, filmstrip, coloring book, and instruction guide is designed to help prepare the child of between ages four and eight for elective surgery.

Pediatric Conferences with Sydney Gellis
    Reye's Syndrome, Glick, T. H.

Trainex Corporation

Preparing the Child for Procedures
    35mm filmstrip, audio-tape cassette, 33⅓ LP, color.
This program is designed to help health care personnel minimize emotional trauma that a child could experience as a result of hospitalization. Shows ways in which the child might interpret hospital surroundings and procedures, and techniques employed in helping him to make correct interpretations. Included is a discussion of the value of structured play activities.

°Complete addresses are given in the Appendix.

Chapter Twenty-Four

CONDITIONS OF THE SCHOOL CHILD REQUIRING LONG-TERM CARE

REHABILITATION OF THE SCHOOL CHILD

The process of rehabilitation begins as soon after recognition of the illness as possible and continues throughout illness until the child is rehabilitated to the fullest possible extent. Rehabilitation in our culture is based on the belief that all persons should be helped to maintain or regain their best possible physical or mental health. Whether the child has multiple handicaps or a chronic disease, rehabilitation is geared to averting further preventable damage, and to helping him gain his maximum physical potential while bolstering his psychologic defenses for the future. If the members of the health team and the nursing team do not make a positive effort to rehabilitate their patients, these children may *regress* in their abilities and interpersonal relations. Thus rehabilitation becomes one goal in the comprehensive care of pa-

tients. The nurse must work closely with other members of the interdisciplinary health team to achieve this end.

By school age and adolescence the child must assume increasing responsibility for his own rehabilitation after illness. His cooperation must be gained through understanding the necessity for this. The nurse has an important role in interpreting this need to him and in helping him to assume this responsibility.

In order to help the child achieve the goal of rehabilitation, his own goals must be considered. Thus the nurse has the responsibility of investigating these goals through discussions with him and relaying pertinent information to other members of the health team. In our society it is our privilege and responsibility to help prepare each child, whether normal or handicapped, to take his rightful place in the world of tomorrow.

School in the Hospital. In our culture going to school has become identified with the mainstream of child growth and development. It is of utmost importance that the hospitalized child be assured of a continuing relation with this mainstream. When the child cannot go to school, the school must come to him. School to the older child is his "life work." He is usually just as serious about it as an adult is about his employment. For this reason many hospitals maintain a school program for hospitalized children. Although the program may include the acutely ill child, the majority of children attending class are the chronically ill and convalescent children.

The purpose of the school program is, first, to keep the child up with his grade group academically; second, to keep the child with his peer group socially; third, to act as a supportive factor in the child's total adjustment to his hospitalization. Attendance at school gives him an opportunity to express himself and to use his time in a constructive manner. It brings some of the familiar outside world into the hospital.

766

Many times the chronically ill child needs individual or remedial help. School in the hospital presents an excellent opportunity for the child to receive such help.

With the liberalization of visiting privileges parents see their children more frequently. This provides a unique opportunity for parent-teacher communication. Parents become the link between the child's home-school and his hospital-school.

Attitudes toward school and school work can be important factors in understanding the child. Sometimes these attitudes have implications for the physicians, nurses, and all other personnel who work with the child. They provide clues to his motivation, his potential, the satisfaction he derives from his work, and the degree to which he has learned to function effectively. They reflect his self-image as well as the quality of his home and school backgrounds.

In many hospitals the child is taught by a visiting teacher, either at his bedside or in a group of children in a classroom made to accommodate wheelchairs and even beds on wheels. The classroom should have the usual equipment, including blackboard and movable tables and chairs. The hours spent in study are short, and no child is under pressure to learn. His program is suited to his condition.

Hospitalized school children miss not only school, but also many opportunities for learning which other children have. They should be given what opportunities are available in the hospital setting. They can learn facts about their own bodies and something about preventing

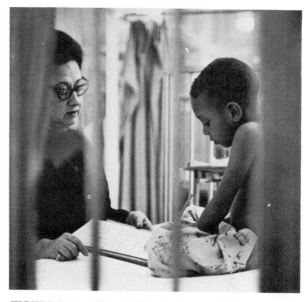

FIGURE 24-2. This child is on bed rest and cannot be taken to the classroom in the hospital with the other children. The school teacher therefore visits him in his room and helps him to gain the satisfaction of keeping up with his class. (Courtesy of Children's Hospital of Philadelphia, Public Relations Department.)

disease. Convalescent children may be taken on picnics and sightseeing trips. Those who cannot leave the hospital may have motion pictures and exhibitions brought to them. School children become bored and withdrawn if they are not given an opportunity to learn.

A child discharged from the hospital may have to convalesce at home for weeks or months. If he lives in a community which has a school-to-home telephone or closed-circuit television service, he may be able to participate in his regular classes. Thus he can continue his education without feeling left out. If such a service is not available, a visiting teacher may come to the home to tutor him so that he will be able to return to his class when he is fully recovered.

LONG-TERM CONDITIONS

RHEUMATIC FEVER

Collagen Diseases. Collagen diseases are a group of diseases characterized by damage to the ground substance of connective tissue, followed by changes in collagen fibrils. The connective tissue of all organ systems is usually affected, and the small blood vessels are frequently involved. The following are collagen diseases (they are heterogeneous from the clinical point of view, but have certain symptoms in common): rheumatic fever, juvenile rheumatoid arthritis (JRA), periarteritis nodosa, systemic

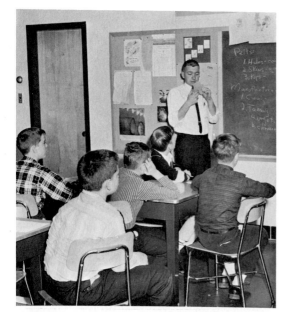

FIGURE 24-1. Attendance at school is an essential part of the rehabilitation program. (H. Armstrong Roberts.)

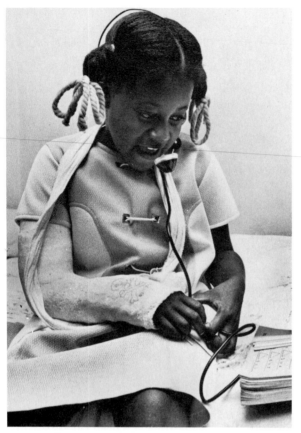

FIGURE 24–3. "Tele-classes" permit homebound students to talk with other shut-in students, to listen to their answers, and to hear instructions from the teacher in the classroom. (Courtesy of International Telephone and Telegraph Company.)

lupus erythematosus (SLE), scleroderma, and dermatomyositis. All these diseases appear to be like allergic responses of the child and respond symptomatically to corticotropin (ACTH) or cortisone during some stage. The basic problem in these conditions is the deposition of fibrinoid material in the tissues. Histopathologically, fibrinoid is extensively deposited in the lumen and walls of blood vessels and in the surrounding connective tissues.

Etiology, Incidence, and Pathology. Rheumatic fever is a general systemic disease characterized by frequent recurrences following infection with group A beta hemolytic streptococcus. The etiologic importance of this organism is based on clinical epidemiology, as shown by its association with a sore throat preceding rheumatic fever by one to three weeks, and by immunologic response seen in the antigen-antibody reaction. A streptolysin which causes a clear zone of hemolysis around bacterial colonies on blood agar plates causes an antibody response in the patient's blood which can be measured as the antistreptolysin-O

titer (ASO titer). The level of this antibody response reflects the intensity of tissue reaction and is an aid in diagnosis. The common origin of infection is in the throat (possibly followed by scarlet fever) or skin.

The pathologic sequence in rheumatic fever is (1) the initial infection with group A beta hemolytic streptococcus, (2) usually a latent or nonsymptomatic period lasting one to three weeks, and (3) the onset of rheumatic fever.

Rheumatic fever is one of the leading causes of chronic illness and death in children. It has its highest *incidence* between the ages of five and 15 years; the majority of first attacks occur between six and eight years. It is most prevalent in the temperate zones. Climate is a more important factor than racial susceptibility. The incidence varies with the season and geographic location, but it always follows the curve of incidence of streptococcal infections. It is most common in the spring months in the United States, but in the later months of the year in England. Overcrowded living conditions and general lack of hygiene among the lower socioeconomic groups in large cities are predisposing factors. The disease has a high family incidence; hereditary predisposition is possible.

The characteristic lesions of rheumatic fever are found in the connective tissue of the heart, subcutaneous tissue and in the arteries. Collagenous structures become edematous and may form granulomas or *Aschoff bodies*. These bodies are usually found in the wall of the left ventricle and interventricular septum. Structures resembling Aschoff bodies may also be found as *subcutaneous nodules*. These lesions may develop exudative manifestations. Such rheumatic effusions are usually absorbed, but adhesions may be found, especially in the pericardium. They are found in the hearts of the majority of children who succumb to acute carditis. Valvular lesions which form scars as they heal may result in thickening of the leaflet and shortening of the chordae tendineae. Such deformities of the valves result from repeated infection.

The heart may be impaired after rheumatic fever, owing to damage to the myocardium, the endocardium (including the valves) or the pericardium. The effects of the contracting scar tissue may not be evident for several years after the initial attack of rheumatic fever. Chronic valvular heart disease results.

Clinical Manifestations. The symptoms and course of the disease are variable. The three principal clinical manifestations, however, are carditis, migratory polyarthritis, and Sydenham's chorea. The typical attack may present any one of the clinical manifestations, which tend to recur at varying intervals. The onset may be acute or insidious with symptoms of "growing pains," pallor, nosebleed, malaise, and attacks of abdominal pain. Attacks last from one to three months, and recurrence may follow if the child acquires a streptococcal infection.

Carditis tends to occur in younger children. It is a more serious manifestation than arthritis or chorea, since it may lead to permanent disability or death. The pathologic changes include exudation and proliferation. The pericardium, myocardium and endocardium may be affected with subsequent scarring. The temperature may rise to 104° F (40° C.). Tachycardia which is disproportionate to the fever even during sleep persists after the elevation of temperature is under control. The pulse is of poor quality. Leukocytosis, anemia and severe pallor may occur. The respirations are rapid. In severe cases the following manifestations may be seen: prostration, weakness, orthopnea, cyanosis, precordial pain, and cardiac decompensation and dilatation. Cardiac murmurs are present and may change in quality.

Arthritis of a migratory polyarthritic type is usually seen in older children. The larger joints—hips, knees, ankles, shoulders, wrists, and elbows—are characteristically involved. The duration of involvement varies, and the pain moves from one joint to another. In older children the affected joint is hot, tender, red, and swollen. Permanent deformities do not follow this type of arthritis.

There is moderate leukocytosis, and the erythrocyte sedimentation rate is increased. The child's temperature usually runs from 101 to 102° F. (38.3 to 38.8° C.). Cardiac involvement may follow polyarthritis. So-called growing pains may be distinguished from migratory polyarthritis because they tend to occur only at night, are not associated with other manifestations of rheumatic fever, and are generally muscular rather than joint pains.

Sydenham's chorea (St. Vitus's dance) is a disorder of the central nervous system. It usually occurs in older children. See page 775 for a discussion of this condition.

There are other clinical manifestations of rheumatic fever (Fig. 24–4): (1) subcutaneous nodules of varying size which may be found on the extensor tendons of the hands and feet, on elbows, scapulae, scalp, patella, and vertebrae. The skin moves freely over these nodules; they are not painful, and they disappear gradually. (2) Pericarditis, in which there is pain in the precordial area and a friction rub heard over the precordium. (3) Muscle and joint pains (the so-called growing pains) may indicate rheumatic fever, and the child should be examined to rule out this disease and also orthopedic problems.

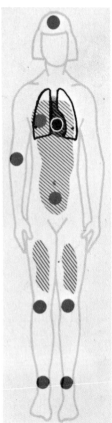

FIGURE 24–4. Sites of involvement in acute rheumatic fever. (From Disease Panorama on Rheumatic Fever. Courtesy of the Schering Corporation.)

(4) Epistaxis is a common manifestation of the onset of rheumatic fever. (5) Abdominal pain may be severe and may be mistaken for appendicitis. It is usually located in the epigastrium and may be due to enlargement of the mesenteric lymph nodes or to inflammation of the peritoneum. (6) There may be low-grade fever in the afternoon. If the diagnosis is uncertain, the erythrocyte sedimentation rate should be determined. (7) There may be skin manifestations. Various types of erythema may appear, e.g., erythema marginatum (Fig. 24–5) or erythema multiforme. Erythema marginatum is a pink eruption with serpiginous outline, occurring mainly on the trunk. These lesions may appear and disappear for years. (8) Pleurisy and rheumatic pneumonia may be complications. (9) The child tires easily, loses weight, and is pale and anorectic.

Diagnosis. The diagnosis may be difficult because many other conditions show clinical manifestations similar to those of rheumatic fever. Each laboratory test must be interpreted in the light of other test results and of the child's total clinical picture.

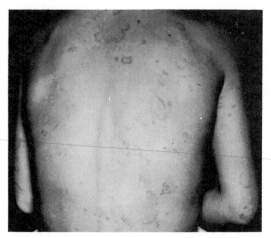

FIGURE 24–5. Erythema marginatum. (Nadas and Fyler: *Pediatric Cardiology.* 3rd edition. Philadelphia, W. B. Saunders Co., 1972.)

Laboratory tests are of value in diagnosing rheumatic fever and in evaluation of the disease. (1) There are several abnormal proteins found in the serum of children having rheumatic fever, as in other inflammatory states. C-reactive protein is never present in normal blood. This protein disappears as the child's condition improves. (2) The erythrocyte sedimentation rate is almost always elevated in children who have rheumatic carditis and polyarthritis, thereby indicating the presence of an inflammatory reaction. The sedimentation rate may remain elevated after clinical manifestations have subsided, showing that the rheumatic process is still active.

The rheumatic process should not be considered over until the white blood cell count is below 10,000 per cubic millimeter. Leukocytosis indicates inflammation. As long as anemia persists, the infection is probably still active.

Streptococci may be present in the upper respiratory tract of the child, a member of his family, or others whom he contacts. The organism may not be present if treatment has been given, but certain antibodies formed against streptococcal products may be present. Laboratory examinations may detect antifibrinolysin, antistreptolysin or antihyaluronidase.

Electrocardiograms may provide evidence of carditis. The P–R interval is often prolonged in the presence of carditis.

Treatment. Treatment of a child having rheumatic fever involves especially the following members of the health team: physicians, nurses in the pediatric unit, public health or community nurses, social worker, teacher, and Play Lady or recreational therapist.

No specific treatment will stop the rheumatic process. Bed rest is essential until the C-reactive protein is negative, the pulse rate normal, the erythrocyte sedimentation rate decreasing, the pain gone, and the hemoglobin level normal. The child should begin to gain weight before activity is permitted. If the work of the heart is reduced until the healing process occurs, a minimum of scar tissue in the heart results.

Penicillin is given only to eradicate group A streptococci from the body. It does not alleviate symptoms. Salicylates quickly relieve fever, joint pains and swelling. Symptoms of toxicity such as tinnitus, hyperpnea, purpuric manifestations, nausea, and vomiting are recorded. Salicylates are usually given orally. Aspirin (acetylsalicylic acid) or sodium salicylate is given. This therapy is continued until C-reactive protein is negative and the erythrocyte sedimentation rate is decreasing. If the child cannot tolerate salicylates, aminopyrine or phenylbutazone (Butazolidin) may be used.

Therapy with corticoids produces the same effects as salicylates. ACTH, prednisone or cortisone may be used. Prednisone is preferred because it may be given orally and causes less sodium retention than cortisone. Laboratory findings tend to return to normal more quickly than with the use of salicylates. Corticoids are considered by many to be beneficial in the treatment of rheumatic carditis, especially in extremely acute phases of the condition or if life-threatening failure is present. These drugs do not terminate the rheumatic process, but suppress it. There may be a mild recurrence of symptoms when the drug is discontinued.

Steroid therapy masks symptoms; thus it is necessary to watch the child closely for symptoms of infection or complications. These children do not have a fever when they have infections. The blood pressure should be taken daily and the drug discontinued if the diastolic pressure rises to 100 mm. or above. The salt intake should be moderately restricted.

A side effect of steroid therapy is the production of a *Cushing-like syndrome* characterized by acne, moon face, increased pigmentation, hirsutism, and abnormal fat distribution. This disappears when therapy is discontinued.

Morphine is given to control precordial pain, and sedatives such as phenobarbital to allay apprehension. Oxygen may be necessary. Digitalis may be indicated if cardiac failure is present (see p. 292).

Responsibilities of the Nurse. ACUTE PHASE. In the acute phase of rheumatic fever, rest is all-important in order to reduce the work of the heart. The need for absolute bed rest is explained to the child, and he is reassured that it will be a restriction only as long as necessary.

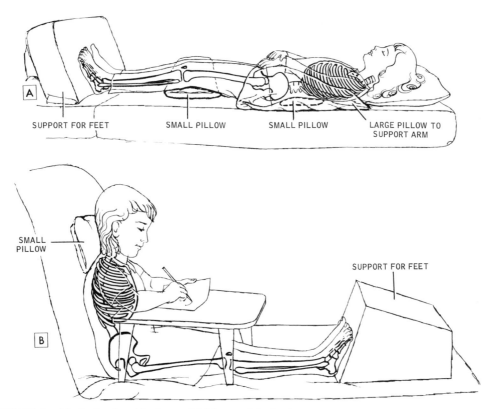

SUPPORT FOR FEET   SMALL PILLOW   SMALL PILLOW   LARGE PILLOW TO SUPPORT ARM

SMALL PILLOW

SUPPORT FOR FEET

FIGURE 24–6.   Methods of positioning a child for good body alignment. A, Flat in bed. B, In a sitting position.

The bed must have a firm mattress, since this promotes good posture and is less uncomfortable than a mattress which sags. If the child is dyspneic, or if the position provides comfort for him, the head of the bed may be elevated. During the period of complete bed rest when the head of the bed is elevated, the child's arms are supported at his sides with pillows to reduce their weight from the shoulders. If the pillows are of the proper height, the child will find it easier to expand his chest, and his arms will not bring pressure on his abdomen when he folds them across his body. The child's legs are in proper alignment, and his feet supported with a footboard to prevent foot drop and external rotation of the hips. A bed cradle may be used to prevent pressure from the bedclothes on his toes.

Nursing care is given at appropriate times so that the child can have long periods of complete rest without being disturbed. Since bodily movement causes pain, he is moved unnecessarily as little as possible. The nurse's movements must be smooth, sure, and unhurried; this helps to inspire confidence of the child in his nurse. If he is hurt, he becomes anxious and does not want to be touched. The nurse explains what will happen, e.g., insert the thermometer or lift him. What the child may be permitted to do for himself depends upon the physician's orders. If the child becomes irritable and more restless in bed than he would be out of it, the physician may permit a limited amount of activity in spite of the fact that laboratory findings are not normal.

The nurse is responsible for providing the child not only with physical comfort, but also with emotional rest. His needs must be anticipated and met in order to alleviate his anxiety.

In a child with rheumatic fever who is on bed rest pressure areas may develop, owing to constant pressure on his skin which is edematous, wet with perspiration, and very warm because of his fever. He should have frequent skin care, especially of the back and buttocks. An alternating pressure mattress may be used to prevent skin breakdown. If one is not available, a rubber ring may be used to prevent pressure on the sacrum and buttocks, since these children may be constantly in a sitting position. The child's elbows are massaged with lotion lest they become irritated by rubbing on the sheets. They may be further protected by dressing him in a garment having long sleeves. His position is changed frequently in order to prevent breakdown of the skin, to increase expansion of the lungs, and to prevent his extremities from becoming stiff. Sore joints are handled carefully when he is moved. The child is helped to use the bedpan as necessary.

If the child breathes through his mouth or has a limited fluid intake, good mouth care is essential.

Small, frequent feedings of light, nourishing food are better than meals served at the usual intervals. Although steroid therapy is usually accompanied by an increase in appetite, it may be necessary to cater to the child's appetite. He is not forced to eat, nor allowed to overeat, since without exercise he might become obese. When food is brought, he is placed in a comfortable position for eating and, if he is unable to help himself, is assisted by the nurse. If the child's appetite is poor, small blood or plasma transfusions may become necessary.

If oxygen is ordered, it may be given in a tent. The procedure is explained to the child. The school child is not likely to be frightened as is the younger child. He is given a bell so that he can summon his nurse. He should wear adequate clothing so that he does not become chilled.

Nursing records must be full and specific. The rate and nature of the pulse are indicative of the child's progress. If the physician so orders, the pulse is taken when the child is sleeping as well as when he is awake. The pulse rate is counted for a full minute, before the thermometer is inserted. The temperature and respiration rate are also taken and accurately recorded.

If digitalis is ordered, the nurse counts the pulse rate before the administration of each dose (see p. 292 for a discussion of digitalis therapy). If the rate has decreased or the quality of the pulse has changed, the dose is withheld until the physician can examine the child. Criteria by which improvement can be measured include the quality of the pulse rate when the child is resting and its ability to return to its former rate after mild exertion. If heart damage is evident, the child's activity must continue to be limited.

In general, an intake and output record is required. If possible, the child is allowed to keep his own record. If fluids are limited, he should have a schedule to follow. The reason for limiting fluid intake and for keeping the intake and output chart are explained to him. The amount and kind of food taken are also charted.

The nurse also observes and records the emotional state of the child, fatigue, respiratory excursion, orthopnea, venous distention in the neck, dyspnea, cough, pain, color of the skin, lips or nails, skin lesions, and edema.

The personnel caring for the child should understand the parents' attitude toward the child and his illness. The nurse and the physician

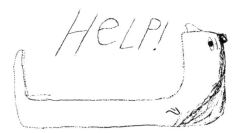

FIGURE 24–7. This plea for "HELP" was drawn by a long-term hospitalized, seriously ill school child whose deep needs for love and acceptance could not be met. Although he was not able to express his needs verbally, he could put his feelings into one word on paper. (Courtesy of Miss Mary Brooks.)

begin early in the illness to evaluate the family's attitude, which may vary from apparent unconcern to extreme anxiety. Parents must be helped to a more positive approach to the illness if the child is to be successfully rehabilitated.

CONVALESCENT CARE. Probably the first requisite in successful nursing of the convalescing child is to keep him happy and contented. These children become depressed because they see other acutely ill children admitted, recover, and be discharged, while they themselves remain in the hospital. The child's activities must be confined to the limits permitted by the physician. There is a gradual increase in the child's ability to care for himself (bathing, feeding, and so on) as he improves.

If schoolwork is permitted, the child has this interest and the satisfaction of feeling that he is keeping up with his class. This helps him to look forward to the time of his discharge from the hospital. Recreational and occupational therapy helps him by teaching him new skills which he is interested in learning and which are related to the physician's plan for his care while in the hospital. Suitable activities include finger painting, making beads from macaroni and stringing them, or making other kinds of jewelry, making puppets or cuddly toys, soap carving, spatter prints, spool knitting, making model airplanes and boats, leather construction, clay modeling, knitting, and so on. Making collections of items which interest children of his age is also appropriate. These children enjoy guessing games, many of which have educational value. Acceptance of activities within the limits set by the physician helps the child to understand and accept quiet games or a physically inactive role in an active game when he plays with his friends after his discharge.

The play period in the hospital is short and is followed by periods of music, story telling or reading, during which the child relaxes.

The time out of bed is gradually increased. A

comfortable chair (not a wheelchair because the child is likely to wheel himself around in it) may be placed by the window, and the child may be given playthings which interest him and ensure quiet activity. A wheelchair is used when the nurse pushes him about to explore his environment. After several weeks or months he is allowed to walk, but he must be closely supervised so that he does not overdo it.

Home is the best place for the convalescent child, but if this is not possible because of overcrowding and general lack of facilities, he may be sent to a convalescent hospital where the environment is planned to give him the emotional security he needs, opportunities for play, education, work, and group life, as well as continued supervision of his physical health. The community or public health nurse or home care personnel may make an evaluation of the home as to the adequacy of facilities prior to the child's discharge from the hospital. In some cases the child may be sent to a foster home, but it is extremely difficult to find such a home.

Resumption of normal activities is gradual over a period of several weeks to months.

If the child is sent to a convalescent hospital or a foster home, he should help to make plans, know about total plans, and meet his foster parents before he leaves the hospital. His parents should remain in contact with him, since such arrangements are only temporary.

It is necessary to work out a plan with the parents or foster parents for the child's care when he leaves the hospital. Not only his physical but also his psychologic needs must be met. Gradual independence must be given and behavior disorders prevented. All aspects of his care are discussed. If any equipment is needed, e.g., overbed table, back rest, or footboard, the parents may be shown how to make these from wooden crates and suitcases, or, if they cannot be made at home and the parents cannot afford to buy them, they may be provided through some community agencies.

The home atmosphere should be cheerful. The child should have the same kind of quiet recreation which was provided in the hospital. In some cities a visiting school teacher will be sent by the school board, or a telephone connection may be made between his room and the classroom of the school he has attended. This enables him to hear the instruction given his class and their responses. The child may also be sent to a day hospital where he can get an education and have supervised activity with his peers.

Not too much attention should be directed toward the child's heart condition. The whole child is helped to develop confidence. He learns how to set his own standards for activity. The ultimate aim is kept in mind: to restore the child to his place in society with the least possible emotional trauma. When he returns to school, the health team, including teacher and school nurse or school nurse practitioner, must know the health plan to be carried out. They should understand his illness and thus help other children to understand and accept the difference in his routine; e.g., he will use the elevator, but they will not; his hours in school may not be as long as theirs.

The parents and the child are helped to understand the need for visits to the clinic or his private physician for prophylactic medications and to his dentist for dental care. The social service department may be helpful in arranging for transportation for these visits. Parents should understand and accept his daily routine and also be able to recognize respiratory infections and skin infections, possibly caused by streptococci, and to get adequate medical care when these occur.

Caring for the child in the home is difficult for the mother, especially if she has other children who need her attention, if the home is crowded, or if the mother must work outside the home to supplement the family income. Another problem is that of keeping appointments for regular follow-up care for the child when transportation is difficult and when there are small children for whom a baby-sitter must be found. A more subtle problem emerges when the child is well enough so that he requires little professional care. The mother no longer has the support of physicians, nurses, and social workers at a time when she needs increasing psychologic help in coping with the child's convalescence. The public health or community nurse who visits in the home can help the mother find solutions to many of these problems as they emerge.

The parents of an adolescent who has had rheumatic fever may worry about what will happen when he reaches adulthood. They may try to persuade him to enter a sedentary occupation against his own desire. They may doubt his suitability for marriage. If the adolescent is a girl, her parents may be concerned about the strains of pregnancy and childbirth. Such concerns should be discussed with the physician so that the adolescent can lead as normal a life as possible.

Prognosis and Prevention. The mortality rate is declining from both initial attacks and recur-

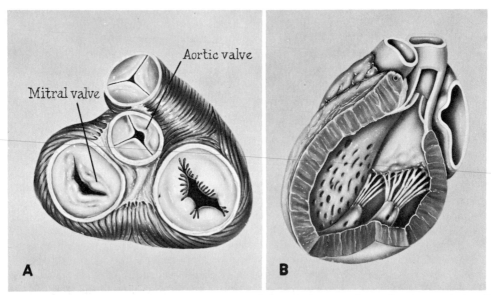

FIGURE 24–8. Chronic rheumatic heart. *A*, Superior view of chronic rheumatic heart showing aortic insufficiency and mitral stenosis. *B*, Dissection of chronic rheumatic heart showing fibrosis of mitral valve and thickened chordae tendineae. (From Disease Panorama on Rheumatic Fever, Courtesy of the Schering Corporation.)

rences of rheumatic fever. Recurrences are most common during childhood and decline after puberty.

Serious cardiac damage results from repeated, severe rheumatic attacks (Fig. 24–8). The *prognosis* for children who have their first attack before six years of age is graver than for those who have it later, because they usually have carditis with residual cardiac damage. If the child has chronic valvular disease resulting from rheumatic carditis, his heart will become hypertrophied, owing to the increased work load. When his heart is compensated, the only finding may be a cardiac murmur. When the heart is decompensated, the circulation is inadequate, and blood accumulates in the venous system. Edema, ascites, congestion of the lungs and liver, dyspnea and cyanosis result. The treatment of cardiac decompensation in the child is similar to that in the adult and includes reduction of the work of the heart by keeping the child in bed and rested by the use of sedatives (see p. 292). Further treatment includes the administration of oxygen to relieve dyspnea, digitalis to slow the heart rate and diuretics to relieve edema. The diet usually ordered is one low in salt. Fluids may or may not be limited. Often the residual heart condition may be so severe that it handicaps the adolescent or adult in his home and community life.

The prognosis is good for children who have no evidence of cardiac involvement. Death in childhood is apt to be due to further rheumatic infection rather than mechanical failure of the heart. Operation to place artificial valves like those used in the affected hearts of adults is not usually done in children.

Rheumatic polyarthritis does not result in permanent joint changes, and chorea does not produce permanent changes in the central nervous system.

The *prevention* of rheumatic fever lies in the prevention of infection with group A beta hemolytic streptococci. Streptococcal throat screening, in which throat cultures are done on children in elementary schools with follow-up care, is important in the prevention of rheumatic fever. Prevention of the first attack is through elimination of streptococci from the upper respiratory tract when the child has pharyngitis or scarlet fever. Penicillin is given for ten to 14 days, preferably by mouth except in those instances in which the certainty of the patient's maintaining his own prophylaxis is questionable.

Recurrence must be prevented, since each attack increases the threat of additional cardiac damage. The child should be kept from persons with upper respiratory tract infections. If he does acquire a respiratory illness, a throat culture should be taken, possibly by the school nurse practitioner or school nurse. Ideally, he should live in a warm climate and an uncrowded environment. As a prophylactic measure, benzathine penicillin is given monthly by intramuscular injection, or penicillin or sulfadiazine is given by mouth daily indefinitely after the initial attack. It is essential for the nurse to stress the importance of taking this preventive medication to both the parents and the child. These drugs may be obtained either free of charge or at minimal cost, depending on the ability of the parents to pay. The responsibility for the full cost of the drug may be assumed by the health department, the heart association, the welfare department, the crippled children's agency, or a combination of these. This eases the financial burden for the parents and facilitates oral prophylaxis.

If it is necessary for the child to have a tonsillectomy and adenoidectomy or undergo dental work, an increased dose of penicillin should be given to prevent bacterial endocarditis.

Public Health Aspects. There is need for a community program of control, case finding, and preventive work. There should be long-range programs for the care of these children. Improved living conditions of the lower-income group and better health programs in the schools would do much to prevent this serious disease. In some cities the coordination of team efforts for the benefit of these patients needs to be improved.

SYDENHAM'S CHOREA (ST. VITUS'S DANCE)

Incidence, Clinical Manifestations, and Diagnosis. Sydenham's chorea is one of the clinical manifestations of the rheumatic process. It is primarily a disorder of the central nervous system. It is most common in girls during later childhood and early adolescence—from seven to 14 years of age. The highest *incidence* is at eight years. Some authorities believe that the disease occurs in certain families more than in the general population (thus heredity would appear to be important) and that nervous persons are most liable to have the disease. It is seldom seen after puberty.

Sydenham's chorea is characterized by involuntary, purposeless, irregular movements involving any part or all of the voluntary musculature.

The *clinical manifestations* may vary from mild to severe. The onset is gradual. The child becomes increasingly nervous, and his jerking, spasmodic, purposeless, incoordinated, irregular movements cause him great discomfort. These movements are different from, and more severe than, those of tic. The first symptom of the condition may be clumsiness, and the child may be reprimanded for dropping something or spilling food at the table. Although he knows that he is doing this, he cannot control his movements. The movements of the facial muscles produce grimaces which often may appear to the adult as rude and to other children as silly. The child's handwriting shows lack of muscular control and may become almost illegible. The child cannot suppress his spasmodic movements, which be-

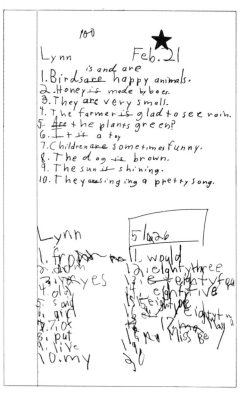

FIGURE 24–9. The deterioration of this child's writing ability led to a medical diagnosis of chorea. (From Myklebust, H. R.: *Progress in Learning Disabilities.* Vol. 2. New York, Grune & Stratton, Inc., 1971. Used by permission.)

come worse with excitement and embarrassment, but cease when he is asleep. Muscular weakness may become so great that he is unable to walk or even sit up. He talks with difficulty, and it is often impossible to understand his speech. He is "jittery," and slovenly in his personal habits, and may be unable to dress himself, having greatest difficulty in buttoning his clothes and tying his shoelaces. He may be unable to feed himself and may have difficulty in swallowing. Some children become incontinent. Emotional instability is shown in giggling, crying, fretfulness, and rapid shifting from depression to elation. Usually the child does not have fever. The school teacher is apt to recognize the early signs of chorea: the child's lack of ability to sit still in school, his grimacing, and the obvious changes in his handwriting. Teachers should be educated about the early signs of illnesses such as chorea which affect school children.

The *diagnosis* is based on the clinical manifestations, the most important of which are increase of choreiform movements when tense, increased dysfunction of speech, and rapid changes of facial expression from a grin to tears. Laboratory tests such as the sedimentation rate, the leukocyte count and the antistreptolysin O titer may give normal results, and the C-reactive protein may be negative.

Treatment, Responsibilities of the Nurse, and Prognosis. Both *treatment* and *nursing care* are based on the relief of symptoms. Since there is no really effective treatment, nursing care is of central importance.

Drugs are given as ordered. The child has absolute mental and physical rest. He should have a private room or be with a few carefully chosen children who meet his need for companionship. Prolonged, warm baths may have a sedative effect, and tranquilizers and phenobarbital may be given. He must be fed by his nurse. He is protected from injury by padded sideboards for his bed; blankets, sheets, or pillows may be used for this purpose. His toys are those with which he will not hurt himself. The nurse must anticipate his needs. Waiting for a bedpan or urinal increases his nervousness.

Gradual exercise, both physical and mental, is given in accordance with the physician's orders as the child's condition improves. Improvement in the child's condition can be noted by having the child write his name each day on a sheet of paper. This record can be kept on the child's chart.

Since these children move constantly, they need adequate nourishment. They are fed frequently with a light, nourishing diet, high in protein and iron. Vitamin supplements are provided. The child is fed with a spoon rather than a fork, because he might injure himself upon the prongs.

Skin care is important. Soothing baths to relieve his nervousness are also part of good skin care. Constant motion is likely to produce abraded surfaces on his elbows and knees. His skin is massaged with a soothing lotion or ointment, and his pajamas are of soft material to protect his skin from friction on the bedclothes. If he is incontinent, the bed is changed as soon as it is soiled or wet, and the skin of the buttocks and the genitalia is washed and dried thoroughly.

Psychologic care is as important as physical care. The nurse must be patient and understanding because the child's movements constantly interfere with care, and also because he is emotionally unstable and irritable. He is allowed to help himself as much as the physician permits, since this gives him a feeling of independence. He needs both love and happiness in his contacts with his parents and nurses. The nurse should help the parents to give him these essentials.

Child-parent relations may have been strained by the child's behavior before his condition became so evident that he was taken to a physician. Some parents will feel guilty at having blamed him for clumsiness he could not help, and others will find it difficult to understand that his irritating behavior was and is due to his disease, and not under his control. They doubt whether his recovery will bring a return to good behavior. The nurse's understanding attitude will help them to see the situation objectively and to give the child the emotional support he badly needs.

The convalescent child may be taught at home or in a special school where the hours of study are short and the whole educational plan is adapted to his needs. During his convalescence, play material appropriate to his needs should be provided. At first toys which exercise large muscles should be given, and then those which promote the use of small muscles. In this way the child will learn muscle control again.

The *prognosis* is good. There is spontaneous recovery in eight to ten weeks. Attacks may recur, but recovery is eventually complete. The disease is seldom fatal, but death may occur from exhaustion or cardiac disease.

JUVENILE RHEUMATOID ARTHRITIS (JRA) (STILL'S DISEASE)

Juvenile rheumatoid arthritis (JRA) is found in three forms: *polyarticular* disease, in which there are many joints involved, *pauciarticular* disease, in which only a few joints are involved, and *systemic* disease, in which there is a high fever with a rheumatoid rash and polyarthritis.

Etiology, Incidence, Epidemiology, and Pathology. The cause of rheumatoid arthritis is unknown. Chronic arthritis occurs in patients having an IgA deficiency and hypogammaglobulinemia, so that an immunodeficiency may predispose to rheumatoid arthritis. No definite immunodeficiency has been found, however. Juvenile rheumatoid arthritis is not a hereditary disease. There may be exacerbations of this condition after psychic stress or intercurrent illness.

Although onset may be during the preschool years, JRA during the school period is especially important because of the possible development of deformities that may have a crippling effect on the child and may prevent normal growth and development. It is especially seen in children between 8 and 12 years of age.

The characteristic pathologic finding in juvenile rheumatoid arthritis is chronic nonsuppurative inflammation of the synovium. Joint effusions result from the secretion of increased amounts of joint fluid. The articular cartilage may become progressively destroyed as the disease progresses. Many children with JRA, however, never develop permanent joint damage

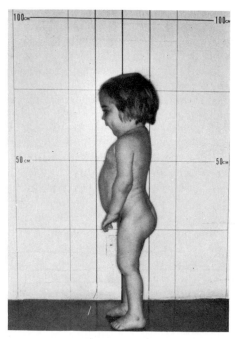

FIGURE 24–10. A six-year-old girl with classical systemic polyarthritis and severe joint involvement. Note the short stature and classical rash. At the age of 12 years, after receiving daily doses of prednisone and therapeutic aspirin, the child is still short, but medication dosages have been reduced. (From Boone, J. E., Baldwin, J., and Levine, C.: *Pediatr. Clin. N. Am.*, 21:898, November 1974.)

despite prolonged synovitis. Rheumatoid nodules are less frequent in children than in adults. The pleura, peritoneum, and pericardium may show nonspecific serositis.

Clinical Manifestations. Clinical manifestations of *polyarticular* disease involve multiple joints, especially the small joints of the hands. Girls are affected primarily.

The onset of polyarticular disease may be gradual, with the slow development of joint stiffness, loss of motion, and swelling. It may occur suddenly, however, with symptomatic arthritis. The affected joints are rarely red, but they are swollen and warm. They are painful and have limited motion. Stiffness following inactivity is common among children having JRA. Affected children are anxious and irritable, guarding themselves against being touched.

Arthritis often begins symmetrically in the knees, ankles, wrists, and elbows. The inflammation of the proximal interphalangeal joints results in spindling changes of the fingers. Arthritis of the cervical spine, temporomandibular joints, and hips may occur. Severe hip disease is a major cause of disability. Overgrowth or undergrowth of tissues adjacent to the inflamed joints may result in growth disturbances.

These children may have anorexia, general malaise, mild anemia, and a low-grade fever. A slight hepatosplenomegaly and lymphadenopathy may be present. Although growth may be retarded during periods of exacerbation, growth spurts may occur during periods of remission.

Clinical manifestations of *pauciarticular* disease include arthritis that affects only a few large joints such as the knees, ankles, and elbows. Other joints may occasionally be affected. About one third of children having JRA have this form of the disease; girls are affected more than boys. This form of arthritis may be recurrent or chronic, but serious disability does not usually occur.

One of four children having pauciarticular disease runs the risk of having *iridocyclitis* (inflammation of the iris and ciliary body) at some time during the course of the illness. Iridocyclitis is usually chronic and not associated with the activity of arthritis or with an elevated sedimentation rate. Symptoms include redness, photophobia, pain, or decreased visual acuity in one or both eyes. Children having iridocyclitis many times have positive tests for antinuclear antibodies. Loss of vision or permanent blindness may result (see p. 589). If early diagnosis is made and treatment is given before scarring, vision may be preserved. All children having pauciarticular disease with or without arthritis must therefore have slit lamp examinations every three or four months for the first five years of the disease.

Other clinical manifestations of this type of JRA include general malaise, low-grade fever, mild anemia, lymphadenopathy, and hepatosplenomegaly.

Clinical manifestations of *systemic* disease are largely extra-articular and include an intermittent high fever to 103° F. (39.4° C) or higher and a rheumatoid rash. Boys and girls are affected equally. About one quarter of children having JRA have systemic disease.

Elevations of temperature with shaking chills occur usually in the evenings, but they may occur at other times of the day. When the fever is present, these patients are very ill, but they feel well when the temperature returns to normal. The rheumatic rash consists of small pale, red-pink macular lesions often with central pallor, usually found on the trunk and proximal extremities. Generalized lymphadenopathy and hepatosplenomegaly also are present. Leukocytosis and anemia may be found.

Polyarticular joint manifestations occur within a few months of onset. Chronic arthritis may persist after the systemic symptoms have gone into remission, possibly even into adulthood.

Diagnosis. There are no specific laboratory tests for JRA. The sedimentation rate may be elevated during active disease. Anemia is common. The white blood cell count may be elevated. Urine is normal. Any of the serum immunoglobins may be elevated. Positive agglutination tests for rheumatoid factors are found more frequently with increasing age of onset.

Synovial fluid is cloudy, may clot spontaneously, and contains increased amounts of protein. Radiographic changes occur in the affected joints.

Treatment and Responsibilities of the Nurse. *Treatment* of JRA must involve the whole child because of the long-term nature of this condition and the lack of a specific cure. Treatment and nursing care require patience and understanding. The family may move from physician to physician looking for a cure, and the child may end up being treated by a quack, thus permitting unnecessary crippling to occur.

The major purposes of treatment are to preserve the functioning of the joints and to care for the extra-articular manifestations of JRA without causing additional problems. Support is provided for family members, including the child, so that normal growth and development are maintained and the disease can be accepted. The treatment team includes the physician, physiotherapist, orthopedist, rheumatologist, orthodontist, ophthalmologist, social worker or psychiatrist, and nurse.

Drugs used include the salicylates, corticosteroids, and gold salts. Aspirin is the drug of choice, since it is the safest. The nurse must watch constantly for symptoms of aspirin toxicity if very large doses are given. Drowsiness or

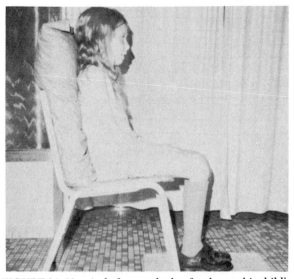

FIGURE 24–11. A platform under her feet keeps this child's feet from dangling despite the height of the chair. A pillow shortens the depth of the chair, so that her feet are at right angles to her legs. (From Pendleton, T., and Grossman, B. J.: *Am. J. Nursing,* 74:2224, December 1974.)

other central nervous system changes and rapid or heavy breathing are early indications of toxicity in children. Aspirin should be given with food to prevent irritation of the stomach.

Systemic corticosteroids may be given because they suppress the symptoms, but they do not prevent joint damage. In addition to suppressing growth, however, they cause many other undesirable side effects. If severe systemic disease is unresponsive to salicylates or if iridocyclitis does not respond to topical steroids, prednisone may be given. This drug is discontinued as soon as possible, and aspirin is again given.

Gold salts are used in the treatment of children as they are in adults—by weekly intramuscular injection. It is important to watch for indications of toxicity such as mucosal ulcers, skin rash, leukopenia, thrombocytopenia, and proteinuria.

Chloroquine or hydroxychloroquine may be of some help in therapy, but they are not usually used because of the possibility of retinal toxicity.

The physical therapist can outline a daily exercise program to maintain and improve the motion and muscular strength around affected joints. Swimming and riding the tricycle are especially helpful forms of exercise. Night splints for knees and wrists may prevent joint deformity. Prolonged bedrest is not beneficial for these children. They may exercise as they wish, avoiding prolonged exercise that leads to joint pain or overtiring. Orthopedic surgery is done to correct joint deformities.

Prompt diagnosis and therapy are required to preserve vision if the child has iridocyclitis. Parents should report decreased visual acuity or any other eye symptoms immediately. If symptoms occur, topical steroids and dilating agents are used. Frequent examinations of the eyes are required over a prolonged period of time.

The *nursing care* during the acute phase of JRA includes complete physical care including feeding, bathing, and dressing the child if his hands are severely involved. Later, the child should be encouraged to be as active as possible, since inactivity may lead to permanent deformity.

Physiotherapy is essential in the care of these children. If joints are held in flexion, muscles may become shortened. After inflammation in the joints has been reduced, they are put through the full range of motion at least once a day. The child is encouraged to lie flat on a firm mattress rather than curling up on his side. Half-shell splints applied to the legs at night help to prevent foot drop.

The parents are taught how best to care for these children. Warm tub baths in the morning reduce the stiffness of joints that develops through the night. In addition, warm compresses may facilitate joint movement at any time. The nurse can teach parents and child what to anticipate, that the disease is unpredictable and may have a course of several years. Support and encouragement of parents and child are necessary during this period. The child can learn to be as self-sufficient as possible in the home and at school. Children having residual handicaps may need help in the future to plan their vocations.

The community or public health nurse is responsible for the early detection of this disease and for follow-up care of these patients. Follow-up care of these children in the home includes the giving of gold intramuscularly and the observation of side effects of any medication that has been ordered. The nurse encourages the parents to observe for further symptoms of the disease and to report these immediately. The nurse also encourages the parents to continue follow-up care with the ophthalmologist if the child has iridocyclitis and with other members of the team as necessary.

Prognosis. In polyarticular and systemic JRA the major problem is chronic joint disease; in pauciarticular disease it is chronic iridocyclitis. This disease is rarely life-threatening. Exacerbations and remissions may continue for years, possibly into adulthood. Three quarters of affected children go into long remissions without severe deformity or loss of function.

SYSTEMIC LUPUS ERYTHEMATOSUS (SLE)

Etiology, Incidence, Pathology, Clinical Manifestations, and Diagnosis. Systemic lupus erythematosus (SLE) is a systemic disease that typically affects many organ systems. Lupus in children is usually more acute and severe than in adult patients. It may begin insidiously and it may be familial. Symptoms sometimes are present for years before the condition is diagnosed. This disease may be progressive and end in the death of the child if untreated. One fifth of adult cases begin in childhood, usually after the age of eight years. The ratio of affected females to males is 8:1 in all age groups. Members of any race may be affected.

The *etiology* is unknown. Systemic lupus erythematosus may be a disease of altered immune reactivity, possibly genetically determined. Viruses may be involved. Levels of immunoglobins in the serum are increased, and several immune phenomena occur.

The initial phase or an exacerbation may be related to intercurrent infections or there may be increased susceptibility to infections on the basis of faulty immune mechanisms.

A lupus-like disease may follow exposure to certain drugs, but it is generally mild and reversible when the drug is withdrawn. Sunlight may lead to exacerbation of the cutaneous and sometimes systemic manifestations of this disease.

Pathologic changes occur in many organ systems at various sites. Numerous autoantibodies are developed, and reactions to these antibodies cause most of the laboratory findings and clinical manifestations.

The early *clinical manifestations* are fever, arthritis or arthralgia, anorexia, malaise, weight loss, and rash. The rash occurs especially as erythematous or scaly patches involving the malar or cheekbone areas and extending over the bridge of the nose. It may spread from the face to the scalp, neck, extremities, and chest and may become secondarily infected. Other lesions may occur on the palms, soles of the feet, and fingertips.

Arthralgia and joint stiffness are common; tenosynovitis and myositis may occur. Anemia, thrombocytopenia, hyperglobulinemia, leukopenia, hepatomegaly, inflammation of serous membranes with effusions, generalized adenopathy, and cardiac involvement may be present. Signs of renal involvement such as nephritis occur in at least 75 per cent of children having SLE.

There may be personality changes, seizures, peripheral neuritis, and cerebral vascular accidents because of the involvement of the nervous system. Gastrointestinal manifestations and ocular changes may also be present. The disease may appear like any rheumatic disease and like many other illnesses, as well.

Antinuclear antibodies (ANA) can be found in all patients having active SLE. This is the best screening test for this condition. Antibodies to DNA are specific to SLE and are associated with active disease, especially with nephritis. Levels of serum gamma globulin are usually elevated. The presence of idiopathic thrombocytopenic purpura (see p. 686) may be the first manifestation of SLE. Red and white cells may be present in the urine, as well as casts and protein. If the blood urea nitrogen or creatinine are elevated and abnormal renal function studies are found, renal insufficiency can be diagnosed.

Treatment, Responsibilities of the Nurse, and Prognosis. *Treatment* is based on the severity of the disease in the individual child. The type and severity of kidney involvement can be determined by a renal biopsy.

Salicylates are used to provide symptomatic

relief of arthritis. Chloroquine and hydroxychloroquine are used but may cause retinal toxicity. The facial rash may be suppressed by using topical steroid preparations. Corticosteroids, which are potent inflammatory agents, may be given and tapered to the lowest suppressive dose effective for the child. In patients with SLE with severe nephritis, treatment is given to suppress the renal disease as reflected in the reduction of circulating antibodies to DNA and by the return of serum complement levels to normal. Seizures and other central nervous manifestations are treated with large doses of prednisone.

Careful follow-up is necessary for children having SLE since there is no cure. These patients must be evaluated and treated for years, possibly for life.

Helping parents to anticipate long-term medical supervision in the care of their child may be difficult. Parents should not be led to expect spontaneous remissions or sudden cures. Parents should be assisted in providing good general hygiene and a balanced diet for their child. These children can benefit from active physical activity to maintain joint range-of-motion and muscle tone.

Parents need to be taught about applying topical steroids to the rash and giving corticosteroids or other drugs as ordered. Prevention of secondary infections in the affected cutaneous areas is important. The child who has cutaneous manifestations must be protected from strong sunlight, especially during the summer months. Sun-screening lotions and creams that are effective in excluding ultraviolet light should be used on exposed skin areas.

Parents should know the potential side effects of prolonged steroid therapy such as problems associated with the child's body image, as well as indications of when medical care is required. The child treated with prednisone must be observed for the development of infections including tuberculosis and fungal infections, among others.

The nurse or parents should observe for indications of renal disease such as the presence of edema, altered intake and output, and changes in the color and characteristics of the urine.

Adolescent females who have SLE should be made aware that exacerbations of their disease may occur if they use some birth control agents or if pregnancy occurs. The nurse may answer questions concerning these matters or they may be referred to the physician.

The *prognosis* for SLE in children in the past was considered poor; however, some children having a milder form of the disease without severe nephritis are being treated and helped. Spontaneous exacerbations and remissions do occur. Prolonged spontaneous remissions are unusual. Corticosteroid and antibiotic therapy improve the overall prognosis. The risks of long-term immunosuppressive therapy are not known, although it may result in the increased occurrence of malignancy at an early age or possibly infertility. Death is usually caused by nephritis.

INFECTIOUS NEURONITIS (GUILLAIN-BARRÉ SYNDROME; INFECTIOUS POLYNEURITIS)

Etiology, Incidence and Clinical Manifestations. There is no known origin for infectious neuronitis. It is a condition involving the nervous system, with varying degrees of motor and sensory disturbances. Infectious neuronitis may be a hypersensitivity phenomenon or it may represent a toxic effect of an original infection. The original infection may have been influenza, a respiratory infection, infectious mononucleosis, or any of a number of communicable diseases. This condition has been diagnosed after the administration of some vaccines.

The *incidence* of this condition seems to be increasing in children. It can occur in either sex and is seen especially in children between the ages of four and ten years.

Clinical manifestations include an acute ascending motor paralysis and motor and sensory disturbances. Several days after an infection peripheral neuritis may develop symmetrically in the legs. Cutaneous reflexes are maintained, but the muscles become tender and the deep tendon reflexes are diminished or abolished. Paresthesias and cramping pains may be felt by the child. The abdominal and thoracic muscles may be involved as may the facial and bulbar musculature. Muscular atrophy does not usually occur. Other areas of the nervous system are not affected.

There are pathologic changes in the peripheral nerves and nerve roots. There is degeneration in the myelin and in the axis cylinders. No typical central nervous system changes are noted. Lesions in the viscera consist of focal necroses with round cell infiltration in the adrenals, kidneys, and liver. There are characteristic findings in the cerebrospinal fluid of elevation of protein, primarily albumin, and a normal cell count.

Treatment, Responsibilities of the Nurse, and Prognosis. Treatment and nursing care are symptomatic. There is no specific therapy, although steroids have been tried.

If there is impaired respiratory function due to

involvement of the diaphragm and the intercostal muscles, postural drainage and mechanical suction are used as needed. It is important to monitor vital capacity, blood gases, and respiratory rate and depth. If respiratory function deteriorates, oxygen by mask or endotracheal intubation with intermittent positive pressure may be utilized or a tracheotomy may become necessary. If pneumonia develops, antibiotic therapy is given. The swallowing function may also be impaired.

If cardiovascular functioning is impaired, cardiac monitoring and frequent observation of vital signs may become necessary. Autonomic dysfunction with manifestations of hypertension, orthostatic hypotension, cardiac arrhythmias, ileus, and urinary retention may be life-threatening.

Since an elevation of temperature is not typical in this syndrome, a fever may be an indication of infection, a disturbance in temperature regulation, or dehydration. Adequate nutrition and fluids may be provided by nasogastric tube feeding or by a gastrostomy.

Frequent changes in position and good skin care are necessary to avoid decubitus ulcers. Irritability, fatigue, and mood changes may be present even after the recovery of motor function. A physical therapy program is carried out with active and passive exercises to prevent contractures.

The *prognosis* is good for complete recovery of most patients, but some may have residual weakness, contractures, and areflexia. Adequate neural function may be restored in a few months to a few years. A few patients may die during the acute phase of this disease.

DIABETES MELLITUS

Incidence and Pathology. In diabetes mellitus the body is unable to metabolize carbohydrates, owing to insufficient production of insulin, an internal secretion of the pancreas. There is also abnormal metabolism of fat and protein. Diabetes occurs in 1 of every 2500 children under the age of 15 years. Approximately 5 per cent of all people with diabetes show the first symptoms in childhood. The disorder is not common among children, but it tends to be more serious than in later life. The disease is inherited as a recessive characteristic. Genetic counseling may help the parents of an affected child to understand the hereditary aspects of this condition.

Diabetes mellitus having its onset before 15 years of age is called *juvenile diabetes*. This disease must be distinguished from *diabetes insipidus*, which is a disease of the pituitary or the hypothalamus.

Since there is a deficiency of insulin, or since its effect is inhibited in diabetes mellitus, diabetic acidosis, coma, and death may result. Hyperglycemia is produced, which, when it exceeds the normal threshold, causes glycosuria. Hyperglycemia initiates diuresis, and as a result excess glucose is excreted. In addition to glucose, electrolytes and water are lost from both the intracellular and extracellular compartments of the body.

Tissue breakdown is due in part to osmotic forces and in part to tissue catabolism because of the body's inability to use glucose for fuel. Protein and fat are oxidized more rapidly than is normal. Because of the increased rate of breakdown of fats, ketonuria results. Ketonuria, dehydration, and kidney dysfunction result in acidosis.

In uncontrolled diabetes, hyperglycemia is found; body water, electrolytes and fixed base are lost; the plasma carbon dioxide content is lowered; acidosis develops; and glycogen stored in the muscles and liver is lost.

Nurses must be alert for evidence of diabetes in children, especially if there is a family history of the illness. They should educate the family about potential danger signals, such as a child's unusual thirst and frequent need to void.

Clinical Manifestations, Laboratory Studies, and Diagnosis. Diabetes may develop slowly or may first be recognized when the child is in coma. The onset in children is generally more rapid than in adults, and the child is likely to be underweight at the onset. Obesity does not appear to be a factor in juvenile diabetes.

The *symptoms* are increased thirst and appetite, weight loss, polyuria (this may be the cause of bed wetting in children who had achieved night control of urination), possibly weakness and, over a period of time, pruritus, dry skin, and excessive hairiness.

Nurses and all others responsible for the daily care of chidren should know the symptoms of *diabetic coma* or *acidosis*. Coma usually follows an infection in untreated diabetics who are not able to burn up carbohydrate and therefore utilize fat for energy. The symptoms are drowsiness, dry skin, cherry red lips and flushed cheeks, hyperpnea, acetone odor to the breath, abdominal pain, nausea, and vomiting. The child in coma has Kussmaul breathing or severe hyperpnea, a rigid abdomen, rapid and weak pulse, lowered blood pressure and temperature, and soft, sunken eyeballs.

Laboratory studies show a lowered carbon

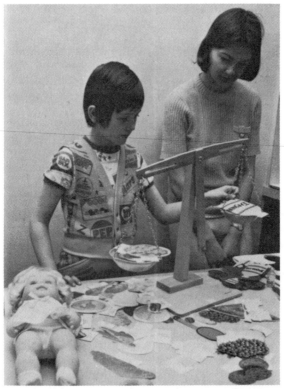

FIGURE 24–12. This diabetic child attempts to balance food intake with adequate insulin, using the toy scale and cardboard models. (From Leahey, M.D., Logan, S. A., and McArthur, R. G.: *The Canadian Nurse*, 71:19, October 1975.)

dioxide content of the blood and a shift of pH to the acid side. Albumin and casts may be present in the urine when the child has acidosis.

The *diagnosis* is based on the family history and the history of the child's previous health, and on the clinical manifestations and laboratory studies. A fasting hyperglycemia with glycosuria is diagnostic of diabetes mellitus. Other conditions, however, may have to be ruled out. Whenever glycosuria is found, a blood sugar determination is made. If the blood sugar level is more than 200 mg. per 100 ml., a diagnosis of diabetes mellitus is tentatively made. A glucose tolerance test may show prolonged, high levels of sugar in the blood, indicating that the body cannot burn carbohydrates. A high white blood cell count may be present with diabetic acidosis.

Treatment. Management of the preadolescent diabetic is usually not too difficult if he and his parents understand the disease and his care. Management of the adolescent diabetic is more difficult because of his desire to rebel against the authority of his parents and the physician. If he is adequately treated, the diabetic should be able to compete with his peers in physical, mental and social development.

Treatment includes a *diet* which supports normal growth and development and satisfies the child's appetite, and the administration of insulin in sufficient amount to maintain glycemic equilibrium. An important aspect of treatment is instruction of the child and his parents so that they can manage the treatment in the home. This requires acceptance by the child and his family of the fact that he is essentially a normal child.

Should *diabetic acidosis* develop, treatment involves close cooperation of the physician, nurse and laboratory personnel. Laboratory examinations are needed to determine the blood sugar level and carbon dioxide-combining power or carbon dioxide content, and urinalysis for sugar and acetone. Intravenous therapy is used. Electrolytes, carbohydrate, and water are given with insulin. Vitamins may also be given. If the child is in severe acidosis, with a pH of less than 7.1 and a carbon dioxide measurement of less than 12 mEq. per liter, sodium bicarbonate may be given. Urine should be collected each hour in order to guide modification of the dosage of insulin and carbohydrates as therapy progresses. Warmth and comfort are essential for the child with acidosis. The nurse should watch for changes in color, type of respiration, and degree of consciousness. Gastric aspiration may be carried out to relieve distention, to prevent pulmonary aspiration of vomitus and to hasten the time when the child can take fluids by mouth. Sodium bicarbonate solution may be introduced through the tube into the stomach after the stomach has been emptied. Large doses of appropriate antibiotics may be given if infection is present. Oral feedings may be started when the child regains consciousness, usually after 12 to 16 hours of parenteral therapy, and then carbohydrate and electrolyte mixtures are given. This dietary stage is followed with an adequate fluid diet. Small doses of insulin are given to cover the oral intake of carbohydrates; the amount is based on the amount of sugar in the urine. While taking oral feedings the child should be checked for symptoms of insulin shock or diabetic acidosis. An average diet may be given in a few days if he shows no untoward symptoms.

Management of the child in whom diabetes was not adequately controlled or after correction of the acidosis requires the same teamwork that is necessary in the acute crisis, but nursing care becomes the center of the program. Treatment must be individualized; each child needs a satisfactory diet and insulin dosage. The diet is approximately that of a normal child and similar to the family's diet. The specific requirements of the diet are that it supply caloric intake for activity and growth, sufficient protein intake for growth, and the required vitamins and minerals. An appointment with the dietitian for the child and his family is planned for clarification of the diet.

One of two types of diets may be ordered. (1) Quantities of food may be *measured.* Many parents find that children feel more secure when a definite dietary program is ordered and exactly followed. (2) The so-called *unrestricted* or *free diet* is that of a normal child. It is restricted only in that excesses, such as high carbohydrate intake, are avoided. On this diet the child feels as free as a normal child because he may eat practically whatever he wishes. The present trend in therapy appears to be toward the unrestricted diet.

In general, the child is on a stabilized, measured diet only at the beginning of treatment. Upon discharge from the hospital he and his parents are given a list of foods which are exchangeable in planning his meals for the day. For such a diet gross household measures are adequate. They are not as rigid as in a weighed diet. Occasional deviations are not important. The child on such a diet receives a satisfactory intake with adequate distribution of caloric intake at various meals. He learns to manage his diet himself as he grows older.

The child is stabilized on his diet and the amount of insulin he needs while he is in the hospital. The health team must know the child's normal exercise pattern at home in order to plan for his care before discharge. Since the amount of exercise he takes changes his needs, for several days before his discharge he takes about the same amount of exercise as he will when he is at home. The child may be taken on tours in the hospital or for walks outside. Arrangements may be made, if possible, for him to eat in the hospital cafeteria where the dietitian or nurse can help him select his diet. The diet is planned so that his appetite is satisfied and his growth and development are normal when he is leading the same kind of life his friends lead.

Insulin is a specially prepared extract of the pancreas. Injected into the body, it enables the body to burn sugar. All juvenile diabetics need insulin. Although adult diabetics have profited from sulfonylureas (orally administered hypoglycemic agents) and the biguanides (Phenformin-DBI), these do not provide a reliable replacement for insulin in the treatment of diabetic children. Sulfonylureas stimulate the production of insulin. They are not used in children because the capacity to produce insulin is quickly and to a large extent lost. The biguanides lower blood glucose levels by altering carbohydrate metabolism in adults, but these are not useful in children and the incidence of side effects when they are given is high. Retardation in growth may also occur.

Insulin administered on a daily basis is required in practically all children who have diabetes. There are several insulin preparations available, falling into three categories, depending upon their length of action. Insulin that has a *rapid action of short duration* is either regular or crystalline and Semi-Lente. The onset of effect of these insulins is about a half hour, reaching a peak in two to four hours, with a duration of effect of six to eight hours for regular insulin to 10 to 12 hours for Semi-Lente insulin. Insulin that is *intermediate in rapidity of action and is relatively long in duration* includes NPH (isophane), Lente, and Globin insulin. The onset of effect of these insulins is two hours, reaching a peak in approximately 8 to 16 hours, and having a duration of effect of about 20 to 30 hours. Insulin that has a *delayed action and a long duration* includes protamine zinc (PZI) and Ultra-Lente. The onset of effect of these insulins is four to eight hours, reaching a peak in 14 to 24 hours, and having a duration of effect from 24 to 36 hours or more. Although insulin was supplied in the past in either 40 units/ml. (U40) or 80 units/ml. (U80), in the future it will be available only in one concentration: 100 units/ml. (U100). Commercial insulin will be available in a more highly purified preparation that will reduce the problems of insulin allergy and of local reactions to injections. Insulin is usually given subcutaneously. When the child is in acidosis, insulin may be given intravenously or intramuscularly.

The dose of insulin is estimated on the basis of qualitative tests of the urine for sugar. Urine specimens should be collected at the following hours: before breakfast, at 7 or 8 a.m., before lunch, at 11:30 to noon, before the evening meal, at 5 to 6 p.m., and before bedtime, at 7 to 9 p.m. Actually, another specimen obtained approximately 30 minutes after the initial specimen will be more accurate when tested than the first. Obtaining the second specimen from a young child may be difficult, however; therefore it is probably wise to test the urine each time the child voids. Usually Clinitest tablets are used in preference to other methods. If too large a dose of insulin, too little food or too much exercise is taken, insulin shock may result. With an even balance between the diet and the dosage of insulin, the urine is essentially sugar-free. Some physicians prefer to have recorded a trace of sugar but no acetone in the urine, since the danger of insulin shock from a constantly negative result would be prevented.

Several factors are important in varying the

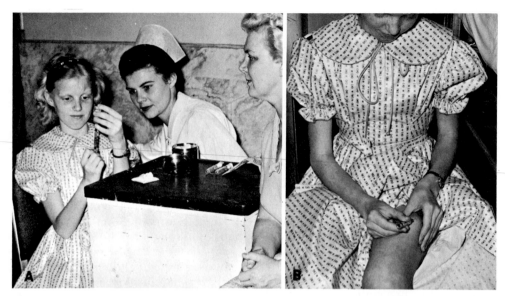

FIGURE 24–13.   Diabetes. A, This 11-year-old girl is learning how to prepare her dosage of insulin. Her mother, who has already learned the procedure, is interested in her progress. B, Having practiced the procedure, this child is now able to inject the insulin and thus to assume more responsibility for her own care.

need for insulin. Adjustment must be made periodically in the relation of *diet* to insulin dosage. All children need *exercise*, but diabetics must take exercise that requires a relatively definite amount of energy expenditure. Exercise pro-

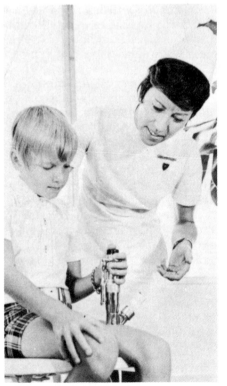

FIGURE 24–14.   The Medi-jector is a newer device to give insulin without the use of a needle and syringe. (Courtesy of Derada Corp., St. Paul, Minn.)

duces a lowering of the blood sugar level and may cause shock in children taking insulin. Only when the diet and exercise are standardized is it possible to give the requisite amount of insulin. Changes in diet and in energy output makes adjustment of the dose to the child's needs essential. This is difficult because of the difference in the child's activity on school days and on vacation days, and in wet and sunny weather. The child should always carry sugar with him and take it if he feels the symptoms of shock. If unusually strenuous activity is planned, insulin dosage must be reduced proportionally. Some physicians maintain diabetic children on an insulin dosage which permits some spilling of sugar daily so that their margin of safety is a little greater with changes in the amount of exercise they have. Some physicians also teach these children to alter their insulin dosage slightly, based on the results of their urine tests.

Since *infection* increases the need for insulin, the child may go into acidosis easily if he has an infection. During such periods additional amounts of insulin may be needed to prevent glycosuria. The mother should receive instructions on the care of the child when he has an infection or is vomiting. The amount of insulin is reduced during convalescence.

Emotional disturbances also increase the child's need for insulin. Diabetic children who are emotionally stable can be regulated more easily than those who are easily upset.

Adjustment in dosage may also need to be made on the basis of *body growth*. Some children require more insulin as they approach puberty and adolescence, but some do not.

Responsibilities of the Nurse. After the parents and the child have learned what diabetes is and how it affects the body, an important part of the nursing care of the diabetic child is helping him and his parents to develop positive attitudes toward his condition. The members of the health team stress the fact that the child who has diabetes is not significantly different from other children of the same age. It is important, therefore, that the patient not be referred to as "the diabetic," a term which labels the child as potentially ill.

Probably the central problem is to help the parents accept the fact that the child can be healthy and active if dietary rules are followed and insulin is given in adjustment to his needs. Their initial attitude is likely to be that restriction is necessary only when the child is sick. The parents and the child must learn that constant care is necessary. The nurse listens to the parents when they express their feelings about the illness and tries to reconcile both parents and child to maintaining the prescribed diet and dosage of insulin, together with regular exercise.

As with other illnesses, the child having diabetes is encouraged to express his feelings about his disease and his treatment. Many children believe that they are being punished because of the dietary restrictions and the use of injections in treatment. The child's questions are answered, and he is encouraged to reduce some of his anxiety through play.

If a free diet is ordered, the child will have little problem in controlling his food intake. If a measured diet is ordered, the nurse must condition the child to self-control and make it easy for him, and instruct the mother in the need for, and the means of, helping the child conform to his regulated life. He should have exercise *after* meals. All tempting but restricted food should be kept out of the way as far as possible. Nevertheless school children must learn to go without, while others eat, the foods they are denied. The diet can be made attractive. Snacks are permitted and planned for at bedtime and between meals. The child should understand that if he reports breaks in dietary rules, he will not be punished or scolded, but that unreported breaks may cause sudden sickness.

The parents and child are usually taught only one method of determining whether there is sugar or acetone in the urine. A record of the results is kept on a chart. They are taught what the results of the tests should be and what must be done if results differ. It is important that parents and child strictly adhere to the directions enclosed in the package of the reagent used. Observations include the time interval required for reading the results of the particular test and the Clinitest reaction for "pass through" phenomenon. The correct color chart is used for the brand of reagent selected and the method

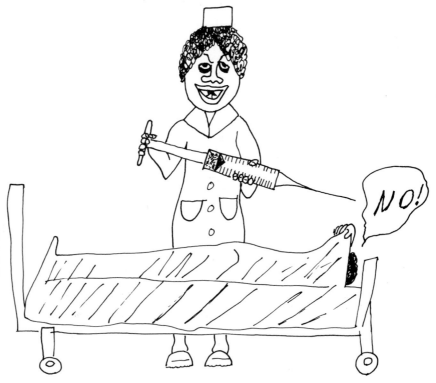

FIGURE 24–15. A ten-year-old diabetic child's view of his nurse. When asked about this picture, he said, "The nurse sticks me a lot with that needle!"

used, whether the two-drop or the five-drop method, is charted. The directions in the package are also followed for the correct handling of the reagent and the necessity of using unexpired reagent only.

No attempt should be made to hide the fact that the child is a diabetic. He and those about him should know this so as to understand his restriction of diet and need for a regular life. But he should not be permitted to use illness as a defense against accepting the role of a well child. He should be encouraged to assume his share of family responsibilities. He should also participate on an equal basis with his peer group, not looking on his diabetes as a handicap.

Table 24–1 presents material which nurses will find useful in understanding the child's treatment in the hospital and care at home. The general headings of the list can also be used as a check list for teaching purposes. This information supplements, but does not take the place of, individual instruction which the physicians, nurses, and dietitians will give the parents and the child. Understanding the care given the child in the hospital not only brings about better cooperation between the child, his parents, and the nurses, but also is the basis for the acceptance and following of the program for his care at home. The nurse should be thoroughly familiar with the information in the table.

Juvenile diabetes presents a tremendous teaching challenge to the members of the health and nursing teams (see p. 90 for a review of the principles of teaching and learning). When the child and his parents are ready to learn, repetition is important. Teaching aids such as film strips, visual aids, tapes, booklets and demonstrations may be used. The effectiveness of learning of the child and his parents should be evaluated.

The teacher and the school nurse can be aware of the child's illness and the manifestations of shock and coma so that they can help him in such emergencies. The child's parents and the school nurse can keep emergency kits containing glucagon available for use in case the child becomes unconscious from insulin shock. The school personnel, parents, and the child must realize that readmission to the hospital will be necessary for evaluation and adjustment of the diet and insulin dosage.

The school nurse or school nurse practitioner can also help the child in school by providing a place for him to collect and test urine specimens privately. The child should be taught to record the results of his urine tests on a homemade or

TABLE 24–1. CARE OF THE DIABETIC CHILD

SYMPTOMS OF INSULIN SHOCK AND DIABETIC COMA

Insulin Shock (Due to overdose of insulin, reduction of diet or increase in exercise)		*Diabetic Coma* (Acidosis)
Early manifestations:	Pallor Weakness Dizziness Changes in disposition* Sweating Tremor Sudden hunger Dilated pupils	Changes in mental state (lethargic)* Vomiting Abdominal pain
Severe reactions:	Semiconsciousness Later: convulsions, coma, death Low blood sugar Urine sugar-free Acetone absent	Acetone odor on breath Dehydration Hyperpnea Face flushed Lips cherry red Little perspiration Blood sugar high, low carbon dioxide Sugar and acetone present in urine

*The emotional reaction of the child is characteristic of him. He may cry, be hostile or appear happy.

The child and his parents should recognize the need for immediate assistance if symptoms of shock or acidosis occur. (Some physicians have induced mild insulin reactions in their patients so that both child and parents can learn the symptoms and treatment of this condition.) In case of shock the child should be given fruit juice or sugar. The child should carry a lump of sugar with him and, if he recognizes symptoms of shock, take the sugar. If the child becomes unconscious, he should be kept warm. The parents or school nurse should inject glucagon in the amount of 0.5 to 1 mg. intramuscularly. (Glucagon is normally produced by the pancreas. Its purpose is to increase blood sugar levels by changing glycogen in the liver back into glucose.) When the child regains consciousness, sugar can be given by mouth. If the child does not respond, he should be seen by a physician, who will administer glucose intravenously. Recovery after treatment for shock is usually rapid.

TABLE 24–1. *CARE OF THE DIABETIC CHILD (Continued)*

GENERAL CARE

1. Skin care to prevent infection
   a. Give frequent baths, at least every other day. Use lotion to keep the skin soft
   b. Provide properly fitted shoes (not of vinyl or plastic materials that prevent evaporation) that may be discarded when the child outgrows them
   c. Cut and trim the toenails correctly
   d. Teach the child to report any break in the skin and treat it promptly

2. Maintenance of resistance to infection
   a. Dress the child appropriately according to the temperature, not the season of the year
   b. Keep the child away from anyone who has an upper respiratory tract or other infection
   c. Report infections promptly to the physician
   d. Immunize the child against common communicable diseases

3. Proper elimination

4. Regulation of exercise
   a. In the hospital keep him as busy as he would be at home
   b. At home encourage him to take moderate exercise regularly each day

5. Accuracy in saving of urine specimens
   a. Save and test a specimen of urine at prescribed hours. Parents and child can be taught to test urine specimens
   b. Be careful that the child does not dilute the urine to cover a break in adhering to his diet

6. Diet
   a. Let the child eat with other diabetics in the hospital, for he is then more likely to accept his diet
   b. Teach the child to keep to the diet ordered by the physician. Give the child the list of allowed exchanges of food if such is ordered
   c. Make adherence to the diet as easy as possible by varying it as much as is permitted
   d. Teach the child to manage his own diet as early as possible

7. Administration of insulin
   a. Both child and parents should learn the reason for and the procedure of administration of insulin
   b. Children 7 to 10 years of age can usually be taught to give insulin to themselves (even an intelligent younger child can learn). The earlier the responsibility is given the child, the better it is for him. The public health nurse can provide assistance with this procedure to parents and child at home
      (1) Make the explanation simple. After the nurse has explained the procedure initially, another diabetic child can assist him better than an adult can, perhaps because he has more time to spend on showing how and why each step is done
      (2) Let the child practice frequently under supervision
         (a) Use routine sites of injections: upper right arm, upper left arm, left thigh, right thigh (each extremity may be used for several weeks if injections are given ½ inch apart). The outer areas of the abdomen, the upper back and the buttocks may also be used. These injection sites are rotated
         (b) Check the dose measured by the child until his accuracy is proved
         (c) Pinch the skin, or teach the child to do so, when using a site on the thigh, because this minimizes the pain of injection
         (d) Do not give insulin too near the surface of the skin

8. Records
   a. The child should be taught to keep daily records of the insulin dose, diet, and urine test findings until he learns about his illness and it is under control

9. The child's part in his recovery
   a. Keep the child under supervision as long as necessary, but give him independence as soon as possible
   b. Get his cooperation in
      (1) Voluntary self-control in diet so that other children cannot tempt him
      (2) Taking regular exercise
      (3) Honest reporting if he transgresses against the physician's orders
      (4) Not fooling his parents with faked symptoms of insulin shock
      (5) Avoiding self-pity or exaggerating his handicap
      (6) Carrying on his person at all times an identification card or tag which reads "I HAVE DIABETES" and gives his name, address, telephone number and his physician's name and number where he can be reached
   c. Guide the child to normal adolescence by understanding his aggressiveness, withdrawal or rebellion against restraint. Bring him, through understanding of his problem, to normal adulthood in which he can take his place in society

commercially available chart. The importance of honesty in keeping this record should be stressed.

Children who have diabetes may learn more about their disease by attending a summer camp for diabetics. Programs vary from camp to camp, but all attempt to develop the child's self-confidence, self-esteem, and independence.

As the child approaches preadolescence and the rapid growth spurt, his need for food increases. Since at this time his need to be like his peers is great, the child may eat what they eat even though he knows that he should not do so. The preadolescent diabetic then needs support and understanding so that he can keep his disease under control. If the child is threatened or punished for eating food he should not eat, further dietary indiscretions may result. The diet may need to be readjusted so that the preadolescent gets the food he needs.

Adolescence may be a difficult period for the diabetic youth and for his parents. While the young person may wish to become independent and rebel against restraints such as are involved in his own care, his parents may seek to protect him, thus keeping him dependent on them. Girls may be concerned about the effect of their diabetes on dating, marriage, and motherhood. Boys worry about the effect of their disease on their chances for employment and for marriage. Both girls and boys are concerned about being different from their peers. The social worker and genetic counselor with other team members can help both parents and child in their struggles so that the adolescent can reach adulthood and take a productive place in society. Psychiatric assistance may be necessary to achieve this goal.

Complications, Course, and Prognosis. *Complications* are uncommon except in children who have been inadequately treated or have had the condition for a long time. The following may possibly result from diabetes: lack of develop-

ment, stunted growth, amenorrhea, and lack of development of secondary sex characteristics. Children may also suffer cataracts, gangrene, and arteriosclerosis after the disease has been present for years. Infections are common and heal more slowly than is normal in the poorly treated diabetic child. These include infections of the skin, respiratory tract, and lower urinary tract. Dental caries is also common.

Complications which may occur as a result of insulin injections include atrophy of the subcutaneous fat and allergy to insulin.

The *course* and *prognosis* depend on the accuracy of control measures. Serious degenerative lesions appear in young adults who have had diabetes mellitus for ten to 20 years. These include arteriosclerosis with hypertension, nephropathy and retinal changes.

PRECOCIOUS SEXUAL DEVELOPMENT (PRECOCIOUS PUBERTY)

Etiology, Treatment, and Prognosis. Precocious sexual development can be diagnosed when secondary sexual characteristics appear before the child is eight to ten years of age.

These children may be divided into two groups: those with *true* or *idiopathic precocious puberty,* and those with *precocious pseudopuberty,* in which secondary sexual characteristics appear, but no sperm or ova are formed.

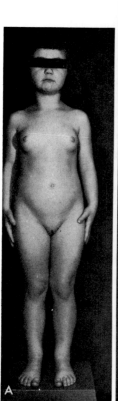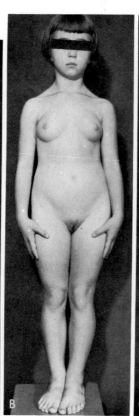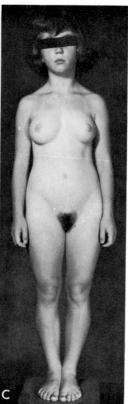

FIGURE 24–16. Idiopathic precocious puberty. Patient *(A)* $3^{11}/_{12}$ years, *(B)* $5^{8}/_{12}$ years, and *(C)* $8^{1}/_2$ years. Breast development and vaginal bleeding began at $2^{1}/_2$ years of age. Osseous age was 14 years at 8 years of age. Intelligence and dental age are normal for chronologic age. Growth was completed at 10 years; ultimate height was 142 cm. (56 in.). (From Vaughan, V. C., III, and McKay, R. J. (Eds): *Nelson Textbook of Pediatrics.* 10th ed. Philadelphia, W. B. Saunders Co., 1975.)

Most cases of true precocious puberty are due to a constitutional premature maturation of the endocrine control of the genital tissues. This may be either sporadic or familial. In this condition the hypothalamic mechanism is precociously activated and the changes of puberty begin. In girls the breasts develop and pubic hair appears. Later the external genitalia develop, axillary hair becomes evident, and menstruation begins. In boys the penis and testes enlarge, pubic hair appears, acne develops, and erections occur. The production of sperm may occur as early as five years of age.

Although the appearance of the child may be embarrassing, other children eventually catch up with the preadolescent in development. There is a decided spurt in physical growth resulting in early epiphyseal closure of the long bones. The eventual height of these children therefore tends to be below average on maturity. The physician will explain this condition to the parents and to the child. These children should

be guarded against sexual abuses, which, in a girl, may lead to pregnancy. No treatment is necessary for this condition.

Precocious puberty may also be due to a central nervous system infection such as encephalitis, hydrocephalus, or a lesion which usually involves the hypothalamus or the floor of the third ventricle. Convulsions or mental retardation may also be present in these children. In girls tumors of the ovaries, feminizing adrenal cortical tumors, McCune-Albright syndrome, or the accidental ingestion of estrogens may cause precocious puberty. In boys cerebral lesions, the adrenogenital syndrome, a Leydig-cell tumor, or accidental ingestion of androgens may cause precocious puberty.

Treatment is concerned mostly with the psychological adjustment of the child and his parents. The physician should discuss the child's condition with his parents, emphasizing that other children will catch up to him in development by the age of 14 years. Further treatment is directed to the cause itself.

The ultimate *prognosis* depends upon the cause and treatment of the condition.

HEAD TRAUMA

Active school children acquire head injuries usually as a result of automobile accidents, falls from bicycles, falls when climbing, or being hit on the head when playing.

CEREBRAL CONCUSSION

Clinical Manifestations, Treatment and Responsibilities of the Nurse. The term *cerebral concussion* means a temporary disturbance of cerebral functioning. The *clinical manifestations* of cerebral concussion following a sudden blow on the head include a transient loss of consciousness, headache, pallor, vomiting, apathy, and irritability. If the child is unconscious for a prolonged time with varying degrees of amnesia, the diagnosis of *cerebral contusion* or *laceration* is made. Convulsions may occur.

The *treatment* and *nursing care* for the first 12 to 24 hours after a head injury include the following: careful observation at least every two hours of the level of consciousness, recording of the vital signs, and notation of the movement of the eyes and equality of the pupils, including their size and reaction. Any change in these signs or deepening of the level of unconsciousness may indicate intracranial bleeding. If the child is very restless, a sedative such as chloral hydrate may be ordered. The side rails are padded to prevent injury in case a convulsion occurs. The child's bladder is examined for overdistention, which may be a cause of continued restlessness.

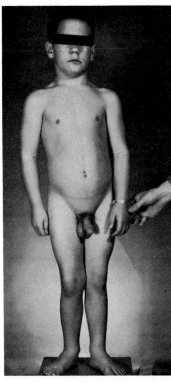

FIGURE 24–17. Precocious puberty without a demonstrable lesion in a 3½-year-old boy. Height age was 5 years and bone age 8 years. Note well-developed testes; testicular biopsy revealed Leydig cells and well-developed tubules with adult spermatogonia. At 5 years of age the boy had a height age of 10 years and osseous maturation of 14 years. Growth ceased at 9 years; ultimate stature was 148.6 cm. (58½ in.) He had no neurologic abnormalities and was bright-normal in intelligence and well-adjusted emotionally. (From Vaughan, V. C., III, and McKay, R. J. (Eds.): *Nelson Textbook of Pediatrics,* 10th ed. Philadelphia, W. B. Saunders Co., 1975.)

Pt.					
Date					
Tour					
	Person	Orienta-tion	Levels of Consciousness		Nursing Assessment for Increasing Intracranial Pressure
	Place				
	Time				
	Recent	Memory			
	Remote				
	Insight				
	Distinct	Speech			
	Coherent				
	Flowing				
	Small	Size	Pupillary Signs		
	Medium				
	Large				
	Equality				
	Brisk	Reactivity			
	Moderate				
	Sluggish				
	Spontaneous	Upper Extremities	Extremity Movement, Strength and Sensation		
	Command				
	Decort.				
	Decereb.				
	Strong				
	Moderate				
	Weak				
	Touch				
	Pressure				
	Pain				
	Spontaneous	Lower Extremities			
	Command				
	Decort.				
	Decereb.				
	Strong				
	Moderate				
	Weak				
	Touch				
	Pressure				
	Pain				
	Temp		Vital Signs		
	Pulse				
	Blood Pressure				
	Rate	Respir			
	Adequacy				
	Abnormal				
Signature					

FIGURE 24–18. Nursing assessment for increasing intracranial pressure. (From Jimm, L. R., *Nursing Digest*, 3:7, July–August 1975.)

SKULL FRACTURE

Clinical Manifestations, Diagnosis, Treatment and Responsibilities of the Nurse. The *clinical manifestations* of a basilar fracture include blood in the external auditory canal, a discolored tympanic membrane, periorbital ecchymosis, epistaxis or bleeding from the mouth, subconjunctival hemorrhage, or facial weakness. The *diagnosis* of fracture may be made on the basis of roentgenograms of the skull.

The *treatment* of a depressed fracture includes elevation of the depressed area of the skull. Children having linear fractures usually require treatment similar to that for those having cerebral concussion. Repair of the dura must be considered. Antibiotics may be given as necessary.

The *nursing care* of these children includes careful observation for changes of vital signs indicating increased intracranial pressure. If cerebrospinal fluid is leaking from the nostril or ear, the nares or the external auditory canal are not irrigated or plugged with cotton.

EPIDURAL HEMORRHAGE (EPIDURAL HEMATOMA)

Clinical Manifestations, Treatment, and Responsibilities of the Nurse. The *clinical manifestations* of extradural hematoma are usually seen within 24 hours after the injury even if the child has no skull fracture. The child may have been unconscious immediately after the injury, become conscious, then lapse into a stupor or coma. He may have signs of increased intracranial pressure, ipsilateral dilatation of the pupil, and hemiparesis.

The *treatment* consists in immediate neurosurgery to prevent compression of the brain stem. Post-traumatic epilepsy may follow head injury.

The *nursing care* of a child who has sustained a severe head injury is not unlike that for a child having a brain tumor (see below). If the parents feel guilty that the injury was partially their fault, the members of the health team can support them and help them work through their feelings.

BRAIN TUMOR

Etiology, Incidence, Clinical Manifestations, and Types. The majority of brain tumors in children are due to abnormal growth of cells already present in the brain; few are due to metastases from noncerebral neoplasms. Generally these tumors are located beneath the tentorium cerebri. (Most brain tumors in adults are located above it.)

The *incidence* of brain tumors among children in only one sixth of that among adults. Tumors increase in incidence up to six years of age and then remain at a uniform level during the school period.

Most of the *symptoms* are due to increased intracranial pressure. Such symptoms include *vomiting*, usually in the morning, at first nonprojectile, but later projectile; *headache, diplopia,* and *head enlargement,* if the tumor occurs before the sutures are firmly united; and *changes in mental awareness,* such as lethargy, behavioral changes, drowsiness, stupor, coma, and ultimately death. Many times the initial personality changes are first noted by the child's school teacher or the school nurse practitioner or school nurse, who may encourage the parent to have the child evaluated medically. Changes in *vital signs* are important in diagnosing increased intracranial pressure. Convulsions are rare with infratentorial tumors, but may occur in some children having these lesions.

Other clinical manifestations depend on the type and location of the tumor.

Five types of tumors may be seen.

Medulloblastoma is a fairly common tumor in children. The incidence is greatest during school age and reaches its highest point at five to six years. It is a highly malignant, rapidly developing tumor usually found in the cerebellum. Clinical manifestations are unsteadiness when the child walks, anorexia and vomiting, and headache, usually in the morning. Papilledema and ataxia are present. The child is drowsy, and nystagmus can be observed. If untreated, death usually results in less than a year. Recently, surgery followed by irradiation and chemotherapy has held hope for the survival of some children having medulloblastoma.

Astrocytoma may occur at any age, but the peak incidence is at eight years. The tumor is usually located in the cerebellum. The clinical manifestations differentiate this tumor from others. The onset is insidious, and the course is slow. Signs of focal disturbance or increase in intracranial pressure may occur. The child may have ataxia, hypotonia, diminished reflexes and nystagmus. Papilledema is present. Without operation the prognosis is poor. Total surgical removal with complete cure is possible.

Ependymoma is located in the fourth ventricle or in one of the lateral ventricles of the brain. Increased intracranial pressure and other manifestations are present, depending on the location of the tumor. The child will have vomiting, headache, enlarged head, and unsteady gait. Hydrocephalus may occur. The treatment is by incomplete internal compression and roentgen therapy.

Craniopharyngioma occurs in late childhood. The tumor is near the pituitary gland. There is pituitary or hypothalamic dysfunction. The most common hormonal disturbance is *diabetes insipidus,* the inability to concentrate urine due to the absence of antidiuretic hormone. The child may be stunted in growth and may have myxedema or delayed puberty. The cerebral disturbance results in defects of the visual fields. Later there may be memory or personality disturbances. There is evidence of increased intracranial pressure due to obstruction of the flow of cerebrospinal fluid. Headache and vomiting are noted. A roentgenogram of the skull reveals separated sutures. Surgical removal of the entire tumor is usually impossible. Roentgen therapy may control for years a tumor which was not surgically removed.

Brain stem gliomas have a peak incidence among children about seven years old. The clinical manifestations are multiple cranial nerve palsies, ataxia of the trunk and little sensory loss, without indications of increased intracranial pressure. The course is slow, but the tumor is inoperable. Roentgen therapy may permit the child to survive for a while.

Diagnosis and Treatment. Early *diagnosis* of brain tumor may be impossible because of its insidious beginning. The diagnosis is based on the history of symptoms of increased intracranial pressure or focal cerebral disturbances, and the findings on physical examination. If the child can comprehend verbal explanations, he should be adequately prepared before diagnostic procedures are done. For a discussion of the diagnostic procedures which may be used see p. 293. An electroencephalogram assists in locating superficial supratentorial tumors. Pneumoencephalogram may be done, but this procedure is not without danger. A positive *Macewen's sign* is associated with separation of the sutures. Roentgenograms may show splitting of the suture lines or calcification within the tumor. Ventriculograms and arteriograms help to localize the tumor. Lumbar puncture should not be done when increased intracranial pressure is present, because of the possibility of pushing the medulla into the cervical spine. Brain scans performed on children may be useful as diagnostic screening procedures for suspected intracranial neoplasms. Computerized axial tomography (CAT) is of value as a diagnostic screening procedure for suspected intracranial neoplasms and may prevent these children from needing other diagnostic tests.

The symptoms listed under the different types of tumors may also be found in children with encephalitis, brain abscess, or some degenerative brain disease, and such conditions must be ruled out before a diagnosis of brain tumor is made unqualifiedly.

The *treatment* may be surgical or with deep radiation. In surgery as much of the tumor as possible is excised. Most brain tumors cannot be removed completely. Deep radiation may be of value in some cases. With recent advances in anesthesiology and with improved endocrinologic therapy, especially with the corticosteroids, the results of neurosurgery have been improved. Even when complete cure is not possible, symptoms may be relieved and the child may be able to enjoy life for a variable time.

Responsibilities of the Nurse. EMOTIONAL SUPPORT. Both the parents and the child should become familiar before operation with the nurse who will care for the child postoperatively. The relation can be one of mutual trust. The parents are naturally anxious. They as well as the child should be prepared for neurosurgery, for how the child will look postoperatively, and for the treatment and procedures which will be necessary after operation. Conversation that is anxiety-producing is not carried on where the child can hear what is said, even though he appears to be unconscious. Parents need continued understanding and support from the nurse during the preoperative and postoperative periods. Maintenance of his general nutrition and of his and his parents' morale and outlook about the condition is important.

PREOPERATIVE CARE AND OBSERVATIONS. Preoperative care consists in placing the child in a bed with crib sides or, if he is too large for a crib, side bars, because of the danger of his being confused or drowsy and falling out of bed.

The child should have a nourishing diet. If he vomits, he can be refed, because usually he is not nauseated. Enemas are not given because of the danger of increasing the intracranial pressure.

Observations by the nurse in order to help the physician in localizing the tumor and appraising the increasing intracranial pressure are of the utmost importance. The nurse should listen to the complaints or comments of the older child and observe children of all ages. Both complaints and observations are charted fully, with the conditions under which they occurred. Specifically noted are lowering of the pulse rate and change in its nature, gradual or sudden change in body temperature, decrease in the respiratory rate and change in the nature of respiration, especially irregular respiration, and any change in blood pressure, particularly a rise in the systolic pressure with widening pulse pressure.

The nurse records vomiting, and indications of headache, lethargy, and drowsiness. Any convulsions are recorded in full. (Seizure precautions are followed—see page 474.) If possible, the nurse ascertains whether there is limitation of the visual field or whether the child sees a double image of a single object. The nurse records the degree and situation of muscular weakness. Fecal and urinary incontinence or retention is routinely recorded. All complaints of pain and discomfort are noted.

The nurse should know where emergency equipment—such as oxygen, aspirator, sterile gloves, ventricular tap tray, emergency drugs, and other supplies and equipment—is kept in case it is needed. Whenever the nurse is in doubt, the supervisor or clinical instructor can be called for instructions and explanations of the care the child requires or the procedure to be used for a specific treatment.

Prior to surgery both the parents and child are prepared for the child's head being shaved. This may be done in the child's room or in the operating room.

If the child will be taken to another room or to the intensive care unit after surgery, the nurse can prepare both the parents and him for the move so that when he awakens in a strange place he will not be fearful that his parents will not find him.

POSTOPERATIVE CARE. Postoperative care is exacting and requires both skill and experience in the nursing care of children undergoing brain surgery. The child may evidence varying degrees of consciousness, depending on his level of consciousness prior to surgery and the extent of the operative procedure. After surgery he may need respiratory assistance.

Parenteral fluid therapy is given when the child cannot take fluids by mouth. Any difficulties with the intravenous setup are reported at once. The rate of absorption of fluid is noted carefully. Too rapid administration may produce a dangerous increase in intracranial pressure. Mouth care is essential to prevent parotitis and monilia infection.

The child's position immediately postoperatively is lying flat on the unaffected side. After the danger of vomiting has passed and the nasopharynx no longer needs to be aspirated, his position is changed frequently from side to back in order to prevent pressure areas and hypostatic pneumonia. The surgeon may prefer that the head be slightly elevated. For turning the child who has had surgery in the cerebellar area the nurse's movements are slow, and his body is kept in a straight line; the position of the head is not changed or turned. In moving the child the head, neck, and shoulders are well supported so that no twisting of these parts of the body occurs (Fig. 24–19). Two nurses are needed to move the child of school age. Further measures to prevent the formation of pressure areas on the child's head or body include the use of a sponge rubber pad over the mattress and the use of cotton doughnuts under pressure areas such as the ears or the side of the head.

The patient is kept clean and dry at all times.

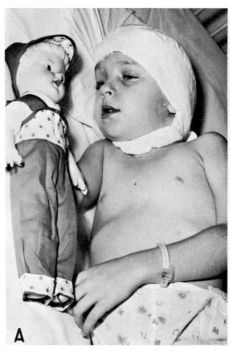
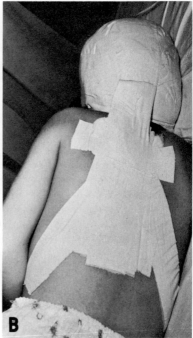

FIGURE 24–19. Suboccipital craniectomy dressings assist in keeping the head in correct alignment with the child's body even when the child is turned. A, Front view; B, back veiw.

Back care is given frequently, and the area around pressure points is massaged. If paralysis or spasticity of the extremities occurs, pillows or other support are used. Foot drop must be prevented by adequate support.

The vital signs are taken as ordered by the physician—every 15 minutes at first and then less frequently as the condition warrants—to determine indications of rising intracranial pressure.

The nasopharynx is aspirated as necessary. The child is encouraged to breathe deeply at regular periods, hourly or as ordered.

If shock occurs, warm blankets are applied. Emergency stimulants, fluids for intravenous therapy, and oxygen are kept on hand for immediate use. The foot of the bed is usually not raised because of the danger of increasing intracranial pressure. The nurse must be alert for, and immediately report, urinary incontinence or retention.

Restraints are not used unless absolutely necessary, because the child may struggle against them and increase intracranial pressure. They can be used if the child pulls at his dressings, tries to dislodge the intravenous or gavage tube or in any way tries to injure himself. Elbow restraints, mitts for the hands or clove hitch restraints (see p. 256) may then be used.

If the head dressing becomes wet with drainage, the area is circled with gentian violet. If there is rapid enlargement of the stained area or if bright red blood appears on the dressing, the surgeon is notified immediately. The nurse may reinforce the dressings with sterile pads held in place with a bandage. Meningitis may result from contamination of the surgical area.

Edema of the face, eyelids, and brain may result from injury during operation. Because lacrimal secretion cannot circulate over the eyes when edema is present, the conjunctivae may become dry and infected. Warm saline irrigations of the eyes, eye drops, or the application of cold compresses to the swollen eyelids may be ordered to prevent this complication. Some physicians recommend that the eyelids be taped closed with small pieces of cellophane or covered with eye shields. Corticosteroids or other hormonal substitutes may be given preoperatively and postoperatively to lower intracranial pressure by reducing edema.

Hyperthermia may be caused by intracranial edema, bleeding, or disturbance of the heat-regulating center. The temperature is taken at least every half-hour when it is elevated. Methods to reduce fever include undressing the child and covering him with a sheet or only a diaper over the pubic area, reduction of room temperature, tepid sponge bath, cold water mattress, ice or cold water enemas or small retention enemas, or rectal suppositories containing aspirin. The body temperature is usually not brought down to normal, but it may be kept fairly low.

If the child cannot swallow, gavage feedings may be given. If they are given, distention should be noted. As soon as the child has ceased to vomit and shows signs of being able to swallow, small amounts of water may be given. Nourishing liquids and a soft diet are added gradually. Fluids and foods are not encouraged too much because vomiting, which increases intracranial pressure, may result. Solid foods are given as soon as the child can tolerate them.

As the child recovers from operation he can be helped to gain greater independence in his own care. He can be given opportunities to play alone and with other children. Parents need assurance that he should continue to be given independence after he returns home. They should also understand that the child needs continued medical supervision after discharge.

Course and Prognosis. The *course* depends on the type of tumor involved. Illness may last from a few weeks to several years. The *prognosis* for living into adulthood is very poor.

Response of Nurses to the Prolonged Care of Comatose Children. Nurses who care for comatose children over a period of time may respond with personal feelings of frustration, anger, anxiety, guilt, and sorrow, yet they feel hope for the recovery of their patients. These nurses need opportunities to share their experiences with others and to give and receive support from other staff members.

MINIMAL CEREBRAL DYSFUNCTION (THE BRAIN-DAMAGED CHILD) AND SCHOOL UNDERACHIEVEMENT

Incidence, Etiology, Clinical Manifestations, Diagnosis, Treatment, and Prognosis. The term *minimal cerebral dysfunction* is applied loosely to an extremely heterogeneous, chronically disabled group of children. It is not a clear-cut entity or specific diagnosis. This condition may be due to actual brain damage, but it may also be due to genetic, cytogenic and morphogenic developmental defects or maturational irregularities of the nervous system. The number of these children appears to be increasing either because of improved diagnostic skill or because more of these children are living because of improved medical science.

During the preschool years these children may have unpredictable variations in behavior, a very short or a longer than average attention span, a low level of frustration, and awkwardness.

Children having minimal cerebral dysfunction may have behavioral and learning disabilities which are observed only after they enter school. These children are characterized by psychologic, behavioral, academic, and neurologic deviations from the normal. They may have one or many of the following problems: difficulty in paying attention in class, and problems in the general areas of remembering, language, conceptualization and perception, impulsivity, and sensory and motor function such as hyperactivity, underactivity, or awkwardness. These children have normal, near-normal, or above-normal intelligence, although they may have difficulty in learning; therefore they can be distinguished from the mentally retarded group. Since they may realize that they are different from their peers, they may develop adverse emotional reactions.

When the child becomes older, he may show secondary behavioral manifestations. He may be immature emotionally and may have unusual fears and anxieties. He may act impulsively and may then feel deep remorse about his behavior. He may also have mild hearing or visual impairment. On intelligence testing the child may have scattered results and thus not do well on an overall score.

Management of the child having minimal cerebral dysfunction is best accomplished through the efforts of all involved: the parents, pediatrician as leader of the team, specialized physicians, psychologists, school administrator, teachers, social workers, school nurse practitioner or

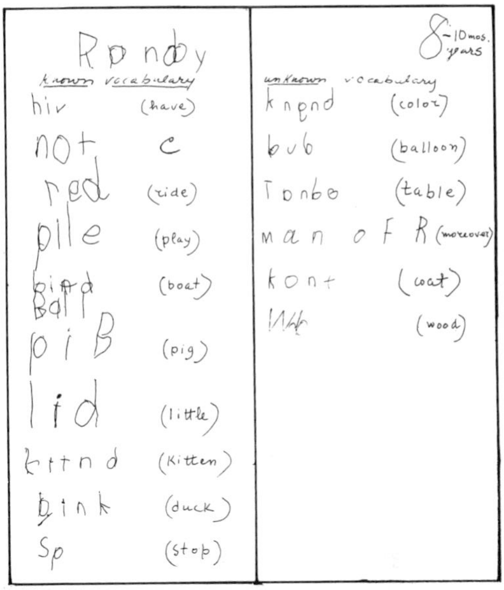

FIGURE 24–21. Clues to physical health problems may appear in schoolwork. This child's paper revealed a perceptual problem diagnosed as severe developmental dyslexia. (From Boder, E. *in* Myklebust, H. R.: *Progress in Learning Disabilities*, Vol. 2. New York, Grune & Stratton, Inc., 1971. Used by permission.)

school nurse, and nurses in the hospital when he is admitted for diagnosis or treatment.

Evaluation of the child is made on the basis of behavior, academic performance, psychologic evaluation, a carefully taken medical history, and medical and neurologic examinations, including an electroencephalogram. Positive therapeutic results require detailed evaluation of the child's status and a plan based upon the assets and liabilities of the patient and his environment. Establishment of a firm, consistent environment with attention to the social problems of the family probably contributes more to therapy than reliance on drugs. The use of amphetamines or a remote relative, methylphenidate (Ritalin), tends to prolong the attention span and to reduce behavioral outbursts. Tranquilizing drugs may lessen irritability and decrease impulsiveness. Care must be taken that these children are under medical supervision while taking such drugs. The potential for overuse and even abuse is always present.

Special school classes may be provided for children having learning disabilities. The frustrations which these children experience can also be reduced by environmental changes, including the use of various teaching techniques which translate abstract concepts into concrete terms and provide for individual attention and parental counseling on an individual or a group basis. Psychotherapy may also be considered when other methods of dealing with the problem have not been successful.

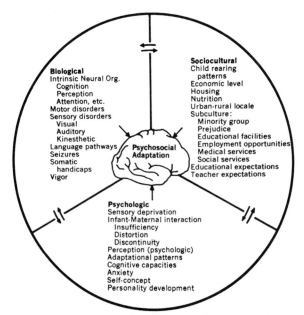

FIGURE 24–20. Multiple factors affecting psychosocial adaptation. (From Walzer, S., and Richmond, J. B.: *Pediatr. Clin. N. Am.*, 20:551, August 1973.)

The *prognosis* for these children depends upon the attitudes and guidance of the adults responsible for their care, the age when treatment was begun, and the emotional adjustment of the family to the situation. Some children may become delinquent, mentally retarded or psychotic. If they can develop self-confidence, they may be able to make a good adjustment as adults.

Responsibilities of the Nurse. The nurse's role in the care of the child having minimal cerebral dysfunction includes early case finding and cooperation in the efforts of the team caring for the child. These efforts involve diagnosing, and providing counseling for the parents, including the need for appropriate teaching techniques and occasional psychotherapy.

Nursing intervention when the child is hospitalized is directed toward controlling an overstimulating environment and providing a stable structured environment in which he can achieve success. Since the child has difficulty in adjusting to changing conditions, the nurse provides continuity of care and avoidance of tension-producing situations, possibly through the consistency of nurses assigned to his care or by the mother's staying with the child. The nurse tells the child in a simple, direct manner what is expected of him and praises him when he accomplishes desired behaviors. He will respond to understanding guidance and approval. A confident attitude toward his abilities and liabilities will improve his self-image.

If the mother lives in the hospital with the child, the nurse can observe the mother-child relations for emerging emotional problems. The social growth of a child having perceptual disorders is poor if the parents refuse to recognize his problems and consider him just a "bad child." The nurse should also have knowledge of the community agencies to which the family can be referred. The parents are told what to expect from their child now and in the future and that he will probably improve with maturation and therapy.

DYSLEXIA (READING DISORDER)

Definition, Causes, Treatment, Responsibilities of the Nurse, and Prevention. Dyslexia or reading disorder exists when a significant discrepancy is present between a child's performance on a standardized reading test and the usual expectation for his age and grade level. Reading is a complex process. The ability to use spoken words usually precedes the acquisition of reading skills. More boys than girls have reading disabilities.

The *causes* of dyslexia are sociopsychologic and psychophysiologic. The sociopsychologic causes include deficiencies in cognitive readiness (the child from an illiterate home who has not been exposed to books), deficiencies in teaching (insufficient attendance at school or a poor level of teaching), and deficient motivation resulting from social problems or individual psychopathology. Conduct disturbances (see p. 803) may be secondary to poor reading ability because of the individual's low level of self-esteem and his pessimism about his possibilities for success.

Psychophysiological causes of dyslexia include general debility (the malnourished child or the one who is chronically ill), sensory defects (visual impairment or a lack of auditory perception), brain injury, mental retardation, and "specific reading disability" or "developmental dyslexia" (failure to learn to read despite the ability to do so).

The *treatment* may require rectifying the underlying social causes (poverty and discrimination), reducing absences from school, improving the level of teaching, supplementing early life experiences, and relieving emotional disturbance.

If the child has poor visual or auditory perception or is chronically ill or malnourished, medical measures can be taken to improve the situation.

Prepared remedial reading teachers use a wide variety of instructional techniques: perceptual, kinesthetic, and operant among others. The child is taught individually or in a group over a period of years. If the teacher can evoke a cooperative and enthusiastic response from the child, there is a chance for success. Many children can learn to read with minimal competence if they have a severe disability. Others learn to draw attention from their disability by developing other talents.

Responsibilities of the nurse include assessing school-age children for their visual and auditory abilities as part of their health evaluation. The school nurse or the school nurse practitioner should evidence interest in the academic achievement of the children as well as in any behavioral disturbances they may show. The nurse can refer any children having problems to school authorities: the school principal, physician, or psychologist. The nurse can become familiar with sources of remedial reading help in the community. As a citizen, the nurse can provide the necessary leadership in securing the resources for helping such children receive adequate diagnosis and treatment.

Prevention of dyslexia requires the removal or the remedying of its causes if they can be identified.

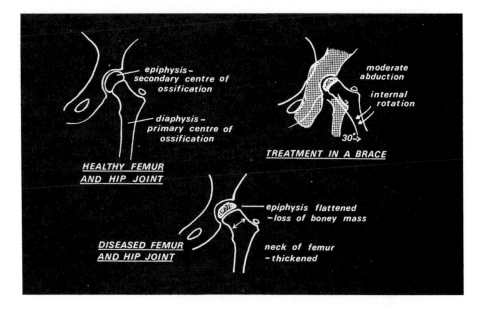

FIGURE 24–22. A healthy femur and hip joint as compared with a femur and hip joint of a child having Legg-Perthes disease. (From Nichol, C.: *The Canadian Nurse*, 72:31, June 1976.)

LEGG-CALVÉ-PERTHES DISEASE (PERTHES'S DISEASE, COXA PLANA)

Etiology and Incidence. Perthes's disease is an aseptic necrosis of the head of the femur. The cause is unknown. It is a self-limited disease occurring in children between four and ten years of age. The usual course of this disease is from three to four years. The condition affects boys more frequently than girls, possibly as a result of trauma to the hip.

Pathology, Clinical Manifestations, Treatment, Responsibilities of the Nurse, and Prognosis. The *pathology* may be divided into three stages, each lasting about nine months to a year. The first stage is an aseptic necrosis. Roentgen films show a relative opacity of the epiphysis. The bone becomes necrotic. The second stage is revascularization. On roentgen study the epiphysis is shown as fragmented and mottled. The third stage is reossification. Roentgen examination shows the head of the femur to be gradually re-forming.

If weight is placed on the leg, the head of the femur tends to become flattened and mushroom-shaped. Later in life degenerative changes occur because of discrepancies in shape between the acetabulum and the head of the femur.

The *clinical manifestations* are those of synovitis, i.e., a limp, and pain in the hip. The pain is often referred to the knee. Muscle spasm is not commonly severe. Motion is usually restricted only in relation to abduction and rotation.

The most important point in *treatment* is avoidance of weight bearing, although some physicians disagree with this. Some physicians believe that the child should have complete rest and traction on the leg during the course of the disease. Others immobilize the hip by surgery,

casts or braces to prevent the deformity resulting from weight bearing.

The *nursing care* includes stressing to both the child and the parents the importance of not bearing weight on the extremity for several months. The child is kept in bed on a firm mattress and bed board. If the child is in traction, he may be either supine or prone. He is turned at least every four hours. He must be encouraged to move his joints and to maintain good muscle tone. If a cast is applied, he is cared for as outlined previously (see p. 322).

One of the most difficult aspects in the care of the very active school child who has Perthes's disease is the necessity of prolonged immobility. If the child is to be confined to bed for a long time, the home can be evaluated and guidance given to the family for implementation of their facilities for his care. The ingenuity of the

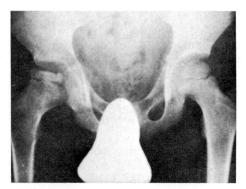

FIGURE 24–23. Standing (anterior-posterior) view showing Legg-Perthes disease, right hip. Note the changes of avascular necrosis and revascularization; the flattening and appearance of "fragmentation" of the femoral head (due to bony resorption and deposition; the subluxation tendency; and the slightly broadened metaphysis (femoral neck). (From Nichol, C. *The Canadian Nurse*, 72:34, June 1976.)

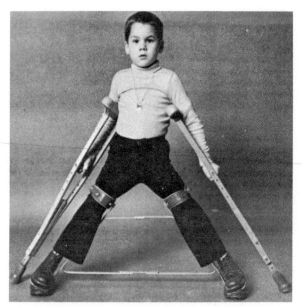

FIGURE 24–24. A child with Legg-Perthes disease in an A-frame brace demonstrates the stance of the swing-through gait. (From Nichol, C.: *The Canadian Nurse:* 72:35, June 1976.)

mother or nurse may be taxed in providing activities which will keep him occupied. The child might possibly be referred to an institution for the care of convalescent children.

The younger the child at the onset of the condition, the more likely is he to retain a spherical than to acquire a deformed, flattened head of the femur. Complete recovery depends on when treatment was given and whether gross deformity of the hip occurred.

JUVENILE MYASTHENIA GRAVIS

Juvenile myasthenia gravis is a long-term condition that was discussed in Chapter 12, although this type becomes more apparent after the age of 10 years (see p. 317).

DENTAL PROBLEMS

Pedodontia has as its main purposes the maintenance of healthy teeth, the prevention of disease, the treatment of defects, and the restoration of function. Common dental problems include dental caries, malocclusion, traumatic injuries, and discolored teeth.

Dental caries is the leading dental problem of children (see also "Nursing-bottle mouth" syndrome, p. 571). There seems to be a positive correlation between parental dental health education and the incidence of dental caries in children. Thus children from socioeconomically deprived areas have more dental caries than those from other groups. Genetic factors, adequate diet, good oral hygiene, and the use of fluoride are important in the incidence of this condition. Dental caries in children is treated much as it is in adults.

Malocclusion is a term applied to irregular positioning of the teeth and the improper coming together of the teeth when the jaws are closed. The causes of malocclusion may be inherited, such as the size of teeth and jaw, or may be acquired, such as due to harmful habits or early loss of teeth through decay. This condition results in decreased masticatory functioning and possibly a disfigured mouth, facial deformities, faulty speech, nutritional disturbances and emotional problems. The dentist should evaluate a child's occlusion as it develops. An orthodontist, a dentist who is especially trained to diagnose and treat malocclusion, should be consulted if malocclusion is evident. If the deciduous teeth are lost prematurely or if there is congenital absence of teeth, treatment should be begun early in order to prevent malocclusion. Treatment may include either placement of space-maintaining appliances or actual movement of the teeth. Preventive orthodontics may save many children from becoming dental cripples.

Children having *traumatic injuries* to the teeth are examined immediately after the accident. The treatment given depends on whether it is a deciduous or permanent tooth, the stage of tooth development, the nature of the fracture and the status of the dental pulp.

The permanent teeth are usually darker than the deciduous teeth; thus parents become anxious lest their child's teeth be permanently *discolored*. They should be told that when all the permanent teeth have erupted, their color will probably be uniform. Teeth may be stained by extrinsic agents. These stains can usually be removed by cleansing and polishing by the dental hygienist.

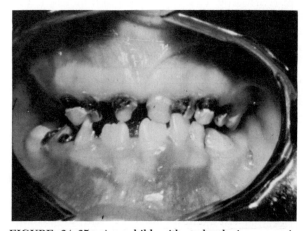

FIGURE 24–25. Any child with malocclusion or caries should be referred for examination. Together, parents and health personnel sometimes need to discuss available community resources for orthodontic care or other dental treatment. (Courtesy of Stanley Horwitz, D.D.S.)

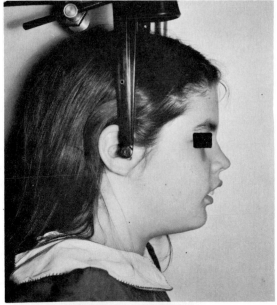

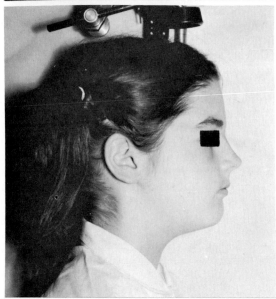

FIGURE 24–26. Profile of a child before and after ortho-dontic treatment for malocclusion. (From Mayne, W. R., in Graber, T. M., and Swain, B. F.: *Current Orthodontic Concepts and Techniques*, Vol. I. 2nd ed. Philadelphia, W. B. Saunders Co., 1975.)

SEXUAL AGGRESSION AGAINST THE CHILD

Sexual aggression against a child may include assault by a stranger or a known individual and incest.

ASSAULT OF A CHILD

Girls between the ages of 6 and 11 years are usually the victims of forcible sexual attempts on children. Either an adolescent or an adult male may be the perpetrator. This act most often occurs during the summer months. The incident may include undressing the child, fondling, choking, beating, fellatio, cunnilingus, mastur-bation, vaginal or anal intercourse, or mutilation. Major genital lacerations may occur. The child may die before being found and cared for.

If the child survives a forcible assault, she may either be acutely frightened, in a daze, or may show little emotion. Sometime later the child may scream and appear to become hys-terical. When questioned these children are usually vague about the attack. Psychiatric con-sultation may be needed to help in questioning the child and evaluating the situation.

After the attack the child needs to have her mother stay with her in quiet surroundings to reduce her fear and agitation. A complete physi-cal examination must be done in order to assess the extent of the injury, the presence of semen, and the treatment necessary. Such children may have sustained injuries to various parts of the body such as the head, ribs, spine, genitalia, and peritoneal cavity. The examination is also required as a medicolegal procedure.

A gynecologic examination is also necessary. The mother and child should have the proce-dure explained to them. The mother remains with the girl during the procedure. A general an-esthesia may be required if the genitalia are traumatized—reddened, bleeding, bruised, or lacerated. There may be vulvar midline tears from the urethra to the perineum.

If the assailant is not known and therefore cannot be examined, the child should be given prophylaxis against gonorrhea and syphilis using procaine penicillin G in aqueous suspension.

Since the child probably feels more secure at home than in the hospital, hospitalization is avoided whenever it is not essential. The little girl is encouraged to resume her usual activities as soon as possible. If playmates or neighbors question her about the incident, she should dis-courage them from discussing it.

Parents may need counseling in order to ven-tilate hostile feelings against the child's aggres-sor. They may need guidance in order to pre-vent them from being overly suspicious and overly protective of the child. The parents should not produce in the child unfounded feel-ings of anxiety and guilt. The child's fears such as being permanently injured, diseased, or un-able to marry or have children must be corrected so that they do not create problems later in life. The parents, physician, counselor, or nurse should answer any questions the child may ask concerning these matters.

If the attacker is found to be a friend, relative, or neighbor, he should be removed from the area in which the child lives. Although the parents may wish to move from the neighborhood themselves, this is not usually wise.

Parents should be encouraged to cooperate with the legal authorities in order to apprehend the attacker and thus prevent future injury to other children. Everything possible is done to prevent the child from becoming embarrassed or upset over the incident and the legal efforts required. There must be close cooperation between law and medicine so that justice is served and at the same time the child's emotional health is protected.

Responsibilities of the Nurse. When counseling parents of sexually abused children, the most important principle to remember is that the child must be protected from further trauma. Over-reaction and over-response can cause increased difficulties for the child. The thoughtful and empathetic handling of the child by the parents and other concerned adults can reduce or prevent the long-term harmful effects of the situation. Parents may be very distraught because of guilt feelings over not protecting the child more adequately. The parents themselves may have had traumatic sexual experiences earlier and may be reliving those events through the current incident.

The nurse must help the parents discuss the incident with the child in an understanding, open, and calm manner, helping the child describe the assailant and exactly what happened. The nurse must understand that although the experience may have been traumatic, the child may also feel guilty because exciting and stimulating emotions may have been aroused through such contact.

The parents need help in discussing the situation with the police and they also need reassurance that the incident is not one that always scars the child for life. The child is not encouraged to 'forget' about the situation; by talking about it she will become desensitized to it.

Before the gynecologic examination the nurse prepares both the mother and child for the procedure. The mother stands at the child's head during the examination. The nurse reassures the child that although it may be unpleasant it usually is not painful. The nurse explains what sensations the child can expect to feel such as the urge to have a bowel movement during the digital rectal examination. If specula or other instruments are to be introduced, they are warmed to body temperature and well-lubricated before use.

Children may exhibit nightmares, eating disturbances, regressive behavior, crying spells, and expressions of fear after the attack. The nurse can counsel the parents about handling these behaviors. If reassurance is not enough, consultation with a child psychologist or psychiatrist may be of value.

Sexual abuse of children is horrifying for the majority of adults, including nurses. It is difficult to accept. Nurses are, however, in a position in the health care delivery system where they may be the first to detect and assess behavior problems in children that need investigation.

In most states it is mandatory to report a case of sexual abuse to the Child Protective Service Agency in the community or state. Every nurse should be familiar with the law and act accordingly.

FATHER-DAUGHTER INCEST

The term incest means sexual intercourse between two members of the immediate family. There are legal prohibitions against incest that protect all underage or minor children against sexual abuse by others. Offenders are punished everywhere by imprisonment if the charge is proven.

In the nuclear family the most frequent kind of incest occurs between a brother and a sister, but incest between a father and his daughter is more frequently reported. Mother-son incest is extremely rare.

An incestuous relationship between father and daughter usually continues for five to ten years, starting when the female child is nine to ten years of age. The majority of these situations are not reported. The fathers are usually employed, of average intelligence and education. Incest occurs in fathers of all social classes; it is not typically an upper-, middle- or a lower-class problem.

Incest usually occurs in a home where disturbed family relations exist. The mother is usually infantile and dependent. She has many times given up her role as sex partner to her husband and as mother to her daughter. A type of mother-daughter role reversal occurs in which the mother subtly manipulates the situation and pushes adult responsibilities on one or more of her daughters, rushing them toward a kind of pseudomaturity. The mother in this situation is at the base of the family disease. The father is usually a passive, immature man who was deprived of affection as a growing child.

The young daughter is initiated into this incestual relationship at first by fondling and mutual erotic sex play. The daughter gradually accepts and cooperates with coital activity over the years without complaining to her mother. The girl tends to hate and resent her mother, perhaps even wishing her dead.

Usually while the incestuous relationship continues the girl shows little emotional illness. When the relationship ends, however, self-destructive suicidal depression, or adolescent psychosis may occur. The girl may run away from home. As a woman she may be incapable of a normal heterosexual love relationship. One must use caution, however, in generalizing these negative effects to a specific individual and situation.

When an incestuous relationship is brought into the open, the help of a children's aid organization or a youth-protective service is needed. Family therapy and individual therapy should be initiated. Neither separation nor punishment is a suitable substitute for treatment. The young girl may be placed in an institution such as a boarding home or school for rehabilitation purposes. She needs a great deal of emotional support during this period of time. Preventive psychotropic medication may be given.

An infant born of an incestuous relationship with either the father or brother many times has genetic defects, a degree of mental retardation, and the possibility of death in infancy.

In addition to the possibility of pregnancy during the period of incest, an incestuous father also exposes his daughter to a greater risk of developing lesions of the cervix later in life. Squamous cell carcinoma of the cervix is now believed to be a sexually transmitted disease. The crucial time for this to be transmitted is at menarche and one year following it and at the time of the first pregnancy. The younger the girl is at the time of her first coitus, the greater the risk of cancer in the future. The fact that she has multiple sexual partners may be an additional aggravating factor in the causation of this disease.

In summary, the emotional sequelae of incest vary with the degree of severity, chronicity, and disruption of functioning of family members. The family and individual factors that generate incest vary in their psychopathological potential.

Responsibilities of the Nurse. Incest is the most common and most difficult type of sexual abuse to handle. A mother many times knows what is happening in her family and will bring the child to the physician or nurse, not for the problem of incest, but for a complaint of headache, refusal to attend school, stomachache, enuresis, nightmares, or some other problem. During the visit the nurse may incidentally learn of the sexual abuse. This must be reported according to the respective laws of various states.

Since the mother is aware of the incest, she is usually reluctant to take an active role in protecting her child from another member of her family. It is helpful to have the active support of the Child Protective Service Agency in dealing with such a family.

The nurse must help parents of sexually abused children to realize that the traumatic reactions to these incidents are intensified by parental response. Through supportive and warm therapy parent-child interaction can resolve the child's confusion and fears in a healthful manner.

EMOTIONAL DISTURBANCES

By the time the child is six years of age his personality is fairly well established. He should be free to gain further skill in the use of his body and mind and to develop both stronger inner controls and relations with children and adults outside his family. He needs time to achieve these goals; during the same period he is making a good adjustment at school.

If the child shows behavior problems which are symptoms of emotional disturbances during the school years, his response usually resembles some adult reactions to difficulties. The child may present neurotic symptoms such as nervousness, finger-sucking, nail-biting, and fears; school phobia; conduct disorders (the problem child); language disorders such as stuttering; and psychosomatic illnesses including anorexia nervosa, overeating, abdominal pain, peptic ulcer, constipation, chronic ulcerative colitis, and enuresis.

These disorders, serious in themselves, may also prevent the child from making a good adjustment at school. *Failure in school may thus be due to emotional disturbance as well as to mental retardation.* The child who is overanxious and tense cannot concentrate on learning even if he has the intellectual capacity to achieve.

The teacher and the school nurse practitioner or school nurse should be aware of such problems as they arise. They should be able to work with parents and other team members in order to help the child.

Neurotic Symptoms

Physicians often find it difficult to differentiate between normal behavior and neurotic behavior of children. Some behavior, however, when it is consistent, must be classified as neurotic.

NERVOUSNESS

Etiology and Clinical Manifestations. Nervousness is not a separate condition in itself, but represents a group of symptoms. Nervous children are physically and mentally restless, over-excitable, timid, and easily fatigued.

The inciting cause of nervousness may be a continued heavy load of anxiety or stress, or severe illness. Some children become nervous because of parental pressure to achieve. Children may also be nervous because they feel inferior to others, are overstimulated at play or acquire anxiety from their parents.

The *manifestations* are easily recognized. The child is tense and restless, the pulse and respiration rates are increased, the movements are jerky, and the child's responses are too rapid.

Treatment and Prognosis. *Treatment* may be given by a physician or a psychiatrist, depending upon the severity of the problem. The child should have adequate nutrition and sleep without excessive excitement, discipline, or stimulation to achieve in either motor ability or school work. The nervous child needs support and a well-planned routine. Sometimes he may need to be placed in a new environment away from an anxiety-producing home.

The *prognosis* depends upon the cause and the management of the child and his problems.

FINGER-SUCKING

The average child gives up thumb- and finger-sucking by the time he is two years old; others relinquish it by five or six years of age. If a child continues past this time and into the school age, investigation should be made into the life of the child and his parents to find out the cause of his neurotic behavior. Punitive measures or those producing physical prevention of the sucking activity, e.g., splints on the arms and bandages on the fingers, or making the practice unpleasant, such as putting bad-tasting lotions on the thumb or fingers, should be avoided.

If a child stopped sucking his fingers at an early age and resumed the habit at seven or eight years, he probably met an unsolvable difficulty in his development and regressed to gain satisfaction. Such difficulties include the birth of a sibling, divorce, the mother's leaving home to work, the death of a loved parent or grandparent or moving to a new home. The treatment is to learn and correct the child's attitude toward the traumatic event.

NAIL-BITING

Nail-biting is an indication of tension. If the parents resist his attempts to gain satisfaction by nail-biting too traumatically, a parent-child conflict is begun. Severe nail-biting may become an attempt by the child to humiliate and annoy his parents. It is physically painful; thus the child punishes himself for his hostility to his parents.

He should be given a manicure set as soon as he is able to use it and praised for his well kept hands. He should be helped to express his hostile feelings so that he no longer needs to bite his nails. His self-confidence in the home situation should be increased.

Imitation may also be important in nail-biting. The child may be simply imitating a parent who has the same habit. The parent may accept the behavior in himself, but not in the child.

FEARS

Children must develop certain fears based on dangers that exist in the real world. Such things as bonfires and sharp knives should arouse a degree of fear in children that they will be harmed unless they take necessary precautions.

Fear of the dark, one of childhood's most common fears, is due to the fact that in the dark the child feels alone and deserted. The dark may be peopled for him with dangerous persons of his fantasy. Parents should assure him that they have not deserted him and that they do not fear the dark.

Crippling anxiety replaces fear when there is an unconscious distortion of reality. The distortion occurs because the real situation is equated with an unconscious conflict or an anxiety-charged previous experience. Usually the exact meaning of the previous experience is repressed.

If anxiety persists in spite of the child's experience which should disprove it or of the passage of time which should weaken the fear, some symbolic significance is attached to what is feared, and professional help should be sought.

Children should not be exposed thoughtlessly to situations which generate anxiety. If they are exposed, they can handle the anxiety best if they have secure relations with their parents and can talk about their fears or act out their feelings in relation to the fear.

SCHOOL PHOBIA

School phobia is a term which indicates a symptom and not a disease, since many of these children are not phobic (see p. 700). These children may refuse to go to school. They may prefer either to remain at home or to become truant away from home. This latter category will not be included in this discussion. Manifestations of this problem may be the development of somatic complaints, fear of the teacher or children, or some situation at school. This problem may also be an indication of psychosis. Actually, these children are afraid to leave their parents, especially the mother, and their parents do not want their children to leave them. Central to the problem, therefore, is an exaggerated dependency on the parents.

School phobia may indeed be a "cry for help" by the child. The cooperation of various professionals such as the school nurse practitioner or school nurse, teacher, principal, counselor and social worker, the pediatrician, and the psychologist or psychiatrist is essential. A coordinated plan of action which includes the parents must be evolved in which all persons understand their functions.

The aim in therapy of children having a school phobia is to have them return to school immediately, with the use of force if necessary. Failure to have them returned to school is the responsibility of the parents as much as of the children themselves. After these children have returned to school, therapy is aimed at correcting the underlying family relation problems in order to prevent a recurrence. If the child, as indicated by other manifestations, is very emotionally ill or psychotic, he should be referred to a child psychiatrist for therapy.

Conduct Disorders

THE PROBLEM CHILD

Etiology, Types, Management, and Prognosis. The child whom the parents and teachers call a problem child is usually merely trying to solve a problem with his behavior. Such behavior may occur in any socioeconomic group. It usually occurs because the child's basic emotional needs have not been met. The problem generally arises because his methods of expressing his distress are limited. Such children may steal, be truant from school, hurt smaller children, tell dirty stories, or engage in prolonged sex play.

In recent years some of these children have found that glue-sniffing provides a form of intoxication which they enjoy. Under the influence of glue vapors some of them commit misdemeanors. Recent research has also raised the possibility that glue-sniffing may alter chromosomes and even increase susceptibility to leukemia. Children also inhale aerosol propellent from the spray cans in which various kinds of household products are packaged. This is a deadly game, because the highly concentrated fluorocarbon gas sensitizes the heart muscle, and fibrillation can occur quickly, or else the gas may freeze the air passages and cause death. If untreated, these children who have learned to enjoy the experience of becoming intoxicated may turn to alcohol, narcotics, or other drugs (see p. 892) during their later school years or

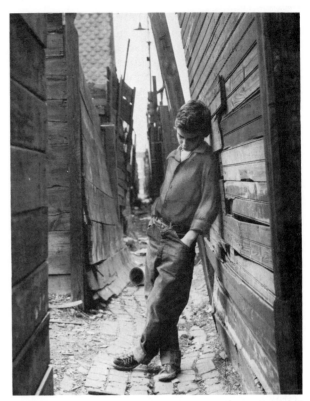

FIGURE 24–27. The child who is truant from school and lonely may turn to drugs in order to gain a place for himself in his peer group. (H. Armstrong Roberts.)

their adolescent years. Behavior may be, but is not always, directed toward those who, the child feels, are responsible for his problems.

In the *management* of this problem the psychiatrist first of all gains the child's confidence. He does not blame the child for his behavior. He encourages the child to tell his own story. *Treatment* must be extended in every phase of the child's life. It may require a team approach to the whole problem, including parents, physician, teacher, spiritual adviser, scout leader, social worker, and nurse. The child also should be a partner in making the therapeutic plan. Treatment is usually directed at the parent-child relations and at the child's feelings of inferiority over a variety of problems.

The outlook is usually good if these children are given the understanding help which they need.

Language Disorders

Etiology and Incidence. The cause of any language disorder is usually complex. The *incidence* of speech defects is greatest between the ages of four and 11 years. Boys are more frequently affected than girls. Any type of disturbed communication in childhood can cause many difficulties and later disorders in communication as a skill in relating to others.

Types, Diagnosis, and Management. There are three *types* of speech disorders: functional disorders such as stuttering, defects due to anatomic malformations such as cleft palate (see p. 274) and cleft lip, and defects due to central nervous system lesions such as cerebral palsy (see p. 578). The whole child must be considered when the *diagnosis* is made and management is planned. *Management* depends on the basic problem causing the speech disorder.

STUTTERING

Stuttering is the most common functional speech disorder. The child is unable to speak freely because of incoordination and spasmodic action of the muscles involved in speech. Although there is some question about the cause, there is increasing evidence that stuttering is a symptom of a profound emotional disturbance. Some experts believe that the emotional disturbance may be due to an enforced change of handedness. Before treatment can be planned the child's physical, intellectual, and emotional status must be ascertained.

Management consists in reducing the child's anxiety about his stuttering, and treatment of any other problem found in the evaluation. The child should receive adequate health care and be helped to gain insight into, and understanding of, his disorder. Usually the services of a psychiatrist and a speech therapist are needed.

Psychosomatic Illness

Etiology. Psychosomatic illness is a physical disturbance that has a psychologic origin. There may also be an organic basis for such illness, but the element of emotions enters into the causation. Every child may have emotional reactions which interfere with his bodily functions. The degree of interference and the location of the problem vary with the individual child. In school children several psychosomatic illnesses arise in connection with the gastrointestinal tract, including anorexia, overeating, abdominal pain, peptic ulcer, constipation, and ulcerative colitis. Enuresis (see p. 807) and asthma (see p. 689) may also be classified as psychosomatic illnesses in children. The diagnosis and treatment of psychosomatic illnesses are the joint responsibilities of the physician and the psychiatrist.

ANOREXIA NERVOSA

The child who has anorexia nervosa seems to have a relentless drive toward self-destruction

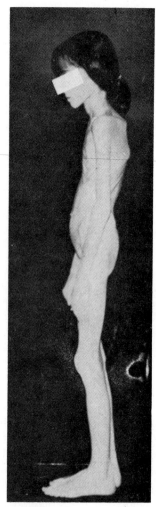

FIGURE 24–28. Anorexia nervosa. (From Seligmann, J. A.: *Newsweek*, September 9, 1974.)

through starvation. This condition is most often seen in girls. Such a child at first deliberately refuses food, even though he has an excellent appetite. Anorexia nervosa occurs only if he has some deep emotional problem. There is often an intense conflict between mother and daughter. The girl is likely to have misconceptions about pregnancy and indulges in sexual fantasies. As the period of starvation is prolonged, real anorexia and self-induced vomiting of food directly after it has been eaten produce rapid weight loss and bodily changes due to food deprivation. The child may gain sympathy from the family because of these symptoms.

Treatment includes correcting any electrolyte imbalance and increasing the diet. The child is usually hospitalized for diagnosis and initial treatment. The use of operant conditioning within the context of structural family therapy has produced improvement in some patients. Family involvement tends to promote weight gain. Continued family involvement in therapy facilitates the necessary restructuring of the family to prevent relapses. Further psychiatric consultation may become necessary.

Anorexia nervosa is a chronic condition, and the ultimate prognosis is questionable.

OVEREATING

Overeating which results in extreme obesity is usually thought to be due to the child's need for love, which he equates with food. It may also be due, however, to his wanting to grow big in size or to other emotional factors. Treatment is generally difficult. Many times the services of both a physician and a psychiatrist are necessary to curb the child's desire for food.

ABDOMINAL PAIN

Recurrent abdominal pain without organic cause is frequent in older school children. It occurs with little regularity in relation to meals, evacuations, or time of day. The intensity varies from mild discomfort to severe pain. Appendectomy or exploratory laparotomy procedures are of no benefit.

These children generally seem to be older and more pleasant and responsible in their behavior than their peers. Their parents have a high expectation of themselves and their children or they may fear that the child cannot cope with the usual process of development. The child, not being able to handle the anxiety of his parents, looks for direction and safety and does not then achieve as well as other children his age. This behavior only reinforces the parental anxiety over the child. The services of a physician and a psychiatrist may be necessary in the treatment of such children.

PEPTIC ULCER

Incidence, Etiology, Clinical Manifestations, and Diagnosis. Peptic ulcer of the adult type is not common in children, but gastric and duodenal ulcers may be seen at any age in childhood. An ulcer is a lesion on the surface of the gastric or duodenal mucosa caused by inflammation. Gastric ulcers are more common during infancy. Duodenal ulcers are seen with greater frequency in later infancy and childhood. Adolescent boys are also prone to develop ulcers.

Ulcerations of the upper gastrointestinal tract are usually acute and may be secondary to the following conditions: severe burns (Curling's ulcer, see p. 562), intensive treatment with adrenocorticosteroids, neurologic lesions (Rokitansky-Cushing ulcer), severe infections and marasmus (see p. 435).

Children who have ulcers are usually highly competitive and intense individuals who strive very hard to achieve in school. They have emotional conflicts with others in their homes. Peptic ulcer may coexist with other functional disorders such as constipation in the same patient.

The *clinical manifestations* include vomiting, possibly with bleeding (hematemesis and melena), or with abdominal distention caused by perforation. Persistent intermittent abdominal pain may also be present. In the school-age child the major complaint may be epigastric pain during the night or before meals. Eating may relieve this pain. Younger children may not complain about these typical symptoms.

The *diagnosis* is made on the basis of the roentgenographic findings. These studies, however, may not always be helpful. Gastric analysis is also not usually of value. Fiberoptic endoscopy may be used. This procedure involves the insertion of a flexible endoscope into the stomach and duodenum in order to visualize the area directly.

Treatment, Responsibilities of the Nurse, Complications, and Prognosis. The treatment of acute perforation of an ulcer is immediate surgical closure. When acute hemorrhage occurs, nasogastric suction, iced saline lavage, and blood transfusions are indicated. Infants who have mild hemorrhage but no perforation can be given milk feedings, while older children are given a bland diet. Bed rest is not usually necessary. These patients are hospitalized for diagnosis and initial therapy. A thorough investigation must be made of the interactions of the patient with his family members.

As soon as possible a freer bland then regular diet is given with gastric antacids or small feedings between meals and at bedtime. Children soon learn not to eat foods which cause pain. Anticholinergic drugs may be given shortly before meals. Further roentgenographic studies should be done from four to eight weeks after the beginning of treatment to determine the progress of the patient.

One of the major *responsibilities of the nurse* is to teach the child and his parents about nutrition. A wholesome diet is important, but coffee, tea, carbonated beverages, and spices should not be given. Helping the parents and child to understand the necessary diet is done slowly over a period of time.

The child and his family must receive education and support in an attempt to prevent further occurrence of this problem since emotional factors are important in the etiology of this condition. The nurse can assess the family situation and support the coping methods of all the family members. Psychotherapy or a form of psychiatric care may become necessary.

Peptic ulcers during childhood usually heal

well without surgery. Surgical intervention is necessary for the possible *complications* of massive hemorrhage, intractability, obstruction, or perforation. The usual surgical procedures used are vagotomy and pyloroplasty.

The *prognosis* is poor among infants having perforated peptic ulcers. Most ulcers during childhood, however, heal within three to four weeks. One half of the patients who have chronic ulcers during childhood have ulcer-like pain or even recurrent ulcers during adult life.

CONSTIPATION

Many cases of so-called constipation in children exist only in the minds of the parents. They feel that their child is constipated because he does not have evacuations as often as the parents think he should. Nevertheless, children do have true constipation, and on occasion it is due to emotional factors.

There are two main kinds of constipation. One occurs in children who show disgust at any form of dirt, especially excreta. These children, in the toddler and preschool ages, before control of elimination was definitely established, feared that their parents would punish them even if they defecated at socially approved times and places, and hence became afraid of *all* defecation. This early fear conditioned them to feel anxiety about defection even after control was thoroughly established, with the result that they restrained the normal need to have bowel movements. The usual treatment for this sort of constipation is to add a small amount of bulk to the diet and to praise the child whenever he becomes dirty during play periods. The older child may have the hygienic aspect of regular evacuation explained to him.

The other kind of constipation is due to excessive early toilet training and results in the child's feeling that excreting is a hostile act against his parents. Such a child needs psychiatric help in order to uncover and remove his fear of his own emotional reactions.

CHRONIC ULCERATIVE COLITIS

Etiology. This is a chronic and serious inflammatory disease of the large intestine. During exacerbations the mucous membrane is hyperemic; it bleeds easily and may develop ulcers and pseudopolyps, the latter tending to malignant changes. Several theories have been advanced about the cause, that it is due to an allergy or an infection, or is a psychosomatic illness. It may occur in more than one person in a family. The child having ulcerative colitis is usually a dependent, fearful, and passive patient who is closely attached, although with ambiva-

lent feelings, usually to the mother. The mother may have ambivalent feelings toward the child, yet she may remain unhappily married for "his sake."

Pathology and Clinical Manifestations. Part or all of the colon may be involved, as may be the ileum. The mucosa may be largely denuded, and multiple longitudinal ulcers may form a network over the colon. There may be fibrosis, and the colon may be decreased in size.

The onset may be insidious or acute. The most important symptom is frequent passage of small stools containing mucus, blood and pus. Diarrhea may occur on occasion. There is usually no fever, abdominal pain, or vomiting, although these may occur during exacerbations of the condition. Hemorrhage from the bowel or rectal prolapse may be a complication. Emaciation, anemia, nutritional edema, and vitamin deficiencies may also be present.

Diagnosis, Treatment, and Responsibilities of the Nurse. The *diagnosis* is made on the basis of the history, lack of causative organisms in the stools, and finding of ulceration and inflammation on proctoscopic examination. When the condition is prolonged, the colon becomes a smoothly outlined tube.

The diet should be soft and bland with a low residue. Additional vitamins and minerals should be given. Blood transfusions may be given for anemia. Sulfasalazine (Azulfidine) may be given orally. Relief may be achieved with one of the corticosteroids, sometimes given by enema. Ileostomy or colectomy may be done. The most encouraging plan of therapy is that carried out jointly by the pediatrician, the psychiatrist, and the surgeon. Emotional and environmental stresses should be relieved. To this end, the parents as well as the child may require psychotherapy. The nurse must become skillful in motivating the parents and the child not only to seek the help of a psychiatrist, but also to continue in the therapeutic plan.

After the child has become bowel-trained any illness associated with fecal incontinence is physically and emotionally distressing to him. Good *nursing care* can reduce the child's concern over this problem.

If the child is very thin, good skin care is essential, especially over bony prominences. The child must be kept clean and warm. The nurse may find it necessary to tempt the child's appetite, because often there is a real distaste for food. The nurse must also be alert to any side effects of drugs given the child.

The nurse's recording of observations is important, especially of the number, amount, and nature of the bowel movements. An accurate record of intake and output is essential. The nurse should also note the child's own report and any observations of anything that seems to stimulate peristalsis and cause frequency of bowel movements. The nurse must be aware of the possibility of complications and report any signs of distention, severe nausea, vomiting, and bleeding.

Physical and emotional rest is essential. The nurse can ease the child's interpersonal relations with others by being warm and sincere in efforts to help the child and his family.

Since the child may seem to accept his disease rather stoically, but not be able to conform to his treatment, the nurse must be alert for any possible problems which may occur after discharge from the hospital. The nurse can help the mother with planning for the intestinal needs of the child, with his medications, with his response to his illness, and with the observations to be made should a relapse occur.

Course and Prognosis. The chronic *course* is interrupted by periods of remission and exacerbations. The disease may continue for years. Death is usually caused by exhaustion, perforation, or, in later years, cancer.

ENURESIS

Enuresis is bed wetting, especially at night, after the age when toilet training should have been completed. Boys are usually more enuretic than girls. Although these children are usually normal, they should have a physical examination to rule out such conditions as diabetes, pyelitis, or nocturnal epilepsy.

Inadequate bladder capacity has been implicated as a cause of nocturnal enuresis. Delayed bladder development makes it physically impossible for some children to store urine throughout the night. Therapy in this situation consists in increasing bladder capacity by having the child retain progressively larger amounts of fluid during the day. Medications may be given to reduce the tone of the muscle wall of the bladder, thus decreasing the amplitude and frequency of contractions and allowing the bladder to dilate. Other problems involving the genitourinary tract may also cause enuresis.

A serious emotional cause of enuresis is a personality or character maladjustment. These children need psychiatric help for their emotional problem. Other less serious causes of enuresis may perhaps be due to jealousy of a new sibling, revenge enuresis because of lack of love from parents, or a regressive neurosis. Treatment of these types consists in changing the parents' attitudes toward the child so that they can give him more love. Treatment using behavior modifica-

tion techniques may be of value. Treatment by restricting fluids before bedtime, with charts of achievement, or by mechanical devices to waken the child may cure the enuresis, but not the basic problem.

Additional causes of enuresis in the school child include retardation, lack of toilet training, profound sleep, or a situation in which the child's bedroom is too far from the bathroom. Treatment here is easier than for the child with a severe emotional problem who may require psychiatric care.

Parents many times are concerned about a chid who has enuresis because they believe that friends and neighbors may feel they have not reared the child well. The nurse can support them by listening to their feelings concerning the child and his problem. Sometimes such support will improve the parent-child relationship and produce an improvement in the child's behavior. Upon assessing the family situation and finding a more complex problem, the nurse can assist in referral of the family to sources for further counseling.

Therapy

Parents may make mistakes, and the child may not be too much affected. Too many mistakes, however, will affect the child's behavior. Parents are too close to the situation to see what is really happening. They may be bothered by the child's behavior, but may not realize the basic problem involved.

Sometimes a child's behavior is upsetting to parents even though it is only a manifestation of his development. All that such parents need is an explanation of the normal growth and development of a child. Usually no therapy is required.

Professional help may be needed, however, if the cause of the problem is deep-seated and not understood by the parents. Such help may be required if the child is afraid to leave his level of development and advance toward maturity, is not growing and developing according to the usual pattern of maturation, is oversubmissive, overaggressive or not learning at a rate commensurate with his ability, cannot deal with frustrations or challenges in a way socially acceptable for a child of his age or shows socially unacceptable behavior characteristics.

Sources and Types. Outside help may be gained from the family physician, pediatrician, psychologist, psychiatrist, parent study group, teachers, or guidance counselors.

Parents often hesitate to seek help for emotionally disturbed children. They feel that they should know all the answers. A psychiatrist would want a detailed history of the parents' development and problems, as well as a history of the child. He would also want to know the relations between the parents and other family members.

The psychiatrist may believe that the problem is typical for a child of this age and will help the parents handle the particular problem; he may believe that it is largely the parents' problem and recommend a change of environment for the child or secure help for the parents; or he may believe that it is largely the child's problem and ask to see him frequently in order to help him gain an understanding of his problem and see other ways to handle it.

Prolonged therapy may be necessary. At times during such therapy the child's behavior may seem to become worse in that he may act out impulses that previously were under control. Parents need the help of the psychiatrist to understand what is happening in the parent-child relations and to know how to deal with the child's behavior. The psychiatrist does not divulge the material which the child gives him without the child's permission. This is difficult for the parents to understand, but it is essential that they accept this element in the counseling situation. In addition to therapy for the child, the parents may also be involved in psychotherapy. Family therapy, which involves the child and his parents as an educational and therapeutic experience, is becoming more widely used.

The emotionally disturbed child may be placed in a foster home, a day school, a boarding school, or a structured residential treatment center or psychiatric hospital. These facilities provide children who have emotional problems a way of receiving therapy outside the setting of their own homes.

Responsibilities of the Nurse. The nurse who cares for children having psychosomatic illnesses or emotional disturbances must be able to observe their behavior accurately and record what she hears, feels and sees. Such observations help those who are treating these children, as well as helping the nurses themselves in the care of the children.

Close cooperation with the therapist is essential. The therapist can help nurses to understand the meaning of the behavior they observe and to provide the kind of nursing care skills these children need. Therapists are interested in the child's relations with his parents, his peers, and other adults. They would also like to know his adjustment to the hospital, to school and to play activities.

More nurses who have been educationally prepared as clinical specialists in the area of child psychiatry are needed to improve the care of emotionally disturbed children by working closely with the children's therapists.

Group conferences of all team members, including physicians, social workers, school teachers, play therapists, nurses, aides, and other auxiliary personnel who have contact with these children, are necessary. They help everyone to understand the care of the child, as well as the cause of his illness. Such conferences often also help the nurse to understand his or her own personality and thus improve relations with the children under care.

CLINICAL SITUATIONS

Marsha Dullin, a nine-year old girl, has been admitted to the pediatric unit with a diagnosis of rheumatic fever. She lives with her parents, three brothers, and two sisters in an apartment in a tenement house. Her father is a manual laborer, and the family income is $200.00 a week. On admission Marsha's temperature was elevated, and she complained of joint pains.

1. When Marsha was admitted to the hospital, the nurse found nits in her long blond hair, but could see no pediculi. The physician ordered an application of gamma benzene hexachloride. The nurse removed the nits by
   a. Washing Marsha's hair daily with soap containing hexachlorophene.
   b. Sliding each nit off its hair shaft.
   c. Applying benzyl benzoate lotion and brushing the nits out of the hair.
   d. Combing her hair with a fine-tooth metal comb dipped in hot vinegar.

2. Marsha had been ill at home only a brief time before her admission to the hospital. She is fortunate that her illness was diagnosed and treated early because
   a. Cardiac damage can be minimized or prevented.
   b. Manifestations of chorea can be prevented.
   c. Spread of this infection to her siblings is minimized.
   d. Large amounts of medications will not be necessary in her treatment.

3. The most important point in providing nursing care for Marsha during the acute phase of her illness is
   a. Maintaining contact with her parents.
   b. Physical and psychologic rest.
   c. A nutritious diet.
   d. Maintaining her interest in school.

4. The physician has ordered sodium salicylate for Marsha. The nurse should be aware that some of the toxic symptoms of this drug are
   A. Tinnitus and nausea.
   b. Dermatitis and blurred vision.
   c. Unconsciousness and acetone odor of the breath.
   d. Chills and an elevation of temperature.

5. Significant instructions which Marsha's mother will receive before the child is discharged will concern
   a. A high protein diet, adequate immunization, and avoidance of contact with anyone having an upper respiratory tract infection.

b. Routine immunizations, limited activity, and adequate nutrition.

c. Adequate nutrition, avoidance of contact with anyone having an upper respiratory tract infection, and prophylactic medication.

d. Limited activity, administration of sodium salicylate, and a high vitamin diet.

6. Marsha's one desire before the onset of rheumatic fever was to be a ballet dancer. Now that she may possibly have some cardiac involvement, the team in long-range planning for her rehabilitation would

a. Avoid all reference to dancing in their discussions with her.

b. Investigate Marsha's feeling about her future and help her to consider other career interests.

c. Assure Marsha that a career in dancing would be possible if she promised to take care of herself.

d. Ignore her questions related to dancing because this problem can be discussed later.

Elaine Watson, an 11-year-old child, was admitted to the pediatric unit four weeks ago in diabetic coma. Both her parents and her two older sisters have shown a deep interest in her condition. Elaine is in the sixth grade in school. Her teachers are proud of her level of achievement.

7. In the management of juvenile diabetics, which one of the following factors is considered the *least important?*

a. Taking of regular daily exercise.

b. Prompt treatment of all infections.

c. Maintenance of emotional stability.

d. Treatment of allergies.

8. In evaluating Elaine's ability to care for herself the nurse believes that

a. Elaine is too young to give herself insulin.

b. A visiting nurse should teach Elaine to give herself insulin after she is discharged.

c. Elaine should be taught to give herself insulin while she is in the hospital.

d. Elaine's mother should assume the responsibility for insulin administration until Elaine is an adolescent.

9. When Elaine returns to school, she should certainly remember to carry with her at all times

a. A lump of sugar.

b. A bag of salted nuts.

c. Her insulin and a syringe.

d. Sufficient money to telephone her mother in case she feels ill.

10. Mrs. Watson asks the nurse whether Elaine should join the Girl Scouts of America. Although the mother should make her own decision, the nurse could base comments on a belief that

a. If her closest friends are members of the troop, she should join regardless of whether she wants to or not.

b. The leader will teach her many things a young girl should know.

c. Elaine will meet many girls her own age who share her interests.

d. If Elaine joins, she will probably lose interest in her school work.

11. Mrs. Watson is concerned because Elaine's friends have recently begun to use lipstick. Elaine has expressed a desire to use it also. The nurse believes that

a. Mrs. Watson should forbid the use of lipstick for another year at least.

b. Mrs. Watson should permit Elaine to use it, but that she should teach her to apply it correctly.

c. Mrs. Watson should explain to Elaine that the use of lipstick at her age is not refined.

d. Mrs. Watson should degrade the mothers of Elaine's friends because they have permitted their daughters to use lipstick.

GUIDES TO FURTHER STUDY

1. The children's clinic in your hospital does not have a playroom. Plan the room, including the furniture and the equipment (creative materials, toys, records, and books) that would be needed. Indicate the personnel necessary. In your planning indicate your knowledge of safety factors for children of various ages who will be using the room.

2. Eight-year-old Rebecca Schwartz was recently admitted to the pediatric unit with a diagnosis of diabetes. She is the only child of older parents. Her father has a small grocery business of his own. Rebecca is in the third grade in school and has average scholastic ability. Discuss in seminar that guidance this child and her parents will need. Role-play with another student the process of teaching this child regulation of diet, testing of urine and administration of insulin. Discuss the principles of learning to be considered as well as the content to be presented.

3. Discuss with a school nurse practitioner or school nurse in your community the total program in relation to prevention of disease, treatment of illness, rehabilitation of the handicapped and health education of children. Is the program based on the level of growth and development and understanding of the children in the school? Has the nurse taken into consideration the cultural backgrounds and the socioeconomic levels of these children and their families? What is the role of this nurse in relation to the children's parents? In your discussion of this question in seminar give specific illustrations to support your answers.

4. During your experience in the pediatric unit you have been caring for a school-age child with a diagnosis of ulcerative colitis. Incorporate in your plan of care the recommendations of his psychiatrist. Did your patient show any change in behavior as a result of your altered approach? Discuss any problems you had in attempting to carry out the recommendations of the therapist.

5. You are providing care for two eight-year-old boys whose oral fluid requirements are greater than normal. On the basis of your understanding of growth and development, suggest ways by which you could help these children to cooperate with you in meeting this particular need.

TEACHING AIDS AND OTHER INFORMATION*

American Academy of Pediatrics

Children with Learning Disabilities.
Early Identification of Children with Learning Disabilities.
Eye and Learning Disabilities.
Use of d-Amphetamine and Related Central Nervous System Stimulants in Children.

American Dental Association

Orthodontics: Questions and Answers.

American Diabetes Association, Inc.

Facts about Diabetes.
Favorite Foods for Youngsters.
Food Values for Passover Dishes.
Glucagon: Prompt Relief from Insulin Reactions.
Good Eating from South of the Border.
Hypoglycemic Reactions from Insulin or Oral Compounds.
Identification Cards.
Meal Planning with Exchange Lists.
The Care and Handling of Insulin Syringes.
The Diabetic Looks at His Feet.
Treatment of Infection in Diabetes Mellitus.
Urine Testing—Its Methods and Its Importance.
What Does Sugar in the Urine Mean?
What School Personnel Should Know about the Student with Diabetes.
What You Need to Know about Diabetes, 1976.
When Diabetics Marry.
Your Child Can Live a Normal Life with Diabetes.

American Heart Association

Children with Heart Disease, 1971.
Have Fun...Get Well!
Home Care of the Child with Rheumatic Fever.
Protect Your Child's Heart.
You, Your Child, and Rheumatic Fever.

The Arthritis Foundation

Arthritis in Children.

Medic Alert Foundation International

What is Medic Alert?

The National Easter Seal Society

Bloodstein, O.: A Handbook on Stuttering, Revised 1975.
Denhoff, E.: The Responsibility of the Physician, Parent, and Child in Learning Disabilities, 1974.
Henscheid, H.: View of Life, 1975.
Neishloss, L.: Swimming for the Handicapped Child and Adult, 1973.

Public Affairs Committee

Barman, A., and Cohen, L.: Help for Your Troubled Child.
Bryant, J. E.: Helping Your Child Speak Correctly.
Drugs—Use, Misuse, Abuse: Guidance for Families.
Family Lifestyle, Parents' Own Drug Habits, Have Strong Influence on Whether Children Become Drug Users.

United States Government

A Long Dark Hallway (To Inform Mexican-American Youth and Their Parents of the Dangers of Drug Abuse), 1972.
Drug Abuse Prevention Materials for Schools, Revised 1972.
Drugs and Family/Peer Influence, 1974.
Growing Up in America: A Background to Contemporary Drug Abuse, 1973.
Juvenile Delinquency and Youth Crime, Reprinted 1975.
Runaway House: A Youth-Run Service Project, 1974.
Tips on Drug Abuse Prevention, For the Parents of a Young Child, 1972.

*Complete addresses are given in the Appendix.

REFERENCES

Books

American Diabetes Association, Inc.: *Diabetes Mellitus.* 4th ed. New York, American Diabetes Association, Inc., 1975.
Anderson, C. M., and Burke, V. (Eds.): *Paediatric Gastroenterology.* Philadelphia, J. B. Lippincott Company, 1975.
Anderson, R. P., and Halcomb, C. G. (Eds.): *Learning Disability/Minimal Brain Dysfunction Syndrome.* Springfield, Ill., Charles C Thomas, 1975.
Baer, P. N., and Benjamin, S. D.: *Periodontal Disease in Children and Adolescents.* Philadelphia, J. B. Lippincott Company, 1974.
Baller, W. R.: *Bed Wetting: Origins and Treatment.* Toronto, Pergamon Press, Inc., 1975.
Buscaglia, L.: *The Disabled and Their Parents: A Counseling Challenge.* Thorofare, N.J., Charles B. Slack, 1975.
Catzel, P.: *A Short Textbook of Paediatrics.* Philadelphia, J. B. Lippincott Company, 1976.
Cavan, R. S., and Ferdinand, T. N.: *Juvenile Delinquency.* 3rd ed. Philadelphia, J. B. Lippincott Company, 1975.
Commission on Emotional and Learning Disorders in Children: *One Million Children—The CELDIC Report: A National Study of Canadian Children with Emotional and Learning Disorders.* Toronto, Canada, 1970.
Cull, J. G., and Hardy, R. E. (Eds.): *Problems of Disadvantaged and Deprived Youth.* Springfield, Ill., Charles C Thomas, 1975.
Ellingson, C.: *Speaking of Children: Their Learning Abilities/Disabilities.* New York, Harper & Row, 1975.

Fagin, C. M. (Ed.): *Readings in Child and Adolescent Psychiatric Nursing.* St. Louis, The C. V. Mosby Company, 1974.
Farmer, T. W. (Ed.): *Pediatric Neurology.* 2nd ed. New York, Harper & Row, 1975.
Foster, T. D.: *Textbook of Orthodontics.* Philadelphia, J. B. Lippincott Company, 1975.
Francis, D. E. M., and Dixon, D. J. W.: *Diets for Sick Children.* 3rd ed. Philadelphia, J. B. Lippincott Company, 1975.
Gardner, L. I. (Ed.): *Endocrine and Genetic Diseases of Childhood and Adolescence.* Philadelphia, W. B. Saunders Company, 1975.
Gross, M. D., and Wilson, W. C.: *Minimal Brain Dysfunction.* New York, Brunner/Mazel, 1974.
Illingworth, R. S.: *Common Symptoms of Disease in Children.* 4th ed. Philadelphia, J. B. Lippincott Company, 1973.
Lettieri, D. J. (ed.): *Predicting Adolescent Drug Abuse: A Review of Issues, Methods and Correlates.* Washington, D.C., National Institute on Drug Abuse, 1975.
Mason, R. L., Jr., Richmond, B. O., and Fleurant, L. B.: *The Emotionally Troubled Child: A Guide for Parents and Teachers in the Early Recognition of Mental and Nervous Disorders in Children.* Springfield, Ill., Charles C Thomas, Publisher, 1976.
McCollum, A. T.: *Coping with Prolonged Health Impairment in Your Child.* Boston, Little, Brown & Company, 1975.

McIntyre, H. M. (Ed.): *Heart Disease: New Dimensions of Nursing Care.* Garden Grove, Calif., Trainex Press, 1974.

Menkes, J. H.: *Textbook of Child Neurology.* Philadelphia, Lea & Febiger, 1974.

Millichap, J. G.: *The Hyperactive Child with Minimal Brain Dysfunction.* Chicago, Year Book Medical Publishers, 1975.

Oakley, W. G., Pyke, D. A., and Taylor, K. W.: *Diabetes and Its Management.* 2nd ed. Philadelphia, J. B. Lippincott Company, 1975.

Ross, A. O.: *Psychological Aspects of Learning Disabilities and Reading Disorders.* New York, McGraw-Hill Book Company, Inc., 1976.

Silver, H. K., Kempe, C. H., and Bruyn, H. B.: *Handbook of Pediatrics.* 11th Ed. Los Altos, California, Lange Medical Publishers, 1975.

Swaiman, K. F.: *The Practice of Pediatric Neurology.* St. Louis, The C. V. Mosby Company, 1975.

Till, K., and Hoare, R. D.: *Paediatric Neurosurgery.* Philadelphia, J. B. Lippincott Company, 1975.

Vince, D. J.: *Essentials of Pediatric Cardiology.* Philadelphia, J. B. Lippincott Company, 1974.

Weiss, C., and Lillywhite, H.: *Recognition and Early Intervention in Communicative Disorders.* St. Louis, The C. V. Mosby Company, 1976.

Periodicals

Anonsen, D. C.: The Hyperkinetic Child. *The Canadian Nurse,* 71:27, May 1975.

Bellam, G.: The Nursing Challenge of the Child with Neurological Problems. *Nursing Forum,* 11:396, No. 1, 1972.

Block, S. R.: Juvenile Rheumatoid Arthritis. *Nursing Digest,* 4:50, Summer 1976.

Burgess, A. W., and Holmstrom, L. L.: Sexual Trauma of Children and Adolescents. *Nursing Clin. N. Am.,* 10:551, September 1975.

Cohen, M. W.: Enuresis. *Pediatr. Clin. N. Am.,* 22:545, August 1975.

Denhoff, E.: The Best Management of Learning Disabilities Calls for Pediatric Skills of a Special Sort. *Nursing Digest,* 2:49, March 1974.

Dixon, G., and Rickard, K.: Nutrition Education for Young Patients. *Children Today,* 4:7, January-February 1975.

Doyle, E. F.: Rheumatic Fever—A Continuing Problem. *Nursing Digest,* 3:23, January-February 1975.

Fajans, S. S., et al.: The Various Faces of Diabetes in the Young. *Arch. Intern. Med.,* 136:194, February 1976.

Feighner, A. C., and Feighner, J. P.: Multimodality Treatment of the Hyperkinetic Child. *Am. J. Psychiatry,* 131:459, April 1974.

Forsythe, W. I., and Redmond, A.: Enuresis and Spontaneous Cure Rate: Study of 1129 Enuretics. *Arch. Dis. Child,* 49:259, April 1974.

Friedland, G. M.: Learning Behaviors of a Preadolescent With Diabetes. *Am. J. Nursing,* 76:59, January 1976.

Gomez, M. R., and Reese, D. F.: Computed Tomography of the Head in Infants and Children. *Pediatr. Clin. N. Am.,* 23:473, August 1976.

Greenfield, D., Grant, R., and Lieberman, E.: Children Can Have High Blood Pressure, Too. *Am. J. Nursing,* 76:770, May 1976.

Guthrie, D. W., and Guthrie, R. A.: Diabetes in Adolescence. *Am. J. Nursing,* 75:1740, October 1975.

Heisel, J. S., et al.: The Significance of Life Events as Contributing Factors in the Diseases of Children: *J. Pediatr.* 83:119, July 1973.

Jackson, R., et al. III A Study of Pediatric Patients. A Teenager's Torment: Rheumatic Heart Disease. *Nursing '74,* 3:51, March 1974.

Jaffe, A. C., et al.: Sexual Abuse of Children. *Am. J. Dis. Child,* 129:689, June 1975.

Jimm, L. R.: Nursing Assessment of Patients for Increased Intracranial Pressure. *Nursing Digest,* 3:4, July-August, 1975.

Johnson, A.: A Continuing Threat: Rheumatic Fever. *Nursing '74,* 3:57, March 1974.

Kiester, E. Jr.: Explosive Youngsters: What To Do About Them. *Today's Health,* 52:48, January 1974.

Kosidlak, J. G.: Improving Health Care for Troubled Youths. *Am. J. Nursing,* 76:95, January 1976.

Kryk, H., et al.: Grand Rounds on Brain Tumors. *The Canadian Nurse,* 71:42, September 1975.

Laugharne, E.: Insulin Goes Metric: A Time for Review. *The Canadian Nurse,* 71:22, February 1975.

Leahey, M. D., Logan, S. A., and McArthur, R. G.: Pediatric Diabetes: A New Teaching Approach. *The Canadian Nurse,* 71:18, October 1975.

Lieberman, E.: Children with Hypertension. *Am. Fam. Physician,* 12:99, October 1975.

Liebman, R., Minuchin, S., and Baker, L.: An Integrated Treatment Program for Anorexia Nervosa. *Am. J. Psychiatry,* 131:432, April 1974.

Lorich, M. L., and Kaiser, S. A.: A Diabetic Child is Still A Child—With Diabetes. *RN,* 38:39, October 1975.

McAnarney, E. R., et al.: Psychological Problems of Children with Chronic Juvenile Arthritis. *Pediatrics,* 53:523, April 1974.

McFarlane, J.: Children With Diabetes: Special Needs During Growth Years. *Am. J. Nursing,* 73:1360, August 1973.

Mitchell, P. H., and Mauss, N.: Intracranial Pressure: Fact & Fancy. *Nursing '76,* 6:53, June 1976.

Nader, P. R., Bullock, D., and Caldwell, B.: School Phobia. *Pediatr. Clin. N. Am.,* 22:605, August 1975.

Nichol, C.: Legg-Perthes Disease. *The Canadian Nurse,* 72:31, June 1976.

Pendleton, T., and Grossman, B. J.: Rehabilitating Children with Inflammatory Joint Disease. *Am. J. Nursing,* 74:2223, December 1974.

Reeves, K. R.: This CAT Is a Revolutionary Scanner. *RN,* 39:40, August 1976.

Stein, S. P., and Charles, E. S.: Emotional Factors in Juvenile Diabetes Mellitus: A Study of the Early Life Experiences of Eight Diabetic Children. *Psychosom. Med.,* 37:237, May-June 1975.

Stewart, M. A.: Treatment of Bedwetting. *Nursing Digest,* 4:90, Summer 1976.

Surveyer, J. A.: Coma in Children: How It Affects Parents. *The American Journal of Maternal Child Nursing.* 1:17, January-February 1976.

Surveyer, J. A.: The Emotional Toll on Nurses Who Care for Comatose Children. *The American Journal of Maternal Child Nursing,* 1:243, July-August 1976.

Tealey, A. R.: Getting Children to Keep Still During Radiotherapy. *The American Journal of Maternal Child Nursing.* 2:178, May-June 1977.

Wahl, S.: Only A Concussion. *Nursing '76,* 6:44, August 1976.

Waizer, J., Hoffman, S. P., Polizos, P., and Engelhardt, D. M.: Outpatient Treatment of Hyperactive School Children with Imipramine. *Am. J. Psychiatry,* 131:587, May 1974.

Waldron, S.: The Significance of Childhood Neurosis for Adult Mental Health: A Follow-up Study." *Am. J. Psychiatry,* 133:532, May 1976.

Walker, M. D.: Diagnosis and Treatment of Brain Tumors. *Pediatr. Clin. N. Am.,* 23:131, February 1976.

Winslow, E. H.: Digitalis. *Am. J. Nursing,* 74:1062, June 1974.

AUDIOVISUAL MEDIA

The American Cancer Society, Inc.

Meeting Highlights: The American Cancer Society's National Conference on Childhood Cancer
  Album with two standard C-60 audio cassettes.

The participants discuss the progress being made in the diagnosis and treatment of childhood cancer. Topics include: environmental, immunologic, genetics and familial factors involved; management of Wilms' tumor, neuroblastoma, and other abdominal tumors; role of surgery, chemotherapy, radiation therapy and immunotherapy; diagnosis and treatment of brain tumors; radiation therapy of central nervous system tumors; treatment of Hodgkin's disease and lymphomas; etiology, diagnosis, and treatment of leukemia.

CIBA

Cerebral Dysfunction in Children
  25 minutes, film, sound, black and white.

This film shows and describes a 10-year-old patient with hyperkinetic behavior, short attention span, lack of social sense, etc., and what can be done to help such children by physicians, parents, and medication. Recommended for general practitioners and pediatricians, as well as school personnel dealing with children of this type.

McGraw-Hill Book Company

The Diabetic: Series of 4 Film Loops
  Remillet, J. G.
  7 minutes each, 4 16mm films or Super-8mm filmloops, sound, color.

For use by the nurse in the education of the person who has diabetes. The four topics covered are Diabetic Diet, Self-Administration of Insulin, Foot Care for Diabetics, and Urine Testing for Sugar and Ketones.

W. B. Saunders Company

Pediatric Cardiology
  Schmidt, R., and Khoury, G. H.
  Four 35mm filmstrips totaling 145 frames, two tape cassettes, color, booklet.

A combination of lucid line drawings, photographs of unusual clarity, and actual taped auscultatory findings help you recognize both rare and common pediatric heart disorders. The presentation comprises two units — Cardiac Examination of the Child, and Rheumatic Fever in Children.

Pediatric Conferences with Sydney Gellis
  Hyperactivity, Eisenberg, L.
  Juvenile Rheumatoid Arthritis, Calabro, J. J.
  The Role of the Pediatrician in Learning Disorders, Reed, H. B. C.

Trainex Corporation

Diabetes and Inheritance
  35mm filmstrip, audio-tape cassettes, 33 1/3 LP, color.
  Explains to the diabetic how he inherited the disease and informs those with a history of diabetes of the possibilities of recurrence in their families.

Diabetes Mellitus — Pathophysiology
  35mm filmstrip, audio-tape cassettes, 33 1/3 LP, color.
  The general pathophysiology of diabetes mellitus is described. Long-range complications and patient attitudes are discussed.

Pathology of Diabetes
  35mm filmstrip, audio-tape cassettes, 33 1/3 LP, color.
  A comprehensive overview of the pathogenesis of diabetes. Examines the gross pathologic and histologic abnormalities of the pancreas in juvenile-onset and maturity-onset diabetes. An extensive discussion of diabetic ketoacidosis, retinopathy, nephropathy, neuropathy, ophthalmopathy, cardiovascular disease, and skin disorders is included.

Rheumatic Diseases in Children and Young Adults
  35mm filmstrip, audio-tape cassettes, 33 1/3 LP, color.
  A comprehensive overview of juvenile rheumatoid arthritis and rheumatic fever. Covers the clinical manifestations of the acute stage, the permanent deformities and abnormalities of growth that may occur in affected individuals, diagnosis, and therapy. A special section is concerned with surgery of diseased heart valves.

Testing the Urine for Glucose and Ketones
  35mm filmstrip, audio-tape cassettes, 33 1/3 LP, color.
  Demonstrates various techniques for testing urine for the presence of glucose and ketones. Each test method is explained in sequence, with full-color photography of testing materials and reactions visually reinforcing each explanation.

The Hyperactive Child
  35mm filmstrip, audio-tape cassettes, 33 1/3 LP, color.
  The behavior of a hyperactive child, his parent's decision to seek medical help, and the subsequent medical treatment are illustrated and explained in this program. Included is a concise description, supported by appropriate visuals, of the test given to help determine the diagnosis of hyperkinesis, such as the Meeting Street School Screening Test (MSSST).

United States Government

Curious Alice
  Producer: USNIMH
  14 minutes, 16mm film, optical sound, color.
  Portrays an animated fantasy based upon the characters in *Alice in Wonderland*. Shows Alice touring a strange land where everyone has chosen drugs — the Mad Hatter uses LSD, the Dormouse uses sleeping pills, and the King of Hearts represents heroin. Alice concludes that drug abuse is senseless. Fun for grade school children to watch, but also communicates effectively the seriousness of drug abuse.

°Complete addresses are given in the Appendix.

UNIT SEVEN

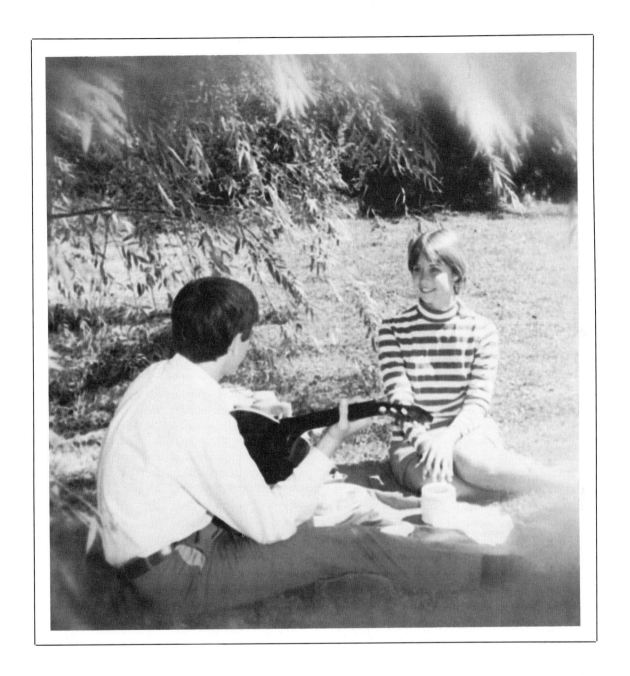

THE PUBESCENT
AND THE
ADOLESCENT

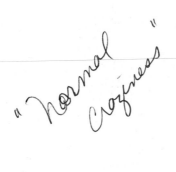

"normal" craziness

"Our adolescents now seem to love luxury. They have bad manners and contempt for authority. They show disrespect for adults and spend their time hanging around places gossiping with one another . . . They are ready to contradict their parents, monopolize the conversation in company, eat gluttonously, and tyrannize their teachers."

—Socrates
5th Century B. C.

Chapter Twenty-Five

THE NORMAL PUBESCENT AND THE NORMAL ADOLESCENT: THEIR GROWTH, DEVELOPMENT, AND CARE

When their child reaches the pubescent and adolescent years, the parents must take still another step in their own development. Their teenager, in trying to build a *sense of identity* of his own, may tend to separate himself to some degree physically and emotionally from his family. His parents must then learn to build a new life of their own and, standing in the background, watch their adolescent with increasing maturity proceed to shape his own life.

Adolescence is unique to human beings and is thought by some to be especially unique to our culture. All other mammals achieve sexual maturity early, but man, with his long period of dependency, achieves sexual maturity much later. Thus the sexual function takes on certain features peculiar to man. This refers to the point that man is a social animal and in his highest state of maturity is able to find a balanced integration between his social responsibility and his sexual nature. Adolescence, then, is the period when the young person is struggling to find this balance within himself.

A host of possibilities enter into the success or failure of this struggle: genetic factors, health, family constitution and attitudes, economic level, the culture of the group to which the adolescent belongs, and the various educational, recreational and vocational opportunities afforded him by society at local, state, and national levels.

In order to differentiate the terms used in this chapter, the following definitions are given. The *prepuberty* or *prepubescent* period refers to the period of rapid physical growth when secondary sex characteristics appear. *Puberty* may be said to have occurred when the girl begins to menstruate and the boy to produce spermatozoa. *Menarche* refers more specifically to the time of the first menstrual period. *Adolescence* begins when the secondary sex characteristics appear and ends when somatic growth is completed and the individual is psychologically mature, capable of taking his place as a contributing member of society. It is a period of conflict, stress and anxiety, as well as one of self-realization and accomplishment.

By about ten to 12 years of age the child begins the last period of life before adulthood. Before that time the child should have developed a sense of trust in others, a sense of autonomy in that he is a human being with a mind and a will of his own, a sense of initiative in that he wants to learn to do what he sees others doing, and, during school age, a sense of duty, industry, or accomplishment of real tasks which he can carry through to completion. The young

815

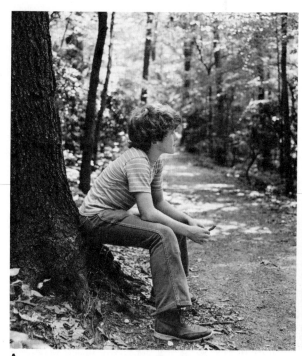 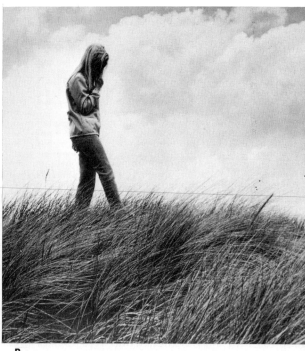

A   B

FIGURE 25–1.   The adolescent questions, "Who am I?" The search for a sense of identity is important for the individual. (Courtesy of H. Armstrong Roberts.)

person who approaches puberty and adolescence has two additional strides to make in his personality development. These can be termed a *sense of identity* and a *sense of intimacy*. Adolescence ends gradually with the beginning of adult life—about 18 years in our culture. The termination of adolescence may be evident early, owing to the individual's assuming the social and economic responsibilities of the adult, or it may be prolonged to the mid-twenties or later when the college education has been completed.

Although the chronologic age of ten years may be given as the beginning of prepubescence and the chronologic age of 18 years or an indefinite age according to the individual as the end of adolescence, few specific times when definite changes occur may be given for this period. As the youth grows older, the span of time in which a specific step in development occurs becomes wider. It is therefore possible to describe only the overall changes in growth and development which occur during prepuberty, puberty, and adolescence. Adolescence is basically a time when the individual battles for recognition of his adulthood, and yet at the same time desires unconsciously to remain a child.

Many young people at some time during these years reach a period of emotional crisis or change, with the outcome not easily assured. Such a crisis may lead to backtracking in development or to further growth and maturing. This crisis provides a new chance to resolve emotional problems which were not resolved before and have remained quiescent.

OVERVIEW OF EMOTIONAL AND SOCIAL DEVELOPMENT

Puberty

The pubescent period may be considered a pause of two or three years between childhood and adolescence. It is basically the organic phenomenon of adolescence. It is a period of rapid physical change and personality growth when the individual achieves nearly his adult bodily stature. Girls begin their preadolescent growth spurt by about ten years and boys by about 12 years. Between 12 and 14 years for girls and one or two years later for boys, they approach the end of puberty. Children who, during school years, resembled each other in body build now show definite indications of belonging to one or the other sex, of becoming taller, shorter, thinner, or more obese than others.

The child during pubescence shows strides in personality development as well as physical growth. He becomes increasingly more adaptable, approaching his peer group and problem situations at home and at school with greater confidence. He enjoys games that involve not only physical skills but also team cooperation. Although there is a revival of love for the parent of the opposite sex, he argues with his parents frequently. He is able to assume increasing responsibility in what to him is reality. Because the young teenager has grown up in a rapidly moving society, has been influenced by the mass media, and has greater communication with an enlarging peer group, his parents may not have the same values that he holds during this period. The parents may want him to assume greater responsibilities around the home, but he may feel that his responsibility lies in helping his friends with a game or in completing a project he has started.

The pubescent seems able to handle important emotional problems easily. If a parent, grandparent, or sibling dies, or if his parents are separated or divorced, the child may appear on the surface to adjust very well, turning rapidly to other activities in his environment. Later, however, he may have to face the problem again because it was not worked through satisfactorily; it was only hidden from his own as well as an observer's view.

Parents become aware that during pubescence the hostility which previously existed between boys and girls is gradually disappearing. There is an interest in "dating," in going to mixed parties, especially dances, and in talking about members of the opposite sex. Such activities do not really mean that the children have become emotionally mature. They merely indicate that the youngsters are trying to leave childhood and to assume the pattern of behavior of the adolescent or adult group.

The child realizes that he is inadequate in these initial attempts to be grown up. He knows that he is not mature and that most of his activity still centers around school, friends, play, and home. Unfortunately, many parents try to capitalize on this step in development and urge more rapid development of interest in the opposite sex than the child is ready for. There may be reasons for parental pressure in this area, not the least of which is their wish that the child be popular with both sexes, that he be well accepted in his peer group. Severe pressure of this sort usually does not achieve the positive goal that parents might wish.

On the whole, however, puberty is a period of comparative quiet for the child and for the adults in his environment. He seems now to be a relatively independent person. Parents can reason with him and come to some kind of solution for their problems. Both the school and society expect him to understand the mores of his group. Behavior such as lying and stealing, which were not punished too severely in earlier years because of his immaturity are now unacceptable because he is presumed to know what behavior society expects. Adults expect the child during puberty to make a fairly adequate adjustment to the demands of reality in our society.

Adolescence (the Sense of Identity and the Sense of Intimacy)

The transition from childhood to adulthood is not a smooth one. Adolescence is a period of stress for young people and parents alike. The adolescent must learn who he is and must modify his conscience for his adult role in life. He now questions many of the beliefs that he held as certain and true. Besides this intellectual and emotional upheaval, his rapid body growth causes him anxiety, and the cultural pressures of today's world add futher stress to his uncertainty.

Adolescents today are faced with many pressures which the older generation did not have. The rapid rate of social change, the threat or presence of war, increase in the speed of travel and rapid technological progress pose problems unknown in previous generations.

Perhaps more important is the fact that adolescents are faced with a problem of finding employment at a time when they seek independence from home. Child labor laws, which greatly restrict adolescents in terms of employment, have had beneficial effects, but have also made problems. This in turn makes for great problems for schools in that compulsory education laws become exceedingly difficult to administer in view of the increasing number of adolescents who are actually uneducable. This refers not only to mentally retarded children, but also to those having emotional difficulties.

Erikson has called the central problem of the early period of adolescence the establishment of a *sense of identity*. In the words of a modern adolescent girl: "I could never begin to discuss my feelings and conflicts because of their confusing order. My ideas on life and people are always changing because I am going through that process of trying to find myself."

The adolescent wonders how he appears and will appear to others in the future. Does he fit what society expects him to be? This is really a question about the continuity of the individual, from early childhood to adult years.

Adolescents in primitive societies have an

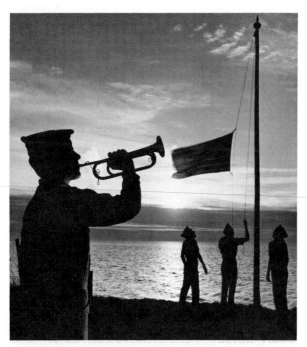

FIGURE 25–2. Ceremonies and activities of young peoples' organizations help adolescents to understand their roles in our society. (Courtesy of H. Armstrong Roberts.)

easier time defining their role than do those in our culture. They have initiation rites which symbolize to themselves and to others that they are young adults. For instance, in the Navajo religion the ceremonial of the Blessing Way is performed for girls at puberty. In our society confirmation, or acceptance into the Church, graduation from school, and the ceremonies of various youth organizations may mean the same thing to the adolescent who belongs to them. Although these ceremonies are important, they do not have the significance that initiation rites have in primitive societies. Probably of greater importance to the youth of today is the age when he can vote and enter the military service.

Nevertheless, even though the rites in primitive societies do add a measure of security to the individual youth's life, they take away the freedom of choice which the youth of our culture have.

Since our society does not have rigid rules, mores, customs, and taboos which govern the behavior of adolescents, they themselves must organize them. Patterns of dress, behavior, or prejudice are set by the group and tend to make the members feel worthwhile. Unfortunately, such limits on behavior tend to form groups from which many young people are excluded. Those who are excluded then have a much more difficult time in gaining a sense of security and of identity.

The young person in our society may be dis-turbed not only because he is not certain of himself, but also because he is not certain of who he is to become. There are so many choices to be made in growing up, so many opportunities ahead, that instead of being comforting, they are confusing.

The adolescent who is not able to face himself and life squarely, who has a feeling of *self-diffusion,* may become delinquent, neurotic, or psychotic. The outcome of the adolescent's struggle to establish his sense of identity is dependent largely on what his personality development was during childhood. The problem is further complicated in our society for the individual who belongs to a minority group.

The child whose personality development was not adequate may be helped during pubescence and the adolescent years through psychiatric therapy or helpful guidance of teachers and others. Less fortunate is the child whose security during his early years was based on the mores of a minority group. During adolescence he may decide to reject his past and try to become a true American middle-class citizen. This step may be too difficult, and he may falter and become delinquent. Although many professional persons are trying to find an answer for this problem, it has no easy solution.

Although the sense of identity is difficult to achieve, the young person must gain it in order to be saved from emotional turmoil. He must be able to find for himself a meaning to life; he must be able to see clearly that life has continuity for him individually. Probably never before in history has youth faced the difficulty that it faces today in a world of rapidly changing values and ideas, a world facing destruction at the same time that the youth is trying to save himself.

After the youth has developed a sense of identity during early adolescence he should be able to develop a *sense of intimacy* with himself and with persons of both sexes. Intimacy is the capacity to commit oneself to another or to others and to continue the commitment even when to do so is difficult. If the individual has a weak ego, if he is not certain of himself, he will not be able to form close ties of friendship or love with other people.

Although closer relations between boys and girls begin during pubescence, they are not intimate relations and serve only as settings for discussion of what they think and feel. During later adolescence these relations serve another purpose. They help to resolve the individual's preoccupation with the integration of the sexual function. They help one young person to unite with another. If the young person cannot do this because of his lack of a valued personality, he

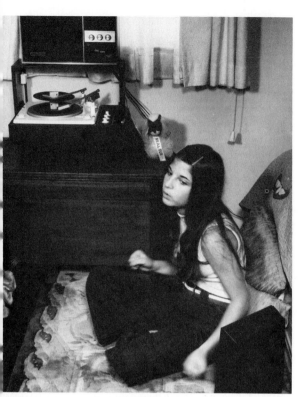

FIGURE 25–3. "I believe I know a little more about myself now, but how can I learn about you?" The adolescent gradually develops a *sense of intimacy.* (Courtesy of James L. Dillon & Co. Inc.)

may enter a state of *isolation,* keeping his relations with others on a cool, rigid, formal basis. If such a person rushes into an early heterosexual relationship, it will probably fail because, lacking the ability to know himself, he is not able to know and love another. If intimacy cannot be achieved, his sexual relationships are distorted, with resulting frustration caused by a lack of total gratification.

While the healthy adolescent is establishing his sense of intimacy he has a real struggle with sexual feelings. This new force drives him to his peers. In the healthy adolescent this does not lead to the sexual act, although some physical expressions of affection are common. Such an adolescent does not usually want to proceed with the sexual act, because this involves a feeling of loss of independence. Sexual promiscuity in adolescence is usually an attempt to find an infantile relation rather than a mature form of psychosexual development.

Unfortunately our culture places less emphasis on the young person's developing a sense of intimacy than on his becoming independent and industrious. In our materialistic society the emphasis is often on success, not in interpersonal relations, but in the competitive world of work. For this reason many "successful" young people

and adults have not developed the ability to understand the personality of others. They tend to be unhappy even though to the world they appear to be highly successful.

DEVELOPMENTAL NEEDS OF THE ADOLESCENT

The adolescent must face five important developmental needs and find a solution to them if he is to gain a sense of identity and a sense of intimacy and to reach some degree of emotional maturity as an adult: (1) *integration of his personality for future responsibility,* (2) *emancipation from his parents and family,* (3) *creation of satisfactory relations with the opposite sex,* (4) *acceptance of a new body image after the rapid physical changes of this period,* and (5) *a decision about the vocation he will follow as an adult.* If his development to puberty has been satisfactory, these goals will not be too difficult, provided parents and other adults give him the help and guidance he needs. All too frequently, however, much friction and misunderstanding between parents and their adolescent children exists, making the process of growing up more difficult than it might be.

Integration of Personality. By the time the child reaches adolescence he should already have made a beginning toward the integration of his personality. He should have some consistent ways of acting in certain situations. He should have a healthy way of meeting reality, of doing something constructive in problem situations. If he has not reached this point in development, he may enter adolescence shy, anxious and with a desire to retreat and isolate himself when a problem arises. He may avoid social contacts and responsibilities whenever possible. He may, without help, complete adolescence poorly equipped to face life.

In order to achieve integration of personality the adolescent must participate in society as a whole, not only in relation to himself as an individual. He must be able to accept people—friends, and later his spouse, children, neighbors, and those of cultures other than his own. He should refrain from being too critical of others and should try to see their point of view. He should take part in the life of the larger community. He must have a deep feeling of willingness to help others in order to achieve a feeling of social unity and thus gain social strength. As one adolescent said: "By giving of myself I receive satisfaction and contentment. But by giving I also receive much more. It is a chance to mature and understand myself through others."

The Adolescent and His Family. Parents, teachers and other adults may not be as impor-

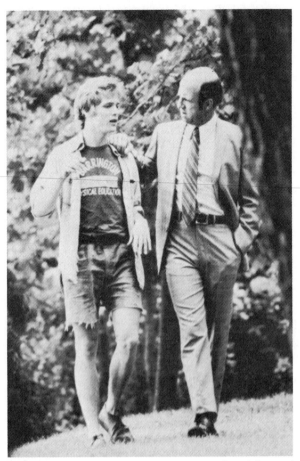

FIGURE 25–4. Adults should recognize the adolescent's growing feelings of maturity but also accept his occasional need for guidance and help. (From Robinson, R.: *Today's Health*, 51:12, August 1973.)

younger adolescent thus makes some of the characteristics—a trait, a manner of speaking, a skill—of the adult a part of his own personality. Often the adult, whether a teacher, Scout leader, relative, minister, priest, rabbi, physician, nurse, or someone in public life, never realizes the effect he has had upon these young people. Many times parents who do not wish their child to grow up resent the fact that another adult is imitated in this way.

On the other hand, such relations may be extremely helpful for the adolescent and his family. A trusted, respected adult outside the family can help the adolescent find himself and his role in life more easily than can the parent, who may be less objective. Such an adult can help the adolescent clarify his thinking, work out his solution and find more mature patterns of behavior. When an adolescent reaches this point, his behavior gradually becomes determined by his own judgment rather than by controls imposed from outside. His parents and friends become less frustrating, and his hostility toward them diminishes.

Some parents need as much help and understanding as their adolescents do. Having had stormy periods of adolescence themselves they may have acute apprehension over the trials of their children. If they do not get the help they need, they may be either too strict or too lenient in setting limits to their children's behavior. Neither of these extremes provides the help which youth needs at this crucial time. The adolescent needs acceptance and guidance as a growing individual. Only in this way can he discover his limitations and powers.

The adolescent's relations with his siblings may become exceedingly strained. This is especially true of a boy whose younger sister has already reached puberty and left him behind in growth. Yet both the brother and the sister should feel more confident about approaching the problems of adolescence, especially in adjusting to the opposite sex, because they have learned the acceptable patterns of behavior from each other.

In some families younger siblings may place an adolescent sister or brother in the role of a parent-substitute. This kind of identification is probably not harmful if it does not interfere too much with the adolescent's own development and social activities.

The battle for independence is fought in practically every family. The parents fight to maintain authority and prestige in the eyes of the young person, and the young person fights for liberty. The youth who fights such a battle should probably be less a source of worry than one who causes no conflict over his strivings to

tant to the adolescent as they were previously. He may be hostile to them and resent their authority. He is torn between his need for support and acceptance, to be dependent as a child, and his need for independence. He must defend himself against his unconscious love for the parent of the opposite sex and resolve his ambivalence toward the parent of the same sex. Although parents may consider the adolescent unmanageable and say that they cannot understand him, they should recognize his growing feelings of maturity and also his occasional need for help.

The adolescent, instead of wishing to be like the parent of the same sex, may attempt to be as different as possible. He may even ridicule his parents at home, but still value them highly outside the home. Affection is turned from the parents to adults outside the family. This begins a series of brief *"crushes"* typical of adolescence. The adolescent loves the adult, desires to please him, and identifies with him. The

become independent. The latter will probably stay emotionally in childhood and not weather the storm of the adolescent period.

Adolescence is the ideal time for children to begin to have their own lives. Unfortunately parents often say that they want their children to mature, but block them at every turn. The greatest harm parents can do is to expect the worst from their children, because they will probably get it. If parents expect the best, children are more apt to live up to this expectation.

Emancipation from the family is difficult because both sides have problems. The adolescent is often reluctant to accept responsibility and fears criticism if he does accept it. At the same time that he needs to feel cared for he lacks a desire to cooperate with adults who could give him this feeling of security. Parents also usually unconsciously have their problems. They have great difficulty sharing the adolescent's love with others. They tend to underestimate his strength to function away from them. They may desire to continue dominating the adolescent. They may say that they fear that he will be harmed if he leaves home. The mother may feel these problems more than the father if she does not work outside the home.

Any activity of daily living may be the basis of conflict; the time of leaving or coming home, whether the car may be used, whether the adolescent may have a key to the house, the selection of clothes, and the like. The adolescent should gain emancipation slowly. Just as his parents should try to understand his role in this conflict, so he should attempt to understand their problems.

If parents and child build a good foundation during the first six years of life, if the parents have given of *themselves* and not only material things to their children, these battles will not wreck the adolescent's life. Parents must let the youth develop his judgment and skills, tell him the truth, and avoid attacking or ridiculing him.

There has been a tendency in recent years to be too permissive with adolescents, perhaps as a reaction to the former trend to handle all young people too rigidly. Some limits are still important. A tolerant parent need not condone everything the adolescent does. One of the most difficult problems parents face is the establishment of a relation that enables them to give their children the freedom they need while assuring their acceptance of guidance.

Eventually the adolescent's anxiety decreases, and his return to the more immature relation with his parents is no longer necessary. He is then able to have a mature, interdependent relation with them and others because his independence is more confidently maintained.

The Adolescent and His Friends. The young

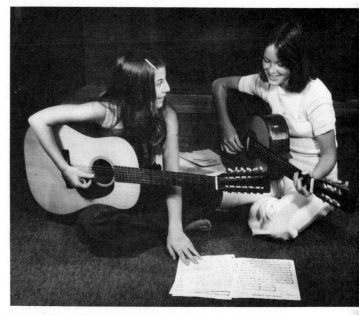

FIGURE 25-5. The adolescent's friends are very important. They may share aspects of their lives such as musical and literary interests as well as personal possessions such as clothing.

adolescent who becomes a group member is fortunate because then the whole group tends to strengthen the individual's concept of his own capabilities. Groups which the adolescent may join are those organized by his friends for social or, unfortunately, antisocial purposes (see p. 889 for a discussion of juvenile delinquency), and those organized by adults for community activities. His ideas are dominated by the social and ethical codes in the group. Fads are important whether they involve clothes or behavior. The adolescent must be accepted by his group to feel secure. He may not express his individuality beyond the limits imposed by the group.

As a result of mutual soul-searching by individual members of the group, standards for basic concepts of living are worked out. Attitudes about morality, ethics, religion, and social customs are formulated and adopted by group members. The group thus plans how the individual member should behave and becomes an island of security in what seems to be a confused world.

As soon as an *authoritarian* adult leader is introduced, this function of the group is lost. The young people are no longer fully able to develop themselves as individuals or to learn how to get along with their peers.

The child who does not reach puberty at the same time as others may have emotional problems that are difficult for him to solve. He may find himself alienated from his peer group, yet not accepted by a younger or older group.

Children who reach puberty late are especially at a disadvantage because feeling weak and less capable physically and physiologically hurts their pride and self concept.

Adolescents may develop a strong bond of friendship with just one or possibly two other adolescents of their own sex. This relation is based on similarities in interest, age, and personality factors. Such friendships are important to personality development. These friends are devoted to each other and become inseparable. They have a relatively mature understanding and appreciation of each other's needs, reacting without the selfishness evident in earlier periods of development. They share each other's ideas, deepest secrets, and troubles, and thus develop a sense of responsibility and loyalty to others that had not existed before. A great deal of whispering is evident in these friendships.

These relations help the adolescent girl especially to break away from her attachment to her mother. Boys do not seem to have the intense friendship with other boys that girls have with other girls. Boys work out their feelings in horseplay, teasing, and wrestling. They use the peer group more as a loyal band offering them support and having an authority of its own.

Gradually short-term attachments develop with members of the opposite sex which tend to break up the intense friendships with members of the same sex.

Adjustment to the Opposite Sex. When interest develops in the opposite sex, great secrecy surrounds it at first. When the boy sees a group of girls, he may perform physically in a way to attract their attention. He may say to himself and others that he was "just getting some exercise." The girls may giggle in response to attract the boy's attention.

Later, real interest and romantic love affairs develop, usually between a girl and a boy one or two years older than she because of the difference in physical maturation rates of the two sexes. These attachments are usually short-lived, but they do give those concerned some knowledge of the personality characteristics of the opposite sex which will help later when each is in a better position to fall in love.

To establish heterosexual relations the adolescent must rebel against and free himself from the forbidding infantile conscience. If he reduces his inner standards too rapidly, his anxiety becomes intolerable, and he tries even harder to control himself. Although he resents his parents' authority, the adolescent may at this time seek their control. He may also turn to religion or to the pursuit of intellectual interests to reduce his conflict. Ultimately his fear of his instincts will lessen, he will learn to control

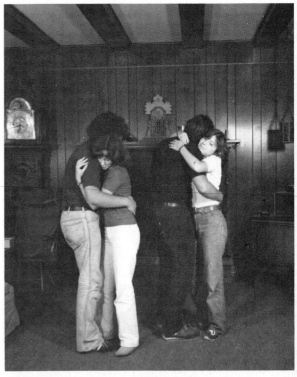

FIGURE 25–6. Pubescents and adolescents enjoy attending mixed parties. In addition to learning to dance, adolescents learn to get along with their peers.

himself, and he will be able to enjoy pleasures which are needed for his growth.

Since marriage and parenthood lie just ahead for many adolescents, the two sexes must become accustomed to each other and learn to know each other well. Adolescents get practice in this by participation in dances, picnics, and the like. Physical expressions such as hand holding, kissing, and embracing are normal functions of a person preparing for marriage.

In their efforts to develop an understanding of the other sex, adolescents are often inhibited by adults. Parents are afraid that if young people are too much interested in the opposite sex, they will marry too soon and be unable to finish their education or support themselves well. They are afraid of pregnancy out of wedlock, disease, and disgrace to the family. The adolescent needs help from parents in accepting a masculine or feminine role and in understanding sex drives. Parents often do not remember that if good parent-child relations have existed, if the young person has been given adequate sex education and has been taught social responsibility and consideration for others, he will usually abide by his parents' wishes about sexual behavior. Young people should have an opportunity to mix with each other without anxiety and shame.

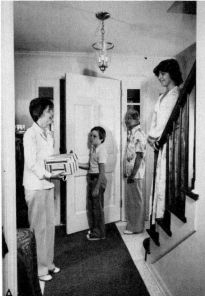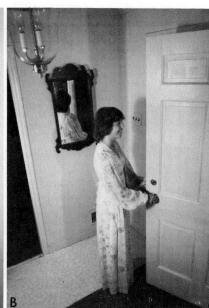

FIGURE 25-7. The adolescent attends her first formal dance. *A,* The arrival of the floral corsage may be a family affair. *B,* "His" arrival may be a moment long to be remembered.

Many parents in the past discouraged young people from "going steady." They were afraid that the adolescents would be hurt when the friendship ended because the relationship seemed to be a demimarriage. More recently adolescents consider themselves to be "going steadily" instead of "going steady." In our socially mobile society many are wary of entangling alliances and are more convinced that a relationship depends on what emotions the couple invest in it, not on what the relationship is called.

If the child has had adequate sex education, if he was taught respect for others in these matters, and if he has had religious education on which he can base his decisions about his conduct, few problems are likely to arise during the adolescent years. Adolescents may need guidance, however, on specific problems that may arise in relation to assuming an adult role. The adolescent must be helped to understand the moral and social customs that should govern his conduct in the matters of "dating" and sexual intercourse. He should be helped to find socially acceptable outlets for his interests.

Threatening the adolescent does more harm than good and may serve to encourage the very behavior that adults term undesirable. The adolescent can thus rebel against adult authority and standards in a way that may be disastrous to him. Since the conduct of adolescents is controlled not only by what adults say, but also by what the group dictates, it is vitally important that the individual be a member of a group that upholds society's standards of conduct.

Ultimately each young adult will learn as he matures that although everyone has sexual needs, "love" of another human being is not composed only and constantly of passion. Some individuals substitute heavy petting and intercourse or physical closeness for real, emotionally close relationships. As the adolescent develops a full sense of who he is, as he is able to love and accept himself, then only is he able to form a lasting, loving relationship with another. As he is able to use his emotions fully, he must understand the consequences of his so doing and answer the questions: Will I like myself, or will I hurt myself or someone else as a result of my actions? Love is built over a period of time upon identification with and compassion for another. Only when the youth can relate to another human being in this way and have realistic expectations will he be able to provide a firm foundation for marriage and the beginning of a family of his own.

EMOTIONAL MATURITY

No one ever really becomes emotionally mature in all facets of his personality. There is always some development of the past that is incomplete, although the stages of development are the very cornerstones upon which a mature personality is built.

Theoretically, an emotionally and physically mature person is able to face reality, to use good judgment, to select a mate, to provide a home, and to rear his children wisely. He should be able to meet responsibilities and get pleasure from activities participated in alone or with others. He should be able to balance responsibility and pleasure in a way that keeps him free

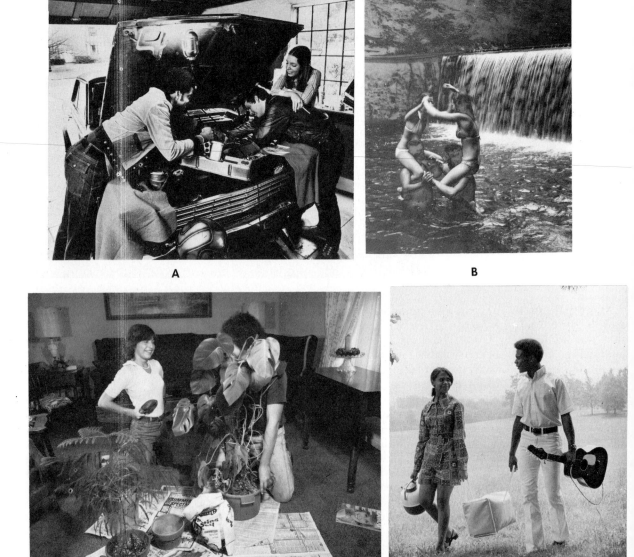

FIGURE 25–8. Close friendships are formed during adolescence, characterized by a more mature understanding of each other's needs than was possible during earlier periods of development. These opportunities for cooperation help adolescents to know members of the opposite sex. (*A*, Courtesy of International Telephone and Telegraph Corporation; *D*, Courtesy of H. Armstrong Roberts.)

from tension. Yet while he is master of himself and of his world, he should be humble, recognizing his own limitations as well as those of reality.

The mature person should be able to accept dependency, both of others and of himself, when necessary. This capacity for mutual dependency is a crucial part of social living.

A mature person believes in himself and in others who love him and whom he loves. He is able to deal wisely with those who dislike him and whom he dislikes.

Toward this goal the adolescent must work. He must formulate his own code of behavior and philosophy of life. These must be based on his individual decisions, but both are greatly influenced by previous family life, by teaching in school and church, by all his contacts in his lifetime and by all the experiences he has lived through.

OVERVIEW OF PHYSICAL AND MENTAL DEVELOPMENT

During puberty and adolescence the young person not only makes great strides toward emotional maturity, but also reaches physical maturity, although the sequence of signs of physical maturation may vary in individuals. Various factors may influence sexual development, such as broad socioeconomic factors (nutrition and urban vs. rural living among others), genetic background, body build, and state of health. During the past hundred years there has been an acceleration of sexual development in the youth of certain areas of the world. Changes in appearance as a result of physical development may cause disturbances in emotional well-being.

Puberty

Pubescence is associated with reaching sexual maturity. During the year or two preceding puberty rapid changes occur in the rate of growth in weight and height, in body contours and in the physiology of the body as a result of maturation of the gonads and hormonal activity. These changes usually continue to puberty, which occurs by about 12 to 14 years, with a range of 11 to 15 years in girls and a year or two later for boys. Girls tend to develop more rapidly than boys and to maintain their lead until they reach adult maturity.

The specific physiologic explanation for the onset of puberty is unknown; however, it is believed that it may begin in the hypothalamus with a resultant neurohumoral stimulation to the pituitary gland. Gonadotropic hormones from the pituitary stimulate the Leydig cells of the testes, which secrete testosterone, and the follicles of the ovary, which secrete estradiol. Simultaneously the adrenal cortex increases the production of androgen. The action of these hormones results in the production of secondary sex characteristics.

The secondary sex characteristics that develop depend on which hormone is produced in the greatest amount, since both male and female hormones are produced by each person. The androgens produce the male configuration and the estrogens the female configuration of the body. Both male and female gonadal hormones stimulate the fusion of the epiphyses by repression of the pituitary growth hormone. This results in a slowing of physical growth.

Physical changes in the boy include, in order of appearance, (1) increase in the size of the genitalia, (2) swelling of the breasts, (3) growth of pubic, axillary, facial, and chest hair, (4) voice

[handwritten annotations: "estrogen"; "nothing to do ē reproduction"; "seperate boy + gurls"; "↑ ht + wt"; "growth in larynx"; "groin, thighs, chest"; "PH & odor change of sweat (Apocrine Sweat Glands)"]

FIGURE 25-9. Developmental stages in adolescence (after Tanner). (Faigel, H. C.: *Pediatr. Clin. N. Am.*, 21:355, May 1974.)

STAGE	MALE Genital	MALE Extragenital	FEMALE Genital	FEMALE Extragenital
I	Prepubertal	Prepubertal	Prepubertal	Prepubertal
II	Long fine straight hair at base of penis; testes larger; penis thicker; scrotal skin thinning.	Axillary and facial hair absent; voice childlike.	Sparse long fine straight hair on labia; labia majora thickens; vaginal epithelium thickens; vaginal pH falls.	Breast and papilla elevated; areola enlarges; axillary hair absent.
III	Hair longer, coarser, spreading laterally; testes larger; penis growing longer; scrotal skin thin.	Facial hair on upper lip; axillary hair may be present; voice cracking.	Coarse curly hair over pubes; uterus enlarging; vaginal pH low; labia enlarged; menses.	Breast enlarged without separation of contours; axillary hair may be present.
IV	Coarse curly hair at base of penis; testes nearly adult; varicocele may be present; penis nearly adult.	Upper lip hair coarser; chin hair present; perianal hair present; axillary hair starting; voice deepening.	Adult hair over smaller area; vaginal rugae; uterus enlarging; ovulation.	Papilla and areola project and separation of breast contour begins; axillary hair begins.
V	Adult	Adult	Adult	Adult

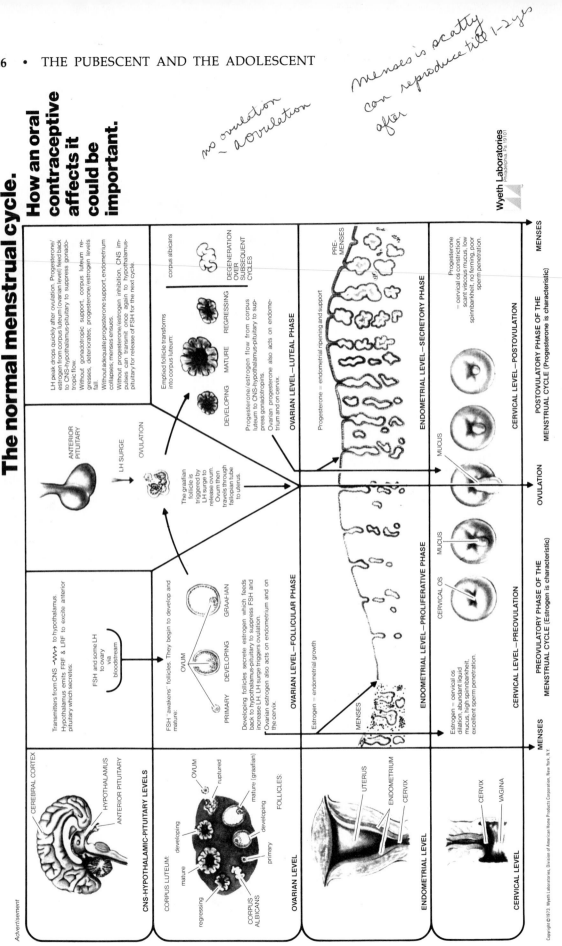

FIGURE 25-10. Changes during the normal menstrual cycle are of great interest to the adolescent. (Courtesy of Wyeth Laboratories, Philadelphia, Pa.)

first ejaculation 13-16 yrs.

process that mature sperm are formed about (15 yrs)

changes, and (5) production of spermatozoa. Boys grow rapidly in shoulder breadth from about the age of 13 years③ *Spermatogenesis*

Boys can become disturbed by ① *nocturnal emissions*, the loss of seminal fluid during sleep. If they have not been told that this is normal, they may regard it as a disease, or a punishment because of masturbation or thinking too much about sex. They may also believe that it is devitalizing. Nocturnal emissions are due to the activity of the sexual glands, and occasional release of spermatic fluid during sleep should cause no concern. If boys are not adequately prepared for this phenomenon, they ask either their father or their friends about it. Boys generally are able to talk more freely among themselves than girls are and therefore usually find a solution to this problem.

Changes in the girl, in order of appearance, include (1) increase in the transverse diameter *rounder* of the pelvis, (2) development of the breasts, (3)PH change in the vaginal secretions, *alkaline → acid*, and (4) growth of pubic and axillary hair. Menstruation has its onset between the appearance of pubic hair and that of axillary hair. Girls begin to have broad hips from about the age of 12 years on *(average 13)*

In the girl the gonadotropic hormones of the pituitary stimulate the production of estrogen by the ovary and the maturation of ova. When the ovum starts to ripen, its follicle secretes an increased amount of estrogen. This increased estrogen production results in further growth and vascularity of the inner lining or endometrium of the uterus. After the ovum is completely matured, it is extruded. Under the stimulus of a luteinizing hormone from the pituitary the follicle site is filled with cells which form the corpus luteum, which in turn produces the hormone progesterone. Progesterone causes further increase in thickness and vascularity of the endometrium, thus preparing it for the fertilized ovum. If the ovum is not fertilized, the corpus luteum atrophies and progesterone is no longer produced. When the progesterone is decreased, the hypertrophied endometrium sloughs off, resulting in menstruation.

Because of lack of adequate information, girls may have ambivalent feelings about menstruation. They may resent the fact that they cannot completely control all their bodily functions, and may therefore consider menstruation a burden.

Many parents do not adequately explain to girls the various changes in body contour indicative of puberty. Before puberty and adolescence the child should be well oriented as to the anatomic and functional differences between the sexes. The girl should have a clear conception of ovulation, fertilization, pregnancy, and birth. She should certainly have been told about menstruation before it occurs. Especially in discussing menstruation, adults are likely to pass on to their children the same beliefs and taboos which were told to them. They may say that the girl should rest or not participate in social activities during the menstrual period, thus implying that she is not well.

Menstruation is a normal physiologic phenomenon. There is no reason why women should curb their normal activities at this time. Menstruation is not debilitating. The blood loss is quickly made up. If mothers would only stress that menstruation is a normal phenomenon, young women would have fewer problems.

In discussions about sex, parents should impress upon their children that the realities of sex are far more complex than the image presented by sensation-seeking media and pornographic materials, which are likely to contain more fiction than fact. Parents should provide guidance to counteract the false information many adolescents obtain from such sources. They should also encourage discussion of sexual matters, allowing sex its proper place as a healthy part of life.

Other physical changes also occur in children of both sexes at adolescence. The sebaceous glands of the face, back, and chest become more active. If the pores are too small, sebaceous material cannot escape, so that it collects beneath the skin and produces pimples or acne (see p. 849). Perspiration is increased. Vasomotor instability produces blushing.

Growth in height tends to decrease each year from birth, but with the onset of pubescence there is a rapid increase, and the child becomes tall. Gain in weight is proportionately greater than gain in height during early adolescence; therefore the adolescent appears to be stocky. This obesity has an important effect from both a physical and a psychologic standpoint.

There are differences in the rate of growth of various organ systems. The skeletal system often grows faster than its supporting muscles. This difference in growth rate tends to cause clumsiness and poor posture. Since large muscles may grow faster than small ones, the youth is likely to lack coordination. His extremities, hands, and feet, may grow out of proportion to the rest of his body and cause more problems in coordination.

Since the heart and lungs usually grow more slowly than the rest of the body, the supply of oxygen may be inadequate, and the pubescent may feel constantly tired.

The youth, and sometimes the parents, not

realizing that this is a stage every adolescent must go through, may feel inferior and socially embarrassed by these bodily changes. The youth may try to compensate for his supposed inferiority by ridiculing others, by trying to force his body to behave and to appear better by exercising and dieting, by attracting attention to himself by giggling and fidgetiness or by developing his intellect so that his physical appearance can be tolerated. Other pubescents may withdraw so that they cannot be compared with others. Parents should not scold or ridicule a child at this stage. Further growth will correct many of the problems. Instead, children should get from their parents reassurance and help to face the conflict between the image of themselves as they would like to be and as they are.

At puberty the child is flooded with new sensations and feelings which he cannot understand. This is one of the reasons why the youth may be alert and interested in everything for a time and then shortly after be bored, withdrawn, and disinterested. By withdrawing, he is able to assimilate and digest the incoming sensations. This developmental phenomenon may occur about the time he is 13 years old. He may do poorly in school for about a year at this time. Parents and teachers can help him by being patient and by explaining to him that this is just a period in his growth. He should not be ridiculed.

Motor behavior is influenced by the rapid changes taking place in the body. The young adolescent may appear awkward in his gross body movements because of his difficulty in adapting to these changes and because of his fear of ridicule, although he is actually gaining in strength and skill. As a result of rapid growth, pubescents may not have sufficient energy left for activity; therefore they may tire easily.

Girls do not usually develop the gross motor ability that boys do. This may be partially due to the fact that girls may have many interests other than sports.

When rapid physical changes and changes in motor skill occur, the pubescent may become intensely interested in his physical appearance. During preadolescence he had an image of what he would be like as an adult. If what he is becoming is unlike his previous image, he may become uncertain of himself and of his body. Parents should help the young adolescent to make a realistic appraisal of his appearance and to make the most of his outstanding qualities.

Adolescence

After the pubescent years growth slows, and the change in body proportions occurs more

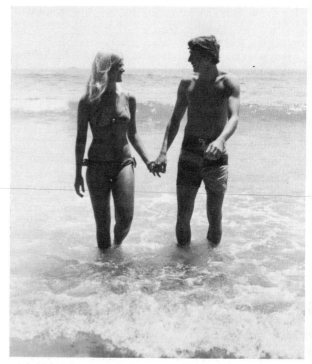

FIGURE 25–11. After the pubescent years the rate of growth slows, and changes in body proportions occur more gradually. These young people have nearly achieved their adult size. (H. Armstrong Roberts.)

gradually. The adolescent must continue to live with organ systems and functional capacities of widely varying levels of maturity. Usually by 15 to 16 years the secondary sex characteristics have developed fully, and adolescents are capable of reproduction. During the first year or longer of menstruation, periods are frequently missed or are irregular. Conception is unlikely until a year after periods have begun and usually does not occur until around the sixteenth year.

By this age the adolescent's motor abilities are similar to those of adults; thus adolescents can perform tasks which require muscular control and skill. Parents must guard against the adolescent's trying to live up to that part of his development which is most advanced, such as stature. They must try to help him set limits to his behavior as a result of understanding the problems involved.

At the end of adolescence the young person appears physically like an adult. His head is approximately one eighth of his body length. When his wisdom teeth erupt, between 17 and 21 years of age, he has his full set of 32 permanent teeth (see Fig. 22–4).

In summary, the stages of puberty and adolescence are on a continuum along which many changes occur, so that the 13-year-old is very different from the 19-year-old. Stress and anxiety may occur with these physical, emotional, social and intellectual changes in the young maturing person.

MENTAL DEVELOPMENT

The *formal operational stage* (11 to 15 years), according to Piaget, is the final stage of cognitive development.

While the younger child needed real situations in order to deal with problems, the adolescent can deal with problems not having a basis in the here and now. He is able to solve purely abstract problems and those on a verbal level. Unlike the younger child, the adolescent can solve the following problem: "Tom is shorter than Joe; Tom is taller than Ted. Which boy is the tallest?" The solution to this problem involves scientific and verbal reasoning. The adolescent can make use of assumptions while thinking. He can formulate hypotheses and construct theories. He can also do systematic experimentation. The adolescent can solve problems that require purely abstract thinking in a flexible manner. He can have many ideas about a problem at the same time and can predict a variety of possible solutions. Reality to the adolescent is only one of a number of areas in which to think.

The adolescent can also think about problems in the social area of life in terms of abstract ideas. He can see possibilities for action that lie beyond the constraints of reality. This ability is the basis for the *idealism* found so characteristically among adolescents. The adolescent does not see realistic limitations as he goes forth to champion an idealistic cause. Since he looks only at what *he* believes is possible, he criticizes adults, including his parents, for not measuring up to his expectations. Thus criticism of his parents may occur for their lack of worldly goods, of better educational achievements, and of their acceptance of limitations about what they can accomplish. The egocentrism of the adolescent is embodied in the power he gives to the world of the abstract. In the coming years of adulthood, the adolescent will learn to live within the world of reality in a more mature way.

Since the adolescent can utilize *hypothetical deductive reasoning*, he may question and perhaps argue the rules that others impose on him. If he is not satisfied with their rationale and logic, he may reject the authority of others on these grounds.

Adolescents dream and plan into the future. Since learning continues for the individual through his whole life span, these dreams and plans may change. The individual, nevertheless, will continue to think and learn and to develop his cognitive abilities through continued use.

DEVELOPMENT OF SEXUALITY IN THE ADOLESCENT

It is during adolescence that the child passes through the *genital period* of development from approximately 11 to 16 years of age. Puberty and adolescence are periods during which there is a great surge of genital sexual development. The secondary sexual characteristics appear (see p. 825). Masturbation and sexual fantasies are common during this period.

The child entering adolescence is not sexually fully matured, yet he or she is genitally mature and capable of reproduction. Stress results when the adolescent is physically ready for heterosexual genital expression but is denied it. Some cultures permit this to a greater extent than ours. The heightened sexual tension during adolescence necessitates a mode of expression that usually becomes a pattern for adult life.

The male is, from the beginning, more aware of his genitals and much more aware of genital responsiveness. Erections occur almost daily. The male's penis is the anatomical distinction that makes him clearly a male. This awareness is intensified during adolescence by the production of semen in ejaculation. Spermatogenesis is usually evident by 13 years of age.

Overt awareness of sexual feelings is a more diffuse process in the female than in the male and generally occurs at a later age. This awareness is less obviously associated with physiologic changes; learning arises more from the young girl's social and sexual contacts, especially with males.

Masturbation is a central concern in early adolescence, especially in boys who almost universally engage in the practice to some extent during the teen years. Girls may do it to a lesser extent. Adolescents should be informed that masturbation is a normal response to an increase in sexual development. This is necessary for the control of new urges and the working out of new relationships through fantasy.

Through experience the adolescent learns that sexual excitement and erection of the penis or the clitoris can occur as a result of masturbation. This occurrence can be controlled through the manner of masturbation. This can contribute to a developing sense of mastery over sexual impulses and capacities and helps the adolescent prepare for heterosexual relationships.

During puberty and immediately following this period many youths become involved in genital examination, sexual play, and experimentation with members of their own sex. These experiences may be called homosexual in nature, but undue importance is given to this behavior. These experiences are part of the developmental process; the adolescent learns something about what may be expected sexual manifestations in himself and others. Usually in our culture, most young adolescents move on to some kind of heterosexual behavior. The age at which heterosexual behavior is started is occurring earlier.

Adolescent boys frequently apply intense pressure on girls to engage in sex. Strangely enough, when they succeed, the boys often lose interest or disappear after they have had coitus two or three times. Girls are very disturbed by this behavior, since they believe they have done something wrong to upset the boys. This wish for sexual experimentation among adolescent boys is fulfilled and because they believe that another kind of relationship would be better, they move on to someone else. Boys who have reached a maturational stage in which they are able to be loving are more likely to have a longer relationship with the girl with whom they first had intercourse. Since girls look forward to a permanent loving relationship with a partner, they may verbally imply permanence in their relationships. Young men become frightened by this possibility and may physically or psychologically withdraw.

Premarital sexual experience among teenage girls is increasing, possibly because of the use of contraceptives. Most young women, however, do not begin to use contraceptives until after their first sexual experience and most are ignorant of the time of the month when they are likely to conceive. The irony of this is that pregnancies among unmarried adolescents are at an all-time high at a time when contraceptive use is on the upswing.

Three of every ten teenage girls who have had sexual intercourse have at least one out-of-wedlock pregnancy. Three quarters of all teenage pregnancies occur outside of marriage. Even if the mother and baby at birth are in good physical health, the chances are that the immature mother and the unwanted infant will later experience serious psychologic scars.

Persons who marry as teenagers are more likely than others to have already conceived a child prior to the wedding ceremony. They have more than likely never experienced autonomous functioning before and they grasp for someone else on whom to depend. These teenagers have also probably had a limited dating experience. Individuals who marry as teenagers tend to be less educated than those who marry later, thus they may have lower levels of annual income. A couple's chances of marital dissolution, discord, or dissatisfaction increase precipitously if they choose marriage at an early age.

The genital period signals the end of the individual's previous stages of psychosexual development. If the infant, toddler, preschool child, and school-age child did not resolve the crises at their appropriate levels of development, problems may arise in later adolescence or adult life in the areas of sexual expression, interpersonal relationships with others, and activities in work or career situations.

EDUCATION REGARDING SEXUALITY

Pubescents and adolescents have a great need for education about sexuality. The time and the way in which such education is given are both vitally important.

Three primary conditions are essential for normal heterosexual development: (1) the parent of the same sex must not be so weak or so punishing that the child cannot identify with that parent, (2) the parent of the opposite sex must not be so seductive, punishing, or emotionally erratic that the child cannot trust members of the opposite sex, and (3) the parents must not systematically reject the child's biologic sex or try to teach the child cross-sex behavior.

Sex education should probably be provided by the parents. Practically, however, not all parents have the ability to teach their pubescent or adolescent sons and daughters, nor do all parents know enough about their own bodies to be able to teach someone else.

The changes at puberty often cause concern about normalcy. Preadolescents often compare themselves to their peers, many of whom are at different stages of maturation. Young adolescents need reassurance that there are individual differences and that lags and spurts are normal.

Lack of information regarding the physical and emotional changes that they face during puberty and adolescence is a serious problem for them. Girls are concerned about irregular menstruation and what to them is atypical breast development. Boys are concerned about masturbation, nocturnal emissions, and what to them is atypical penile size.

Many adults have suppressed or have forgotten their own childhood. They may also be too embarrassed to talk about sexuality, and thus they do not answer the hinted questions or the evident worries that trouble teenagers about their emerging sexuality.

The nurse who deals with adolescents can be of the most help to them by offering to answer any questions they may wish to discuss. Unsolicited advice is seldom welcomed at any age, but during adolescence it may be very disruptive. The nurse is one of the most likely adults outside of the home to be asked about sex by adolescents. The nurse is considered by most children to be nonjudgmental and not to have a disciplinary role as do teachers.

Sometimes children may deliberately use an obscene word in the proximity of the nurse. If the nurse is calm and tells the adolescent that he used a word that upsets others instead of threatening punishment, this acceptance may give him courage to ask questions which are bothering him.

Some children may ask a sexual question, but say that they are asking for a friend. Others approach the nurse with somatic complaints such as stomach cramps or a headache. When they have sufficient confidence in the nurse, they will then reveal their true concerns.

In regard to sexual molestation during the pubescent and adolescent years, parents and nurses must shift their emphasis from that used with younger children to discover ways of handling the young person's growing independence. Both boys and girls profit from more detailed knowledge about how sexual molesters are likely to approach them. A blanket prohibition during adolescence is much less effective than an open discussion of the realistic risks of hitchhiking or long trips away from home.

As is true in all counseling, the nurse should not attempt to identify a problem concerning sexuality during the adolescent years unless he or she is also willing to discuss it with the individual.

LIFE PERSPECTIVE

The adolescent has the ability to think and plan into the future. He has the ability not only to make tentative plans for a family and a vocation and to formulate possible solutions to problems in other areas of life but also to frame the concept of personal mortality. His thoughts about the proposition "I will die" are intimately related to his sense of futurity. The individual as an adolescent, and later as an adult, needs to integrate the concepts of more time—new and fresh time—and trust, hope, and uncertainty with the concept of certain ultimate death.

Adolescence is the time when the developing individual seriously begins to create his own life perspective. He had notions about his life to some extent previously, but during adolescence he has the intellectual equipment to forge all aspects of this thinking into a perspective. He also has the psychosocial readiness to venture forth as his own self. The late adolescent can think about his own thoughts and to some extent compare the ideal with reality. He can shatter the world as it is presented to him with his new found abilities of intellectual analysis and then at least attempt to assemble the pieces in a more satisfying manner.

The adolescent has a strong sense of his movement into the future, a restless feeling of a developmental current running within himself. However, the adolescent projects his thoughts and feelings strongly into a fairly narrow sector of the future at one time. He is concerned about the eventful time that is just around the corner. Old age to him is remote. At the same time that the adolescent looks ahead, however, he also wages an active battle against the past, attempting to place psychologic distance between the "me-I-used-to be" and the "me-I'm-going-to become."

In all of this, the adolescent does come to terms with finality. He may try to gloss over the idea of death, kid about it, avoid it. Many adolescents are extremely concerned about death, however, in the sense of fathoming its nature and in confronting the actual prospect of their own demise. A foreshortened life perspective is not the special prerogative of the aged individual; the behavior of many adolescents is influenced by the expectation that they may die at an early age.

INTERRELATIONS OF PHYSICAL, EMOTIONAL, SOCIAL, AND MENTAL DEVELOPMENT

Pubescence and adolescence are best understood if considered as a period of accelerated maturation and not a span of a certain number of years with specific steps in development to be accomplished each year. To subdivide this span of years is artificial, since development proceeds at varied rates. The rate of growth and development depends on all the factors mentioned throughout this text: heredity and constitutional make-up, racial and national characteristics, sex, environment—including prenatal environment—socioeconomic status of the family, nutrition, climate, illness and injury, exercise, position in the family, intelligence, hormonal balance, and emotions.

SCHOOL

Adolescents as a group can think much more abstractly than they did when they were in the lower school grades. As their school subjects become more complex, there is a period of rapid increase in vocabulary and language development. Unfortunately, mental growth is not exactly correlated with increase in size. Parents and teachers should therefore not expect more mentally from a young person simply because of his rapid increase in physical size.

Adolescents have some difficulties in adjustment to school. They may spend more time in extracurricular activities than in academic work. They may be so disturbed by the problems inherent in adolescence that they may not be able to concentrate long enough to study. The school, recognizing that such problems exist, should offer activities that will help them find answers to their problems and satisfy their social needs.

There is great variation in academic ability and interest. A few adolescents excel in all areas, more excel in a few areas, and some excel in no areas. Often the degree of interest in school is based on the ultimate goal the adolescent has set for himself. If he needs further academic preparation leading to a profession, he will apply himself to his studies. If his goal is to be an unskilled laborer requiring no additional preparation, he may not see the necessity of achieving excellence in his high school work.

Besides academic preparation for adult life, high school offers the adolescent opportunities in extracurricular activities for satisfying his needs for security, recognition, and success for himself and his group. Adolescents should have opportunities to develop intellectual and physical skills and to satisfy their interests in areas such as crafts, music, and art.

School programs should take into consideration the stage in development each pupil is going through. This is especially essential since the students in any one class may be prepubescent, pubescent, or early adolescent, depending on their rate of growth.

Parents should continue to take an interest in the school life of the adolescent. They should also invite him to some of the social activities of adults in the community. It has been said that high school activities such as sports events, dances, and parties are too expensive and that this is one reason why some children develop feelings of inferiority in their group and a desire to leave school before graduation. Adults in the community can help such children by providing opportunities for them to make their own money for these purposes.

Adults may also assist adolescents in their selection of a vocation by being willing to talk to groups about their own vocational choices.

PLAY AND WORK

During pubescence and adolescence, sex makes more of a difference than ever in play and work interests.

Girls may develop interests in social functions such as parties and dances, romance, housekeeping, and child-rearing responsibilities.

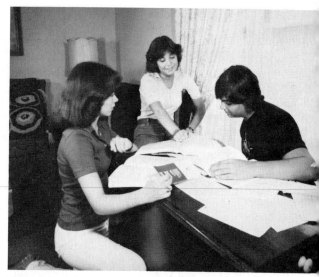

FIGURE 25–12. These high school students are able to think more abstractly than they could when in elementary school. They involve themselves deeply in subjects that interest them, in this case studying college catalogues.

They often enjoy romantic motion pictures and television programs. They may spend hours making themselves more attractive, experimenting with hair styles, cosmetics, and new clothes. They may learn to cook, clean, and sew. Their interests widen in such fields as art, poetry, and music. They, as well as boys, may spend a long time talking on the telephone to someone they have just seen a short time before the conversation began.

Boys are usually interested in competing and excelling in sports. They develop team loyalty and spirit. They are interested in mechanical or electrical devices as hobbies. Their acceptance in the group depends not so much on personal appearance as on manliness, physical abilities, and ability to complete a job.

In recent years a blurring has occurred in the activities of adolescents of both sexes. Many adolescent girls are interested in competitive and noncompetitive sports and many adolescent boys are interested in activities concerning family life. Girls have become participants on traditional boys' teams in sports, and boys have learned to cook and to assume responsibilities for baby-sitting.

Adolescents enjoy part-time work by which they can earn spending money for themselves. They may deliver newspapers, mow lawns, shovel snow, or care for young children. Although these activities have little relation in most cases to their ultimate work in life, the way they carry out their responsibilities gives some indication of their level of industry in whatever work they perform as adults. The adolescent

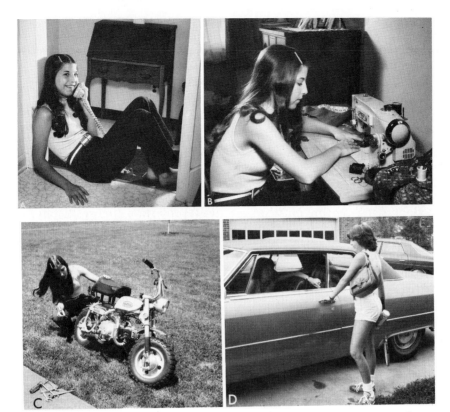

FIGURE 25–13.   The interests of adolescents vary from seemingly endless telephone conversations (*A*), to sewing (*B*) to repairing a minibike (*C*), to going to play tennis (*D*) in her own new car.

thus learns to work with others, to cooperate even with those to whom he has no real personal attachment. He should find satisfaction in knowing that he has done a job well and that he can contribute in some way to society.

Adolescents gain great satisfaction from working for a worthwhile cause. Feelings of altruism are well developed at this age, and the individual and the group can make valuable contributions to a worthwhile effort.

CHOICE OF VOCATION

Three kinds of vocation face the young person: the vocation of citizenship, the vocation which will make a living for himself and his family, and the vocation of parenthood. Parents should be honest with their children and tell them the problems involved in each.

Probably the vocation which the adolescent believes is most immediately important is a career. The attitude among some groups that ev-

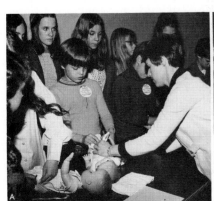
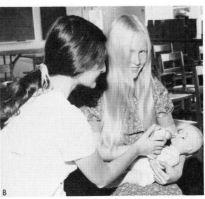

FIGURE 25–14.   Some adolescent boys and girls may wish to earn money by babysitting. In preparation for this responsibility, each may take a short course at a local school or hospital. *A*, Diapering is one technique that the students must master. *B*, A nurse teaches proper feeding technique. (Courtesy of Norma L. Heid, New England Memorial Hospital.)

eryone will be taken care of, that adolescents need not worry about working, is an unhealthy one. The adolescent should probably prepare for both a career and marriage.

It is important for the adolescent to begin his vocational choice with self-knowledge. No career choice can be valid without a realistic appraisal about what one is capable of doing. Adolescents must evaluate what they have already accomplished in life. They must determine their major classroom and leisure interests. They must ask themselves what is most important to them: adventure, prestige, money, security, or personal satisfaction. Each person must assess his or her own actual and potential abilities when selecting a career.

The adolescent should be guided in vocational preparation with consideration for his limitations and capacities. Simply because the father wanted to be a physician all his life is no reason why the child should be encouraged to study medicine. The young person can make his best contribution to society by doing something he is sincerely interested in. It is unfortunate if an adolescent's desires about his future must be changed because of his socioeconomic status or level of intelligence. Guidance in vocational choice is essential if the young person is to avoid such a disappointment or is to make plans so that he can achieve his goal.

Guidance of the Adolescent

PRINCIPLES OF GUIDANCE

Many times parents struggle with adjustments to their pubescent and adolescent sons and daughters alone. Sometimes they seek guidance in their management from physicians and nurses who know them. Several broad principles of management can be offered as suggestions, but each must be molded to the individual adolescent by his parents.

Privacy. Adolescents need privacy, especially at home. They should be given as much privacy as possible in the family dwelling. The adolescent should have his own room to decorate as he sees fit, even though the decorations may displease his parents. It is helpful if he can have his own telephone, paid for by the parents, or better still, paid for by the earnings of the adolescent himself. The adolescent can enjoy his long telephone conversations in privacy, and the rest of the family can enjoy their peace of mind. Parents can show an interest in what the adolescent does but should not be too intrusive into matters that concern him alone.

Communication. Parents many times have little conversation with their adolescents outside of a few shared words in the morning, at mealtimes, and possibly at night. Parents should talk to adolescents and spend time with them, but of even greater importance, they should listen to them. This is often difficult for parents because they and their adolescent tend to agree on so few topics. If the parents can say, "I can see your point of view," or "I never thought of that before in quite the same way," the adolescent may appreciate their effort of communicating with him.

Praise, Reassurance, and Criticism. Adolescents question their own physical attractiveness and abilities, but they often cover up their doubts with overwhelming self-confidence and appear arrogantly self-assured. Parents who praise and reassure such adolescents do not increase the unwanted behavior. Instead, reassurance helps the adolescent to be more moderate in his activities.

A frequent problem in many homes is the adolescent's striving to improve his physical appearance. Parents who nag about the time spent in this activity usually do not achieve their goal. Peer pressure in such matters is stronger than the strident voices of the most disapproving parents. Praise for the result or a portion of the result, depending on the current fad in hair styling and clothing, can help the adolescent to relax.

Ridiculing an adolescent does not achieve the desired results. When parents want to make constructive criticism, they should make their comments brief and then stop. Ridicule and nagging often lead to further rebellion instead of acceptance. If criticism is necessary, it should be made so that the adolescent is not alienated from his family. Each criticism should be linked with a compliment; this increases the chances that the criticism will be taken seriously. The parent may say, for example, "Mary, you really do have lovely eyes, but that heavy makeup detracts from their appearance."

The adolescent, after his attention has been turned to the opposite sex, becomes very much aware of how he appears to others. Parents are usually amazed at the change in the young person's behavior at this time. He becomes unusually clean, neat in dress, and careful of grooming. Appearance is of the utmost importance socially. After this time parents need have little concern about the daily care of the adolescent, other than to see to it that he gets adequate rest and a balanced diet. Adolescents require about eight to nine hours of sleep a day. They require a higher caloric intake than ever before because of their rapid growth.

Privileges and Restrictions: Liberties and Responsibilities. Adolescents need certain restrictions, but too many restrictions arouse resentment and resistance. If each new restriction can be imposed, however, when a new privilege is given, the adolescent is more likely to accept both graciously. The same principle holds true in relation to a responsibility. When a liberty is given, a responsibility can be imposed at the same time. The parent may say, "Jack, if you want to use the family car tonight for a date, it is your responsibility to clean it up and fill it with gas." In the same manner, as the adolescent begins to date, he has the liberty to enjoy himself, but he also has the responsibility to tell his parents where he will be going, whom he will be with, and what he will be doing. This conduct is not old-fashioned. It shows a common courtesy and respect, both of which are important in the maintenance of good parent-child relationships.

When pubescents or adolescents begin to date, parents should encourage them to bring their friends home for meals, picnics, parties, or just good fun. On such occasions, other than at mealtimes, the parents would be wise to provide whatever food and entertainment is desired and then to remove themselves from sight. The young people have the liberty to enjoy themselves, but they also have the responsibility to clean up the area when they are done.

Earning versus Spending. Many parents are overwhelmed by the amounts of things their teenager wants: clothes, records, stereo, a ten-speed bicycle, and eventually a car. These things may cost more than the family budget allows. If parents can discuss these hard facts with their adolescent, they can then realistically point out that they can share a part of the expense of what he wants, but that he will have to add the rest from his earnings. The parents can thus not deny the adolescent his wishes if he shares in the cost. Such a mutual facing of the reality of a situation fosters growth in parent-child relations.

AREAS FOR GUIDANCE
Breast Self-Examination (BSE). Adolescent girls should learn to examine their breasts monthly during the week following menstruation. The method of procedure advised by the American Cancer Society (see Fig. 25–15) can give women of all ages the confidence that they are doing breast self-examination correctly. If the young woman learns what her breasts feel like in their normal state, she should be able to recognize a thickening or a lump easily.

Pelvic Examination. The Papanicolaou method of examining exfoliated cells from the uterine cervix is an inexpensive and simple method of identifying patients at risk for developing life-threatening stages of cervical carcinoma early. Since the early onset of sexual activity seems to be a critical factor associated with this condition, all sexually active adolescent females should undergo Pap smear screening.

The Pap smear is not enough to evaluate young women with a possible *in utero* exposure to diethylstilbestrol. The incidence of vaginal adenocarcinoma in female offspring of mothers who took this medication during pregnancy is well known (see p. 879). Further examination of such young women is necessary.

In adolescence it is important for any female who has had sexual intercourse to have a pelvic examination. It is important also if the adolescent has signs or symptoms referrable to the genitourinary system or who has undiagnosed abdominal complaints. Before contraception is given, a pelvic examination and a Pap smear should be done.

Because the adolescent's concerns regarding her body image and her sexual functioning are important to her, prior to the examination the physician or nurse is responsible for ascertaining in a nonjudgmental way her psychosocial and sexual history including: menstrual history (age of menarche and menstrual pattern); age when sexual activity began; current pattern of sexuality; use of contraception; and the history of pregnancy and its outcome. The components of the pelvic examination should be explained, using pamphlets or a model of the pelvis and the equipment to be used. The focus is on health maintenance and the importance of periodic pelvic examinations in the future. Also, should the adolescent become pregnant, she will know that an immediate pelvic examination is necessary. The adolescent must be assured of the confidentiality of the details of her sexual history and examination.

EDUCATION FOR PARENTHOOD

The word "parenting" covers a full range of concerns and activities in addition to all the knowledge and skill that being a parent requires, regardless of life style. While adolescents are interested in their involvement with heterosexual activities, they know little about caring for the families they may some day produce.

Education for parenthood has been lacking in the past within families, schools, and in other community agencies. This lack of education is evident in statistics on the high rate of infant mortality, preventable congenital conditions, accidents, lack of dental care, and child abuse, among other dire results. Other factors besides the lack of parenting skills influence some of these statistics; nevertheless, each presents a problem area that could be alleviated by increased parental competencies developed through improved parent education.

SAFETY EDUCATION

Although much effort in the home, schools, and youth organizations has gone into safety education for young people, the accident rate among adolescents continues to be distressingly high. In the teen-age group the greatest cause of accidents is motor vehicles. In an effort to reduce mortality and morbidity from this cause, many schools offer driver-training and safety programs for older children. Adolescents must learn to discipline themselves in order to become safe and courteous drivers, to save their own lives as well as those of others.

Pubescents and adolescents are especially susceptible to injury when riding on minibikes, snowmobiles, or motorcycles, a sport which is increasing in popularity. Girls who ride behind the driver of a motorcycle may burn their legs on the exhaust pipe. The persistent noise when riding on a motorcycle for long periods of time may result in some decrease in the ability to hear. Adolescents may be thrown from the motorcycle for many reasons. Since most motorcycle deaths are caused by head injuries, any person who drives a motorcycle, motor scooter, or motorbike should wear a safety helmet for protection in case of accident.

Other causes of accidental death during the adolescent years are drowning and firearms. Such accidents are largely preventable. Young people should learn to swim and should be taught to use firearms safely, if they are interested in using them at all. They should be cautioned against playing with a loaded weapon, especially against playing the game Russian roulette.

Many young adults are injured each year when playing in competitive sports. Investigation is currently being made on the value of sports such as football during the adolescent years. Consideration is also being given to the kind of shoes, equipment, and turf used and their relations to the injuries that occur.

To a degree adolescents must be safeguarded to prevent injury when they want to do something beyond their physical endurance.

Emergency Care in the Event of Choking. Thousands of children and adults die by choking on food or foreign objects each year. Among infants, choking is due to a lack of chewing ability and the natural inclination to put food and

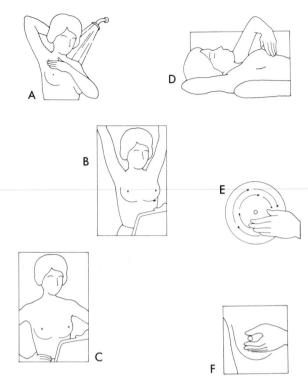

FIGURE 25–15. Did you examine your breasts this month? The American Cancer Society has suggested an easy procedure for breast self-examination: *A*, Examine breasts in the bath or shower; hands glide easier over wet skin. Fingers flat, move gently over every part of each breast. Use right hand to examine left breast, left hand for right breast. Check for any lump, hard knot or thickening. *B*, Before a mirror inspect breasts with arms at sides; then raise arms overhead, looking for changes in contour of each breast, a swelling, dimpling of skin, or changes in nipple. *C*, Rest palms on hips and press down firmly to flex chest muscles. Left and right breasts will not exactly match—few women's breasts do. *D*, Lying down. To examine right breast, put a pillow or folded towel under right shoulder. Place right hand behind head. With left hand, fingers flat, press gently in small circular motions around an imaginary clock face. *E*, Begin at outermost top of breast and move around a full circle. A ridge of firm tissue in the lower curve of each breast is normal. Then move in an inch, toward the nipple, and repeat circling to examine every part of breast, including nipple. Repeat procedure on left breast. *F*, Finally squeeze the nipple of each breast gently between thumb and index finger. Any discharge, clear or bloody, should be reported to a doctor immediately. (Courtesy of the American Cancer Society.)

objects into their mouths (see p. 403). Some children choke because they do not chew properly or inhale food or objects into their throats while playing. Among adolescents and adults, choking may be caused by difficulty in chewing or gulping huge pieces of food while eating. Alcoholic intake that affects judgment and numbs the senses of the throat and swallowing mechanisms can also produce choking.

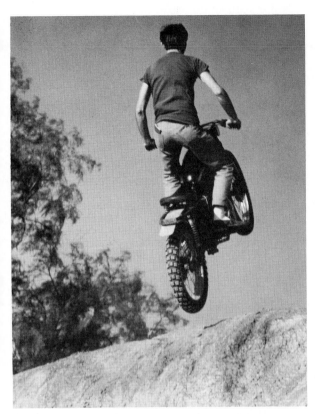

FIGURE 25–16. The sport of motorcycle riding is especially dangerous when the driver does not wear a safety helmet. (H. Armstrong Roberts.)

Adolescents are often present when an emergency such as this arises. They should be taught how to give emergency care to the victim. If the victim is conscious but unable to talk or make sounds, he is probably choking. The steps to be taken in providing care include the following: (1) send for help, but do not wait for it to arrive; (2) open the mouth and grasp the tongue with a firm grip, pulling it forward as far as possible; (3) if an obstruction can be seen, using the index and middle fingers, grasp the object and pull it out; (4) if unsuccessful, use the Heimlich procedure (see Fig. 25–17); (5) administer artificial respiration to restore breathing if necessary; (6) keep the victim quiet and warm and seek medical assistance.

EDUCATION ON DEATH

Death, a topic that many people would like to ignore, has become an increasingly popular subject for students in high schools. The subject of death may be integrated into various courses in the curriculum or it may be discussed in one course particularly. The need for such emphasis has arisen because students have been generally isolated from the facts of death that used to be learned naturally at home.

NUTRITION

Adolescents must receive adequate nutrition, especially at the time of their greatest growth. Appetite usually poses no problem; adolescents are known for their propensity to raid the refrigerator.

Because of rapid growth the girl may need 2400 calories daily and the boy 3000 calories. Table 25–1 gives the nutritional requirements of adolescent boys and girls at different ages. The difference in requirements between the sexes is due largely to the difference in ultimate size.

As soon as interest in personal appearance develops, young women especially may resent the fact that they seem to be gaining too much weight. They may go on a diet or develop food fads which may endanger their health. Parents should supervise the diet without being obvious about it. The adolescent may have practice in planning meals, in marketing and in balancing a day's meals, and thereby learn the essentials of an adequate diet. This is especially important so that the young woman may be in a state of adequate nutrition when she is married and begins her childbearing period.

Both parents and school personnel should educate young people in the essentials of a good diet, because often adolescents tend to drink too many carbonated beverages and to eat too many pizzas and French fries. Between-meal snacks may not be as detrimental to health as was previously thought. Although the calories supplied to teenagers by between-meal foods are far from empty, there is an overall dietary deficiency in calcium and iron contained in these foods. The teenager should eat snack foods with various nutrients, especially those containing calcium and iron. Vending machines in schools should contain nutritious foods such as fruits and nuts instead of only candies, sodas, and other sweet and starchy foods. Since group consciousness is strong, at times a whole group must be helped toward an understanding of better eating habits. They should learn that only by eating a diet that includes meat and other protein foods, vegetables, fruits, whole grain cereals, and milk will they achieve the health status in adulthood that is desired. The teenager's interest in his own health and appearance can be used to encourage wholesome food practices. Adolescent boys many times eat properly because of their interest in being in good physical condition for competitive sports.

During this period approximately 15 per cent of the total calories should be derived from protein so as to maintain a positive nitrogen balance. This means that the adolescent should re-

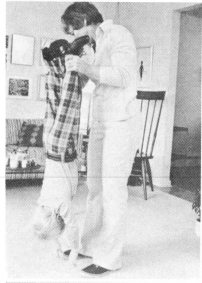

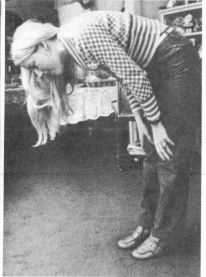

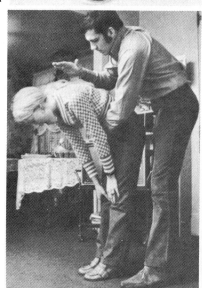

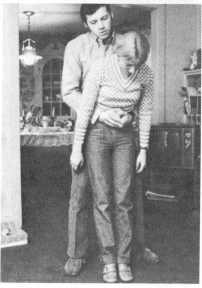

A

B

C

D

FIGURE 25–17. Emergency care for a person who has aspirated an object leading to airway obstruction. *A*, If the victim is a small child, suspend him by his ankles and let his arms dangle below his head. *B*, If the victim is an adult, have him continue to cough as he bends over. *C*, If the object is not dislodged, administer a sharp thump between his scapulae. The object may be forced out by the air pressure from his lungs. *D*, The Heimlich procedure. Have the victim bend over while you put your arms around his waist. With your hands in a clenched fist, quickly compress and release his epigastric area. If the object is not expelled, but is visible in the victim's throat, remove it manually, being careful not to push it deeper into the respiratory passages. (From Rinear, C. E. and Rinear, E. E.: Reprinted with permission from the April, 1975, issue of *Nursing '75*, Intermed Communications, Inc. Further reproduction in whole or part expressly prohibited by law.)

ceive up to 60 gm. of protein a day. This may be obtained from milk, eggs, meat, and cheese. He needs at least two to four glasses of milk to provide calcium. He also needs about 400 International Units of vitamin D a day to absorb adequately and retain calcium in his body.

EFFECTS OF SEPARATION

The pubescent child and the adolescent may be separated from their parents and home for long periods of time with little problem if their emotional development has been sound. Young adolescents may spend a few nights at the homes of friends under the supervision of their parents. They may go to camp in summer for several weeks at a time. Others may spend the school year at boarding schools some distance from home. Although homesickness may be a complaint at the beginning of a separation, even when the young person goes to college, activities in the new environment quickly seize upon his interest.

TABLE 25–1. *RECOMMENDED DAILY DIETARY ALLOWANCES FOR PUBESCENTS AND ADOLESCENTS (11 TO 18 YEARS)*

	BOYS		GIRLS	
Weight Height	11–14 Years 44 kg. (97 Pounds) 158 cm. (63 Inches)	15–18 Years 61 kg. (134 Pounds) 172 cm. (69 Inches)	11–14 Years 44 kg. (97 Pounds) 155 cm. (62 Inches)	15–18 Years 54 kg. (119 Pounds) 162 cm. (65 Inches)
K calories	2,800	3,000	2,400	2,100
Protein	44 g.	54 g.	44 g.	48 g.
Fat-soluble vitamins				
Vitamin A activity	5,000 I.U.	5,000 I.U.	4,000 I.U.	4,000 I.U.
Vitamin D	400 I.U.	400 I.U.	400 I.U.	400 I.U.
Vitamin E activity	12 I.U.	15 I.U.	12 I.U.	12 I.U.
Water-soluble vitamins				
Ascorbic acid	45 mg.	45 mg.	45 mg.	45 mg.
Folacin[a]	400 μg	400 μg	400 μg	400 μg
Niacin[b]	18 mg.	20 mg.	16 mg.	14 mg.
Riboflavin	1.5 mg.	1.8 mg.	1.3 mg.	1.4 mg.
Thiamine	1.4 mg.	1.5 mg.	1.2 mg.	1.1 mg.
Vitamin B_6	1.6 mg.	2.0 mg.	1.6 mg.	2.0 mg.
Vitamin B_{12}	3.0 μg	3.0 μg	3.0 μg	3.0 μg
Minerals				
Calcium	1,200 mg.	1,200 mg.	1,200 mg.	1,200 mg.
Phosphorus	1,200 mg.	1,200 mg.	1,200 mg.	1,200 mg.
Iodine	130 μg	150 μg	115 μg	115 μg
Iron	18 mg.	18 mg.	18 mg.	18 mg.
Magnesium	350 mg.	400 mg.	300 mg.	300 mg.
Zinc	15 mg.	15 mg.	15 mg.	15 mg.

[a]The folacin allowances refer to dietary sources as determined by *Lactobacillus casei* assay. Pure forms of folacin may be effective in doses less than ¼ of the RDA.

[b]Although allowances are expressed as niacin, it is recognized that on the average 1 mg. of niacin is derived from each 60 mg. of dietary tryptophan.

From the Food and Nutrition Board, National Academy of Sciences–National Research Council: Recommended Daily Dietary Allowances (1974).

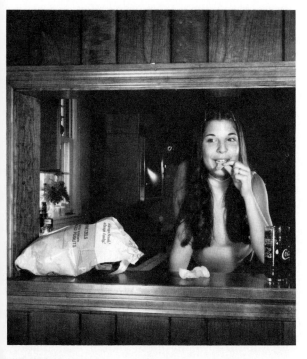

FIGURE 25–18. Because pubescence and adolescence are periods of rapid growth, adequate nutrition must be received. Carbonated beverages and potato chips and pretzels provide mainly empty calories.

HEALTH SUPERVISION AND GUIDANCE

Adolescents frequently cannot find a place where they can receive care in the traditional medical delivery system. They may have been cared for by a pediatrician when they were younger and may be seen by an internist or an obstetrician when they are older. In addition to the usual health problems, the characteristics of adolescents predispose them to a range of experiences: early sexual activity, venereal disease, pregnancy, experimentation with drugs and alcohol, and emotional disorders such as suicidal states.

Ephebiatrics (from the Greek *ephebos,* meaning youth, puberty) is a growing new specialty whose purpose is to help teenagers solve their problems. Adolescents as a group have special needs, and not all physicians are comfortable dealing with them. *Ephebiatrists,* then, are physicians who work with adolescents, many of them in adolescent clinics.

In recent years *adolescent clinics* have been organized in many sections of this country. In these clinics all sorts of problems are seen and treated. They are general-practice clinics de-

This is a part of your medical evaluation. Please circle YES or NO. Your doctor will go over this form with you.

1. Do you have frequent headaches?		Yes	No
2. Do you seem to tire easily?		Yes	No
3. Do you get short of breath or wheeze?		Yes	No
4. Do you often have stomach aches?		Yes	No
5. Do you often have backaches or sore bones or joints?		Yes	No
6. Are you allergic to anything? _____		Yes	No
7. Do you sleep well most of the time?		Yes	No
8. Do you have frequent dreams or nightmares?		Yes	No
9. Are you concerned about your weight?		Yes	No
10. Are you worried about your height?		Yes	No
11. Do you get easily upset?		Yes	No
12. Do you think something is wrong with your heart?		Yes	No
13. Are you worried you might have cancer? Where? _____		Yes	No
14. Are you satisfied with your progress in school?		Yes	No
15. Do you think something is wrong with your eyes?		Yes	No
16. Are you having problems with your parents?		Yes	No
17. Do you think something is wrong with your skin?		Yes	No
18. Does it burn when you urinate?		Yes	No
19. Do you have questions about contraception?		Yes	No
20. Is there any question about sexual matters you would like to ask?		Yes	No
21. Are there any questions about pregnancy you would like to ask?		Yes	No
22. Do you have any questions about discharge or venereal disease?		Yes	No
23. Do you think something is wrong with your health?		Yes	No
24. Are you concerned about your sexual development or sexual feelings?		Yes	No
25. Do you have any questions about drugs or alcohol?		Yes	No
26. Are there any other questions or concerns that you would like to discuss with the doctor?		Yes	No

FIGURE 25–19. Screening medical inventory. (From Hammar, S. L.: *Pediatr. Clin. N. Am.*, 20:787, November 1973.)

voted to an age group instead of to a particular kind of illness or a specific problem. Specialists' help is available if the adolescent needs it.

Usually youths between 12 and 21 years of age are offered help regardless of their complaint, whether emotional, physical, social, or intellectual. A physician interested in the total adolescent and his problems sees the young person and establishes a close relation with him. The parents may be interviewed initially and as necessary, but the primary relation is between the physician and the adolescent. The adolescent is expected to take the responsibility for his own health.

Physicians in these clinics see illnesses common to young people (see Chap. 26). The focus in management should be on the young person himself, not on the specific problem he presents.

Physicians trained in these clinics do not necessarily become specialists in the treatment of adolescents. But whether they are essentially pediatricians or internists, they develop insights into the problems of this age group which will help them in their treatment of adolescents.

An alternative means of health care for adolescents is the nontraditional *free clinic*, which is democratically operated and staffed by volunteers. These clinics can offer a wide range of services to adolescents and to the community. Many free clinics have a highly transient population consisting of diverse groups, embracing a wide variety of lifestyles and values. Such a

clinic may have a 24-hour switchboard that is a communication center where information is given out concerning their own and other community agencies and services. Usually such a clinic provides medical services, first-aid treatment, possibly dental care, a place for "rap" sessions of groups, emergency psychiatric care, and health information and education. These clinics thus provide services in response to expressed community needs. Those who receive care are encouraged to become actively involved in their own health and to develop their own potential for health, whatever that may be.

Adolescents need someone to talk with about their problems. They also need measures to protect them against disease after their childhood immunizations have worn off (see the immunization schedule given in Chapter 13).

Certain physical problems may be prevented by proper care during adolescence. Because adolescents spend increasingly longer time at night studying, they need frequent re-examination of their eyes. Also, because adolescents are more athletic and subject to foot injuries and because they are style-conscious and wear ill-fitting shoes, both sexes should be cautioned about the proper care of their feet. Both sexes also should have frequent dental examinations because caries, prevalent during the second decade of life partly because of a diet high in carbohydrate and erratic dental hygiene habits, should be treated promptly. They should also learn of the methods of the new preventive dentistry. The adolescent should assume responsibility both for his own general medical care and for his visits to the dentist.

Adolescents must develop a good attitude toward health so as to profit from factual information gained from various sources. Education about growth and development, accident prevention, nutrition, sex education, and mental hygiene is of special interest to them. Facts about the effects of smoking on health should be given to adolescents, since many of them acquire this habit during this period of their lives.

The nurse who guides adolescents either individually or in a group will succeed more because of a liking for young people, honesty and objectivity, respect for others as human beings with a right to privacy, and use of self than because of the specific techniques of counseling learned and mastered. The nurse who regards each adolescent as a person in his own right and values any relationship with that adolescent and who is willing to listen acceptingly and understandingly to problems will help the adolescent find his own answers rather than depending only upon the solutions of others. It is important that the nurse understand the meaning of the language adolescents use so that effective communication is possible. In counseling, if both the nurse and the adolescent respond openly to each other, they can work through their differences and modify their behavior to meet each other's needs. The adolescent can learn that it is normal to have feelings and fears and that it helps to talk about them. Mutual respect is of great importance. Such a counseling relationship can be a healthy one because it is mutually satisfying. The nurse remains a health educator and is not identified as a parent, *in loco parentis*.

The nurse learns that beneath the surface of many routine questions and complaints that young people have are the real concenrs with which they are struggling. The specific problems which concern adolescents and the appropriate behavioral choices available to them must be seen against the background of the adolescent in relation to his parents, pressures from his own community, society, and his subculture, and the interaction of all these. Problems usually concern the physical and emotional changes occurring at puberty and ways of coping with these, relations between young men and women, independence from the family, and educational and vocational planning.

Nurses in conference with adolescents have an opportunity to provide factual information to help clarify distorted ideas about menstruation, venereal disease, pregnancy, and the dangers of smoking, alcoholic beverages, and experimentation with other drugs. In spite of the availability of written material on these subjects, many young people are confused about the basic facts.

Many pubescents are embarrassed by their development of secondary sex characteristics. Girls are upset about their developing breasts, and boys are concerned about their penile and scrotal development, especially if they are different from their peers. After an exploration of the adolescent's feelings about his development, factual information concerning the changes that are occurring can help to alleviate anxiety.

Both young men and women may ask questions about dating, petting, premarital sex, and contraceptive devices. Members of each sex should understand how frightened the other usually is about these topics also. Honest discussion of these issues is a necessary step in helping them to face the choices open to them in their relations with the opposite sex. Such choices are dependent on their parents' attitudes, their religious beliefs, the beliefs of the society of which they are a part, and the health consequences of their actions. Each choice must be considered in the light of what it will mean to them and to others as individuals in the future.

Discussions concerning the adolescents' emerging drives toward independence from their families can lead them to look at their rebellious feelings. They can be helped to recognize their confusion and lack of readiness for some of the experiences they are already encountering. Certainly in the question of money the best way to have learned how to handle finances reasonably and confidently is by having parents who set a good example in the home.

Many adolescents, especially those who come from economically deprived families, may think about dropping out of high school before graduation. The nurse can help such young people consider possible alternatives to this action and what each will mean to them in the future. If the youth does graduate from high school and goes on to college, his success will be dependent upon his motivation, his intellectual potential, his academic interest, and his past scholastic preparation. If he decides that college is not what he really wants, the nurse should support him in his right to decide for himself on another career goal.

The sort of counselor or nurse who has charisma for young people bases actions on personal beliefs and yet has an intensely private inner nature from which inspiration comes. The adolescent can learn from the adult who has the muscle to give courageous support, a value system based on experience, the ability to laugh, and the goal of treasuring personal rights as well as those of youth.

TEACHING AIDS AND OTHER INFORMATION*

American Academy of Pediatrics

Salt Intake and High Blood Pressure.
Selected References on Low Cost Sex Education Publications.

The American Cancer Society, Inc.

A Breast Check—So Simple—So Important.

American Dental Association

Between You and Me Is Your Smile.
Cleaning Your Teeth and Gums.
Cómo Limpiar los Dientes y las Encías (Cleaning Your Teeth and Gums).

American Heart Association

Healthy Eating for Teenagers.

Child Study Association of America

Olds, S. W.: Your Child and Alcohol, 1976.
Levinsohn, F., and Kelly, G. L.: What Teenagers Want to Know, 1975.

Consumer Product Information

An Adolescent in Your Home, 1975.
Breast Self-Examination, 1974.
Pocket Guide to Babysitting, 1974.
Unless You Decide to Quit, Your Problem Isn't Going to Be Smoking; Your Problem's Going to Be Staying Alive, 1973.

Department of National Health and Welfare: Ottawa, Canada

Birth Control Facts for Teenagers.
Breast Self-Examination.
Table of Heights and Weights of Canadians.

Kimberly-Clark Corporation

Getting Married.
Growing Up Young.
The Life Cycle Center.
The Miracle of You.
The Years of Independence.
Your First Pregnancy.
Your Years of Self-Discovery.

Maternity Center Association

Organs of Human Reproduction.
Shape and Structure of Breasts.
The Female Pelvis.

National Council on Alcoholism, Inc.

Blakeslee, A., and Sullivan, B.: Alcohol: The New Teen-Age Turn On, 1975.
Hornik, E. L.: You and Your Alcoholic Parent, 1974.
Milgram, G. G.: What Is Alcohol? And Why Do People Drink?, 1975.
Strictly for Teenagers, Revised 1975.

Personal Products Company

Boys: Have You Wondered What Happens When Girls Grow Up?
Strictly Feminine.

Planned Parenthood Federation of America, Inc.

To Be a Mother... To Be a Father.

Public Affairs Committee

Bienvenu, M.: Parent-Teenager Communication.
Bienvenu, M.: Talking It Over Before Marriage.
Hill, M.: Parents and Teenagers.
Landis, P. H.: Coming of Age: Problems of Teenagers.
Milt, H.: Young Adults and Their Parents.
Ogg, E.: Preparing Tomorrow's Parents.
Schwartz, J. V.: Health Care for the Adolescent.
Shiller, A.: Drug Abuse and Your Child.

United States Government

Adolescent in Your Home, 1975.
Approaches to Adolescent Health Care in the 1970's.
Behavior Patterns in School of Youths 12–17 Years, U.S., Reprinted 1975.
Height and Weight of Youths 12–17 Years, U.S., 1973.
Jones, P. S.: Parenthood Education in a City High School, 1975.
McKigney, J. I., and Munro, H. N.: Nutrient Requirements in Adolescence, 1976.
Publications of the Office of Child Development, 1976.
The Man Who Cares, 1975.
The Pocket Guide to Babysitting, Reprinted 1975.
Un Adolescente en su Hogar (An Adolescent in Your Home, 1976.

---

*Complete addresses are given in the Appendix.

REFERENCES

Books

Browning, M. H., and Lewis, E. P.: *Human Sexuality: Nursing Implications.* New York, American Journal of Nursing Company, 1973.
Button, L.: *Developmental Group Work with Adolescents.* New York, Halsted Press, 1975.
Cohn, F., and Moritz, C. E.: *Understanding Human Sexuality.* Englewood Cliffs, N.J., Prentice-Hall, 1974.
Cole, L., and Hall, I. N.: *Psychology of Adolescence.* 7th ed. Toronto, Holt, Rinehart and Winston, 1970.
Comer, J., and Poussaint, A.: *Black Child Care.* New York, Simon & Schuster, 1975.
Densen-Gerber, J., and Baden, T.: *Drugs, Sex, Parents and You.* Philadelphia, J. B. Lippincott Company, 1972.

Gallagher, J. R., Heald, F. P., and Garell, D. C. (Eds.): *Medical Care of the Adolescent.* 3rd ed. New York, Appleton-Century-Crofts, 1976.
Hall, R. H.: *Food for Nought.* New York, Harper & Row, 1974.
Hill, J. P., and Shelton, J. (Eds.): *Readings in Adolescent Development and Behavior.* Englewood Cliffs, N.J., Prentice-Hall, Inc., 1971.
Huenemann, R. L., et al.: *Teenage Nutrition and Physique.* Springfield, Ill., Charles C Thomas, 1974.
Johnson, W. R., and Belzer, E. G., Jr.: *Human Sexual Behavior and Sex Education: With Historical, Moral, Legal, Linguistic, and Cultural Perspectives.* 3rd ed. Philadelphia, Lea & Febiger, 1973.

Kalafatich, A. J. (Ed.): *Approaches to the Care of Adolescents*. New York, Appleton-Century-Crofts, 1975.

Lief, H. I.: *Medical Aspects of Human Sexuality*. Baltimore, Williams & Wilkins Company, 1975.

Pierson, E. C., and D'Antonio, W. V.: *Female and Male: Dimensions of Human Sexuality*. Philadelphia, J. B. Lippincott Company, 1974.

Pierson, E. C.: *Sex is Never an Emergency: A Candid Guide for Young Adults*. 3rd ed. Philadelphia, J. B. Lippincott Company, 1973.

Rachman, A. W.: *Identity Group Psychotherapy With Adolescents*. Springfield, Ill., Charles C Thomas, 1975.

Recommended Dietary Allowances. 8th ed. rev. Washington, D.C., National Academy of Sciences–National Research Council, 1974.

Reinhardt, A. M., and Quinn, M. D. (Eds.): *Family-Centered Community Nursing: A Socio-Cultural Framework*. St. Louis, The C. V. Mosby Company, 1973.

Sauer, G. C.: *Teen Skin*. Springfield, Ill., Charles C Thomas, 1973.

Selye, H.: *The Stress of Life*. Revised Ed. New York, McGraw-Hill Book Company, 1976.

Shope, D. F.: *Interpersonal Sexuality*. Philadelphia, W. B. Saunders, 1975.

Smith, D. W., and Bierman, E. L. (Eds.): *The Biologic Ages of Man: From Conception Through Old Age*. Philadelphia, W. B. Saunders Company, 1973.

Smoyak, S. (Ed.): *The Psychiatric Nurse as a Family Therapist*. New York, John Wiley & Sons, 1975.

Sugar, M. (Ed.): *The Adolescent in Group and Family Therapy*. New York, Brunner/Mazel Publishers, 1975.

The Health Law Center, and Streiff, C. J. (Eds.): *Nursing and the Law*. 2nd ed. Rockville, Maryland, Aspen Systems Corp., 1975.

Udry, J. R.: *The Social Context of Marriage*. 3rd ed. Philadelphia, J. B. Lippincott Company, 1974.

White House Conference on Youth, Estes Park, Colorado, April 18–22, 1971; *Report of the White House Conference on Youth*. Washington, D.C., Government Printing Office, 1971.

Willgoose, C. E.: *Health Teaching in Secondary Schools*. 2nd ed. Philadelphia, W. B. Saunders Company, 1977.

Woods, N. F.: *Human Sexuality in Health and Illness*. St. Louis, The C. V. Mosby Company, 1975.

Periodicals

Barnes, H. V.: Symposium on Adolescent Medicine. *Med. Clin. N. Am.*, 59:1279, November 1975.

Bayer, A. E.: Early Marriage in the United States. *Medical Aspects of Human Sexuality*, 7:208, August 1973.

Byles, J. A.: Teenagers' Attitudes Toward Parenting. *Health Educ.*, 6:15, September-October 1975.

Caghan, S. B.: The Adolescent Process and the Problem of Nutrition. *Am. J. Nursing*, 75:1728, October 1975.

Chard, M.: An Approach to Examining the Adolescent Male. *The American Journal of Maternal Child Nursing*, 1:41, January-February 1976.

Diekelmann, N. L.: The Young Adult: The Choice is Health or Illness. *Am. J. Nursing*, 76:1272, August 1976.

Duyff, R. L., Sanjur, D., and Nelson, H. Y.: Food Behavior and Related Factors of Puerto Rican–American Teenagers. *J. Nutr. Educ.*, 7:99, July-September 1975.

Ehrman, M. L.: Sex Education for the Young. *Nursing Outlook*, 23:583, September 1975.

Elder, R. G.: Orientation of Senior Nursing Students Toward Access to Contraceptives. *Nursing Research*, 25:338, September-October 1976.

Fiedler, D. E., Lang, D. M., and Carlson, J. M.: Pathology in the 'Healthy' Female Teenager. *Am. J. Pub. Health*, 63:962, November 1973.

Fine, L. L.: What's a Normal Adolescent? *Clinical Pediatrics*, 12:1, January 1973.

Finkel, M. L., and Finkel, D. J.: Sexual and Contraceptive Knowledge, Attitudes and Behavior of Male Adolescents. *Fam. Plan. Perspec.*, 7:256, November-December 1975.

Garvin, B. J.: Values of Male Nursing Students. *Nursing Research*, 25:352, September-October 1976.

Giuffra, M. J.: Demystifying Adolescent Behavior. *Am. J. Nursing*, 75:1724, October 1975.

Hill, D.: Sex Education Background of Selected Students in Louisiana. *J. Sch. Health*, 40:473, October 1975.

Hofmann, A. D.: Health Care of Inner-City Adolescents. *Clinical Pediatrics*, 13:570, July 1974.

Hofmann, A. D., and Pilpel, H. F.: The Legal Rights of Minors. *Pediatr. Clin. N. Am.*, 20:989, November 1973.

Irving, J. E.: Friends Unlimited: Adolescents as Helping Resources. *Children Today*, 4:14, July-August 1975.

Kelson, S. R., Pullella, J. L., and Otterland, A.: The Growing Epidemic. A Survey of Smoking Habits and Attitudes toward Smoking among Students in Grades 7 through 12 in Toledo and Lucas County (Ohio) Public Schools – 1964 and 1971. *Am. J. Pub. Health*, 65:923, September 1975.

Kruger, W. S.: Education for Parenthood and the Schools. *Children Today*, 2:4, March-April 1973.

Lawrence, R.: Exploring Childhood on an Indian Reservation. *Children Today*, 5:10, September-October 1976.

Lief, H. I., and Payne, T.: Sexuality-Knowledge and Attitudes. *Am. J. Nursing*, 75:2026, November 1975.

Manisoff, M.: Family Planning Democratized. *Am. J. Nursing*, 75:1660, October 1975.

Mercer, R.: Becoming a Mother at Sixteen. *The American Journal of Maternal Child Nursing*, 1:44, January-February 1976.

Muhich, D. F., and Johnson, B. J.: Youth and Society, Changing Values and Roles. *Pediatr. Clin. N. Am.*, 20:772, November 1973.

Opp, M.: The Confidentiality Dilemma. *Nursing Digest*, 4:17, Fall 1976.

Oppenheimer, R. P., and Reid, L.: Hearing Loss Due to Minibikes. *Am. Fam. Physician*, 8:125, October 1973.

Parlee, M. B.: Stereotypic Beliefs About Menstruation: A Methodological Note on the Moos Menstrual Distress Questionnaire and Some New Data. *Psychosom. Med.*, 36:229, May-June 1974.

Paulshock, B. Z.: Birth Control: What I Want My Daughter to Know. *Today's Health*, 53:20, February 1975.

Rasmussen, C. M., and Lochner, F. E.: How Immune Are Our Teenagers? *Am. Fam. Physician*, 10:100, July 1974.

Rinear, C. E., and Rinear, E. E.: Emergency! Part 3: On-The-Spot Care for Aspiration, Burns, and Poisoning. *Nursing '75*, 5:40, April 1975.

Roberts, M. E.: Health Information and the College Student. *J. Am. Coll. Health Assoc.*, 21:221, February 1973.

Robinson, A. M.: Confidential Health Care for the Teenager. *RN*, 37:58, November 1974.

Rodgers, J. A.: Struggling Out of the Feminine Pluperfect. *Am. J. Nursing*, 75:1655, October 1975.

Root, A. W.: Endocrinology of Puberty. *J. Pediatr.*, 83:1, July 1973.

Roznoy, M. S.: The Young Adult: Taking a Sexual History. *Am. J. Nursing*, 76:1279, August 1976.

Speca, J. M., and Cowell, H. R.: Minibike and Motorcycle Accidents in Adolescents. *J.A.M.A.*, 232:55, 1975.

Stromborg, M. R.: Relationship of Sex Role Identity to Occupational Image of Female Nursing Students. *Nursing Research*, 25:363, September-October 1976.

Suskin, E., and Bouhys, A.: Acute Airway Responses to Hairspray Preparations. *N. Engl. J. Med.*, 290:660, March 1974.

Tifft, M., and Stanton, J. B.: Nutrition Misconceptions of

Secondary School Youth. *Sch. Health Rev.*, 3:12, November-December 1972.

Warren, C. L., and St. Pierre, R.: Sources and Accuracy of College Students' Sex Knowledge. *J. Sch. Health*, 43:588, November 1973.

Whisnant, L., and Zegans, L.: White Middle-Class Adolescent Girls' Attitudes Toward Menarche. *Nursing Digest*, 4:52, September-October 1976.

Wuerger, M. K.: The Young Adult: Stepping into Parenthood. *Am. J. Nursing*, 76:1283, August 1976.

AUDIOVISUAL MEDIA*

American Dental Association

Teeth Are Good Things to Have
   13½ minutes, 16mm, sound, color.
   An entertaining and educational film for both young adults and adults. In a light but meaningful way, the film relates the necessity of a personal in-home program of preventive oral hygiene.

American Lung Association

Is it Worth Your Life?
   24½ minutes, 16mm, sound, color.
   Powerful presentation by Dr. Charles Tate of Miami on the effects of cigarette smoking. For high school and college students and adults.

Canadian Cancer Society

Breast Self-Examination and Time and Two Women
   21 minutes, 16mm, color.
   Demonstrates the technique of breast self-examination and explains the importance of the Pap smear in cervical cancer detection.

Harper & Row, Publishers

The Biological Aspects of Sexuality
   Allen, J. M.
   35mm slides, 22 minutes each, audio-tape cassette, sound, color, guide.

   The Nature of Human Sexuality
   Pervasive nature of sexuality; reproductive phase of the life cycle; physiologic significance of puberty; sexual anatomy; sex inheritance mechanisms; genetics of sex determination; mechanisms of sex differentiation in vertebrates; duality of sexual anatomy as evidenced by differentiation of external genitalia.

   Conception Control
   Major methods of contraception discussed against background of human sexual anatomy; mechanics and statistical effectiveness of each method; importance of contraception in regulating population; individual responsibility; sterilization and abortion.

   Hormones and Reproduction
   Endocrine regulatory mechanisms; hormones as messenger molecules; nature of feedback regulation; roles of hypothalmus, pituitary, and gonads in human reproduction control; menstrual cycle and its regulation by hormonal interactions; biological basis of pregnancy tests; mechanism of "the pill" in the context of hormonal factors; interrelation of hormonal and neural factors in control of reproduction.

McGraw-Hill Book Company

Conflict and Awareness
   Producer: CRM Educational Films
   Series of 9 films, 16mm, color.
   Separation and Divorce—"It Has Nothing to Do with You"
   Parent-Child Relationships—"It's My Decision as Long as It's What You Want"
   Therapy—"What Do You Want Me to Say?"
   Frustration and Aggression—"It's Not Fair"
   Adolescent Sexual Conflict—"Are We Still Going to the Movies?"

Young Marriage—"When's the Big Day?"
Self-Identity/Sex Roles—"I Only Want You to be Happy"
Group Conformity/Rejection—"How's Your New Friend?"
Job Interview—"I Guess I Got the Job"

Paramount Oxford Films

How to Save a Choking Victim: The Heimlich Maneuver
   11 minutes, 16mm film.
   Dr. Heimlich demonstrates his life-saving techniques in detail. Most importantly, he shows how to avoid the danger of choking in the first place.

W. B. Saunders Company

Pediatric Conferences with Sydney Gellis
   Legal Problems in Dealing with Adolescents, Hofmann, A.
   Pediatric Gynecology, Mitchell, G.

Tampax Inc.

The Menstrual Cycle
   Chart, color.
   Depicts the changes that take place inside the uterus during a menstrual cycle. It shows the location of the female reproductive organs, the ripening of the ovum, and includes the famous Dickinson anatomical drawings.

Telstar Productions, Inc.

Interpersonal Competence Series—Unit I, Self
   Concept of Self
   29 minutes, videotape, sound, color.
   Variety of answers to question "who am I?" Stresses two concepts—need to be loved, and man becomes what surrounds him.

Trainex Corporation

Cancer Detection: Self Examination of the Breast and Pap Smear
   35mm filmstrip, audio-tape cassettes, 33 1/3 LP, color, available in Spanish.
   Discusses the necessity for self-examination of the breasts, where and how to look, and what to do if a lump is found. It also discusses cancer of the cervix and the Pap smear.

United States Government

Social Seminar Series
Brian at Seventeen
   Producer: USNIMH
   30 minutes, 16mm film, optical sound, black and white.
   Presents an adolescent's view of his educational needs and how school is and is not fulfilling them. Gives perspective of his educational experience, his parents, and life in general. Especially for the teacher and parent who find the current scene confusing.

Wayne State University

DENT: Directions for Education in Nursing Via Technology
   30 minute lessons, 16mm film, videotape and videocassette, color.
   Human Sexuality Series
   Psychosocial Sexual Development

---

*Complete addresses are given in the Appendix.

Chapter Twenty-Six

PROBLEMS OF PUBESCENCE AND ADOLESCENCE RELATED TO THE PROCESS OF GROWTH AND DEVELOPMENT

One of the common concerns of adolescents is the question "Am I growing up the way I should?" This concern with themselves and their own bodies must be recognized and utilized to advantage by medical and nursing personnel if the adolescent is to be helped. Professional personnel must be more willing to listen to concerns than to advise, and to show the young person *respect* as he approaches adulthood.

Since the adolescent is much more concerned than his parents usually are about some of the typical problems of adolescence such as menstruation, size of the sex organs, masturbation, postural defects, acne, fatigue, styes, and obesity, it is he or she as an individual who should receive directly the guidance, medical assistance, and directions for care needed from the physician or nurse. Although the parents may be informed of such actions, direct responsibility for following medical advice belongs to the young person himself. *The experience of illness may thus help the adolescent not only to conquer present handicaps, but also to manage his future life better by himself.* In this process many times parents with guidance also learn that their job is to produce an adult, not a child.

The adolescent, in addition to seeking help with medical problems, may also need an adult who has no close ties with him, as his parents have, one who can discuss emotionally charged concerns such as sex, religion, death, or school in an objective way. Such concerns or anxieties may result eventually in physical symptoms if they are not alleviated. If the physician or nurse has a warm, interested, neither disapproving nor approving manner, the confidence of the adolescent can be gained, and he can be helped with problems which concern him. If the adolescent does not receive such assistance and guidance when he needs it, he will probably be less able to accept it and profit from it as he grows older. If medical and nursing personnel refuse to rec-

ognize the adolescent as an individual in a particular stage of life, neither adult nor child, he will not continue treatment or will rebel and refuse to cooperate.

The *legal aspects* of care of the adolescent without parental consent are not clearly defined or the same in all states. Some states have enacted laws declaring that a person reaches his majority or age of emancipation at 18 years and is therefore entitled to sign agreements. Other states may rule that an individual under 21 years is emancipated if he is self-supporting or married. Some states grant minors self-consent for

845

medical care if they understand the nature of the treatment to be given. It is, therefore, essential that the nurse know the law in the state in which care is to be given to adolescents.

In summary, many of the symptoms of physical distress complained of by pubescents and adolescents are the manifestations of normal physical and physiologic changes occurring in their bodies and of inner emotional turmoils they are experiencing. Treatment of these problems often requires the close cooperation of the patient, his parents, physician, teacher, counselor, school nurse practitioner or school nurse, and community, or public health nurse.

These problems cannot be clearly divided into physical or emotional groups, since each may be caused by a mixture of both.

CONCERNS OF ADOLESCENTS

Many adolescents boast about how sexually liberated their generation has become. Just because an adolescent is sexually active, however, does not mean that he or she is knowledgeable about his or her own sexuality. Some adolescents who appear to be the most sophisticated are in reality the individuals who are most confused and concerned about problems related to the process of sexual growth and development.

PREMENSTRUAL SYNDROME

Premenstrual tension is a syndrome with identifiable cross-cultural symptoms. It is a treatable syndrome, based on individual symptoms.

The premenstrual period is the period immediately preceding the menses, from one to three or up to 12 days before the period starts. Common symptoms of the premenstrual syndrome are nervous tension, depression, irritability, anxiety, bloated feeling of the abdomen and breasts, leg pains, tightness of the skin, and swollen fingers and legs. Headaches, dizziness, and palpitations may also occur. Symptoms are varied in intensity in individuals and in individual menstrual cycles.

The actual causes of the premenstrual syndrome are a mystery because it is so complex in nature. Investigation of its etiology is ongoing.

The effects of the premenstrual syndrome on the individual's performance during adolescence include poor achievement in high school, problems in the home, and an increase in emotional upsets. Because of the possibility of decreased utilization of mental ability, critical competitive examinations should not be taken during this period if they can be avoided.

The young woman should have a complete physical examination to rule out abnormalities. The teenager may be unwilling to disrobe for a pelvic examination (see p. 834). Usually a pre-examination discussion using line drawings of the processes of ovulation, menstruation, pregnancy, and labor and delivery will make the adolescent feel more at ease because of her personal involvement in this normal feminine cycle. The need for determining whether her own body is maturing as it should can be explained to her.

Therapy for this condition consists of explanation, reassurance, diversionary activities, and reduction of the individual's workload. Diuretics and tranquilizers can be used to relieve fluid retention and irritability. Ovarian hormones may also be used. Until the cause of the premenstrual syndrome is better understood, therapy must be based on the relief of symptoms.

Students many times seek the counsel of nurses for the prevention and care of this problem. Prevention begins during the prepubescent years by adequately preparing each child for the process of menstruation, a normal bodily function. The development of a healthy attitude toward menstruation will prevent minor symptoms from developing into a major problem. Exercise during the premenstrual phase decreases undesirable symptoms; the elimination of stress, fear, and tension has a similar effect.

In the care of an adolescent having premenstrual tension, the role of the nurse lies in the areas of counseling, support, education, and referral if necessary.

MENSTRUATION

A great deal of mythology exists around the subject of menstruation. Many societies in the past considered menstrual blood to be dangerous, especially to men. Common taboos have prevented menstruating women from cooking or preparing food for men and from having intercourse with them. Many societies like the Arapesh of New Guinea isolate women in small specially built menstrual huts—the menstruating woman must remain in a crouched position during the period of isolation; she is not permitted to touch her body, nor to eat, sleep, or bathe; no man would dare to go near her for fear of his life.

In the United States the superstition has long been held that the menstruating woman is unclean. Women go to great lengths to avoid any sign of menstruation. Great pressure is placed on women to maintain high standards of "good feminine hygiene."

Many premenarcheal and postmenarcheal girls perceive themselves as being knowledgeable about menstruation. They can describe the anatomy and physiology of menstruation using the correct terminology. They may still, however, have erroneous ideas about the reason why women menstruate. Some answers to questions on this subject include, "Your body doesn't need all its blood so it's wasted" and "When the egg doesn't get fertilized, it changes to blood and comes out."

DYSFUNCTIONAL UTERINE BLEEDING

Menstruation begins, on the average, at 12 to 13 years of age, although the range of onset is from 11 to 15 years. Since the cycles at first are anovulatory, absence or irregularity of menstrual periods, or scanty or increased flow, may be expected. This is due to imbalance in the secretion of hormones that usually control menstrual functioning. It may also be due to the responsiveness of the target organs in the pubescent and adolescent. The cycles may take from a few months to a few years to achieve maturation. Anovulatory cycles are considered normal for one to three years after the menarche, producing a period of relative infertility.

Dysfunctional uterine bleeding is normal and self-limited in most adolescents. In some, however, a physical examination and a pelvic examination are necessary to rule out more serious problems such as hypothyroidism and local organic causes, including pregnancy. Excessive menstrual bleeding may be the first symptom of thrombocytopenic purpura.

If no organic cause for dysfunctional uterine bleeding can be found, the adolescent should be given a high protein diet with vitamin and iron supplements. If anemia occurs, iron therapy may be necessary. Since the cycles are anovulatory, there may be persistent estrogen stimulation of the endometrium with a lack of progesterone. The administration of potent oral progestins may be helpful. In prolonged severe bleeding, dilatation and curettage may become necessary. Reassurance can be very helpful. When the cycles become ovulatory, menstrual irregularities will no longer occur.

DYSMENORRHEA

Dysmenorrhea ("menstrual cramps") is not uncommon. There are two types of dysmenorrhea: primary, by far the most common type, in which the pelvic organs are normal, and secondary, which is associated with known organ pathology such as endometriosis or pelvic inflammatory disease. The treatment for secondary dysmenorrhea is directed toward the cause.

Primary dysmenorrhea is believed to be due to muscle spasms of the uterus compounded by nervous tension, possibly related to sexual conflicts, or it may be due to vascular changes associated with menstrual flow. It may also be due to hormone imbalance, cervical obstruction, or poor posture. Symptoms of dysmenorrhea include abnominal discomfort, nausea, vomiting, pallor, sweating, and syncope. Usually a warm bath, a heating pad applied to the abdomen or lower back, exercise, good posture and a mild analgesic or sedative will help to decrease the discomfort. Diuretics may be given if signs of premenstrual tension and fluid retention are present. The use of oral contraceptives may be successful in treating primary dysmenorrhea. An anovulatory cycle can be produced with the use of estrogen alone or estrogen and progesterone in combination. In rare cases, surgical intervention may become necessary. Psychotherapy may occasionally be warranted.

MITTELSCHMERZ

Fourteen days before the onset of the menstrual period the young woman may experience a dull pain in the pelvic area. This discomfort may accompany ovulation. Both dysmenorrhea and mittelschmerz may become less of a problem after the woman has borne her first child.

BREAST SIZE DURING THE MENSTRUAL CYCLE

The breast responds to the action of several hormones. Estrogen and progesterone are essential for the development and function of the alveolar and ductal systems. As estrogen levels increase throughout the menstrual cycle, and particularly during the luteal phase with the secretion of progesterone, the breasts increase in size and the alveolar components become easily palpable. In addition, fluid retention, characteristic of the postovulatory phase of most cycles, contributes to a change in breast size. Breast examination should, therefore, be done in the early cycle phase, because with the perimenstrual decline in estrogen and progesterone, along with diuresis, greater palpatory acuity is permitted.

GYNECOMASTIA

An enlargement of mammary tissue in the male is termed *gynecomastia*. It occurs in about two thirds of boys to some degreee at puberty (*physiologic pubertal gynecomastia*). It may be due to excessive secretion of estrogens as well as androgens by the testis at puberty. Gynecomastia may occur before other signs of pubertal development appear and usually disappears within two years. Enlargement and tenderness of one or both breasts may occur. Hormonal treatment is not necessary. If excessive enlargement occurs, surgery may be indicated to prevent emotional disturbance.

Gynecomastia may be inherited as a male-limited autosomal dominant trait *(familial gynecomastia)*, or infrequently it may be associated with interstitial cell tumors of the testis or feminizing tumors of the adrenal gland. It may also occur with Klinefelter's syndrome as well as other types of testicular failure and, in older children, with hepatic disease and paraplegia. If the young man is exposed to estrogens accidentally or therapeutically, he may acquire this condition.

Pseudogynecomastia is a condition caused by an increased amount of fat on the anterior chest wall of obese boys.

Nursing care of a young man having physiologic pubertal gynecomastia involves reassuring the youth and his parents that the condition is transient. If the nipples are tender, a soft covering over them will reduce the discomfort.

SIZE OF THE PENIS

Since the adolescent is extremely concerned with his physical self, any deviation from what he considers to be normal can be a source of excruciating self-consciousness. Also, since his cognitive development is becoming more analytical and introspective, and his thoughts and behavior seem egocentric, he is sure that everyone's eyes are on his physical appearance and activities.

Although the adolescent may understand that sexual maturation varies widely among teenagers, he may still glance furtively at the anatomy of his classmates in the locker and shower rooms. The size of his penis, depending on the norm he has established, may either enhance his self-esteem or make him very sensitive about his genitalia.

Many adolescent boys are therefore concerned about the size of the penis. The question is: what is the normal size? There is a wide variation in size among healthy young males. The adolescent can be informed that the size of the genital organs has no relationship at all with sexual drives or the ability to give sexual pleasure to the opposite sex during intercourse. This knowledge can, in many instances, help to alleviate his anxiety.

MASTURBATION

Masturbation is normal during adolescence and has a role in the process of physical and emotional development (see p. 828). The nurse who observes the act or is questioned about it examines the behavior for clues it may give in understanding the individual and in uncovering significant problem areas. An adolescent who has learned from his parents to feel guilty about masturbating, and at the same time has experienced pleasurable release following the act, will be in conflict. In trying to solve his dilemma he may attempt to avoid all sexual stimuli and to use extreme self-control. If he fails in his attempts, he experiences even more guilt and self-disgust. His conflict may be expressed in physical symptoms such as severe weakness and fatigue or numerous aches and pains. Some adolescents sublimate their sexual needs through fantasy or by preliminary sexual activity with members of the opposite sex. Excessive masturbation is a symptom that the needs of the individual in the matter of interpersonal relations are not being met. Nursing intervention based on an identification of the unmet needs is directed toward aiding the young person toward more effective methods of attaining gratification. Parents may give the young person more love, affection and attention, attempt to engage him in other activities, and set reasonable limits to his behavior. He also needs increased activity with his peers. As soon as he can attain gratification by other means, the masturbatory activity lessens.

POSTURAL DEFECTS

The erect posture of the adult is usually attained during adolescence. There may be a period, however, during pubescence and early adolescence when posture is poor. There may be four reasons for this. Physically, since the bony structure of the body develops more rapidly than the muscles do, the child may appear clumsy and have poor posture. Another reason may be the emotional reaction of the youth who suddenly finds himself much taller than his peers. Since he does not want to appear different from them, he slumps so that he can be more nearly their size. Both boys and girls may have this difficulty. Some girls may resent their developing breasts, and slump to hide this manifestation of sexual development. Young people of both sexes may develop a forward-thrust head and round shoulders from watching television for years. The muscles of the chest and front of the neck become tight, and the muscles of the back of the neck and between the shoulders become weak.

If the cause of faulty posture is slow growth of muscles, a period of waiting until strength is gained may be all that is required for treatment. If faulty posture is due to embarrassment over rapid growth or sexual development, the problem is discussed realistically with the adolescent. Ridicule, shaming, or threatening is never used.

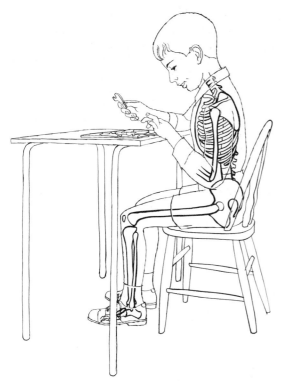

FIGURE 26–1. Throughout the period of physical growth the child, the pubescent and the adolescent need furniture that encourages them to maintain correct posture.

FATIGUE

Pubescents and adolescents frequently complain of being tired. They may be tired because of extremely rapid physical growth, overactivity, lack of sleep, faulty nutrition, anemia, or an emotional problem. If fatigue seems excessive or is prolonged, the underlying cause should be found and corrected.

ANEMIA

Before puberty the hemoglobin level is the same for both sexes. After puberty the level in girls is approximately 2 gm. below that in boys. Although the incidence of anemia is less than it was in the past, hypochromic anemia may occur and may be the cause of fatigue and fainting in this age group.

EAR PIERCING

Young women may have their ears pierced because the practice is a part of their culture, their friends are having it done, or, if they have small ear lobes, they do not want to lose valuable earrings. Unfortunately in some cases, they have their mothers, friends, or jewelers pierce their ears or they may do it themselves.

The complications that may arise after this procedure include metal allergic dermatitis, crust formation, inflammation, bleeding, or cyst

or keloid formation. There is also a possibility that viral hepatitis may be spread by the use of nonsterile earlobe-piercing instruments. Because of the possibility of these complications, young women who have diabetes, a history of keloid formation, skin disorders or other physical problems should have this procedure done only by a physician. Earrings which contain nickel or another skin-sensitizing metal should not be used.

ACNE VULGARIS

Etiology, Incidence, Clinical Manifestations, and Factors Influencing the Condition. Acne vulgaris is an inflammatory condition of the skin that occurs in and around sebaceous glands during adolescence especially. The condition results from a combination of hereditary and endocrine factors. The sebaceous glands become overactive, secreting increased amounts of sebum; they then become plugged. When the plug is exposed to the air, a blackhead is formed because the surface turns black or dark brown. If the gland has produced increased sebum but does not open onto the surface of the skin, a whitehead is formed. This closed comedo is the characteristic lesion of acne. When the walls of the comedo rupture and fatty acids, irritating components of sebum, come in contact with the surrounding skin, an inflammatory reaction occurs. These eruptions generally heal without scarring. If they are deep in the dermis, a papule forms that is likely to develop into an abscess-like lesion. Scar formation may result. Postacne scarring is determined by the severity of the acne and the depth of the inflammatory response.

Acne occurs in both sexes so commonly that it can almost be called a normal manifestation of sexual development. The areas most commonly affected are the forehead, chin, and cheeks. The back, shoulders, and chest may also be involved. Itching may or may not be present. Acne may lead to the youth's withdrawal from social contact and ultimately to emotional problems.

A specific type of acne (*acne conglobata*) occurs only in males in late adolescence. It is characterized by burrowing abscesses, draining sinus tracts, and severe scarring. Systemic signs and symptoms such as temperature elevation, general malaise, and arthralgia may occur. It runs a chronic course.

Factors that provoke acne include diet, climate, emotional problems, and external occurrences. Some physicians believe that carbohydrates and fats, for instance nuts, chocolate, and cola drinks, in general produce exacerbations of acne. Other physicians feel there is little proof that adolescents having acne respond specifically to these foods. Acne is a year-round problem in temperate climates, but it worsens during the cold months of the year. Exposure to ultraviolet light in the summer may improve acne.

Emotional stress exacerbates the condition. An evaluation must be made as to the extent of this relationship in producing the typical lesions. External factors include habitual manipulation of the skin and the application of irritating cosmetics. Topical corticosteroids under an occlusive dressing may aggravate existing acne or produce acne in a predisposed adolescent.

Treatment, Responsibilities of the Nurse, and Prognosis. Acne is treated as early as possible. The parents and the adolescent are encouraged to seek medical attention if acne occurs, since this skin condition can produce permanent scars.

An important responsibility of the nurse in acne care is an assessment of how the individual feels about his appearance, and his relationship with his peers. It is important also to determine how he feels about his treatment for acne.

The nurse assesses the adolescent for the extent of the lesions and the depth to which the skin is involved. The effectiveness of various treatments used is ascertained through discussions with the patient.

The purposes of the plan of care for the adolescent are to help him develop a positive self-image and to prevent permanent scarring of the affected areas. The adolescent wants to be attractive and popular with his peers. Any skin condition can decrease his self-confidence and cause social withdrawal due to shyness and anxiety He may look into the mirror and believe that his skin condition is worse than it really is.

Acne is a condition that may have remissions and exacerbations. The adolescent can be helped to understand the reasons why acne occurs, the factors influencing it, and the reasons for the treatment suggested. He must understand that successful treatment can only occur with his full cooperation. He is encouraged to help in planning his own care and to make suggestions for improvements in therapy if he can. An adult who really *listens* to the adolescent can hear what he is trying to say about his care even if he is hesitant and self-conscious in his approach.

The general health can be improved through dietary management, provision of adequate sleep, exposure to natural sunlight or ultraviolet light in winter, reduction of emotional tension and anxiety, and adequate cleanliness. Foods with a high carbohydrate or fat content should be eliminated; otherwise a well-balanced diet can be eaten. Sports and exercise may be helpful, since profuse perspiration loosens blackheads plugging sebaceous glands and encourages the flow of sebum. The adolescent should bathe properly after perspiring.

The affected skin is cleansed thoroughly at least three times a day with a washcloth, soap, and hot water to remove oil, bacteria, and dirt. A soap substitute containing sulfur and salicylic acid (Fostex) may be better tolerated and more effective than soap. The aim of topical treatment is to gently peel and degrease the skin, thus preventing comedone formation. Topical therapy may consist in the application of preparations containing sulfur or sulfur and salicylic acid, benzoyl peroxide, and resorcinol, a keratolytic or peeling agent. The frequency of application depends on the degree of dryness produced. Vitamin A may be applied topically to reduce comedone formation. When a new preparation is used, it is applied to one side of the face for several nights to determine whether it produces improvement in the condition of the skin.

Ultraviolet irradiation is given weekly to produce peeling of the stratum corneum. Comedones and pustular lesions can be removed with a comedo extractor. Infiltration of the lesion after evacuation with triamcinolene helps to clear the inflammatory nodule.

Preparations that are cosmetically acceptable have been developed to hide the lesions. The physician or nurse warns the adolescent against picking or squeezing the pimples, since this practice may lead to scarring. Other creams and lotions such as suntan lotion are not applied to the affected areas because the grease or oil in these substances may plug the follicles.

In severe acne, systemic antibiotic therapy may be advantageous. A broad-spectrum antibiotic such as tetracycline is used to reduce the bacteria on the skin. Monilial vaginitis can occur occasionally as a result of antibiotic therapy. Sensitivity to sunlight may occur if Vitamin A and tetracycline are used.

Anovulatory drugs may be used only after 16 years of age to decrease the amount of sebum produced. If given to boys these drugs may produce feminizing effects in time. A newer treatment for acne involves the use of erythromycin in lotion form in conjunction with a topical preparation of Vitamin A.

Seborrhea of the scalp may occur because of marked oiliness of the skin. If the hair is shampooed two to three times a week, the excess oil can be removed. Some commercial shampoos contain agents that can assist in controlling seborrhea. When necessary, topical lotions may be applied to the scalp.

If postacne scarring is severe, dermabrasion

may be used; however, the results of this therapy are many times disappointing, and many physicians no longer utilize it.

Acne vulgaris is usually relieved as adolescence is completed at about 20 years of age, although it may persist into the fourth or fifth decade of life.

HORDEOLUM (STYE) AND CHALAZION

Etiology, Incidence, Clinical Manifestations, and Treatment. *Hordeolum* (stye) is common in children and adolescents. It is an inflammation of one or more of the sebaceous glands of the eyelids. A meibomian stye is an inflammation of a meibomian gland at the posterior surface of the lid. A zeisian stye is an inflammation of a zeisian gland, occurring at the edge of the lid. The hordeolum is almost always caused by a *staphylococcal* infection. There is a localized pyogenic inflammation with abscess formation at the site.

Treatment involves localizing the infection and encouraging drainage. Topical ophthalmic antibiotics may be used, but the usual treatment consists of hot wet dressings applied every four hours. If drainage does not occur, a test for culture and sensitivity can be done to determine the appropriate antibiotic to be used. A vaccine can also be of value in the treatment of persistent recurrences.

A *chalazion* is a chronic granulation tissue tumor of the meibomian glands. Therapy is given to shrink this tumor with the purpose of letting it absorb. Hot wet dressings are applied every four hours. Appropriate topical antibiotic ointment and drops may be used to keep the area soft and to prevent secondary infection. Treatment may be prolonged to several weeks. If the lump remains after eight weeks, excision of the granuloma is recommended.

Responsibilities of the Nurse. Styes and chalazions may occur at any age. They are common among adolescents because of the hormonal changes at puberty and among girls because they do not adequately remove cosmetics at night. The nurse can teach affected adolescents the procedures for instilling eye drops and applying hot wet dressings and antibiotic ointment to their eyes. Pressure should not be applied to the eye during treatment. It is also important for the nurse to stress good eye care.

OBESITY

Incidence. Obesity is a generalized and excessive accumulation of fat in subcutaneous tissue. It is relatively common during pubescence and adolescence in both sexes. It is more frequent in the lower socioeconomic classes because of dietary habits involving foods containing large amounts of starch and fat. Children with moderate obesity in the pubescent years usually require no treatment, since this may be considered normal. Many children and adolescents, however, who are obese because of overeating will continue to be obese as adults. This is unfortunate, since adolescence is a critical period for the possible development of a distorted body image.

Society, especially the peer group, stigmatizes the child or adolescent who is obese by not fully accepting him. When a young person sees a distortion in the body of another, he feels threatened, probably because distortion reminds him of his own vulnerability. When an adolescent stigmatizes another, he is denying his own vulnerability. A young person with a strong ego probably has less need to reject those different from himself than does one with a weak ego.

Unfortunately, the obese person may respond to the reactions of his peers by becoming withdrawn and passive. In time he develops a poor self-image.

Etiology, Clinical Manifestations, and Diagnosis. The amount of food a person needs is determined by the energy needed for basal metabolism, growth, and activity. The amount of food an adolescent requires and the amount he takes are influenced by a number of factors. Among the common causes of obesity are overeating with inactivity; hereditary, familial, or racial factors; and emotional difficulties. An unhappy, withdrawn adolescent may develop an excessive appetite in order to try to escape from a difficult environment. Often the obesity makes the problem even more difficult, however. In other cases some overprotective mothers may force food upon their children. The children continue to be dependent upon their mothers and are likely to turn to eating as a comforting device for any deprivation.

Obesity due to endocrine problems such as hypothyroidism or hyperadenocorticism, which results in Cushing's syndrome, is rare.

Intracranial lesions may cause obesity as in Froelich's syndrome, but this too is rare.

The *clinical manifestations* are many. Obese adolescents are usually taller than the average for their age. The adolescent's appearance is a better criterion by which to judge obesity than is an arbitrary standard for normal and excess weight. These adolescents are usually inactive. Their facial features often appear fine or small. There may be collections of adipose tissue in the breast region, and they may have pendulous abdomens with striae. In boys the external genitalia may seem small, but only because they are buried in pubic fat.

The upper arms and the thighs may appear

obese. These adolescents are often clumsy and unable to take part successfully in competitive games. Slipping of the epiphysis of the head of the femur may occur. Flat feet and knock-knees are common.

Emotional disturbances are also common.

In making a *diagnosis* of the cause of obesity, the possibility of endocrine or other physical disturbance must be ruled out. The diet must be recorded to determine whether overeating is really present. Many of these adolescents eat normally at meals, but overeat between meals. An evaluation of the emotional status must be made.

Treatment, Responsibilities of the Nurse, and Prognosis. The cooperation of the adolescent and his family in the *treatment* of obesity is essential. If the cause is dietary, the dietary intake is reduced. Often the diet of the entire family must be adjusted. The diet can be based on nutritional needs, but the caloric intake may be reduced to 1000 to 1200 calories for children ten to 14 years of age. The protein content should be high, and the fat and carbohydrate content low. The diet should contain as much bulk as possible. Vitamin concentrates, especially those containing vitamin D, for growth may also be given. Since adolescents often desire a midafternoon or an evening snack, these can be calculated in the diet. The energy output is increased through exercise. The objective is burning of body fat to provide energy. A weight loss of 1 or 2 pounds a week is desirable.

If the child overeats because of emotional difficulties, the emphasis in treatment is not on diet, but on the management of problem areas. Unconditional acceptance of the person is essential. The child is helped to make a more adequate adjustment in his home, school, and community. School or camp personnel can often be of value in helping the child to form better relations with his peers. Psychotherapy may be necessary along with drug therapy.

The *prognosis* depends on the extent of cooperation among parents, child, and physician. If even the best treatment ordered is not followed, there will be no weight reduction.

FOOD FADDISM

Food faddism of adolescents may result in inadequate nutrition even in those whose families can financially afford an adequate diet. Currently the trend is for "natural foods" or other special diets to lose weight. Some adolescents follow a food fad because it promises to help them reduce, because it is popular or simple, or because it promises beauty or strength.

Eating is an emotional experience: from the day of birth it requires the cooperation of at least one other person. In addition to this, some adolescents are constantly searching for something new to do. This may help them to tolerate feelings of unrest and dissatisfaction they have with life in general, and thus to find peace of mind.

Adolescents must be educated to the need of a well-balanced diet if they are to avoid the hazards of nutritional deficiencies. Nurses can help to teach young people that the four basic foods should be eaten each day. The teenager should be involved in making his decision to eat a good diet after he has as much information as possible as to its necessity.

HYPERTHYROIDISM

The basal metabolic rate generally decreases from early infancy to the end of the growth period. There is a relative increase, however, during the period of rapid growth preceding puberty. This temporarily elevated metabolic rate is probably related to the hyperthyroidism noted at this age.

Treatment includes a high caloric diet, reduction in school schedule and activity, and administration of iodine This type of hyperthyroidism disappears when sexual maturity is reached.

Hyperthyroidism or exophthalmic goiter with excessive liberation of thyroid hormone is uncommon in children or adolescents.

MINOR NEUROSES

Mildly neurotic symptoms are present in many adolescents. These are usually short-lived and may result from some stress or challenge the youth has had. They persist only if he finds that the symptoms bring rewards from others in his environment.

The adolescent may show symptoms of tension over unpopularity, poor athletic ability, or poor school work. Failure to participate in recreational activities or to gain a degree of independence from his parents, guilt about masturbation, and fear of sexual development or of being unsuccessful may cause neurotic manifestations.

The parents and the adolescent may complain specifically that he has insomnia, nightmares, headaches, difficulty in concentration, and gastrointestinal or menstrual problems.

Treatment of these mild neuroses consists in helping the adolescent to appreciate the basic cause of the problem The physician should have good rapport with the parents and with the adolescent so that they will accept the plan of treatment and cooperate. The family physician or the pediatrician can usually treat these young people successfully If there is a question of a deeper difficulty, however, consultation with a psychiatrist can be sought.

TEACHING AIDS AND OTHER INFORMATION*

American Academy of Pediatrics

A Model Act Providing for Consent of Minors for Health Services.

The Treatment of Acne with Antibiotics.

American Dietetic Association

Food Facts Talk Back.

Consumer Product Information

Myths about Vitamins, 1974.

National Dairy Council

The Food Way to Weight Reduction.

Public Affairs Committee

Irwin, M. H. K.: Overweight—A Problem for Millions.
Irwin, T.: The Rights of Teenagers as Patients, 1972.
Margolius, S.: Health Foods: Facts and Fakes, 1973.

United States Government

Approaches to Health Care for Adolescents in the 1970's, 1975.
Calories and Weight: The USDA Pocket Guide, 1974.
Food and Your Weight, Revised 1973
We Want You to Know What We Know about Cosmetics, 1973.

*Complete addresses are given in the Appendix.

REFERENCES

Books

Arndt, K. A.: *Manual of Dermatologic Therapeutics.* Boston, Little, Brown & Company, 1974.

Bowes, A. D., and Church, C. F.: *Food Values of Portions Commonly Used.* 12th ed. Philadelphia, J. B. Lippincott, 1975.

Bray, G. A., and Bethune, J. E. (Eds.): *Treatment and Management of Obesity.* New York, Harper & Row, 1974.

Cunliffe, W. J., and Cotterill, A.: *Acne.* Philadelphia, W. B. Saunders Company, 1975.

Edinburg, G. M., Zinberg, N. E., and Kelman, W.: *Clinical Interviewing and Counseling: Principles and Techniques.* New York, Appleton-Century-Crofts, 1975.

Garb, S.: *Food: High Nutrition, Low Cost.* New York, Springer Publishing Company, 1975.

Gellis, S. S., and Kagan, B. M.: *Current Pediatric Therapy 7.* Philadelphia, W. B. Saunders Company, 1976.

Guyton, A. C.: *Textbook of Medical Physiology.* 5th ed. Philadelphia, W. B. Saunders Company, 1976.

Heald, F. P. (Ed.): *Adolescent Nutrition and Growth.* New York, Appleton-Century-Crofts, 1969.

Howe, P. S.: *Basic Nutrition in Health and Disease.* 6th ed. Philadelphia, W. B. Saunders Company, 1976.

Kalogerakis, M. G. (Ed.): *The Emotionally Troubled Adolescent and the Family Physician.* Springfield, Ill., Charles C Thomas, 1973.

Kline, M. V., Coleman, L. L., and Wick, E. E. (Eds.): *Obesity.* Springfield, Ill. Charles C Thomas, 1975.

Parrish, J. A.: *Dermatology and Skin Care.* New York, McGraw-Hill Book Company, Inc., 1975.

Sauer, G. C.: *Manual of Skin Diseases.* 3rd ed. Philadelphia, J. B Lippincott Company, 1973.

Stewart, W. D., Danto, J. L., and Maddin, S.: *Dermatology: Diagnosis and Treatment of Cutaneous Disorders.* 3rd ed. St. Louis, the C. V. Mosby Company, 1974.

Vaughan, V. C., III, and McKay, R. J. (Eds.): *Nelson Textbook of Pediatrics.* 10th ed. Philadelphia, W. B. Saunders Company, 1975.

Wallace, H. M., Gold, E. M., and Lis, E. H. (Eds.): *Maternal and Child Health Practices: Problems, Resources, and Methods of Delivery.* Springfield, Ill., Charles C Thomas, 1973.

Wasserman, E., and Slobody, L. B.: *Survey of Clinical Pediatrics.* 6th ed. New York, McGraw-Hill Book Company, Inc., 1974.

Weinberg, S., Shapiro, L., and Leider, M.: *Color Atlas of Pediatric Dermatology.* New York, McGraw-Hill Book Company, 1975.

Winick, M. (Ed.): *Childhood Obesity: Current Concepts in Nutrition.* New York, John Wiley & Sons, Inc., 1975.

Ziai, M. (Ed.): *Pediatrics.* 2nd ed. Boston, Little, Brown & Company, 1975.

Periodicals

Barnes, H. V. (Ed.): Symposium on Adolescent Medicine. *Med. Clin. N. Am.,* 59:1279, November 1975.

Brown, F.: Sexual Problems of the Adolescent Girl. *Pediatr. Clin. N. Am.,* 19:759, August 1972.

Caghan, S. B.: The Adolescent Process and the Problem of Nutrition. *Am. J. Nursing,* 75:1728, October 1975.

Fielding, J. E., and Nelson, S. H.: Health Care for the Economically Disadvantaged. *Pediatr. Clin. N. Am.,* 20:975, November 1973.

Guthrie, A. D., and Howell, M. C.: Mobile Medical Care for Alienated Youths. *J. Pediatr.,* 81:1025, November 1972.

Hammer, S. L.: The Approach to the Adolescent Patient. *Pediatr. Clin. N. Am.,* 20:779, November 1973.

Heald, F. P., and Khan, M. A.: Teenage Obesity. *Pediatr. Clin. N. Am.,* 20:807, November 1973.

Hofmann, A. D., and Pilpel, H. F.: The Legal Rights of Minors. *Pediatr. Clin. N. Am.,* 20:989, February 1973.

Jackson, D. W.: The Adolescent and the Hospital. *Pediatr. Clin. N. Am.,* 20:901, November 1973.

Jacoby, A., Altman, D. G., Cook, J., and Holland, W. W.: Influence of Some Social and Environmental Factors on the Nutrient Intake and Nutritional Status of Schoolchildren. *Br. J. Prev. Soc. Med.,* 29:116, June 1975.

Johnson, C. J., Anderson, H., Spearman, J., and Madson, J.: Ear Piercing and Hepatitis. *J.A.M.A.,* 227:1165, March 11, 1974.

Kalisch, B. J.: The Stigma of Obesity. *Am. J. Nursing,* 72:1124, June 1972.

Kenny, T. J.: The Hospitalized Child. *Pediatr. Clin. N. Am.,* 22:583, August 1975.

Kline, J., and Schowalter, J. E.: How To Care for The 'Betweener-Ager.' *Nursing '74,* 4:42, November 1974.

Leveille, G. A., and Romsos, D. R.: Meal Eating and Obesity. *Nursing Digest,* 4:18, March-April 1976.

Lore, A.: Adolescents: People, Not Problems. *Am. J. Nursing,* 73:1232, July 1973.

Loxsom, R.: Changing Obesity Patterns. *Nursing Outlook,* 23:711, November 1975.

McCormick, W. O.: Amenorrhea and Other Menstrual Symptoms in Student Nurses. *J. Psychosom. Res.,* 19:131, April 1975.

Madsen, K. O.: Frequency of Eating and Dental Health. *Nursing Digest,* 4:80, Summer 1976.

Mahoney, M. J., and Mahoney, K.: Fight Fat With Behavior Control. *Psychology Today,* 9:39, May 1976.

O'Boyle, C. M.: Sports Injuries in Adolescents: Emergency Care. *Am. J. Nursing,* 75:1732, October 1975.

Reisner, R. M.: Acne Vulgaris. *Pediatr. Clin. N. Am.,* 20:851, November 1973.

Skeen, C.: We Made Teen-Age Health Care Free: But It Wasn't Easy. *RN,* 39:38, July 1976.

Sloan, D.: Pelvic Pain and Dysmenorrhea. *Pediatr. Clin. N. Am.,* 19:669, August 1972.

Sternlieb, J. J., and Munan, L.: A Survey of Health Problems, Practices, and Needs of Youth. *Pediatrics,* 49:177, February 1972.

Trowbridge, F. L., Matovinovic, J., McLaren, G. D., and Nichaman, M. Z.: Iodine and Goiter in Children. *Pediatrics,* 56:82, July 1975.

Ujhely, G. B.: Two Types of Problem Patients...And How To Deal With Them. *Nursing 76,* 6:64; May 1976.

Williams, E. R.: Making Vegetarian Diets Nutritious. *Am. J. Nursing,* 75:2168, December 1975.

Wunderlich, R. A., et al.: The Ponderous Problems of Severely Obese Patients...(And of Their Nurses). *Nursing '72,* 2:10, December 1972.

AUDIOVISUAL MEDIA*

Harper & Row Publishers

The Adolescent Patient
   126 slides, 1 cassette, 25 response books.
   Discusses such basic adolescent developmental problems as acceptance of a changing body. Also illustrates the ways in which an adolescent's growth and development can be affected by the stress of illness and hospitalization.

W. B. Saunders Company

Pediatric Conferences with Sydney Gellis
   Obesity in Children, Gellis, S.
   Rhinoplasty in Adolescence, Bloom, S. M.

Trainex Corporation

Clinical Dermatology

35mm. filmstrip, audio-tape cassette, 33⅓ LP, color.
   A brief description of the anatomy and physiology of the skin and its accessory organs. Various forms of inflammatory skin eruptions involving the epidermis are illustrated and discussed.

United States Government

Acne Vulgaris—Its Pathogenesis
   Producer: USNMAC
   15 minutes, 16mm. film, optical sound, color.
   A detailed presentation of the many causes that bring on acne. It attempts to explain the pathogenesis of an individual acne lesion.

*Complete addresses are given in the Appendix.

Chapter Twenty-Seven

EFFECT OF ILLNESS ON ADOLESCENTS

Serious or prolonged illness during infancy or childhood may have negative effects on the personality of the adolescent unless special care has been taken to prevent this. Illness or accident may interfere with the child's sense of trust that his own body or the outside world is really dependable. Illness or accident may prove to the child that he is loved only when he is not well. Prolonged illness may lead the child whose sense of autonomy is not fully developed into overdependency on others. Illness may also in later years so curb the development of a sense of initiative or of industry that the adolescent is unable to gain satisfaction from seeking the answers to questions or from starting or completing a project. Malnutrition, alone or in relation to a disease, may result in apathy and listlessness.

Adolescence is difficult enough for normal young people, but more so for the handicapped person. Accepting his sex role, finding himself, emancipating himself from his family, and selecting a career are difficult. The social aspects of his handicap are much greater during adolescence than they were earlier. If he did not accept the reality of his handicap earlier, he may be emotionally disturbed about it in adolescence.

The effects of a handicap such as impaired hearing, blindness, cardiac disease, diabetes, or cerebral palsy tend to make children of any age overdependent on adults and to warp their personality development in several ways. Such conditions tend to limit both their social contacts with other children and their ability to relieve their pent-up emotions through physical activity, and to cause various degrees of rejection in themselves, their parents and peers. The adolescent, because of his feelings of guilt about his

LONG-TERM CONDITIONS OF THE ADOLESCENT

illness or handicap, may develop feelings of mistrust, self-doubt, and inferiority. He either may give up in the battle for healthy personality development or may seek to punish others for his failure.

On the other hand, if handicapped or chronically ill children have been given the opportunity to master themselves and their environment within the limits of reality, to become independent, they will probably succeed in the battle of life. They must be given the opportunity to try; if they fail, they must be helped in their effort so that they can achieve success. If the adolescent cannot achieve success in the use of his legs, for instance, he can be helped to achieve by using his head or hands. Many people, even so-called normal people, have limitations which only they know. They have been able to use what they have to such advantage that the world is unaware of their handicaps. They have developed a sense of security in their achievements with the help of their parents and other adults. Both they and their parents, facing the handicap realistically together, have been able to build parent-child relations which many normal children and parents might envy.

Long-term illness during adolescence may

have disastrous effects. During illness the youth is unable to discover the kind of person he really is or what his role in the future will be, much less develop the sense of intimacy which is important to his later adjustment.

THE ROLE OF THE NURSE IN CARING FOR THE HOSPITALIZED ADOLESCENT

Adolescents at times complain about vague physical discomforts. Much of this is due to the fact that they have sensations in their changing bodies that they had not noticed before. Adolescents should be examined for pathologic changes. If none are present, the physician or nurse can take advantage of the opportunity to discuss with them problems which may lie behind their complaints. Knowing that they are physically sound or that something can be done about their problems may help to reduce their anxiety.

If the adolescent is to be hospitalized, he can be prepared well for his hospitalization. Any treatments or surgical procedures to be done are explained thoroughly. He is given the opportunity to participate in making decisions which will affect his therapy.

The adolescent, depending on his degree of maturity, can adjust well to the hospital, remembering what he did prior to his admission and what he may do on discharge. He can trust his family and friends to visit him while he is hospitalized. He is able to handle moderate anxiety and to relate to new adults he meets much better than he could when he was younger.

The adolescent, however, may resent the fact

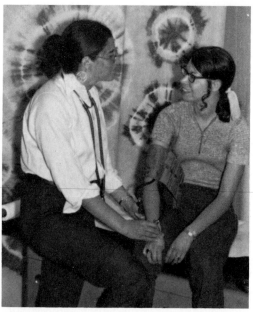

FIGURE 27–1. The noise, color, mod props, and casual atmosphere attract adolescents to a free clinic in Pittsburgh. (From Amenta, M. A.: *Am. J. Nursing*, 74:285, © February 1974. The American Journal of Nursing Company. Reproduced with permission from *The American Journal of Nursing*.)

that his illness interrupts his school and social life. He may be so overburdened with the usual problems of adolescence that he feels overwhelmed by his disease. The adolescent wants to keep the self-image of strength he had created, but with illness he fears that he will no longer be the same, that irreparable damage will be done to him. Like the school-age child (see p. 744), the adolescent may feel that his illness is a punishment for wrongdoing and in an exaggerated way feel that it will affect his life forever,

TABLE 27–1. *HEALTH PROBLEMS MOST OFTEN IDENTIFIED AMONG ADOLESCENT PATIENTS AT MONTEFIORE HOSPITAL AND MEDICAL CENTER*

PRIMARY PROBLEMS OF ADOLESCENCE	PROBLEMS MADE WORSE BY ADOLESCENCE	PROBLEMS WITH ORIGIN DURING ADOLESCENCE
Scoliosis	Tuberculosis	Obesity
Slipped epiphysis	Automotive injuries	Alcoholism
Acne	Unwed pregnancy	Duodenal ulcer
Sports injuries	Suicide	Hypercholesterolemia
Mononucleosis	Diabetes	Labile hypertension
Body image	Inflammatory bowel disease	Irritable colon syndrome
Drug abuse	Menstrual dysfunction	Migraine
Venereal disease	Dental caries	Marital conflicts
Goiter	Abortion	
Sexual dysfunction	Gynecomastia	
Delinquency	Mental retardation	
Tumors	Dying	
Anorexia nervosa		
Hepatitis		
Primary amenorrhea		
School-learning problems		

Adapted from Michael I. Cohen. Iris F. Litt, et al., "Health care for adolescents in a traditional medical setting." Youth, Health and Social Systems Symposium. Washington, D.C., April 1974.

destroying the tentative plans he had made. During illness the adolescent who had appeared to be strong and self-confident may feel weak and threatened. Since he does not want others, especially his peers, to know of these feelings, he may try to hide them even from himself.

If the adolescent is admitted to an adult unit, he may annoy other patients with his noisy activities. He may sustain considerable emotional damage because he is exposed to erroneous information given by adult patients. He may see sights or hear noises that may cause him to be terrified, since the adolescent has increased imagination and a tendency to introspection.

When the adolescent is hospitalized on the adult unit, the question arises as to whether to call him by his first name or to address him as Mr. or Miss or Ms. Such a decision can be made by the adolescent himself. When he has an adult roommate, the adolescent may be at a disadvantage because he is naive about such things as selecting his own diet and planning his own leisure time activities. Embarrassment due to the lack of privacy behind only drawn curtains may lead to the adolescent's taking only partial bed baths or to his becoming constipated because he does not want to use a bedpan. Also the adolescent may want and need "someone to talk to," especially if he has a roommate who is much older than he.

Visitors to a teenage patient on an adult unit may cause some problems for the nursing staff. Although limitations are usually placed on visiting privileges, an adolescent may want to have several of his friends come at once. Usually an explanation as to why he cannot entertain such a group is sufficient, that the noise level would be too much for seriously ill patients and that a group would interfere with the nursing care of patients. If obstreperous groups of young people try to "crash" the unit, usually a firm "No" will restrain them and administrative intervention will not be necessary. The teenager who has no visitors from his peer group should concern the nursing staff more than the one who has too many.

If the adolescent is admitted to the children's unit, he may be annoyed with the crying of younger children, feel isolated because no other adolescents have been admitted, and become embarrassed because of his lack of privacy. He may be concerned about what his friends might think of his being cared for with a group of "babies." He may be annoyed also if the equipment with which he is provided is not of adult size. This is especially true if he is assigned to a large crib in which he cannot fully extend his legs.

In recent years *adolescent units* have been opened in some hospitals. In these units adolescents are comfortable with others in their own age group. Physicians and nurses are also likely to give more understanding care to their patients because they enjoy working with them. It is believed that adolescents need a continuing relation with their pediatricians until they reach maturity and find their place in the world.

In adolescent units the environment of the patients is important. It should be as homelike and informal as possible. A phonograph and a television set in the lounge will encourage the patients to congregate together. A telephone beside each bed enables the adolescent to keep in contact with his friends at home. Certainly liberal visiting hours should be provided, since relations with peers are important at this age. Also, adolescents with their usually large appetites should be permitted to select their menus unless they are on restricted diets. Snacks should be available as needed. Group meetings can be held to expedite understanding between the adolescents and the staff and to encourage communication between the members of each group.

When adolescents are hospitalized in any kind of unit, they are usually mature enough to admit that they are sick and to be aware of the adjustments required by their illness. They may protest, however, about restrictions such as special diets and the necessity for bed rest. They want information about their illnesses and procedures which must be done to them. They need reassurance about their medical progress and condition. Hospitalized adolescents need contact with their peers, diversion, and respect as individuals. The nurse is responsible, therefore, for providing the special kind of care these young people need.

Young adolescents from a deprived socioeconomic group may respond differently to hospitalization from those of middle-class backgrounds. After admission they may shut out their new environment and become unresponsive and sullen. They may not make any effort to engage in self-expressive activity, and not attempt to fill their empty hours with reading or conversation with others. They frequently are disinclined to ask questions abut their condition and do not ask the professional personnel for assistance. Many seem to prefer to suffer in silence and alone, withdrawn except for their eyes, which actively follow any activity around them.

The role of the nurse includes understanding the emotional impact of illness on the individual adolescent, helping him to be actively involved in the solution of his problems, providing the

Text continued on page 861

NURSING ADMISSION HISTORY   12-21 YEARS

DIAGNOSIS: _____

T_____ P_____ R_____ B.P._____

HT._____ WT._____ ALLERGIES_____

PHYSICAL DESCRIPTION: _____

_____

_____

_____

_____

USE PLATE
OR PRINT

M.R. No._____ DATE_____

PT. NAME_____

PARENT_____

ADDRESS_____

_____

DATE OF BIRTH_____ B.C. No._____

M.A. No._____

DIV _____ CLIN._____ P.P. DR._____

Nickname_____ Age_____

Hist. From_____ Lang._____

THE CHILDREN'S HOSPITAL MEDICAL CENTER, BOSTON, MASSACHUSETTS 02115

1. **FAMILY:**

Household composition (i.e., parents, siblings, grandparents, etc.) _____

_____

Names and ages of siblings _____

_____

How can parents usually be reached _____

Language spoken by parents _____

Any additional problems or changes in the family that might affect the patient (i.e., births, deaths, illness, etc.) _____

_____

2. **EATING PATTERNS:**

☐ Yes
Special diet ☐ No   Explain _____

Any food likes and dislikes _____

_____

Example of typical day's meals:

Breakfast @_____	Lunch @_____	Supper @_____	Snacks @_____
_____	_____	_____	_____
_____	_____	_____	_____
_____	_____	_____	_____
_____	_____	_____	_____
_____	_____	_____	_____

3. **SLEEPING:**

☐ Yes
Any problems sleeping at night ☐ No   Explain _____

How many hours of sleep a night _____

03301M 11-74

FIGURE 27–2.   Nursing admission history, 12 to 21 years. (Courtesy of the Children's Hospital Medical Center, Boston, Mass.)

4. ELIMINATION:

How often do you normally have a bowel movement _____

Do you get up to go to the bathroom at night ☐ Yes ☐ No _____

5. PERSONAL HYGIENE:

Do you prefer a shower or tub bath _____

How often do you shampoo your hair _____

Any dental or other appliances _____

6. TEMPERAMENT AND RECREATION:

How would you describe your own temperament (i.e., outgoing, nervous, quiet, etc.) _____

_____

What kinds of recreational activities do you enjoy _____

_____

Any hobbies _____

Responsibilities in home and/or outside of home _____

_____

Smoking habits _____

Do you expect family and/or friends to visit _____

7. SCHOOL:

Name of school _____ Grade _____

Course _____ Performance: ☐ Good ☐ Fair ☐ Poor

8. PAST AND PRESENT HEALTH CARE:

Have you been hospitalized before ☐ Yes ☐ No   When _____

Where _____ Why _____

Can you remember any difficulties encountered with that hospitalization _____

_____

Primary Care recieved from _____

Are there any other health agencies involved with you or your family (i.e., Visiting Nurse Association) _____

_____

Have you been or are you presently involved with any CHMC facility (i.e., clinics, etc.) _____

FIGURE 27–2 *Continued.*

Illustration continued on following page.

9. <u>ADJUSTMENT TO ILLNESS:</u>

What is your understanding of your illness _____

_____

_____

Has anyone explained any possible procedures to you yet   ☐ Yes   ☐ No   Who _____

Explain _____

How has your illness changed your daily routines _____

_____

What questions do you have now about your illness _____

_____

Do you now take medication at home   ☐ Yes   ☐ No   What _____

What medications have you taken today _____

What aspects of your care do you do yourself _____

_____

Who else assists in your care _____

10. <u>ADDITIONAL QUESTIONS ASKED BY PATIENT OR FAMILY:</u>

_____

_____

_____

11. <u>ADDITIONAL OBSERVATIONS DURING INTERVIEW:</u>

_____

_____

_____

12. <u>INITIAL NURSING PROBLEMS FOR CARE PLAN:</u>

1. _____

2. _____

3. _____

4. _____

COMMENTS: _____

_____

_____

_____

Date: _____ Nurse Interviewer: _____

FIGURE 27–2 *Continued.*

physical care which he cannot complete himself, and remaining calm in the face of the defenses he may use to make others believe that he is in control. If the nurse is successful, the adolescent may be able to continue to respect himself and have the courage to face the future.

The nurse may find working with adolescents a difficult matter if he or she does not understand them and does not remember the professional role in working with them. The adolescent may feel embarrassed when being given personal care by a nurse just a few years older than he. He may also be shy about exposing portions of his body to someone near his own age. Many times adolescents relate more easily to an older, more mature person; however, it is ultimately the responsibility of the nurse to work out personal feelings in order to provide professional care to these patients.

By being aware of an adolescent's problem about acceptance of his newly developing body, the nurse may be of great help to him at the time of a physical examination or when he is receiving treatments. The adolescent girl, when examined by a male physician, and the adolescent boy, when examined by a female physician, need support to lessen their embarrassment. The nurse should stay if the adolescent indicates that he or she would feel more comfortable. The nurse can also explain what the physician will do and afterward can help the patient understand what has been found. Adolescents will often feel more comfortable with a nurse of their own sex.

If the nurse recognizes the fears characteristic of this phase of growth, the meaning behind some of the adolescent's seemingly purposeless questions can be sensed. The nurse can help him by explaining that fears of this sort are common and are understandable. Adolescents need assurance that they are normal males or females. For a nurse to say to a pubescent girl, "Your genitalia must be abnormal, because I cannot locate the meatus," during a catheterization is inexcusable.

The nurse must understand that adolescents are frequently unpredictable, and that they may be emotionally unstable and torn between their desires to be dependent and independent. The nurse must also remember their great need for security, to love and be loved, to be an accepted group member and to be approved. Sometimes these very needs make it difficult for them to verbalize their anxieties and feelings about illness and hospitalization. In addition, their language may be such that adults may not be able to understand the real meaning of what they say.

The nurse must be able to detect hostility and rejection in these patients. Adolescents may resent hospital rules and regulations because these may represent an extension of parental authority from which they are trying to emancipate themselves. When such feelings are evident, the nurse must often alter the approach completely in order to gain cooperation from them. The nurse must remember not to argue with them, to avoid giving rigid orders to them, and to let them be as independent as possible. They should be trusted and treated as if they were grown up. If an adolescent placidly accepts the rules and regulations without question, the nurse should wonder whether this is good adjustment or evidence of regression and denial.

The nurse in the hospital must provide the young person with freedom but with guidance and restrictions when necessary. The limits established on behavior must be flexible, according to the capacity of the individual patient to handle situations. Restrictions must be related to privileges, and privileges must be related to responsibility. For example, although visiting hours may be over routinely at 9 P.M., if the friends of an adolescent patient who has a birthday wish to give him or her a party lasting until 9:30, they might be permitted to do so. They must realize, however, that excessive noise may disturb other patients; therefore they must assume the responsibility of remaining relatively quiet. They should also assume the responsibility of straightening up the area when the party is over.

Adolescents in the hospital tend to form peer groups just as they would at home. These groups are generally composed of patients of a wide age range and are less stable than in the nonhospitalized group because of admissions and discharges. Within such a peer group adolescents with similar problems tend to find common interests in relation to the parts of their bodies affected. An example of this is the close bond adolescents having scoliosis form when hospitalized together. The nurse must be aware of the structure of such a group, its leader, and its followers. The group can be influenced if its leader believes in the value of the nurse's ideas.

The nurse must also remember the emotional development of the persons involved. One of the greatest fears of adolescents is that of losing control of themselves in front of others, especially their peers. The nurse can see that this does not happen by handling them in a firm, consistent but fair manner. If an adolescent boy or girl, but particularly a boy, is to face a painful treatment, it might be better to remove him from the group so that he can express his feelings

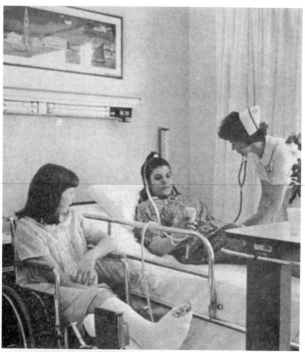

FIGURE 27-3. Relationships with nursing personnel and peer groups are very important to the hospitalized adolescent, especially if on bedrest. (From Weinberg, S., Schonberg, C. E., and Grier, D. Y.: *Nursing Outlook*, 17:18, December, 1968.)

openly rather than have him cry in the presence of others and be humiliated.

The nurse may feel that simply because the patient is not a child he should understand that whatever is done is for his good and may fail to explain treatments to him. The adolescent, who is keenly interested in himself, his body, and his illness, needs detailed explanations frequently.

In giving such explanations the nurse must be willing to answer questions and to offer reassurance just as for younger children. The nurse should be willing to spend time with the adolescent and to provide support when he needs it.

The adolescent who is scheduled for surgery under general anesthesia faces a period of maximum helplessness. During adolescence the psychologic effects of surgery are often greater than the physical ones. It is not until the adolescent is 19 years of age or older that his terror of surgery may be reduced. Adolescents usually behave like young adults, but during stress they regress and revert to childlike behavior.

Adolescents are obsessed with their own bodies. They have a fear of physically surrendering their bodies to another as in surgery. Adolescent girls are very concerned with disfigurement, especially of their faces, while boys are concerned, perhaps on a subconscious level, with a loss of sexual potency. Loss of hair is very upsetting to members of both sexes. Adolescents may find reassurance by talking with others who have already had such a surgical procedure, as well as utilizing the support given by the nurse.

The adolescent subjected to enforced limitation of motion may have adverse physical and emotional responses. He may have feelings of shame and loss of self-esteem and become insecure, anxious, dependent, aggressive, and hostile. He may complain of physical discomfort and may show changes in his pattern of sleep. The anxiety of the adolescent may be reduced by sharing with him his medical condition, the progress he is making, and any procedures which must be done. If the adolescent is dependent on others for his total care, he may

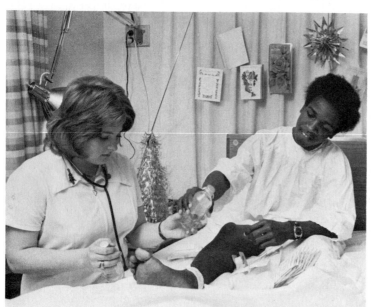

FIGURE 27-4. An adolescent shows independence in care as he dresses his own leg ulcer. (Courtesy of Esther Bubley, photographer, New York, N.Y. © 1973, The American Journal of Nursing Company. Reproduced with permission from *The American Journal of Nursing*, Vol. 73, No. 12.)

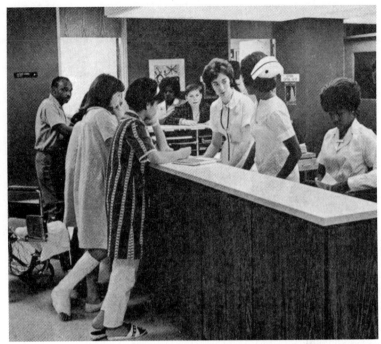

FIGURE 27–5. The nurses' station on the adolescent unit is a favorite hangout for ambulatory patients. They listen with interest to instructions about x-rays, diets, and the school program. (From Weinberg, S., Schonberg, C. E., and Grier, D. Y.: *Nursing Outlook,* 17:18, December, 1968.)

make excessive demands, evidence irrational fears, and reject therapy when it is given, or he may become totally dependent and helpless. Such an adolescent needs reassurance and encouragement to do as much self-care as is possible.

Adolescent girls are interested in making themselves as attractive as possible. Lipstick and other cosmetics are important to them. The nurse must understand that helping a young girl comb her hair in an attractive way, even though she is immobilized in a body cast, is an important part of nursing care.

Many times adolescents seek physical contact from the nurses who care for them. They may want to hold hands or may request repeated backrubs. Touch in this situation, as in infancy, has implications for physical survival as well as for emotional self-esteem. In such a situation the patient may represent a threat for the inexperienced nurse. The nurse, especially if near the patient's age, must consider how such physical closeness is perceived personally and how the adolescent perceives it. The nurse may find it helpful to discuss this sort of situation in conference so that it does not become too disturbing. Since the adolescent usually respects the nurses who care for him, he will respond best if all of them handle his requests in a consistent manner.

The hospitalized adolescent needs help in the task of developing social competencies which include self-help skills and socialization. He is helped to continue with his school work, even though he is ill, so that he can feel that he is achieving and can join his group at school when he is discharged. The teenager's mind must be occupied with recreational interests when he is not doing school work. He enjoys watching television, listening to the radio, or helping with the care of others or with their school work.

The physician and the nurse can help the adolescent by keeping the school teacher in the hospital and the school nurse in the community informed of the adolescent's disability and thereby help them to gain insight into his physical and psychologic needs in relation to his illness. They can also interpret to members of the community the fact that his basic needs are like those of normal adolescents.

In summary, if adolescents are given love, with limitations on their behavior, and with increasing amounts of responsibility for themselves and others in the hospital as well as at home, they will continue in their growth toward the goal of the independence of adulthood.

ILLNESS DURING ADOLESCENCE

The fact that children grow rapidly, physically and emotionally, during pubescence and adolescence makes them particularly vulnerable to certain illnesses which may result in significant effects on the developmental process. Accidents, however, are the principal cause of death. The death rate from illness in this age group is relatively low.

TABLE 27-2. DEATHS AND DEATH RATES
FOR THE 10 LEADING CAUSES OF DEATH
FOR SPECIFIED AGE GROUPS, BY SEX:
UNITED STATES, 1975

RANK ORDER	AGE, SEX, AND CAUSE OF DEATH	NUMBER	RATE
	15–24 Years—Male		
	All causes	35,508	176.8
1	Accidents	19,416	96.7
	Motor vehicle accidents	12,244	61.0
	All other accidents	7,172	35.7
2	Homicide	4,258	21.2
3	Suicide	3,787	18.9
4	Malignant neoplasms, including neoplasms of lymphatic and hematopoietic tissues	1,626	8.1
5	Diseases of heart	631	5.1
6	Influenza and pneumonia	417	2.1
7	Congenital anomalies	381	1.9
8	Cerebrovascular diseases	310	1.5
9	Diabetes mellitus	90	0.4
10	Anemias	80	0.4
	All other causes	4,512	22.5
	15–24 Years—Female		
	All causes	12,037	60.5
1	Accidents	4,705	23.7
	Motor vehicle accidents	3,428	17.2
	All other accidents	1,277	6.4
2	Homicide	1,235	6.2
3	Malignant neoplasms, including neoplasms of lymphatic and hematopoietic tissues	1,075	5.4
4	Suicide	949	4.8
5	Diseases of heart	414	2.1
6	Influenza and pneumonia	272	1.4
7	Congenital anomalies	265	1.3
8	Cerebrovascular diseases	238	1.2
9	Complications of pregnancy, childbirth, and the puerperium	151	0.8
10	Diabetes mellitus	88	0.4
	All other causes	2,645	13.3

Rates per 100,000 estimated population in specified groups.
Department of Health, Education, and Welfare, Public Health
Service, National Center for Health Statistics.

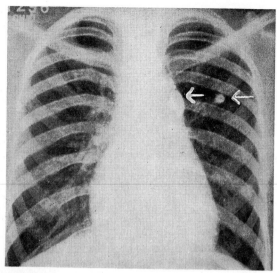

FIGURE 27-6. Calcified tuberculous focus (right arrow) and calcified tracheobronchial lymph node (left arrow) in a young girl. (From Vaughan, V. C. III, and McKay, R. J. (Eds.): *Nelson Textbook of Pediatrics.* 10th ed. Philadelphia, W. B. Saunders Co., 1975.)

Illnesses may occur in adolescents which are more closely related to their *emotional* development than to their physical growth. Although some of these illnesses are discussed in this chapter, it must be remembered that most adolescents reach normal levels of maturity for their age and ultimately become contributing members of their communities and positive models for their children, the next generation, to emulate.

TUBERCULOSIS

Tuberculosis is a world-wide disease. Although its incidence has decreased in the more advanced countries, it is still prevalent in underdeveloped countries. The methods used to control tuberculosis in this country have brought excellent results, but they cannot be applied with equal success in other countries. Each country must find methods which can be utilized successfully with its own people in the areas of ed-

ucational programs, better standards of living, earlier diagnosis and the best methods of treatment. The World Health Organization is working to help countries to bring this infection under control.

Incidence. Although tuberculosis was at one time a leading cause of death, its incidence has been reduced in recent years. It is still true, however, that adolescents seem more susceptible to this disease than persons in other age groups. The fact that adolescent girls seem to be more susceptible at an earlier age than boys may be related to their earlier maturation. The incidence is high in slum areas where overcrowding and poor health conditions are prevalent. There is also a higher incidence in areas with periods of flood or famine.

Early discovery and improved methods of treatment provide these young people with a good chance of cure.

Etiology and Epidemiology. Tuberculosis is caused by an acid-fast bacillus, *Mycobacterium tuberculosis.* Disease in man is produced by organisms causing either the bovine or the human form of the disease. A person may contract tuberculosis by drinking contaminated milk, although this method of infection has been almost completely eliminated in this country, owing to the practices of killing diseased cattle, forbidding the sale of contaminated milk, pasteurization of milk, and testing milk handlers for tuberculosis.

The bacillus enters the body through the respiratory or the gastrointestinal tract. It is spread today chiefly by droplet infection or by direct contact with infected human beings. Entrance into the body may also take place by ingestion.

Children most frequently contract tuberculosis from an infected adult in the home. This is the reason why newborn infants should be removed from mothers who have the disease; the mothers cannot then contaminate the children by breathing or coughing on them while feeding or caring for them. Older children and adolescents may contract the disease in their own homes or in the homes of friends or from close contact with their peer groups. Children of any age may put contaminated objects into their mouths. The unhygienic practice of sharing taffies, candy, or drinking or eating utensils may help spread the disease.

Predisposing Factors, Types of Infection, and Pathology. Chronic illness, fatigue, or undernutrition may predispose to tuberculosis.

A *primary infection* occurs when the tubercle bacillus enters the body, usually in the tissues of the lungs. Individual resistance and the number of organisms entering the body determine the extent of the disease. The reaction of the invaded tissue is basically one of inflammation and repair with later calcification, which may be noted on an x-ray film. The primary focus usually heals spontaneously.

The primary (Ghon) complex includes the initial lesion and lesions in the regional lymph nodes. The disease process may extend to other parts of the lung and to the gastrointestinal tract because of swallowed infected sputum. In some cases the organisms may produce symptoms of mild pneumonia. The organisms may enter the lymph nodes, lymph vessels, and blood vessels. Foci of infection then occur in various organs and in serous membranes.

When widespread infection occurs, the child is said to have *miliary tuberculosis*. This type generally occurs in the infant or very young child. Its onset is usually acute, with an irregular fever, rales in the chest, possibly an enlarged spleen, distended abdomen, prostration, dyspnea, cough and cyanosis. The mortality rate has been reduced through the use of newer drugs.

If the acid-fast bacillus affects the meninges, *tuberculous meningitis* may result. Tuberculosis of the mesenteric or cervical lymph nodes, peritoneum, bones, and joints may also occur. The bones most frequently involved include the head of the femur (*tuberculous coxitis*), fingers and toes (*tuberculous dactylitis*), and vertebrae (*tuberculous spondylitis* or *Pott's disease*).

If the child's resistance is good, healing of a primary lesion and calcification may take place. Later, because of lowered resistance, the latent lesion may again become active.

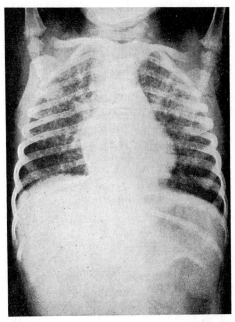

FIGURE 27–7. Miliary tuberculosis of the lungs in a boy 3 years of age. His mother had pulmonary tuberculosis. The physical findings were fine, crackling rales throughout both lungs. Death occurred shortly after this roentgenogram was taken. The tuberculin reaction was positive. (From Vaughan, V. C., III, and McKay, R. J. (Eds.): *Nelson Textbook of Pediatrics*. 10th ed. W. B. Saunders Co., Philadelphia, 1975.)

Secondary infections usually occur during adolescence or early in adult life either from the original focus or from reinfection. They differ from the primary type because of the allergic response of the body. Reinfection is a much more destructive process than the primary lesion. Secondary infection may include extensive inflammatory reaction with tissue destruction and cavitation. Healing in secondary infections is largely by means of scar tissue or fibrosis. The pulmonary lesion in a secondary infection is likely to be in the apex of the lung.

Clinical Manifestations and Diagnosis. In *primary* tuberculosis the *manifestations* of a pulmonary lesion may or may not be evident. The child may complain of malaise, fatigue, and anorexia, have a weight loss, and be irritable. If tuberculosis is suspected, but no symptoms are evident, the *diagnosis* may be made with a tuberculin test and an x-ray film of the chest.

The clinical manifestations of *secondary* tuberculosis may resemble those of infected adults. The disease may become chronic, progressive pulmonary tuberculosis with cough and expectoration, fever, hemoptysis, weight loss, and night sweats.

For diagnostic testing two types of tuberculin are available: old tuberculin (O.T.) and purified protein derivative (P.P.D.). The tests used in the diagnosis of tuberculosis are the Mantoux test and the Heaf multiple puncture test or the tine test.

MANTOUX TEST. About six weeks after infection of a tuberculin-negative person the presence of allergy or hypersensitivity to tuberculoprotein may be observed by a positive skin test reaction to tuberculin. A known amount of tuberculin is injected intracutaneously. The test should be read in 48 to 72 hours. In a positive reaction an area at least 5 mm. in diameter with erythema and definite induration occurs. The exact measurement of the reaction should be recorded. The larger the area of reaction, the greater is the risk that the child has a tuberculous infection. This is a most accurate test.

HEAF MULTIPLE PUNCTURE TEST (OR ITS MODIFICATION, THE TINE TEST). In the tine test a stainless steel disk with four prongs precoated with concentrated old tuberculin is pressed firmly against the cleansed (using alcohol or acetone) volar surface of the forearm. The tines penetrate the skin, depositing the tuberculin in the outer layer. The test should be read in 48 to 72 hours. The reaction is considered positive if the induration around one or more of the puncture sites is 2 mm. or more in diameter. Any person having doubtful reactions should be tested with a Mantoux test.

MEANING OF REACTIONS. A positive tuberculin reaction is usually evidence that the person has been infected with the tubercle bacillus and is allergic or hypersensitive to its protein. It does not necessarily mean that the person has an active lesion at the time of testing. The size of the skin reaction indicates whether the result is positive or negative.

Tuberculin tests should be done on the advice of the physician, depending on the risk of exposure of the child and the prevalence of tuberculosis in his geographic area. This would help in locating the source of infection.

Every child who shows a positive reaction to tuberculin should have a physical examination, have his temperature checked, and have a chest roentgenogram, blood cell count, and sedimentation rate done. Contacts, whether parents, grandparents, siblings, or friends, should be located and checked for tuberculosis.

A positive diagnosis of tuberculosis is made if the tubercle bacillus is found in the gastric contents or sputum. Young children seldom expectorate. Since sputum is swallowed, examination of the stomach contents obtained by gastric aspiration is of value.

Before breakfast a lavage tube is passed. After a few cubic centimeters of water have been injected a sample of the stomach contents is withdrawn by means of a syringe. The sediment in the return is examined for the tubercle bacillus by culture or guinea pig inoculation, or both. The test should be repeated three times before the result is considered negative.

Treatment and Responsibilities of the Nurse. Whether the patient is given care at home or in a hospital, the plan for his care depends on the total situation. If someone in his environment is infected, the patient is removed from continued contact with this source of infection.

The patient should have mental and physical rest. Rest in bed may be necessary. A daily schedule to which he adheres is essential. Too much activity must be avoided. He must be kept out of school for his own sake and for the safety of other pupils. Adequate health supervision is essential.

The emotional attitude of the child and his family can be optimistic. The child is isolated from close contact with other family members to prevent the spread of infection and also for his own protection from exposure to other infections which would tend further to drain his bodily resources. Measles is especially dangerous for a child with tuberculosis.

The patient requires an adequate diet, high in protein, calcium, and vitamins, particularly B, C, and D. Feeding should not be forced, but the child is encouraged to eat sufficient food. Fresh air and sunshine may aid in his recovery and add to his sense of well-being.

The patient resumes his usual activities gradually as the lesion heals. He is encouraged to do whatever he can for himself in order to prevent invalidism. He is encouraged to plan with his parents and counselor for the future. The adolescent and even the older grade school child can be a member of the health team which plans for his care and rehabilitation. This team also includes his parents, physician, social worker, public school or visiting teacher, and school nurse practitioner or school nurse. Even during convalescence the child is helped to keep in contact with his friends. A telephone near his bed and active correspondence with relatives and friends are of great value in helping him feel that he is still a part of his group and will return to them.

Several drugs have been used successfully in the treatment of tuberculosis, although no one specific drug will cure the disease. Prolonged treatment, from six months to a year or longer, is usually necessary.

Isoniazid (INH) is the most effective drug in common use against tuberculosis. It is administered with one or more antituberculosis drugs if the patient has an active disease, in order to reduce the chance of emergence of resistant mycobacterial strains. It has a low toxicity, can control progressive lesions, and is effective in preventing hematogenous dissemination. It may be given orally or parenterally. Stimulation of the central nervous system by the drug may result in excitement or convulsions which can be controlled by the administration of pyridoxine.

Streptomycin (SM) is given intramuscularly. Long-term treatment may be complicated by labyrinth disorders and possibly deafness. Streptomycin is not used alone against tuberculosis, since streptomycin-resistant organisms rapidly emerge. Another tuberculostatic agent should be given at the same time.

Aminosalicylic acid (para-aminosalicylic acid or PAS) is given orally. It is not as effective as streptomycin or isoniazid. The usual toxic reaction is gastric irritation. PAS is valuable because it inhibits the development of resistance by the bacilli to both streptomycin and isoniazid and it enhances the effectiveness of isoniazid. This drug must be given in such large dosage that it may create a problem when it is ordered for a young child.

These drugs in various combinations have reduced the length of tuberculous infection and also certain secondary forms of the infection.

Other drugs which may be used include rifampin, cycloserine and possibly pyrazinamide, ethionamide, and ethambutol. Rifampin is probably one of the best drugs discovered for tuberculosis. These drugs may be used when there is mycobacterial resistance or patient-sensitivity to standard drugs. Whether cortisone and corticotropin therapy is used depends on the type of lesion present.

Surgical treatment of tuberculous lesions other than bronchoscopy is rarely indicated in children.

If the child or adolescent is properly motivated, he will stay on his therapy for the full course. Enthusiastic encouragement must be given by the members of the health team after the patient and his parents have been taught the facts about the disease. The nurse in the community should visit with the family regularly to reinforce the teachings.

If the patient does not take the prescribed medication, the therapy will fail. An adolescent especially must be helped to develop ways to remind himself to take his drugs daily, since it is his responsibility. The nurse can give the adolescent individual attention to secure his cooperation. Sometimes parents ignore the problem because they do not want anyone to know of the treatment even when it is only prophylactic for a tuberculin-positive patient. The school nurse practitioner or school nurse can often help such an adolescent to remember appointments with

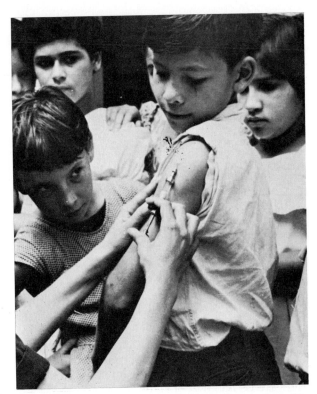

FIGURE 27–8.   BCG vaccine is being used to vaccinate this child against tuberculosis. The World Health Organization has used BCG vaccination for the immunization of millions of children throughout the world in an effort to eliminate tuberculosis. (Byrd: *Health*, 4th ed. W. B. Saunders Co., Philadelphia, 1966.)

his physician and to take the medications as ordered. Nurses caring for the patient in the hospital and in the community must help the child or adolescent and his family to understand the disease, to continue therapy, and to resolve any sense of guilt they may have about this infection.

Prognosis, Prevention, and Methods of Control.   In general the mortality rate is higher in infancy and adolescence than in childhood.

The primary lesion, usually benign, may become an extensive infection. The younger the child, the greater is the danger. During adolescence, however, there is an increased risk of development of chronic, progressive pulmonary tuberculosis, either from the primary focus or from reinfection. With secondary lesions the prognosis depends on the severity of the lesion, and sex, age, and environment of the child.

In recent years antimicrobial treatment has prevented the development of miliary tuberculosis and tuberculous meningitis in infants and toddlers who have been infected with tuberculosis. It has also prevented older children who have recently become tuberculin-positive from acquiring the disease. When isoniazid is given to such children for one year, the localized lesion usually does not progress, and hematogenous dissemination usually does not occur.

If the child or adolescent having a positive tuberculin reaction contracts measles or pertussis, he should receive chemoprophylactic therapy.

The only effective means to prevent tuberculosis is to avoid contact with infected persons. Widespread education of the public is essential. In order to build their resistance to the tubercle bacilli, persons should be taught to maintain adequate nutrition and to avoid fatigue and debilitating infections. They are taught to drink only pasteurized milk from cows free of tuberculosis. They can be helped to understand the disease and the value of early diagnosis and treatment. Communities can organize tuberculin-testing and case-finding programs and also public health programs for control of the disease. These programs should include treatment of infectious patients, case-finding, examination of contacts, supervision of inactive cases, x-ray screening and measures to improve community health.

Ways to develop artificial immunity against tuberculosis have been attempted. Vaccination with BCG (Bacillus of Calmette and Guérin) has been used. This vaccine may be given intradermally. The actual period of resistance to infection after the use of BCG is not known. Because BCG vaccine changes nonreactors to tuberculin tests into reactors, tests subsequent to its administration are of no value.

INFECTIOUS MONONUCLEOSIS

Definition, Etiology and Epidemiology. Infectious mononucleosis is an acute, world-wide illness, the cause of which is usually considered to be a virus. A herpes-type virus known as the EB (Epstein and Barr) virus has appeared to be implicated in this disease. This condition occurs chiefly in older children and adolescents, although it may appear at any time in life. Although it is only mildly contagious, it may appear in epidemic form; however, sporadic cases are more commonly seen.

The incubation period is from one to two weeks. The period of communicability is not known. The mode of transmission is by direct contact with patients or by droplet infection. This disease is commonly believed to be spread by kissing and is therefore sometimes called the "kissing disease."

Pathology, Clinical Manifestations, Diagnosis and Differential Diagnosis. Infectious mononucleosis is a generalized disease which causes enlargement of lymphoid tissue throughout the body. *Clinical manifestations* vary markedly, but may include fever, pharyngitis, tonsillitis, generalized lymphadenopathy, especially of the cervical glands, splenomegaly, atypical lymphocytes, and the presence of heterophil antibodies. Anorexia and general malaise may occur. Skin rashes may occur early in the disease. Hepatitis with jaundice may be a common manifestation. Neurologic manifestations may include severe headache, nuchal rigidity, mental confusion, blurring of vision, and perhaps convulsions. Pneumonitis, myocarditis, and pericarditis may also occur.

Diagnosis is based on laboratory findings: the peripheral blood smear reveals the presence of atypical lymphocytes, the leukocyte count may be normal or low, and the polymorphonuclear cells may increase initially. Lymphocytic leukocytosis develops which may reach leukemoid levels during the first days of the disease.

The heterophil antibody test is useful in the diagnosis, but positive results may or may not be obtained. An accurate two-minute slide test using a small amount of fingertip blood has been developed for the diagnosis of infectious mononucleosis. It is an extremely specific and sensitive test.

Treatment, Responsibilities of the Nurse, Prognosis, and Prevention. *Treatment* and *nursing care* are not specific and consist of symptomatic management, including bed rest and a high caloric diet. Bland, cool liquids are given to increase fluid intake when the adolescent has a severe sore throat. The patient must be observed for unusual manifestations of the disease. Steroid hormones, as well as other drugs, may be used to treat complications such as severe dysphagia, myocarditis, pericarditis, hepatitis, or hemolytic anemia.

The *prognosis* is usually good unless complications develop. Recovery is usually slow; complete return to full strength may not occur for several weeks. This inactivity is difficult for the adolescent to accept because of his involvement in various school and extracurricular activities. The nurse can assist him to make arrangements to continue his studies in bed until he has recovered. This necessary change in lifestyle may lead to resentment and depression. The nurse can listen to the expression of these feelings and thus help to reduce the anxiety of the adolescent.

There is no known means of *prevention*, although research is currently being done on a vaccine to protect against infectious mononucleosis.

ATHEROSCLEROSIS

Since atherosclerosis has seemingly increased in incidence in middle-aged adults, interest has been focused recently on the possible origin of the condition in children and adolescents. Attention has been given to the known risk factors in adults: hypertension, hyperlipidemia, and cigarette smoking.

In infants, *fatty streaks*, an abnormal lipid accumulation in the intima of large elastic and muscular arteries, may begin to appear in the aorta. These may disappear, remain unchanged, or later develop into atherosclerotic plaques. Black and female children have a greater proportion of aortic intimal surface involved with fatty streaks than do white and male children. Before 20 years of age, *raised atherosclerotic lesions* may be present in both the coronary arteries and the aorta. These lesions tend to narrow the arterial lumen so that later thrombosis and occlusion may occur. Prevention of this sequence of events and early recognition are important in relation to the risk factors noted.

The prognosis of children with *hypertension* is dependent on the height of either the systolic or diastolic blood pressure. A family history that includes close relatives who have hypertension is important in the case-finding and identification of children who will possibly be hypertensives as adolescents and adults. Such children should have yearly blood pressure measurements through adult life. When hypertension does develop, the recommended treatment includes the restriction of salt, weight reduction, and appropriate drug therapy. The individual may have to change his lifestyle to reduce his blood pressure.

Familial *hyperlipidemia* can be diagnosed in children by determining their level of total serum cholesterol. This is especially important for children in a family where a parent has had a coronary problem before the age of 50 years. Treatment of hyperlipidemia in children is usually unsatisfactory; however, alterations in diet may be recommended.

Cigarette smoking is related to the development of coronary atherosclerosis. Young men who smoke heavily are especially at risk. It is important, therefore, for both physicians and nurses to make a major effort through education to prevent adolescents from beginning to smoke and to assist those who have already started the habit to stop.

Environmental factors, not yet clearly defined, may also predispose the adolescent to atherosclerosis.

HYPERTENSION

Etiology, Incidence, Clinical Manifestations, Diagnosis, and Prognosis. A variety of acute and chronic illnesses of childhood have hypertension as a clinical manifestation. Essential hypertension may occur, but usually hypertension is a secondary manifestation of such conditions as coarctation of the aorta (see p. 281), glomerulonephritis (see p. 664), pheochromocytoma, Wilms' tumor (see p. 311) or neuroblastoma (see p. 477), and the taking of oral contraceptives (see p. 885), among others.

From infancy through adolescence blood pressure normally increases. It is not known precisely what level of blood pressure should be considered abnormal for any specific age; however, a child whose diastolic blood pressure is 90 mm. Hg or above could be considered hypertensive. Hypertension can also be defined as systolic and diastolic pressures that are repeatedly between the 90th and 95th percentiles for their age on at least one testing occasion.

Hypertension is more common in the black population than among whites in this country. Since the *incidence* of hypertension appears to be increasing, it is important that blood pressure be measured during routine physical examinations on all children from toddler age through the adolescent years.

The *clinical manifestations* of hypertension include frequent headaches (frontal in nature), possible changes in vision, and dizziness. Anorexia, lethargy, and failure to thrive may be additional problems. Vomiting may occur if hypertensive encephalopathy is present in addition to seizures, stupor and coma. Sustained systemic hypertension may cause deterioration of renal functioning and heart failure.

Mild hypertension may cause no clinical manifestations in children and adolescents. It is important, however, to obtain a family history with particular emphasis on close relatives who have hypertension, heart disease, and stroke.

The *diagnosis* of the exact cause of hypertension in children and adolescents may be difficult. The *prognosis* of individual hypertensive patients depends on the underlying cause of the condition and its treatment.

Treatment. *Treatment* may be through the use of antihypertensive drugs. The dose depends on the needs of the individual patient. The goal of treatment with hypertensive drugs is to achieve normotension during the day without inflicting problems on the individual due to the side effects of the drug. Usually the patient is given only one drug at a time until its effect is known.

The drugs usually used in the treatment of *acute hypertension* in the pediatric age group include hydralazine (Apresoline) and reserpine (Serpasil), each given alone or in combination. Hydralazine decreases peripheral resistance and increases cardiac output, thus lowering blood pressure. This drug may be given orally or parenterally. Side effects include headaches, which may respond to antihistamine medication, and nausea. Side effects of reserpine may include depression, nasal congestion, sedation, and bradycardia.

Diuretics may be given for their action of reducing extracellular fluid volume. Their use, therefore, is combined with a reduced sodium intake. Thiazide diuretics or chlorthalidone may be given. Diazoxide (Hyperstat) also lowers blood pressure in acute hypertension.

These drugs, in addition to intravenous methyldopa (Aldomet) and ganglion blocking agents, may be used in emergency situations. The side effects of methyldopa include emotional lability, bradycardia, postural hypotension, and drowsiness.

In the treatment of *chronic hypertension* guanethidine (Ismelin) may be used. Since this drug has little effect when the child is in the supine position, he should sleep with several pillows or with the head of his bed elevated. Hydralazine may also be given. Postural hypotension may be observed early in the morning when these drugs are used. This can be prevented if the patient gets out of bed slowly, sitting on the side of the bed for awhile before rising. Mild diarrhea may be a complication. Activity may be restricted when guanethidine is used because of postexercise syncope or postural hypotension.

Oral methyldopa may be given for long-standing hypertension. Drowsiness may result, but side effects are rare. Reserpine and methyldopa are incompatible when given simultaneously.

The use of diuretics and a reduced salt intake may also be effective in the treatment of chronic hypertension. Hypertensive children are usually not otherwise restricted in their activity or their diet.

Surgery may be done for specific diagnoses such as coarctation of the aorta, hydronephrosis, renal artery stenosis, and pheochromocytoma. It is likely that surgery can result in a permanent cure.

Responsibilities of the Nurse. Since hypertension appears to be increasing among children and adolescents, it is important that nurses in all settings take the blood pressure when doing nursing assessments on well children over the age of two years and on adolescents. It is also the responsibility of the school nurse or school nurse practitioner to screen students for hypertension during their school years. The nurse can assume an active role in referral and follow-up when a child having a blood pressure above normal is found.

The nurse is responsible for using a cuff of the correct size when taking blood pressure readings on children. The bladder of the cuff should be large enough to cover two thirds of the upper arm without covering the antecubital fossa. The length of the bladder of the cuff should be long enough to encircle the upper arm so that all adipose tissue overlying the brachial artery is evenly compressed.

Blood pressure readings are taken when the child or adolescent is at rest and accustomed to his surroundings. Agitation, anxiety, and the use of a blood pressure cuff that is too small may result in falsely elevated blood pressure values. A cuff that is too large may result in erroneously low readings.

In order to take blood pressure readings on their own child, many parents purchase a sphygmomanometer. The nurse is responsible for teaching them the method of measuring the blood pressure accurately. Taking measurements correctly at home and reporting them can reduce the frequency of visits to the physician's office.

If the child or adolescent has chronic hypertension, too rapid correction of the condition may result in hypotensive symptoms, in spite of the fact that the blood pressure reading may still be above normal. The nurse must be aware of this possibility and report any changes in the patient's condition.

Nursing intervention includes health teaching. Knowledge about the predisposing factors of hypertension such as obesity, smoking, excessive salt intake, and chronic frustration and stress can form a basis for teaching parents and children how to improve their health and possibly prevent hypertension in later years. Since adolescents need to participate in their health care and assume responsibility for it, they especially should learn the predisposing factors of hypertension.

The treatment of hypertension in the pediatric group does not show short-term benefits. It is important, therefore, for the nurse to discuss with the parents and children the reasons for long-term therapy and the possible side effects of the drugs used. Emphasis is placed on the need for follow-up care even when the patients feel well.

Orthopedic Disorders

SCOLIOSIS

Incidence and Types. Scoliosis is an S-shaped lateral curvature usually associated with rotation of the spine. Scoliosis is most frequent

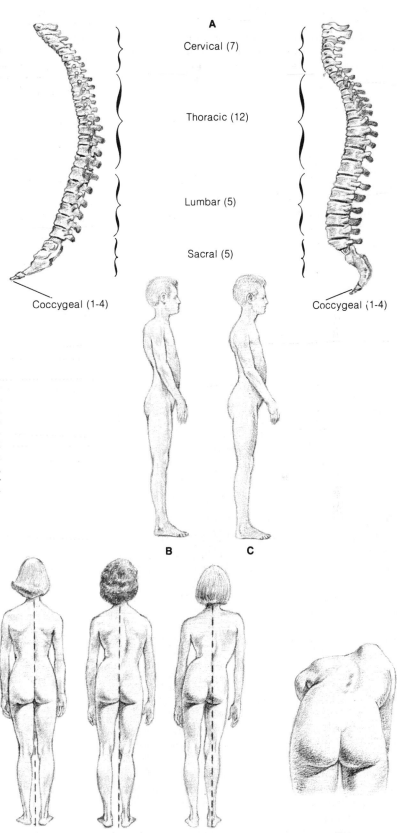

A

Cervical (7)

Thoracic (12)

Lumbar (5)

Sacral (5)

Coccygeal (1-4)

Coccygeal (1-4)

FIGURE 27–9. *A*, Normal spinal curve of the infant (left) and adult (right). *B*, Kyphosis. *C*, Lordosis. *D*, Normal spine in balance. *E*, Mild scoliosis in balance. *F*, Severe scoliosis, uncompensated, not in balance. *G*, Rib hump and flank asymmetry seen in flexion due to rotatory component. (From Alexander, M. M., and Brown, M. S.: Reprinted with permission from the April 1976 issue of *Nursing 76*, Intermed Communications, Inc. Further reproduction in whole or part expressly prohibited by law.)

B

C

D

E

F

G

between the ages of 12 and 16 years, a period of rapid growth.

There are two *types:* correctable or functional scoliosis and fixed or structural scoliosis. Correctable or *functional* scoliosis is usually caused by poor posture. It is seen especially in young persons who sit slumped over desks. Such persons can correct their scoliosis by bending toward the side of the curvature. If faulty posture is not corrected, structural changes may rarely occur, and the curvature is then not fully correctable.

Fixed or *structural* scoliosis is due to changes in the shape of the vertebrae or thorax. The patient cannot correct the deformity by bending.

Structural scoliosis most frequently is idiopathic and is usually found in young girls. Other causes may be congenital deformities (fusion of the ribs or vertebrae, hemivertebrae), infections of the vertebrae such as occur in Pott's disease caused by tuberculous infection, or paralytic diseases such as poliomyelitis.

Clinical Manifestations and Diagnosis. *Clinical manifestations* usually occur during periods of spinal growth such as at pubescence.

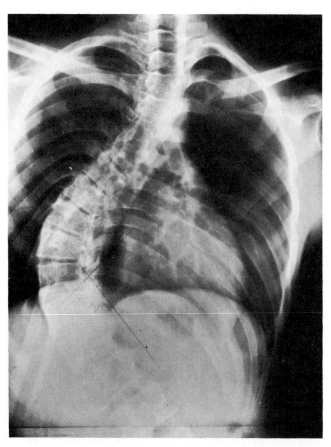

FIGURE 27–10. X-ray film from a patient presenting for the first time at a scoliosis clinic. He had been vaguely aware of "something" wrong with his back for about a year. (From Hungerford, D. S.: *Med. Clin. N. Am.,* 59:1521, November 1975.)

The child or adolescent has no pain until the later stages of the disease. One shoulder is elevated, one hip may be prominent, or the spinal curve itself may be obvious.

The *diagnosis* is made on physical examination. An x-ray picture of the entire spine is taken with the patient in a standing position. Roentgenograms may also be taken with the patient bending as far as possible to the right and to the left.

Treatment. The child should receive a well-balanced diet high in proteins, vitamins, and minerals. Postural curves with no structural changes may be corrected by improving sitting habits and general health, by getting more rest and by doing appropriate exercises. The physiotherapist may teach the child exercises to correct the condition. The child can be appealed to through his desire to improve his appearance. If the scoliosis is not caused merely by faulty posture, the primary condition must be corrected before structural changes occur in the vertebrae.

Bracing is used to prevent the degree of curvature from increasing. A pressure device known as the Milwaukee brace may be used as a conservative method of therapy. This brace may also be used for postoperative immobilization for those patients who require spinal fusion.

A plaster cast with wedging may be used to obtain maximal correction. The scoliosis turnbuckle plaster jacket including the head and leg is designed in such a way that it can be cut at the apex of the primary curve and wedged to overcome the deformity. Application of such a cast is exhausting to the patient. In a few days the cast is cut, and the turnbuckle is placed on the side of the concavity. The turnbuckle is turned each day. The wedge-shaped opening on one side becomes smaller, and the opening on the side where the turnbuckle is becomes larger. The primary deforming curve is then fused.

Although the turnbuckle cast was used for many years, a newer device called the Risser localizer jacket has replaced it. When the localizer cast is used, the corrective forces are applied by pelvic and head distraction. Lateral pressure is also made so that when the cast is completed, the correction has been accomplished. This is a lightweight cast in which the patient can walk. It is removed for operation, but must be reapplied afterwards. Spinal fusion may be done after maximum growth has occurred. For extensive surgery, fusion may have to be done in more than one stage. The orthopedist, the physiotherapist, the nurse, the parents, and the patient must work closely together.

Severe curves can be treated by the use of skeletal traction or halofemoral distraction be-

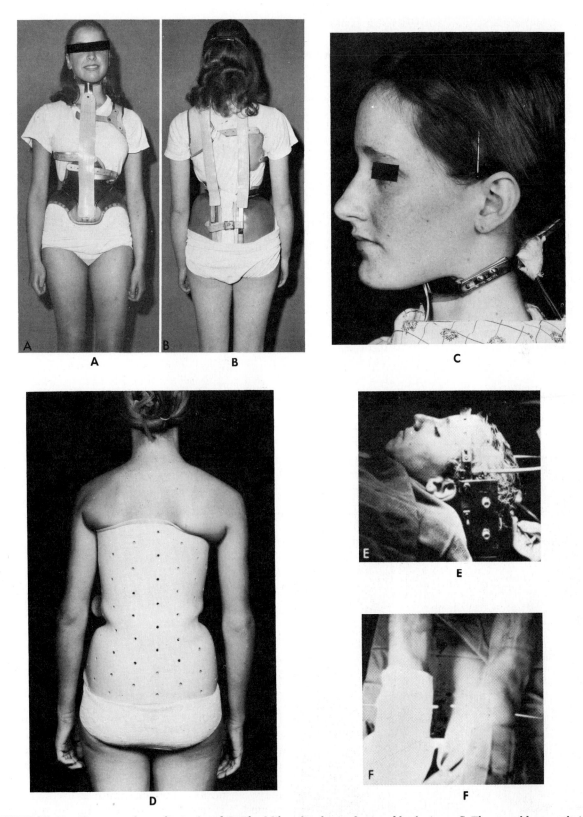

FIGURE 27–11. Treatment for scoliosis. *A* and *B*, The Milwaukee brace, front and back views. *C*, Throat mold currently in use. *D*, Plastic molded body jacket. *E*, Halofemoral traction. Positioning of halo ring with two posterior and two anterior pins. *F*, Steinmann pins inserted into distal end of the femur to provide countertraction. (From: *A* and *B*, Sells, C. J., and May, E. A.: *Am. J. Nursing*, 74:60, January 1974; *C* and *D*, Hungerford, D. S.: *Med. Clin. N. Am.*, 59:1522, 1524, November 1975; *E* and *F*, Treadway, B., et al.: *Nursing 74*, 4:51, August 1974.)

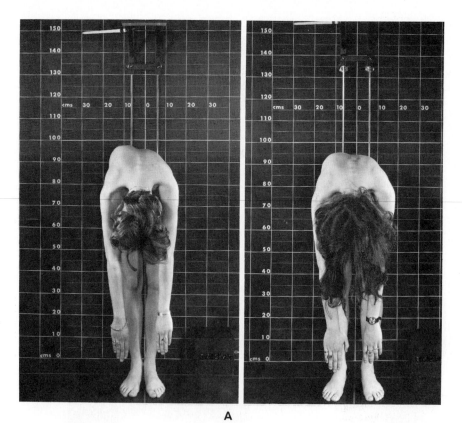

A

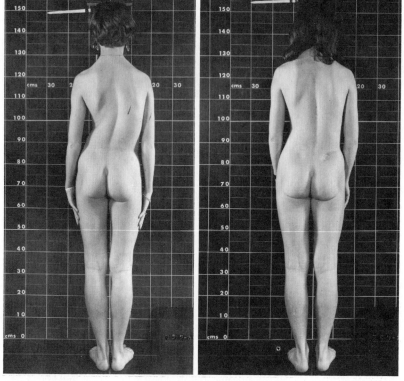

B

FIGURE 27–12. *A*, Internal correction with Harrington rods. *B*, The scar on the right hip corresponds to the opening made for spinal grafting by arthrodesis. (Courtesy Saint Justine Hospital, Montreal.)

fore and after spinal fusion. Skeletal traction is applied through the lower end of both femurs. Countertraction on the skull is applied with the use of a halo. When the traction is removed, the adolescent may be placed in a modified Milwaukee brace.

The use of Harrington rods is a method of internal instrumentation which consists of distraction and compression rods that assist in correcting the curves of scoliosis. This instrumentation or internal fixation is based on the principle of applying a distracting force on the concave side of the curve and a compression force on the convex side. A spinal fusion of the involved segment of the spine must be done at the time of application of the Harrington rods.

Research is being done on the use of a "spinal pacemaker," an implantable device, to correct scoliosis.

Responsibilities of the Nurse. The nurse assists with therapeutic exercises designed to promote realignment of the body, to increase the vital capacity and to improve muscle tone. Since these patients tire easily, periods of exercise are alternated with periods of rest. Rest positions may be specified by the physician or physiotherapist and can be as valuable as exercises. The adolescent is encouraged to sleep on a firm bed without a pillow. Breathing exercises may also be ordered. The nurse should know the exercises to be carried out so that they can be supervised properly.

The young patient in a thick, heavy turnbuckle or lighter cast requires comprehensive nursing care.

Some adolescents fear being encased in a brace or cast, some fear that their further growth will be prevented, and some fear the partial helplessness that inevitably results. Such immobilization may divert the adolescent's attention from interests outside himself and focus them on his own body with a subsequent change in self-image. He cannot master the natural developmental tasks when he is ready to do so. Immobilization exposes the adolescent to feelings of rage, grief, fear of bodily harm, abandonment, and guilt, with the concomitant feelings of despair and self-depreciation. If the adolescent ordinarily coped with his aggression through bodily activity, he may be threatened with a fear of disorganization and ultimate separation from reality.

The nurse and the family can provide information, encouragement, and support to reduce these fears. If another adolescent who has had a brace or cast applied can share his experiences with him, he can help reduce his anxiety and thus keep him in contact with the real world and its activities.

Skin care is important. Problems associated with the use of mechanical aids which forcefully correct scoliosis include the breakdown of skin around the edges of the cast and the creation of pressure areas beneath the cast. The nurse must observe and explore the skin with the fingers for pressure areas, especially over the ribs. The nurse must check for the cause of all complaints of pain or discomfort. The nurse must not permit the adolescent to reach under his own cast to scratch, since in doing so he may injure his skin. Drug therapy may be used if the itching persists, but powder should not be applied.

All exposed edges of the cast must be covered with large adhesive petals (see p. 321), or stockinet should be pulled over the edges of the cast and securely fastened to it. The exposed skin should be rubbed frequently. Slight padding may be used to allay discomfort from pressure by the cast, but too much padding may cause extra pressure. The cast around the buttocks and genitalia must be protected with waterproof material. The skin is cleansed thoroughly after soiling.

It is necessary to place some adolescents with scoliosis into halofemoral skeletal traction prior to spinal fusion. The nurse's role in teaching the patient is very important because the possibility of being immobilized with pins in the head and legs and being completely dependent on other persons for food, hygienic measures, warmth, communication, and the relief of pain may be quite frightening. The adolescent may also be placed on a frame when in traction. For the adolescent who is struggling to gain control of his new body image and of his environment, this relinquishing of all control can be devastating. The need to know what will happen to him is the adolescent's main source of anxiety. Thus preoperative teaching and emotional support are extremely important.

Preoperatively the adolescent needs to learn about skeletal traction, its purposes, how it is applied, and how he can function after it has been applied. It is important that the adolescent be included in the discussion between the surgeon and his parents: he must know what to expect after surgery.

The nurse's goals in caring for the patient who has had a spinal fusion include: (1) promotion of wound healing, (2) maintenance of good aeration of the lungs, (3) monitoring of movement and assessing sensation in the extremities, and (4) alleviation of pain and anxiety. If the spinal fusion includes the insertion of a Harrington rod, the patient will probably be on a Stryker frame for more than a week. The use of prism glasses is helpful during this period. After wound healing has occurred, the adolescent is put into a localizer cast. The physiotherapist can assist the patient to walk when the cast is dry and has been properly trimmed.

After spinal fusion, immobilization in casts or braces may be continued for six to 12 months. If a tibial graft has been taken, the limb should be handled carefully for at least eight weeks until healing has taken place. Immobility and lack of control are frustrating for the patient having a spinal fusion. During this time the adolescent, even though he understands his treatment, may exhibit demanding behavior.

Whenever the adolescent is examined, the nurse must be certain that he is adequately draped in order to avoid embarrassment.

Comprehensive nursing care is planned to meet the patient's needs during the long-term treatment of scoliosis. The patient may be cared for at home and taken to the outpatient department before and after hospitalization. The orthopedist, the physiotherapist, and the nurse must work closely together. Crippled children's services in many states provide physiotherapy follow-up in the home. The child should continue exercises for months or years.

The public health or community nurse can give the child encouragement. An adolescent girl may not want to wear a brace because she is "too tired" or thinks that it ruins her appearance. She may not want to do her exercises because she is "too busy." Parents can be warned of such complaints and be given support in insisting that the physician's orders be carried out for the girl's future welfare.

If a cast or brace is worn for a prolonged time, the adolescent may isolate himself from his peer group. Parents may need assistance in helping him to maintain contact with his friends. Continuation in a school program may provide the contacts with peers that the adolescent needs.

If the adolescent exercises before a full-length mirror, he will become more conscious of his posture and be more able to see the correction which the use of his muscles creates. Dancing exercises are also of value for developing better balance. The adolescent should wear shoes that support him well.

Early recognition and treatment are vitally important to prevent serious deformity. The school or nurse in the community should make observations on the posture of children. The tendency to postpone treatment while waiting to see whether the adolescent will outgrow the condition is dangerous.

SLIPPED FEMORAL EPIPHYSIS

Etiology and Incidence. Epiphyseal closure, which marks the completion of skeletal growth, also coincides with the attainment of sexual maturity. This is related more to physiologic than to chronologic age. This fact of development is especially important in the occurrence of slipped epiphysis, which is one of the outstanding osseous disturbances of adolescence. Exactly why this condition occurs is not known, but trauma and hormonal changes may be factors.

The phase of maximum growth is, on the average, for girls 12 years and for boys between 14 and 15 years. Usually the adolescent in whom slipped femoral epiphysis occurs is tall and heavy, but not fat. Such a person needs larger than average amounts of calcium and vitamin D during the preadolescent growth spurt.

Clinical Manifestations, Diagnosis, and Treatment. In the early stages, signs and symptoms of synovitis are present. The adolescent may have a slight limp to the affected side. Later the femoral portion of the epiphysis may slide farther upward. Finally the epiphysis may slip extensively upward with increased eversion of the limb. There is increased limitation of abduction and internal rotation. Pain in the hip (sometimes referred to the knee) causes the child to limp. The symptoms are similar to those in Legg-Perthes disease in school children (see p. 797). The onset is insidious. The condition is frequently bilateral.

The *diagnosis* is based on roentgen examination. A lateral view shows that the femoral capital epiphysis has slipped posteriorly and inferiorly. The neck of the femur assumes a horseneck appearance. Early diagnosis and treatment are essential.

The main objective of *treatment* is to arrest slipping by immobilizing the hip in a spica cast or by internal fixation of the epiphysis to the metaphysis of the neck of the femur.

Since this condition may be bilateral, the adolescent should be observed carefully for any indication of a problem with the other hip.

MALIGNANT TUMORS OF BONE

The most frequent primary malignant bone tumors are osteosarcoma and Ewing's sarcoma. These occur most often between ten and 20 years of age and in boys more often than in girls.

The cause is unknown, but heredity may be a factor.

Roentgenographic features resemble those of non-neoplastic lesions of bone. Careful diagnosis must be made on the bases of roentgenographic examinations and surgical biopsy.

Osteosarcoma (osteogenic sarcoma)

Clinical Manifestations, Diagnosis, Treatment and Prognosis. Osteosarcoma occurs more frequently than Ewing's sarcoma and usually involves the metaphyseal end of a long bone—the lower end of the femur or the upper end of the tibia or humerus. It may also occur in other locations. The *clinical manifestations* are pain and swelling of the affected part. The *diagnosis* is made on roentgenographic examination, which reveals destruction of bone and new bone formation. *Treatment* in the past consisted only of amputation of the affected extremity. The neoplasm

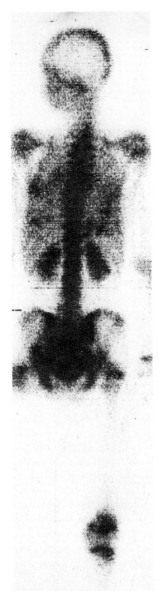

FIGURE 27–13. Osteogenic sarcoma multiple metastases. The whole body scan shows that the right leg has been amputated just below the intertrochanteric region. There are multiple areas of increased activity throughout the ribs, seen posteriorly. (From Gilday, D. L.: *Pediatr. Clin. N. Am.*, 23:42, February 1976.)

may involve the medullary cavity, the cortex, and the adjoining soft tissue. The sarcoma commonly metastasizes to the lungs, although other organs may be involved.

Today, one or more chemotherapeutic agents are given to control osteosarcoma. High doses of methotrexate and citrovorum factor (folinic acid), which counteracts the toxic effects of methotrexate, along with several other drugs, are used. These drugs destroy the malignant cells so completely that the affected femur becomes necrotic and can be replaced with a metallic prosthesis. This therapy is appropriate only in hospitals, where the adverse effects of treatment can be controlled. Hydration is an important part of therapy due to the side effects of chemotherapeutic agents. Hair loss due to chemotherapy causes anxiety in the adolescent who is trying to deal with his body image.

Responsibilities of the Nurse. Nursing care is similar to that of patients having Ewing's sarcoma.

Ewing's sarcoma

Clinical Manifestations, Diagnosis, Treatment, Responsibilities of the Nurse, and Prognosis. Ewing's sarcoma usually involves the shaft of a long bone. It may also involve the flat bones and ribs. The *clinical manifestations* are similar to those of osteosarcoma. Fever and leukocytosis may also be present. Usually at the time of diagnosis only one bone is involved, but other bones become affected. The *diagnosis* is made on roentgenographic examination and by histologic study of the tumor. *Treatment* is unsatisfactory. The neoplasm usually responds to supervoltage irradiation and chemotherapy, but few young people are cured. Radiation therapy to the affected bone in addition to systemic chemotherapy has produced some measure of therapeutic success. Amputation is the only other treatment used.

When a nurse sees an adolescent with the symptoms of a malignant tumor of the bone, a medical examination is suggested without alarming him or his parents by telling them that a tumor of the bone is suspected.

As the disease progresses, the patient will become anemic and look pale and tired. The optimism the patient shows at the onset of the condition changes to depression. Parents, visitors, and nurses should try to provide emotional support to help the patient face the probable outcome of the disease.

Since a pathologic fracture may occur at or near the site of the tumor, the nurse should be gentle with the extremity when making the bed or bathing the patient. If he is ambulatory, he is protected from falling. Such fractures may be painless; therefore the nurse must observe carefully for evidence of fracture if the patient falls or otherwise sustains any trauma which could result in a fracture of the diseased bone.

The diet is high in protein and vitamins to counteract the progressive anemia.

The nurse watches for indications of lung involvement such as pain in the chest, coughing, and expectoration of blood, and reports findings immediately. As with osteogenic sarcoma, metastases to the lungs occur frequently.

RETICULUM CELL SARCOMA

Ewing's sarcoma must be differentiated from reticulum cell sarcoma (medullary canal tumor), which is diagnosed by a biopsy, since its roentgen appearance may be variable. Irradiation and chemotherapy are the treatments of choice. Amputation may also be necessary. While the patient is undergoing roentgen therapy the limb should be protected by bracing or by a bivalved plaster cast in order to prevent fractures. After roentgen therapy the adolescent may experience problems with his skin, pain, nausea and vomiting. Intravenous therapy may be necessary to maintain hydration.

Gonadal Disorders

FAILURE OF SEXUAL DEVELOPMENT

Delayed puberty, like precocious puberty (see p. 788), may occur in both sexes. Parents may be much concerned when puberty is delayed in their child. The child may also be much concerned, since prolonged delay usually means that friends have outgrown him or her physically and emotionally. The child may feel alone and unloved. His self-image and self-respect may be distorted.

DELAYED PUBERTY IN THE FEMALE

Etiology, Clinical Manifestations and Treatment. At the normal age of puberty *clinical manifestations* become evident. There is failure of body hair growth and of the characteristic breast development. The genitalia remain infantile, and menstruation does not occur. There is retarded physical growth, and the epiphyses are late in closing.

In *primary hypogonadism* there is ovarian agenesis or destruction. This may be due to surgical removal or destruction by roentgen therapy. *Turner's syndrome* (gonadal dysgenesis) has as its symptoms sexual infantilism and a webbed neck. These persons do not develop sexually at puberty. Their gonads contain no germinal elements. They have 45 chromosomes

instead of 46 which is normal. They have only one X chromosome and no Y chromosome. *Treatment* for primary hypogonadism consists of replacement therapy with estrogens after the child has reached puberty. Although the secondary sex organs develop and function, the affected young woman is sterile. There are positive psychologic benefits from therapy in addition to the fact that premature senility from lack of estrogen is prevented.

Secondary hypogonadism is due to failure to secrete normal levels of gonadotropins. It may be due to destruction of or defect in the pituitary gland or in hypothalamic connections with the pituitary gland or to a severe systemic disease causing secondary pituitary deficiency. *Treatment* for secondary hypogonadism consists of substitution therapy with estrogens. Ovulation in these women can be induced with human pituitary gonadotropin when they want to become pregnant.

DELAYED PUBERTY IN THE MALE

Etiology, Clinical Manifestations, Treatment, and Prognosis. In *primary hypogonadism* of the male there is a decreased production of androgen and impaired spermatogenesis. If the testes are missing or have been destroyed, there is no abnormality until puberty, when the genitalia fail to enlarge, pubic hair is sparse or absent, the voice remains childlike, and epiphyseal closure is slow. The 17-ketosteroid excretion is usually low.

In *Klinefelter's syndrome* the affected child usually has a chromosomal aberration, having two or more X and one or more Y chromosomes in some of their cells. The XXY chromosomal pattern is the most common. Mental retardation may be present.

In all young boys having primary hypogonadism the *treatment* consists in substitution therapy with a testosterone preparation given intramuscularly.

In *secondary hypogonadism* there exists a deficiency of the follicle-stimulating hormone or of the luteinizing hormone of the anterior pituitary gland. The testes may be normal, but do not develop because they are not stimulated by gonadotropic hormones. In *Fröhlich's syndrome* a lesion of the hypothalamus causes obesity and sexual infantilism. These patients may also have growth retardation and diabetes mellitus. *Treatment* consists in the administration of maintenance therapy with androgen.

Responsibilities of the Nurse. The nurse can help the child whose puberty has been delayed to obtain medical diagnosis and treatment and with the psychologic problems that emerge. The nurse can emphasize the positive factors in the child's growth such as beginning evidence of the development of secondary sex characteristics. The nurse can also support the child and encourage his participation in school activities through which he can gain recognition from his peers but that do not require the physical development of others his age. Such activities may include editing the school newspaper or designing costumes for the class play. The child's parents need support in allaying their anxieties about the child's lack of development.

ADENOSIS AND CLEAR CELL ADENOCARCINOMA OF THE VAGINA

Etiology, Incidence, Clinical Manifestations, and Treatment. Adenocarcinoma of the vagina or lower genital tract occurs in young females whose mothers were advised to take diethylstilbestrol (DES) or related nonsteroidal synthetic estrogens during their pregnancy. Stilbestrol was used in an attempt to prevent loss of pregnancies, especially in the mid-1940s and mid-1950s. The risk to children of mothers having taken this drug is believed to be small. These tumors are seen relatively infrequently.

An adenocarcinoma is a malignant tumor that is locally invasive. It occurs primarily as a vaginal, cervical, or endocervical tumor, especially at puberty when ovarian hormonal stimulation occurs. The most frequent symptoms are vaginal discharge and irregular bleeding, although some pubescents or adolescents may have no symptoms. These lesions may be nodular, polypoid, or papillary. The Pap smear (vaginal cytology) is not as reliable for the detection of these tumors as it is for squamous cell carcinoma of the cervix. Vaginal and cervical smears are done at the time of pelvic examination. Rectovaginal palpation is carried out for the possible location of nodular lesions. A biopsy must be done if anything abnormal is found.

The *treatment* of adenocarcinoma of the vagina is an aggressive surgical approach. Total pelvic exenteration may be necessary, depending on the location of the lesion. Radiotherapy may be used for advanced cases.

Responsibilities of the Nurse. Early case-finding is important in the care of these adolescents, since success is dependent on early treatment of the adenocarcinoma. Irregular vaginal bleeding may occur not only with this form of malignancy but also in normal pubescents and adolescents following menarche. The nurse must encourage parents to seek early medical evaluation for their child if vaginal discharge or irregular bleeding occurs. If adenosis, a cellular change that may or may not be a forerunner of cancer, is found, the young woman should have a pelvic examination every 3 to 12 months to determine whether any changes are occurring.

If the diagnosis of a malignancy is made, the nurse can support the parents and their child by listening to their concerns and helping them to understand the physician's description of the condition and its therapy. The parents and possibly the child, if she is old enough, will be anxious about future reproductive ability after surgery. This depends on the extent of surgery that is necessary.

The nursing care of the patient following the operation is based on the same principles of care as for any postoperative gynecologic patient, with due consideration being given for the age and the degree of maturity of the individual. After her discharge from the hospital the community or public health nurse can help the child and her family in resolving their concern and anxieties.

Recently it has been learned that a significant number of sons of women who had taken diethylstilbestrol during their pregnancies have displayed cystic changes of the testes. Although no evidence of malignancy has been found, these young men should also have periodic examinations to determine whether any changes have occurred.

The Rebellious and Impulsive Adolescent

Rebellious and impulsive adolescents usually have parents who grew up in the years of economic depression and war and ultimately wanted only to achieve comfortable economic success. They wanted also that their children have minimal frustration and that they would be permitted to do what they desired without limits on their behavior. These parents wanted their children to have material advantages they never enjoyed themselves when they were young. At the same time, they wanted their children to achieve in academic pursuits, personal beauty, and social popularity. These children as they became older expected that they would be catered to by society since they had so few demands made on them as they were growing up at home. Certainly many of them were never required to work for remuneration, nor were they permitted to do so.

Many of these adolescents, then, wish to do nothing except sleep, eat, and enjoy themselves. Their impulsive and rebellious behavior leads them to act solely as their whims dictate, many times recklessly and without concern for others.

A typical parent-child relationship is one of oversubmission by parents to their child's impulsiveness and then overcoercion by them in order for the child to achieve. Parents become more anxious, especially over scholastic performance, and the adolescent develops an even more pronounced "I don't care" attitude. The adolescent becomes oversubmissive to his own impulses and develops an impulsive desire for freedom. Without adequate self-control such a young person will give his impulses free rein as he becomes prematurely independent of parental control. He may display outward defiance and flout all authority, especially that of his parents.

Responsibilities of the Nurse. Nurses, because of their knowledge of normal growth and development, can many times observe rebellious behavior and assist parents who face the problem of such an adolescent. These children may need professional help from physicians or psychiatrists. Parents may need to separate themselves physically from their adolescent youth for a short time, to cease providing money and other luxuries without the youth's earning them through honest effort, and to discontinue doing those personal chores such as ironing his clothes which the adolescent can do for himself. Parents should not scold, lecture, or criticize such an adolescent, because these will only produce more rebellion and family disharmony.

Problems of Sexuality in the Adolescent

RAPE (FORCIBLE INTERCOURSE)

Rape is coitus without the consent of the victim. *Statutory rape* is coitus with a female who is below the age of consent. This age limit may be 16 years, but it differs in various states. The issue of lack of consent is of prime importance in the definition of rape. *Sexual molestation* is noncoital sexual contact without consent.

Incidence. The incidence of reported rape is increasing at an alarming rate. Not all rapes are reported because of feelings of fear and shame of the victim. How many of the ones reported are real is a question that cannot be accurately answered. For example, an adolescent who finds that she is pregnant out-of-wedlock may tell her parents that the pregnancy was the result of a rape.

Rape may occur almost anywhere, at any time. Most rapists, however, attack in their own neighborhoods. Rapes occur usually in the late-evening or early-morning hours. They may occur on isolated streets, dark lots, empty laundromats, parking lots, or restrooms in public places. The rapist looks for someone who is alone and who appears vulnerable to attack such as an adolescent girl, a mentally retarded individual, a female under the influence of alcohol or drugs, a handicapped person, or an elderly woman. Friendly adolescents or women who freely give help to others are particularly vulnerable to attack. The rapist treats his victim as an object, not as a human being.

The fear of rape, of attack, mutilation, loss of control, and possible loss of life is universal in adolescent females and adult women. The violence of the assault is not only against the body, but also against her sense of autonomy as well. It is an insult to her personal integrity.

Rape is a crime of aggression or violence, not of sex. Rapists reach their goals with more than the necessary force; they use the penis as a weapon; they may attack with or without a gun, knife, or other weapon. Rape can be an outlet for the hostilities of the attacker. Gang rape tends to be more common by teenage males. It is often a misguided attempt to establish a sense of masculine identity—the adolescent needs the reassurance of friends that he can perform rape, an act that he would not be likely to commit by himself. Gang rape that starts in adolescence may continue when the individuals become adults.

Response of the Victim. The initial reaction of a victim of rape is one of shock and disbelief. The adolescent, depending on her age, feels terror, that she will be killed whether she resists or not. Feelings of vulnerability, that she is powerless over the situation, arise, and then feelings of disgust with both her attacker and herself surface.

A victim who resists faces a greater risk of injury *during* the attack. Since rapists are unsure of themselves at the beginning of an attack, however, fierce resistance such as scratching, "screaming bloody murder," pulling hair, kicking in the crotch, or biting, and then running toward a populated area is the best protection. The potential victim should shout "Fire!" or "Call the police!" This usually gets a better response from others than shouting "Help!" or "Rape!"

The adolescent should refuse to permit her attacker to intimidate her, especially since the rapist needs to intimidate his victim in order to continue the attack. Disagreement exists about whether the potential victim should try to calm a rapist by talking to him. If she does, she should not show fear or submissiveness. A clear refusal to cooperate is the best way to repel a potential rapist. If the adolescent plays along with an assailant to calm his anxiety and then kicks him in the genitals, there is nothing but the assailant's inadequate ego to stop him from maiming or murdering her.

Each adolescent or woman must use her own common sense and judgment about fighting back. If the individual chooses to resist, she must act quickly, without hesitation, and with all the strength possible.

If the attacker threatens violence, has a weapon, or if it is impossible to talk him out of it or to flee, quiet submission is possibly the best choice. Most rapists are not violent unless they are enraged at their victims. They usually disappear after the attack.

In the final analysis, the victim must make the decision about what to do at the beginning of an attack and then she must live with it. No one can tell her what approach to use at that time. The proof as to whether she made the right decision is the fact that she is still alive to talk about it.

After the attack is over and the rapist leaves, the adolescent, a member of her family, or a friend should call the police for two reasons: so that the assailant will be apprehended and so that the police can take her to the hospital or to her physician for treatment. The victim will be able to give the police the information and possibly the evidence they will need for a successful court prosecution.

Police officers usually see the victim initially. To protect the defendant against a false charge, special evidence is needed in many jurisdictions to support the victim's testimony, such as physical injury, semen in the vagina, or a witness.

Treatment. To protect physicians and nurses in a private office or in the emergency room of a hospital, written and witnessed consent must be obtained for the following procedures if possible: examination, collection of specimens, photographs, and permission to release information to the proper authorities. Every reported rape is a potential court case.

The question of whether rape has occurred is a legal matter for the decision of the court; it is not a medical diagnosis. In addition to obtaining consent from the victim or a responsible person, the medical personnel must get a written history in the adolescent's own words, record the findings of the examination, evaluate and treat any bruises or injury, obtain necessary laboratory work, save the victim's clothing, and protect her against venereal disease, pregnancy, and psychic trauma.

In many cities there are crisis centers where the adolescent and her parents can obtain advice about police procedures and where to get medical and psychologic help. Rape prevention and crisis centers that are staffed by women who are counselors and victim advocates are being organized increasingly all over the country.

In the emergency room of the hospital counselors talk with the victim, parents, and friends who accompany the adolescent. They assist the police to gain as much information as possible to assess the crisis. To guard against pregnancy the gynecologist may prescribe diethylstilbestrol, the morning-after pill, or another drug as soon after the attack as possible. If pregnancy occurs as a result of rape, its interruption rests on the decision of the adolescent, depending on her age, and her parents. To prevent venereal disease procaine penicillin may be administered intramuscularly or oral antibiotics may be prescribed. Adolescents should be examined again approximately six weeks after the attack to be certain that these measures have been effective.

When and if the case is brought to court, it is often the victim who appears to be on trial through the creation of an impression that she had encouraged the rapist. This is because rape is a crime that is susceptible to false accusation. The parents or the adolescent can receive guidance concerning the legal maze involved by consulting with their local chapter of the National Organization for Women or a similar association. If the case is brought to court, the adolescent may experience additional emotional trauma and possibly increased guilt by having to review the events of the attack before strangers. The nurse can assist the adolescent to verbalize her feelings and help her deal with them realistically.

The initial physical and mental harm to the victim may be less debilitating than the long-range psychologic effects. It is difficult to forget an act of rape. For about two days after the attack a period of normalcy occurs. The adolescent tries to deny that it occurred as she goes about her daily routine. During the following weeks, however, a period of depression may occur, with a lowered level of self-esteem. The adolescent may have a loss of trust in male-female relationships and have a diminution in self-respect. Nightmares about sexual assault may occur. Finally, and with psychologic counseling if necessary, the final phase of resolution and integration occurs.

Responsibilities of the Nurse. The nursing care of a rape victim is built on three assumptions: (1) the rape provokes a situational crisis for the victim, (2) the victim is a consumer in need of medical and psychologic services, and (3) the way in which the rape victim is treated and counseled is the practice of primary prevention of possible later psychiatric problems.

The nurse in the physician's office or in the emergency room of a hospital must know the procedures necessary to help the victim so that they are carried out as quickly and smoothly as possible. The adolescent victim is not left alone if at all possible. Parents, other family members and friends can stay with her to provide emotional support.

Privacy during the medical and gynecologic examinations is important. If the victim is made to feel guilty about the attack during the examination or the counseling period, medical personnel will not be able to develop a therapeutic relationship with her. The nurse is, under no circumstances, judgmental, but records accurately and completely the adolescent's physical and emotional status. The victim must be encouraged to talk about her experience. Listening and understanding are important skills in counseling.

The nurse needs to determine prior to the examinations whether the adolescent has ever been examined before. If this is the first pelvic examination the adolescent has had, the nurse must explain what is expected of her and the reasons for what the physician will be doing. After the examination the adolescent may request a place to wash because she may feel "dirty." Mouthwash may also be provided for those adolescents who have been forced to have oral sex.

The nurse is responsible for health education, such as emphasizing the importance of taking the prescribed medications, the reasons for taking them, and making certain that she or her parents know the side effects of the drugs ordered. The adolescent should also learn how to care for any physical injuries she may have suffered. Emphasis must be placed on follow-up care by her private physician or a clinic physician and referral to other sources of help as needed. It is essential that all nurses have the counseling skills necessary to talk with victims of rape. Emotional support and sympathetic understanding of the adolescent and her family are important.

The attitude of the adolescent's parents is vitally important in determining her ultimate adjustment to the crisis of rape. Some parents cannot understand why the adolescent is upset and anxious about the incident, thus they give her little or no emotional support. Other parents may heighten the girl's anxiety, fear, and guilt because of their own rage at her attacker and the event. Finally, overprotective parents may reinforce the adolescent's denial and may limit her social activity with her peers, thus making it more difficult for her to recover emotionally from the event. Because of the various attitudes parents may demonstrate, it is important for the nurse to observe the parent-adolescent interaction and to discuss with the parents their feelings about the attack.

The nurse in the emergency room can assist in referring the adolescent and her family to the community or public health nurse for follow-up care. As with any referral, adequate information is shared with the nurse who will visit the home so that appropriate care and counseling can be given.

Prevention. The nurse can help to educate parents and adolescents in ways to prevent rape. The adolescent should be certain that the doors and windows of her home are locked securely, especially when she is alone or babysitting. The door should not be opened to any stranger. The adolescent should refuse to help or to be helped by a strange man.

Hitchhiking or accepting rides from strange men makes an adolescent female especially vulnerable to attack. She should not walk alone at night in high-crime areas of town, on dark streets or other areas such as parking lots. If she drives a car, she should check the back seat before entering it.

If away from home, the adolescent may carry a device that makes noise such as a whistle on her watch bracelet, charm bracelet, or on a chain around her neck. An alarm siren is available that comes in two parts that can be separated and thrown on the ground to start the device screeching. These devices should be used only if the attacker is unarmed and only to gain sufficient time to run away.

Carrying a concealed weapon is a crime in most states. An assailant could take a weapon from an adolescent and use it against her. The adolescent can, however, carry a substance to spray in the attacker's face and eyes such as perfume, hairspray, or concentrated lemon juice from a plastic lemon to temporarily blind him. Any articles of this type should be accessible and not carried in the bottom of the handbag.

The nurse must be familiar with the laws, regulations, and customs regarding rape in the area where care is given. It may be necessary to make a report under the battered child laws (see p. 481).

PREMARITAL SEX

The major task of adolescence is the development of a sense of identity and the avoidance of identity confusion (see p. 817). The individual must formulate a consistent self-image that is in accord with his perception of his personal and mental capacities. The adolescent derives his self-image from his environment and his peer group. He searches constantly for models after which to pattern himself. In order to develop his own identity the adolescent must, to a certain extent, reject parental and adult values. The stage of "falling in love" then becomes an attempt to arrive at a definition of his own identity by projecting a diffuse image of his ego onto another and then seeing it reflected and clarified.

Confusion results when the adolescent cannot incorporate the many sources of input about himself into a consistent self-image. If he does not develop a self-image, the adolescent finds it difficult to make decisions about his future regarding such things as his education and his career. The adolescent also finds it difficult to relate to his parents, other adult figures, and peers. If this identity confusion persists, he will also have a diminished ability to develop intimate relationships with others. If the youth cannot establish normal one-to-one boy-girl relationships, he is likely to become promiscuous.

Many adolescents have a transitory period of role confusion before they develop a self-image and a sense of identity. This period may be intense and prolonged. These adolescents are the ones who are vulnerable to performing sexually for nonsexual reasons. Nonsexual motivation reflects underlying social and psychologic conflicts and needs.

The importance of the sociocultural milieu must be considered in determining this behavior pattern. Reasons why the adolescent acts this way include: to obtain peer approval, to express rebellion against parental and adult values, to express hostility against parents, and to escape from his own life situation. Sexual activity in the adolescent may be his attempt to bring attention to himself and his needs. It may also be viewed as an attempt at self-destruction by depressed teenagers.

Sexual behavior that is motivated not by erotic pleasure, curiosity, or the establishment of a meaningful relationship represents the misuse of sex. This misuse is detrimental to the development of true intimate relationships in adolescents and young adults.

Girls who were raised in unaffectionate homes may want to become pregnant in order to have a child to love. After the birth of the infant, however, the adolescent is disappointed because it is the infant who is dependent and is unable to meet the mother's needs. The adolescent then is unable to mother the infant, leading to ambivalent and negative feelings towards him. The needs for which the pregnancy was planned are therefore unfulfilled.

Adolescents who have grown up in an affectionate home where the daughter can identify with her mother who is loved and esteemed and can be close to her father in a nonthreatening sexual relationship without excluding her mother usually do not become promiscuous. In an overwhelmingly disastrous parental marriage the adolescent is not likely to wish to enter a sexual relationship in which an unwanted pregnancy may occur.

If the adolescent does not like her mother or consider her a good role model as a woman and if she does not have another woman who is a good surrogate mother, the adolescent is likely to have a low level of self-esteem. This is especially true if the mother and daughter were close during childhood but became alienated during the early years of adolescence. In an effort to compensate for her low level of self-esteem, the adolescent may become promiscuous. Through her behavior she feels that she is sought after and wanted.

The adolescent who has negative feelings about her mother and a quasiseductive relationship with her father may turn to sex with other men. She does this in order to move emotionally further from her father and to redirect her possibly incestuous feelings for him toward others. If the parents evidence a moderate level of hostility toward each other, the daughter, feeling unloved and alone, may become sexually active at an early age.

Attitudes toward standards in regard to sex are varied among adolescents: some believe that chastity before marriage is an absolute requisite; some believe that chastity is right for girls but not for boys (double standard); some believe that there should be sexual freedom for those who love each other; some believe in sexual permissiveness; and some believe in total sexual irresponsibility.

UNWED ADOLESCENT PARENTS

It is unfortunate that in our society many thousands of unmarried adolescents are bearing children each year. For these young people the change from being an immature adolescent to being a parent may be overwhelming. Professional personnel of several disciplines can contribute to providing services and care for these teenagers in order to help them find solutions to their problems, the intensity of which may vary, depending upon the culture to which the adolescents belong.

Pregnancy out of wedlock occurs at every social, economic, and intellectual level, although most often the teenager who is seen by a public health worker has been socially and eco-

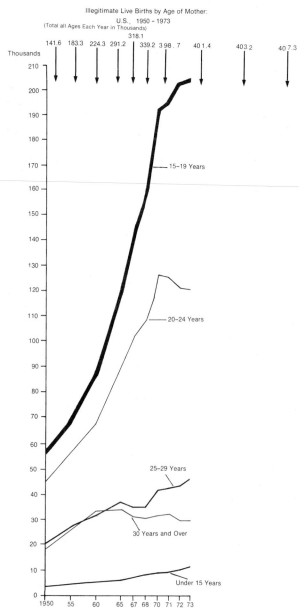

Illegitimate Live Births by Age of Mother:
U.S., 1950 - 1973
(Total all Ages Each Year in Thousands)
318.1
141.6 183.3 224.3 291.2 339.2 398.7 401.4 403.2 407.3

FIGURE 27–14. The number of illegitimate live births has been steadily increasing.

nancy out of wedlock include the presence of frustrations and pent-up emotions which seek an outlet, loss of inhibitions due to the use of alcohol or drugs, and a lack of knowledge about sex. These adolescents may also have been rebellious and impulsive prior to their pregnancies.

Some approaches to the prevention of pregnancy out of wedlock include the development in the female of a positive self-identity (see Chap. 25), the ability to postpone immediate desires in order to achieve long-range goals, and sufficient confidence in herself so that she does not have to conform to the wishes of her group. Parents can support their daughters in this regard by setting limits on their dating, by not forcing them to become "popular" at an early age, and by providing the kind of sex education that goes beyond the usual "facts of life."

The unmarried pregnant adolescent needs professional counseling. Many adolescent girls are afraid to seek advice, however, because they are afraid that their parents will find out that they are pregnant. The adolescent needs help in dealing with her feelings of guilt, in deciding whether to have the baby or not, in planning for prenatal care and admission to a shelter or hospital, in planning for financial assistance, and in deciding whether to keep her infant or to relinquish him for adoption. The putative father also needs help in determining his role and, like the mother, needs guidance for the future.

Pregnancy at an early age carries significant medical risks such as increased infant mortality and prematurity, and increased susceptibility to toxemia of pregnancy for the mother. The unmarried adolescent many times has inadequate prenatal care and an unbalanced diet, which contribute further to these risks. Her nutritional status has been lowered by poor dietary habits and her increased nutritional demands for growth and development have depleted her reserves making her poorly prepared for pregnancy. Although the dietary habits are many times poor, they may be worsened by eating compulsions arising from fears and anxiety associated with pregnancy. Instructions concerning diet given to these young women must be kept simple and practical in order for them to understand and to follow them properly.

The nurse in the community, the school nurse or school nurse practitioner or the nurse in the hospital may be the initial contact the unmarried pregnant girl may have with the community health services. This relation between the nurse and the unwed teen-age mother is vital. The

nomically deprived. Some of the underlying causes of pregnancy in the typical unwed adolescent may be conflict between her parents and herself, resulting in her feeling rejected and insecure at home, and lack of satisfactory adjustment in other areas of living. The unwed teenager is basically struggling with her desire for independence and her need for dependence on her parents.

A few reasons among others given for preg-

nurse must establish a relation of trust with the adolescent by being understanding and nonjudgmental and then help her to transfer this feeling of trust to the physician who will provide medical care for her. The nurse must know the resources in the particular community to care for such a patient. Interagency communication and cooperation are essential if the adolescent is to have continuity of care.

Most adolescent girls fear the birth process itself because of a lack of understanding of the physiologic process and because of their lack of experience in coping with crisis situations. The nurse is many times the one to whom such an adolescent will turn for support. After the infant is born the nurse with other team members must support the mother in her decision as to whether or not she plans to keep the infant.

Attention has recently turned to the unmarried adolescent father and his needs in establishing his future relationships and goals. Male high school counselors and social workers are especially valuable in helping such young people.

If sufficient assistance and guidance are given to unmarried adolescent parents, much of the tragedy of broken lives, both those of the parents and the child, can be averted. If the decision is made not to keep the infant, he should be placed for adoption through a reputable agency instead of being placed on the black market.

The nurse is a vital member of the health team in both urban and rural areas and can with the physician and social worker assume leadership in the drive to provide unwed pregnant adolescents with good prenatal care and to help with their rehabilitation. Certainly continuation of the education of such adolescents is essential if they are to become socially productive human beings. Formal education must be made available to them.

THE USE OF CONTRACEPTIVES

It is possible to identify high risk adolescents who need birth control services without referring to their sexual behavior. There are psychologic factors such as their level of self-esteem, their feelings about each of their parents, and their parents' marriage that are important indicators of their probable level of sexual activity.

Counseling. The goals of counseling are to strengthen the adolescent's self-concept, especially in areas relating to sexual identity and to help the high-risk adolescent to use responsible adult contraceptive methods.

Counseling an adolescent concerning sexuality requires an application of counseling principles and techniques and a knowledge of the characteristics and problems of the adolescent. Counseling must be done in an atmosphere of privacy; what the adolescent says is privileged information, to be kept in strict confidence. The counselor must be a good listener and recognize each adolescent as an individual.

The concerns of an adolescent can be explored by using open-ended questions such as "Please explain how you feel." Reflection can be used as an indication of a need for elaboration about a subject. Verbal and nonverbal skills can be used. It is important that the counselor be nonjudgmental, stable, and possess integrity when working with adolescents.

Birth control methods can prevent, by natural or artificial means, the union of the female ovum and the male sperm when the adolescent is not pregnant. Nurses can provide adolescents with knowledge about birth control methods through the use of charts, simplified explanations, and take-home pamphlets. Devices such as the intrauterine device and diaphragm can be demonstrated in a pelvic model.

Adolescents select the type of contraceptive to use on the basis of ready availability, ease of use, and effectiveness. Although they may learn about more effective means of contraception, they often use the condom or withdrawal methods to prevent conception. Many adolescents do not choose a contraceptive such as the pill, which would indicate that they had planned on intercourse. The majority of adolescent intercourse is impulsive and occurs without foresight and planning for contraception.

The methods of contraception that may be used are given in order from the most effective to the least effective; birth control pill, intrauterine device (IUD), diaphragm, condom, spermicides, coitus interruptus (withdrawal), rhythm method, and douching. Naturally, the most effective method is abstention.

The *birth control pill* is a hormonal type of contraceptive made of synthetic compounds similar to the natural progesterone and estrogen produced by the female and is very effective. The pill prevents pregnancy because it prevents ovulation. Pills, of which there are many types, are prescribed on an individual basis. The physician who does the original examination prior to prescribing the medication provides follow-up medical supervision while the adolescent is taking the pill. It must be stressed that there is danger involved if the adolescent forgets to take the pill regularly. She should take the pill at the same time each day.

Advantages of taking the pill, in addition to

protection from pregnancy, are that it may regulate the menstrual flow, clear up complexion problems, and relieve dysmenorrhea. Disadvantages of taking the pill include nausea and vomiting, breast tenderness, weight gain, and the need for continued medical supervision. No one really knows the possible long-term effects of the pill on growth and development, but it is known that there is an increased risk of blood clots, migraine headaches, high blood pressure, and strokes when the pill is taken for prolonged periods.

The *intrauterine device* (IUD) is a small piece of flexible material that is inserted into the uterus to prevent pregnancy. The IUD must be changed periodically, depending on the type used. The adolescent must have periodic follow-up care when an IUD is in use. She must check to see that the strings which are attached to the device and which protrude into the upper vagina are in place since the device may slip or be expelled. When the IUD is in place, no prior planning for intercourse is necessary; its rate of effectiveness is high. The disadvantages in the use of this device are that it can cause heavy menstrual bleeding, spotting between periods, and cramping. These symptoms should be brought to the attention of the physician.

The *diaphragm* is a thin, soft rubber dome that has a flexible metal ring within its rim. This covers the cervix by fitting between the back wall of the vagina and the pubic bone. It is used with a spermicide cream or a jelly. The diaphragm is not a practical type of contraceptive for an adolescent since it requires individual fitting and follow-up care. It may be difficult to insert properly. Infection may occur if it is left in place for more than a day.

The *condom* (rubber) is a sheath worn over the penis to prevent contact of semen with the vagina during intercourse. The male has the responsibility for using the condom as a contraceptive method. The condom also provides protection against venereal disease. When applied, the condom should allow for expansion of the penis prior to orgasm. If the condom is of good quality and if it is used correctly, it has a favorable rate of effectiveness.

Spermicides contain chemicals that kill sperm without harming vaginal tissues. They act by lowering the pH of the vagina, thus making it a more acidic environment, which is unsuitable for sperm. Having to apply a spermicide into the vagina prior to intercourse takes the spontaneity out of sexual relationships. Spermicides are most effective when used as a foam in combination with the condom or diaphragm.

Coitus interruptus (withdrawal) means that the penis is withdrawn from the vagina prior to ejaculation. This requires self-control on the part of the male and may cause psychologic problems during adolescence. Since semen can escape before ejaculation and since the girl can become pregnant even if it is deposited on her external genitalia, coitus interruptus is not regarded as a good method of contraceptive.

The *rhythm method* depends on restricting sexual activity to the period of the month when it is safe, that is, during the nonfertile days of the menstrual cycle. Because of the irregularity of the menstrual cycle, it is difficult for adolescents to use this method. This method of birth control is approved by all religions.

Douching immediately after intercourse is not an effective means of birth control. Since some sperm are in the cervical canal within a minute and one half following intercourse and since douching may propel more sperm towards the cervix, it is obvious that the failure rate for this method is high.

When counseling an adolescent regarding contraceptive use or abortion, it is vitally important that the nurse present the facts objectively and encourage the client to make her own decision regarding the problem. The nurse should not be judgmental nor inflict personal ideas regarding the problem on the client or her family.

Some nurses, because of their religious beliefs and value systems, may find it difficult, if not impossible, to counsel teenagers about the use of contraceptives or about abortion. This is understandable. It is necessary, however, for these nurses to refer such adolescents to appropriate sources of help where guidance can be given.

ABORTION

Adolescents accounted for more than one quarter of the nation's more than 900,000 abortions in 1975. Nurses who deal with members of the childbearing population have a responsibility for teaching them that abortion is only one and possibly the least desirable way of making a decision about childbearing. The operation is still potentially life-threatening, and the risks increase with each month of delay. The utilization of a sound knowledge of the reproductive process and contraceptive methods are much more desirable than resorting to abortion.

The effects of abortion on the adolescent may be both physical and emotional, mild or severe. There are several aspects of an adolescent's decision-making process that are crucial in relation to an abortion. Adolescents who are the most settled about their decision to have an abortion usually have the smoothest time after surgery. The fact that the individual decided for herself to have the surgery bodes well for her future adjustment. If the adolescent is unable or reluctant to make the decision concerning abortion for herself, symptomatic emotional responses can be expected in the postabortion period. A vulnerable adolescent who is forced into having an abortion and accepts this decision while really wanting the child is also likely to have emotional problems after the surgery.

After an abortion a mild, transient negative emotional response including regret, grief, sadness, and guilt can be expected. This is a normal response to abortion and may be increased by social attitudes toward the procedure. Psychiatric symptoms from sexual dysfunction to psychotic decompensation may appear after an abortion. These symptoms may or may not be a continuation of a pre-existing illness.

Nurses must be aware of their own feelings about abortion and how these feelings can affect their clients. They must also know about the social and legal conditions relating to adolescent contraceptive use and abortions in the areas in which they practice.

VENEREAL DISEASES: SYPHILIS, GONORRHEA AND GENITAL HERPES

Venereal disease is present to an alarming degree among adolescents, especially those 15 to 19 years old. These adolescents are from all socioeconomic groups. Many engage in sexual intercourse because they are lonely or want status, not because they have a deep relation with their partners. Some who have lost a fear of pregnancy because they are taking a contraceptive medication may increase the dissemination of veneral disease. Since adolescents are prone to worry about their bodies, their concern over subsequent venereal disease often prompts them to seek treatment. Some may not seek treatment, however, for fear that their behavior will become known.

Treatment must be undertaken by a large health team if success is to be achieved. Many of the aspects of adult treatment and control apply equally to adolescents, though special problems are present in the younger group.

The two most common venereal diseases are syphilis and gonorrhea. The incidence of gonorrhea especially has reached epidemic proportions, ranking first among reportable communicable diseases. These diseases follow the adult pattern in adolescents. The medical aspects will not be discussed here fully, since they have already been discussed (see pp. 262 and 653).

The early signs and symptoms of acquired *syphilis* (lues) either are absent or may go unnoticed by the infected person. In the primary stage a single painless sore or chancre may occur where the spirochete entered the body. This may look like a pimple or blister and appears usually about 21 days after exposure. The secondary stage of syphilis may appear two to six months after contact and may go unnoticed even though a rash may be present or sores may appear in the mouth or throat. A fever may be present. A darkfield microscopic examination or

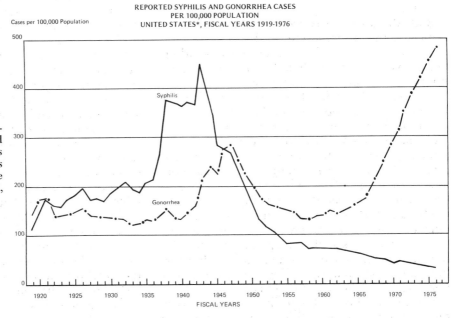

FIGURE 27–15. While the incidence of syphilis had dropped in recent years, gonorrhea has reached epidemic proportions in this country. (Courtesy of the Center for Disease Control, Atlanta, Ga.)

REPORTED SYPHILIS AND GONORRHEA CASES
PER 100,000 POPULATION
UNITED STATES*, FISCAL YEARS 1919-1976

Cases per 100,000 Population

Syphilis

Gonorrhea

FISCAL YEARS

*Beginning in 1939 all states are included in the reporting area
(Military cases included 1919-1940 excluded thereafter)

serologic tests may be done for diagnostic purposes. If the primary and secondary signs go untreated, the spirochetes may cause congenital syphilis in the infants of infected mothers (see p. 262), may damage vital organs, and in later years may cause paralysis, crippling, cardiovascular disease, blindness, or paresis. Although research is being done on an antisyphilis vaccine, it will probably not be ready for use with human patients for several years.

Gonorrhea, commonly called "clap," causes a discharge of purulent material and burning pain of the penis when an infected male urinates within two to six days after exposure. The woman who has contracted gonorrhea may or may not have an increased vaginal discharge, pain, or urinary frequency. She may therefore without knowing it infect others and allow her own infection to progress into serious complications such as salpingitis, pelvic inflammatory disease, peritonitis, and sterility. The organism may cause gonococcal ophthalmia neonatorum (see p. 260) in the newborns of infected mothers. In males infection may occur in the posterior urethra and prostate gland, among other sites. Ultimately, scarring of the seminal ducts and sterility may occur. In both sexes arthritis, conjunctivitis, and endocarditis may occur.

A simple, inexpensive blood test has been developed for diagnosing gonorrhea, although it is not yet available commercially. Research is continuing in this area and in the development of a vaccine against gonorrhea. Diagnosis can be made in the male by a stained smear or culture of the purulent urethral exudate, and in the female by a culture using a Thayer-Martin VCN medium.

Both diseases are contracted through sexual promiscuity. The important problems in adolescents are treatment of the disease, case-finding, and prevention by the health team. Early case-finding is especially important if the young girl is pregnant, in order that treatment may be completed before delivery of the infant.

Although the mortality rates from these diseases have decreased as a result of treatment, the infections persist and are being seen increasingly in the adolescent group. The social problem, a violation of sexual mores, is perhaps a greater problem than the morbidity.

The fact that adolescents turn to such an extent to promiscuous heterosexual relations may be a reflection of social maladjustment. Other indications of the same problem include increasing parenthood out of wedlock, juvenile delinquency, and emotional problems.

Several members of the health team must work together to help control the problem of venereal disease: (*a*) the parents, who have contributed to the adolescent's forming a philosophy of life or life perspective and his concept of other people, and have given approval to his selection of friends. Often it is the friends who initially lead the adolescent into this behavior. (*b*) The teacher, who helps to build proper attitudes toward these diseases through counseling, can disseminate information about venereal disease and help to guide troubled adolescents to appropriate sources for aid. (*c*) The clergyman, who appreciates the fact that religious motives have a great effect on the degree of inhibition exercised in subordinating unacceptable sexual expression, is an important team member. Apparently, the more active adolescents are in religion, the less they engage in promiscuity. (*d*) The social worker, working with nurses in helping these adolescents, can help the nurse appreciate the probable causes of such antisocial behavior and what disease means to the patient. (*e*) The family physician can teach his young patients about venereal disease, treat and report cases, and locate their contacts. (*f*) The venereal disease investigator is a trained interviewer who interviews patients with an aim to locating contacts.

Although other sources of help are available, many adolescents utilize the "hot line," "storefront clinics," free clinics, or youth clinics available to them for problems related to venereal disease, drug use, suicidal ideation, or any type of crisis situation. These are staffed by young people along with professional personnel who avoid the use of shame and stigma in their relations with the adolescents. All members of the health team should develop a frank, honest, and nonjudgmental approach to these persons and give information pertinent to the particular problems presented.

Genital Herpes (Herpes Progenitalis). Genital herpes is being diagnosed with greater frequency than before among sexually active adolescents. The condition is caused by the type 2 virus and is spread venereally. In a small percentage of patients the causative agent is HVH-1.

The clinical manifestations if the adolescent has no antibody to either type of herpes include elevation of temperature, dysuria, and regional adenopathy. The typical painful ulcerations may be difficult to distinguish from the lesions of chancroid. Recurrence of this condition is common and may be subclinical in nature. If the adolescent is pregnant and has this disease, the infection can easily be acquired by the newborn during the process of birth (see p. 264). Herpesvirus may also be a possible factor in the etiology of cervical dysplasia and carcinoma of the cervix.

In males, ulcers or vesicles due to the herpesvirus can be seen on the glans penis, prepuce, or shaft of the penis. The scrotum is not usually involved.

Symptomatic relief can be obtained with local compresses of aluminum acetate (Borow's solution). There is no known specific therapy for herpes.

A pelvic examination should be performed early on a teenager following a herpes infection because of the possible development of a malignancy of the cervix.

Responsibilities of the Nurse. The nurse must understand and appreciate the roles of other members of the health team, in order to assist in case-finding.

The school nurse practitioner or school nurse should be aware of signs and symptoms of venereal disease as of other communicable diseases in students. The nurse should be able to evaluate complaints and refer such adolescents to the physician. Adequate health records must be kept on all students in order to know their individual problems. The nurse must have a nonjudgmental attitude about these diseases and may function as a teacher of health and as a counselor for the students on such matters.

The hospital nurse works in conjunction with the school nurse or school nurse practitioner. Although syphilis, gonorrhea, and genital herpes are usually treated on an outpatient basis, the nurse caring for adolescent patients in the hospital units must remember that because the incubation period of syphilis is about three weeks and of gonorrhea about five days, some adolescents recently admitted may manifest symptoms during the early part of a hospitalization period.

The primary chancre of syphilis and the pustular discharge of gonorrhea are highly infectious. Isolation technique to protect other patients as well as personnel is thus necessary.

The treatment of choice for syphilis and gonorrhea is penicillin. Some strains of organisms develop a high resistance to penicillin and very large doses are required for some patients; in these instances or if there is an allergy to penicillin alternative antibiotics must be used. The nurse must watch for signs of untoward reactions to the drugs used.

The clinic or office nurse can encourage the adolescent to obtain therapy. The nurse must know the diagnostic and therapeutic measures in order to interpret these to the patients and reassure them. Adolescents want answers to their questions, especially those in relation to their own bodies. The nurse can also be active in case-finding. One problem in the medical treatment of infected minors has been that of the need for parental permission. Such permission is no longer required in some states.

The nurse in the community can do a great deal in controlling venereal disease among adolescents by knowing local families well, by guidance, case-finding, and by helping infected persons understand their responsibility in controlling the spread of infection to others.

The only way to control venereal disease in the adolescent group is by a multidisciplinary approach. The nurse should understand the responsibility as a cooperating member of the health team in order to reduce the incidence of this social tragedy of youth.

Emotional Disorders

JUVENILE DELINQUENCY (DEVIANT BEHAVIOR)

Incidence and Etiology. A delinquent is one who does not behave in accordance with standards set by his society or community. Basically, delinquent behavior is antisocial, aggressive behavior usually due to anxiety and frustrations. Included under the category of delinquent behavior, among others, are shoplifting, which is almost becoming a national epidemic in persons under 21 years of age; truancy from school; running away from home; damage to and theft of property, especially automobiles; destruction of property appearance by graffiti using spray-paint or felt-tipped markers; and violence, including sex offenses, against other persons. Juvenile delinquency in the United States has increased for more than 20 consecutive years.

There is usually a combination of causative factors in any one problem of delinquency.

DELINQUENCY DUE TO FORCE OF CIRCUMSTANCES. An example of this kind of delinquency is stealing so that the adolescent can have necessities, e.g., food. Spending money such as their friends have appears to many adolescents as a necessity. They may steal so that they can remain in the group. This sort of adolescent is essentially normal and dislikes stealing from others. He needs the help of the sociologist, the educator, and the economist.

DELINQUENCY DUE TO POOR HOME AND COMMUNITY ENVIRONMENT. The adolescent whose insecurity at home, in his community, and in society is very great may become delinquent. As a child he may have felt rejection or lack of understanding. As an adolescent he may engage in criminal activity such as robbery, sex orgies, addiction to narcotics or alcohol, and even apparently unmotivated murder. Actually,

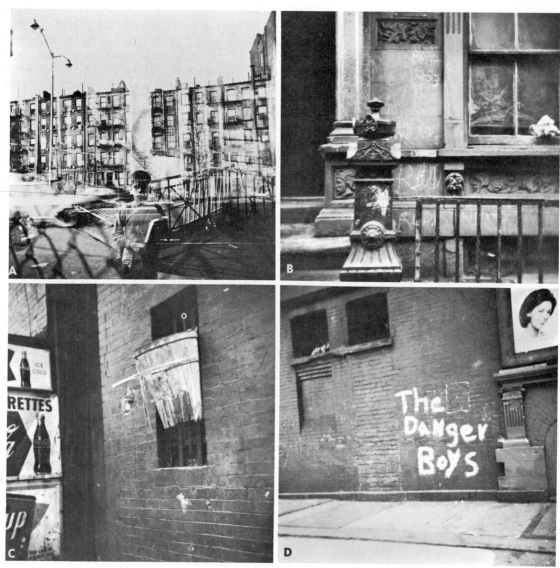

FIGURE 27–16. *A*, This is a lower East Side youth surrounded by urban problems: poverty, slum housing, physical and emotional neglect, lack of adequate educational opportunities and the endless lines of cars passing by his house. *B*, This is the place where he lives, *C*, this is the place where he plays, and *D*, this is what he may become—a danger to society. (From *T C Topics*, Vol. 12. Photographs by Joseph Deitch.)

when he gets into trouble with the law, he harms his parents more than he does himself, because he gains a stronger position in his peer group by his delinquencies. He is thus likely to do anything the gang says so as not to be rejected by them. Treatment may be very difficult, since the basis of the insecurity is in the home and the community. Treatment lies in education and helping these adolescents to accept the mores of a new group.

A child who has been brought up according to one set of mores and then is transplanted to another society may be considered normal in his original society, but delinquent in the new one. In other words, the child who has been reared in a poor neighborhood may not be termed a delinquent when he steals an apple from a fruit stand, because this is fairly normal behavior. If he moves to a neighborhood having a higher socioeconomic standing and steals fruit from a store, he is apprehended and held as a delinquent. The treatment again lies in education and helping the youth to accept the mores of his new group. At the same time his new social group should be helped to understand the adolescent's problem.

DELINQUENCY DUE TO MENTAL RETARDATION. A mentally retarded adolescent depends on other persons for emotional support and therefore is easily lead by them. He is not

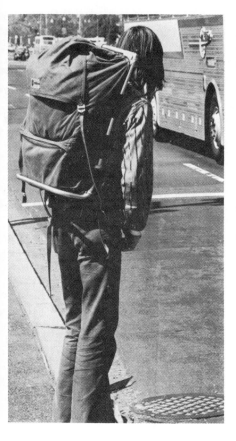

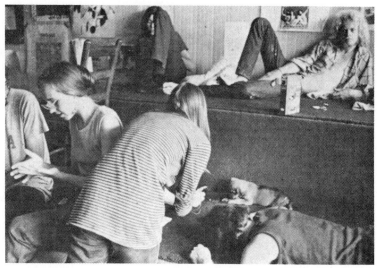

FIGURE 27–17.   Runaways. *A*, Running away from home may not be the best answer. (From Shore, M. F.: *Children Today*, 5:23, January-February 1976.) *B*, In many cities local helping groups have established "crash pads" for teenage runaways. There is usually a time limit for any stay, as well as rules regarding sex and drug use. A special toll-free telephone service has also been set up so runaways can assure their parents that they are all right without revealing where they are. (From *Newsweek*, October 26, 1970.)

able to distinguish clearly what property does not belong to him or what will happen to him as a result of asocial acts. Often he has not been able to develop a conscience, so that he does not know right from wrong. Since he probably has not received adequate love, he may develop an aggressive reaction pattern. He may be used by intelligent delinquents and many times is the one who is caught by the authorities. He needs protection, training, and supervision.

DELINQUENCY DUE TO NEUROSIS Some adolescents become delinquent because they have a need to be punished, since they feel guilty over something in the past. They carry out delinquent acts in order to be punished.

DELINQUENCY DUE TO CHARACTER DISORDERS. Delinquents may have character disorders which result in behavior similar to that of adults who have psychopathic personalities. They cannot learn from experience. They cannot establish meaningful relations even with those persons who try to help them with their problems. They cannot control their desire to do exactly what they want without regard for the consequences to others or to themselves. They may require institutionalization and treatment in order to protect society from their acts. Many

such delinquents could have been recognized in early childhood and given adequate treatment. Unfortunately, too often they are not given help until they come in conflict with the law, and then only if the court has facilities for treatment other than confinement in the outdated home for delinquents. Such institutions often have no psychiatrist or counselor, or so few in proportion to the number of inmates that individual treatment of only a small number of selected patients is possible.

DELINQUENCY DUE TO EMOTIONAL DISTURBANCES (PSYCHOSES). Emotionally disturbed or psychotic adolescents may become delinquent. Their behavior would be normal if the world of reality were like their world of delusions. This kind of delinquency is relatively rare in adolescence, but when it does occur, psychiatric treatment is necessary.

Treatment, Prevention, and Responsibilities of the Nurse. If the delinquent adolescent is to be given adequate *treatment*, emphasis should not be on the delinquent act alone, but must be placed on the total individual in his home and community and on the reasons why he committed the act.

The delinquent adolescent can best be managed by personnel in the juvenile instead of the adult courts. The objectives of juvenile courts are basically diagnostic, protective, and educational. After a study of the total individual, management is planned on the basis of his fundamental problem and what is best for him and for society.

Many suggestions for *prevention* have been made: more and better schools, playgrounds and recreational facilities, and better housing. The gang influence should be replaced with other activities such as those planned by established facilities if they could be kept open in the evenings and over weekends and holidays. Authorities have also recommended that more attention be paid to children of minority groups (see p. 11) and to their economic and social status in their communities. The basic problem confronting all growing children in our society must be better understood if delinquency is to be prevented. If the living situation could be stabilized for all children, there would probably be less delinquency. If more mature adults from the community could take an active interest in the adolescents who do not have adequate parental figures, a positive influence would be brought to bear on these young people.

Broadly, prevention lies in relation not only to individual delinquents, but also to the causative factors operating in communities which lead adolescents into asocial acts. The sociologist, the educator, the economist, the psychologist, and the psychiatrist must make efforts to alter customs and mores which our culture seems to have outgrown. Any preventive effort must combine the skills of many disciplines if it is to be successful.

The school nurse, school nurse practitioner, or nurse in the community may see children who have frequent expressions of physical distress or frequent serious accidents and may seem to be socially distant from their peers, being either more aggressive or more submissive than others in their age group. Such children may later become involved in delinquent acts.

The nurse may be called upon to care for delinquent adolescents. The nurse must recognize that the patient is first of all an individual and must accept him as such without emphasis on his asocial acts. The nurse must make accurate observations of his behavior, provide him with support and work closely with other members of the health team in his treatment.

The nurse must also use professional insight in working with others in the community to help prevent the formation of personality traits which lead to delinquency. In such an endeavor it is not sufficient to assume that a desire to help is enough to make that work effective. The professional person is likely to have deeply rooted misconceptions, stereotypes, and values about those from cultural, ethnic, or socioeconomic backgrounds different from his or her own. The nurse must develop an open and sensitive attitude toward others in order to deliver care that is both socially and medically oriented.

DRUG DEPENDENCE OR ABUSE

Some adolescents or even younger children may become physically addicted to or psychologically dependent on drugs because in society today there is a general breakdown in communications among people. Even among family members who appear genuinely fond of each other, the youths may not feel really loved. They may feel alienated from society. They may

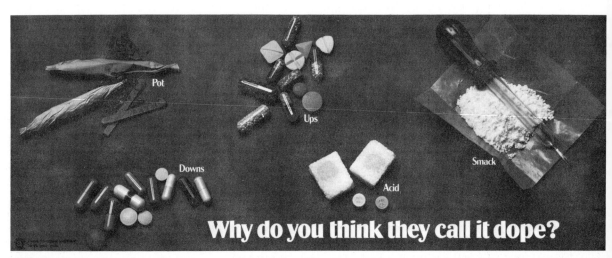

FIGURE 27–18. Drug dependence is a complex crippler. Why do you think they call it dope? (Courtesy of Advertising Council – Transit Advertising for the Public Good.)

therefore begin to take any drug for the comfort and pleasure it gives. Many have seen their parents become pleasure-seekers themselves through their consumption of alcohol and pills. These parents at the same time do not set limits on their children's behavior. Prevention of youthful drug addiction lies largely, therefore, in the improvement of family structure and in relations between parents and their children, the establishment of personal values, and the setting of limits on the behavior of the young. Adolescents especially must also be helped to find their own identity and purpose in life.

A broad definition of an addict is a person who abuses any drug because of its effect on his behavior or mood. The substances to which physical addiction or psychologic dependence may occur vary from nicotine, to glue, to Freon, to alcohol, and to drugs including amphetamines, barbiturates, marihuana, lysergic acid diethylamide (LSD), and narcotics.

Nicotine. Much publicity has been devoted to the dangers of smoking cigarettes, especially their potential effect on the health of the young person. Some children still, however, begin to smoke when they are students in elementary school or during their adolescent years. Recently there has been an alarming increase in incidence and amount of smoking among teenage girls and young women. Both the schools and parents have a responsibility for educating children concerning the dangers of this habit.

Many schools and parents have cracked down on students who smoke. Some school administrators do not permit smoking on school grounds and require students to attend lectures on the harmful effects of smoking. Parents can best influence their child against smoking if they do not smoke themselves. If the child argues that, "If I don't smoke, I won't fit in with the gang," parents should point out that they have tried to teach him to follow his own beliefs, to be independent, even though this requires strong will power. An adolescent who does not follow the advice of his parents may take such guidance more seriously if given by a respected teacher, physician, religious advisor, or nurse.

Glue-Sniffing. Some school-age children and adolescents have become psychologically dependent on inhaling the toxic fumes from rubber cement and model airplane glue, among other commonly used products. Increased amounts are needed for the addict to get the response he desires. The use of large amounts of this substance may lead to intense exhilaration, intoxication, hallucinations, crime, and even death. Unfortunately, some adolescents in time turn from the use of glue to stronger drugs.

In order to attempt to prevent the adverse effects resulting from glue-sniffing, a type of glue is being developed which is vaporless and nontoxic to the human body. Storekeepers should report any sudden increase in sales of glue to young people to the appropriate health department in their community. Parents should have a physician examine their child if they suspect that he has sniffed glue. Teachers should strongly suspect this habit if any of their students are irritable or inattentive, or become excessively drowsy in class. Also, community leaders should make intensive efforts to alert the public about the practice and hazards of glue-sniffing.

Freon-Sniffing. The sniffing or inhalation of a glass-chilling gas which contains one of the Freons and is marketed in aerosol cans is a possible hazard to health. When the gas comes in contact with the skin, it can produce frostbite. When in contact with an open flame or a very hot surface, Freons can decompose into highly irritant and toxic gases. When inhaled in high concentrations, Freons have a narcotizing effect in addition to other reactions thought to be freezing damage to the lungs, laryngeal spasm, or anoxia. Death may result from the inhalation of this substance.

Alcohol. Alcohol can become a problem for anyone using it who has lost the ability to prevent himself from taking a drink or to control the amount he consumes. He develops a physiologic addiction along with a psychologic compulsion which destroys his ability to control his drinking. Alcoholism is a progressive and ultimately fatal disease if the addict does not learn to live without this drug.

Alcohol when consumed is absorbed rapidly into the blood stream. Its most pronounced physiologic effects are on the brain, resulting, depending on the amount taken, in compulsiveness, loss of inhibitions, loss of control of the body as in walking, and ultimate stupor.

The belief that alcoholism can occur only after adult status has been achieved is a fallacy. It is not chronologic age, nor how many years the person has been drinking, that determines whether he is an alcoholic. The important point in making this decision is whether he can control his drinking or whether he is dependent on alcohol and cannot control the amount he consumes. A small percentage of alcoholics are alcoholic from their first drink. Loss of control or alcoholism may occur as early as 15 years of age or even earlier in some persons. For the person who has lost control of his drinking, it is commonly believed that there is no compromise with abstinence.

TABLE 27–3. COMPARISON CHART FOR MAJOR SUBSTANCES USED FOR MIND ALTERATION
(Courtesy of Joel Fort, M.D.)

		1	2	3	4	5	6	7	8
		Official name of drug or chemical	Slang name(s)	Usual single adult dose	Duration of action (hours)	Method of taking	Legitimate medical uses (present and projected)	Potential for psychological dependence[1]	Potential for tolerance (leading to increased dosage)
A		Alcohol Whisky, gin, beer, wine	Booze Hooch	1½ oz. gin or whisky, 12 oz. beer	2–4	Swallowing liquid	Rare. Sometimes used as a sedative (for tension).	High	Yes
B		Caffeine Coffee, tea, Coca-Cola No-Doz, APC	Java	1–2 cups 1 bottle 5 mg.	2–4	Swallowing liquid	Mild stimulant. Treatment of some forms of coma.	Moderate	Yes
C		Nicotine (and coal tar) Cigarettes, cigars	Fag	1–2 cigarettes	1–2	Smoking (inhalation)	None (used as an insecticide).	High	Yes

D		Sedatives
		Alcohol—see above
		Barbiturates
		  Nembutal
		  Seconal
		  Phenobarbital
		Doriden (Glutethimide)
		Chloral hydrate
		Miltown, Equanil
		  (Meprobamate)
			Yellow jackets
			Red devils
			Phennies
			Goofers
				50–100 mg.
				
				500 mg.
				500 mg.
				400 mg.
					4	Swallowing pills or capsules	Treatment of insomnia and tension. Induction of anesthesia.	High	Yes

E		Stimulants
		Caffeine—see above
		Nicotine—see above
		Amphetamines
		  Benzedrine
		  Methedrine
		  Dexedrine
		
		Cocaine
			Bennies
			Crystal
			Dexies or Xmas trees (spansules)
			Coke, snow
				2.5–5.0 mg.
				
				Variable
					4	Swallowing pills, capsules or injecting in vein.
						
						Sniffing or injecting.
							Treatment of obesity, narcolepsy, fatigue, depression.
							
							Anesthesia of the eye and throat.
								High	Yes

F		Tranquilizers
		Librium (Chlordiazepoxide)
		Phenothiazines
		  Thorazine
		  Compazine
		  Stelazine
		Reserpine (Rauwolfia)
				5–10 mg.
				
				10–25 mg.
				10 mg.
				2 mg.
				1 mg.
					4–6	Swallowing pills or capsules	Treatment of anxiety, tension, alcoholism, neurosis, psychosis, psychosomatic disorders and vomiting.	Minimal	No

G		Cannabis (marihuana)	Pot, grass, tea, weed, stuff	Variable—1 cigarette or 1 drink or cake (India)	4	Smoking (inhalation) Swallowing	Treatment of depression, tension, loss of appetite, sexual maladjustment, and narcotic addiction	Moderate	No
H		Narcotics (opiates, analgesics) Opium Heroin Morphine Codeine Percodan Demerol Cough syrups (Cheracol, Hycodan, etc.)	Op Horse, H	10–12 "pipes" (Asia) Variable—bag or paper w. 5–10 percent heroin 15 mg. 30 mg. 1 tablet 50–100 mg. 2–4 oz. (for euphoria)	4	Smoking (inhalation) Injecting in muscle or vein. Swallowing	Treatment of severe pain, diarrhea, and cough.	High	Yes
I		LSD Psilocybin Mescaline (Peyote)	Acid, sugar Cactus	150 micrograms 25 mg. 350 mg.	12 6 12	Swallowing liquid, capsule, pill (or sugar cube) Chewing plant	Experimental study of mind and brain function. Enhancement of creativity and problem solving. Treatment of alcoholism, mental illness, and the dying person. (Chemical warfare)	Minimal	Yes (rare)
J		Antidepressants Ritalin Dibenzapines (Tofranil, Elavil) MAO inhibitors (Nardil, Parnate)		10 mg. 25 mg., 10 mg. 15 mg., 10 mg.	4–6	Swallowing pills or capsules	Treatment of moderate to severe depression.	Minimal	No
K		Miscellaneous Glue Gasoline Amyl nitrite Antihistaminics Nutmeg Nonprescription "sedatives"		Variable 1–2 ampules 25–50 mg. Variable	2	Inhalation Swallowing	None except for antihistamines used for allergy and amyl nitrite for some episodes of fainting.	Minimal to Moderate	Not known

[1] The term "habituation" has sometimes been used to refer to psychological dependence; and the term "addiction" to refer to the combination of tolerance and an abstinence (withdrawal) syndrome.

[2] Drug Abuse (Dependency) properly means: (excessive, often compulsive) use of a drug to an extent that it damages an individual's health or social or vocational adjustment; or is otherwise specifically harmful to society.

TABLE 27–3. COMPARISON CHART FOR MAJOR SUBSTANCES USED FOR MIND ALTERATION (Continued).

9	10	11	12	13	14
Potential for physical dependence	Overall potential for abuse [2]	Reasons drug is sought by users (drug effects and social factors)	Usual short-term effects [3] (psychological, pharmacological, social)	Usual long-term effects (psychological, pharmacological, social)	Form of legal regulation [4] and control
Yes	High	To relax. To escape from tensions, problems and inhibitions. To get ''high'' (euphoria). seeking manhood or rebelling (particularly those under 21). Social custom and conformity. Massive advertising and promotion. Ready availability.	CNS depressant. Relaxation (sedation). Sometimes euphoria. Drowsiness. Impaired judgment, reaction time, coordination and emotional control. Frequent aggressive behavior and driving accidents.	Diversion of energy and money from more creative and productive pursuits. Habituation, Possible obesity with chronic excessive use. Irreversible damage to brain and liver with severe withdrawal illness (D.T.s).	Available and advertised without limitation in many forms with only minimal regulation by age (21, or 18), hours of sale, location, taxation, ban on bootlegging and driving laws. Some ''black market'' for those under age and those evading taxes. Minimal penalties.
No	None	For a ''pick-up'' or stimulation. ''Taking a Break''. Social custom and low cost. Advertising. Ready availability.	CNS stimulant. Increased alertness. Reduction of fatigue.	Sometimes insomia or restlessness. Habituation.	Available and advertised without limit with no regulation for children or adults.
No	Moderate	For a ''pick-up'' or stimulation. ''Taking a Break''. Social custom. Advertising. Ready availability.	CNS stimulant. Relaxation (or distraction) from the process of smoking.	Lung (and other) cancer, heart and blood vessel disease, cough, etc. Habituation. Diversion of energy and money. Air pollution. Fire.	Available and advertised without limit with only minimal regulation by age, taxation, and labeling of packages.
Yes	High	To relax or sleep. To get ''high'' (euphoria). Widely prescribed by physicians, both for specific and nonspecific complaints. General climate encouraging taking pills for everything.	CNS depressants. Sleep induction. Relaxation (sedation). Sometimes euphoria. Drowsiness. Impaired judgment, reaction time, coordination and emotional control. Relief of anxiety-tension. Muscle relaxation.	Irritability, weight loss, addiction with severe withdrawal illness (like D.T.s). Diversion of energy and money. Habituation, addiction.	Available in large amounts by ordinary medical prescription which can be repeatedly refilled or can be obtained from more than one physician. Widely advertised and ''detailed'' to M.D.s and pharmacists. Other manufacture, sale or possession prohibited under federal drug abuse and similar state (dangerous) drug laws. Moderate penalties. Widespread illicit traffic.
No	High	For stimulation and relief of fatigue. To get ''high'' (euphoria). General climate encouraging taking pills for everything.	CNS stimulants. Increased alertness, reduction of fatigue, loss of appetite, insomnia, often euphoria.	Restlessness, irritability, weight loss, toxic psychosis (mainly paranoid). Diversion of energy and money. Habituation. Extreme irritability, toxic psychosis.	Amphetamines, same as Sedatives above. Cocaine, same as Narcotics below.
No	Minimal	Medical (including psychiatric) treatment of anxiety or tension states, alcoholism, psychoses, and other disorders.	Selective CNS depressants. Relaxation, relief of anxiety-tension. Suppression of hallucinations or delusions, improved functioning.	Sometimes drowsiness, dryness of mouth, blurring of vision, skin rash, tremor. Occasionally jaundice, agranulocytosis.	Same as Sedatives above, except not usually included under the special federal or state drug laws. Negligible illicit traffic.
No	Moderate	To get ''high'' (euphoria). As an escape. To relax. To socialize. To conform to various subcultures which sanction its use. For rebellion. Attraction of behavior labeled as deviant. Availability.	Relaxation, euphoria, increased appetite, some alteration of time perception, possible impairment of judgment and coordination. (Probable CNS depressant.)	Usually none. Possible diversion of energy and money.	Unavailable (although permissible) for ordinary medical prescription. Possession, sale, and cultivation prohibited by state and federal narcotic or marihuana laws. Severe penalties. Widespread illicit traffic.
Yes	High	To get ''high'' (euphoria). As an escape. To avoid withdrawal symptoms. As a substitute for aggressive and sexual drives which cause anxiety. To conform to various sub-cultures which sanction use. For rebellion.	CNS depressants. Sedation, euphoria, relief of pain, impaired intellectual functioning and coordination.	Constipation, loss of appetite and weight, temporary impotency or sterility. Habituation, addiction with unpleasant and painful withdrawal illness.	Available (except heroin) by special (narcotics) medical prescriptions. Some available by ordinary prescription or over-the-counter. Other manufacture, sale, or possession prohibited under state and federal narcotics laws. Severe penalties. Extensive illicit traffic.
No	Moderate	Curiosity created by recent widespread publicity. Seeking for meaning and consciousness—expansion. Rebellion. Attraction of behavior recently labeled as deviant. Availability.	Production of visual imagery, increased sensory awareness, anxiety, nausea, impaired coordination; sometimes consciousness-expansion.	Usually none. Sometimes precipitates or intensifies an already existing psychosis; more commonly can produce a panic reaction when person is improperly prepared.	Available only to a few medical researchers (or to members of the Native American Church). Other manufacture, sale or possession prohibited by state dangerous drug or federal drug abuse laws. Moderate penalties. Extensive illicit traffic.
No	Minimal	Medical (including psychiatric) treatment of depression.	Relief of depression (elevation of mood), stimulation.	Basically the same as Tranquilizers above.	Same as Tranquilizers above.
No	Moderate	Curiosity. To get ''high'' (euphoria). Thrill seeking. Ready availability.	When used for mind-alteration generally produces a ''high'' (euphoria) with impaired coordination and judgment.	Variable—some of the substances can seriously damage the liver or kidney.	Generally easily available. Some require prescriptions. In several states glue banned for those under 21.

[3] Always to be considered in evaluating the effects of these drugs is the amount consumed, purity, frequency, time interval since ingestion, food in the stomach, combinations with other drugs, and most importantly, the personality or character of the individual taking it and the setting or context in which it is taken. The determinations made in this chart are based upon the evidence with human use of these drugs rather than upon isolated artificial experimental situations or animal research.
[4] Only scattered, inadequate health, educational or rehabilitation programs (usually prison hospitals) exist for narcotic addicts and alcoholics (usually outpatient clinics) with nothing for the others except sometimes prison.

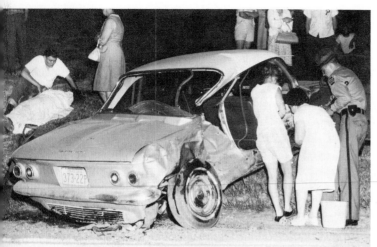

FIGURE 27–19. The teenage driver of this car had been drinking. His passenger, a 17-year-old girl, was killed instantly. (Courtesy of Citizens Ambulance Service, Indiana, Pa.)

For the alcoholic, alcohol is a drug rather than a beverage. He drinks because he is depressed, lonely, angry, or nervous. Compulsive behavior in regard to the use of a chemical is a good indication of addiction. Continued excessive use of alcohol affects the person's power of reason and level of functioning, seriously impairs his ability to make critical judgments, and destroys his ability for self-evaluation.

Teenage alcoholism is a major social problem today. In adolescence, recurrent drinking occurs more frequently among boys than among girls. Excessive drinking occurs among adolescents in large metropolitan areas, and is also occurring more frequently among adolescents in suburbia in the United States and in many countries throughout the world. Excessive drinking, whether the person is an alcoholic or not, is responsible for many fatal highway accidents.

Guidance for therapy of alcoholics of any age may be obtained from the group known as Alcoholics Anonymous. Assistance for members of families of alcoholics may be obtained from Al-Anon, a group which helps relatives understand the scope of the problem. The National Council on Alcoholism, Inc., also provides the professions and the community with knowledge needed to prevent alcoholism and rehabilitate alcoholics.

The aim of modern alcohol education is to produce more intelligent approaches to the drinking experience itself and to alcohol as a drug. We live in a drinking culture, which generally approves of drinking and in which many young people will accept the prevailing pattern and use alcohol. Society is therefore concerned more with what kind of drinkers they will become, rather than with the simple fact of whether they do or do not drink. When alcohol is used as a beverage, an appetizer or as a religious or cultural symbol, its effects will probably be benign. When it is used as an intoxicant or drug as a means of escaping stress, it becomes a problem.

Amphetamines and Barbiturates. *Amphetamines* are drugs known to combat sleepiness and fatigue because they are stimulants to the central nervous system. They may also be used medically to suppress appetite. The amphetamines most commonly used are amphetamine (Benzedrine), methamphetamine, and dextroamphetamine (Dexedrine). To those persons who use slang terms for these drugs, they are called "pep pills," "speed," "bennies," and "uppers."

Amphetamines can produce a feeling of well-being and alertness, but overdoses can cause irritability and tension. These drugs cause tachycardia, increase in the blood pressure, rapid respirations, headache, diarrhea, and increased perspiration. These effects are due to the fact that in the body these drugs stimulate the release of norepinephrine, a substance stored in nerve endings, and concentrate it in higher centers of the brain.

These stimulants may be misused by people of all ages. Abusers may take them orally or intravenously; however, this practice is dangerous. Taking drugs intravenously is known as "speeding." As a result of injecting "speed" into the vein, serum hepatitis, abscess, and long-term personality disorders or death may occur. A common saying in certain parts of the country is that "Speed kills."

Stimulant drugs do not produce physical dependence; however, the body can develop a tolerance to these drugs so that larger and larger doses are required to achieve the desired effect. Psychologic dependence on these drugs can occur.

Barbiturates are sedatives commonly used to relax the central nervous system. These drugs include the fast-acting pentobarbital (Nembutal) and secobarbital (Seconal) and the long-acting phenobarbital (Luminal), butabarbital (Butisol) and amobarbital (Amytal). Slang terms for the fast-acting barbiturates are "downers" and "barbs."

Barbiturates depress the action of the heart muscles, skeletal muscles, and nerves; thus they reduce the heart and respiratory rates and lower the blood pressure. Increased dosages of these drugs, however, cause confusion, slurred speech, staggering gait, and decreased ability to concentrate and work, and may ultimately produce anger, assaultive behavior, or a deep sleep.

Barbiturates, especially when taken with alcohol, may be the cause of automobile accidents. They are also, because they are readily obtained, one of the main ways people choose to commit suicide.

These drugs are physically addicting; thus increasingly higher doses are needed before the body can feel their effects. Rapid withdrawal from the use of these drugs may cause nausea, convulsions, and death. Withdrawal under medical supervision may take several weeks or months on gradually reduced doses.

Both amphetamines and barbiturates are regulated nationally by the Food and Drug Administration. They may be obtained legally by prescription from a physician; however, all too often adolescents obtain them illegally. Research is currently being done to determine how young people learn to abuse drugs and what can be done once this occurs.

Methaqualone (Quaalude, Parest). Methaqualone is a nonbarbiturate, sedative hypnotic that is used for sedation in order to produce sleep. It is attractive to drug abusers because its effects are rapid and long-lasting. It tends to lower inhibitions for those who seek successful social encounters and at the same time, has an aphrodisiac effect. Heroin addicts supplement their habits with methaqualone to increase the effects of heroin and to make withdrawal from it easier.

Methaqualone is a dangerous drug and must be used with caution in persons having impaired hepatic function and anxiety states, especially if there is evidence of an impending depression or when tendencies to suicide exist. Its effects can prove fatal. This drug can lead to psychologic and physical dependence. When the individual stops taking the drug he may experience progressive anxiety, involuntary muscle twitching, tremor of the hands and fingers, dizziness, weakness, fatigue, headaches, nausea, weight loss, sleeplessness, grand mal seizures, and a delirium not unlike alcoholic delirium tremens. Withdrawal therapy consists of cross-substituting pentobarbital for methaqualone. The dose of pentobarbital is decreased by 10 per cent each day until complete detoxification occurs.

Marihuana. Marihuana is a drug found in the Indian hemp plant, *Cannabis sativa*, which grows in countries around the world having a mild climate. The flowers and leaves of this plant are dried and rolled and smoked in cigarettes or pipes. This substance can also be taken in food or sniffed. The cigarettes, termed "joints," "sticks" or "reefers," have a sweetish odor when smoked.

The use of marihuana ("pot," "grass") has increased rapidly in the United States in recent years. When marihuana is smoked, it enters the blood stream quickly and acts on the nervous system and brain. Physical reactions to the drug include tachycardia, reddening of the eyes, lowered body temperature, and an increase in appetite. Persons who use marihuana may become loud, very talkative, or drowsy with an inability to coordinate their movements. They may feel excited or depressed and have a distortion of their sense of distance, time, color, and hearing ability. They may find it difficult to think clearly and thus to make decisions.

In larger doses or higher strengths, marihuana may be termed a "hallucinogen" because it may cause visual hallucinations, illusions or delusions. Paranoia is the most common untoward reaction to this drug.

Marihuana at present is classified as a drug which causes dependence rather than true addiction. It does not cause physical dependence as do narcotics. The body probably does not develop a tolerance to the drug, nor does withdrawal of the drug result in physical illness. Psychologic dependence, it is thought, may develop if it is used regularly.

Persons using marihuana may or may not ultimately use narcotics. Although no link has been found between these drugs, those who abuse one drug may abuse others or may be led to use them through their contacts with other users or sellers.

In most of the United States, possessing or selling marihuana is against federal law. If adolescents break the laws regarding this drug, their education may be interrupted and they may have a shadow cast on their future by having a police record. In addition to the legal aspects, a young person who experiments with drugs which may have an effect on his personality development may find it increasingly difficult to develop a sense of identity, to adjust to life as an adult, and to develop a value system.

Lysergic Acid Diethylamide (LSD). Lysergic acid diethylamide is a man-made chemical which is classed as a "hallucinogen," a drug which affects the mind. It produces bizarre mental reactions in people, with severe distortions in their physical senses of seeing, smelling, hearing, and touch. Other drugs which are also powerful hallucinogens, or psychedelic drugs, include mescaline, psilocybin, peyote, DMT, and STP.

Although the use of LSD ("acid") is illegal in the United States except for government-approved use, many persons use it on either an experimental or regular basis. LSD may be taken on a sugar cube, cookie, or other food, or it can be licked off a postage stamp on which the drug has been placed. The physical response to this drug includes tachycardia, irregular respirations, rise in blood pressure and temperature, shaking of the extremities, dilatation of the pupils, flushed or pale face, chills, nausea, and anorexia. This drug is not physically addicting; therefore there is no physical illness when it is withdrawn.

The psychologic effects of this drug include changes in the physical senses, but it does not make people more creative, nor does it help them to find themselves. Colors may seem more brilliant, strange patterns may emerge before the eyes, and walls of rooms may appear to move. The senses of taste, smell, hearing, and touch may seem more acute than usual. The sense of time may be disturbed, although consciousness is not lost. Users of this drug may feel happy and depressed at the same time. They may also lose the normal appreciation of the difference between their bodies and space; therefore they sometimes feel that they can fly or float through air. Individual users may explain, depending on their sensation, that they have had a "good" or a "bad" trip.

Long-continued use of this drug may impair the person's ability to concentrate, especially on a goal in life, and eventually cause him to leave what the usual person calls "society."

Certain dangers are involved in the use of LSD. The user may experience panic because he feels that he cannot stop the action of the drug once he has taken it, or he may become paranoid. For the youthful users especially, the effect of this drug can be extremely frightening, since they are not yet mature in their emotional development. The user may have a recurrence of the effects of the drug long after he has taken it. He may become depressed or mentally deranged. The use of the drug may also contribute to acts of murder or suicide. Some persons may suffer acute or long-term mental illness after taking this drug.

Of more serious consequence is the possibility that the use of LSD may affect the chromosomes, causing chromosomal breakage and damage and possibly abnormalities in the children of those who have used this drug, or malignancy in the user. Research is being done to determine how these changes occur, since total genetic and psychologic damage caused by LSD to the human population may not be evident for some time to come.

The most important danger associated with the use of LSD is accidental death because the person under the effects of this drug may jump from a height, believing that he can float or fly, or jump in front of a moving vehicle, believing that no harm can come to him.

There are severe penalties, including imprisonment or fines, for anyone who illegally produces, sells, or otherwise distributes LSD.

Research is currently being done to determine the drug's action and value for human beings, the ways to treat those who suffer from the side effects of the drug, the extent of use of the drug, and the culture of those who use it.

Narcotics. Narcotics is a term usually used to refer to opium, a product of the poppy flower, or drugs made from opium, including heroin and morphine. Cocaine made from cocoa leaves as well as other drugs may also be considered a narcotic. Heroin (Horse, Smack, H) currently appears to be the most widely used narcotic, so that this is the drug which will be discussed more fully.

The person who becomes addicted ("hooked") to a narcotic craves repeated and larger doses of the drug because his body develops a tolerance for the substance taken. When the drug is withdrawn, physical illness occurs with symptoms of sweating, shaking, vomiting, diarrhea, and severe abdominal pains. Psychologic dependence also occurs because the addict uses the drug as a means to escape facing the reality of life. If sufficient drug is taken, death may result.

When heroin is taken initially, the person may feel a reduction of his fears, a relief from his worries and a degree of inactivity which may result in stupor. The drug has the effect of depressing certain parts of the brain and nerves. It reduces thirst, hunger, the sex drive, and feelings of pain. Malnutrition may result when this drug is used over a period of time. When the drug is discontinued, withdrawal symptoms appear in approximately 18 hours.

Heroin addiction occurs chiefly among young men in large cities. Narcotic addiction unfortunately also occurs among young women who may also be pregnant. Infants born to these mothers may be narcotic addicts at birth (see p. 269) who must go through a period of withdrawal during the neonatal period or who may die from their addiction.

In recent years serum hepatitis has been acquired increasingly by adolescents through the habitual use of narcotics. The physician who ex-

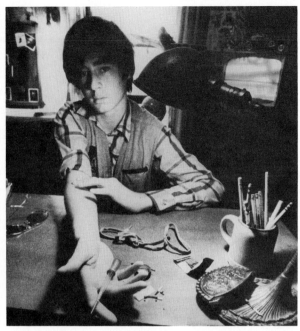

A

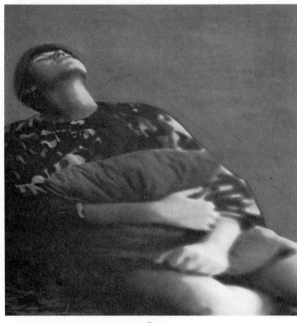

B

FIGURE 27-20. Drug addiction. *A*, A "junkie's" parents should not be the last to know. *B*, Withdrawal. (*A*, Courtesy of Metropolitan Life Insurance Company. *B*, From *Education Age*, January-February, 1969.)

amines these young people and finds signs and symptoms of hepatitis should have a high index of suspicion and rule out intravenous use of drugs as the mode of transmission. Research is currently being done on a vaccine to immunize against this disease.

Once a person is addicted, the main objective of his life is to obtain a continued supply of drugs. His education and his working in gainful employment may be discontinued because he may be frequently ill from either withdrawal or overdosage of the drug. He may have difficulties with both his family and the law. Continuing his habit leads him into crime, chiefly thefts or other crimes against property, because his addiction is so costly. Illegal possession or sale of narcotics is punishable by fines or imprisonment.

Drug addiction is a medical illness, and therefore treatment is needed. If treatment resulting in withdrawal of the drug is successful, the person returns to his community, where he may find it difficult not to resume his use of drugs. Therapy, including physical, mental, social, and vocational rehabilitation efforts, has been attempted in order to prevent the person from returning to the drug and wasting his life.

Research is currently being done on the effects of narcotics, the users themselves, and on the antidotes which can be used for heroin addiction. In recent years, a treatment for heroin addiction has been developed using methadone, a synthetic drug that takes the place of the narcotic in the system. Many major cities support methadone clinics in which addicts are treated on a voluntary basis. Methodone, although also addictive, can turn a heroin addict into a socially acceptable, physically comfortable, responsible member of society.

Responsibilities of the Nurse. The role of the nurse in relation to the adolescent who is taking drugs which may cause physical addiction or psychologic dependence is complex. Certainly the first obligation of the nurse is to be alert to the possibility that addiction may exist in this age group and to be knowledgeable about the signs and symptoms of the various forms of addiction. The nurse must be able to recognize certain personality or behavioral changes which occur with the use of certain drugs. The nurse must also be cognizant of the treatment of various forms of drug addiction, which is increasingly being considered a medical instead of a moral problem.

The nurse, whether in the hospital or in the community, must be prepared to answer questions about the use of drugs, whether these questions are asked by anxious parents or the adolescents themselves. The nurse must know sources of help in the community to which such persons can be referred, should the need arise. The nurse should also know of educational materials such as those listed at the end of this chapter which can be used to educate the public.

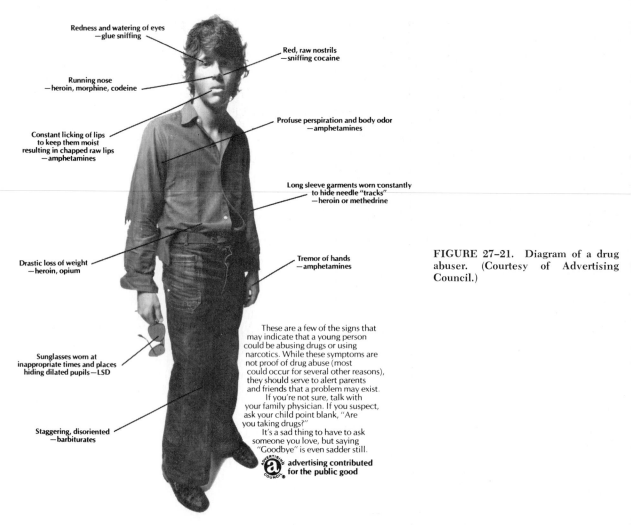

Redness and watering of eyes
—glue sniffing

Red, raw nostrils
—sniffing cocaine

Running nose
—heroin, morphine, codeine

Profuse perspiration and body odor
—amphetamines

Constant licking of lips
to keep them moist
resulting in chapped raw lips
—amphetamines

Long sleeve garments worn constantly
to hide needle "tracks"
—heroin or methedrine

Drastic loss of weight
—heroin, opium

Tremor of hands
—amphetamines

Sunglasses worn at
inappropriate times and places
hiding dilated pupils—LSD

Staggering, disoriented
—barbiturates

These are a few of the signs that
may indicate that a young person
could be abusing drugs or using
narcotics. While these symptoms are
not proof of drug abuse (most
could occur for several other reasons),
they should serve to alert parents
and friends that a problem may exist.
If you're not sure, talk with
your family physician. If you suspect,
ask your child point blank, "Are
you taking drugs?"
It's a sad thing to have to ask
someone you love, but saying
"Goodbye" is even sadder still.

advertising contributed
for the public good

FIGURE 27–21. Diagram of a drug abuser. (Courtesy of Advertising Council.)

The school nurse or nurse in the community may be asked to present classes in the school or community on the methods of identification of adolescents taking drugs, as well as on the dangerous aspects of the use of various drugs. Certainly the nurse would need to be knowledgeable in this area if such a challenge is to be accepted.

The nurse may also play an extremely important role in the prevention of addiction and in case-finding of adolescents who have become addicts. Empathy and understanding must be shown for the problems of these young people and the nurse must not talk down to them or sit in judgment on them. The nurse can listen to their comments attentively and try to help them, but when necessary can refer them to sources such as individual physicians or to clinics where further help can be obtained.

It is especially necessary for youth and their parents to recognize the fact that addiction to drugs except nicotine may result in rejection of an application for admission to a college, rejection by prospective employers, legal action

against them for crimes committed under the influence of drugs, or ultimate death from the drug itself or from irresponsible actions while using the drug, such as careless driving of an automobile or motorcycle.

Since the actual therapy and nursing care of the adolescent who is addicted are not too different from those of the adult addict, details of rehabilitation will not be discussed in this text. The common denominator in the treatment and care of persons addicted to drugs is that of reducing anxiety through quiet, calm reassurance and support given in a controlled environment by a warm, understanding human being. A team approach to the rehabilitation of these young persons has been found helpful in many centers devoted to their care.

The nurse as a member of the community should be knowledgeable about the current laws relating to drugs in the area. The nurse should actively strive to have legislation passed to protect those too young to protect themselves from the possibility of physical addiction or psychologic dependence on drugs. If the nurse suspects that drugs are being peddled in the schools or elsewhere in the area, school authorities or the police should be notified. The nurse should know also, however, that legal action is only part of the answer to the use of drugs by juveniles. The ultimate cure for the drug menace lies in the home and in the community, where many parents presently are not sufficiently concerned to provide guidance and control for their youths.

SEVERE PSYCHONEUROSES

Adolescents may have manifestations of severe neuroses similar to those seen in adults. They may show symptoms of severe depression, hysteria, anxiety, or withdrawal. The patient usually has a mixture of these symptoms. Older adolescents may become anxious and show a deep concern about their physical health. Although this may be an extension of their normal concern about their health, they resist reassurance from their physician. They may also evidence highly organized compulsions and phobias. The physician and the nurse may need guidance from a psychiatrist in the care of such patients.

ADOLESCENT SCHIZOPHRENIC REACTIONS

Incidence and Etiology. Although schizophrenic reactions are not too common in children, they are the most important kind of mental illness during the adolescent years.

There are several theories about the causes of schizophrenic reactions. No one cause has been proved. It is not certain to what extent heredity is a factor. There may also be a basic biochemical or neurologic defect in schizophrenics. Environmental and developmental stresses may cause a defect in interpersonal relations. The schizophrenic has never in his life felt accepted by others or gained satisfaction from what he attempted to do. Usually, as a child he received too little love and affection. Too much was expected of him, and too little happiness or reward was given in return.

Clinical Manifestations and Diagnosis. The onset may seem acute, but personality changes have probably been going on for months or years. The following behavior may be shown: (a) Rigidity in adjustment to various persons or situations in the environment. The child cannot tolerate any kind of life other than his own. He abides by his rituals in his daily life and cannot change them quickly. (b) He begins to draw a curtain between himself and others. He becomes reserved and seems to have only brief periods of contact with reality. His personality becomes disorganized to a degree. (c) There is an emotional and intellectual split between the

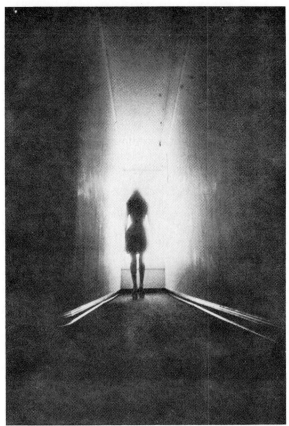

FIGURE 27–22. The schizophrenic withdraws from the world of reality to a world of his or her own making. (From Wiley, L. (Ed.): Reprinted with permission from the February 1976 issue of *Nursing 76*, Intermed Communications, Inc. Further reproduction in whole or part expressly prohibited by law.)

meaning of the act itself and his response to it. He may laugh when a tragedy occurs. He appears odd in his behavior. (d) He becomes careless, untidy and tardy and finally is satisfied just to sit alone. At last he retreats into his own world because the world of reality is intolerable. Delusions and hallucinations occur. Speech becomes irregular and illogical.

Mental illness is difficult to *diagnose* in adolescence because normal children and adolescents at one time or another in the developmental process may show similar behavior. It is the degree to which abnormal behavior occurs that is important in making a diagnosis.

Treatment, Responsibilities of the Nurse, and Prognosis. Psychiatric *treatment* is given as promptly as possible. Care, to be effective, must be given by accepting, warm adults who give the young person their undivided attention. The adolescent must be provided with love and acceptance and recognition given to his need for appropriate experiences with gratification and mastery of frustration. His physical condition should be improved. Institutional care is provided as necessary.

Before the age of 12 years it is difficult to be certain of the *prognosis*. Even with therapy and institutional care the prognosis has been poor. In recent years some success has been achieved with intensive therapy. Cure occurs rarely, but a satisfactory social adjustment can be made. More and more work is being done so that treatment of these adolescents can be more successful.

SUICIDE

Suicidal attempts and suicide are not rare in children and adolescents. The rate of these deaths has almost doubled in recent years. This problem is less common in grade-school children than in adolescents; however, it may be seen in children as young as the early school years. Suicide is more common in males than females. Females, however, make more suicidal attempts than males. Suicide occurs most often in the spring of the year. It is surpassed in the age group from 12 to 19 years only by accidents, homicides, and malignant neoplasms as causes of death. Many suicides are disguised as accidents such as poisoning, falls, electrocutions, or motorcycle and automobile crashes.

Some physicians believe that the increased rate of suicide among adolescents can be blamed on the general permissiveness in modern society which, combined with a sexual revolution, results in the destruction rather than the strengthening of the egos of young people. More specifically, most children and adolescents who contemplate or commit suicide are "social isolates," come from disorganized homes and are under intolerable stress, having a sense of failure, feeling unloved, unwanted, and bad. They react with anger, usually against their parents. These feelings produce guilt which leads to a suicidal effort and, in a way, results in their punishing their parents. Some adolescents may commit suicide as a result of efforts to manipulate others, as a signal of distress, or because they are schizophrenic (see p. 901). Adolescents who threaten or commit suicide are in general impulsive and immature persons who tend to overreact to even minor stresses. They are restless, bored, hyperactive persons who many times have a history of truancy from school, absence from the home, sexual promiscuity, and depression.

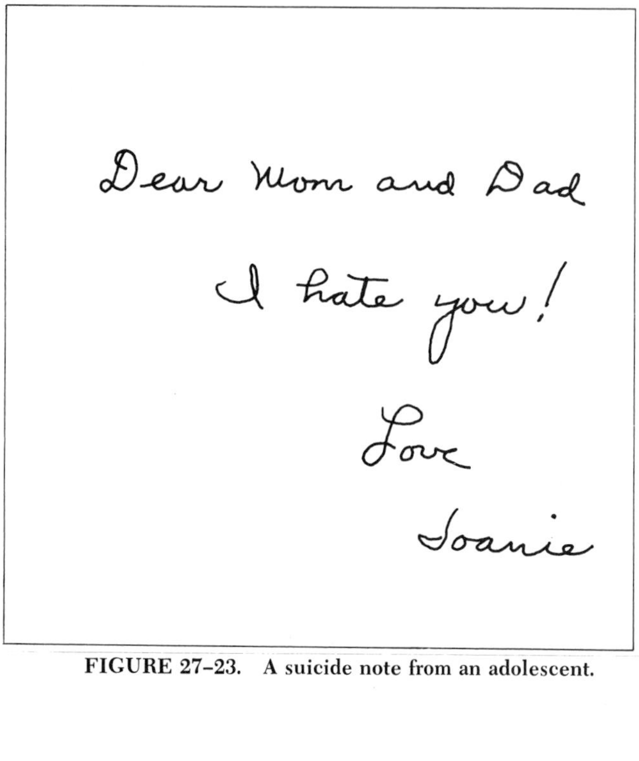

In the grade-school and adolescent groups depression is often evidenced by disobedience, boredom, continued temper tantrums, restlessness, running away from home and school, and accident proneness. Many such adolescents act out their feelings through the use of drugs, alcohol, and sexual promiscuity. They may evidence failure in school, inability to concentrate, isolation from others, weight loss due to anorexia, insomnia, and somatic complaints, a common one of which is overwhelming fatigue. They may also be preoccupied with the meaninglessness of their lives and a wish for death. The person's actual thought of death (see p. 107) depends on his age. This accounts in part for the lower incidence of suicide among children younger than adolescents.

Prior to a suicide attempt there is usually, but not always, a triggering event such as a serious crisis involving discipline, punishment which the person considers unfair, jealousy in love, loss of a parent by divorce or death, or pregnancy out of wedlock. Suicidal attempts almost always occur when the person feels extremely lonely.

Adolescents who are depressed or who have threatened suicide require a thorough physical, neurologic, and psychiatric evaluation. Often significant persons in the adolescent's life such as parents, teachers, religious advisors, and Scout leaders can contribute observations helpful in understanding his emotional adjustment. The adolescent should also be observed carefully for his behavior after admission to the hospital, especially for self-destructive behavior.

After a period of observation, both parents and the patient should be engaged in the process of therapy, given either by a pediatrician experi-

FIGURE 27–23. A suicide note from an adolescent.

enced in this clinical area or by a child psychiatrist. The physician must help the adolescent to build sufficient ego strength to face his serious emotional problems. If the adolescent does not trust his physician, he may resist therapy, deny his illness, and act out his feelings as a way of escaping from what he considers an intolerable situation. These patients should receive care and close observation for at least three months. The period of after-care is often more important than the immediate emergency therapy.

Responsibilities of the Nurse. Since adolescents commit suicide during an emotional crisis at a time when there is no one for them to talk to, the nurse who is in contact with this age group must be alert to changes in behavior evidenced by depression, disorientation, defiance and dissatisfaction with life which could lead to a suicidal act. The nurse must observe such behavior and take steps to obtain help for the person as soon as possible. This is especially true of those who give definite verbal warnings of suicidal intent. Nurses must also help parents to understand more about suicide and to spot presuicidal warning signs. Many suicide-prevention centers have been formed in cities across our country in order to provide assistance when needed.

Because of their extreme feelings of loneliness, many would-be suicides are easy to talk back to life. They are never totally certain that they want to die. If someone says, "Don't," they many times will not go through with the act. An interested person must answer the cry for help and help the person to cope with his loneliness and provide a hopeful, positive attitude toward life.

The responsible nurse when giving care to such a young person must respect and accept him as a person, and provide protection against self-destruction by reducing environmental hazards until he is able to assume this responsibility for himself. The nurse must bolster his self-confidence and self-esteem. When he expresses feelings of worthlessness, the nurse can guide him into doing therapeutic tasks such as helping others. The nurse can also provide diversional activities for him in order to help him express his feelings of aggression and hostility constructively and outwardly rather than destructively turning them inward on himself. The adolescent should be encouraged to participate in making plans for such activities and other aspects of his care.

Probably the most important factor for the nurse in helping the suicidal young person is in maintaining a therapeutic relation with him. The nurse must evidence support and protection

of him through sincere interest, warmth, and understanding until he can manage his self-destructive urges for himself.

CLINICAL SITUATIONS

Mrs. Horter brought her 14-year-old daughter, Barbara, to the adolescent clinic because she had "pimples on her face" which she persisted in picking. After an examination of the lesions the physician made the diagnosis of acne vulgaris. Barbara is a well developed and attractive adolescent whose menarche occurred when she was 12 years of age. Both Barbara and her mother appeared to be alert and interested in the activities of the clinic.

1. Acne vulgaris is caused primarily by
a. The erratic diet of the adolescent.
b. Changes in the skin during adolescence.
c. Irritation of the skin due to the habit of picking the face.
d. Allergy to foods containing chocolate.

2. Several weeks later the nurse, who had previously established a good relation with Barbara, met her in the clinic and commented on the improvement of the acne. During the conversation Barbara said, "I'm glad my mother didn't come with me today. She's always telling me what to do, and when I refuse to do what she says, she threatens to tell my father." In response to this expression of feeling the nurse would answer
a. "Your mother did seem to be a domineering type of woman. Perhaps if you do what she says, she won't bother you so much."
b. "If you would act your age, your mother wouldn't have to tell you what to do."
c. "Why don't you talk to your father about this situation and see how he feels about your mother?"
d. "Your mother may be having difficulty in remembering that you are almost grown up now. Perhaps if you would talk with her about this problem, you both would understand each other better."

3. Mrs. Horter confides in the nurse her deep concern because she has observed Barbara daydreaming on occasion. Some of the mothers of Barbara's friends are equally disturbed about this behavior in their adolescents. The nurse should realize in order to answer this comment that
a. Adolescents daydream because they want to evade doing their homework or helping with the housework.
b. They are showing early indications of becoming schizophrenics and should be examined by their physicians as soon as possible.
c. They need time to formulate their philosophies of life, to learn to know themselves and to plan for their futures.
d. They are growing rapidly and are too fatigued to engage in activities such as sports.

Fifteen-year-old Carmella Nignari has been admitted to the hospital with a diagnosis of pulmonary tuberculosis. Her father is a guard at a local warehouse, and her mother before Carmella's hospitalization worked as a waitress in the evenings and over the weekends to supplement the family income. When her mother worked, Carmella had cared for the six younger siblings. Now her mother must stay home from work to assume this responsibility.

4. As a result of Carmella's illness all the other members of her family had tuberculin tests and chest x-rays to deter-

mine whether they also had the infection. The infant and the toddler were examined thoroughly to determine the presence of:

a. Miliary tuberculosis.

b. Pott's disease.

c. Tuberculosis of the cervical lymph nodes.

d. Tuberculous dactylitis.

5. A positive reaction to a tuberculin skin test indicates that the person

a. Has an active lesion of pulmonary tuberculosis.

b. Has never had tuberculosis or come in contact with the disease.

c. Has been infected with *Mycobacterium tuberculosis* and is hypersensitive to its protein.

d. Has not been infected with the disease, but is allergic to *Mycobacterium tuberculosis.*

6. Carmella is concerned about her health and asks many questions about her condition. The nurse would

a. Ask the physician to talk with her about each question she asks.

b. Explain that worrying about her health is harmful for her. Assure her the physician knows how to care for persons having tuberculosis.

c. Ignore most of her questions because Carmella only wants attention.

d. Answer her questions to the best of her ability and refer those which she cannot answer to the physician.

7. Carmella asked why she could not be treated with only one kind of medication. To answer her question the nurse would need to know that streptomycin should not be used alone in the treatment of tuberculosis because

a. Streptomycin-resistant organisms emerge rapidly.

b. The eighth cranial nerve may be damaged.

c. The drug is not very effective against *Mycobacterium tuberculosis.*

d. Treatment with more than one drug hastens recovery.

8. The nurse who cared for Carmella had had a negative reaction to the Mantoux test on entrance to the school of nursing. The physician had recommended that the nurse be protected against *Mycobacterium tuberculosis* by

a. Bacillus of Calmette and Guérin vaccine.

b. Plague vaccine.

c. Salk vaccine.

d. Pertussis vaccine.

GUIDES TO FURTHER STUDY

1. Observe a group of adolescents in high school, a recreation center or a neighborhood meeting place. Describe the general activity of the members of the group. Were any adolescents paired off in couples? What activity, if any, were those doing who did not mix with the others? Observe their posture when sitting and standing. Observe their manner of dress and their grooming. Compare your observations with your knowledge of the normal behavior patterns of adolescents.

2. What is your understanding of the function of a clinic for adolescents? How many adolescent clinics have been organized in your state or community?

3. What are the most recent statistics in your state on the causes of mortality in the adolescent age group? What preventive measures could be taken to reduce these tragedies?

4. What rehabilitative services are available for physically and mentally handicapped adolescents in your hospital, your community and your state? Evaluate these services to determine whether they are adequately meeting the need.

5. Bob, a 13-year-old delinquent, has been admitted to the pediatric unit with a diagnosis of bilateral fractured legs. This injury resulted from a fall from a third floor window while he was experiencing a bad trip from LSD. What would be your approach to this adolescent and his parents? What would be your role and responsibility as a member of the

health team in providing care for this young person? Investigate the agencies in your community which could assist in his rehabilitation.

6. In class role play an evening situation in a "hot line" office during which calls come in from (a) Marcia, a 13-year-old adolescent, who fears she is pregnant; (b) Richard, a 16-year-old, who asks, "I think I got 'clap!' What should I do?"; (c) Jennifer, a 16-year-old, who says, "My boyfriend and I have a ten-pill-a-day habit with 'barbs.' I want to kick it!" and (d) David, a 15-year-old youth, who says, "I cut my wrists open. I thought I wanted to get out of everything, but I'm afraid." With your classmates taking turns making the calls and answering them, tape record the class so that you can evaluate with your teacher the responses made.

7. What facilities are available in your state for the care of adolescents having a diagnosis of schizophrenia? Are these facilities adequately meeting the need?

8. Select the three experiences which were most disturbing to you and the three experiences which were most satisfying to you in providing care for children. State for each incident the age of the patient, his diagnosis and a description of the situation. Analyze each of these incidents to determine why they were disturbing or satisfying to you and discuss them in seminar.

TEACHING AIDS AND OTHER INFORMATION*

Al-Anon World Services, Inc.

The Mother and Father of an Alcoholic.

This Is Al-Anon.

American Academy of Pediatrics

A Model Act Providing for Consent of Minors for Health Services.

Drugs and Sports.

Infectious Diseases (Red Book).

Stilbestrol and Adenocarcinoma of the Vagina.

Teenage Pregnancy and the Problem of Abortion.

The American Cancer Society, Inc.

Nursing Problems of Children with Cancer, 1974.

_____

*Complete addresses are given in the Appendix.

American Lung Association

For TB Patients.
Fundamentals of Tuberculosis Today.
Lo que Todo el Mundo Necesita Sabe Acerca de Tuberculosis.
Me Quit Smoking? How?
¿Se Preocupa Usted Porque Pudiera Tener Tuberculosis?
TB Outside the Lungs Facts.
Treatment and Control of Tuberculosis.

Department of National Health and Welfare: Ottawa, Canada

Annotated Guide to Venereal Disease Instructional Materials Available in Canada.
A Parents' Guide to Drug Abuse.
VD (venereal disease).

The National Association for Mental Health, Inc.

Drug Abuse: Answers to the Most Frequently Asked Questions.

National Council on Alcoholism, Inc.

Blakeslee, A., and Sullivan, B.: Alcohol: The New Teen-age Turn On, 1975.
Davis, F. T., Jr.: Alcoholism: The Needs of Minorities, 1973.
Hornik, E. L.: You and Your Alcoholic Parent, 1974.
It's Best to Know.
Let's Get the Problem Drinker Off Our Highways, 1974.
Thinking about Drinking.
Young People and AA.

Public Affairs Committee

Ayrault, E. W.: Helping the Handicapped Teenager Mature.
Bienvenu, M.: Talking It Over at Home.
Dealing with the Crisis of Suicide.
Drugs—Use, Misuse, Abuse; Guidance for Families.
Henley, A.: Schizophrenia: Current Approaches to a Baffling Problem.
Irwin, T.: The Rights of Teen-agers as Patients.
Ogg, E.: Homosexuality in Our Society.

Saltman, J.: El Abuso de las Drogas—¿Qué Podemos Hacer? (Drug Abuse—What Can Be Done?).
Saltman, J.: The New Alcoholics: Teenagers.
Saltman, J.: VD—Epidemic Among Teenagers.
Shiller, A.: Drug Abuse and Your Child.
Shiller, A.: The Unmarried Mother.

Rainbow Hospital Youth Spine Center

What if You Need an Operation for Scoliosis?

SIECUS Publications Office

Homosexuality.

United States Government

Comprehensive Emergency Services, 1975.
Drugs of Abuse, 1976.
Marihuana and Health, 1974.
Millar, H. E. C.: Approaches to Adolescent Health Care in the 1970's. 1975.
NICHD Answers Your Questions About Family Planning, Infants and Children, 1976.
Outpatient Drug-Free Treatment Manual, 1974.
Residential Drug-Free Manual, 1974.
Suicide, Homicide, and Alcoholism Among American Indians: Guidelines for Help, 1973.
Teenage Delinquency in Small Town America, 1974.
The Contemporary Woman and Crime, 1975.
The Hassles of Becoming a Teenage Parent, 1975.
The Maternity and Infant Care Projects; Reducing Risks for Mothers and Babies, 1975.
The Philadelphia Neighborhood Youth Resources Center, 1975.
What's New on Smoking in Print and on Film.
White Paper on Drug Abuse, 1975.
You're Young, You're Female, and You Smoke, 1974.
Food for the Teenager During Pregnancy, 1976.
Sexually Transmitted Diseases, 1976.
The Whole College Catalog about Drinking, 1976.

REFERENCES

Books

Aguilera, D. C., and Messick, J. M.: *Crisis Intervention: Theory and Methodology.* 2nd ed. St. Louis, The C. V. Mosby Company, 1974.
American Medical Association: *Human Sexuality.* Chicago, American Medical Association (OP 139).
Archer, S. E., and Fleshman, R.: *Community Health Nursing: Patterns and Practice.* Scituate, Mass., Duxbury Press, 1975.
Arieti, S.: *Interpretation of Schizophrenia.* 2nd ed. New York, Basic Books, Inc., 1974.
Baker, A. A. (Ed.): *Comprehensive Psychiatric Care.* Philadelphia, J. B. Lippincott Company, 1976.
Barber, V., and Skaggs, M. M.: *The Mother Person.* Indianapolis, Bobbs-Merrill, 1975.
Beck, A. T., Resnik, H. L. P., and Lettieri, D. J.: *The Prediction of Suicide.* Bowie, Md., Charles Press Publishers, Inc., 1974.
Blachly, P. H.: *Seduction: A Conceptual Model in the Drug Dependencies and Other Contagious Ills.* Springfield, Ill., Charles C Thomas, 1973.
Brownmiller, S.: *Against Our Will: Men, Women and Rape.* New York, Simon and Schuster, 1975.

Burgess, A. W., and Holmstrom, L. L.: *Rape: Victims of Crisis.* Bowie, Md., Robert J. Brady Company, 1974.
Burkhalter, P. K.: *Nursing Care of the Alcoholic and Drug Abuser.* New York, McGraw-Hill Book Company, 1975.
Cailliet, R.: *Scoliosis: Diagnosis and Management.* Philadelphia, F. A. Davis Company, 1975.
Carter, F. M.: *Psychosocial Nursing: Theory and Practice in Hospital and Community Mental Health.* 2nd ed. New York, Macmillan Company, 1976.
Catterall, R. D.: *A Short Textbook of Venereology.* 2nd ed. Philadelphia, J. B. Lippincott Company, 1974.
Copeland, A. D.: *Textbook of Adolescent Psychopathology and Treatment.* Springfield, Ill., Charles C Thomas, 1974.
Cull, J. G., and Hurdy, R. E. (Eds.): *Problems of Runaway Youth.* Springfield, Ill., Charles C Thomas, 1976.
Cutter, F.: *Coming to Terms with Death.* Chicago, Nelson-Hall Company, 1974.
Demarest, R. J., and Sciarra, J. J.: *Conception, Birth and Contraception: A Visual Presentation.* New York, McGraw-Hill Book Company, 1976.
Dreyer, S. O., Bailey, D., and Doucet, W.: *A Guide to Nursing Management of Psychiatric Patients.* St. Louis, The C. V. Mosby Company, 1975.
Ferguson, A. B., Jr. (Ed.): *Orthopaedic Surgery in Infancy*

and Childhood. 4th ed. Baltimore, Williams & Wilkins Company, 1975.

Filstead, W. J., Rossi, J. J., and Keller, M. (Eds.): Alcohol and Alcohol Problems: New Thinking and New Directions. Philadelphia, J. B. Lippincott Company, 1975.

Freeman, T.: Childhood Psychopathology and Adult Psychoses. New York, International Universities Press, 1976.

Fulton, R., and Bendiksen, R.: Death and Identity. Bowie, Maryland, Robert J. Brady Company, 1976.

Garcia, C. R., and Rosenfeld, D. L.: Family Planning. Philadelphia, F. A. Davis Company, 1976.

Gianturco, D. T., and Smith, H. L.: The Promiscuous Teenager. Springfield, Ill., Charles C Thomas, 1974.

Glade, P. R. (Ed.): Infectious Mononucleosis. Philadelphia, J. B. Lippincott Company, 1973.

Goldstein, B.: Human Sexuality. New York, McGraw-Hill Book Company, 1976.

Hilt, N. E., and Schmitt, E. W., Jr.: Pediatric Orthopedic Nursing. St. Louis, The C. V. Mosby Company, 1975.

Howard, M.: Only Human: Teenage Pregnancy and Parenthood. New York, The Seabury Press, 1975.

Hudgens, R. W.: Psychiatric Disorders in Adolescents. Baltimore, Williams & Wilkins Company, 1974.

Kübler-Ross, E.: Death: The Final Stage of Growth. Englewood Cliffs, N.J., Prentice-Hall, Inc., 1975.

Kugelmass, I. N.: Adolescent Medicine: Principles and Practice. Springfield, Ill., Charles C Thomas, 1975.

Lasagna, L.: The VD Epidemic: How It Started, Where It's Going, and What to Do About It. Philadelphia, Temple University Press, 1975.

McInnes, M. E.: Essentials of Communicable Disease. St. Louis, The C. V. Mosby Company, 1975.

Morton, B. M.: VD: A Guide for Nurses and Counselors. Boston, Little, Brown & Company, 1976.

Ray, O. S.: Drugs, Society, and Human Behavior. St. Louis, The C. V. Mosby Company, 1974.

Richter, R. W. (Ed.): Medical Aspects of Drug Abuse. New York, Harper & Row, 1975.

Schiller, P.: Creative Approach to Sex Education and Counseling. New York, Association Press, 1973.

Silverstein, A., and Silverstein, V. B.: Alcoholism. Philadelphia, J. B. Lippincott Company, 1975.

Tripp, C. A.: The Homosexual Matrix. New York, McGraw-Hill Book Company, Inc., 1975.

Usdin, G. (Ed.): Schizophrenia: Biological and Psychological Perspectives. New York, Brunner/Mazel Publishers, 1975.

Vaughan, V. C., III, and Brazelton, T. B. (Eds.): The Family—Can It Be Saved? Chicago, Year Book Medical Publishers, 1976.

Youmans, G. P., Paterson, P. Y., and Sommers, H. M. (Eds.): The Biological and Clinical Basis of Infectious Diseases. Philadelphia, W. B. Saunders Company, 1975.

Zackler, J., and Branstadt, W. (Eds.): The Teenage Pregnant Girl. Springfield, Ill., Charles C Thomas, 1975.

Periodicals

Abernethy, V.: Illegitimate Conception Among Teenagers. Nursing Digest, 4:8, Summer 1976.

Alexander, M. M., and Brown, M. S.: Physical Examination. Part 16: The Musculoskeletal System. Nursing 76, 6:51, April, 1976.

Amenta, M. M.: Free Clinics Change the Scene. Am. J. Nursing, 74:284, February 1974.

Anderson, C.: The Lengthening Shadow: A Case Study in Adolescent, Out-of Wedlock Pregnancy. JOGN Nursing, 5:19, July-August 1976.

Arieti, S.: Anxiety and Beyond in Schizophrenia and Psychotic Depression. Nursing Digest, 2:67, March 1974.

Arnold, H. M.: Working With Schizophrenic Patients: Four A's—A Guide to One-to-One Relationships. Am. J. Nursing, 76:941, June 1976.

Babcock, J. L.: Spinal Injuries in Children. Pediatric. Clin. N. Am., 22:487, May 1975.

Bahra, R. J.: The Potential for Suicide. Am. J. Nursing, 75:1782, October 1975.

Barnes, A., Jr.: Infectious Mononucleosis. Nursing Digest, 4:51, January-February 1976.

Barnes, H. V. (Ed.): Symposium on Adolescent Medicine. Med. Clin. N. Am., 59:1279, November 1975.

Berg, I., Butler, A., and Hall, G.: The Outcome of Adolescent School Phobia. Br. J. Psychiatry, 128:80 January 1976.

Blume, S. B.: A Psychiatrist Looks at Alcoholism. Nursing Digest, 4:36, Summer 1976.

Braverman, S. J.: Homosexuality. Am. J. Nursing, 73:652, April 1973.

Brown, M. A.: Adolescents and VD. Nursing Outlook, 21:99, February 1973.

Brown, M. S.: Syphilis and Gonorrhea. Nursing 76, 6:71, January 1976.

Bruggen, P., and Pitt-Aikens, T.: Authority As a Key Factor in Adolescent Disturbance. Br. J. Med. Psychol., 48:158, June 1975.

Burgess, A. W., and Holmstrom, L. L.: Crisis and Counseling Requests of Rape Victims. Nursing Research, 23:196, May-June 1974.

Cates, W., and Rochat, R. W.: Illegal Abortions in the United States: 1972–1974. Fam. Plan. Perspect., 8:86 March-April 1976.

Cohen, D., and Richards, C. V.: Youths As Advocates. Children Today, 1:32, March-April 1972.

Coleman, J. C.: Life Stress and Maladaptive Behavior. Nursing Digest, 1:4, December 1973.

Cunningham, R.: What Do Nurses Do To Help Patients Who Attempt Suicide? The Canadian Nurse, 71:27, January 1975.

DeGrave, G., and Riordan, B.: Sex Education for Delinquent Boys: Unveiling the Taboo. Nursing 76, 6:22, June 1976.

DeLong, J. V.: The Methadone Habit. Nursing Digest, 4:84, Fall 1976.

Distasio, C., and Nawrot, M.: Methaqualone. Am. J. Nursing, 73:1922, November 1973.

Donovan, C. M., Greenspan, R., and Mittleman, F.: Post-abortion Psychiatric Illness. Nursing Digest, 3:12, September-October 1975.

Eiduson, B. T.: Looking At Children in Emergent Family Styles. Children Today, 3:2, July-August 1974.

Evans, R. L., et al.: Multidisciplinary Approach to Sex Education of Spinal Cord-Injured Patients. Phys. Ther., 56:541–545, May 1976.

Gallagher, U. M.: Changing Focus on Services to Teenagers. Children Today, 2:24, September-October 1973.

Gay, G. R.: Treatment of Acute Drug Reactions and Overdose. Nursing Digest, 3:32, November-December 1975.

Gedan, S.: Abortion Counseling with Adolescents. Am. J. Nursing, 74:1856, October 1974.

Gilday, D. L.: Nuclear Medicine and Pediatric Neoplasia. Pediatr. Clin. N. Am., 23:41, February 1976.

Goldmeier, H.: School-Age Parents and the Public Schools. Children Today, 5:18, September-October 1976.

Gottheil, E., McGurn, W. C., and Pollak, O.: Truth and/or Hope for the Dying Patient. Nursing Digest, 4:12, March-April 1976.

Hammer, S. L.: The Approach to the Adolescent Patient. Pediatr. Clin. N. Am., 20:779, November 1973.

Hamric, A., Allen, V. A., Yoon, P., and Windsor, N.: Caring for the Totally Dependent Patient: Some Traps—Some Guidelines. Nursing 76, 6:38, July 1976.

Herbst, A. L., et al.: Clear-Cell Adenocarcinoma of the Genital Tract in Young Females. *New Engl. J. Med.* 287:1259, December 1972.

Hofmann, A. D., and Pilpel, H. F.: The Legal Rights of Minors. *Pediatr. Clin. N. Am.*, 20:989, February 1973.

Holmstrom, L. L., and Burgess, A. W.: Assessing Trauma in the Rape Victim. *Am. J. Nursing*, 75:1288, August 1975.

Hungerford, D. S.: Spinal Deformity in Adolescence: Early Detection and Nonoperative Management. *Med Clin. N. Am.*, 59:1517, November 1975.

Hurwitz, A., and Eadie, R. F.: Psychological Impact on Nursing Students of Participation in Abortion. *Nursing Research*, 26:112, March-April, 1977.

Isler, C.: Newest Treatment for Cancer: Immunotherapy. *RN*, 39:29, May 1976.

Jackson, D. W.: The Adolescent and the Hospital. *Pediatr. Clin. N. Am.*, 20:901, November 1973.

Kress, H.: Adaptation to Chronic Dialysis: A Two-Way Street. *Nursing Digest*, 5:26, Spring 1977.

Lenocker, J. M., and Dougherty, M. C.: Adolescent Mothers' Social and Health-Related Interests: Report of a Project for Rural, Black Mothers. *JOGN Nursing*, 5:9, July-August 1976.

Luckmann, J., and Sorensen, K. C.: What Patients' Actions Tell You About Their Feelings, Fears and Needs. *Nursing 75*, 5:54, February 1975.

Mardosa, S. A.: Difficult Patients: Rebecca was a Primipara... Unmarried, Retarded, 14 years Old and Hostile. *Nursing 74*, 3:34, March 1974.

McGreevy, A., and Van Heukelem, J.: Crying: The Neglected Dimension. *Nursing Digest*, 5:61, Spring 1977.

Opp, M.: The Confidentiality Dilemma. *Nursing Digest*, 4:17, Fall 1976.

Packer, J., and Cooke, C. W.: The Interdependent Team Approach in Caring for the Pregnant Adolescent. *JOGN Nursing*, 5:18, July-August 1976.

Popoff, D., and Nursing 75: What Are Your Feelings About Death and Dying? Part 2. *Nursing 75*, 5:55, September 1975.

Price, V.: Rape Victims—The Invisible Patients. *The Canadian Nurse*, 71:29, April 1975.

Raynolds, N.: Teaching Parents Home Care After Surgery for Scoliosis. *Am. J. Nursing*, 74:1090, June 1974.

Razzell, M.: No Thanks, I've Quit Smoking. *The Canadian Nurse*, 71:23, September 1975.

Reid, U. V.: Screening for Adolescent Idiopathic Scoliosis. *The Candian Nurse*, 71:13, November 1975.

Rementeria, J. L.: Janakammal, S., and Hollander, M.: Multiple Births in Drug-Addicted Women. *Am. J. Obstet. Gynecol.*, 122:958, August 15 1975.

Reynolds, D. K., and Farberow, N. L.: The Suicidal Patient—An Inside View. *Nursing Digest*, 2:58, October 1974.

Robins, J.: Failures of Contraceptive Practice. *N.Y. State J. Med.*, 76:361, March 1976.

Rosen, G.: Management of Malignant Bone Tumors in Children and Adolescents. *Pediatr. Clin. N. Am.*, 23:183, February 1976.

Runnels, J. B., et al.: Manipulative Adolescent. *Nursing 73*, 3:36, July 1973.

Schmid, N. J., and Schmid, D. T.: Nursing Students' Attitudes Toward Alcoholics. *Nursing Research*, 22:246, May-June 1973.

Sells, C. J., and May, E. A.: Scoliosis Screening in Public Schools. *Am. J. Nursing*, 74:60, Janurary 1974.

Shore, M. F.: Youth Advisory Services in Six European Countries. *Children Today*, 5:23, January-February 1976.

Smith, M.: A Young Pregnant Girl Tells Her Story. *The Canadian Nurse*, 71:30, October 1975.

Staudt, A. R.: Femur Replacement. *Am. J. Nursing*, 75:1346, August 1975.

Steiger, T. B.: Shadow Child. *Am. J. Nursing*, 73:2080, December 1973.

Stewart, B. M.: Biochemical Aspects of Schizophrenia. *Am. J. Nursing*, 75:2176, December 1975.

Tiedt, E.: The Adolescent in the Hospital: An Identity-Resolution Approach. *Nursing Forum*, 11:120, No. 2, 1972.

Treadway, B., et al.: Scoliosis: Affectionate Yet Firm Postoperative Nursing Care. *Nursing 74*, 4:49, August 1974.

Vincent, P. J., Smith, J., and Danglasan, E.: Treatment of Patients with Spinal Cord Injuries. *The Canadian Nurse*, 71:26, August 1975.

Welch, M. S.: Rape and the Trauma of Inadequate Care. *Nursing Digest*, 5:50, Spring 1977.

Wiley, L. (Ed.): Salvaging an Unwilling Life. *Nursing 76*, 6:54, February 1976.

AUDIOVISUAL MEDIA*

The American Cancer Society, Inc.

Primary Cancer of Bone
21½ minutes, color.

Surveys the five most important classes of malignant bone tumors and how they are differentiated, emphasizing the importance of early diagnosis and treatment in improving the chance of successful outcome. The relative frequency of bone cancer among adolescents is pointed out, and the criteria for biopsy are discussed.

The American Journal of Nursing Company

How Many Children Do You Want?
15 minutes each filmstrip, three 35mm filmstrip series, audio-tape cassettes, 33⅓ RPM records, sound, color.

How Babies Begin
A discussion of the reproductive organs and conception.
Drugstore Methods and Least Effective Methods of Birth Control
Evaluates methods of birth control and explains the most common misunderstandings about contraception.

Doctor Methods of Birth Control
Provides basic information about birth control pills, IUD, diaphragm, vasectomy, tubal ligation and hysterectomy.

Drug Abuse and Therapy
30 minutes, 16 mm film, sound, black and white.
Two nurses employed at a drug addiction treatment facility and two former drug addicts explore the issues involved in drug abuse and therapy.

Psychiatric-Mental Health Nursing
Series Instructor: Mitchell, M.
30 minutes, videotape, sound, color, guide.

The Crisis of Loss
Guest Participants: Werner-Beland, J., and Mercer, R. The commonly encountered nursing problem of loss and mourning is examined within the framework of crisis theory. Examples support the importance of the patient's perception of control and responsibility in coping with loss events.

Psychosocial Assessment (Part I)
A descriptive overview of aims, content areas, and methods of obtaining data for a nursing psychosocial assess-

ment. The central importance of the initial interview is illustrated.

Psychosocial Assessment (Part II)
A more detailed illustration of the initial psychiatric interview as an investigative and therapeutic method. The use of assessment data in the nurse's plans for care is explained.

Suicide Intervention
The nurse's potential to contribute to suicide intervention is examined. Two representative patient-nurse interactions, of varying lethal risk, point up assessment and therapeutic opportunities.

Acute Alcoholic Intoxication
Guest Participant: Covert, C. The emphasis is on ways the nurse can facilitate involvement in treatment for alcoholism by skilled interventions in the initial, more acute phase of the illness. Critical assessment factors are outlined and portrayed.

Adolescent Drug Abuse
Guest Participant: Shick, F. Identifies the knowledge and skills needed to recognize and treat the patient who has overdosed on psychotropic drugs, emergency treatment of patient, and counseling with family and peers.

Facilitating Self-Disclosure
Guest Participant: Carlson, C. Examines the personal qualities and interviewing skills that facilitate patients' expression of feelings and information. Both psychiatric and nonpsychiatric clinical settings are discussed in terms of facilitating self-disclosure.

American Lung Association

Be Proud! Be Well! Fight TB!
Poster, 11″ × 15″, 2 colors.
For black community.

The Elusive Enemy
22 minutes, 16 mm, sound, color, English and Spanish sound track, guide.
Documentary showing young people who had TB or were positive reactors.

Audio Visual Narrative Arts, Inc. (AVNA)

Abortion: A Rational Appraisal
Two filmstrips, two cassettes or two 12″ LP records, guide.
This program is designed to provide teachers with a factual framework in which the subject of abortion and the implications of the U.S. Supreme Court's landmark decision of 1973 can be discussed with students and parent-teacher groups.

Contraception: A Matter of Choice
Two filmstrips, two cassettes or two 12″ LP records, guide.
This two-part program traces the history of man's efforts to control fertility; summarizes state laws governing birth control; describes and evaluates medically-accepted means of contraception.

Homosexuality: Thursday's Child
Two filmstrips, two cassettes or two 12″ LP records, guide.
This program offers students a straightforward discussion of current attitudes, opinions, and theories on homosexuality. Discovering that one is, or might be, a homosexual is a difficult and frightening experience for a young person and, unfortunately, it is often made more painful by a lack of sound data and sympathetic understanding.

Canadian Film Institute

About Conception and Contraception
12 minutes, film, color.

Illustrates reproductive physiology, sexual intercourse, conception, and methods of contraception.

Purposes of Family Planning
18 minutes, film, color.
Demonstrates the positive purposes of family planning—health, emotional stability, a child's need for individual love and attention—presented simply for all ages and income levels.

Charles Press–Prentice-Hall, Inc.

Adolescent Suicide . . . A Documentary
54 minutes, tape.
Included are interviews with young men and women who have attempted suicide, a discussion of the impact of suicide on survivors, and some observations on suicide prevention and intervention.

Venereal Disease
20 overhead transparencies, color, guide, pre- and posttests.
Details the way VD is transmitted, and illustrates the symptoms, diagnosis, dangers, and results of gonorrhea and syphilis. Features material on the cure and prevention of these diseases. Stresses the importance of early detection and the tracing of sexual contacts to break the VD cycle.

National Council on Alcoholism, Inc.

The Doctor Talks to You About Alcoholism
Audio-tape cassette.
Dr. F. A. Seixas discusses alcoholism. The tape is brief, to the point, practical, down to earth, straightforward, informative, and scientifically sound.

Planned Parenthood Federation of America, Inc.

Basics of Birth Control
Chart
All the methods in chart form. Explains each and allows easy comparison. Gives use, effectiveness, acceptability, where obtained, and average costs.

W. B. Saunders Company

Current Topics in Obstetrics and Gynecology
Director: Tyson, J. E.
Diagnosis and Treatment of Herpes Vulvitis, Friedrich, E. G.
Gonorrhea, Tyson, J. E.
Update: Stilbestrol and Adenocarcinoma, Herbst, A. L.

Pediatric Conferences with Sydney Gellis
Infectious Mononucleosis and the Epstein-Barr Virus, Henle, W.
Scoliosis In Infancy, Childhood and Adolescence, Goldberg, M.

The Royal College of General Practitioners, Medical Recording Service

Psychiatric Medicine in Family Practice
Schizophrenia—The Divided Mind
27 minutes, 8 slides 2×2 35 mm, sound.
Describes the nature and causes of schizophrenia. Evaluates various theories of the part that family relationships have in the development of the psychosis.

Trainex Corporation

Crisis Intervention with a Rape Victim: Interviewing Techniques
Audio-tape cassettes.
Covers the theory of crisis intervention techniques. In addition, it defines the three stages of a therapeutic relationship—the dependency stage, the stage of interdependence,

and the stage of independence or separation. Includes a dramatization of three interviews with a rape victim during the three separate stages of her crisis and step-by-step analysis of the interviews by the nurse counselor.

Drug Dependency — Alcohol
35mm filmstrip, audio-tape cassettes, 33 1/3 LP, color.
A detailed discussion examines the role in society of this most widely abused drug. Those persons susceptible to alcoholism are identified, and programs of treatment, maintenance, withdrawal, and rehabilitation are discussed.

Drug Dependency — Narcotic Analgesics
35mm filmstrip, audio-tape cassettes, 33 1/3 LP, color.
An exploration of reasons for addiction and the life style of abusers; also describes hospitalization of the addict, including care during withdrawal. Rehabilitation techniques, maintenance programs, and therapeutic community programs are discussed.

Drug Dependency — Stimulants, Depressants, and Psychedelics
35mm filmstrip, audio-tape cassettes, 33 1/3 LP, color.
Illustrates differences between oral and IV users and details the role of the nurse in treating the hospitalized stimulant abuser. Nursing care during hospitalization and withdrawal of the depressant-dependent patient are shown. Observations and nursing measures involved in caring for the psychedelic drug abuser are discussed in detail.

Family Planning
35mm filmstrip, audio-tape cassettes, 33 1/3 LP, color, English and Spanish narration.
Advises the viewer about six methods of birth control. It briefly discusses problems of not using birth control measures and how the physician decides which device is right for each patient.

Hallucinations
35mm filmstrip, audio-tape cassettes, 33 1/3 LP, color.
Focuses on the experience of one patient whose mental disorders are accompanied by false sensory perceptions, those for which external stimuli do not exist. The program provides the learner with an understanding of the disorder and an awareness of the importance of nursing care for the hallucinating person. The impact of the hallucination upon the life of the patient is discussed.

Pathogenesis of Tuberculosis
35mm filmstrip, audio-tape cassettes, 33 1/3 LP, color.
This program portrays the typical course of untreated pulmonary tuberculosis from its transmission through the stages of early tuberculosis, latency, and advanced disease. Stress is placed on the importance of identifying and treating all infected persons if this health threat is to be eradicated.

Syphilis and Gonorrhea
35mm filmstrip, audio-tape cassettes, 33 1/3 LP, color.
This program provides an overview of these two major venereal diseases. Each is discussed separately, including data on the epidemiology, causative organism, modes of transmission, signs, and symptoms, and an outline of diagnostic procedures.

The Human Reproductive System
This series is meant to be used for patient education. Presents simple, basic concepts.

The Nurse's Role in Tuberculosis
35mm filmstrip, audio-tape cassette, 33 1/3 LP, color.
Infection control methods, the role of X-ray and laboratory tests, and the principles of chemotherapy are illustrated and explained. Provides the nurse with the information needed to teach and motivate the tuberculosis patient in the treatment of his disease.

The Nursing and Medical Management of the Rape Victim
Audio-tape cassettes.
Discusses the nursing and medical management of rape victims, provides some preventive measures against possible rape assaults, and concludes with a Bill of Rights for victims of sexual assault.

The Psychological Crisis of Rape
Audio-tape cassettes.
An overview of the theory of crisis, the concept of anxiety, the stages of rape, and the psychology of the rapist are given. A woman who was a victim of rape discusses her reactions, the signs and symptoms she experienced, and how she recovered with the support and guidance she received from a nurse.

Tuberculosis Skin Testing
35mm filmstrip, audio-tape cassettes, 33 1/3 LP, color.
The nature of delayed hypersensitivity and of an induration, the differences between Old Tuberculin and Purified Protein Derivative, the Multiple Puncture Skin Test and the Mantoux Skin Test are illustrated and discussed. Giving, reading, and interpreting both the Mantoux Skin Test and the Multiple Puncture Skin Test are shown and explained in detail with particular emphasis on the patient's history during interpretation.

United States Government

Are Drugs the Answer?
Producer: USNIMH
20 minutes, 16mm film, optical sound, color.
Discusses the nature and harmful effects of various kinds of drugs, such as the psychedelics, speed and marihuana.

Blue
Producer: USNIMH
24 minutes, 16mm film, optical sound, color.
Shows what addiction is like for the black person. Reconstructs the past of a young black addict, portraying the hardships, misery and despair connected with the life of a drug addict.

Human Reproduction: How Reproduction Is Controlled
Producer: USNMAC
35mm filmstrip, audiotape, color.
Discusses control of conception to include the rhythm method, mechanical blockage, chemical blockage, and contraceptive pills.

Slow Death
Producer: USNIMH
23 minutes, 16mm film, optical sound, black and white.
Dramatizes the life of heroin users in the inner city. Made by a group of black young people in Philadelphia.

---

*Complete addresses are given in the Appendix.

WHEN I WAS ONE-AND-TWENTY

When I was one-and-twenty
    I heard a wise man say,
"Give crowns and pounds and guineas
    But not your heart away;
Give pearls away and rubies
    But keep your fancy free."
But I was one-and-twenty,
    No use to talk to me.

When I was one-and-twenty
    I heard him say again,
"The heart out of the bosom
    Was never given in vain;
'Tis paid with sighs a-plenty
    And sold for endless rue."
And I am two-and-twenty,
    And oh, 'tis true, 'tis true.

A. E. Housman
1859–1936

APPENDIX I

THE NURSING PROCESS

PREPARED BY EVELYN N. BEHANNA AND SHEILA M. PRINGLE

PREMATURE INFANT

TODDLER AGE—NEPHROSIS

PRESCHOOL AGE—TONSILLECTOMY AND ADENOIDECTOMY

PREMATURE INFANT*

DATA		ASSESSMENT		PROBLEM IDENTIFICATION	PLANNING	INTERVENTION	EVALUATION
Mark	History Taking and Examination	Comparison and Contrast	Strengths and Weaknesses				
Sex: Male	Weight: 1800 gm. (4 lb.)	abnormal: normal is 3200 gm. (7 lb.)	weakness	1. Nutrition and hydration: needs 60 to 80 calories and 3 to 4 gm. of protein per pound of body weight and sufficient carbohydrates and fluids.	1. Offer frequent small feedings to avoid tiring / Start with sterile water, then glucose water, then formula as ordered to assure ability to suck and swallow / Provide a minimum of 240 ml. per day and 60 calories per pound per day to assure weight gain / Bubble frequently to reduce regurgitation	1. Offer 1 to 2 ounces every 3 hours	1. Sucking reflex improves / Infant gains weight slowly, but steadily
	Length: 16.5 in. (42 cm.)	abnormal: normal is 18 in. to 21 in. (45 cm. to 52 cm.)	strength				
	Gestational age: 34 weeks	premature: should be 40 weeks	weakness				
Cry: present	Cry: weak	should be lusty	minimal strength				
	Eyes: clear, blink reflex present	normal	strength				
Respirations: rapid	Rapid and shallow; 65 per minute	should be 35 to 60 per minute	weakness	2. Maintain patent airway / Respirations difficult and irregular. Lungs are immature, incomplete development of the alveoli and weakness of thoracic cage and of the respiratory muscles / Cyanosis is evidence of inadequate oxygenation of arterial blood	2. Position infant on side or with head to side to prevent aspiration of fluids / Change position frequently to decrease chance of hypostatic pneumonia / Monitor pulse and respiration and record to provide baseline of knowledge and provide indication of respiratory distress	2. Turn infant from side to back to side every hour. / Take vital signs q 2 hours. Report immediately if P ↑ 170, R ↑ 60.	2. Patent airway maintained. / Lungs remain clear.
Skin: covered with lanugo	Skin: wrinkled, thin, red, absence of subcutaneous fat and little vernix caseosa	normal: covered with vernix caseosa and small amounts of lanugo; subcutaneous fat deposits; color of skin, pink	weakness				
	Temp.: 36°C. (96.8°F.) at birth	below normal 36.4°C. to 37°C. (97.5°F. to 98.6°F.)	weakness				
	Pulse: 165 per minute; normal 100 to 180 at birth	above normal, 130 to 160 per minute within 24 hours	weakness				

Head circumference: 30 cm. (12 in.) Demonstrates head lag	below normal: 34 cm. to 35 cm. (13.6 to 14 in.) is normal range; in proportion with body	weakness and strength	3. Temperature control: Heat regulatory center is immature. Skin surface is great in proportion to weight. Lacks the insulation of the subcutaneous fat layer	3. Maintain body temperature within range of 97°–98° (36–37)	3. May use isolette, which can be thermostatically controlled. Decrease external stimuli (over and beyond feeding, cleanliness and required procedures) to reduce BMR. Organize activities to reduce heat and energy expenditures	3. Temperature is maintained. Progress from isolette to crib and maintain temperature
Fontanels: open and palpable	normal	strength				
Hair: fuzzy and a small amount	fuller amount of hair	weakness				
Swallowing reflex: difficult	normal: present and consistent ability	weakness				
Arms: extended—observe when infant is quiet and in a supine position	normal position is flexed	weakness	4. Maintenance of skin integrity	4. Keep skin clean and dry, avoid irritation via rubbing or use of soap	4. Bathe when necessary; use minimal soap; pat dry gently	4. Skin integrity maintained
Hands: some cyanosis. Grasp reflex is weak	normal: strong grasp, reflex; acrocyanosis is normal	weakness	5. Immaturity of muscular system	5. Support head and body when moving baby due to immaturity of muscular system. Passive range of motion to extremities to increase circulation to peripheral areas	5. Perform at least once each shift but with gentleness and care	5. Muscular coordination and strength increases
Legs: beginning of some flexion at hips and knees. Thin, muscles small	normal: total flexion	minimal strength				
Feet: Babinski response is difficult to elicit	normal: toes should curl downward		6. Neurologic Immaturity	6. Test for reflexes; note responses. Do not feed if swallowing reflex missing	6. Observe for excess mucous—note lack of swallowing	6. Will mature as infant matures
Abdomen: protrudes	normal	strength				
Genitalia: small in size	appear normal	strength	7. Emotional support; instruction and referral: Short time for in-hospital instruction. Refer to nursing service within the community for home follow-up and private physician	7. Instruction on feeding, bathing, and diapering. Include parents in all aspects of care	7. Individual and group discussion with demonstrations as review of knowledge with parents	7. Infant gains strength and weight; health maintained
First-born infant. Attended prenatal classes.		strength				
Parents: Father—20 years old Mother—17 years old						

*This example of the nursing process is not inclusive of all care that an individual child might require.

TODDLER AGE—NEPHROSIS*

	DATA COLLECTION	ASSESSMENT		PROBLEM IDENTIFICATION	PLANNING	INTERVENTION	EVALUATION
Jeff	History Taking and Examination	Comparison and Contrast	Strengths and Weaknesses	Obtained from Strengths and Weaknesses Areas			
2½-year-old brought in by parents. Jeff is pale and ex-atous. His eyes are almost swollen shut, his abdomen is distended, his extremities and scrotum are very swollen	Weight: 38 lb. Mother states his usual weight is about 30 lb. Height: not obtained. Carried by father; could not stand alone at this time. TPR: 98⁴-130-32	abnormal	weakness	1. Maintenance of nutrition	1. a. Weigh daily to assess gain or loss	1. a. Same time, same scale, same weight clothing	1. Anticipate weight loss
			weakness		b. High protein diet to replace lost protein and provide tissue building blocks. High in vitamins to provide elements for skin integrity. Restrict salt to minimize fluid retention. Provide potassium since excreted daily	b. Diet attractively presented	Anticipate improved appetite
						c. Include favorite foods where possible	
						d. Small, frequent feedings	
	B/P: 80/55	abnormal					
	temperature is normal; pulse and respirations slightly elevated; blood pressure normal for age		elevated pulse and respiration may be a potential weakness				
	Chest: normal	normal	strength				
	Motor: Difficulty with standing, walking, sitting and fine motor skills Parents state that prior to this time, Jeff was extremely active and into everything		weakness	2. Maintenance of hydration	2. Fluid intake may be restricted due to edema and medical regimen	2. Ensure allocation of fluids over the 24 hour period	2. Anticipate diuresis
		abnormal			Maintain accurate intake and output to provide a baseline of information for future intake levels	Report and record I and O levels every eight hours	Return to normal I and O ratio
	Speech: Responds to questions with one- or two-word answers. Parents state he talks a blue streak at home	previously within normal range	strength		Report and record inability to void or urinary output below 15 ml./hr, as this could indicate renal shutdown		
		normal					
	Social: Responds to directions. Tried to help change his clothes. Brought favorite toy car with him.	normal	strength	3. Maintenance of skin integrity and comfort	3. Provide periods of rest to reduce BMR and conserve energy Wash without soap to prevent drying of skin	3. Plan activities Bathe once daily	3. No skin breakdown
	Head: Eyes almost swollen shut Face puffy and edematous Pallor noted Skin shiny and taut	abnormal eyes should be clearly visible, facial characteristics should be readily identifiable, skin usually soft and pliable	weakness		Wash carefully and gently to prevent abrading the tissue Dry gently but thoroughly particularly in skin folds to prevent intertrigo	Use long, smooth strokes Pat dry	Return of skin turgor Decrease in edema everywhere
	Abdomen: Abdominal distention noted: Skin shiny and taut, pitted areas noted at waist line where pants belt made indentation marks Bowel sounds can be heard	it is normal to hear bowel sounds and for liquids to be taken and retained.	strengths		Bathing cleanses the skin— refreshes the individual— increases circulation and provides comfort	Powder or ointment may be used if skin has not broken down Do early in a.m.	Able to open eyes easily
	Palpation of organs difficult Parents state Jeff has been incontinent of urine and feces today Has eaten nothing since the previous day, though he drank and retained some orange juice They also state he cries when he urinates	abdominal size is greater than that usually seen in the toddler; organs readily palpated. Jeff's parents state he has been totally toilet trained for over a month and never complained of pain on voiding	weaknesses		Irrigate eyes with warm saline to prevent collection of exudate Separate skin surfaces that are in contact, to prevent rubbing, intertrigo, and skin breakdown	Provide scrotal (or labial) support Place cotton between skin surfaces Provide pillows to support arms and legs or between knees when on side	Decreased need for scrotal (or labial) support Decreased need for pillows

Assessment Data			Nursing Diagnosis	Nursing Interventions	Nursing Interventions	Expected Outcomes
Genital: Scrotum extremely swollen and tender to touch. Skin taut, almost translucent	abnormal – testes usually easily palpable within scrotal sac	weakness		Turn frequently to prevent skin breakdown. Elevate the head to reduce the discomfort from facial edema	Turn every two hours. Pillows may be used or head of bed elevated.	Able to change own position
Anus: Anal sphincter intact	normal	strength				
Extremities: Arms and legs very edematous. Pitting edema noted in arms, legs, ankles, feet, and hands. Fingers and toes also edematous. Could not make a fist nor pick up a pencil	abnormal	weakness	4. Prevention of infection	4. Maintain integrity of skin as body's first line of defense. Monitor vital signs for baselines of knowledge	4. Take vital signs and blood pressure every four hours.	4. Anticipate stable temperature and blood pressure and decrease in pulse and respiration as child improves
Skin: Shiny and taut over entire body	abnormal	weakness		Change position frequently to prevent stasis pneumonia. Avoid contact with others who have known infection due to debilitation and decreased resistance to infection	Turn every two hours. Place in rooms with children who do not have known infections	
25 ml. of foamy urine obtained from Jeff. Cried while urinating	abnormal	weakness	5. Maintenance of elimination	5. Monitor elimination patterns. Encourage intake of fruits and vegetables allowed on diet to assist in solid waste elimination	5. Record status every eight hours	5. Normal Elimination pattern resumes. Return to continent patterns
Dipsticked: Positive for protein			6. Maintenance of diversional activities	6. Spend time reading and talking to child since activities will be limited by edematous process. Prevent fatigue. Plan activities that can be accomplished while on bed rest. Make referral to play therapist (when available)	6. Talk to child during bath. Encourage parent participation in diversional activities. Plan with parents times for rest as well as diversion	6. Provides or participates in diversional activities
Tentative medical Diagnosis: Nephrosis			7. Maintenance of emotional support to child and parents	7. Provide explanation of plan of care as well as procedures to parent and child to decrease anxiety and gain cooperation. Encourage parent visitation and participation in care. Encourage verbalization of concerns of parent and child. Refer to spiritual advisor	7. Gear explanations to level of understanding	7. Decrease in anxiety
			8. Maintenance of treatment regimen	8. Be knowledgeable of the treatment regimen, desired effects, side effects and untoward effects. Corticosteroids and diuretics may be given	8. Watch for Cushingoid symptoms. Anticipate diuresis	8. Progression from bed rest to activities of daily living. Reduction in medications

*This example of the nursing process is not inclusive of all care that an individual child might require.

PRESCHOOL AGE–TONSILLECTOMY AND ADENOIDECTOMY*

	DATA — History Taking and Examination	ASSESSMENT — Comparison and Contrast	ASSESSMENT — Strengths and Weaknesses	PROBLEM IDENTIFICATION	PLANNING	INTERVENTION	EVALUATION
Sue — 5-year-old girl brought to hospital by mother for scheduled tonsillectomy and adenoidectomy	Weight: 45 lb.	within normal range	A relatively healthy child with many strengths	1. Preoperative	1. Child should have been prepared for hospital experience early.	1. Preparation decreases anxiety and assists in gaining cooperation.	
	Height: 38 inches	within normal range					
	Vital Signs: TPR: 98–104–26 B/P: 90/60	within normal range normal for age		a. Preoperative teaching	a. Determine base-line of knowledge before giving information	a. Use language that is appropriate for level of understanding. Suggest parent(s) be present	a. Child will be able to repeat verbally what is going to take place preoperatively and postoperatively
	Chest: lungs sound clear Heart beat strong and regular Mother states she had a cold two weeks ago.	normal	The reason for hospitalization is based on need for tonsillectomy and adenoidectomy		Prepare child for site of surgery, for going to the operating room and for going to sleep (anesthesia) Prepare child for preoperative medications	Use doll for giving example of site of surgery, for going to the operating room and for receiving anesthesia	
	Abdomen: Bowel sounds heard Palpation finds no abnormal masses, nor tenderness	within normal range			Prepare child for a sore throat post-surgery. Knowledge of what to expect decreases fear Give reason for withholding food Include parents in all aspects of care	Use doll for demonstrating how medication is given with parents in support Use language that can be understood	Involve child in question and answer game to elicit understanding
	Head: Ears symmetrical Eyes clear–PERLA† Breathes through mouth at all times No evidence of glandular enlargement Enlarged tonsils noted	normal in all areas except: a. a mouth breather b. enlarged tonsils					
	Skin: Clear, clean; good turgor	normal		b. Preparation for OR	b. Operative permit must be signed Lab report must be on the chart	b. Check chart for signed permit and lab results Be sure that Hematocrit is above 30% and WBC is below 10,000. If either is unusual, report to physician and anesthesiologist	b. Anticipate that child will be able to undergo surgery
	Extremities: Symmetrical No problems noted	normal					
	Motor Speech and Social: Nothing abnormal noted	normal			Check for loose teeth to prevent aspiration Remove jewelry to prevent loss Remove nail polish to provide a visible area for circulatory check	Have child assist in removing nail polish or have parent assist	
	Mother states Sue.has had repeated colds, ear infections and sore throats over the past two years	the average preschooler has occasional colds or sore throats; rarely has ear infections		c. Emotional support to child and parents	c. Give preop injections in treatment room rather than bedroom to avoid upsetting other children	c. After injection is given, keep in bed with side rails up to provide for safety. Involve parent(s) by inviting their quiet presence with child in room	c. Child will attempt to cooperate, may need to be assisted by parents or others
	No known allergies	normal			Have child void before going to OR to empty bladder.		

a. Maintenance of patent airway	a. Facilitate drainage of secretions and to prevent aspiration of blood or vomitus	a. Place child partially on her side and partially on her abdomen with the knee of the uppermost leg flexed to hold her in position	a. Positioning and supervision will maintain a patent airway
b. Monitor vital signs	b. Observe for degree of restlessness. Take vital signs and blood pressure since changes may be indicative of hemorrhage	b. Vital signs and blood pressure every 15 to 30 minutes until stable and child is fully awake. Report if bright red bleeding occurs, if pulse increases, and if child swallows repeatedly	b. Anticipate that temperature, pulse, and respiration will stabilize for age of child
c. Maintenance of hydration	c. Plan for minimum of 1400 ml. intake in a 24-hour period	c. Small amounts of clear liquids every 15 to 30 minutes	c. Able to take and retain clear liquids. Anticipate taking and retaining 300 ml. as of 6 hours postoperatively
d. Maintenance of elimination	d. Encourage voiding within 8 to 10 hours postsurgery	d. Offer bedpan 4 hours postoperatively and every hour to maximum of 10 hours	d. Child voids within 4 hours
e. Maintenance of nutrition	e. Try to maintain the minimum normal basal metabolic requirement of 200 to 400 calories over a 24-hour period	e. Offer small amounts of clear liquids (iced popsicles), and progress to sherbets and jello	e. Anticipate retention of minimal fluid intake and progress to full diet at home in 5 to 7 days
f. Prevention of infection	f. Prevent exposure and contact with persons with infectious disease	f. Prevent contact with persons with cold and upper respiratory infections	f. Child kept free of infection
g. Promotion of health	g. Encourage hydration, maintenance of nutrition, and gradual increase in activities	g. Plan quiet periods of play to reduce overexertion. Involve parents with planning for long-range immunization protection	g. Child gradually returns to activities of daily living without incidence. Immunization levels are maintained and updated

This example of the nursing process is not inclusive of all care that an individual child might require.

† Pupils equal, react to light and accommodate

APPENDIX II

ADDRESSES FOR SOURCES OF TEACHING AID MATERIALS LISTED AT THE ENDS OF CHAPTERS

Al-Anon World Services, Inc.
P.O. Box 182, Madison Square Station
New York, N.Y. 10010

Alexander Graham Bell Association for the Deaf
1537 35th St., N.W.
Washington, D.C. 20007

Allergy Foundation of America
801 Second Ave.
New York, N.Y. 10017

American Academy of Pediatrics
1801 Hinman Avenue
Evanston, Ill. 60204

The American Cancer Society, Inc. (next page)

American Celiac Society
45 Gifford Ave.
Jersey City, N.J. 07304

American Dental Association
211 E. Chicago Ave.
Chicago, Ill. 60611

American Diabetes Association, Inc.
1 W. 48th St.
New York, N.Y. 10020

American Dietetic Association
430 N. Michigan Ave.
Chicago, Ill. 60611

American Foundation for the Blind, Inc.
15 W. 16th St.
New York, N.Y. 10011

The American Humane Association (next page)

The American Journal of Nursing Company (next page)

American Heart Association
7320 Greenville Avenue
Dallas, TX 75231

American Lung Association
1740 Broadway
New York, N.Y. 10019

American Medical Association
535 N. Dearborn St.
Chicago, Ill. 60610

American National Red Cross
17th and D Streets, N.W.
Washington, D.C. 20006

The American Nurses' Association
2420 Pershing Rd.
Kansas City, Missouri 64108

The Arthritis Foundation (see page 921)

Breakthru Inc.
777 W. Glencoe Place
Milwaukee, Wis. 53217

Blue Cross Association: Local Offices

Canadian Mental Health Association
52 St. Clair Ave. East
Toronto 7, Ontario, Canada

The Children's Hospital Medical Center (see p. 921)

Child Study Association of America
c/o Dr. J. R. Goldberg, Executive Director
School of Social Work
New York University,
New York, N.Y. 12206

Child Welfare League of America, Inc.
67 Irving Place
New York, N.Y. 10003

Consumer Product Information
Pueblo, Colorado 81009

Department of National Health and Welfare
Brooke Claxton Building
Ottawa, Ontario, Canada K1A OK9

Dysautonomia Foundation, Inc.
370 Lexington Ave.,
Suite 1508
New York, N.Y. 10017

Epilepsy Foundation of America
1828 L St. N.W.
Suite 406
Washington, D.C. 20036

Johnson & Johnson
501 George St.
New Brunswick, N.J. 08903

Kimberly-Clark Corporation
Neenah, Wis. 54956

La Leche League International, Inc.
9616 Minneapolis Ave.
Franklin Pk., Ill. 60131

Leukemia Society of America, Inc.
211 E. 43rd St.
New York, N.Y. 10017

Maternity Center Association
48 East 92nd St.
New York, N.Y. 10028

Mead Johnson & Company
2404 W. Pennsylvania Street
Evansville, Ind. 47721

Medic Alert Foundation International
1000 North Palm
Turlock, Calif. 95380

Muscular Dystrophy Associations of America, Inc.
810 Seventh Avenue
New York, N.Y. 10019

The National Association for Mental Health Inc.
  (see p. 921)

National Association for Retarded Citizens
2709 Avenue E., East
P.O. Box 6109
Arlington, Texas 76011

National Council on Alcoholism, Inc.
2 Park Ave.
New York, N.Y. 10016

National Cystic Fibrosis Research Foundation
3379 Peachtree Rd. N.E.
Atlanta, Ga. 30326

National Dairy Council
111 N. Canal St.
Chicago, Ill. 60606

The National Easter Seal Society for Crippled
  Children and Adults

The National Foundation — March of Dimes

The National Hemophilia Foundation (see p. 921)

National Kidney Foundation
116 E. 27th St.
New York, N.Y. 10016

National League for Nursing
10 Columbus Circle
New York, N.Y. 10019

National Society for the Prevention of Blindness, Inc.
79 Madison Ave.
New York, N.Y. 10016

National Sudden Infant Death Syndrome Foundation
(formerly National Foundation for Sudden Infant
Death.)
310 S. Michigan Ave.
Chicago, Ill. 60604

Personal Products Company
Box S-6
Milltown, N.J. 08850

Planned Parenthood Federation of America, Inc.
810 Seventh Ave.
New York, N.Y. 10019

Play Schools Association, Inc.
120 West 57th St.
New York, N.Y. 10019

Public Affairs Committee
381 Park Ave. S.
New York, N.Y. 10016

Rainbow Hospital Youth Spine Center
2065 Adelbert Road
Cleveland, Ohio 44106

ROERIG: A Division of Pfizer Pharmaceuticals
235 E. 42nd St.
New York, N.Y. 10017

Ross Laboratories
Division of Abbott Laboratories
Columbus, Ohio 43216

SIECUS Publications Office
1855 Broadway
New York, N.Y. 10023

Southern Regional Council, Inc.
52 Fairlie St. N.W.
Atlanta, Ga. 30303

The American Cancer Society, Inc.
219 E. 42nd St.
New York, N.Y. 10017

The American Humane Association
Children's Division
P.O. Box 1266
Denver, Col. 80201

The American Journal of Nursing Company
10 Columbus Circle
New York, N.Y. 10019

The Arthritis Foundation
1212 Avenue of the Americas
New York, N.Y. 10036

The Children's Hospital Medical Center
300 Longwood Ave.
Boston, Mass. 02115

The National Association for Mental Health, Inc.
1800 N. Kent St.
Rosslyn, Va. 22209

The National Easter Seal Society for
    Crippled Children and Adults
2023 W. Ogden Ave.
Chicago, Ill. 60612

The National Foundation — March of Dimes
1707 H Street, N.W.
Washington, D.C. 20006

The National Hemophilia Foundation
25 W. 39th St.
New York, N.Y. 10018

The Touchstone Center
141 E. 88th St.
New York, N.Y. 10028

United Cerebral Palsy Association
66 E. 34th St.
New York, N.Y. 10016

United States Government

United States Department of Health, Education,
    and Welfare
Superintendent of Documents
U.S. Government Printing Office
Washington, D.C. 20402

United States Metric System Association
Sugarloaf Star Route
Boulder, Col. 80302

ADDRESSES FOR SOURCES OF AUDIOVISUAL MATERIALS LISTED AT THE ENDS OF CHAPTERS

American Academy of Pediatrics
1801 Hinman Avenue
Evanston, Ill. 60204

The American Cancer Society, Inc. (see p. 924)

American College of Nurse-Midwifery
330 W. 58th St.
New York, N.Y. 10019

American Dental Association
211 E. Chicago Ave.
Chicago, Ill. 60611

The American Journal of Nursing Company (see p. 924)

American Lung Association
1740 Broadway
New York, N.Y. 10019

Audio Visual Narrative Arts, Inc. (AVNA)
P.O. Box 398
Pleasantville, N.Y. 10570

Bandera Productions
11071 Ventura Blvd.
Suite 103
Studio City, Calif. 91604

Canadian Cancer Society
22 Davisville Ave.
Ontario Province
Toronto, Canada

Canadian Film Institute
303 Richmond Rd.
Ottawa, Ontario

Carousel Films
1501 Broadway
Suite 1503
New York, N.Y. 10036

Charles Press–Prentice-Hall, Inc.
Englewood Cliffs, New Jersey 07632

Childbirth Education Films, Inc.
648 Riverside Rd.
North Palm Beach, Florida 33408

Children's Hospital, National Medical Center
Washington, D.C. 20014

Churchill Films: 6671 Sunset Blvd.
Los Angeles, Calif. 90028

CIBA
Summit, New Jersey 07901
(Request from local office of Association Films, Inc.)

CIBA and Wayne State University
Summit, New Jersey 07901

Concept Media
1500 Adams Ave.
Costa Mesa, Calif. 92626

Department of National Health and Welfare
Brooke Claxton Building
Ottawa, Ontario K1A OK9

Education Development Center, Inc.
Distribution Center
39 Chapel St.
Newton, Mass. 02160

Film & Videotape Library, National Institute on
  Mental Retardation
Kinsmen NIMR Building
York University Campus
4700 Keele St.
Downsview, Ontario, Canada M3J 1P3

Greater Cleveland Hospital Association
1021 Euclid Ave.
Cleveland, Ohio 44115

Harper & Row, Publishers
Media Department
10 E. 53rd St.
New York, N.Y. 10022

Health Sciences Communication Center
Case Western Reserve University
University Circle
Cleveland, Ohio 44106

Hospital Audio Visual Education
606 Halstead Ave.
Mamaroneck, N.Y. 19543

International Film Bureau, Inc.
332 S. Michigan Ave.
Chicago, Ill. 60604

LaDoca Project and Publishing Foundation, Inc.
E. 51st Ave. and Lincoln
Denver, Colorado 80216

J. B. Lippincott Company
Audiovisual Department
Division of Higher Education
East Washington Square
Philadelphia, Pa. 19105

Long Island Film Studios
P.O. Box P
Brightwaters, New York 11718

Maternity Center Association
48 E. 92nd St.
New York, N.Y. 10028

McGraw-Hill Book Company
College Division
1221 Avenue of the Americas
New York, N.Y. 10020

Medical Electronic Educational Services, Inc.
1802 West Grant Rd.
Suite No. 119
Tucson, Ariz. 85705

Metropolitan Life Insurance Company
1 Madison Ave.
New York, N.Y. 10010

National Communicable Disease Center
1600 Clifton Road N.E.
Atlanta, Ga. 30333

National Council on Alcoholism, Inc.
2 Park Ave.
New York, N.Y. 10016

National Cystic Fibrosis Research Foundation
3379 Peachtree Rd. N.E.
Atlanta, Ga. 30326

The National Easter Seal Society for Crippled
  Children and Adults (see p. 925)

The National Hemophilia Foundation (see p. 925)

National Institute for Burn Medicine
909 East Ann St.
Ann Arbor, Michigan 48104

National Society for the Prevention of Blindness, Inc.
79 Madison Ave.
New York, N.Y. 10016

New York University Medical Center
Institute of Physical Medicine and Rehabilitation
New York, N.Y. 10016

Ottawa-Carleton Regional Health Unit
1827 Woodward Dr.
Ottawa, Ontario K2C 0R5

Paramount Oxford Films
A Subsidiary of Paramount Pictures Corporation
5451 Marathon St.
Hollywood, Calif. 90038

Parents' Magazine Films, Inc.
Dept. F0979
52 Vanderbilt Ave.
New York, N.Y. 10017

Perkins School for the Blind
Guidance Information Center
Saxtons River, Vt. 05154

Personal Products Company
c/o Association-Sterling Films
Milltown, N.J. 08850

Planned Parenthood Federation of America, Inc.
810 Seventh Ave.
New York, N.Y. 10019

Public Affairs Committee
381 Park Ave.
New York, N.Y. 10016

Ross Laboratories: Columbus, Ohio 43216

The Royal College of General Practitioners (see p. 925)

W. B. Saunders Company
West Washington Square
Philadelphia, Pa. 19105

Tampax, Inc.
5 Dakota Dr.
Lake Success, N.Y. 11040

Telstar Productions, Inc.
366 N. Prior
St. Paul, Minnesota 55104

The American Cancer Society, Inc.
219 E. 42nd St.
New York, N.Y. 10017

The American Journal of Nursing Company
Educational Services Division
10 Columbus Circle
New York, N.Y. 10019

The National Easter Seal Society For Crippled
Children and Adults
2023 W. Ogden Ave.
Chicago, Ill. 60612

The National Hemophilia Foundation
25 W. 39th St.
New York, N.Y. 10018

The Royal College of General Practitioners
Medical Recording Service
London, England

Trainex Corporation
Subsidiary Medcom Inc.
P.O. Box 116
Garden Grove, Calif. 92642

United States Government
Washington, D.C.

USBEH: Bureau of Education for the Handicapped
(Department of Health, Education, and
Welfare)
20014

USDA: Department of Agriculture
20250

USDHEW: Department of Health, Education,
and Welfare
National Institutes of Health
20014

USN: Department of the Navy
(Department of Defense)
20301

USNIMH: National Institute of Mental Health
(Department of Health, Education, and Welfare)
20014

USNMAC: National Medical Audiovisual Center
(Department of Health, Education, and Welfare)
General Services Administration
20409

USOEO: Office of Economic Opportunity
20506

USPHS: Public Health Service
(Department of Health, Education, and Welfare)
20014

USSRS: Social Rehabilitation Service
(Department of Health, Education, and Welfare)
20014

V.C.I. Studios, C.B.S.
201 No. Occidental
Los Angeles, Calif. 90026

Wayne State University
Rm. 323 Cohn Bldg.
5557 Cass Ave.
Detroit, Mich. 48202

Yale University School of Medicine
New Haven, Conn. 06520

INDEX

Note: *Italicized* numbers indicate illustrations; numbers followed by (t) indicate tables.